*A Pharmacologic Approach
to Gastrointestinal Disorders*

A Pharmacologic Approach to Gastrointestinal Disorders

Edited by

James H. Lewis, M.D.

Associate Professor of Medicine
Division of Gastroenterology
Georgetown University
School of Medicine
Washington, D.C.

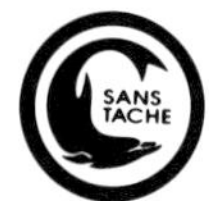

Editor: David C. Retford
Managing Editor: Molly L. Mullen
Copy Editor: Carol Zimmerman
Designer: Ann Feild
Illustration Planner: Ray Lowman
Production Coordinator: Kimberly S. Nawrozki
Cover Designer: Dan Pfisterer

Copyright © 1994
Williams & Wilkins
428 East Preston Street
Baltimore, Maryland 21202, USA

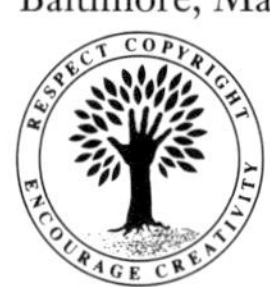

Accurate indications, adverse reactions, and dosage schedules for drugs are provided in this book, but it is possible that they may change. The reader is urged to review the package information data of the manufacturers of the medications mentioned.

Printed in the United States of America

Chapter reprints are available from the Publisher

Library of Congress Cataloging-in-Publication Data

A Pharmacologic approach to gastrointestinal disorders / edited by
  James H. Lewis.
     p. cm.
   Includes index.
   ISBN 0-683-04970-4
   1. Gastrointestinal system—Diseases—Chemotherapy.   I. Lewis,
James H.
   [DNLM: 1. Digestive System Diseases—drug therapy. WI 100 P536
1993]
   RC802.P48   1993
   616.3'3061—dc20
   DNLM/DLC
   for Library of Congress   93-13185

94 95 96 97 98
1 2 3 4 5 6 7 8 9 10

To Hyman J. Zimmerman, M.D.,
for his enduring inspiration to
generations of physicians and students,
and
to my wife, Stephanie, with love,
for her encouragement and support.

FOREWORD

A Pharmacologic Approach to Gastrointestinal Diseases represents what I believe to be the first major textbook concerning the drug treatment of diseases of the gastrointestinal tract. One cannot say that the book is overdue, because it is only recently that effective treatment has become available for many of these clinical problems. I was a clinical medical student when Avery-Jones, Gummer, and Lennard-Jones published the second edition of *Clinical Gastroenterology* in 1968. The book placed great emphasis on clinical features, diagnostic tests, and surgical management—much of the medical management was expectant, and it was rarely of decisive benefit. It is interesting to recall the small number of drugs that were available only a quarter of a century ago. For example, the management of a pelvic abscess was either surgical drainage or treatment with hot rectal wash-outs at a temperature of 108°C. There was no mention of antibiotics—metronidazole was recommended as an experimental treatment for amebic colitis, but its role in anaerobic sepsis had yet to be identified. The other important drugs surviving from that era are remarkably few—for example, prednisone, codeine phosphate, cholestyramine, salicylazosulphapyridine (sulfasalazine).

The rate of pharmacologic discovery over the last quarter of a century is clearly demonstrated by the first section of *A Pharmacologic Approach to Gastrointestinal Diseases*. The histamine H_2-receptor antagonists provided physicians with the opportunity to control gastric acid secretion for the first time. The drugs were effective, acid-related disorders were common, and cimetidine followed by ranitidine rapidly became the most successful drugs around the world. However, they are not ideal for every indication and the H^+, K^+-ATPase inhibitors, in particular, omeprazole, have a role for patients with aggressive duodenal ulceration or severe reflux esophagitis. All three drugs have proved to be commercial successes as well, and this must be part of the reason why so much pharmacologic attention is now paid to the gastrointestinal tract, realizing that diseases in this area are common and few specific remedies are available. Today the success of gastric acid antisecretory drugs is being challenged by the surprising discovery of *Helicobacter pylori*, a bacterium that was seen but ignored for many years. However, the passing of 10 years and the publication of 2500 papers has not produced a decisive regimen for the eradication of this chronic infection.

Disorders of gastrointestinal motility are also common, but mostly misunderstood. The irritable bowel syndrome is a priority area for research in terms of morbidity and high prevalence. At the moment, treatment is heavily dependent upon the charisma of the prescribing physician. The answer may lie in the peptide and opioid transmitters that are abundant within the wall of the gastrointestinal tract—they behave rather like the members of an orchestra: we can now identify individual players, but are unable to get the orchestra to play a tune.

It is interesting that three drugs used to treat inflammatory bowel disease a quarter of a century ago have continued in use. In terms of suffering, patients with inflammatory bowel disease deserve a decisive pharmacologic breakthrough. Mortality has declined over the last quarter of a century, due mainly to the benefits of antimicrobial therapy and improved nutrition; aggressive immunosuppression will often help but it is associated with appreciable morbidity.

Spironolactone is one of the few drugs used in hepatology to have survived the last 25 years, but there are now a range of pharmacologic interventions that delay the downhill progress of many diseases of the liver and biliary tract. The treatments for viral hepatitis B and C are the most successful examples. Conversely, enormous ingenuity was applied to the chemical dissolution of gallstones, only for surgeons to regain leadership using laparoscopic surgery.

The sixth section of this book explores a number of general topics that relate to the treatment of gastrointestinal disorders. My textbook of gastroenterology a quarter of a century ago offered the patient requiring endoscopy either a blindfold or a general anaesthetic—things have changed a great deal during a very short time. This section also lays emphasis on prescribing for patients with renal disease, for patients during pregnancy and lactation, or for children with gastrointestinal disease—all very relevant topics, particularly when read in conjunction with the final chapter, which assesses medical-legal aspects of prescribing for our patients.

Chapter 29 discusses prescribing for patients with gastrointestinal malignancy, an area where slow progress is beginning to offer measurable clinical benefit.

A Pharmacologic Approach to Gastrointestinal Diseases is an excellent textbook that describes an area where there has been dramatic recent progress. We now have a range of truly effective treatments for many of our patients with gastrointestinal disorders. Areas of need, in particular, for those patients with functional bowel disorders, inflammatory bowel disease, or gastrointestinal malignancy are identified. It will be fascinating to record progress through future editions of this important contribution to the literature of modern gastroenterology.

PROFESSOR ROY POUNDER, M.A., M.D., D.Sc. (MED), F.R.C.P., F.A.C.G.
Professor of Medicine
Royal Free Hospital
and School of Medicine, London
Co-Editor,
Alimentary Pharmacology and Therapeutics

Preface

Advances in drug therapy continue to revolutionize the practice of gastroenterology— some might say, to the same extent, that endoscopic developments have redefined therapeutic approaches to the specialty. Many of these pharmacologic advances have been achieved through an improved understanding of the pathophysiology of disease states and a more refined appreciation of the mechanisms by which drugs can influence gastrointestinal disorders. Given the constant introduction of new agents into the field, as well as the use of existing agents for new clinical indications, *A Pharmacologic Approach to Gastrointestinal Disorders* was conceived as an innovative means to provide the busy practitioner or student with a compendium to keep abreast of the current practices and ongoing developments in the ever-widening field of gastrointestinal pharmacotherapeutics. The goal was to write a complete yet practical guide that incorporates the ease and utility of a handbook with the expertise and authority of a full-scale reference text. This is accomplished by dividing the book into five main disease sections, with each chapter providing a comprehensive review of current drug therapy for gastrointestinal problems based on pathophysiologic mechanisms. The reader is presented not only with the personal insights, expertise, and extensive clinical experience of the contributing authors, but also with a look to the future of drugs for GI therapy through discussions of investigational agents and other areas of ongoing and future research.

A Pharmacologic Approach to Gastrointestinal Disorders is intended for use by physicians, pharmacologists, nursing staff, students, and others in need of a quick yet in-depth source of drug treatment approaches for GI diseases. A collection of chapters dealing with the use of GI drugs in renal disease, in pregnancy and lactation, and in pediatric patients, as well as drugs for endoscopic conscious sedation and drug interactions encountered with specific gastrointestinal agents, provides the reader with unique single-source reference material not generally found in medical texts of this genre. In addition, a discussion of the medical-legal concerns involved in the drug treatment of GI disorders is included. Every attempt has been made by the authors and the editor to ensure that the information, references, and advice are as up-to-date as possible. The practitioner is urged to continually evaluate the appropriateness of any medical opinion depending on the clinical circumstances, mindful of new developments in the field. In this context, *A Pharmacologic Approach to Gastrointestinal Disorders* provides the necessary foundation in pathophysiology of disease and clinical gastrointestinal pharmacotherapy so the reader can confidently take full advantage of the changes in drug therapy that are occurring now and that are predicted for the future.

JAMES H. LEWIS, M.D.

Contributors

Firas H. Al-Kawas, M.D.
Associate Professor of Medicine
Department of Gastroenterology
Georgetown University Medical Center
Washington, D.C.

Bruce R. Bacon, M.D.
Professor of Internal Medicine
Director, Division of Gastroenterology & Hepatology
St. Louis University School of Medicine
St. Louis, Missouri

Stanley B. Benjamin, M.D.
Professor of Medicine
Chief, Division of Gastroenterology
Georgetown University Medical Center
Washington, D.C.

William M. Bennett, M.D.
Professor of Medicine & Pharmacology
Head, Division of Nephrology, Hypertension and
    Clinical Pharmacology
Oregon Health Sciences University
Portland, Oregon

Richard V. Benya, M.D.
Clinical Associate
Digestive Diseases Branch
National Institutes of Health
Bethesda, Maryland

Nora V. Bergasa, M.D.
Assistant Professor
Rockefeller University
New York, New York

Lawrence J. Brandt, M.D.
Professor of Medicine
Albert Einstein College of Medicine
Director, Division of Gastroenterology
Montefiore Medical Center and North Central Bronx
    Hospital
Bronx, New York

Scott R. Brazer, M.D., M.H.S.
Assistant Professor of Medicine
Division of Gastroenterology
Duke University Medical Center
Durham, North Carolina

Gerald G. Briggs, Pharm.D.
Lead Pharmacist/Clinical Coordinator
Women's Hospital
Long Beach Memorial Hospital
Long Beach, California
Assistant Clinical Professor of Pharmacy
University of California, San Francisco
Adjunct Associate Clinical Professor of Pharmacy
University of Southern California

Paul E. Buse, M.D.
Consultant in Gastroenterology
Department of Medicine
St. Luke's Hospital and Missouri Baptist Medical
    Center
St. Louis, Missouri

Harris R. Clearfield, M.D.
Professor of Medicine
Director, Division of Gastroenterology
Hahnemann University
Philadelphia, Pennsylvania

Angel R. Colón, M.D.
Professor of Pediatrics
Department of Pediatric Gastroenterology &
    Nutrition
Georgetown University Medical Center
Washington, D.C.

Joan A. Culpepper-Morgan, M.D.
Director, Gastroenterology and Nutrition Research
Norwalk Hospital
Norwalk, Connecticut
Assistant Clinical Professor
Department of Medicine
Yale University
New Haven, Connecticut

Geert D'Haens, M.D.
Department of Medicine/Gastroenterology
University Hospital "Gasthuisberg"
Leuven, Belgium

Dennis L. Decktor, Ph.D.
Assistant Director
Clinical Research
Johnson & Johnson and Merck Consumer Pharmacy
    Company
Ft. Washington, Pennsylvania
Scientific Director
Oklahoma Foundation for Digestive Research
Oklahoma City, Oklahoma

Robert J. DeLap, M.D.
Assistant Professor of Medicine
Division of Medical Oncology
Georgetown University Medical Center
Washington, D.C.

Adrian M. Di Bisceglie, M.D.
Chief, Liver Diseases Section
National Institute of Diabetes and Digestive and
  Kidney Disease
National Institutes of Health
Bethesda, Maryland

Anna Mae Diehl, M.D.
Associate Professor of Medicine
Gastroenterology Division
The Johns Hopkins University School of Medicine
Baltimore, Maryland

Andre DuBois, M.D., Ph.D.
Professor and Chief
Laboratory of Gastrointestinal and Liver Studies
  of Medicine
Uniformed Services University of the Health Sciences
Bethesda, Maryland

David E. Fleischer, M.D.
Professor of Medicine
Chief of Endoscopy
Division of Gastroenterology
Georgetown University Medical Center
Washington, D.C.

Gerald Friedman, M.D., Ph.D.
Clinical Professor of Medicine
Department of Medicine
The Mount Sinai School of Medicine
New York, New York

Gregory G. Ginsberg, M.D.
Assistant Professor of Medicine
Division of Gastroenterology
Hospital of the University of Pennsylvania
Philadelphia, Pennsylvania

Edgar R. Gonzalez, Pharm.D.
Associate Professor of Pharmacy and Pharmaceutics
Department of Pharmacy and Medicine
Medical College of Virginia
Virginia Commonwealth University
Richmond, Virginia

Sherwood L. Gorbach, M.D.
Professor of Community Health and Medicine
Tufts University School of Medicine
Boston, Massachusetts

Joanne Grainger, Pharm.D.
Manager, Drug Information
Glaxo, Inc.
Research Triangle Park, North Carolina

Stephen B. Hanauer, M.D.
Professor of Medicine
Department of Medicine/Gastroenterology
University of Chicago
Chicago, Illinois

Philip D. Hansten, Pharm.D.
Professor of Pharmacy
School of Pharmacy
University of Washington
Seattle, Washington

Christopher J. Hawkey, M.D.
Professor of Gastroenterology
Department of Medicine
Division of Gastroenterology
University Hospital
Queen's Medical Center
Nottingham, England

Colin W. Howden, M.D.
Professor of Medicine
Department of Medicine/Gastroenterology
University of South Carolina
School of Medicine
Columbia, South Carolina

Nicholas Hudson, M.R.C.P.
Senior Registrar
Department of Gastroenterology
Western General Hospital
Edinburgh, United Kingdom

Richard H. Hunt, M.D.
Professor of Medicine
Division of Gastroenterology
McMaster University
Hamilton, Ontario
Canada

E. Anthony Jones, M.D., D.Sc
Department of Health
London, England

Louis Y. Korman, M.D.
Chief, GI Physiology Research
Veterans Administration Medical Center
Clinical Associate Professor of Medicine and
  Physiology
George Washington University Medical Center
Washington, D.C.

Mary Jeanne Kreek, M.D.
Associate Professor & Physician
Laboratory on the Biology of Addictive Diseases
Rockefeller University
New York, New York

Robert S. Levine, M.D.
Fellow
Division of Gastroenterology
George Washington University
Washington, D.C.

James H. Lewis, M.D.
Associate Professor of Medicine
Division of Gastroenterology
Georgetown University Medical Center
Washington, D.C.

Spencer C.Y. Li, M.D.
Subspecialty Resident
St. Louis University Medical Center
St. Louis, Missouri

Paul N. Maton, M.D.
Associate Clinical Professor of Medicine
College of Medicine
University of Oklahoma
Associate Medical Director
Oklahoma Foundation for Digestive Research
Oklahoma City, Oklahoma

Mary M. Meyer, M.D.
Assistant Professor of Medicine
Department of Medicine & Pharmacology
Division of Nephrology & Hypertension
Oregon Health Sciences University
Portland, Oregon

Kevin D. Mullen, M.B., F.R.C.P.I.
Associate Professor of Medicine
MetroHealth Medical Center
Division of Gastroenterology
Case Western Reserve University
Cleveland, Ohio

Cuong C. Nguyen, M.D.
Assistant Professor of Medicine
Division of Gastroenterology
Georgetown University Medical Center
Washington, D.C.

Walter L. Peterson, M.D.
Professor of Medicine
Director, Fellowship Training in Digestive Diseases
University of Texas Southwestern Medical Center
VA Medical Center
Dallas, Texas

Peter A. Plumeri, D.O., J.D., L.L.M.
Associate Professor of Medicine
Director, Section of Medical Jurisprudence
Department of Medicine
University of Medicine and Dentistry of New Jersey
Partner, Lofft & Plumeri
Sewell, New Jersey

Joel E. Richter, M.D.
Professor of Medicine
Director of Clinical Research
Gastroenterology Division
University of Alabama at Birmingham
Birmingham, Alabama

Malcolm Robinson, M.D.
Clinical Professor of Medicine
College of Medicine
University of Oklahoma
Medical Director
Oklahoma Foundation for Digestive Research
Oklahoma City, Oklahoma

Leonard B. Seeff, M.D.
Professor of Medicine
Georgetown University School of Medicine
Chief, Division of Gastroenterology, Hepatology &
 Nutrition
VA Medical Center
Washington, D.C.

Douglas Simon, M.D.
Associate Professor of Medicine
Division of Gastroenterology
Albert Einstein School of Medicine
Bronx, New York

Gary L. Simon M.D., Ph.D.
Professor of Medicine, Biochemistry and Molecular
 Biology
Associate Chairman, Department of Medicine
George Washington University Medical Center
Washington, D.C.

William M. Steinberg, M.D.
Professor of Medicine
Division of Gastroenterology & Nutrition
George Washington University Medical Center
Washington, D.C.

Scott Tenner, M.D., M.P.H.
Department of Medicine
George Washington University Medical Center
Washington, D.C.

Thomas G. Tietjen, M.D.
Fellow in Gastroenterology
The Johns Hopkins University School of Medicine
Baltimore, Maryland

Paul V. Woolley III, M.D.
Clinical Professor of Medicine
University of Pittsburgh Medical Center
Director
Laurel Highlands Cancer Program
Johnstown, Pennsylvania

Sumner J. Yaffe, M.D.
Director, Center for Research for Mothers &
 Children
National Institute of Child Health and Human
 Development
National Institutes of Health
Bethesda, Maryland

Gary R. Zuckerman, D.O.
Associate Professor of Medicine
Digestive Disease Clinical Center
Washington University School of Medicine
St. Louis, Missouri

Contents

SECTION I.

ACID-PEPTIC AND RELATED DISEASES

SECTION II.

DISORDERS OF GASTROINTESTINAL MOTILITY

SECTION VI.

MISCELLANEOUS TOPICS

ACID-PEPTIC AND RELATED DISEASES

1

Peptic Ulcer Disease

COLIN W. HOWDEN and RICHARD H. HUNT

INTRODUCTION

Peptic ulcer remains a prevalent condition affecting up to 10% of the population and is responsible for considerable morbidity and loss of time from work. There are currently a variety of pharmacologic agents approved for the treatment of peptic ulcer. This chapter will attempt to appraise each of these and place them in current context with respect to the pathophysiology.

The increasing awareness of the importance of the eradication of *Helicobacter pylori* in the long-term management of patients with duodenal ulcer, and perhaps also gastric ulcer, and the increasing acceptance of the use of effective eradication regimens are likely to alter significantly our current concepts about the pharmacotherapy of peptic ulcer (1). Although it is relatively easy to heal ulcers with appropriate drug treatment, ulcer relapse after healing has, until now, been a persistent problem. With the exception of treatments that truly eradicate *H. pylori*, the natural tendency of ulcers to relapse after initial healing has not been influenced by currently available drugs. The importance of *H. pylori* in current thinking about the treatment of peptic ulcer cannot be overestimated, and this subject is dealt with in greater detail elsewhere in this book.

PATHOPHYSIOLOGY OF PEPTIC ULCERS: RATIONALE FOR TREATMENT

Most peptic ulcers form in the first part of the duodenum or in the body of the stomach. These duodenal and gastric ulcers have some different pathophysiologic characteristics.

Gastric acid and pepsin secretion are of central importance in the formation of peptic ulcers, although infection with *H. pylori* is increasingly recognized as crucial to the production of an environment that promotes or facilitates ulceration by acid and pepsin. The precise role of *H. pylori* has not yet been elucidated. *H. pylori* infection may be detected in 95–100% of patients with duodenal ulcer and 70–80% of patients with gastric ulcer. In patients with gastric ulcer, the distribution of the bacterium in the gastric mucosa is heterogeneous, so evidence of it may by missed on routine biopsy unless a number of samples are taken from the antrum, body and fundus. This suggests that the quoted rates of prevalence in gastric ulcer could be an underestimation. Furthermore, the prevalence of *H. pylori* in patients with gastric ulcer is confounded by the widespread use of nonsteroidal anti-inflammatory drugs (NSAIDs).

Even with the increasing interest in *H. pylori*, drugs whose sole or principal pharmacologic property is to suppress the secretion of gastric acid are still the most widely used form of therapy for both duodenal and gastric ulcer. Some drugs, including sucralfate, (discussed in greater detail below), do not suppress gastric acid secretion yet can heal ulcers effectively. Their precise mode(s) of action is unknown but stimulation of mucosal defensive factors is clearly another approach to the process of accelerating ulcer healing. It is worthwhile considering aspects of gastric acid secretion. Detailed accounts of the cellular mechanisms of gastric acid secretion are dis-

Table 1.1
Healing Agents for Peptic Ulcer[a]

Generic name	Trade name	Dosage schedules	Half-life (hr)[b]
Antacids	Many	Many	Not applicable
H_2-receptor antagonists			
Cimetidine	Tagamet	800 mg qhs 300 mg qid 400 mg bid	2.0
Ranitidine	Zantac	300 mg qhs 150 mg bid	2–3
Famotidine	Pepcid	40 mg qhs	3.8
Nizatidine	Axid	300 mg qhs	1.3
Proton pump inhibitors			
Omeprazole	Prilosec	20 mg qam	1.0
Lansoprazole[c]	Prevacid		
Sucralfate	Carafate	1 g qid 2 g bid	NA
Misoprostol[d]	Cytotec	200 μg qid	NA

[a]All are currently available agents of proven value in accelerating the healing of peptic ulcer. Key to abbreviations: qhs, every night; qid, four times daily; bid, twice daily; NA, not applicable.
[b]In patients with renal impairment, all were prolonged.
[c]Not approved for use in the United States.
[d]Only approved by FDA for prevention of nonsteroidal anti-inflammatory drugs (NSAID)-induced gastric mucosal damage.

cussed elsewhere (2, 3). Absolute levels of gastric acid secretion are increased in patients with duodenal ulcer (4–6), especially in some individuals with ulcers resistant to early healing (7, 8). However, there is such a degree of overlap with healthy control subjects without ulcers that knowledge of an individual's gastric acid secretion is of no diagnostic value in determining the presence of an ulcer. Acid secretion is increased in duodenal ulcer patients in the basal, unstimulated state, such as occurs with overnight fasting in most patients and also in response to food ingestion (5). The high levels of acidity overnight when acid is normally unbuffered by food is also very characteristic of duodenal ulcer (9). Typically, patients with untreated duodenal ulcer will complain of their pain awakening them from sleep at night. That this is due to unbuffered acid seems logical, particularly since most patients report alleviation of the pain following the ingestion of food or antacids that can buffer or neutralize acid.

Excess basal acid secretion overnight has been ascribed to an increased vagal drive to the parietal cell mass in duodenal ulcer patients. The initial observation of this phenomenon by Dragstedt and Owens in 1943 led to the widespread use of vagotomy, an acid-lowering surgical operation, as treatment for duodenal ulcer. Since then, the advent of a variety of effective pharmacologic agents to suppress gastric acid secretion has greatly reduced the demand for and the practice of elective acid-lowering surgical procedures for duodenal ulcer. Pharmacologic suppression of gastric acid secretion accelerates the healing of duodenal ulcer. A complex mathematical relationship has been established between degree and duration of acid secretion and rates of healing of duodenal ulcer (10) as well as gastric ulcer (11, 12). This is discussed in greater detail later in this chapter.

Patients with gastric ulcer may have normal or even reduced levels of gastric acid secretion (4, 6). There is no excessive nocturnal acid secretion in gastric ulcer as there is in duodenal ulcer (6, 13).

Antisecretory drugs are widely used for the treatment of gastric ulcer and have been the most successful form of medical therapy employed (12). Despite the differences in acid secretory profiles between duodenal ulcer and gastric ulcer patients, antisecretory drugs are used in similar regimens for both conditions. Drugs that suppress gastric acid secretion to the greatest extent are associated with the most rapid healing of gastric as well as duodenal ulcer. There is a mathematical relationship between acid suppression and gastric ulcer healing rates (12, 14), but the overall duration of treatment with an antisecretory drug is the single most important factor. Furthermore, the therapeutic gain in healing rates of gastric ulcer for increased levels of suppression of acidity is less marked and less well-defined than it is for duodenal ulcer (10, 12, 15).

One additional factor in the pathogenesis of gastric ulcer that has attracted considerable attention is the use of aspirin or other NSAIDs. There are numerous epidemiologic and clinical data supporting a causal relationship between high-dose aspirin ingestion and gastric ulcer formation, and a number of observational and interventional studies support the contention that other NSAIDs may also induce gastric ulcers (16). The area of NSAID-induced gastric mucosal damage and its prevention and treatment are discussed in greater detail elsewhere in this book (see Chapter 3).

AGENTS TO HEAL PEPTIC ULCERS

Table 1.1 lists those agents of proven value in accelerating the healing of peptic ulcer. Not all of these currently have FDA approval for all indications, but all have been shown in controlled clinical trials to heal peptic ulcers faster than placebo.

Antacids

Although there is a huge market for proprietary antacids in the United States, these are most often used for symptomatic relief of dyspepsia or heartburn. However, antacids can heal peptic ulcers if given in appropriate amounts. A liquid antacid containing both aluminum and magnesium given in a dosage of 30 ml seven times daily, equivalent to an acid-buffering capacity of >1000 mmol, was more effective than placebo in healing duodenal ulcer in a multicenter Veterans' Administration study (17). Such a dosage schedule, however, is impractical for routine clinical use, and side effects were common in this

study, particularly diarrhea, in view of the high magnesium content of the antacid.

Much lower doses of antacids, either in liquid or tablet form, are also superior to placebo in healing duodenal ulcer (18, 19). In fact, antacid with a buffering capacity of only 120 mmol daily was as effective as cimetidine 800 mg at night in healing duodenal ulcer (20). In addition, pain relief in the first week of treatment was better in the antacid-treated patients. However, an antacid regimen equivalent to 320 mmol/day buffering capacity was no more effective than placebo in healing benign gastric ulcer (21).

The observation that low doses of antacid are sufficient to heal duodenal ulcer has led to speculation that their efficacy is not entirely explained by an effect on acid neutralization. Other properties of antacids that might also be involved include the stimulation of local endogenous prostaglandin production (22). At present, it is only the very high dose of liquid antacid that has been shown in a U.S.-based trial to increase duodenal ulcer healing rates. However, such a therapeutic approach cannot be recommended, since more effective and convenient forms of therapy are available.

Histamine H₂-Receptor Antagonists

Currently, four H_2-receptor antagonists (H_2RAs) are licensed in the United States; these are listed in Table 1.1. The H_2RA are among the most widely used drugs in the world and have been acknowledged as both highly effective and safe for the management of peptic ulcer disease (23). In pharmacologic terms, they are competitive antagonists for histamine at the H_2-receptor. This receptor is expressed on many different tissues throughout the body, but the only proven physiologic function is in regulating the secretion of hydrochloric acid by parietal cells in the oxyntic mucosa of the stomach. The cellular basis for the process of acid secretion has been well-described elsewhere (2). Since the H_2RAs oppose the action of histamine at the H_2-receptor site, their principal pharmacologic action is to reduce the secretion of acid by the parietal cell. However, they are unable to totally

Table 1.2
H$_2$-Receptor Antagonists for Duodenal Ulcer[a]

Drug and dosage (mg)	Healing rate at 4 weeks	Suppression of 24-hour acidity	Suppression of nocturnal acidity
Ranitidine 300 qhs	84	68	90
Famotidine 40 qhs	82	64	95
Cimetidine 800 qhs	80	48	79
Cimetidine 600 bid	80	67	71
Ranitidine 150 bid	79	68	70
Ranitidine 150 qhs	76	45	76
Cimetidine 300 qid	74	65	68
Cimetidine 200 tid + 400 qhs	74	56	72
Cimetidine 400 bid	72	37	54

[a]Suppression of intragastric acidity and duodenal ulcer healing rates of some commonly used dosage regimens are given. Adapted, with permission, from Jones et al. (15). Key to abbreviations: qhs, every night; bid, twice daily; qid, four times daily. Values are given as percentages.

inhibit acid secretion, since this can be stimulated by other mechanisms involving cholinergic and gastrin receptors, which are not directly related to the H$_2$-receptor (2).

The H$_2$RAs are highly effective in suppressing basal acidity such as occurs, for the most part, in the overnight period and the interprandial periods when patients fast. They are much less effective in counteracting the stimulatory effect of food on gastric acid secretion during the day (24, 25). These observations have a number or important consequences for the use of H$_2$RAs in clinical practice. Since overnight acid secretion is more easily controlled by H$_2$RAs, and since there is often inappropriate hypersecretion overnight in patients with duodenal ulcer, the H$_2$RAs can conveniently be given as single evening or nighttime doses in the management of patients with duodenal ulcer (15, 24). This leaves daytime gastric acid secretion relatively unaffected but is sufficient to heal most duodenal ulcers, and overall healing rates are at least as good as those found with the earlier multiple dose regimens of H$_2$RAs (9, 15, 25). Another important consequence from the observation

that standard dose H$_2$RAs cannot overcome the effect of food on daytime acid secretion is that such treatment is often inadequate to treat gastroesophageal reflux disease (GERD), where reflux of acidic gastric contents during the day after meals appears to be of prime importance in the genesis and perpetuation of the disease (26). It is therefore important to adequately control both daytime and nocturnal gastric acid secretion in patients with significant GERD. Single nocturnal doses of H$_2$RAs are seldom adequate, and additional conventional daytime doses often add little extra useful antisecretory effect. If the H$_2$RAs are given only at night, very high doses must be administered before there is any detectable carryover effect on acidity during the following day (24, 27). When food is ingested, the effect of the H$_2$RAs on intragastric acidity is much reduced (28–29, 30). Ranitidine 150 mg twice daily is no more effective in controlling daytime food-stimulated acidity than ranitidine 300 mg nightly in duodenal ulcer patients (25).

There are few important pharmacologic differences between the currently available

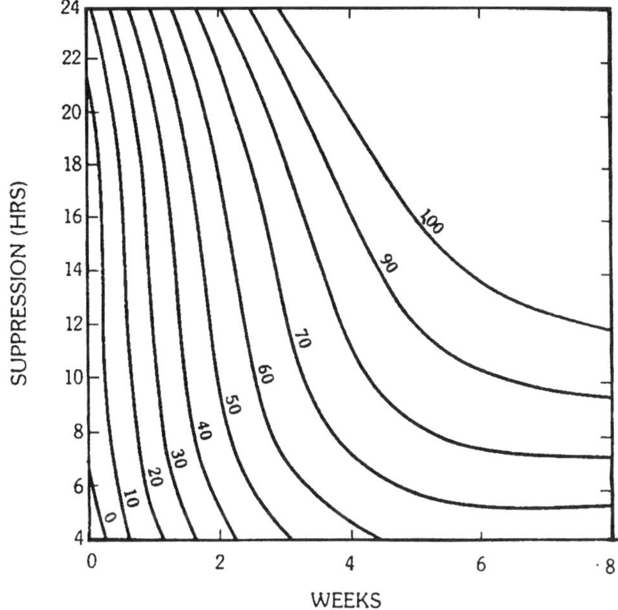

Figure 1.1. Contour plot of duodenal ulcer healing rate predicted by the duration of suppression above a fixed pH threshold of pH 3.0 (*vertical axis*) and duration of therapy (*horizontal axis*).

H_2RAs. All have been extensively studied in clinical pharmacologic studies and in controlled clinical trials in the treatment of patients with peptic ulcer. Different dosage schedules of these drugs have been used at different times and in different countries for the management of duodenal ulcer and gastric ulcer, and the clinical pharmacology of these agents has been extensively reviewed elsewhere (23, 31, 32). Therefore, the following section will deal with the H_2RAs as a class with respect to ulcer healing.

H_2RAs IN DUODENAL ULCER

In the treatment of duodenal ulcer, it is the suppression of overnight gastric acidity that most closely correlates with the therapeutic effect of H_2RA (15). The relationship between suppression of nocturnal intragastric acidity and 4-week duodenal ulcer healing rates for 11 different dose regimens of H_2RAs is shown in Table 1.2. In Figure 1.1, the slope of the regression line relating these two is comparatively slight, showing that the therapeutic gain in overall healing rates at 4 weeks is only about 20%, for an increase in suppression of

nocturnal acidity from about 30% to about 95%. A meta-analysis of duodenal ulcer healing rates for different H_2RAs (15) shows little variability between the different agents, although ranitidine provided slightly better healing compared to cimetidine in a meta-analysis involving these two agents alone (33). When the H_2RAs are given as single doses in the late evening, there are only minor differences in the healing rates between different agents (34).

In addition to their use in healing duodenal ulcers, the H_2RAs have been widely used as continuous maintenance treatment after healing in an attempt to reduce relapse rates (35). They have usually been given, for this purpose, at half of the advocated healing dose (i.e., cimetidine 400 mg, ranitidine 150 mg, famotidine 20 mg, nizatidine 150 mg—all taken every night). When given in this way, the H_2RAs are successful in reducing overall duodenal ulcer relapse rates 12 months after healing from about 80% to about 25% (35). Although the reduction in relapse rates looks impressive, it is likely that many patients with duodenal ulcer do not require such mainte-

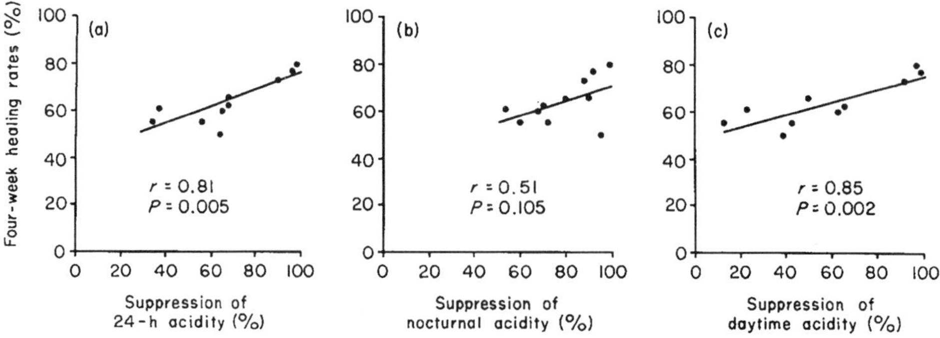

Figure 1.2. Relationship between suppression of 24-hr(*a*), nocturnal (*b*), and daytime intragastric acidity (*c*) and gastric-ulcer healing rates after 4 weeks of treatment.

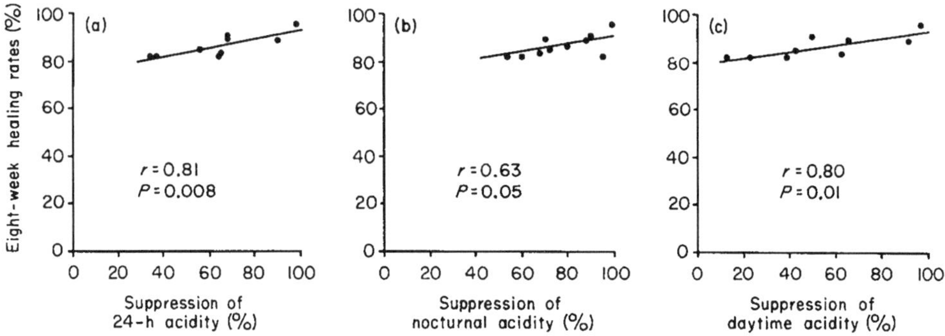

Figure 1.3. Relationship between suppression of 24-hr (*a*), nocturnal (*b*), and daytime intragastric acidity (*c*) and gastric-ulcer healing rates after 8 weeks of treatment.

nance therapy since they have an essentially benign disease process that relapses only once or twice in a year. Such patients can be adequately managed with intermittent courses of therapy when they have episodes of symptomatic relapse. Patients with more aggressive disease (e.g., bleeding ulcers) or more frequently relapsing ulcers may benefit from maintenance treatment, and indeed studies are now emerging that demonstrate a reduction in the rate of recurrent ulcer bleeding among patients receiving daily maintenance therapy (36, 37). It may be even more logical for such maintenance therapy to be at full rather than half dose, particularly if the patients are unwise enough to smoke cigarettes (38). Increasingly, however, such patients may

be managed by treating underlying *H. pylori* infection. If eradication is successful, this is highly effective in reducing and perhaps even eliminating duodenal ulcer relapse (1, 39, 40).

H₂RAs IN GASTRIC ULCER

In the treatment of gastric ulcer, the H₂RAs heal between 50% and 65% of ulcers after 4 weeks (Figure 1.2) and as many as 90% after 8 weeks (Figure 1.3) (12) with only slight differences between the H₂RAs. Suppression of total 24-hour intragastric acidity correlates with healing rates in gastric ulcer. Table 1.3 lists some overall gastric ulcer healing rates for different dosage schedules of H₂RA (12). With H₂RAs, as with other antisecretory drugs, it takes longer to heal gastric than duo-

Table 1.3
H₂-Receptor Antagonists for Gastric Ulcer[a]

Drug and dosage (mg)	Healing rate at 4 weeks	Healing rate at 8 weeks
Nizatidine 150 bid	66	90
Ranitidine 300 qhs	66	91
Nizatidine 800 qhs	65	86
Ranitidine 150 bid	62	90
Cimetidine 400 bid	61	82
Cimetidine 300 qid	60	84
Cimetidine 200 tid + 400 qhs	55	85
Famotidine 40 qhs	50	82

[a]Gastric ulcer healing rates of some commonly used dosage regimens. Adapted, with permission, from Howden and Hunt (12). Key to abbreviations: bid, twice daily; qhs, every night; qid, four times daily. Values are given as percentages.

denal ulcers. Indeed, the duration of effective treatment with antisecretory drugs is the single most important factor in determining gastric ulcer healing rates (11, 14).

In the treatment of gastric ulcers associated with the use of NSAIDs, healing with H₂RAs is more rapid if treatment with NSAIDs can be stopped (41). However, even in this situation, an increased degree of suppression of gastric acidity is more effective in accelerating NSAID-associated gastric ulcer healing, since the proton pump blocker omeprazole was superior to ranitidine in healing gastric ulcers in patients who continued to take NSAIDs (42).

There are fewer data on the use of maintenance treatment with H₂RAs in gastric ulcer than with duodenal ulcer and these drugs are not currently approved by the FDA for such an indication in the United States, although widely used for this purpose in Europe and the rest of the world. (Approval is pending for ranitidine at a dosage of 150 mg every night.)

FURTHER POINTS ABOUT H₂RAs

Despite the enormous amount of attention that these drugs have attracted, there continues to be a great deal of interest in various aspects of their human pharmacology including drug interactions, possible tolerance with their continued use, and possible rebound hypersecretion of acid after stopping treatment. Some of these recent areas of interest are considered below. Drug interactions are discussed in specific detail in Chapter 29.

DRUG INTERACTIONS

Cimetidine is known to bind nonselectively to hepatic cytochrome P450 and to reduce the clearance of a number of different drugs that undergo oxidative metabolism via this pathway (43). The different propensity to interact with other drugs marks one of the differences between cimetidine and ranitidine (44). However, most of these interactions are of purely pharmacokinetic interest. Clinically important interactions with cimetidine are limited to phenytoin, warfarin, and theophylline. Ranitidine may also bind to hepatic cytochrome P450, but the affinity for this is much lower than is seen with cimetidine. There are no convincing, clinically important drug interactions with ranitidine mediated via cytochrome P450 (45). Famotidine, which has the highest affinity for the H₂-receptor, does not bind to cytochrome P450, and no important drug interactions have been described (46). Nizatidine binds weakly to rat hepatic microsomes but no significant drug interactions have been reported in man (47).

One recently described interaction with different H₂RAs that has received considerable attention concerns alcohol (48). Gastric alcohol dehydrogenase (ADH) may be responsible for some of the first-pass metabolism of ingested alcohol, especially when taken in small amounts (49). Cimetidine was first reported to increase blood alcohol levels in 1982 (50), which antedated the isolation and characterization of gastric ADH. The mechanism of cimetidine increasing blood alcohol levels was not known at that time, but since then evidence has accrued that this might be mediated via inhibition of gastric ADH (51). Cimetidine and ranitidine (but not famotidine) show an in vitro concentration-dependent inhibition of two distinct isozymes of gastric ADH (52), although recent studies indicate that the role of gastric ADH in the metabolism of alcohol may, in fact, be negligible (53, 54).

As discussed in detail elsewhere in this book, many of the studies evaluating the interaction of H$_2$RAs are subject to methodologic differences in potential study design and statistical power than cast doubt on their clinical significance. Moreover, when alcohol is administered in low dose over short periods of time in the early morning, the studies may not be directly relevant to or typical of the usual practices of alcohol consumption. Although, one study that attempted to reproduce social drinking habits (55) found a statistically significant effect of cimetidine and nizatidine on peak blood alcohol levels and on the total amount of alcohol absorbed (as judged by the area under the concentration/time curve [AUC]), after a moderately heavy dose of alcohol, other studies have found that H$_2$RAs had no effect on blood alcohol levels (56, 57). Factors contributing to these differing results include variations in basic study design such as the use of parallel groups or crossover designs, differences in the time, dose, and method of alcohol administration, differences in the relationship of alcohol administration to the last main meal consumed by study subjects, and possible interracial differences in alcohol metabolism (56, 58).

Despite these methodologic differences, genuine differences appear among the different H$_2$RAs in their effects on blood alcohol levels, especially at the lowest doses tested. There is evidence for cimetidine increasing blood alcohol levels over a wide range of doses of alcohol (48, 50–52, 55, 59). Famotidine does not appear to influence blood alcohol levels (48, 52, 55), and the data on ranitidine are conflicting, with some studies showing no effect (56, 57, 60) and others showing only a modes effect (48, 55, 61). In most of these studies, the rise in peak blood alcohol levels after a low dose of alcohol was of such low magnitude as to be clinically irrelevant (61) and, to date, no clinical significance has been

attached to the observed interactions between alcohol and certain II$_2$RAs (54, 62).

SAFETY AND POSTMARKETING SURVEILLANCE STUDIES WITH H$_2$RAs

Since the introduction of the first H$_2$RA, cimetidine, in the late 1970s, a huge experience of the safety of H$_2$RAs has accrued (23). Despite the attention placed on drug interactions, the H$_2$RAs are among the safest of drugs. A number of side effects have been reported, but these tend to be mild and self-limiting. Some of the reported adverse events have been identified only as anecdotal case reports. In many formal studies, the H$_2$RA has a similar adverse event profile to placebo.

Cimetidine binds to androgen receptors as well as to histamine H$_2$-receptors. It exerts weakly antiandrogenic effects and its use, rarely, has been associated with gynecomastia, impotence, and diminished libido in male patients. Cimetidine may compete with creatinine for renal tubular secretions sites, but this is not of clinical significance. Cimetidine may also cause reversible confusion in elderly patients (23).

Ranitidine is not associated with antiandrogenic effects in male patients. Headache, mild diarrhea, and a reversible form of drug-induced hepatitis are reported adverse events, but all are rare. Like that of cimetidine, the use of ranitidine has been linked to reversible mental confusion usually seen in sick, elderly patients, especially in the intensive care unit setting, although a causal relationship has not always been proven (23).

Less is known about famotidine and nizatidine since they have been available for a shorter period of time. To date, however, their use has not been associated with any serious adverse events. Because cimetidine was a novel compound at the time of its introduction, it was subjected to extensive postmarketing surveillance studies. The results of these studies (63–65) and subsequent postmarketing surveillance studies performed with ranitidine (66), famotidine (67) and nizatidine (68) have provided much reassurance about the long-term safety of H$_2$RAs in general.

Most importantly, they have demonstrated that prolonged pharmacologic acid suppression with usual doses of H_2RAs are not associated with an increased incidence of gastrointestinal infections or neoplasms (63, 69–71).

TOLERANCE TO H_2RAs

"Tolerance" is frequently used as a term in clinical pharmacology but is seldom adequately defined. It is usually taken to mean a situation where increased doses of a drug are required in order to reproduce an effect that had previously been attained with a lower dose. Using this somewhat arbitrary definition, it cannot by shown conclusively that tolerance develops in patients given oral H_2RAs. However, the effect on suppression of intragastric acidity by H_2RAs is less after some days of continuous treatment than after the first dose (72–76). This does not, however, establish true pharmacologic tolerance and might be explained on the basis of an exaggerated first-dose response. This phenomenon has only been convincingly demonstrated in healthy volunteers and not in patients with acid-related diseases. It is not peculiar to any one H_2RA, having been demonstrated with all currently available competitive H_2RAs (74). It has been more convincingly demonstrated when higher than usual doses or intravenous doses of H_2RAs have been given (72).

Clinical experience with H_2RAs is not consistent with the concept of true or progressive pharmacologic tolerance developing to these drugs. For example, it has been unnecessary to continuously increase the maintenance dose of H_2RA in order to keep patients in remission from duodenal ulceration. The phenomenon labeled as "tolerance" is certainly of scientific interest but is, as yet, of no proven clinical significance.

REBOUND ACID HYPERSECRETION

The possibility of a rebound increase in acid secretion after cessation of treatment with an acid-suppressing drug has long been postulated. However, only recently has there been good experimental evidence to support the notion. A temporary increase in acid output, due to a rise in both acidity and gastric juice volume, to above pretreatment values has been reported after cessation of H_2RAs in both healthy volunteer subjects (77, 78) and in duodenal ulcer patients (79, 80). This finding is also not peculiar to any one H_2RA, although in two studies (77–80) increased acid output or acidity has been demonstrated after stopping some H_2RAs, but not famotidine.

There is some evidence for an up-regulation of the H_2-receptor following treatment with H_2RAs (81). Three months of maintenance treatment with ranitidine 150 mg every night in a group of duodenal ulcer patients was sufficient to increase their acid output in response to stimulation with the specific H_2-receptor agonist impromidine. Furthermore, reversal of impromidine-stimulated acid secretion by intravenous ranitidine was accentuated following 3 months of treatment with ranitidine. This increase in the magnitude of the response to both H_2-receptor agonism and antagonism is suggestive, but is not conclusive evidence for H_2-receptor up-regulation.

Apart from the possibility of receptor up-regulation as an explanation for rebound hypersecretion, the mechanism is unclear. It is unrelated to hypergastrinemia. Gastrin levels are increased following treatment with any acid-suppressing drug, but this is a temporary phenomenon. Gastrin levels also are not correlated with the magnitude of acid rebound, which is, in any case, small, and this interesting phenomenon, like "tolerance," has been of no proven clinical significance.

CURRENT CLINICAL ROLE OF H_2RAs

H_2RAs have held a dominant position in the management of peptic ulcer for almost two decades (23). This prime position however, is likely to be increasingly challenged on two fronts. In the management of duodenal and gastric ulcer, proton pump inhibitors are capable of healing a greater proportion of ulcers than H_2RAs (10, 12, 15, 82, 83) and have been shown in some trials to provide more prompt relief of symptoms (84, 85). However, the therapeutic gain of the proton pump inhibitors over H$_2$RAs in peptic ulcer disease is less than is seen in GERD.

A further challenge to the H$_2$RA is coming from treatment aimed at eradicating infection with *H. pylori*. It is well-recognized that eradication of this organism is associated with a greatly prolonged period of remission from duodenal ulcer, which some have labeled a "cure" (39, 40). Since H$_2$RAs have no activity against *H. pylori* apart from weak in vitro inhibition, ulcer relapse after initial successful treatment is virtually inevitable (38, 86). The main impact of treatment aimed at eradicating *H. pylori* will be on the long-term management of peptic ulcer where there will be an increasing emphasis on eradication rather than on continuous maintenance treatment with half-dose H$_2$RAs (1). However, it is interesting that the addition of ranitidine to a triple-drug regimen aimed at eradicating *H. pylori* resulted in accelerated healing of duodenal ulcer (87). Whether this will be translated into routine clinical practice is uncertain since eradication regimens using three drugs are already complicated enough without the addition of a fourth (1). *H. pylori* is considered in greater detail in a Chapter 6.

The recommendations of the Working Party of the 1990 World Congress of Gastroenterology were that eradication of *H. pylori* should be reserved only for patients with duodenal ulcers that had either been difficult to treat or in whom ulcers had been relapsing frequently (88). It is likely that these recommendations will change as experience with eradication regimens increases and more is learned about the ability of *H. pylori* to acquire resistance to different antibiotics. Indeed, the working party report from the First United European Gastroenterology Week held in Athens in September 1992 recommended that all patients with duodenal ulcer associated with *H. pylori* should be considered candidates for *H. pylori* eradication therapy after their ulcers were healed with standard antisecretory therapy (89). The working party endorsed two major therapeutic approaches for *H. pylori* eradication: (a) standard triple therapy with bismuth, metronidazole, and either tetracycline or amoxicillin; or (b) dual therapy with a proton pump inhibitor and either amoxicillin or clarithromycin. If eradication fails, a combination of triple therapy with a proton pump inhibitor can be tried. Another option is to use maintenance H$_2$RA therapy until more effective therapy becomes available. It should be noted, however, that there was not unanimous agreement on these recommendations, with at least one authority describing the current data on *H. pylori* eradication as being "in chaos" (89).

FUTURE PROSPECTS FOR H$_2$RAs

H$_2$RAs as a class have been extremely successful in clinical practice. They have been well-accepted by prescribers and patients, which reflects confidence in their efficacy and safety (23). Although they have been intensively studied, new aspects to their clinical pharmacology continue to be revealed. "Tolerance" and the "up-regulation" of the H$_2$-receptor are such examples.

The pre-eminence of H$_2$RAs in the management of patients with peptic ulcer is now changing. Increasing acceptance of the proton pump inhibitors over H$_2$RAs as primary treatment for duodenal ulcer will probably continue, as the efficacy and safety of these newer agents is increasingly confirmed. The wider acceptance of the approach of primary eradication of *H. pylori* in the long-term management of duodenal, and perhaps gastric, ulcer may further reduce the use of H$_2$RAs. As previously mentioned, interest is focusing on *H. pylori* eradication rather than long-term continuous maintenance treatment with H$_2$RAs as the optimal treatment strategy for patients with relapsing duodenal ulcer. This will continue to develop, particularly if more simple, safe, and efficacious eradication regimens become available, as seems likely.

There is the possibility that at least some H$_2$RAs may by made available for over-the-counter (OTC) use in the near future. This is already the case for cimetidine in Denmark. The safety record of H$_2$RAs certainly justifies such a development (90).

Table 1.4
Meta-analysis of Omeprazole 20 Mg Daily with Either Cimetidine 800 Mg Daily or Ranitidine 300 Mg Daily in the Healing of Duodenal Ulcer[a]

	At 2 weeks	At 4 weeks
Omeprazole 20 mg	64.1	90.4
Cimetidine 800 mg	43.1	77.7
P value	<.001	<.01
Omeprazole 20 mg	69.3	92.8
Ranitidine 300 mg	52.8	83.1
P value	<.001	<.001

[a]Adapted with permission from Holt and Howden (83). Values are given as percentages.

Proton Pump Inhibitors

At the time of writing, the only member of this class of drugs to be licensed in the United States is omeprazole, although lansoprazole has been launched in France and several other compounds are under development. Aspects of the clinical pharmacology of omeprazole have been reviewed elsewhere (83, 91, 92), and will only be summarized here.

Omeprazole, lansoprazole, and similar agents are irreversible inhibitors of H^+/K^+-ATPase, which is found in the secretory canaliculi of parietal cells (2, 83). This enzyme, the "proton pump" or "acid pump," is responsible for the final step in the process of acid secretion. Omeprazole and other irreversible inhibitors are acid space-dependent prodrugs that, after systemic absorption, are initially widely distributed in the body. However, they become localized and concentrated in the highly acidic environment of the secretory compartment of the parietal cell because they are weakly basic drugs. There, they are protonated and essentially trapped within the acid pump, which is then irreversibly inactivated. The pharmacologic interactions between the irreversible proton pump blockers and H^+/K^+-ATPase have been elegantly discussed by Sachs et al. (2). Non-acid space-dependent reversible inhibitors of the K^+ channel of the H^+/K^+-ATPase are also currently under development.

By virtue of the effect on the final step in the acid secretory process, omeprazole pro-duces an effective reduction in acid secretion in response to all known stimuli. The overall effect of omeprazole on intragastric acidity is proportionately greater than standard dose H_2RA (93, 94). Unlike H_2RAs, omeprazole effectively inhibits meal-stimulated acid secretion during the day as well as basal secretion overnight. In the standard clinical dosage of 20 mg once daily, omeprazole maintains intragastric pH >3.0 for 16–18 hours of the day. Complex meta-analyses and the application of response surface methodology to examine the relationship between various parameters of suppression of acidity and duodenal ulcer healing rates has determined that the duration of time for which intragastric pH is kept above a given pH threshold is the most important determinant of duodenal ulcer healing (10). If a pH threshold of 3.0 is examined, the model predicts that 100% of duodenal ulcers would be healed in 4 weeks by a drug sustaining this for 18–20 hours of the day. Omeprazole 20 mg daily closely approximates this. A meta-analysis comparing standard dose omeprazole (20 mg) with standard doses of cimetidine or ranitidine in the short-term healing of duodenal ulcer is summarized in Table 1.4.

PROTON PUMP INHIBITORS IN DUODENAL ULCER

A variety of clinical trials have shown that omeprazole is significantly superior to placebo or standard dose H_2RAs in the short-term healing of duodenal ulcer (83, 84, 95). In an overview of published controlled clinical trials in duodenal ulcer, omeprazole 20 mg daily produced the highest overall 4-week healing rate—94.2% in a total of 465 patients (92). By contrast, the next most effective drug regiment was ranitidine 300 mg daily with a healing rate of 79.1% of duodenal ulcers in 4551 patients (91, 92).

In addition to higher overall healing rates, many trials have shown that omeprazole is superior to H_2RAs in the rapid alleviation of symptoms in patients treated for duodenal ulcer (84). In most cases, this has been reported as a significantly higher proportion of patients who were completely free of pain after, for

mechanisms of action have been proposed (115). It forms a protective coating over ulcers, thereby preventing further acid-peptic digestion, and this may persist for 12–16 hours after administration (116). It may also stimulate healing through augmenting local endogenous prostaglandin production (117). Sucralfate may promote healing through adsorption of pepsins and bile salts, thereby inhibiting the proteolytic and irritant action on ulcers. Sucralfate may also stimulate local production and release of epidermal growth factor (EGF) (118), as well as bind EGF at the ulcer site. Alternatively, the action of sucralfate could be explained by some combination of these effects or by some mechanism as yet unrecognized. Complete reviews of the clinical pharmacology of sucralfate are available elsewhere (115, 119).

In comparative clinical studies, sucralfate produces duodenal ulcer healing rates comparable to those obtained with H₂RAs (115, 119). Reported 4-week healing rates are 79% for sucralfate and 77% for H₂RAs (120). The standard clinical dose of sucralfate has been 1 g four times daily in most studies, although a simpler regimen of 2 g twice daily may be just as efficacious. At least one study (from Hong Kong) has suggested that the duodenal ulcer healing rates in cigarette smokers treated with sucralfate are about equivalent to those seen in nonsmokers (120). Such a situation is generally not seen with H₂RAs where smokers usually have lower overall initial 4-week healing rates than nonsmokers. This is also true for ulcer healing on placebo where healing rates in smokers are usually about 10% lower than corresponding rates in nonsmokers (121). This difference in healing rates, however, generally disappears during the second four weeks of therapy.

It has been suggested that maintenance of ulcer healing may be more prolonged after treatment with sucralfate in comparison with H₂RAs (122), although the mechanism for this claim, which has not been observed in further studies, is unclear. Sucralfate does not exert any major effects on *H. pylori*. However, triple therapy with sucralfate, metronidazole, and tetracycline was as effective as a triple-therapy regimen with bismuth (123). Furthermore, recent work suggests a dose-dependent inhibition of *H. pylori* lipopolysaccharide damage to gastric mucosa (124) and, also, inhibition of the mucolytic effects of *H. pylori* (125).

Sucralfate 1 g twice daily has been approved by the FDA for maintenance treatment of patients with duodenal ulcer. It maintains remission more effectively than placebo and is generally equivalent to H₂RAs when they are given in half their customary healing dose for maintenance therapy. Sucralfate 2 g daily is associated with a 12-month duodenal ulcer relapse rate of approximately 38% (115, 126).

In the treatment of gastric ulcer, sucralfate is superior to placebo and about equivalent to H₂RAs, with healing rates of approximately 75% at 8 weeks. Fewer data are available on the efficacy of sucralfate in the maintenance treatment of gastric ulcer after successful initial healing, and the drug is not currently approved by the FDA for this indication. One study found it to be significantly less effective than ranitidine (127).

Sucralfate has few side effects. The most frequently reported is constipation, which occurs in about 2% of patients and is due to the aluminum content of the drug (115). Sucralfate may alter the rate of absorption of a number of concurrently administered drugs since it may form insoluble complexes with these drugs within the gut. A large number of drugs have been studied in this regard, including NSAIDs, prednisone, acetaminophen, digoxin, phenytoin, and furosemide. As with H₂RAs, most reported interactions are of no clinical relevance, but there is a potentially important interaction with phenytoin and a few others such as quinolone antibiotics (See Chapter 29). Small quantities of aluminum are absorbed following administration of sucralfate, and use of the drug should therefore be avoided in any patients with a significant degree of renal impairment because of the association between aluminum and dialysis encephalopathy.

Misoprostol (and Other Synthetic Prostaglandins)

Misoprostol is the only synthetic prostaglandin derivative to have been introduced into clinical practice for the management of acid-related disorders. The structure of misoprostol is based on naturally occurring prostaglandin E_1. In the United States the main indication for its use is to limit or prevent new gastric mucosal damage attributable to the use of NSAIDs (128, 129), which is dealt with in detail in Chapter 3.

Misoprostol and other synthetic prostaglandin derivatives have also been studied in the treatment of duodenal ulcer (130–133). However, healing rates have been generally inferior to those obtained with H_2RAs and side effect profiles have shown more adverse events. The prostaglandins have two principal pharmacologic actions that include acid suppression and "cytoprotection." However, cytoprotection does not seem to be involved in their therapeutic effectiveness in duodenal ulcer healing since healing rates are almost exactly those that would be predicted from a knowledge of their antisecretory effect (15). Furthermore, prostaglandins are ineffective in healing duodenal ulcer when given in doses that are not antisecretory but are sufficient to exert cytoprotective effect (131). Enprostil, a synthetic prostaglandin E_2 derivative, was inferior to ranitidine in the maintenance treatment of patients with healed duodenal ulcer (134).

Misoprostol and other synthetic prostaglandins are associated with a high incidence of diarrhea, and the side effect profile is certainly inferior to other agents currently available for the treatment of peptic ulcer (115). In one study (128), diarrhea developed in >42% of patients receiving misoprostol 200 μg four times daily. The diarrhea was usually mild, however, and few patients had to discontinue treatment. In addition, misoprostol and other prostaglandins cannot be given to young women of child-bearing age because they are potentially abortifacient.

The synthetic prostaglandins are not currently recommended for the routine treatment of duodenal ulcer. They have been considered "a promise unfulfilled" in the management of patients with ulcer disease (135). Moreover, the routine use of misoprostol to prevent damage from NSAIDs is not recommended (136).

REFERENCES

1. Chiba N, Rao BV, Rademaker JW, Hunt RH. Meta-analysis of the efficacy of antibiotic therapy in eradicating *Helicobacter pylori*. Am J Gastroenterol 1992;87:1716–1727.
2. Sachs G, Maton PN, Wallmark B. Pharmacology of the parietal cell. In: Collen MJ, Benjamin SB, eds. Pharmacology of peptic ulcer disease. New York: Springer-Verlag, 1991:1–54.
3. Gleeson D. Acid-base transport systems in gastrointestinal epithelia. Gut 1992;33:1134–1145.
4. Grossman MI, Kirsner JB, Gillespie IE. Basal and histalog-stimulated gastric secretion in control subjects and in patients with peptic ulcer or gastric cancer. Gastroenterology 1963;45:14–26.
5. Feldman M, Richardson CT. Total 24-hour gastric acid secretion in patients with duodenal ulcer: comparison with normal subjects and effects of cimetidine and parietal cell vagotomy. Gastroenterology 1986;90:540–544.
6. Lanzon-Miller S, Pounder RE, Hamilton MR, et al. Twenty-four-hour intragastric acidity and plasma gastrin concentration in healthy subjects and patients with duodenal or gastric ulcer or pernicious anaemia. Aliment Pharmacol Ther 1987;1:225–238.
7. Collen MJ, Stanczak VJ, Ciarleglio CA. Refractory duodenal ulcers (nonhealing, duodenal ulcers with standard doses of antisecretory medication). Dig Dis Sci 1989;34:233–237.
8. Lewis JH. Idiopathic gastric acid hypersecretion: treatment implications for refractory acid/peptic disorders. Aliment Pharmacol Therap 1991;5 (suppl 1):15–24.
9. Howden CW, Jones DB, Hunt RH. Nocturnal doses of H_2-receptor antagonists for duodenal ulcer. Lancet 1985;1:647–648.
10. Burget DW, Chiverton SG, Hunt RH. Is there an optimal degree of acid suppression for healing duodenal ulcers? A model of the relationship between ulcer healing and acid suppression. Gastroenterology 1990;99:345–351.
11. Howden CW, Jones DB, Peace KE, Burget DW, Hunt RH. The treatment of gastric ulcer with antisecretory drugs: relationship of pharmacological effect to healing rates. Dig Dis Sci 1988;33:619–624.
12. Howden CW, Hunt RH. The relationship between the suppression of acidity and gastric ulcer healing rates. Aliment Pharmacol Ther 1990;4:25–33.
13. Derodra JK, Howden CW, Burget DW, Hunt RH. Twenty-four-hour intragastric acidity and noctur-

nal gastric secretion in gastric ulcer patients-the effects of cimetidine. Aliment Pharmacol Ther 1990;4:275–281.

14. Howden CW, Burget DW, Hunt RH. A meta-analysis to predict gastric ulcer healing from acid suppression[Abstract].Gastroenterology1991;100:A85.

15. Jones DB, Howden CW, Burget DW, Kerr GD, Hunt RH. Acid suppression in duodenal ulcer: a meta-analysis to define optimal dosing with antisecretory drugs. Gut 1987;28:1120–1127.

16. Soll AH, Weinstein UM, Kurata J, McCarthy D. Nonsteroidal anti-inflammatory drugs and peptic ulcer disease. Ann Intern Med 1991;114:307–319.

17. Peterson WL, Sturdevant AL, Frankl HD, et al. Healing of duodenal ulcer with an antacid regimen. N Engl J Med 1977;297:341–345.

18. Kumar N, Vij JC, Karol A, Anand BS. Controlled therapeutic trial to determine the optimum dose of antacids in duodenal ulcer. Gut 1984;25:1199–1202.

19. Weberg R, Berstad A, Lange O, Schultz T, Aubert E. Duodenal ulcer healing with four antacid tablets daily. Scand J Gastroenterol 1985;20:1041–1045.

20. Weberg R, Aubert E, Dahlberg O, et al. Low-dose antacids or cimetidine for duodenal ulcer? Gastroenterology 1988;95:1465–1469.

21. Isenberg JI, Peterson WL, Elashoff JD, et al. Healing of benign gastric ulcer with low-dose antacid or cimetidine: a double-blind, randomized, placebo-controlled trial. N Engl J Med 1983;308:1319–1324.

22. Hatler F, Lam SK. Antacid therapy of ulcer disease. In: Swabb EA, Szabo S, eds. Ulcer disease: Investigation and basis for therapy. New York: Dekker, 1991;167–188.

23. Feldman M, Burton ME. Histamine₂-receptor antagonists: standard therapy for acid-peptic diseases. N Engl J Med 1990;323:1672–1680, 1749–1755.

24. Gledhill T, Howard OM, Buck M, Paul A, Hunt RH. Single nocturnal dose of an H₂-receptor antagonist for the treatment of duodenal ulcer. Gut 1983;24:904–908.

25. Ireland A, Gear P, Colin-Jones DG, et al. 150 mg twice daily versus 300 mg nightly in treatment of duodenal ulcers. Lancet 1984;2:274–275.

26. de Caestecker JS, Blackwell JN, Pryde A, Heading RC. Daytime gastro-oesophageal reflux is important in oesophagitis. Gut 1987;28:519–526.

27. Kapur B, Mills JG, Glenny H, Burland WL, Lunt M, Bardhan KD. Evaluation of large single night-time doses of cimetidine using continuous 24-hour ambulatory gastric pH monitoring [Abstract]. Gut 1985;26:A559.

28. Kempf M, Kaufmann D, Walt RP, et al. TV snacks are bad for H₂-receptor blockade [Abstract]. Gastroenterology 1988;94:A222.

29. Merki HS, Halter F, Wilder-Smith CH, et al. Effect of food on H₂-receptor blockade in normal subjects and duodenal patients. Gut 1990;31:148–150.

30. Merki HS, Wilder-Smith CH, Walt RP, Halter F. The cephalic and gastric phases of gastric secretion during H₂-antagonist treatment. Gastroenterology 1991;101:599–606.

31. Howden CW, Hunt RH. The histamine H₂-receptor antagonists. In: Swabb EA, Szabo S, eds. Ulcer diseases: Investigation and basis for therapy. New York: Dekker, 1991;189–215.

32. Howden CW. Advances in the therapeutic uses of histamine H₂-receptors antagonists. Balliere's Clin Gastroenterol 1993;7:81–94.

33. McIsaac RL, McCandless I, Summers K, Wood JR. Ranitidine and cimetidine in the healing of duodenal ulcer: meta-analysis of comparative clinical trials. Ailment Pharmacol Ther 1987;1:369–381.

34. Chiverton SG, Hunt RH. Medical regimens in short- and long-term ulcer management. Balliere's Clin Gastroenterol 1988;2:655–676.

35. Sontag JJ and the ACG Committee on FDA-Related Matters. Current status of maintenance therapy in peptic ulcer disease. Am J Gastroenterol 1988;93:607–617.

36. Jensen DM, Machicado GA, Kovacs TOG, et al. Long-term recurrence rates of peptic ulceration and rebleeding with H₂ maintenance, surgery or no maintenance therapy. Gastroenterology 1989; 96:A239.

37. Penston JG, Wormsley KG. Nine years of maintenance treatment with ranitidine for patients, with duodenal ulcer disease. Ailment Pharmacol Ther 1992;6:629–646.

38. Lewis JH. The natural history of duodenal ulcer disease: has it been altered by drug therapy? In: Collen MJ, Benjamin SB, eds. Pharmacology of peptic ulcer disease. New York: Springer-Verlag, 1991:263–300.

39. Rauws EAJ, Tytgat GNJ. Cure of duodenal ulcer associated with eradication of *Helicobacter pylori*. Lancet 1990;335:1233–1235.

40. Graham DY, Lew GM, Klein PD, et al. Effect of treatment of *Helicobacter pylori* infection on the long-term recurrence of gastric or duodenal ulcer: a randomized, controlled study. Ann Intern Med 1992;116:705–708.

41. Lancaster-Smith MJ, Jaderberg ME, Jackson DA. Ranitidine in the treatment of non-steroidal anti-inflammatory drug associated gastric and duodenal ulcers. Gut 1991;32:252–255.

42. Walan A, Bader JP, Classen M, et al. Effect of omeprazole and ranitidine on ulcer healing and relapse rates in patients with benign gastric ulcer. N Engl J Med 1989;320:69–75.

43. Somogyi A, Muirhead M. Pharmacokinetic interactions of cimetidine 1987. Clin Pharmacokinet 1987;12:321–366.

44. Smith SR, Kendall MJ. Ranitidine versus cimetidine: a comparison of their potential to cause clinically important drug interactions. Clin Pharmacokinet 1988;15:44–56.

45. Mitchard M, Harris A, Mullinger BM. Ranitidine drug interactions: a literature review. Pharmacol Ther 1987;32:293–325.
46. Humphries TJ. Famotidine: A notable lack of drug interactions. Scand Gastroenterol 1987;22(suppl 134):55–60.
47. Klotz U. Lack of effect of nizatidine on drug metabolism. Scand J Gastroenterol 1987;22(suppl 136):18–23.
48. DiPadova C, Roine R, Frezza M, Gentry RT, Baraona E, Lieber CS. Effects of ranitidine on blood alcohol levels after ethanol ingestion. Comparison with other H_2-receptor antagonists. JAMA 1992;267:83–86.
49. Caballeria J, Frezza M, Hernandez-Munoz R, et al. Gastric origin of the first-pass metabolism of ethanol in humans: Effect of gastrectomy. Gastroenterology 1989;97:1205–1209.
50. Feely J, Wood AJJ. Effects of cimetidine on the elimination of ethanol. JAMA 1982;247:2819–2821.
51. Caballeria J, Baraona E, Rodamilans M, Lieber CS. Effects of cimetidine on gastric alcohol dehydrogenase activity and blood ethanol levels. Gastroenterology 1989;96:388–392.
52. Hernandez-Munoz R, Caballeria J, Baraona E, Uppal R, Greenstein R, Lieber CS. Human gastric alcohol dehydrogenase: its inhibition by H_2-receptor antagonists and its effect on the bioavailability of ethanol. Alcoholism: Clin Exp Res 1990;14:946–950.
53. Smith T, DeMaster FG, Furne JK, Springfield J, Levitt MD. First-pass gastric mucosal metabolism of ethanol is negligible in the rat. J Clin Invest 1992;89:1801–1806.
54. Levitt MD. Review article: lack of clinical significance of the interaction between H_2-receptor antagonists and ethanol. Aliment Pharmacol Ther 1993;7:131–138.
55. Guram M, Howden CW, Holt S. Further evidence for an interaction between alcohol and certain H_2-receptor antagonists. Alcoholism: Clin Exp Res 1991;15:1084–1085.
56. Fraser AG, Prewett EJ, Hudson M, Sawyer AM, Rosalki SB, Pounder RE. The effect of ranitidine, cimetidine or famotidine on low-dose post-prandial alcohol absorption. Aliment Pharmacol Ther 1991;5:263–272.
57. Raufman JP, Notar-Francesco V, Raffaniello R, Straus E. Histamine-H_2-receptor antagonists do not alter serum ethanol levels in fed, non-alcoholic men. Am J Gastroenterol 1992;87:1344.
58. Tanaka E, Nakamura K. Effects of H_2-receptor antagonists on ethanol metabolism in Japanese volunteers. Br J Clin Pharmacol 1988;26:96–99.
59. Seitz HK, Veith S, Czygan P, et al. In vivo interactions between H_2-receptor antagonists and ethanol metabolism in man and in rats. Hepatology 1984;4:1231–1234.
60. Dobrilla G, de Pretis G, Piazzi L, et al. Is ethanol metabolism affected by oral administration of cimetidine and ranitidine in therapeutic doses? Hepatogastroenterology 1984;31:35–37.
61. Fraser AG, Hudson M, Sawyerr AM, Rosalki SB, Pounder RE. Short report: the effect of ranitidine on the postprandial absorption of a low dose of alcohol. Aliment Pharmacol Ther 1992;6:267–271.
62. Lewis JH, McIsaac RL. H_2 antagonists and blood alcohol levels. Dig Dis Sci 1993;38:569–572.
63. Colin-Jones DG, Langman MJS, Lawson DH, Vessey MP. Cimetidine and gastric cancer: preliminary report from post-marketing surveillance study. Br Med J 1982;285:1311–1313.
64. Colin-Jones DG, Langman MJS, Lawson DH, Vessey MP. Postmarketing surveillance of the safety of cimetidine: 12 month mortality report. Br Med J 1983;286:1713–1716.
65. Colin-Jones DG, Langman MJS, Lawson DH, Vessey MP. Postmarketing surveillance of the safety of cimetidine: 12 month morbidity report. Q J Med 1987;54:253–268.
66. Simon B, Muller P, Dammann HG. Safety profile of ranitidine. In: Riley AJ, Salmon PR, eds. Ranitidine: Proceedings of an international symposium held in the context of the Seventh World Congress of Gastroenterology. Stockholm, 17 June 1982. Amsterdam: Excepta Medica 1982:181–189.
67. Saigenji K, Fukutomi H, Nakazawa S. Famotidine: Postmarketing clinical experience. Scand J Gastroenterol 1987;22(suppl 134):34–40.
68. Cloud ML. Safety of nizatidine in clinical trials conducted in the USA and Europe. Scand J Gastroenterol 1987;22(suppl 136):29–36.
69. Lewis JH. Safety profile of long-term H_2-antagonist therapy. Aliment Pharmacol Ther 1991;5(suppl 1):49–57.
70. Penston JG. The efficacy and safety of long-term maintenance treatment of duodenal ulcer with ranitidine. Scand J Gastroenterol 1990;25(suppl 177):1–104.
71. McIsaac RL, Wilson TH, Mills JG, Euler AR, Lewis JH. Safety profile of higher doses of ranitidine given for up to one year [Abstract]. Gastroenterology 1993;104:A144.
72. Wilder-Smith CH, Ernst T, Gennoni M, Zeyen B, Halter F, Merki HS. Tolerance to oral H_2-receptor antagonists. Dig Dis Sci 1990;35:976–983.
73. Smith JTL, Gavey C, Nwokolo CU, Pounder RE. Tolerance during 8 days of high-dose H_2-blockade: Placebo-controlled studies of 24-h acidity and gastrin. Aliment Pharmacol Ther 1990;4(suppl 1):47–64.
74. Nwokolo CU, Smith JTL, Gavey C, Sawyerr A, Pounder RE. Tolerance during 29 days of conventional dosing with cimetidine, nizatidine, famotidine or ranitidine. Aliment Pharmacol Ther 1990;4(suppl 1):29–46.

75. Misiewicz JJ. Clinical relevance of tolerance to peptic ulcer healing and relapse. Aliment Pharmacol Ther 1990;4(suppl 1):85–96.

76. Nwokolo CU, Prewett EJ, Sawyerr AFM, Hudson M, Lim S, Pounder RE. Tolerance during 5 months of dosing with ranitidine 150 mg nightly: a placebo-controlled, double-blind study. Gastroenterology 1991;101:948–953.

77. Nwokolo CU, Smith JTL, Sawyerr AM, Pounder RE. Rebound intragastric hyperacidity after abrupt withdrawal of histamine H₂-receptor blockade. Gut 1991;32:1455–1460.

78. Prewett EJ, Hudson M, Nwokolo CU, Sawyerr AM, Pounder RE. Nocturnal intragastric acidity during and after a period of dosing with either ranitidine or omeprazole. Gastroenterology 1991; 100:873–877.

79. Fullarton GM, McLaughlin G, MacDonald A, Crean GP, McColl KEL. Rebound nocturnal hypersecretion after four weeks H₂ antagonist therapy. Gut 1989;30:449–454.

80. Fullarton GM, MacDonald AMI, McColl KEL. Rebound hypersecretion after H₂ antagonist withdrawal: a comparative study with nizatidine, ranitidine and famotidine. Aliment Pharmacol Ther 1991;5:391–398.

81. Jones DB, Howden CW, Burget DW, Silletti C, Hunt RH. Alteration of H₂-receptor sensitivity in duodenal ulcer patients during maintenance treatment with an H₂-receptor antagonist. Gut 1988;29:890–893.

82. Poynard T, Pignon JP. Duodenal ulcer: analyses of 293 randomized controlled trials. London: John Libbey, 1989.

83. Holt S, Howden CW. Omeprazole: overview and opinion. Dig Dis Sci 1991;36:385–393.

84. McFarland RJ, Bateson MC, Green JRB, et al. Omeprazole provides quicker symptom relief and duodenal ulcer healing than ranitidine. Gastroenterology 1990;98:278–283.

85. Valenzuela JE, Berlin RG, Snape WJ, et al. U.S. experience with omeprazole in duodenal ulcer: multicenter double-blind comparative study with ranitidine. Dig Dis Sci 1991;36:761–768.

86. Graham DY, Colon-Pagan J, Morse RS, et al. Ulcer recurrence following duodenal ulcer healing with omeprazole, ranitidine or placebo: a double-blind, multicenter, 6-month study. Gastroenterology 1992;102:1289–1294.

87. Graham DY, Lew GM, Evans DG, Evans DJ Jr., Klein PD. Effect of triple therapy (antibiotics plus bismuth) on duodenal ulcer healing: a randomized controlled effect. Ann Intern Med 1991;115:266–269.

88. Tytgat GNJ, Graham DY, Lee A, Marshall BJ, Dixon M, Axon A. Working Party Report of the World Congress of Gastroenterology, Sydney 1990. *Helicobacter pylori*: causal agent in peptic ulcer disease? J Gastroenterol Hepatol 1991;6:103–140.

89. *Helicobacter pylori* Working Party of the First United European Gastroenterology Week, Athens, September 25–30, 1992. Scrip Oct. 5, 1992.

90. Andersen M, Schou RS. Adverse reactions to H₂-receptor antagonists in Denmark before and after transfer of cimetidine and ranitidine to over-the-counter status. Pharmacol Toxicol 1991;69:253–258.

91. Howden CW. Clinical pharmacology of omeprazole. Clin Pharmacokine 1991;20:38–49.

92. Maton PN. Omeprazole. N Engl J Med 1991;324:965–975.

93. Lanzon-Miller S, Pounder RE, Hamilton MR, et al. Twenty-four-hour intragastric acidity and plasma concentration before and during treatment with either ranitidine or omeprazole. Aliment Pharmacol Ther 1987;1:239–252.

94. Walt RP, Gomes MdeFA, Wood EC, Logan LH, Pounder RE. Effect of daily oral omeprazole on 24-hour intragastric acidity. Br Med J 1983;287:12–14.

95. Graham DY, McCullough A, Sklar M, et al. Omeprazole versus placebo in duodenal ulcer healing: the United States experience. Dig Dis Sci 1990;35:66–72.

96. Bianchi Porro G, Bolling E, Barbara L, et al. Maintenance treatment with omeprazole in the prevention of duodenal ulcer relapse: a double-blind comparative trial [Abstract]. Gastroenterology 1990; 98:A21.

97. Lauristen K, Andersen BN, Laursen LS, et al. Omeprazole 20 mg three times a week and 10 mg daily in prevention of duodenal ulcer relapse: double-blind comparative trial. Gastroenterology 1991; 100:663–669.

98. Simon TJ, Bradstreet DC. Comparative tolerability profile of omeprazole in clinical trials. Dig Dis Sci 1991;361:1384–1389.

99. Lindquist M, Edwards IR. Endocrine adverse effects of omeprazole. Br Med J 1992;305:451–452.

100. Wormsley KG. Risk of therapeutic achlorhydria. Scand J Gastroenterol 1988;23 (suppl 153):35–51.

101. Hunt RH, Cederberg C, Dent J, et al. Optimizing acid suppression for the treatment of acid-related disorders. Gastroenterology 1993; in press.

102. Walt RP, Gomes MdeFA, Wood EC, et al. Effect of daily oral omeprazole on 24-hour intragastric acidity. Br Med J 1983;287:12–14.

103. Prewett EJ, Hudson M, Nwokolo CU, et al. Nocturnal intragastric acidity before during and after a period of dosing with either ranitidine or omeprazole. Gastroenterology 1991;100:873–877.

104. Lanzon-Miller S, Pounder RE, Hamilton MR, et al. Twenty-four-hour intragastric acidity and plasma gastrin concentration before and during treatment with either ranitidine or omeprazole. Aliment Pharmacol Ther 1987;1:239–251.

105. Lanzon-Miller S, Pounder RE, Hamilton MR, et al. Twenty-four-hour intragastric acidity and plasma gastrin concentration in healthy subjects and pa-

tients with duodenal and gastric ulcer or pernicious anaemia. Aliment Pharmacol Ther 1987;1:225–237.

106. Lind T, Cederberg C, Olausson M, Olbe L. 24-hour intragastric acidity and plasma gastrin after omeprazole treatment and after proximal gastric vagotomy in duodenal ulcer patients. Gastroenterology 1990;99:1593–1598.

107. Koop H, Klein M, Arnold R. Serum gastrin levels during long-term omeprazole treatment. Aliment Pharmacol Ther 1990;4:131–138.

108. Freston JW, Borch K, Brand SJ, et al. The effects of hypochlorhydria and hypergastrinemia on the structure and function of gastrointestinal cells. A review and analysis. Gastroenterology 1993; in press.

109. Lamberts R, Creutzfeldt W, Struber HG, et al. Long-term omeprazole therapy in peptic ulcer disease: Endocrine cell growth and gastritis. Gastroenterology 1993;10:1356–1370.

110. Holt S, Powers RE, Howden CW. Antisecretory therapy and genotoxicity. Dig Dis Sci 1991;36:545–547.

111. Holt S, Zhu Z-H, Powers RE. Observations on a proposed measure of genotoxicity in rat gastric mucosa. Gastroenterology 1991;101:65–656.

112. Scott D, Reuben RA, Zampighi G, Sachs G. Cell isolation and genotoxicity assessment in gastric mucosa. Dig Dis Sci 1990;35:1217–1225.

113. Labenz J, Gyenes E, Ruhl GH, Borsch G. Amoxicillin—omeprazole treatment for eradication of *Helicobacter pylori* Eur J Gastroenterol Hepatol 1991;3(suppl 1):510.

114. Unge P, Eriksson K, Bergman B, et al. Omeprazole and amoxicillin in patients with duodenal ulcer: *Helicobacter pylori* eradication and remission of ulcers and symptoms during a 6-month follow-up. A double-blind comparative study. Gastroenterology 1992;102:A183.

115. McCarthy DM. Sucralfate. N Engl J Med 1991;325:1017–1025.

116. Nakazawa S, Nagashima R, Samloff MI. Selective binding of sucralfate to duodenal ulcer in man. Scand J Gastroenterol 1981;26:297–300.

117. Crampton JR, Gibbons LC, Rees WDW. Effects of sucralfate on gastroduodenal bicarbonate and prostaglandin E_2 metabolism. Am J Med 1987;3:83–92.

118. Nexo E, Poulsen SS. Does epidermal growth factor play a role in the action of sucralfate? Scand J Gastroenterol 1987;22 (suppl 27):45–49.

119. Hunt RH. Treatment of peptic ulcer disease with sucralfate: a review. Am J Med 1991;91(suppl 2A):102S–106S.

120. Lam SK. Why do ulcers heal with sucralfate? Scand J Gastroenterol 1990;25 (suppl 173):6–16.

121. Kirkendall JW, Evaul J, Johnson LF. Effect of cigarette smoking on gastrointestinal physiology and non-neoplastic digestive disease. J Clin Gastroenterol 1984;6:65–79.

122. Domschke S, Domschke W. Longer relapse-free period after sucralfate than after H_2-blocker treatment of duodenal and gastric ulcers. Am J Med 1991;91 (suppl 2A):74S–83S.

123. Louw JA, Zak J, Lucke W, et al. Triple therapy with sucralfate is as effective as triple therapy containing bismuth in eradicating helicobacter pylori and reducing duodenal ulcer relapse rates. Scand J Gastroenterol; in press.

124. Piotrowski J, Yamaki K, Slomiany A, Slomiany BL. Inhibition of gastric mucosal laminin receptor by *Helicobacter pylori* lipopolysaccharide: Effect of sucralfate. Am J Gastroenterol 1991;86:1756–1760.

125. Slomiany BL, Piotrowski J, Slomiany A. Effect of sucralfate on the degradation of human gastric mucus by *Helicobacter pylori* protease and lipases. Am J Gastroenterol 1992;87:595–599.

126. Bolin TD. Sucralfate maintenance in duodenal ulcer disease. Am J Med 1989;86 (suppl 6A):148–151.

127. Takemoto T, Namiki M, Ishikawa M, et al. Ranitidine and sucralfate as maintenance therapy for gastric ulcer disease: endoscopic control and assessment of scarring. Gut 1989;30:1692–1697.

128. Graham DY, Argrawal N, Roth S. Prevention of NSAID-induced gastric ulcer with the synthetic prostaglandin, misoprostol: a multi-center, double-blinded, placebo-controlled trial. Lancet 1988; 21:1277–1280.

129. Elliott SL, Yeomans ND, Buchanan RRC. Long-term effects of misoprostol on gastropathy induced by nonsteroidal anti-inflammatory drugs. [Abstract]. Gastroenterology 1990;98:A40.

130. Euler AR, Tytgat G, Berenguer J, et al. Failure of a cytoprotective dose of arbaprostil to heal acute duodenal ulcer: results of a multicenter trial. Gastroenterology 1987;92:604–607.

131. Euler AR, Bailey RJ, Zinny MA, et al. Arbaprostil [15(R)-15 methyl prostaglandin E_2] in a single nighttime dose of either 50 or 100 μg in acute duodenal ulcer. Gastroenterology 1989;97:98–103.

132. Birnie GG, Watkinson G, Shroff NE, Akbar FA. Double-blind comparison of two dosage regimens of misoprostol in the treatment of duodenal ulceration. Dig Dis Sci 1988;33:1269–1273.

133. Lauritsen K, Laursen LS, Havelund T, et al. Emprostil and ranitidine in duodenal ulcer healing: double-blind comparative trial. Br Med J 1986;292:864–866.

134. Bardhan KD, Morris P, Hinchcliffe RFC, et al. A comparison of low-dose maintenance treatment with enprostil against ranitidine in the prevention of duodenal ulcer recurrence. Aliment Pharmacol Ther 1989;3:489–497.

135. Hawkey CJ, Walt RP. Prostaglandins for peptic ulcer: a promise unfulfilled. Lancet 1986;2:1084–1087.

136. Walt RP. Drug therapy: misoprostol for the treatment of peptic ulcer and anti-inflammatory drug-induced gastroduodenal ulceration. N Engl J Med 1992;327:1575–1580.

2

The Pharmacologic Treatment of Gastroesophageal Reflux Disease

MALCOLM ROBINSON, PAUL N. MATON, and DENNIS L. DECKTOR

INTRODUCTION

Although the manifestations of gastroesophageal reflux are diverse, heartburn remains the cardinal symptom. An evolving understanding of the pathophysiology of gastroesophageal reflux has made it possible to devise individualized therapeutic measures. These include nonpharmacologic approaches and specific drug therapies to neutralize gastric acid, inhibit acid secretion, increase gastric emptying, and/or elevate esophageal peristaltic amplitude and the resting pressure of the lower esophageal sphincter (LES). Today, surgery has only a limited and diminishing role for the truly refractory patient, although some surgeons now propose that a new story may unfold for laparoscopic fundoplication.

PATHOGENESIS

Gastroesophageal reflux is not necessarily pathologic. A modest amount of reflux often occurs in normal individuals after meals and in the upright position. These reflux episodes tend to be brief and asymptomatic (1). Pathologic reflux ordinarily occurs far less frequently, and episodes tend to last longer and often are associated with heartburn (2, 3). Pathologic gastroesophageal reflux is due to an incompetent or inappropriately relaxing LES. Disease severity appears to be directly related to the duration and timing of reflux. Infrequent but prolonged episodes of acid exposure or frequent short reflux episodes can give rise to reflux disease (4). Secondary factors in producing symptomatic reflux can include the nonacid irritants in refluxed material and the rate of gastric emptying (5, 6).

Lower Esophageal Sphincter Pressure

The normal LES has a basal tone that maintains a barrier to reflux at the gastroesophageal junction, thereby preventing the backward transit of gastric contents. The primary pathophysiologic mechanism in gastroesophageal reflux disease (GERD) seems to be a malfunctioning LES. This malfunction may take the form of persistently hypotensive LES pressure (7) or transient "inappropriate" LES relaxations (1, 8).

Individuals with sphincter pressures greater than 20 to 25 mm Hg are generally well protected from reflux. Patients with LES pressures of 6 mm Hg or less are at increased risk (9). A role for persistently low basal tone in the pathophysiology of reflux disease is supported by the data of Dodds et al. (10), who found that patients with biopsy-proven esophagitis had decreased mean tone of the LES over a 12-hour period compared to healthy volunteers. Episodes of reflux in these patients are often associated with a rise in intra-abdominal pressure caused by physical exertion. Factors that further decrease basal LES pressure include pregnancy (11) and ingestion of fatty foods (12) and coffee (13). Alcohol diminishes LES tone, the amplitude of peristaltic waves, and the frequency of peristaltic contraction (14, 15). Nocturnal ingestion of alcohol followed by recumbency produces particularly prolonged supine reflux (16). Finally, many commonly prescribed medications such as progesterone, isoproterenol, theophylline, calcium channel blockers, and anticholinergics (17) can decrease LES tone.

In patients with normal LES resting pressure, inappropriate relaxations can dramatically reduce or eliminate sphincter pressure. Reflux episodes may be associated with inhalation, coughing, and/or gastric distension. Smoking increases gastroesophageal reflux and apparently is also associated with increased spontaneous esophageal sphincter relaxations (18). The mechanism responsible for these inappropriate relaxations of the sphincter is not understood.

Acid Contact Time

Acid contact time is a product of the frequency of gastroesophageal reflux and esophageal acid clearance time. It was a measure first quantified during prolonged measurement of esophageal pH values popularized by Johnson and DeMeester (19).

Prolonged acid contact increases the risk of complications from gastroesophageal reflux. It has been widely accepted that acid reflux is best defined by the drop in intraesophageal pH below 4 and characterized by the duration of time it remains below 4. In asymptomatic volunteers, ambulatory pH monitoring indicates that single episodes of acid reflux rarely last longer than 9 minutes. During a 24-hour period, normal subjects had three or fewer reflux episodes lasting 5 or more minutes (20, 21). In symptomatic patients, excessive acid exposure in the upright posture occurs primarily because of increased frequency of reflux episodes. These patients may be exposed to acid more than 10% of the time compared with only 2% of the time for controls subjects. Prolonged acid clearance time is not a significant factor in the upright position, since gravity rapidly clears fluid from the esophagus (20, 22) and residual acid is titrated by salivary bicarbonate if salivary function is normal (23).

Conversely, sleep-related or nocturnal gastroesophageal reflux is typically associated with infrequent reflux episodes but with prolonged acid clearance times. Individuals with recumbent reflux demonstrate esophageal acid clearance times as long as 30 minutes. During sleep, both swallowing (24) and saliva production virtually cease, and the influence of gravity is eliminated by the horizontal position.

Pattern of Reflux

A study reported by Johnson (25) indicates that patients can be categorized, based upon 24-hour distal esophageal pH monitoring, as either upright (those who reflux during the daytime), supine (those who reflux while recumbent at night), or combined reflux patients (those with both patterns of reflux). This study strongly suggests that the pattern of reflux influences the incidence and severity of esophagitis. Patients with significant nocturnal reflux and combined reflux exhibited more severe grades of esophagitis, as determined by upper gastrointestinal endoscopy, than did daytime refluxers. Esophagitis occurred in 52% of those with supine reflux and in 66% of those with combined reflux, but no significant mucosal damage was seen in those with upright reflux alone.

Potency of Refluxed Contents

The gastric contents consist of gastric secretion, duodenogastric reflux, and saliva with or without swallowed food, beverages, and medications. A great deal of work has been directed toward elucidating the irritant nature of the specific constituents of refluxed material.

Hydrochloric acid, pepsin, bile acids, and trypsin have been identified as the primary constituents of gastric fluid with the potential to cause injury to the esophageal mucosa (26). The acid concentration of gastric contents alone may cause esophageal injury by protein denaturization. However, pepsin, which is activated by pH <3.5, has been suggested as the most injurious component of gastric content, as even a small amount of pepsin in an acid milieu can produce severe experimental esophagitis (27).

There are some studies indicating that pepsin output and concentration may be increased in patients with esophagitis as compared with control patients (28). Although the role of bile acids remains undefined, experimental studies in animals suggest that bile acids can enhance damage caused by acid and pepsin (29).

On the "defensive" side, considerable evidence exists to support a significant beneficial role for saliva in normal esophageal function and as an endogenous countermeasure to gastroesophageal reflux disease. Saliva neutralizes refluxed gastric acid in the esophageal lumen (30) and facilitates its clearance (23).

Diet

Certain foods can aggravate reflux and thus cause heartburn either by directly irritating the esophageal lining (31) or by lowering LES pressure (32, 33). Some acidic foods and beverages such as citrus fruits and juices, coffee, and tomato products do not affect LES pressure or objectively impair mucosal integrity, but give rise to pain when in contact with inflamed esophageal mucosa. Fats, chocolate, onions, excessive alcohol, and the carminatives (peppermint and spearmint) have no direct irritant action, but decrease LES pressure and increase reflux. Protein meals tend to augment sphincter pressure (20).

Gastric Emptying

A role for increased gastric volume or decreased emptying in the pathogenesis of GERD has been suggested but is yet to be established as critical in more than a minority of patients. Theoretically, it is reasonable that reflux would be increased by gastric retention. Gastric distension is known to compromise LES function by increasing the rate of inappropriate LES relaxations.

Studies by Little et al. (34), McCallum et al. (35), and Collins et al. (36) suggest that emptying may be slowed in many patients with GERD. In contrast, Johnson et al. (37) and Shay et al. (38) found that gastric emptying in a population of patients with GERD was identical to that in healthy individuals. Perhaps the appropriate conclusion is that delayed gastric emptying can be associated with an increased tendency to reflux. For example, the "normal" circadian nocturnal slowing of the rate of gastric emptying observed in the general population may promote nocturnal reflux (39).

Gastric Secretion

A potential role for the hypersecretion of gastric acid has been emphasized in two recent studies of gastric secretion in GERD (40, 41). Standard doses of H_2-receptor antagonists failed to normalize either gastric acid secretion or esophageal acid exposure in these patients. Moreover, Collen et al. (40) have suggested that a significant fraction of patients with refractory GERD hypersecrete acid in the basal state.

The potential importance of hypersecretion of gastric acid in GERD has also been supported by studies of patients with Zollinger-Ellison syndrome (42, 43). These patients, who have exceptionally high levels of gastric acid production, demonstrate a high incidence of GERD. In most of these patients, resolution of their reflux symptoms and esophagitis occurred when acid-suppressive therapy was given in doses large enough to inhibit gastric hypersecretion to levels within the normal range (43). In a minority of patients, however, normal acid outputs were still associated with GERD.

CLINICAL CHARACTERISTICS AND PRESENTATION

Heartburn is the most common symptom of gastroesophageal reflux, although liquid regurgitation into the mouth and dysphagia are also common. Atypical symptoms such as chest pain, cough, hoarseness, and/or sore throat can complicate the clinical presentation. Other symptoms related to reflux include pain on swallowing and frequent belching (20, 22).

Ambulatory 24-hour pH monitoring has proved to be a reproducible quantitative test for gastroesophageal reflux disease. A GERD symptom index has been developed for correlating symptoms and acid reflux events (44). It has been used most widely to correlate the symptoms of heartburn and noncardiac chest pain with acid reflux events.

Heartburn

Heartburn is reported in more than half of patients with gastroesophageal reflux (45) and is typically described as a burning substernal or retrosternal pain that can extend to the mouth. Typically, heartburn occurs in the postprandial state (46, 47), yet some patients have their most severe symptomatic heartburn while lying flat or in relation to sleep (48). Eating, exercise, bending, or lying down may exacerbate heartburn.

Chest Pain

In many patients, recurring pain of esophageal origin is mistaken for cardiac chest pain (49, 50), which, because of its life-threatening implications, often results in cardiovascular assessment. After a cardiac cause has been excluded, investigations should focus on potential esophageal sources. As many as 30% of patients who exhibit anginal syndromes have been found to have normal coronary arteries, and approximately half of these patients were subsequently shown to have esophageal abnormalities (51–53). An esophageal cause of chest pain should be strongly suspected in patients with "atypical" angina that is not induced by effort, occurs after eating or nocturnally, or is exacerbated by the supine position, or is relieved by antacids (54–56).

More recent studies designed to differentiate motility-related and reflux-related chest pain indicate that from 20% to 30% of noncardiac chest pain symptoms are associated with gastric acid reflux into the esophagus (57, 58).

Although every effort should be made to differentiate esophageal and other types of substernal pain, esophageal pain does not preclude concomitant coronary artery disease (CAD). The inter-relationship of reflux and symptomatic heart disease further complicates the differential diagnosis. Svensson et al. (59) reported that esophageal disease was found in as many as 50% of patients with CAD. Subsequently, Mellow et al. (60) suggested that gastroesophageal reflux in patients with CAD might increase myocardial oxygen demand and thus induce chest pain due to myocardial ischemia.

Coughing, Wheezing, and Hoarseness

Although acid reflux may be related to nocturnal coughing, wheezing, and hoarseness (61), its potential role in respiratory-tract disorders is frequently overlooked.

In some cases, respiratory symptoms may be the only indication of GERD (22, 62, 63). Several studies have demonstrated an unusually high incidence of reflux in patients presenting with pulmonary complaints. Abnormal reflux was found during pH monitoring in 82% of patients presenting with asthma (64) and in 62% of patients presenting with chronic bronchitis (65). In another study, 52% of asthma patients had endoscopically verified reflux esophagitis (66). Recent therapeutic trials have shown significant improvement in pulmonary symptoms when gastroesophageal reflux was treated (67, 68).

PHARMACOLOGIC INTERVENTION

Since the pathogenesis of gastroesophageal reflux is multifactorial, therapies have been developed that are directed at various contributing factors such as esophageal and gastric acidity, LES pressure, or esophageal and gastric motility. A better understanding of GERD and the refinement of GI pharmacology have substantially improved treatment.

Antacid Therapy

Antacids are readily available without prescription and are widely used by heartburn sufferers. Antacids have been thought to relieve dyspeptic symptoms by neutralizing gastric acid and thus modifying the irritant nature of material in the stomach and presumably of that refluxing into the esophagus. Consequently, antacid efficacy has been correlated with in vitro acid-neutralizing capacity (69). However, a growing number of studies have called into question the accuracy and/or appropriateness of the in vitro acid-neutralizing capacity test. Studies by Halter et al. (70) and Vatier et al. (71) have highlighted the important influences of co-factors such as individual gastric acidity range, intraluminal variations in secretory and emptying fluxes, and the composition of gastric juice and meal content, especially in terms of protein.

In addition, recent studies from our laboratory (72, 73) indicate that acid-neutralizing capacity (ANC) is not a good predictor of in vivo antacid activity in the esophagus and suggest that antacids demonstrate a surprisingly long-lasting neutralizing effect in the esophagus that is independent of any effect upon gastric pH.

Antacids have been shown to decrease acid reflux into the esophagus (74). However, controlled clinical trial results have been mixed. Both high dose (ANC 85 mEq, seven times daily) and low dose (ANC 30 mEq, four times daily) regimens of aluminum hydroxide and magnesium carbonate-based antacids were superior to a placebo in relieving symptoms of gastroesophageal reflux (75, 76). In contrast, a study comparing a commonly used aluminum and magnesium-based antacid vs. placebo (77) could not demonstrate any significant symptomatic improvement in patients with chronic heartburn after 5 weeks of antacid therapy.

Alginic Acid Preparations

Soluble alginate, when mixed with acid or a soluble metal salt, precipitates as a gel or "raft." The postulated mechanism by which such an alginate raft might alleviate heartburn remains subject to debate. Whether the raft floats and is refluxed in preference to the acidic gastric contents or actually acts as a cork to prevent reflux has not been established (78). Particulate antacids have been added to alginic acid formulations; however, the importance of the resulting acid-neutralizing capacity to the formulation's efficacy is not known.

McHardy (79) reported that Gaviscon tablets and standard antacid were equally effective at reducing symptomatic heartburn. He further postulated that through its foaming/floating action, Gaviscon delivers a minimal dose of antacid directly to the site of acid irritation of the esophageal mucosa. Additional findings from Castell et al. (80) support the floating-action hypothesis by demonstrating that Gaviscon is primarily effective in the upright rather than supine position.

Sucralfate Suspensions

Sucralfate, a sulfated disaccharide complex with aluminum hydroxide, is effective in healing both gastric and duodenal ulcers (81, 82), but has been less frequently studied in patients with reflux esophagitis. It has minimal buffering effect in the stomach and does not alter gastric acid or pepsin secretion appreciably. Sucralfate conceivably might adhere to damaged tissue during passage through the esophagus (83) and may stimulate the regeneration of mucosal prostaglandin E.

European studies have shown sucralfate to be superior to placebo and as effective as standard H_2-receptor antagonist therapy and antacid/alginate preparations in the short-term treatment of reflux esophagitis (84). A recently reported double-blind clinical study found that sucralfate 1 g four times daily and cimetidine 400 mg twice daily were equally effective in causing macroscopic healing in about 60% of esophagitis patients (85).

In a pilot study, Ros et al. (86) found that sucralfate was particularly effective for reflux esophagitis refractory to H_2 antagonists. These surprising findings suggest that esophageal epithelial resistance is important in the persistence of GERD that is refractory to H_2 antagonists. However, a large and well-designed placebo-controlled multicenter U.S. trial of sucralfate in erosive esophagitis failed to establish significant symptom improvement or lesion healing after 8 weeks of treatment (87). Further studies are necessary to settle these discrepancies.

Antisecretory Therapy

H₂-Receptor Antagonists. H$_2$-receptor antagonists remain the most frequently used medications for the treatment of GERD. Cimetidine, ranitidine, nizatidine, and famotidine have each been shown to be effective.

In a controlled multicenter trial of 284 patients with GERD, administration of ranitidine 150 mg twice daily significantly reduced both the severity and frequency of heartburn compared with patients receiving placebo (88). This reduction was sustained throughout the 6-week study period. A significant correlation emerged between improvement in heartburn symptoms and decrease in antacid consumption. Furthermore, there was endoscopic demonstration of mucosal improvement and healing compared to patients receiving placebo treatment. After completion of the early large multicenter ranitidine trial, patients who had at least a 40% improvement in GERD symptoms were enrolled in a new trial to receive ranitidine 150 mg twice daily, ranitidine 150 mg at bedtime, or placebo for as long as 1 year. Ranitidine 150 mg twice daily provided long-term control of heartburn, continued reduction in antacid usage, and significant improvement in the endoscopic appearance of the esophageal mucosa (89).

In two early double-blind placebo-controlled studies (90, 91), cimetidine 300 mg four times daily significantly decreased the frequency and severity of both daytime and nighttime heartburn and reduced antacid consumption. There was no endoscopic or histologic improvement, however. Recent studies have also evaluated the ability of famotidine, the most potent of the currently approved H$_2$-receptor antagonists, to relieve symptoms and heal esophagitis. An open-label study of famotidine 40 mg at bedtime conducted in patients with endoscopically confirmed reflux esophagitis demonstrated symptomatic improvement in 73% of patients after 2 weeks with 81% and 85% improvement after 4 and 8 weeks of therapy, respectively. In addition, complete healing was documented in 50%, 75%, 82%, and 83% of patients, after

4, 8, 12, and 16 weeks of treatment, respectively (92).

A double-blind trial reported by Sabesin et al. (93) compared the efficacy of famotidine 40 mg at bedtime, 20 mg twice daily, and placebo in relieving heartburn and healing documented esophageal erosions. Both famotidine regimens were superior to placebo in producing complete mucosal healing compared to placebo, with the twice daily dosing being numerically superior to the 40-mg bedtime dose. In a separate study, the same twice-daily dosing regimen also relieved gastroesophageal reflux symptoms in patients without erosive esophagitis (94).

Findings reported by Dobrilla et al. (95) indicate that nizatidine 300 mg twice daily improved symptoms and healed endoscopically verified grades II–III esophagitis as defined by the Savary-Miller classification. After 6 weeks of treatment, 71% of nizatidine-treated patients showed complete endoscopic healing compared with 25% of placebo-treated subjects. After 12 weeks, the respective healing rates were 78% and 47%. Additional studies have also shown nizatidine 150 or 300 mg twice daily, but not a 300 mg bedtime dose, was better than placebo at relieving reflux symptoms and healing erosive esophagitis, although 12-week healing rates at the lower doses are only modest (96, 97).

The wide range of comparative studies described above clearly show that H$_2$-receptor antagonists given twice daily are useful in treating erosive and nonerosive gastroesophageal reflux disease. With the introduction of omeprazole and the description of its dramatic effects on symptoms and healing of erosive esophagitis, the effects of larger and/or more frequent doses of H$_2$-receptor antagonists have been carefully assessed. Studies by Russell and colleagues (98) and Jansen et al. (99) have demonstrated a reasonably direct dose-response relationship between acid suppression by ranitidine and the reduction of total esophageal acid exposure. Johnson et al. (100) documented the benefits of reduced acid exposure time, showing that ranitidine 300 mg twice daily significantly accelerated the healing of esophagitis and led to fewer symptoms after both 4 and 8 weeks of treatment when compared with the standard dosage of 150 mg twice daily. Twenty-nine percent of patients treated with ranitidine 150 mg twice daily and 40% of those receiving ranitidine 300 mg four times daily completely healed esophageal erosions. The U.S. dose for endoscopically determined erosive esophagitis, 150 mg four times daily, achieves a 12-week healing rate of >80% (101). With dosages of 300 mg four times daily and higher, Collen and colleagues (40) showed that acid exposure time could be reduced to normal levels and esophagitis healed in a majority of patients previously unresponsive to standard doses of antisecretory therapy.

Proton Pump Inhibitors. Hydrochloric acid secretion by parietal cells ultimately depends on the function of the proton pump. The pump is a H^+/K^+-ATPase, a membrane-spanning enzyme. Over the past 10 years the potent antisecretory properties of omeprazole, the first proton pump inhibitor, have been well described. A second pump inhibitor, lansoprazole, is currently under development and the focus of clinical trials.

Early international studies compared the efficacy of omeprazole and placebo at healing esophagitis. Whereas omeprazole healed >70% of patients, the placebo resulted in healing of only 6% (102). Similarly, symptoms were improved markedly by omeprazole.

In every double-blind study that compared omeprazole 20 mg/day to standard doses of H_2-antagonists (usually ranitidine 150 mg twice daily, but also cimetidine 400 mg twice daily), omeprazole was superior to the H_2 antagonist for symptom relief and for healing the esophageal mucosa. After 4 weeks of treatment, omeprazole abolished heartburn in 71–92%, while H_2 antagonists abolished heartburn in 24–59% (103–106). Omeprazole healed the mucosa in 67–85% after 4 weeks and 85–95% by 8 weeks. Comparable figures for H_2 antagonists were 27–45% and 38–65%. In these studies nearly all patients had erosive esophagitis, but in one study that included grade 1 esophagitis, the advantage of omepra-

zole over H_2 antagonists was more apparent in patients with grade 3 esophagitis than in those with grades 1–2 (107).

Omeprazole has also been given to patients with so-called "resistant esophagitis" who had not healed with standard doses of H_2 antagonists. Initial studies in small groups of patients suggested that omeprazole 40 mg/day would heal esophagitis resistant to standard or even larger doses of H_2 antagonists (108, 109). Klinkenberg-Knol et al. (110) described 73 patients with esophagitis resistant to cimetidine 1600 mg/day or ranitidine 600 mg/day, many of whom had complications of esophagitis. All 73 patients healed after administration of omeprazole 40 mg/day for 4 to 12 weeks. A number of subsequent studies have confirmed these findings. Bardhan et al. (109) gave omeprazole 40 mg/day to 38 patients whose esophagitis had not healed when they were given cimetidine 3200 mg/day, and Lundell (111) gave the same dose of omeprazole to patients who had not responded to ranitidine 450–600 mg/day. Healing occurred in >85% of patients in both studies with 8 weeks of receiving omeprazole.

Although the percentage of patients who were healed treated with omeprazole has been high, often in excess of 85% in the majority of studies cited, an identifiable subset of patients resistent to standard doses of omeprazole can be identified. Resistance to omeprazole varies by study and is not individually predictable. Klinkenberg-Knol and Meuwissen have described a small subset of patients with resistant GERD who require daily doses of 80 mg of omeprazole or more. This highly selected patient population had proven resistant to high doses of H_2-receptor antagonists. Complications such as hemorrhage or stricture, the diagnosis of Barrett's esophagitis, and failed surgical antireflux procedures were common. These patients were found to secrete acid despite treatment with standard dose omeprazole and also had severe esophageal motor abnormalities (112).

Initial study results with the still-investigational proton pump inhibitor lansoprazole indicate that it is also superior to ranitidine

(113) and comparable to omeprazole in treating reflux esophagitis (114). Lansoprazole 30 and 60 mg at bedtime relieved symptoms and healed moderate to severe reflux esophagitis after 8 weeks (115). Symptom improvement was superior to placebo after 2 weeks of treatment. This superiority continued throughout the 8-week treatment period. Endoscopic healing was observed in 94% of patients evaluated. Preliminary data reported by Sontag et al. (116) also indicate that lansoprazole is effective in the treatment of GERD refractory to H_2-receptor antagonists (117).

In another preliminary report of healing of erosive esophagitis with lansoprazole, patients promptly developed symptoms and mucosal erosions after stopping therapy, even when the proton pump blocker was replaced with high dose ranitidine or nizatidine (118) (i.e., double standard doses). It may be difficult to wean patients from proton pump blocker therapy for erosive esophagitis to any less aggressive regimen. Since omeprazole is currently approved for only short-term therapy, this feature of patient response is problematic. Similar restrictions are likely for lansoprazole when approved.

Gastroprokinetic Therapy

Drugs that enhance contractions of the upper gastrointestinal tract can in theory provide an alternative approach to the treatment of GERD. The cholinergic drug bethanechol has been shown to increase LES pressure (119) and may also enhance esophageal clearance (120). Metoclopramide, a dopamine-receptor antagonist, increases both LES pressure (121) and gastric emptying (122), presumably decreasing reflux symptoms by these mechanisms. Further studies by Grande et al. (123) showed that both metoclopramide (40 mg/day) and domperidone (80 mg/day) increased sphincter pressure. However, motility of the esophageal body, duration of esophageal exposure to acid, and esophageal clearance were not changed significantly by either drug.

Guslandi et al. (124) compared the effect of metoclopramide (10 mg three times daily)

with ranitidine (150 mg twice daily) in patients with symptomatic reflux esophagitis. Both drugs induced significant symptomatic and endoscopic improvement. Ranitidine was significantly superior in promoting endoscopic improvement, and unlike metoclopramide, it significantly reduced the severity of histologic changes. Metoclopramide's therapeutic utility in GERD remains limited because of associated side effects such as fatigue, anxiety, confusion, and occasionally severe extrapyramidal reactions.

The recently approved prokinetic compound cisapride has been shown to lower the total duration of acid exposure in the distal esophagus of both volunteers and reflux patients (125). Cisapride (10 mg four times daily) has successfully healed mucosal lesions of esophagitis and reduced associated symptoms (126, 127). Janisch et al. (128) have shown cisapride to be as effective as ranitidine (150 mg twice daily) in healing mucosal lesions in milder forms of reflux esophagitis.

Prokinetic agents may or may not become important primary therapy in reflux esophagitis. Many studies with the currently available agents suggest that the agents have only limited efficacy when used alone. Therefore several studies have been performed to investigate their efficacy when used with H_2-receptor antagonists (129).

Combination Therapy

It has been suggested that combining conventional antisecretory doses of H_2-receptor antagonists with a motor-stimulating agent might be synergistic in therapy of reflux esophagitis. Studies by Galmiche et al. 1988 (130) indicate that patients with erosive esophagitis had better symptomatic and endoscopic response to cimetidine plus cisapride than to cimetidine alone. In addition, Lieberman and Keeffe (131) showed that cimetidine plus metoclopramide was efficacious in the management of chronic reflux esophagitis in those patients who were refractory to cimetidine treatment alone (although side effects due to metoclopramide were frequent). Nevertheless, the data in this area are not con-

Table 2.1
Approaches to Treatment

Phase I
Life-style modifications and maneuvers
—Dietary modifications
—Smoking cessation
—Head of bed elevation
—Avoidance of medications that impair LES pressure, peristalsis, or salivation
—Antacids

Phase II
Pharmacologic therapy
—IIA. H_2 antagonists
—IIB. H_2 antagonists + prokinetic agent
—IIC. H_2 antagonists, high dose/increased frequency
—IID. H^+, K^+-ATPase/proton pump inhibitors (omeprazole)

Phase III
—Antireflux surgery (usually fundoplication)

sistent (129). A report by Singh and Spurrell (132) indicated that the combination of metoclopramide and cimetidine offered no advantage over cimetidine alone.

We have recently completed an 8-week study to determine whether the combination of ranitidine 150 mg twice daily plus metoclopramide 10 mg four times daily was as effective as omeprazole 20 mg daily for the treatment of erosive esophagitis (133). Omeprazole was clearly more efficacious and better tolerated than the combination of ranitidine and metoclopramide. Higher or more frequent doses of H_2-receptor antagonists in combination with newer prokinetic agents have not been studied but might compare more favorably with proton pump blocker therapy of GERD.

MAINTENANCE THERAPY

Irrespective of initial treatment, if esophagitis is healed and then treatment is stopped, the esophagitis almost always recurs (134). Maintenance regimens with low dose H_2-receptor antagonists comparable to effective duodenal ulcer prophylaxis have not always produced esophagitis relapse rates significantly lower than those seen with a placebo (135, 136). More recently, however, Euler et al. (137) were able to demonstrate the superiority of ranitidine 150 mg bid compared to placebo in

preventing esophagitis relapse. An initial report with famotidine 20 or 40 mg at bedtime describes incomplete success in prevention of symptomatic and erosive esophagitis relapse (138).

It appears that higher and/or more frequent doses of the H_2-receptor antagonists are often necessary to prevent disease recurrence. Six-month placebo-controlled trials have demonstrated that both famotidine 20 mg twice daily and 40 mg twice daily were superior to placebo in the prevention of symptom recurrence and relapse of erosive esophagitis (139). The percentage of relapse was 67% in the placebo group, 34% in patients receiving famotidine 20 mg twice daily, and 22% in patients who received famotidine 40 mg twice daily.

Double-blind controlled trials indicate that the investigational prokinetic agent cisapride may also provide effective maintenance therapy. After 12 months, relapse rates were 28% with either cisapride 10 mg twice daily (140) or cisapride 20 mg at bedtime (141), both of which were significantly less than the placebo relapse rate of 49%.

The most impressive remission rates during long-term treatment have come with the use of omeprazole. In patients with healed esophagitis, maintenance treatment with omeprazole 20 mg daily led to 6-, 12-, and 24-month relapse rates of 17%, 26%, and 33%, respectively (142). The importance of a continuous antisecretory effect in preventing relapse was illustrated by the finding that daily treatment with omeprazole 10 mg produced a significantly lower 6-month relapse rate of 21% than did omeprazole 20 mg, taken three consecutive days per week (54%) (143). Omeprazole 20 mg/day was associated with a 12-month relapse rate of 11% compared to relapse rates of 68% with omeprazole 20 mg taken 3 consecutive days per week and 75% with ranitidine 150 mg twice daily (144).

THERAPEUTIC APPROACH

In general, therapy of GERD can be divided into three phases (Table 2.1), incorporating nondrug treatment, drug therapy, and surgical approaches, as required.

Diet and Life-style Modifications

Gastroesophageal reflux is a chronic problem and should be treated accordingly. Phase I therapy is designed to minimize the frequency and duration of reflux episodes with simple maneuvers and life-style changes. These include elevation of the head of the bed, dietary modification, weight loss, cessation of smoking, avoidance of tight garments, and discontinuation of medications that adversely affect LES pressure, salivation, or gastric emptying. Antacids are also included in phase I. These measures should be the primary therapy for all patients with GERD and should be encouraged as adjunctive measures for all patients who require more aggressive pharmacologic therapy.

Elevating the head of the bed with wedges or 4- to 6-inch blocks has been a traditional component of phase I reflux management. Recumbent reflux episodes, though infrequent, can result in prolonged esophageal mucosal exposure to acid. Upper body elevation uses gravity to decrease acid clearance time. Johnson and DeMeester (145) showed that elevating the head of the bed significantly improved nocturnal esophageal clearance time, although the frequency of reflux episodes remained unchanged.

Pharmacologic Therapy

Patients who remain symptomatic despite phase I therapy will require phase II pharmacologic treatment. For reasons discussed above, the primary focus of phase II pharmacologic therapy has been the inhibition of gastric acid secretion. Because acid is critical to most injury from reflux, H_2-receptor antagonists are used most commonly as initial pharmacologic therapy to decrease gastric acid secretion. They are extremely safe and often effective.

If H_2-receptor antagonists alone do not relieve reflux symptoms, a prokinetic or promotility agent could be considered as adjunctive therapy. However, both bethanechol and metoclopramide are of questionable efficacy, and the latter especially produces many unwanted side effects. In the near future, the availability of cisapride may be helpful as adjunctive therapy, at least in selected patients. Currently, however, these patients who typically have more severe esophagitis should be given high-dose H_2-receptor antagonist or omeprazole therapy (101, 146).

Antireflux Surgery

Traditionally, the criteria for surgery have been failure of medical therapy with or without the development of complications such as hemorrhage, chronic aspiration, intractable asthma, stricture formation, or the development of dysplastic epithelium in patients with Barrett's esophagus. However, these criteria will need to be re-examined with the current availability of omeprazole and the evolving medical management of reflux esophagitis that was previously regarded as resistant. Despite the fact that surgery has been performed for many years for GERD, there are relatively few long-term results and only one controlled study. As with any surgical procedure, selection of appropriate patients is crucial. Thus, before surgery, pathologic reflux must be demonstrated, ideally with esophageal pH monitoring. It is also mandatory that esophageal motility be assessed prior to surgery.

Brand et al. (147) described long-term follow-up of 23 patients after surgical antireflux therapy. Eight months postoperatively, 21 patients had symptomatic improvement and 15 had no heartburn. At this relatively early stage, symptomatic and histologic improvements were comparable. By 5 or 6 years postsurgery, deterioration was noted in esophageal histology and acid reflux tests. LES pressures had fallen by the time of the 5-year postoperative assessment. In another study, 12% of patients had recurrent reflux symptoms 10 years after antireflux surgery (148). Finally, Spechler et al. (149) recently reported the results of a large prospective study comparing medical and surgical treatments for reflux disease. Antireflux surgery was significantly more effective than conventional medical therapy in improving the symptoms and endoscopic signs of esophagitis in a predominantly male population of patients with complicated gastroesophageal reflux disease. However, this study lasted only 2 years and did not use either high-dose H_2-receptor antagonist or omeprazole therapy. The role of antireflux surgery as a means to prevent the future development of Barrett's esophagus is currently being more widely considered (150, 151).

SUMMARY

Over the past several years, improvements in the quality and utilization of fiberoptic endoscopy, along with the advent of other imaging and diagnostic techniques such as ambulatory 24-hour pH monitoring have permitted a more thorough characterization of GERD. The continued development of effective antisecretory, prokinetic, and mucosal protective agents affords the clinician a choice of therapeutic approaches to manipulate various contributory factors, such as gastric-acid secretion, LES pressure, and gastric motility. Finally, a clearer appreciation of the pathogenesis of this disease has led to more individualized and presumably more effective treatment. Although standard doses of potent H_2-receptor antagonists are central to current therapy, it seems likely that increasingly effective regimens will become available for those patients whose reflux symptoms are resistant to standard treatment.

REFERENCES

1. Dent J, Dodds WJ, Friedman RH, et al. Mechanism of gastroesophageal reflux in recumbent asymptomatic human subjects. J Clin Invest 1980;65:256–267.
2. Dodds WJ, Dent J, Hogan WJ, et al. Mechanisms of gastroesophageal reflux in patients with reflux esophagitis. N Engl J Med 1982;307:1547–1552.
3. Schindlbeck NE, Heinrich C, Konig A, et al. Optimal thresholds, sensitivity, and specificity of long-term pH-metry for the detection of gastroesophageal reflux disease. Gastroenterology 1987;93:85–90.
4. Little AG, DeMeester TR, Kirchner PT, O'Sullivan GC, Skinner DB. Pathogenesis of esophagitis in patients with gastroesophageal reflux. Surgery 1980;83:101–107.
5. Gillison EW, De Castro VAM, Nyhus LM, et al. The significance of bile in reflux esophagitis. Surg Gynecol Obstet 1972;134:419–424.
6. McCallum RW, Berkowitz DM, Lerner E. Gastric emptying in patients with gastroesophageal reflux. Gastroenterology 1981;80:285–291.
7. Cohen S, Harris LD. Does hiatus hernia affect competence of the gastroesophageal sphincter? N Engl J Med 1971;284:1053–1056.
8. Mittal RK, McCallum RW. Characteristics and frequency of transient relaxations of the lower esophageal sphincter in patients with reflux esophagitis. Gastroenterology 1988;95:593–599.
9. Haddad JK. Relation of gastroesophageal reflux to yield sphincter pressures. Gastroenterology 1970;58:175–184.
10. Dodds WJ, Dent J, Hogan WJ, et al. Mechanisms of gastroesophageal reflux in patients with reflux esophagitis. N Engl J Med 1982;307:1547–1552.
11. Dodds WJ, Hogan WJ, Arndorfer RC. Efficient manometric technique for accurate regional measurement of esophageal body motor activity. Am J Gastroenterol 1978;70:21–24.
12. Nebel OT, Castell DO. Inhibition of the lower oesophageal sphincter by fat: A mechanism for fatty food intolerance. Gut 1973;14:270–274.
13. Thomas FB, Steinbaugh JT, Fromkes JJ, Mekhjian HS, Caldwell JH. Inhibitory effect of coffee on lower esophageal sphincter pressure. Gastroenterology 1980;79:1262–1266.
14. Hogan WJ, Viegas de Andrade SR, Winship DH. Ethanol-induced acute esophageal motor dysfunction. J Appl Physiol 1972;32:755–760.
15. Mayor EN, Grabowski CJ, Fisher RS. Effects of greater doses of alcohol upon esophageal motor function. Gastroenterology 1978;75:1133–1136.
16. Vitale GC, Giedel WG, Patell B, et al. The effect of alcohol and nocturnal gastroesophageal reflux. JAMA 1987;258:2077–2079.
17. Christensen J. Effects of drugs on esophageal motility. Arch Intern Med 1976;136:532–537.
18. Kahrilas PJ, Gupta RR. Mechanisms of acid reflux associated with cigarette smoking. Gut 1990;31:4–10.
19. Johnson LF, DeMeester TR. Twenty-four hour pH monitoring of the distal esophagus. Am J Gastroenterol 1974;62:325–332.
20. Day JP, Richter JE. Medical and surgical conditions predisposing to gastroesophageal reflux disease. Gastroenterol Clin North Am 1990;19:587–607.
21. DeMeester TR, Johnson LF, Guy JJ. Patterns of gastroesophageal reflux in health and disease. Ann Surg 1976;184:459–470.
22. Nebel OT, Formes MF, Castell DO. Symptomatic gastroesophageal reflux: incidence and precipitating factors. Dig Dis 1976;21:953–956.
23. Helm JF, Dodds WJ, Pelc LR, Palmer DW, Hogan WJ, Tecter BC. Effect of esophageal emptying and saliva on clearance of acid from the esophagus. N Engl J Med 1984;310:284–288.
24. Orr WC, Johnson LF, Robinson MG. Effect of sleep on swallowing, esophageal peristalsis, and acid clearance. Gastroenterology 1984;86:814–819.

25. Johnson FL. New concepts and methods in the study and treatment of gastroesophageal reflux disease. Med Clin North Am 1981;65:1195–1222.

26. Dodds WJ, Hogan JW, Helm JF, Dent J. Pathogenesis of reflux esophagitis. Gastroenterology 1981;81:376–394.

27. Goldberg HI, Dodds WJ, Gee S, et al. Role of acid and pepsin in acute experimental esophagitis. Gastroenterology 1969;56:223–230.

28. Coleman S, Hirschowitz BI. Studies of gastric secretion as a risk factor for esophagitis [Abstract]. Gastroenterology 1984;86:1051a.

29. Dubois A. Role of gastric factors in the pathogenesis of gastroesophageal reflux: emptying, acid and pepsin. In: Castell DO, Wu WC, Ott DJ, eds. Gastroesophageal reflux disease. Mt. Kisco, NY: Futura, 1985.

30. Helm JF, Dodds WJ, Hogan WJ, Soergel KH, Egide MS, Wood CM. Acid neutralizing capacity of human saliva. Gastroenterology 1982;83:69–74.

31. Price SF, Smithson KW, Castell DO. Food sensitivity in reflux esophagitis. Gastroenterology 1978;75:240–243.

32. Nebel OT, Castell DO. Lower esophageal sphincter pressure changes after food ingestion. Gastroenterology 1972;63:778–783.

33. Babka JC, Castell DO. On the genesis of heartburn. Am J Dig Dis 1973;18:391–397.

34. Little AG, DeMeester TR, Kirchner PT. Pathogenesis of esophagitis in patients with gastroesophageal reflux. Surgery 1980;88:101–107.

35. McCallum RW, Berkowitz DM, Lerner E. Gastric emptying in patients with gastroesophageal reflux. Gastroenterology 1981;80:285–291.

36. Collins BJ, McFarland RF, O'Hare MTT. Gastric emptying of a solid-liquid meal and GI hormone responses in patients with erosive esophagitis. Digestion 1986;33:61–68.

37. Johnson DA, Winters C, Drane WE. Solid-phase gastric emptying in Barrett's esophagus [Abstract]. Gastroenterology 1985;88:1434a.

38. Shay SD, Eggli D, Van Nostrand D. Gastric emptying of solid food in patients with gastroesophageal reflux [Abstract]. Gastroenterology 1985;88:1582a.

39. Good RH, Moore JG, Greenberg E, Alazraki NP. Circadian variation in gastric emptying of meals in humans. Gastroenterology 1987;93:515–518.

40. Collen MJ, Lewis JH, Benjamin SB. Gastric acid hypersecretion in refractory gastroesophageal reflux disease. Gastroenterology 1990;98:654–661.

41. Barlow AP, DeMeester TR, Ball SC, Eypasch EP. The significance of the gastric secretory state in gastroesophageal reflux disease. Arch Surg 1989;124:937–940.

42. Richter JE, Pandol SJ, Castell DO, et al. Gastroesophageal reflux disease in the Zollinger-Ellison syndrome. Ann Intern Med 1981;95:37–43.

43. Miller L, Vinayek R, Frucht H, et al. Reflux esophagitis in patients with Zollinger-Ellison syndrome. Gastroenterology 1990;98:341–346.

44. Ward BW, Wu WC, Richter JE, et al. Ambulatory 24-hour esophageal pH monitoring: technology searching for a clinical application. J Clin Gastroenterol 1986;8(suppl 1):59–67.

45. Jamieson GG, Duranceau A. Gastroesophageal reflux. Philadelphia: WB Saunders, 1988:65.

46. Fink SM, McCallum RW. The role of prolonged esophageal pH monitoring in the diagnosis of gastroesophageal reflux. JAMA 1984;252:1160–1164.

47. Holloway RH, Hongo M, Berger K, et al. Gastric distention: a mechanism for postprandial gastroesophageal reflux. Gastroenterology 1985;89:779.

48. Orr WC, Johnson LF, Robinson MG. The effect of sleep on swallowing, esophageal peristalsis, acid sensitivity and clearance time. Gastroenterology 1984;86:814–819.

49. Richter JE, Bradley LA, Castell DO. Esophageal chest pain: current controversies in pathogenesis, diagnosis and therapy. Ann Intern Med 1989;110:66–78.

50. Waterfall WE, Craven MA, Allen CJ. Gastroesophageal reflux: clinical presentation, diagnosis, and management. Can Med Assoc J 1986;135:1101–1109.

51. DeMeester TR, O'Sullivan GC, Bermudez G. Esophageal function in patients with angina-type chest pain and normal coronary angiograms. Ann Surg 1982;196:488–498.

52. Kline M, Chesne R, Studevant RL. Esophageal disease in patients with angina-like chest pain. Am J Gastroenterol 1981;75:116–123.

53. Davies HA, Jones DB, Rhodes J. Esophageal angina as the cause of chest pain. JAMA 1982;248:2274–2278.

54. Castell DO. Overview of treatment of gastroesophageal reflux disease. In: Castell DO, Wu WC, Ott DJ, eds. Gastroesophageal reflux disease. Mt. Kisco, NY: Futura, 1985.

55. Vantrappen G, Janssens J, Ghillebert G. The irritable oesophagus: a frequent cause of angina-like pain. Lancet 1987;1:1232–1234.

56. Minami H, McCallum RW. Chest pain: differentiating esophageal disease from angina pectoris. Compr Ther 8 1982;12:50–58.

57. Lam HKT, Dekker W, Kan G, Breedijk M, Smout AJPM. Acute noncardiac chest pain in a coronary care unit. Gastroenterology 1992;102:453–460.

58. Breumelhof R, Nadorp JHSM, Akkermans LMA, Smout AJPM. Analysis of 24-hour esophageal pressure and pH data in unselected patients with noncardiac chest pain. Gastroenterology 1990;99:1257–1264.

59. Svensson O, Stenport G, Tibbling L, Wranne B. Oesophageal function and coronary angiogram in patients with disability chest pain. Acta Med Scand 1976;192.

60. Mellow MH, Simpson AG, Watt L. Esophageal acid perfusion in coronary artery disease. Gastroenterology 1983;65:306–312.

61. Deschner WK, Benjamin SB. Extraesophageal manifestations of gastroesophageal reflux disease. Am J Gastroenterol 1989;84:1–5.

62. Barish CF, Wu WC, Castell DO. Respiratory complications of gastroesophageal reflux. Arch Intern Med 1985;145:1882–1888.

63. Kellogg MP, Allende N. Recurrent pulmonary disease as the presenting problem in cases of gastroesophageal reflux in infants. J Florida Med Assoc 1980;67:842–844.

64. Sontag SJ, Skorodin M, O'Connell S. Ambulatory 24 hour esophageal pH monitoring in patients with asthma. Gastroenterology 1984;86:1261.

65. David P, Denis P, Nouvet G. Lung function and gastroesophageal reflux during chronic bronchitis. Bul Eur Physiol-pathol 1982;18:81–86.

66. Perrin-Fayolle M, Bell A, Braillon G, et al. Asthma and gastro-esophageal reflux (GER): results of surgical treatment of reflux in 50 patients. Poumon Coeur 1980;36:231–237.

67. Gonzalez ER, Castell DO. Respiratory complications of gastroesophageal reflux. Am Fam Physician 1988;38:169–172.

68. Harper PC, Bergner A, Kaye MD. Antireflux treatment for asthma: improvement in patients with associated gastroesophageal reflux. Arch Intern Med 1987;147:56–60.

69. Fordtran JS, Morawski SG, Richardson CT. In vivo and in vitro evaluation of liquid antacids. N Engl J Med 1973;288:923–928.

70. Halter F, Huber R, Hacki WH, et al. Effect of food on antacid neutralizing capacity in man. Eur J Clin Invest 1982;12:209–217.

71. Vatier J, Vallot T, Vitre MT, Mignon M. New approach for the in vitro evaluation of antacids. Drug Res 1990;40:175–179.

72. Decktor DL, Robinson M, Maton PN, Allen ML. Acid neutralizing capacity does not predict antacid efficacy in patients with heartburn [Abstract]. Gastroenterology 1992;102:57a.

73. Decktor DL, Robinson M, Maton PN, Allen ML. Antacids and heartburn: is the "relief" gastric or esophageal? [Abstract] Gastroenterology 1992;102:57a.

74. Deschalliers JP, Galmiche JP, Touchais JY, Denis P, Colin R. Ranitidine, cimetidine, antacids, and gastroesophageal reflux: results of a 24-hour oesophageal pH study. Int J Clin Pharmacol Res 1984;4:217–222.

75. Grove O, Bekker C, Jeppe-Hansen MG, et al. Ranitidine and high-dose antacid in reflux oesophagitis. Scand J Gastroenterol 1985;20:457–461.

76. Weberg R, Berstad A. Symptomatic effect of a low-dose antacid regimen in reflux oesophagitis. Scand J Gastroenterol 1989;24:401–406.

77. Graham DY, Patterson DJ. Double-blind comparison of liquid antacid and placebo in the treatment of symptomatic reflux esophagitis. Dig Dis Sci 1983;28:559–563.

78. Washington N. Antacids and anti-reflux agents. Boca Raton, LA: CRC Press, 1991:210–212.

79. McHardy G. A multicentric, randomized clinical trial of gaviscon in reflux esophagitis. South Med J 1978;71:16–21.

80. Castell DO, Dalton CB, Becker D, Sinclair J, Castell JA. Alginic acid decreases postprandial upright gastroesophageal reflux: comparison with equal-strength antacid. Dig Dis Sci 1992;37:589–593.

81. Asaka M, Takeda H, Saito M, Murashima Y, Miyazaki T. Clinical efficacy of sucralfate in the treatment of gastric ulcer. Am J Med 1991;91:S71–73.

82. Lam SK. Treatment of duodenal ulcer with sucralfate. Scand J Gastroenterol 1991;185(suppl):22–28.

83. Samloff IM, O'Dell C. Inhibition of peptic activity by sucralfate. Am J Med 1985;79(suppl 2C):15.

84. Hameeteman W. Clinical studies of sucralfate in reflux esophagitis: the European experience. J Clin Gastroenterol 1991;13(suppl 2):S16–S20.

85. Elsborg L, Jorgensen F. Sucralfate versus cimetidine in reflux oesophagitis: a double-blind clinical study. Scand J Gastroenterol 1991;26:146–150.

86. Ros E, Pujol A, Bordas JM, Grande L. Efficacy of sucralfate in refractory reflux esophagitis: results of a pilot study. Scand J Gastroenterol 1989;24(suppl 156):49–55.

87. Williams RM, Orlando RC, Bozymski EM. Multicenter trial of sucralfate suspension for the treatment of reflux esophagitis. Am J Med 1987;83(suppl 3B):61–66.

88. Sontag S, Vlahcevic LB, Orr W. Ranitidine versus placebo in long-term treatment of gastroesophageal reflux (GERD). Gastroenterology 1985;88:1595.

89. Sontag S, Robinson M, McCallum RW. Ranitidine therapy for gastroesophageal reflux disease. Arch Intern Med 1987;147:1485–1491.

90. Behar JD, Brand DL, Brown FC. Cimetidine in the treatment of symptomatic gastroesophageal reflux. Gastroenterology 1978;74:441–448.

91. Powell-Jackson H, Barkley, Northfield TC. Effect of cimetidine in symptomatic gastro-oesophageal reflux. Lancet 1978;2:1068–1069.

92. Sekiguchi T, Nishioka T, Kogure M, et al. Once-daily administration of famotidine for reflux esophagitis. Scand J Gastroenterol 1987;22(suppl 134):51–54.

93. Sabesin SM, Berlin RG, Humphries TJ, et al. Famotidine relieves symptoms of gastroesophageal reflux disease and heals erosions and ulcerations. Arch Intern Med 1991;151:2394–2400.

94. Robinson M, Decktor CL, Stone RC, et al. Famotidine (20 mg) b.d. relieves gastroesophageal reflux symptoms in patients without erosive oesophagitis. Aliment Pharmacol Ther 1991;5:631–643.

95. Dobrilla G, Chilovi F, Tafner G, et al. Treatment of erosive reflux oesophagitis: a double-blind multicentre trial with nizatidine 300 mg bid versus placebo. Ital J Gastroenterol 1992;24:338–341.

96. Cloud M, Offen WW, and the Nizatidine Gastroesophageal Reflux Disease Study Group. Nizatidine versus placebo in gastroesophageal reflux disease: a six-week, multicenter, randomized, double-blind comparison. Dig Dis Sci 1992;37:865–874.

97. Cloud M, Offen W. Nizatidine 150 mg relieves symptoms and decreases severity of esophagitis in gastroesophageal reflux [Abstract]. Gastroenterology 1989;96:91a.

98. Russell J, Orr WC, Wilson T, Finn AL. Effects of ranitidine, given t.d.s., on intragastric and oesophageal pH in patients with gastroesophagal reflux. Aliment Pharmacol Ther 1991;5:621–630.

99. Jansen JBN, Baak LC, Lamers CB. Effect of increasing doses of ranitidine on exposure of the oesophagus to gastric acid in patients with gastroesophageal reflux disease. Scand J Gastroenterol 1988;23(suppl 154):2–5.

100. Johnson NJ, Boyd EJS, Mills JG, Wood JR. Acute treatment of reflux oesophagitis: a multicentre trial to compare 150 mg ranitidine b.d. with 300 mg ranitidine q.d.s. Aliment Pharmacol Ther 1989;3:259–266.

101. Roufail W, Belsito A, Robinson M, et al. Ranitidine for erosive oesophagitis: a double-blind, placebo-controlled study. Aliment Pharmacol Ther 1992:6:597–607.

102. Hetzel DJ, Dent J, Reed WD, et al. Healing and relapse of severe peptic esophagitis after treatment with omeprazole. Gastroenterology 1988;95:903–912.

103. Sandmark S, Carlsson R, Fausa O, Lundell L. Omeprazole or ranitidine in the treatment of reflux esophagitis: results of a double-blind, randomized, Scandinavian multicenter study. Scand J Gastroenterol 1988;23:625–632.

104. Van Trappen G, Rutgeerts L, Schurmans P, Coenegrachts JL. Omeprazole (40 mg) is superior to ranitidine in short-term treatment of ulcerative reflux esophagitis. Dig Dis Sci 1988;33:523–529.

105. Zeitoun P, Rampal P, Barbier P, Isal JP, Eriksson S, Carlsson R. Omeprazole (20 mg daily) compared to ranitidine (150 mg twice daily) in the treatment of esophagitis caused by reflux: results of a double-blind randomized multicenter trial in France and Belgium. Gastroenterol Clin Biol 1989;13:457–462.

106. Dehn TCB, Shepherd HA, Colin-Jones D, Kettlewell MGW, Carroll NJ. Double-blind comparison of omeprazole (40 mg qd) versus cimetidine (400 mg qd) in the treatment of symptomatic erosive reflux oesophagitis, assessed endoscopically, histologically and by 24-hour pH monitoring. Gut 1990;31:509–513.

107. Havelund T, Laursen LS, Skoubo-Kristensen E, et al. Omeprazole and ranitidine in treatment of reflux oesophagitis: double blind comparative trial. Br Med J 1988;296:89–92.

108. Fausa O, Aadland E, Lotveit T. Omeprazole in the treatment of patients with severe erosive oesophagitis resistant to treatment with H_2-receptor antag-

onists [Abstract]. Scand J Gastroenterol 1987; 135:38a.

109. Bardhan KD, Morris P, Thompson M, et al. Value of omeprazole in the management of erosive esophagitis refractory to high dose cimetidine [Abstract]. Gut 1987;28:1375a.

110. Klinkenberg-Knol EC, Jansen JBMJ, de Bruyne JW, et al. Long-term efficacy and safety of omeprazole (OME) on healing and prevention of resistant reflux esophagitis [Abstract]. Gastroenterology 1988;94:230a.

111. Lundell L, Backman L, Eckstrom P, et al. Omeprazole or high dose ranitidine in the treatment of patients with reflux esophagitis not responding to 'standard doses' of H_2-receptor antagonists. Aliment Pharmacol Ther 1990;4:145–156.

112. Klinkenberg-Knol EC, Meuwissen SGM. Combined gastric and oesophageal 24-hour pH monitoring and oesophageal manometry in patients with reflux disease, resistant to treatment with omeprazole. Aliment Pharmacol Ther 1990;4:485–495.

113. Robinson M, Kogut D, Jennings D, Greski-Rose P, and the Lansoprazole Study Group. Lansoprazole heals erosive reflux esophagitis better than ranitidine [Abstract]. Gastroenterology 1992;102:153a.

114. Hatlebakk JG, Berstad A, Carling L, Svedberg LE, Unge P, Ekstrom P. Lansoprazole vs. omeprazole in short-term treatment of reflux esophagitis: results of a Scandinavian multicentre trial [Abstract]. Gastroenterology 1992;102:80a.

115. Dorsch E, Jones J, Padgett C, Jennings D, Greski P, and the Lansoprazole Study Group. Lansoprazole heals moderate to severe reflux esophagitis [Abstract]. Gastroenterology 1991;86:1294a.

116. Sontag S, Kurucar C, Murray S, Greski-Rose P, Jennings D, and the Lansoprazole Study Group. Lansoprazole heals erosive esophagitis resistant to histamine H_2-receptor antagonist therapy [Abstract]. Gastroenterology 1992;102:167a.

117. Sontag S, Kurukar C, Murray S, et al. Lansoprazole heals erosive reflux esophagitis resistant to histamine H_2-receptor antagonist therapy [Abstract]. Gastroenterology 1992;102:167a.

118. Antonson CW, Robinson MG, Hawkins TM, McIntosh DL, Campbell DR. High doses of histamine antagonists do not prevent relapses of peptic esophagitis following therapy with a proton pump inhibitor [Abstract]. Gastroenterology 1990;98:16a.

119. Farrell RL, Roling GT, Castell DO. Cholinergic therapy of chronic heartburn. Ann Intern Med 1972;80:573–576.

120. Castell DO. Medical therapy for reflux esophagitis: 1986 and beyond. Ann Intern Med 1986;104:112–114.

121. McCallum RW, et al. Comparative effects of metoclopramide and bethanechol on lower esophageal sphincter pressure. Gastroenterology 1975;68:1114–1118.

122. Fink SM, Lange RC, McCallum RW. Effect of metoclopramide on normal and delayed gastric emptying in gastroesophageal reflux patients. Dig Dis Sci 1983;28:1057–1061.

123. Grande L, Lacima G, Ros E, et al. Lack of effect of metoclopramide and domperidone on esophageal peristalsis and esophageal acid clearance in reflux esophagitis. A randomized, double-blind study. Dig Dis Sci 1992;37:583–588.

124. Guslandi M, Testoni PA, Passaretti S. Ranitidine vs metoclopramide in the medical treatment of reflux esophagitis.Hepatogastroenterology1983;30:96–98.

125. Wienbeck M, Li Q. Cisapride in gastro-oesophageal reflux disease: effects on oesophageal motility and intra-oesophageal pH. Scand J Gastroenterol 1989;24(suppl 165):13–18.

126. Baldi F, Banchi PG, Dobrilla G. Cisapride versus placebo in reflux esophagitis. J Clin Gastroenterol 1988;10:614–618.

127. Dodds W, Champion M, Orr W. Oral cisapride in GERD: a double-blind placebo-controlled multicenter trial [Abstract]. Gastroenterology 1989; 96:126a.

128. Janisch HD. CISRAN Study Group. A double-blind multicenter trial to compare the efficacy of cisapride and ranitidine in GERD. Gastroenterology 1986;90:1475.

129. Ramirez B, Richter JE. Review article: promotility drugs in the treatment of gastro-oesophageal reflux disease. Aliment Pharmacol Ther 1993;7:5–20.

130. Galmiche JP, Brandstatter G, Evreux M, et al. Combined therapy with cisapride and cimetidine in severe reflux oesophagitis: a double-blind controlled trial. Gut 1988;29:675–681.

131. Lieberman DA, Keeffe EB. Treatment of severe reflux esophagitis with cimetidine and metoclopramide. Ann Intern Med 1986;104:21–26.

132. Singh CP, Spurrell JRR. Cimetidine and metoclopramide in oesophageal reflux disease. Br Med J 1983;286:1863–1864.

133. Robinson M, Decktor DL, Maton PN, et al. Omeprazole is superior to ranitidine plus metoclopramide in the short-term treatment of erosive oesophagitis. Aliment Pharmacol Ther 1993;7:67–73.

134. Armstrong D, Nicolet M, Monnier P, Chapuis G, Savary M, Blum A. Maintenance therapy: is there still a place for antireflux surgery? World J Surg 1992;16:300–307.

135. Koelz HR, Birchler R, Bretholz A, et al. Healing and relapse of reflux esophagitis during treatment with ranitidine. Gastroenterology 1986;91:1198.

136. Koop H, Wachtman H, Eissele R, Arnold R. Efficacy and safety of long-term omeprazole maintenance therapy in H_2-blocker-resistant reflux esophagitis healed by omeprazole [Abstract]. Gastroenterology 1990;98:70a.

137. Euler AR, Murdock RH, Brotherton BJ, Silver MT, Parker SE. Ranitidine 150 mg bid prevents erosive esophagitis recurrences [Abstract]. Gastroenterology 1992;102:A65.

138. Berlin R, Ebel D, Cook T. Famotidine 40 mg vs ranitidine 150 mg in the treatment of reflux esophagitis: results of a double blind multicenter trial [Abstract]. Gastroenterology 1989;96:39a.

139. Simon TJ, Berlin RG, Tipping R, et al. Prevention of endoscopic recurrence of erosive esophagitis (EE) with famotidine (F) 20 mg bid and 40 mg bid: results of an international 6 month, randomized, double-blind, placebo-controlled trial [Abstract]. Gastroenterology 1990;100:162a.

140. Blum AL, Verlinden M, and the EUROCIS trialists. Cisapride prevents relapse of reflux esophagitis [Abstract]. Gastroenterology 1990;98:22a.

141. Tytgat GNJ, and the SCAADUS Trialists. Effect of cisapride on relapse of reflux esophagitis healed with an antisecretory drug [Abstract]. Gastroenterology 1991;100:178a.

142. Klinkenberg-Knol EC, Jansen JBMJ, Lamers CBHW, Nelis F, Snel P, Meuwissen SGM. Use of omeprazole in the management of reflux oesophagitis resistant to H_2-receptor antagonists. Scand J Gastroenterol 1989;24(suppl 166):88.

143. Isal JP, Zeitoun P, Barbier P, Cayphas JP, Carlsson R. Comparison of two dosage regimens of omeprazole—10 mg once daily and 20 mg weekends—as prophylaxis against recurrence of reflux esophagitis [Abstract]. Gastroenterology 1990;98:63a.

144. Dent J, Mackinnon M, Reed W, Narielvala FM, Hetzel DJ. Omeprazole prevents relapse of peptic esophagitis. Presentation at the World Congress of Gastroenterology. Sydney: Australia, 1990.

145. Johnson FL, DeMeester TR. Evaluation of elevation of the head of the bed, bethanechol, and antacid foam tablets on gastroesophageal reflux. Dig Dis Sci 1981;26:673–680.

146. Hetzel DJ, Dent J, Reed WD. Healing and relapse of severe peptic esophagitis after treatment with omeprazole. Gastroenterology 1988;95:905–912.

147. Brand DL, Eastwood IR, Martin D. Esophageal symptoms, manometry and histology before and after antireflux surgery: a long-term follow-up. Gastroenterology 1979;76:1393–1401.

148. Negre JB, Markkula HT, Keyrilainen O, Matikainen M. Nissen fundoplication: results at 10 year follow-up. Am J Surg 1983;146:635–648.

149. Spechler SJ and the Department of Veterans Affairs Gastroesophageal Reflux Disease Study Group. Comparison of medical and surgical therapy for complicated gastroesophageal reflux disease in veterans. N Engl J Med 1992;326:786–792.

150. Stein HJ, DeMeester TR. Who benefits from antireflux surgery? World J Surg 1992;16:313–319.

151. Williamson WA, Ellis FH Jr, Gibb JP, et al. The effect of antireflux surgery on Barrett's mucosa. Ann Thorac Surg 1990;49:537–542.

3

Treatment and Prevention of Nonsteroidal Anti-inflammatory Drug-Related Gastroduodenal Ulceration

CHRISTOPHER J. HAWKEY and NICHOLAS HUDSON

INTRODUCTION

Nonsteroidal, anti-inflammatory drugs (NSAIDs) have been available since the mid-1960s. Prescribing of them has increased markedly since then, particularly for the elderly, so that for every thousand elderly women over the age of 65, 1400 prescriptions are issued per annum in the United Kingdom (1). The increased prescription of NSAIDs may well account for epidemiologic changes in ulcer incidence beginning at about the same time. Against a falling background incidence of peptic ulceration in all other groups, several measures suggest a progressive rise in the incidence in old women occurring over the last 25 years.

EFFECTS OF NSAIDS ON GASTRIC MUCOSA

NSAIDs affect three (and possibly four) critical aspects of the ulcer diathesis.

Mucosal Defense

By inhibiting prostaglandin synthesis, NSAIDs interfere with protective mechanisms such as mucus secretion, bicarbonate secretion, surface epithelial hydrophobicity, and mucosal blood flow (2). These agents have other effects on the gastric mucosa that may not necessarily be attributable to reductions in prostaglandin synthesis, including increased margination of neutrophils, production of oxygen-free radicals, and impairment of the gastric mucosal barrier. Recently, patients taking nonsteroidal, anti-inflammatory drugs have been shown to have enhanced synthesis of leukotriene B_4, conceivably because of substrate diversion, as well as reduced prostaglandin synthesis (3). It is not yet known whether this phenomenon accounts for some of the non-prostaglandin-dependent pathology. A consequence of all these actions is that the mucosa becomes more prone to injury, however.

Impaired Ulcer Healing

It is increasingly recognized that NSAIDs impair ulcer healing, as well as rendering the mucosa more vulnerable to injury. Less is known about the underlying mechanisms than about those that predispose to mucosal injury, but NSAIDs have been shown to inhibit cellular proliferation at the edge of ulcers (with restoration toward normal by prostaglandins) (4), to inhibit new blood vessel formation (5) so that the granulation tissue of NSAID ulcers is less vascular than non-NSAID ulcers (6), and to impair contractility of the ulcer base (7).

Impairment of Hemostasis

It is well-recognized that NSAIDs, particularly aspirin, impair platelet aggregation and prolong skin bleeding time. There has been a strange reluctance to accept the fact that the same might be true in the stomach, and several studies have failed to find an effect on hemostasis. We have conducted studies, however, showing that aspirin increases the rate of spontaneous bleeding from mucosal erosions and doubles the amount of bleeding induced by gastric biopsy in a test akin to the skin bleeding time (8).

Pain

Whether, by their analgesic action, NSAIDs interfere with perception of pain and mask ulcer symptoms is uncertain, but is dealt with later in this chapter.

HOW DANGEROUS ARE NSAIDS?

This question can be addressed in a number of ways.

Endoscopic Studies

At first sight, studies in which patients taking NSAIDs chronically have been endoscoped to assess the prevalence of gastric and duodenal ulcers, or where subjects starting on NSAIDs have been endoscoped sequentially to assess the incidence of ulcers developing over a given period of time are alarming. The average prevalence in such studies of gastric ulceration is 15.1% (range 9–21%) and for duodenal ulcer 9.6% (range 2–19%) (9). In studies where patients have been followed prospectively (usually in the placebo arm of a prophylactic study), large numbers have developed ulcers. For example, in a study investigating prophylaxis with misoprostol, 21.7% of subjects taking NSAIDs but receiving placebo prophylaxis developed gastric ulcers over a 3-month period (10). In none of these studies was there a control group of patients, but in two Scandinavian studies extremely low levels of gastric ulceration (0.3% in one study, 0.35% in another) were found among the asymptomatic population of patients not receiving NSAIDs (11, 12). Taking these data as the control group would imply that NSAIDs enhance the risk of ulceration 30- to 70-fold.

Epidemiologic Studies

Epidemiologic studies show a completely different picture with an increased relative risk of only about three (9, 13, 14). This is true for uncomplicated gastric ulceration, as well as gastrointestinal (GI) bleeding from gastric and duodenal ulceration, but not for uncomplicated duodenal ulcer, where no increase has been shown. The paradox of different estimates of risk from endoscopic and epidemiologic studies can be expressed as follows: If patients are endoscoped while taking NSAIDs, there is a very high chance that they will have an ulcer, but about a 10-fold lower chance that they will actually present with a clinically significant end point. Ulcers detected in patients taking NSAIDs are, therefore, common, but are less likely than ulcers detected in patients not taking NSAIDs to develop clinically significant end points, particularly ulcer complications. The reason for this is that in endoscopic studies quite small and superficial lesions are often classified as ulcers. We have conducted blinded interobserver variability studies using video images showing that non-NSAID ulcers are usually classified as deep ulcers and there is a high degree of agreement about their nature. Ulcers seen in patients taking NSAIDs are more often classified as superficial ulcers, however, and there is considerable difficulty in distinguishing erosions from superficial ulcers (15). An important unanswered question is whether and which lesions are predictive of later problems.

Ulcer Complications—Absolute Risks

Both case control and cohort studies suggest, in absolute terms, that the risk of GI hemorrhage or perforation in elderly patients not taking NSAIDs may be around 1 per 300–1000 patient years, and this decreases to approximately 60, or 1 per 600 patient years in those taking NSAIDs (16–24). Because life expectancy in the elderly is limited, most patients will die from other causes without experiencing an NSAID-related problem. For example, women aged 75 and over in Saskatchewan have a life expectancy of 6 years. Interestingly, a subgroup analysis of this study found prolonged rather than reduced life expectancy in subjects receiving NSAID treatment (24). This is plausible, since the GI risks might be offset by cardiovascular and mobility benefits. Obviously, however, independent confirmation is required.

Nevertheless, NSAIDs clearly represent a significant problem to the person who uses them and constitute a substantial problem at a national level because their use is so widespread.

AIMS OF MANAGEMENT

There should be two main aims in the management of patients taking NSAIDs: (*a*) symptom relief and (*b*) prevention of ulcer complications. Clinical trials have concentrated on healing and prophylaxis of endoscopically evident ulcers. However, the predictive value of such endoscopically discovered lesions is uncertain. Therefore, no proactive search for them should not be made in clinical practice. If ulcers are discovered, few would leave them untreated, but it must be appreciated that no study has yet identified a strategy that prevents the important end point of life-threatening consequences and death.

Symptoms

Although half of those taking NSAIDs will experience GI symptoms and as many as 30% may have to change or stop taking NSAIDs because of these symptoms (25), it is surprising that there have not been more controlled studies in this area. One study of patients with NSAID-related nonulcer dyspepsia found a high placebo response rate that was significantly accelerated by cimetidine (26). Alternative approaches to symptoms include switching the NSAID, although systematic data are relatively few. Recently an NSAID toxicity index has been identified that could act as a guide to the strategy of NSAID switching in patients with dyspepsia (27). This has yet to be evaluated prospectively. Another approach is to use enteric coating (28–30). Short-term studies again suggest some value from this, but there are surprisingly few data in the clinical arena.

MANAGEMENT POINTS

1. Choose a drug with a low toxicity index (but note caveats described above).
2. Consider using an enteric-coated preparation.
3. Use an H_2-antagonist for patients with unacceptable dyspepsia.
4. Remember that dyspepsia is no guide to prevalence of ulceration, which is frequently silent.

Ulcer Healing

Gastric and duodenal ulcers can be healed using placebo, H_2-receptor antagonists, sucralfate, prostaglandins, or proton pump inhibitors, while patients continue to take NSAIDs. Four studies suggest, for H_2-receptor antagonists at least, that if the patient's NSAID can be stopped, there will be a substantial placebo healing rate and a significant enhancement of the rate of healing with an active agent (31–34).

H_2-RECEPTOR ANTAGONISTS

For gastric or duodenal ulcers, Davies and colleagues (31) showed a 6-week healing rate of 46% with placebo could be enhanced to 69% with cimetidine 1600 mg daily. Similar results were obtained by Bijlsma (35) and Croker et al. (36), although there was no placebo group in their studies. Analyses restricted to gastric or duodenal ulcer show similar findings, with somewhat higher healing rates for duodenal ulcers than gastric ulcers (34).

SUCRALFATE

Sucralfate increases mucosal prostaglandin synthesis and has been shown to protect against gastric mucosal damage following a single dose of aspirin (37). However, this effect was abolished by pretreatment with indomethacin, and no gastric protection was seen following 2 weeks of aspirin therapy (38). A randomized study in patients with NSAID-associated ulcers has shown that sucralfate was as effective as ranitidine in healing gastroduodenal ulcers following 9 weeks of therapy, although the number of gastric ulcers was small (32). In contrast, in a study examining patients with only NSAID-associated gastric ulcers or erosions, the reduction in damage seen at endoscopy following 6 weeks of treatment was not different from that in the placebo (39). Similarly sucralfate has failed to prevent the development of gastric ulcers in 16% of 131 NSAID users following 3 months of therapy (40).

PROSTAGLANDINS

Data have been reported for misoprostol (41), rioprostil (42), enprostil (43), and arboprostil (44). For example, Roth and his colleagues reported 4 and 8 week healing of gastric ulcers enhanced from 29–62% with misoprostol 800 µg daily. This study, like those for enprostil and rioprostil used anti-secretory doses of misoprostol. Three interesting studies reported by Euler and his colleagues suggest that for arboprostil at least non-antisecretory doses of prostaglandins enhance ulcer healing, probably in a dose-dependent way (44). Thus, for example, 10 µg daily enhanced ulcer healing from 15–38%, the value for 25 µg daily being 43%, and for 50 µg daily, 52%. These data are in contrast to healing of non-NSAID ulcers in which only antisecretory doses have been shown to be effective. There are virtually no published data on healing of duodenal ulcers with prostaglandins.

PROTON PUMP INHIBITORS

Walan and his colleagues (45) reported on gastric ulcer healing by omeprazole 20 and 40 mg daily. They identified a subgroup of patients who continued to take NSAIDs. These patients had lower healing rates than those who did not take NSAIDs when treated by ranitidine 150 mg twice daily or omeprazole 20 mg mane. However, omeprazole 40 mg mane achieved high healing rates that were both significantly better than ranitidine 150 mg twice daily and not significantly different from rates achieved in patients not taking NSAIDs. If confirmed, these interesting data suggest that sufficiently potent ulcer healing can overcome the delay in healing associated with NSAID use.

Two issues should be noted when considering these results. First, many of the ulcers treated were fairly small. Second, while NSAIDs should be stopped if at all possible, there are many patients who are unable to do this without unacceptable deterioration of joint disease, and it is reassuring that healing, albeit retarded, can be achieved under these circumstances. Data from the omeprazole suggest that this retardation can be overcome, although this suggestion requires additional confirmation. However, what is not clear is whether patients remain at increased risk of ulcer complications (and for how long) during the healing period.

MANAGEMENT POINTS

1. NSAIDs retard ulcer healing and, if possible, should be stopped when an ulcer is discovered.
2. Where NSAIDs cannot be reasonably stopped, ulcer healing can still be achieved.
3. Any ulcer-healing drug will accelerate ulcer healing.
4. Published data do not suggest that prostaglandins are particularly effective, but comparisons with H_2-antagonists have not been made.
5. One study suggests that omeprazole 40 mg daily achieves better results than ranitidine, and on this evidence, should be used in patients with significant troublesome gastric ulcers.

PROPHYLAXIS

The ideal prophylactic agent is one with high potency against the end point of interest (in the present case, life-threatening ulcer complications), which is inexpensive and reasonably devoid of significant side effects. Such an agent does not exist. H_2-receptor antagonists are largely free of side effects, but are expensive and appear to be ineffective against gastric ulcers. Misoprostol appears to be effective against both gastric and duodenal ulcers, but has an uncomfortably high incidence of side effects and is not inexpensive. Neither H_2-antagonists nor prostaglandins has yet been shown to prevent life-threatening complications.

H$_2$-RECEPTOR ANTAGONISTS

Two studies from either side of the Atlantic have shown similar results (46, 47). Ehsanullah and her colleagues found that 8% of NSAID patients developed duodenal ulcers over a 2-month period (46). This figure was significantly reduced to 1.5% by twice daily administration of ranitidine 150 mg. However, the incidence of gastric ulcers was 6% whether placebo or ranitidine was given. An American study to almost identical design produced very similar results (47).

PROSTAGLANDINS

By contrast, the first study of misoprostol prophylaxis produced different results. Here, there was a much higher incidence of lesions classified as gastric ulcers (21.7%) and this was reduced to 5.7% by misoprostol 400 μg daily and 1.4% by misoprostol 800 μg daily (10). There was a lower incidence of duodenal ulcer and no obvious effect of the drug on its incidence. In this study, three times as many patients taking misoprostol 800 μg daily developed diarrhea as did those on placebo.

However, in a follow-up study utilizing more than 450 patients and an ulcer definition of $\geq$0.5 cm diameter, misoprostol 200 μg q.i.d. for 12 weeks reduced the development of a duodenal ulcer from 4.6% among placebo recipients to 0.6% among those receiving misoprostol prophylactically ($P = 0.002$). Gastric ulcers were also prevented (7.7 vs. 1.9%, respectively) (48).

Subsequent studies have examined the use of misoprostol over longer periods of time (40, 48–50). In these studies an advantage for misoprostol over placebo was maintained for as much as 1 year, but the differences have not been as great as in the original shorter study. In several of these later studies, patients taking misoprostol have been shown to develop fewer duodenal ulcers than those on placebo, again, in contrast to the initial study results.

Misoprostol has been compared with sucralfate and found to be clearly superior in the prevention of gastric ulcers. At the present time, a role for sucralfate in this respect is not evident (40).

MANAGEMENT POINTS

1. Prophylaxis should be reserved for high risk patients, in particular, those who have already experienced significant ulceration or ulcer complications.
2. On present evidence, prophylaxis can be dictated by the site of previous problems.
3. Ranitidine should be used for those who have had previous duodenal ulceration while taking NSAIDs because it is well tolerated.
4. Misoprostol should be used for those who have had previous gastric ulceration while taking NSAIDs because of its greater effectiveness.
5. It is doubtful whether other patients warrant prophylaxis on present evidence but if the prescriber wants to use a drug, misoprostol 400 μg daily is probably the best choice.
6. There are growing data suggesting omeprazole in prophylaxis.
7. There appears to be no role for sucralfate in prophylaxis.
8. No prophylactic regime has yet been shown to prevent complications or offer increased life expectancy.

COMPLICATIONS AND DEATH

Bleeding is the most common serious complication of NSAID ulcers. It can be calculated that between 2,000 and 10,000 bleeds per annum and between 200 and 1,000 deaths per annum are attributable to use of NSAIDs in the United Kingdom. Several pieces of evidence suggest that bleeding may arise in part because of the antihemostatic effect of NSAIDs discussed above. Thus, there is no increase in uncomplicated duodenal ulcer, but there is an increase in bleeding duodenal ulcer in patients taking NSAIDs (9). There also appears to be an increase in the rate of nonulcer (principally variceal) bleeding. The main risk of presentation is in the first 3 months. Bleeding could arise if provoked by NSAIDs in preexisting silent ulcers (although other explanations are possible). Finally, an increasing number of studies associate the use of aspirin at dosages of 300 mg a day or less with an enhanced risk of melena (51–53), suggesting either that such doses are ulcerogenic and/or that they act to provoke bleeding in prior ulcers. It is possible that bleeding could be a target for prophylaxis—that is, an agent that lowered the risk of an ulcer bleeding without necessarily preventing the ulcer could still be a valuable hemostatic agent. Such agents might include antifibrinolytic drugs such as tranexamic acid, or the less well-defined ethamsylate. However, tranexamic acid is associated with an increased incidence of thrombotic episodes, which would probably counteract any value in prevention of bleeding. An alternative approach is to try to influence local intragastric hemostasis or fibrinolysis. Results in model systems suggest that raising the intragastric pH substantially reduces rates of bleeding from acute lesions (8, 54, 55). In patients not taking NSAIDs who receive H_2-antagonists as maintenance, the proportion of ulcers that relapse as hematemesis and melena appears to be smaller and in those not receiving maintenance (56). Likewise, H_2-antagonists seem to prevent overt stress ulcer bleeding in patients in intensive care units without preventing ulceration itself (57, 58). These data are all consistent with the notion that raising the intragastric pH selectively protects against hematemesis and melena, either by a direct effect on hemostasis or by rendering ulcers sufficiently shallow or benign that bleeding does not occur.

MANAGEMENT POINTS

The idea that acid inhibition might prevent bleeding without preventing ulceration is too theoretical to influence practice, but may nevertheless be yielding unsuspected benefit in patients who take H_2 antagonists together with NSAIDs for other reasons.

CONCLUSION

Much of our advice is fairly pragmatic because data to determine management remain sketchy. Studies of treatment of NSAID-related dyspepsia on the one hand and large prophylactic studies with ulcer complications as the end point on the other are badly needed. At present, the routine use of misoprostol or other agents to prevent damage from NSAIDs in low or average risk individuals is not recommended (60).

REFERENCES

1. Walt R, Katschinski B, Logan R, Ashley J, Langman M. Rising frequency of ulcer perforation in elderly people in the United Kingdom. Lancet 1986;2:489–492.
2. Langman MJS, Brooks P, Hawkey CJ, Silverstein F, Yeomans N. Working party report to the World Congresses Of Gastroenterology, Sydney 1990. Non steroidal anti-inflammatory drug associated ulcer: epidemiology, causation and treatment. J Gastroenterol Hepatol 1991;6:442–449.
3. Hudson N, Balsitis M, Everitt S, Hawkey CJ. Enhanced gastric mucosal leukotriene B_4 synthesis in patients taking nonsteroidal anti-inflammatory drugs. Gut 1993;34:742–747.
4. Levi S, Goodlad RA, Lee CY, et al. Inhibitory effect of non-steroidal anti-inflammatory drugs on mucosal cell proliferation associated with gastric ulcer healing. Lancet 1990;336:841–843.
5. Tarnawski A, Stachura J, Douglass TG, Krause WJ, Gergely H, Sarfeh IJ. Indomethacin impairs quality of experimental gastric ulcer healing: a quantitative histological and ultrastructural analysis. In: Garner A, O'Brien PE, eds. Mechanisms of injury, protection and repair of the upper gastrointestinal tract. New York: Wiley, 1991:521–531.
6. Hudson N, Balsitis M, Hawkey CJ. Reduction in angiogenesis in non-steroidal anti-inflammatory drug associated gastric ulcers. Gut 1991;32:A1246.
7. Ogihara Y, Fuse Y, Okabe S. Effects of indomethacin and prednisolone on connective tissue at the base of acetic acid-induced gastric ulcers in rats. In: Garner A, O'Brien PE, eds. Mechanisms of injury, protection and repair of the upper gastrointestinal tract. New York: Wiley, 1991:455–466.
8. Hawkey CJ, Hawthorne AB, Hudson N, Cole AT, Mahida YR, Daneshmend TK. Separation of aspirin's impairment of haemostasis from mucosal injury in the human stomach. Clin Sci 1991;81:565–573.
9. Hawkey CJ. Non-steroidal anti-inflammatory drugs and peptic ulcers: facts and figures multiply, but do they add up? Br Med J 1990;300:278–284.
10. Graham DY, Agrawal N, Roth SH. Prevention of NSAID-induced gastric ulcer with misoprostol: multicentre, double-blind, placebo-controlled trial. Lancet 1988;2:1277–1280.
11. Jorde R, Bostad L, Burhol PG. Asymptomatic gastric ulcer: a follow up study in patients with previous gastric ulcer disease. Lancet 1986;1:119–121.
12. Bernersen B, Johnsen R, Straume B, Burhol PG, Jenssen TG, Stakkevold PA. Towards a true prevalence of peptic ulcer: the Sorreisa gastrointestinal disorder study. Gut 1990;31:989–992.
13. Bollini P, Rodriguez LAG, Gutthann SP, Walker AM. The impact of research quality and study design

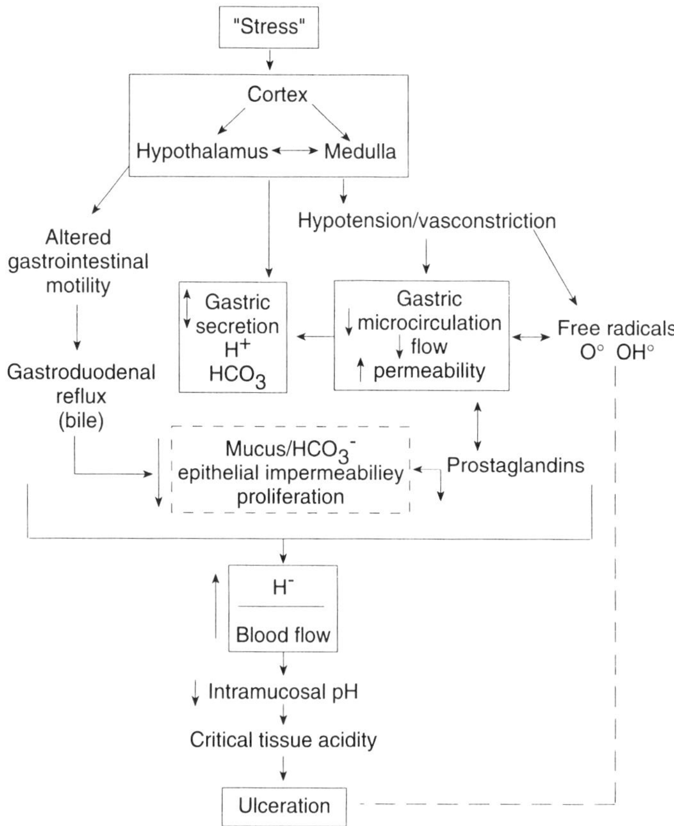

Figure 4.1. Proposed mechanisms for stress ulceration. Stress-related mucosal damage results from complex interaction of multiple systems. Specific relationships depicted remain somewhat speculative.

ity such as post-transfusion hepatitis (1). To date, however, well-designed prospective studies have failed to demonstrate a significant difference in blood transfusion requirements and have not reported on differences in length of hospital stay or other indicators of morbidity. Recently, some concern has been raised that the use of agents for prophylaxis (i.e., antacids and/or H_2-receptor antagonists) might actually increase the incidence of nosocomial pneumonia by neutralizing gastric acidity and allowing bacterial overgrowth in the stomach. (See "Nosocomial Pneumonia".)

PATHOGENESIS OF SRMD

The integrity of the gastric mucosa is highly dependent on the balance of aggressive and defensive factors. The pathophysiological mechanisms of SRMD are not completely understood, but a number of factors have been implicated (19):

- gastric acidity
- mucus production
- mucosal prostaglandins
- mucosal ischemia
- bicarbonate secretion
- epithelial cell renewal/integrity

Aggressive factors include gastric acid and reflux of bile into the stomach. Defensive factors include mucus production, mucosal blood flow and mucosal prostaglandins.

Intraluminal gastric acidity and decreased gastric mucosal blood flow with the development of local ischemia as well as back diffusion of hydrogen ions are considered the major factors involved in the pathogenesis of SRMD

Table 4.1
Risk of GI Bleeding after Medical ICU Admission for 174 Patients

Risk Category	Occult or overt GI bleeding (%)	Overt bleeding only (%)
All admissions	14	6
Length of admission		
<7 days	2	0
≥7 days	48	21
Ventilatory Status		
No mechanical ventilation	3	0
Mechanical ventilation <5 days	16	3
Mechanical ventilation ≥5 days	65	39

Modified from Ref. 10.

(Figure 4.1) (20). Reduced perfusion and/or uptake of oxygen and nutrients to mucosal cells leads to mucosal breakdown and necrosis and an inadequate secretion of mucus and bicarbonate. As a result, the integrity of the gastric mucosal barrier is compromised, leaving the mucosa vulnerable to the effects of luminal acid and pepsin (1, 2, 19, 21–23). Although net acid output may be low or normal, the back diffusion of hydrogen ions from the gastric lumen to the mucosa may cause tissue injury secondary to acidosis and lead to ulceration and hemorrhage (24).

In addition, bile reflux may play a role. Bile refluxes into the stomach more commonly in the critically ill (25), and experimentally, bile reflux plays a role in SRMD in shock models in dogs. In this animal model, neither ischemia nor shock were ulcerogenic in the presence of acid, but in the presence of bile they both produced SRMD (26).

Prostaglandins may play a role since they suppress gastric acid secretion, enhance and maintain mucosal blood flow, and stimulate gastric mucus and bicarbonate secretion. More importantly, prostaglandins mediate adaptive responses that make the gastric mucosa more resistant to noxious stimuli (27). Studies in animals show that stress-induced reductions in mucosal prostaglandin synthesis may render the gastric mucosa more susceptible to acid injury. The reparative cells arising from the neck cells of the crypts help maintain mucosal integrity. Alterations in gastric epithelial cell renewal and migration may lead to acute gastric erosions during periods of stress (28).

Risk Factors of SRMD

Certain risk factors for SRMD apparently predispose a patient to SR-UGIB: Swan first described the association of critical illness with gastroduodenal ulceration and hemorrhage in 1823. Subsequently, Curling described stress ulcers in patients with burns in 1842 and Dieulafoy noted them in patients with pneumococcal pneumonia in 1898 (1).

Bleeding secondary to SRMD appears to be related to the type and number of these risk factors present in an individual patient. Sepsis, in particular, seems to increase the incidence of SR-UGIB significantly in all clinical settings (29). Although the time to onset of bleeding varies, 84% of patients who bled in one prospective study did so within 8 days of ICU admission; the median time of onset was 4 days (10).

Schuster et al. (10) analyzed multiple factors to determine which would best predict the subsequent development of UGIB (Table 4.1). In their prospective study of 174 medical/respiratory ICU patients (179 admissions), the most powerful predictive factors of stress-related bleeding were the need for mechanical ventilation and the presence of a coagulopathy (thrombocytopenia, prolonged prothrombin time or partial thromboplastin time, or the use of an anticoagulant). Of the 25 patients who bled, only three did not have one of these two factors. Of those requiring mechanical ventilation, the risk of overt bleeding was low in those requiring mechanical ventilation for <5 days compared with those requiring mechanical ventilation for longer periods (3% vs. 39%). Sepsis, an underlying malignancy, and acute respiratory illness were also more frequent in those who bled ($P < .05$). Hypotension or shock were more common in those who bled, although not significantly.

Harris et al. (30) reported similar results in a retrospective analysis of patients admitted to a respiratory ICU over a 1-year period. Risk factors associated with bleeding included longer ventilatory support and increased duration of hospital and ICU stays. Thrombocytopenia (defined as a platelet count of less than $100,000/\text{mM}^2$) occurred in a majority of the bleeding patients; thrombocytopenia occurred at some point during the ICU stay in 60% of bleeding patients compared with 3% of those patients who did not bleed ($P < .001$). Bleeding occurred more often in patients with adult respiratory distress syndrome than in those with chronic obstructive pulmonary disease (85% vs. 9%). Ventilatory support, sepsis, or hypotension may have been important for SR-UGIB in the adult respiratory distress group (1).

Macdougall et al. (31) noted a high incidence (53%) of endoscopically documented SR-UGIB in patients with fulminant hepatic failure. In this setting, the development of SRMD and associated severe SR-UGIB is probably a result of the serious underlying deficiencies in the synthesis of clotting factors. The investigators did not evaluate the effects of hypotension, sepsis, or the need for mechanical ventilation in this study (1).

Relationship of SR-UGIB and Severity of Illness

As mentioned, several studies have documented that the incidence of SR-UGIB increases with the number of risk factors per patient commensurate with the severity of illness (17, 18, 32, 33). In a study evaluating treatment with antacids compared with no treatment in 100 surgical patients, Hastings et al. (17) reported that 10 of the 14 bleeding patients had three to six risk factors defined by the investigators. The frequency of bleeding was 9.1%, 20%, and 40% in patients with two, three, or six risk factors, respectively.

Similarly, Zinner et al. (32) used an illness severity index score and found the incidence of SR-UGIB was directly proportional to the severity of illness. The incidence of bleeding was 11%, 34%, and 50%, respectively, for the patients receiving no prophylaxis with an illness score of 0–2, 3–6, and ≥ 7. More than 40% of the patients with the highest score experienced bleeding regardless of prophylaxis compared with only 1–2% of the patients with the lowest score receiving either antacids or cimetidine.

This relationship between multiple risk factors and the incidence of SR-UGIB was confirmed by Priebe and Skillman (33) in ICU patients receiving cimetidine for SRMD prevention. In this study, SR-UGIB occurred in 28% of the cimetidine-treated patients with two risk factors compared with 70% of the cimetidine-treated patients with three to six risk factors.

PATHOPHYSIOLOGIC APPROACH TO TREATMENT

The nearly universal occurrence of SRMD in critically ill patients suggests the need to consider early and effective prophylaxis. To prevent the development of SRMD and its subsequent complications, it is important to first identify and correct the underlying risk factors (23). Preventing shock and improving mucosal blood flow with fluid resuscitation and hemodynamic monitoring, and providing adequate nutritional and ventilatory support are important for minimizing the risk of SRMD. Utilizing a specific pathophysiologic approach, the main principles to be employed are buffering of luminal acid, inhibition of acid secretion, stimulation of protective mechanisms, and maintenance of protective mechanisms.

Role of pH in SRMD

Perhaps the simplest and most readily accessible method for preventing acute SR-UGIB is to reduce luminal acidity (7, 8, 34). A generally accepted endpoint for preventing SRMD and consequent SR-UGIB is maintenance of an intragastric pH value between 3.5 and 5.0 (24, 27, 35).

Animal studies have shown that SRMD develops when intragastric ischemia occurs in the presence of physiologic or even subphysiologic concentrations of gastric acid. There is a close correlation between the occurrence of acute gastric mucosal ulceration and the degree of intramural acidification in experimental animals (36–39). Kivilaakso and associates (38) described the relationship between ulceration and intramural pH of the gastric mucosa during hemorrhagic shock in an animal study: the decrease in intramural pH was significantly greater in the presence of luminal acid than in its absence. These investigators suggested that the capacity of the gastric mucosa to dispose of influxing hydrogen is compromised during hemorrhagic shock and that this may be a critical factor in the pathogenesis of SRMD.

Clearly pH is important in the development of and subsequent bleeding associated with SRMD in humans. Fiddian-Green et al (40), using an indirect method for measuring intramural pH in stomachs of ICU patients, reported that bleeding from ulcers was seen only in patients whose intraluminal pH fell below normal (defined as a pH < 7.24). Of the 103 patients studied, 7 had massive bleeding, and 6 of these 7 died. The best predictor of SR-UGIB was a combination of the number of risk factors for SR-UGIB in a patient and the intraluminal pH.

Not all ICU patients require acid neutralizing or inhibiting therapy, however. Gastric acid secretion is normal in many patients at risk for SR-UGIB. For example, in a study of 144 surgical ICU patients, 15% had persistent hypochlorhydria (41). A preliminary report of 19 patients admitted to a shock/trauma unit revealed persistent hypochlorhydria (median 24-hour pH 7.0) for the first 24 hours of hospitalization in 26% of patients (42). Intragastric pH was measured continuously in these fasted, critically ill patients who were not given any acid-neutralizing or inhibiting treatment. No breakthrough in intragastric pH control was observed during any part of the circadian cycle in these patients (43).

Other studies have provided additional data on the role of pH in gastric bleeding and intragastric hemostasis. The presence of gastric acid and pepsin in this environment may contribute to impaired hemostasis in patients with SRMD. An in vitro study evaluated the effect of pH on the stability and activity of pepsin (44). At a pH of 4.5, 70% of maximum peptic activity was still present; only at a pH of 8 was pepsin irreversibly inactivated. A subsequent in vitro study showed that gastric pH and pepsin influenced clotting and aggregation of platelets (45). As pH values fell below 7.0, blood clotting times (prothrombin time, thrombin time, activated partial thromboplastin time, and plasma recalcification time) decreased. At a pH of 2, all clotting factors were abnormal. The effect of pH on platelet aggregations was similar to that seen with clotting factors. When pH fell below 6.8, platelet aggregation decreased greatly. Coagulation and platelet aggregation were virtually absent at a pH of 5.4. Previously formed platelet aggregates disintegrated when the pH was slightly acidic and pepsin enhanced this process (45).

PHARMACOLOGIC APPROACH TO PREVENTION OF SRMD

Over the last 15 years, the incidence of hemorrhagic SRMD in critically ill patients has declined, even in the absence of prophylactic measures (1, 2). This trend has been attributed to improvements in general supportive care of these patients, such as maintenance of acid-base balance, improved ventilatory support, and use of supplemental parenteral alimentation (1). Controlled studies have shown that prophylactic therapy with antacids or H_2-receptor antagonists reduces the incidence of bleeding secondary to SRMD in critically ill patients.

Pharmacodynamic Data

Regardless of whether the therapeutic focus for SR-UGIB is prophylaxis or treatment, the primary objectives are to promptly restore circulation and to maintain a constant intragastric pH $\geq$ 3.5 and preferably $\geq$4.0. Prompt administration of aggressive fluid resuscitation and institution of other circulatory support measures have contributed to the decrease in severe SR-UGIB over the last decade.

pH Control Criteria in Preventing SRMD

Maintaining an intragastric pH >3.5 has been associated with a decreased frequency of bleeding from SRMD (46). An agent that can inhibit or neutralize gastric acid production should be able to promote gastric hemostasis, and therefore might be useful in treatment of SR-UGIB. Consequently, agents that neutralize or decrease secretion of gastric acid have been used as prophylaxis against bleeding secondary to SRMD. Historically, management of intragastric acidity in the ICU was accomplished with antacids, but current management in the ICU is usually accomplished through the use of H_2-receptor antagonists.

Some investigators have used pH control as a therapeutic endpoint rather than prevention of bleeding, when assessing the efficacy of prophylactic therapy. However, as mentioned earlier, pH control does not always correlate with clinical outcome, and bleeding from SRMD may develop despite apparently adequate pH control with antacids or H_2-antagonists (40, 46).

Drug Therapy for SR-UGIB Prevention

ANTACIDS (TABLE 4.2)

Support for the use of antacids for the prevention of SR-UGIB was initially provided by Hastings et al. (17). Their investigations demonstrated a decrease in the incidence of upper gastrointestinal tract bleeding from 25% to 4% by using antacid titration of intragastric contents. In this study, 100 critically ill patients at risk for developing SR-UGIB were randomized to receive antacid prophylaxis or no specific prophylaxis. The investigators used antacid titration of the intragastric contents; patients received an initial antacid dose of 30 mL via nasogastric tube followed by hourly doses of 30 mL for patients with an intragastric pH of $\geq$3.5 or 60 mL for patients with an intragastric pH <3.5. Efficacy was measured by a guaiac test performed on the gastric aspirate every 4 hours and on stool at least once daily. The pH of the intragastric aspirate was <5 in only two patients who were receiving antacids; it was usually between 7 and 8. In the control group, the intragastric aspirate pH was highly variable in each patient and between patients—ranging from 1 to 8. Only 4% (2/51) of patients given antacid prophylaxis had SR-UGIB compared with 24.5% (12/49) of control patients who bled.

In a similarly designed study, Pinilla et al. (47) found differing results. In their study, the investigators defined a therapeutic failure as macroscopic bleeding and disregarded endoscopic bleeding. Antacids were not found to be beneficial for prophylaxis of macroscopic bleeding. The UGIB that did occur was controlled with the use of an H_2-receptor antagonist and antacids. McAlhany et al. (48) observed a significant reduction ($P < .05$) in the proportion of patients requiring $\geq$3 U of blood per 24 hours in burn injury patients treated with antacids (4%) when compared with patients treated with placebo (25%).

Problems with Antacids. Although antacids are effective in preventing SR-UGIB, these regimens are inconvenient because they require frequent dosing. Antacids frequently clog nasogastric tubes which detract from the care of the patient. Severe diarrhea and electrolyte abnormalities are common problems (even with the combination antacids using both magnesium and aluminum salts). Finally, impaired gastric emptying and lack of peristalsis would preclude their use in some postsurgical patients.

Table 4.2
Selected Studies Evaluating Antacids vs. Placebo in the Prophylaxis of Stress-Related Upper Gastrointestinal Bleeding[a]

Reference	No. of patients	Patient type	Drug/dose	pH target	% Patients achieving pH criteria	Diagnostic SR-UGIB criteria	Incidence of SR-UGIB	Comments
Hastings et al. (17)	100	Surgical	No therapy Antacid (hourly)	NS	NS	Predominantly occult, guaiac	12/49 (24%) 2/51 (4%)	To maintain pH > 5 No difference in mortality
Pinilla et al. (47)	126	Surgical	Placebo Antacid	pH > 5	NS	Overt bleeding	9/61 (15%) 7/65 (11%)	
McAlhaney et al. (48)	48	Burn	Placebo Antacid	pH > 7	NS	Requiring 3 units of blood over 24 hr	6/24 (25%) 1/24 (4%)	Patients with >35% body burned $P > 0.05$ compared with control

[a]Abbreviation: NS, not stated.

H_2-RECEPTOR ANTAGONISTS

Because of the difficulties associated with antacids, H_2-receptor antagonists have been considered an improvement in the control of gastric acid secretion. The H_2-receptor antagonists cimetidine, ranitidine, and famotidine are widely used to prevent SR-UGIB among high-risk patients in intensive care units (11, 12, 14, 16, 18, 29, 31, 32, 46, 49–69) (Tables 4.3–4.4), although cimetidine is the only one currently approved in the United States for this indication. Nizatidine is not available for parenteral use in the United States and therefore is not discussed in the management of SRMD.

Despite the wealth of data comparing antacids, H_2-blockers, placebo, and other agents for the prevention of SRMD, differences between active treatment groups have been difficult to detect, partly because of the low incidence of clinically significant bleeding from SRMD. In addition, most published comparative studies suffer from one or more design weaknesses, including:

- heterogeneous patient populations
- inadequate study designs (e.g., lack of blinding)
- insufficient sample sizes
- inadequate sensitivity and specificity of monitoring techniques
- absence of endoscopy and reliance on nonspecific bleeding endpoints.

Because of the limited statistical power of these individual studies, various meta-analyses have been performed to assess comparative efficacy of the different agents for prophylaxis of SR-UGIB. While meta-analysis is an objective, quantitative method for combining results from a number of separate but similar studies, it is important that only well-controlled studies of similar design are included. When this is done, this methodologic tool increases the statistical power and improves both the precision and accuracy of the estimate of treatment effect.

Meta-analyses of H_2-Receptor Antagonists Compared with Antacids or Placebo

Five-meta-analyses of studies comparing the efficacy of H_2-receptor antagonists with that of antacids show either no clinical difference between treatments or a difference favoring treatment with H_2-receptor antagonists (4, 8, 70, 71, 72). The most recent meta-analysis by Cook and colleagues (4), was the first to examine the differential effect of prophylaxis on clinically important stress-related bleeding (overt bleeding with hemodynamic instability, a fall in hemoglobin by 20 g/l, and a requirement for transfusion) as well as overt bleeding (hematemesis, bloody gastric aspirate, melena, or hematochezia).

This meta-analysis consisted of 42 randomized trials selected according to prospectively defined criteria, and involved 4409 patients at risk (4). The investigators found a 50% reduction in clinically important bleeding and they suggested that this reduction mandated the use of prophylaxis in critically ill patients at risk of SR-UGIB. However, mortality rates in the ICU were not decreased by prophylaxis of SR-UGIB. In this meta-analysis, prophylaxis with antacids or H_2-receptor antagonists was superior to placebo or no therapy in reducing the risk of overt bleeding; H_2-receptor antagonists were superior to prophylaxis with antacids in reducing the risk of overt bleeding; and, most importantly, prophylaxis with H_2-receptor antagonists was more effective than prophylaxis with antacids in reducing clinically important bleeding.

An earlier meta-analysis (8) compared the efficacy of an H_2-receptor antagonist (cimetidine) or antacid in preventing SR-UGIB as compared with either placebo or no treatment by combining the data from 16 randomized trials. Both agents were more effective than placebo in preventing overall, occult, and overt bleeding ($P < .05$). Antacids were superior to cimetidine for prophylaxis of occult bleeding cimetidine ($P < .003$) but both were equally efficacious for overt bleeding.

Lacroix and associates (71) performed a meta-analysis of 15 prospective, randomized trials evaluating antacids and cimetidine in the

Table 4.3

Selected Studies Evaluating Antacids vs. H_2-Receptor Antagonists in the Prophylaxis of SR-UGIB[a]

Reference	No. of patients	Patient type	Drug/dose	pH target	% Patients achieveing pH criteria	Diagnostic SR-UGIB criteria	Incidence of SR-UGIB (%)	Comments
Mcdougall et al. (31)	65	Hepatic failure	Antacid 20 mL q 4 hr Cimetidine Control	pH > 5	NS	Overt bleeding	3/13 (23%) 1/16 (16%) 19/36 (53%)	
Zinner et al. (32)	300	Surgical ICU	Antacid 10–20 mL hourly Cimetidine iv 300 mg q 6 hr Placebo	>4	85 66	Overt Guaiac +4	5/100 (5%)* 14/100 (14%) 20/100 (20%)	$P < 0.05$ compared with control
Basso et al. (18)	168	ICU	Antacid 10 mL hourly Cimetidine iv or po 200 mg q 6 hr Control	NS	NS	Overt	1/52 (2%) 0/60 (0%) 8/56 (14%)	$P < 0.05$ compared with control
Friedman et al. (12)	31	Respiratory failure	Antacid 30 mL q 6 hr Cimetidine iv 300 mg q 6 hr Placebo	NS	NS	Overt	0/6 (0%) 1/11 (9%) 5/14 (35%)	Ventilator dependent
Priebe et al. (46)	75	Surgical ICU	Antacid 30 mL q 1 hr Antacid 60 mL q 1 hr Cimetidine iv 300 mg q 6 hr or po 200 mg q 6 hr	>3.5	76 84 53 76	Occult Guaiac or hemoccult	0/37 (0%) 7/38 (18.5%)	

Table 4.3 Continued

Selected Studies Evaluating Antacids vs. H_2-Receptor Antagonists in the Prophylaxis of SR-UGIB[a]

Reference	No. of patients	Patient type	Drug/dose	pH target	% Patients achieving pH criteria	Diagnostic SR-UGIB criteria	Incidence of SR-UGIB (%)	Comments
Martin et al. (29)	77	Surgical ICU	Antacid 60 mL hourly	>4	76	Occult	2/37 (5.4%)	
			Antacid 120 mL hourly		95			
			Cimetidine iv					
			300 mg q 6 hr		50			
			300 mg q 4 hr		73		3/40 (7.5%)	
Luk et al. (49)	182	ICU	Cimetidine	NS	NS	Overt/occult Endoscopy	4/62 (6%)	
			300 mg q 6 hr					
			Antacid 30 mL q 3 hr			5% decrease in hematocrit	7/59 (12%)	
			Placebo				2/61 (3%)	
Kingsley (50)	249	ICU	Antacid infusion 60 mL/hr	>4	95.3	Macroscopic	(1.5%)	All patients who bled had pH < 4
			Antacid 90 ml q 3 hr		70		(3.1%)	
			Cimetidine iv		55.4		(7.7%)	
			300 mg q 6 hr					
			Cimetidine iv		81.4		(1.7%)	
			50 mg/hr					
Reusser et al. (51)	40	Neurosurgical ICU	Ranitidine iv	>4	76.6	Macroscopic	0/20 (0%)	Stress erosions present in both groups.
			150–200/day					
			+ antacids					
			Placebo		33.3		0/20 (0%)	

[a]*Abbreviations:* NS, not stated; overt, overt bleeding seen; guaiac, bleeding assessed by occult blood.

Table 4.4
Selected Studies Evaluating H_2-Receptor Antagonists vs. Placebo or No Treatment in Prophylaxis of SR-UGIB[a]

Reference	No. of patients	Patient type	Drug/dose	pH target	% Patients achieving pH criteria	Diagnostic SR-UGIB criteria	Incidence of SR-UGIB	Comments
Peura and Johnson (11)	39	Medical ICU	Cimetidine iv 300 mg q 6 hr	NS	NS	Endoscopic	1/21 (5%)	
			Placebo				7/18 (39%)[b]	$P < 0.05$ compared with placebo
Martin et al. (52)	87	ICU	Cimetidine iv 50 mg/hr	NS	NS	Occult/overt Endoscopy	9/65 (14%)	
			Placebo				22/66 (33%)[c]	$P = 0.009$ compared with placebo
Ostro et al. (53)	46	ICU	Cimetidine iv 300 mg q 6 hr	>4	22	NS	1.5	
			Cimetidine iv bolus 300 mg then 37.5 mg/hr		61			
Van den Berg and van Blankenstein (54)	24	Medical/ surgical ICU	Ranitidine 50 mg iv bolus then 0.2 mg/kg/hr	>3.5	75*	Detection of chromium labelled erythrocytes in gastric aspirate	1/13 (7.6%)[d]	Not significant compared with placebo
			Placebo		55		3/11 (27%)	
Hummer-Siegel et al. (55)	?	Head injury	Ranitidine iv 0.2 mg/kg/hr	NS	NS	Overt Endoscopic examinations	No significant difference No decrease in SRMD	
			Placebo					

Table 4.4 Continued
Selected Studies Evaluating H$_2$-Receptor Antagonists vs. Placebo or No Treatment in Prophylaxis of SR-UGIB[a]

Reference	No. of patients	Patient type	Drug/dose	pH target	% Patients achieving pH criteria			Diagnostic SR-UGIB criteria	Incidence of SR-UGIB	Comments
Albin et al. (56)	14	ICU	Ranitidine iv 50 mg bolus then infusion (mean dose 0.2 mg/kg/hr)	>4	78 mean pH 5.4			NS	NS	Ranitidine dose titrated to pH (Maximum dose of 600 mg/24 hr) pH was not controlled in 3 patients with sepsis
Bohrer et al. (57)	6	ICU	Ranitidine iv bolus	3–4.5	pH > 3 = 47.5	pH 3–4.5 = 9.3	pH > 4.5 = 43.5	NS	NS	
			Ranitidine infusion 0.6 mg/kg/day		34	11.6	54.4			
			Ranitidine infusion plus enteral nutrition		31.5	20	48.5			
Rigaud et al. (58)	12	Ventilated patients	Ranitidine iv 0.5 mg/kg then 0.25 mg/kg/hr	>4	65			NS	No significant bleeding	Occult bleeding common
Livingston et al. (14)	167	Head injury	Ranitidine iv 6.25 mg/kg/hr	NS	NS			Overt	3/88 (3%)	
			Placebo						15/79 (19%)	

[a]*Abbreviations:* iv, intravenous; q, every; N/A, data not available.
[b]*P* < .05.
[c]*P* = .009.
[d]Not significant.

overall incidence of bleeding and found congruent results, even though many of the trials were the same as those evaluated above. For overt bleeding, there was no difference in efficacy demonstrated between prophylaxis with antacids and prophylaxis with cimetidine. Of the 1993 patients studied, hemorrhagic shock and death directly related to SR-UGIB occurred in 8 and 5 patients, respectively.

More recently, Karlstadt et al. (72) performed a meta-analysis of cimetidine and placebo to investigate the efficacy of intravenous cimetidine (continuous infusion and intermittent infusion regimens) in the prevention of SR-UGIB in ICU patients. Of the 102 clinical controlled trials studying cimetidine for prevention of SR-UGIB in an ICU setting, 13 trials were identified with overt SR-UGIB used as clinical endpoint. On average, there was a statistically significant reduction in the risk of UGIB in the cimetidine-treated patients relative to placebo (9% vs. 21%, respectively).

Controlled Trials of H_2-Receptor Antagonists by Continuous Infusion Compared with Placebo

H_2-receptor antagonists have generally been administered by bolus injection or by intermittent infusion, resulting in a short duration of pH control after a single dose. Use of continuous infusion has been advocated for maintaining a more consistent serum concentration and intragastric pH control. In placebo-controlled studies in healed duodenal ulcer patients, continuous infusion of ranitidine at a rate of 6.25 mg/hour was more consistent in maintaining gastric pH of 4.0 or more over a 24-hour period than an equivalent intermittent infusion of ranitidine 50 mg every eight hours (73, 74). Likewise, in critically ill patients, ranitidine 6.25 mg/hour produced a mean pH of 4.17 during a 72-hour infusion period compared with 2.14 in the placebo group (75).

Several studies with cimetidine suggest that continuous infusion more reliably maintains intragastric pH at >4.0 than intermittent injection (50, 53). Ostro and colleagues (53) found that intragastric pH was maintained >4 in only 22% of patients receiving intermittent therapy with cimetidine compared with 87% of patients who received cimetidine by continuous infusion (P < .0001). At equivalent doses, all H_2-receptor antagonists will produce similar effects in controlling intragastric pH when infused continuously (76).

Cimetidine and ranitidine are the only H_2-receptor antagonists that have been adequately studied in patients requiring SR-UGIB prophylaxis. Moreover, a number of placebo-controlled studies of cimetidine and ranitidine have been completed in recent years evaluating their efficacy in preventing SR-UGIB (14, 52, 75).

In a multicenter, double-blind, placebo-controlled study of 131 critically ill patients treated with cimetidine (50–100 mg/hr) those receiving the H_2 blocker experienced significantly less SR-UGIB than those receiving placebo (9 [14%] of 65 cimetidine vs. 22 [33%] of 66 placebo patients [P = .009]) (52). Cimetidine-treated patients had higher mean intragastric pH and intragastric pH was maintained >4 for a greater percentage of time: (the mean pH was 5.7 and 3.9 and the mean percentage of time was 82% and 41%, respectively). It should be noted that about half of the cimetidine-treated patients required 100 mg/hr to maintain a pH of ≥4.

This study has been criticized because the study group had few risk factors for SRMD and prophylaxis was stopped within 72 hours in 75% of patients (77). This study was also criticized because the source of bleeding, when it occurred, was not always determined.

Livingston et al. (14) evaluated a continuous infusion of ranitidine (6.25 mg/hr) in a more critically ill patient population for a maximum of 5 days. In this double-blind, placebo-controlled, prospective study, all 167 patients had severe head injury and 72% had three or more risk factors for SR-UGIB (mechanical ventilation, organ dysfunction, major surgery, other trauma). Despite their high risk status, SR-UGIBs occurred in only 3% of (3/88) patients treated with ranitidine compared with 19% (15/79) of placebo-treated patients (P = .002). In addition, ranitidine treatment prevented SR-UGIB in patients with three or more risk factors. Similar results were noted in a smaller study evaluating ranitidine in a similar patient population (75).

H$_2$-receptor antagonists are generally well-tolerated and the frequency of severe adverse reactions is low. The most common adverse reactions are diarrhea, drowsiness, fatigue, headache, muscular pain, and constipation (78). (See discussion on safety concerns in the prophylaxis of SR-UGIB.)

CYTOPROTECTIVE AGENTS

Cytoprotection is the ability of an agent to prevent acute SRMD by a mechanism other than the reduction of gastric acidity. These agents may protect against SRMD by enhancing mucosal defenses and also by stimulating reparative processes (i.e., cellular adaptation) in the gastric mucosa (79).

Comparison of Sucralfate with Antacids and H$_2$-Receptor Antagonists (Table 4.6)

Sucralfate, a basic aluminum salt of sucrose octasulfate, enhances gastric mucosa defenses by forming a protective coat over damaged tissue (19). Sucralfate may also bind pepsin and stimulate endogenous prostaglandin synthesis and mucus secretion.

Studies (16, 66–69a) have compared the efficacy of sucralfate (1 g every 4 hours) vs. 2-hourly antacid suspensions titrated to maintain intragastric pH >4 in critically ill patients requiring stress ulcer prophylaxis (Table 4.5). Bresalier and coworkers (16) observed no significant difference in the incidence of overt or occult bleeding between antacid- and sucralfate-treated patients; despite a significantly (P < .01) greater severity of illness in the sucralfate group. Tryba (69) observed overt bleeding in 2 of 100 patients (one antacid- and one sucralfate-treated patient) in his study. However, the incidence of nosocomial pneumonia was significantly (P < .05) higher in the antacid group (34%) when compared with the sucralfate group (10%). Tryba and coworkers (66) compared the incidence of overt bleeding

among critically ill patients receiving stress ulcer prophylaxis with sucralfate (1 g every 4 hours [n = 34]), 2-hourly antacid suspensions titrated to maintain intragastric pH > 4 (n = 33), or cimetidine (400 mg every 6 hours [n = 33]). All patients received a daily morning dose of intravenous pirenzepine (50 mg), an antimuscarinic agent. Overt bleeding occurred in 2 patients receiving antacids and 2 patients receiving cimetidine. Despite having a significantly (P < .05) lower gastric pH, the sucralfate group did not develop overt bleeding. Cannon and coworkers (69a) compared the incidence of overt bleeding among mechanically ventilated patients receiving stress ulcer prophylaxis with sucralfate (1 g every 6 hours [n = 19]), hourly antacid suspension titrated to maintain intragastric pH >4 (n = 19), or cimetidine (300 mg every 6 hours [n = 21]). Overt bleeding occurred in 4 patients receiving antacids and 1 patient receiving cimetidine. No patient in the sucralfate group developed overt bleeding (P < .05 when compared the antacid group).

These preliminary studies suggest a possible role for sucralfate in patients requiring stress ulcer prophylaxis. Cook et al. (4) conducted a meta-analysis of available data on sucralfate in patients at risk for developing SR-UGIB and concluded that there were insufficient data to show a clear advantage with antacids, H$_2$-antagonists, or sucralfate in preventing clinically important bleeding.

A meta-analysis by Tryba (70) evaluated the efficacy of antacids, H$_2$-receptor antagonists, pirenzepine, and placebo in preventing SR-UGIB. Using macroscopic bleeding as the criteria for SR-UGIB, Tryba found that prophylaxis with antacids reduced the rate of macroscopic bleeds compared with no prophylaxis (6% vs. 15%). Prophylaxis with cimetidine or ranitidine also produced lower rates of bleeding compared with no treatment (5% vs. 16%). There was no difference in the rates of SR-UGIB when prophylaxis with antacids and H$_2$-receptor antagonists were compared. Sucralfate had lower rates of bleeding in comparison with H$_2$-receptor antagonists and in

Table 4.5

Selected Studies Evaluating H_2-Receptor Antagonist Comparisons in the Prophylaxis of SR-UGIB[a]

Reference	No. of patients	Patient type	Drug/dose	pH target	% Patients achieveing of pH criteria	Diagnostic SR-UGIB criteria	Incidence of SR-UGIB	Comments
Barth et al. (59)	193	ICU	Ranitidine iv 50 mg q 6 hr	NS	NS	Overt bleeding	6/98 (6.1%)	
			Cimetidine iv 400 mg q 6 hr				11/95 (11.6%)[b]	Not significant compared to cimetidine
Siepler et al. (60)	227	ICU	Ranitidine iv 50 mg bolus then 8 mg/hr	≥5	70.6 of pH values ≥5	Overt	1/150 (1.6%)	ICU patients on parenteral nutrition with average of 3.2
			Cimetidine iv 300 mg bolus then 50 mg/hr		65.6 of pH values ≥ 5		2/77 (2.5%)[b]	risk factors. Dura- of treatment: 10 days
Ketterl et al. (61)	12	ICU with sepsis	Ranitidine 300 mg/day	NS	NS	NS	0/6 (0%)	
			Cimetidine				0/6 (0%)	
Reid and Bayliff et al. (62)	71	Critically ill	Ranitidine 300 mg/day	NS	NS	Macroscopic	2/33 (6%)	
			Cimetidine				1/38 (2.6%)	
More et al. (63%)	48		Ranitidine iv up to 300 mg/day	>4	50*	Clinically significant	0/20 (0%)	
			Cimetidine iv up to 2400 mg/day		18		0/28 (0%)[c]	$P = 0.04$ compared with cimetidine
Naumann et al. (64)	40	ICU vent-ilated	Ranitidine iv 50 mg q 8 hr	NS	NS	Overt	1/20 (5%)	
			Famotidine iv 10 mg q 8 hr				0/20 (0%)	
Friedl et al. (65)	20	Surgical ICU	Ranitidine iv 50 mg q 6–12 hr	NS	NS	Overt	0/20 (0%)	
			Famotidine iv 10 mg q 6–12 hr				0/20(0%)	

[a]Abbreviation: NS, not stated.

comparison with antacids, although not significantly.

Comparisons between studies are also difficult since different forms of sucralfate have been used in different dosages (e.g., 4, 6, or 9 g/day) as well as different volumes (from 5–20 ml) and different formulations (79). European investigators usually used a commercial suspension, while British and American studies used an extemporaneously prepared suspension. Trials comparing mortality rates in sucralfate-treated patients with those in patients treated with an H_2-antagonist or antacids show no clear statistically significant benefit for sucralfate (79).

Problems Associated with Sucralfate Use. Sucralfate requires enteral administration. This may be problematic in patients who had operations of the upper gastrointestinal tract. In general, sucralfate should be avoided in patients who are fasting after upper gastrointestinal surgery. Reported side effects with sucralfate have been few. However, concommitant use of sucralfate may decrease the absorption of dietary phosphates and of some drugs (e.g., digoxin, tetracycline, quinolones, theophylline, and phenobarbital). Since sucralfate contains aluminum, accumulation and toxicity can occur in patients with impaired renal function.

MISOPROSTOL

Misoprostol, an analog of prostaglandin E_1, is currently marketed for its mucosal protective effects as prophylaxis against NSAID-associated gastric ulcers. Misoprostol and other prostaglandin analogs enhance mucosal defenses by increasing gastric mucus and bicarbonate secretion, stimulating gastric repair and increasing gastric mucosal blood flow. In the prevention of SR-UGIB, misoprostol appears to exert its effect primarily because of its antisecretory properties (3). In one prospective, randomized, multicenter trial, misoprostol 200 μg every 4 hours was compared with antacids for prophylaxis of SRMD (80). Both misoprostol and antacids maintained pH >4 and no clinically significant SR-UGIB occurred with either treatment. Endoscopy re-

vealed no significant difference in the severity of SRMD or in the number of gastric lesions in either group. A relative lack of data for SRMD makes recommendations about the use of misoprostol difficult.

Problems with Misoprostol Use. Misoprostol is generally well-tolerated. Side effects from misoprostol therapy include crampy abdominal pain and diarrhea. Diarrhea is caused in approximately 25% of patients and could cause fluid and electrolyte inbalance as well as increase the need for nursing care in the critically ill patient. The drug is also a recognized abortofascient.

OMEPRAZOLE

Omeprazole is the only proton pump inhibitor currently marketed in the United States. There are no formal clinical studies evaluating this agent for prophylaxis of SRMD or SR-UGIB (3). In the United States, a limitation to its administration to the critically ill patient is its availability only as an enteric-coated capsule for oral administration. Gastric acid in the stomach could inactivate omeprazole if the capsule is opened and its contents administered via a nasogastric tube. In addition, use of a nasogastric tube increases the likelihood of gastric aspiration and chemical pneumonitis. Another important concern is omeprazole's affinity for the cytochrome P-450 mixed function oxidase system and the effects on concurrent drug administration (e.g., warfarin, phenytoin, and diazepam) (90). (See Chapter 27.)

PIRENZEPINE

Pirenzepine, an anticholinergic agent has specific activity against the M_1 muscarinic receptor on the parietal cell. Currently, pirenzepine is not available in the United States. The meta-analysis by Cook et al. (4) found that use of pirenzepine was superior to prophylaxis with H_2-receptor antagonists in reducing the risk of overt bleeding, although relatively few studies have evaluated the efficacy of pirenzepine as prophylaxis for SR-UGIB (81). In one prospective, controlled randomized trial comparing continuous infusions of ranitidine

Table 4.6

Selected Studies Evaluating Sucralfate vs. H_2-Receptor Antagonists and Antacid in the Prophylaxis of Stress-Related Upper Gastrointestinal Bleeding (SR-UGIB)[a]

Reference	No. of patients	Patient type	Drug/dose	pH target	% Patients achieving of pH criteria	Diagnostic SR-UGIB criteria	Incidence of SR-UGIB (%)	Comments
Tryba et al. (66)	100	Medical ICU	Sucralfate 1 g q 4 hr Antacid q 2 hr Cimetidine 2 g/day	NS	NS	Overt Endoscopy	0/34 (0%) 2/33 (6%) 2/33 (6%)	All patients received pirenzepine 50 mg/day
Tryba (69)	100	Medical ICU	Sucralfate 1 g q 4 hr Antacid q 2 hr	NS	NS	Overt Endoscopy	1/50 (2%) 1/50 (2%)	
Driks et al. (67)	130	ICU	Sucralfate 1 g q 6 hr Antacids H_2-antagonist[b] (Ran or Cim) Combination of antacid and H_2-antagonist	NS	NS	Occult/overt	16/61 (26%) NS 26/69 (37.6%) NS	
Bresalier et al. (16)	74	ICU	Sucralfate 1 g q 4 hr Antacid (Maalox)	pH > 4	NS	Overt/occult"	4/38* (10.5%)/ 16/38 (42%) 7/36 (19%)/ 11/36 (30)	Minimum of two risk factors
Borrero et al. (68)	50	Post abdominal aortic surgery	Sucralfate 1 g q 6 hr Antacid 30 ml q 2 hr	pH > 3.5	NS	Overt	1/25 (4%) 2/46 (4.3%)	
Cannon (69a)	59	Ventilator	patients	Sucralfate 1 g q 6 hr Antacid q 1 hr Cimetidine 300 mg q 6 hr	NS	NS	Overt	0/19 (0%) 4/19 (21%) 1/21 (5%)

[a]Abbreviations: q, every; N/A, data not available.
[b]Ranitidine or cimetidine.

and pirenzepine in 400 surgical patients, intragastric pH was significantly lower in patients treated with pirenzepine ($P < .01$) (69). Of those patients in the ranitidine group from whom an intragastric pH measurement could be obtained, only 8.1% showed pH values <4 in more than half the measurements. In comparison, of the patients in the pirenzepine group, this figure was 28.6% ($P < .01$). Nonetheless, macroscopically visible bleeding (hematemesis, blood in the aspirate, melena) occurred in six ranitidine-treated patients and in three pirenzepine-treated patients.

ENTERAL FEEDINGS FOR PH CONTROL

A number of studies have examined the changes in intragastric pH produced by the administration of parenteral and enteral nutrition as protection against the development of SR-UGIB (82, 83). Currently, it is still not known whether administering enteral or parenteral nutrition protects against SRMD by decreasing intragastric acidity or by correcting the catabolic state induced by critical illness (83).

Solem et al. (84) first reported that enteral feeding was useful as prophylaxis against SRMD after reviewing the cases of a selected group of 109 severely burned patients. They concluded that enteral nutrition protected against clinically evident Curling's ulcers when used in the early postburn period and that protection continued until autografting was complete. These results were confirmed by a retrospective study of unselected severely burned patients (85), in which an elemental diet was associated with a noticeable decrease in major SR-UGIB, related to an increased caloric intake.

Although animal studies suggest that intragastric nutrition increases the ability of the gastric mucosa to resist SRMD, at least three clinical studies have shown that enteral nutrition failed to maintain a high intragastric pH (58, 86, 87). In a double-blind, randomized study of 12 critically ill ventilated patients with chronic obstructive pulmonary disease, Rigaud and associates (58) monitored intragastric pH prior to and following sequential

addition of ranitidine or continuous enteral nutrition (CEN), or both. CEN was not effective in raising intragastric pH. In fact, as the dose of CEN increased, the pH decreased. Elmore et al. (86) found similar results when CEN was given with and without an intragastric infusion of cimetidine to 13 critically ill patients. Despite this combination therapy of CEN and cimetidine, 42% of the pH readings fell below pH of 4.0. Likewise, enteral nutrition delivered via intraduodenal or intragastric feeding did not adequately neutralize intragastric acidity as measured by serial pH on 366 gastric aspirates from 20 critically ill patients (87).

A recent study evaluated the effect of continuous intraduodenal nutrition on gastric pH compared with the effects of fasting and of parenteral and standard nutrition containing equal amounts of carbohydrate, protein, and lipid (83). CEN maintained the pH at levels similar to fasting or standard nutrition. Although parenteral nutrition increased intragastric pH compared with CEN, this increase would be inadequate to provide protection against SRMD, as the median 24-hour pH was only 1.9 and 1.4, respectively.

Nevertheless, advantages to enteral feeding include the relative ease of administration and lack of side effects. However, the choice of which nutrition product would provide optimal benefit and safety in a given patient population remains to be determined (83). One complication seen with the use of enteral nutrition includes colonization of the trachea. In contrast, parenteral nutrition can decrease intragastric acidity without providing a source of nutrients at high pH, which might predispose to aspiration pneumonia in critically ill intubated patients. However, parenteral nutrition is costly and requires additional preparation and nursing time.

SAFETY CONCERNS OF SR-UGIB PREVENTION THERAPY

Hematologic System

Blood dyscrasias have been rarely reported with all of the currently marketed H_2-receptor antagonists (88–91). Most published cases of dyscrasias are associated with cimetidine, probably due to the later introduction of the other H_2-receptor antagonists onto the market. Neutropenia and agranulocytosis are reported the most frequently. Interpretation of causality has been complicated in many cases by concomitant illness or the administration of other drugs known to cause blood dyscrasias. Clinical signs and symptoms of blood dyscrasias are often absent, and abnormal hematologic parameters are generally reversible after discontinuation of therapy.

The mechanism for development of the blood cytopenias is not well-defined. Insufficient detail has been provided in most of the published cases to determine which mechanism(s) might be responsible for the blood cytopenias, or whether impaired organ function was a factor. In a review of 85 reported cases of blood cytopoenias attributed to the H_2-receptor antagonists (92), four possible mechanisms related to H_2-receptor antagonist have been identified: (a) a direct inhibitory effect of the H_2-antagonist on pluripotent hemopoietic stem cells, (b) increased proliferation of suppressor T-lymphocytes resulting in granulopoietic failure, (c) autoimmune-mediated toxicity, and (d) inhibition of the metabolism of hematoxic drugs (e.g., cyclophosphamide) resulting in increased hematoxicity. In addition, the authors of this review noted that hepatic cirrhosis, impaired renal function, and bone marrow exhaustion were frequently encountered in the cases reviewed.

Cardiovascular System

Several controlled studies have examined the cardiovascular and hemodynamic effects of intravenously and orally administered cimetidine, ranitidine, and famotidine (88–97). Cardiovascular effects associated with H_2-receptor antagonists include hypotension or hypertension, bradycardia, arrhythmias, and cardiac arrest (93–95). The presence of coexisting disease states and/or concomitant drug therapy makes it difficult to assess causality in many cases (88–91). In patients with underlying cardiac disease, the rapid bolus intravenous administration of cimetidine or raniti-

dine has been associated with hypotension or hypertension, bradycardia, arrhythmias, and rarely cardiac arrest. This effect is usually avoided if the infusion is administered slowly (e.g., over 5 or more minutes) as called for in their respective prescribing information.

Although some differences in cardiovascular effects have been noted among the H_2-receptor antagonists (98), the clinical significance of these findings in selected patient populations is unknown. In addition, other noncomparative trials have reported equivocal findings, perhaps due to differences in study design (e.g., patient types, evaluative procedures, etc.) (99–107). One recent study has suggested that nizatidine may possess negative chronotropic effects (99).

Oral famotidine and quinidine produce similar significant reductions in stroke volume and cardiac output at 1.5 and 3 hours after administration compared with placebo in patients with congestive heart failure (New York Heart Association Class II) using impedance cardiography and Doppler ultrasound. However, no change in blood pressure or cardiac output was observed and the clinical relevance of these observations is unproven (101).

Indeed, other investigators, using other noninvasive methods such as duplex ultrasonography, have found no such effect of famotidine in normal volunteers (102–104) or in hemodynamically stable critically ill patients (105–106).

Central Nervous System

Although rare, central nervous system (CNS) disturbances (e.g., psychosis, mental confusion, agitation, hallucinations, delirium, lethargy, irritability, obtundation, depression, or hostility) have been associated with all H_2-receptor antagonists (108). These disturbances generally occur during the first 2 weeks of therapy and resolve within 3 days of drug withdrawal. The estimated incidence of CNS disturbances ranges from 1.6 to 80% in hospitalized patients, but it should be noted that these disturbances were noted in 15–30% of control patients (109). Cimetidine has been most frequently associated with these disturbances; however, there is no clear evidence of a higher rate of reactions with one H_2-receptor antagonist than another (108). Nevertheless, the incidence of mental status changes has been higher with cimetidine administration compared with ranitidine in some studies evaluating critically ill, hospitalized patients (61, 110, 111).

Proposed risk factors for CNS disturbances include ICU hospitalization, choice of H_2-receptor antagonist therapy, psychiatric disorders and psychotropic drugs, renal or hepatic disease, and advanced age (108). Although CNS disturbances appear to correlate with cimetidine concentrations in some patients, no range of concentrations is predictive for CNS toxicity. In only one (112) of three studies (112–114) was a relationship found between CNS adverse reactions and ranitidine concentration in patients with renal function impairment. However, study design, data collection, inappropriate statistical methods, and questionable pharmacokinetic analysis may have biased these results. This relationship has not been studied for famotidine or nizatidine. There does seem to be some limited data to support advanced age as a risk factor (108). Finally, establishing causality for CNS disturbances is difficult to assess because of the low occurrence of these disturbances, the difficulty involved in determining cause-and-effect relationships in hospitalized patients, and the hypothesis that they could be multifactorial in origin (108).

Hepatic Function

Clinical trials and postmarketing surveillance studies confirm that adverse hepatic events occur infrequently in patients receiving H_2-receptor antagonists (113, 115–119). There are no apparent clinically significant differences between the types of damage caused by either cimetidine or ranitidine (113, 115). Information concerning hepatic effects associated with administration of famotidine and nizatidine is much more limited because of significantly fewer patient exposures to these drugs (115, 116). During clinical trials with famotidine and nizatidine, hepatic injury was reported

but, as with cimetidine and ranitidine, the frequency appears to be quite low (88–91, 115, 116, 119).

The adverse hepatic events reported are generally reversible increases in serum levels of aminotransferase enzymes, mostly in patients receiving large doses of an H_2-receptor antagonist intravenously. These agents are associated with a "mixed" presentation of hepatic injuries (cytotoxic, cholestatic, or a combination of the two) (115, 116). While these case reports frequently have many of the same problems and difficulties inherent in assigning hepatic injury to a particular drug, the pathogenesis of liver injury associated with administration of cimetidine, ranitidine, and famotidine is compatible with an idiosyncratic hypersensitivity-type drug reaction (113, 115, 117).

Nosocomial Pneumonia

A significant controversy has surrounded the prophylactic use of antacids or H_2-receptor antagonists for ICU patients because of the perceived risk for nosocomial pneumonia, especially when compared with other therapies such as sucralfate (67). The incidence of nosocomial pneumonia is considerably higher among patients admitted to ICUs, and mechanical ventilation increases this risk severalfold. Other factors predisposing patients to nosocomial pneumonia include various host factors (advanced age, obesity, coma), the underlying disease state (chronic lung disease, immunosuppression); numerous drugs other than H_2-receptor antagonists; invasive procedures (intubation, tracheostomy, mechanical ventilation, nasogastric intubation); surgery of the head and neck, chest, and abdomen; and prolonged hospitalization (120, 121).

Although it is generally accepted that tracheal colonization is a prerequisite for the development of nosocomial pneumonia (122), the source of organisms colonizing the trachea remains controversial (67, 123–129). Some suggest gastric colonization as a source for tracheal colonization (67, 127) while others suggest gastric colonization as a source for translocation of enteric bacteria (127). Most recently, colonization due to gastroduodenal reflux has been suggested (129). The role of intragastric volume in the development of nosocomial pneumonia has not been well studied.

Attention has been primarily focused on the role of the gastrointestinal tract as a source for upper airway colonization with Gram-negative bacilli, based on the results of a study suggesting that the incidence of nosocomial pneumonia was less with sucralfate than in patients treated with pH-elevating drugs (67). However, the difference in rates of nosocomial pneumonia between patients receiving sucralfate or conventional therapy was not significant ($P = .110$). Nor did the study separate the results of patients treated with antacids from those treated with H_2-receptor antagonists alone. A subgroup analysis revealed that the highest rates of nosocomial pneumonia occurred in antacid-treated patients, suggesting the possible influence of intragastric volume or other factors besides increased pH (5.9% with H_2-receptor antagonists, 11.5% with sucralfate 23.1% with antacids, and 46.2% for the H_2/antacid group) (130, 131).

Recently, several prospective clinical trials have failed to show an increased incidence of nosocomial pneumonia associated with acid manipulation by H_2-receptor antagonists (14, 52, 132). One clinical trial compared a continuous infusion of cimetidine with placebo as prophylaxis for SR-UGIB, and failed to show an increase in the incidence of nosocomial pneumonia associated with cimetidine (52). In this trial, the nosocomial pneumonia rate was 0% (0/56) in the cimetidine group and 7% (4/61) in the placebo group. Although these data have been criticized because this ICU patient population had an overall low severity of illness, duration of H_2-antagonist treatment was short, and few were ventilated (77); a double-blind, placebo-controlled study evaluating ranitidine by continuous infusion (6.25 mg/hr) also provided similar results in the incidence of nosocomial pneumonia in a more severely ill population (14, 132). All 167 patients had a severe head injury with 72% of the patients having three or more risk factors

for SR-UGIB (mechanical ventilation, organ dysfunction, major surgery, other trauma) and 98% having two or more risk factors for nosocomial pneumonia (mechanical ventilation, endotracheal intubation, antibiotic therapy). Development of nosocomial pneumonia (as defined by Centers for Disease Control [CDC] criteria) was less frequent in the patients treated with ranitidine than in the placebo-treated patients—14% (12/84) vs. 19% (15/79), respectively.

In addition, at least two meta-analyses have evaluated this controversial issue, although each reached the opposite conclusion (127, 133). Both meta-analyses, like most studies, suffer methodologically in that nosocomial pneumonia was defined clinically. Quantitative cultures of protected specimen brush or bronchial alveolar lavage specimens would have provided a more accurate diagnosis of nosocomial pneumonia. Further studies using appropriate diagnostic methods of defining nosocomial pneumonia will be needed to settle this controversy.

ACUTE TREATMENT OF SR-UGIB FROM ULCERS

It is easier to prevent SR-UGIB than it is to treat bleeding once it starts. Based on the rationale that blood coagulation and platelet aggregation are extremely sensitive to even minor alterations in pH, and that the corrosive effects of pepsin are attenuated and clot dissolution minimized with increasing pH, antisecretory therapy has been evaluated in the treatment of acute gastrointestinal hemorrhage (AGIH) (134).

Available data indicate that AGIH is unlikely to be arrested by drug therapy, although some data from small trials suggest that antisecretory therapy might be useful in preventing rebleeding. Collins and Langman (135), after conducting a meta-analysis of studies evaluating treatment of AGIH with H_2-receptor antagonists, concluded that treatment with H_2-receptor antagonists might be beneficial in controlling AGIH, especially in gastric ulceration (135).

A small study and a case report series suggested positive results with intravenous omeprazole (136, 137) and with oral omeprazole in a case report of SR-UGIB in a 28-year-old man with a multifactorial coagulopathy (138). However, two recent double-blind, placebo-controlled studies (139, 140) support the argument that a pharmacologic approach to the treatment of bleeding ulcers is not likely to be of major benefit and does not influence the natural history of peptic ulcer hemorrhage (141, 142). A large multicenter trial of 1005 patients with bleeding from peptic ulcer with endoscopic signs of hemorrhage compared the effects of placebo versus a famotidine continuous infusion at a dosage regimen shown to maintain pH near 7 (10 mg bolus followed by 3.2 mg/hr) on ulcer bleeding (139). Mortality, rebleeding, and surgery rates were similar for both treatment groups; specifically, mortality rates were 6.2% for famotidine treatment and 5.0% for placebo, rebleeding rates were 23.9% and 25.5%, and surgery rates were 15.5% and 17.1%, respectively. A similar trial in patients with AGIH treated with intravenous omeprazole followed by oral omeprazole showed a similar lack of efficacy in mortality, rebleeding, and transfusion requirements (140). Thus, there appears to be little justification for the use of antisecretory therapy as a treatment of AGIH. Some suggest, however, that selected subgroups of patients (e.g., patients with varices, portal hypertensive gastropathy, and stress ulcer disease) may benefit from treatment, since AGIH may be a result of various pathologic conditions (142).

CONVERSION FROM INTRAVENOUS TO ORAL THERAPY

Although patients are in improved general condition after leaving ICUs, some SR-UGIB occurs after transfer to hospital wards where stress ulcer prophylaxis may be less than optimal (143). As noted in the clinical and pharmacodynamic studies reviewed above, cimetidine and ranitidine were usually administered intravenously in these studies. Most of the clinical studies were terminated when the patient was discharged from the ICU, the nasogastric tube was removed, or enteral feedings were tolerated. Sometimes, patients were switched from intravenous to oral H_2-receptor antagonist therapy once food or fluids could be taken by mouth (59). Although there are no adequately controlled studies evaluating both the bioavailability and efficacy of the H_2-receptor antagonists administered orally to critically ill patients for SR-UGIB, it seems reasonable to make this intravenous to oral conversion as soon as oral intake is reestablished.

COST BENEFITS

The critically ill patient is at high risk for developing complications, and, as a result, may incur a greater cost of hospitalization and treatment. Although the use of drugs for prophylaxis of SR-UGIB is associated with certain costs of preparation and administration, their use may be associated with clinical benefits such as a reduction in the volume of blood transfused or decreased duration of hospital and ICU stays. SR-UGIB prophylaxis with antacids and H_2-receptor antagonists has significantly reduced the need for surgical management, as documented by a series of studies enrolling 456 patients in which no patients required surgical intervention for SR-UGIB (13, 17, 18). Previous studies had shown that SR-UGIB could prolong ICU stays for up to 6–10 days and increase overall duration of hospitalization (32, 34).

Until recently, little information was available concerning the long-term clinical outcome following treatment with H_2-receptor antagonist in patients at risk for SR-UGIB. In a recent prospective pharmacoeconomic evaluation of continuous infusion ranitidine for prevention of SR-UGIB in head injury patients, continuous infusion therapy with ranitidine provided both clinical and economic benefits (144). In this blinded, retrospective data collection of health care resource use and 6-week outcome data for 167 patients completing a clinical trial for SR-UGIB, patients receiving placebo were 5.29 times more likely to develop a SR-UGIB than patients receiving ranitidine. Patients who did not bleed had a median 2-day shorter stay in the ICU. Bleeding patients receiving placebo required 500 ml more transfused blood. In addition, nonbleeding placebo patients required an additional 300 ml of blood than ranitidine patients. Finally, more placebo-treated patients remained in the hospital or required discharge to rehabilitation services compared with patients treated with ranitidine.

CONCLUSIONS

SRMD occurs frequently in critically ill patients admitted to the ICU, developing rapidly following severe physiologic stress. The natural history of SRMD depends upon the course of the underlying illness, generally improving as the illness improves or worsening as the illness worsens. Although occult bleeding is common, significant SR-UGIB occurs in less than 20% of patients, with a mortality ranging up to 12%.

Patients at high risk for SR-UBIG have been shown to benefit from prophylaxis. Increasing the gastric pH to 3.5–4.0 or more is a primary endpoint (i.e., effective in preventing occult or overt bleeding) when treating patients with antacids or H_2-receptor antagonists. Although antacids were once considered to be the "gold standard" for prophylaxis of SR-UGIB, H_2-receptor antagonists are currently the mainstay of therapy and are as effective as antacids when administered to maintain a pH of ≥ 4. Continuous infusion of an H_2-receptor antagonist maintains the pH >4 for a majority of the day in most critically ill patients and is effective in reducing SR-UGIB. Sucralfate also appears to be effective and safe, although administration to this population may be somewhat inconvenient. The role of enteral feedings and parenteral nutrition as prophylaxis has not been completely defined.

Although prophylaxis does not appear to decrease mortality in the critically ill population, prophylaxis may be of benefit in reducing costs of ICU care by reducing the need for treatment of SR-UGIB. The costs associated with transfusions, surgical intervention, and prolonged hospitalization may be substantial. In addition, AGIH is difficult to treat once it has developed. The decreased incidence in SR-UGIB over the last 10–20 years appears to be a result of the improvement in ventilatory support, nutritional support, and hemodyanamic monitoring as well as the routine administration of prophylactic agents.

REFERENCES

1. Wilcox CM, Spenney JG. Stress ulcer prophylaxis in medical patients: who, what, and how much? Am J Gastroenterol 1988;83:1199–1210.
2. Knight A, Bihari D, Tinker J. Stress ulceration in the critically ill patient. Br J Hosp Med 1985;33:216–219.
3. Durham RM, Shapiro MJ. Management of stress gastritis. J Intens Care Med 1991;6:257–267.
4. Cook DJ, Witt LG, Cook RJ, et al. Stress ulcer prophylaxis in the critically ill: a meta-analysis. Am J Med 1991;91:519–527.
5. Peura DA. Recognizing, setting therapeutic goals, and selecting therapy for the prevention and treatment of stress-related mucosal damage. Pharmacotherapy 1987;7(6 Pt 2):95S–103S.
6. Kitamura T, Ito K. Acute gastric changes in patients with acute stroke, Pt 1: with reference to gastroendoscopic findings. Stroke 1976;7:460–463.
7. Kaplan MM, May JR. The influence of pH control on the prevention and management of gastrointestinal bleeding. J Intens Care Med 1990; 5(suppl):S28–S33.
8. Shuman RB, Schuster DP, Zuckerman GR. Prophylactic therapy for stress ulcer bleeding: a reappraisal. Ann Intern Med 1987;106:562–567.
9. Skillman JJ, Bushnell LS, Goldman H. Respiratory failure, hypotension, sepsis and jaundice: a clinical syndrome associated with lethal hemorrhage from acute stress ulceration of the stomach. Am J Surg 1969;117:523–530.
10. Schuster DP, Rowley H, Feinstein S, et al. Prospective evaluation of the risk of upper gastrointestinal bleeding after admission to a medical intensive care unit. Am J Med 1984;76:623–630.
11. Peura DA, Johnson LF. Cimetidine for prevention and treatment of gastroduodenal mucosal lesions in patients in an intensive care unit. Ann Intern Med 1985;103:173–177.
12. Friedman CJ, Oblinger MJ, Suratt PM, et al. Prophylaxis of upper gastrointestinal hemorrhage in patients requiring mechanical ventilation. Crit Care Med 1982;10:316–319.
13. Groll A, Simon JB, Wigle RD, et al. Cimetidine prophylaxis for gastrointestinal bleeding in an intensive care unit. Gut 1986;27:135–140.
14. Livingston D, Smith JS, Larson GR, et al. Ranitidine 6.25 mg/hr continuous infusion for prevention of stress related upper gastrointestinal bleeding following severe head injury [Abstract]. Gastroenterology 1992;102:A19.

15. Brown RV, Klar J, Teres D, et al. Prospective study of clinical bleeding in intensive care unit patients. Crit Care Med 1988;16:1171–1176.

16. Bresalier RS, Grendell JH, Cello JP, et al. Sucralfate suspension versus titrated antacid for the prevention of acute stress-related gastrointestinal hemorrhage in critically ill patients. Am J Med 1987;83(suppl 3B):110–116.

17. Hastings PR, Skillman JJ, Bushnell LS, et al. Antacid titration in the prevention of acute gastrointestinal bleeding: a controlled randomized trial in 100 critically ill patients. N Engl J Med 1978;298:1041–1045.

18. Basso N, Bagarani M, Materia A, et al. Cimetidine and antacid prophylaxis of acute upper gastrointestinal bleeding in high risk patients: controlled, randomized trial. Am J Surg 1981;141:339–341.

19. Hillman K. Acute stress ulceration. Anaesth Intens Care 1985;13:230–240.

20. Bresalier RS. The clinical significance and pathophysiology of stress-related gastric mucosal hemorrhage. J Clin Gastroenterol 1991;13(suppl 2):S35–S43.

21. Kleiman RL, Adair CG, Ephgrave KS. Stress ulcers: current understanding of pathogenesis and prophylaxis. Drug Intell Clin Pharm 1988;22:452–460.

22. Haglund U. Stress ulcers. Scand J Gastroenterol 1990;25(suppl 175):27–33.

23. Konopad E, Noseworthy T. Stress ulceration: a serious complication in critically ill patients. Heart Lung 1988;17:339–348.

24. Gonzalez ER, Morkunas AR. Prophylaxis of stress ulcers: Antacid titration vs. histamine-2 receptor blockade. Drug Intell Clin Pharm 1985;19:807–811.

25. Gues WP, Lamers CBHW. Prevention of stress ulcer bleeding: a review. Scand J Gastroenterol 1990;25(suppl 178):32–41.

26. Ritchie WP. Acute gastric mucosal damage induced by bile salts, acid, and ischemia. Gastroenterology 1975;68:699–707.

27. Peura DA. Stress-related mucosal damage. Clin Ther 1986;8(suppl A):14–23.

28. Kauffman GL. Mucosal damage to the stomach: how, when, and why? Scand J Gastroenterol 1984;19(suppl 105):19–26.

29. Martin LF, Max MH, Polk, HC. Failure of pH control by antacids or cimetidine in the critically ill: a valid sign of sepsis. Surgery 1980;88:59–68.

30. Harris SK, Bone RC, Ruth WE. Gastrointestinal hemorrhage in patients in a respiratory intensive care unit. Chest 1977;72:301–304.

31. Macdougall BRD, Bailey RJ, Williams R. H_2-receptor antagonists and antacids in the prevention of acute gastrointestinal hemorrhage in fulminant hepatic failure: two controlled trials. Lancet 1977;1:617–619.

32. Zinner MJ, Zuidema GD, Smith PL, et al. The prevention of upper gastrointestinal tract bleeding in patients in an intensive care unit. Surg Gynecol Obstet 1981;153:214–220.

33. Priebe HJ, Skillman JJ. Methods of prophylaxis in stress ulcer disease. World J Surg 1981;5:223–233.

34. Gottlieb JE, Menashe PI, Cruz E. Gastrointestinal complications in critically ill patients: the intensivists' over-view. Am J Gastroenterol 1986;81:227–238.

35. Thompson JC, Walker JP. Indications for the use of parenteral H_2-receptor antagonists. Am J Med 1984;77(suppl 5B):111–115.

36. Kivilaakso E, Barzilai A, Schiessel R, et al. Experimental ulceration of rabbit antral mucosa. Gastroenterology 1981;80:77–83.

37. Kivilaakso E, Fromm D, Silen W. Effect of the acid secretory state on intramural pH of rabbit gastric mucosa. Gastroenterology 1978;75:641–648.

38. Kivilaakso E, Fromm D, Silen W. Relationship between ulceration and intramural pH of gastric mucosa during hemorrhagic shock. Surgery 1978;84:70–78.

39. Kivilaakso E, Silen W. Pathogenesis of experimental gastric-mucosal injury. N Engl J Med 1979;301:364–369.

40. Fiddian-Green RG, McGough E, Pittenger G, et al. Predictive value of intramural pH and other risk factors for massive bleeding from stress ulceration. Gastroenterology 1983;85:613–620.

41. Stothert JC, Simonowitz DA, Dellinger EP, et al. Randomized prospective evaluation of cimetidine and antacid control of gastric pH in the critically ill. Ann Surg 1979;192:169–174.

42. Moore JG. Stress ulceration in the intensive care unit: use of H_2-receptor antagonists. Aliment Pharmacol Ther 1991;5(suppl 1):111–119.

43. Sanders SW, Moore JG, Buchi KN, et al. Circadian variation in the pharmacodynamic effect of intravenous ranitidine. Annu Rev Chronopharmacol 1988;5:335–338.

44. Piper DW, Fenton BH. pH stability and activity curves of pepsin with special reference to their clinical importance. Gut 1965;6:506–508.

45. Green FW, Kaplan MM, Curtis LE, et al. Effect of acid and pepsin on blood coagulation and platelet aggregation. Gastroenterology 1978;74:38–43.

46. Priebe HJ, Skillman JJ, Bushnell LS, et al. Antacid versus cimetidine in preventing acute gastrointestinal bleeding. N Engl J Med 1980;302:426–430.

47. Pinilla JC, Oleniuk FH, Reed D, et al. Does antacid prophylaxis prevent upper gastrointestinal bleeding in critically ill patients? Crit Care Med 1985;13:646–650.

48. McAlhany J, Czaja A, Pruitt B. Antacid control of complications from acute gastroduodenal disease after burns. J Trauma 1986;16:645–648.

49. Luk G, Summer W, Messersmith J, et al. Cimetidine and antacid in the prophylaxis of acute gastrointestinal bleeding: a randomised double blind controlled study. Gastroenterology 1982;82:1121A.

50. Kingsley AH. Prophylaxis for acute stress ulcers: antacids or cimetidine. Am Surg 1985;51:545–547.

51. Reusser P, Gyr K, Scheidegger D, et al. Prospective endoscopic study of stress erosions and ulcers in critically ill neurosurgical patients: current incidence and effect of acid-reducing prophylaxis. Crit Care Med 1990;18:270–274.

52. Martin LF, Booth FV McL, Karlstadt RG, et al. Continuous intravenous cimetidine decreases stress-related upper gastrointestinal hemorrhage without promoting pneumonia. Crit Care Med 1993;21:19–30.

53. Ostro MJ, Russell JA, Soldin SJ, et al. Control of gastric pH with cimetidine: Boluses versus primed infusions. Gastroenterology 1985;89:532–537.

54. Van den Berg B, van Blankenstein M. The prevention of stress-induced upper gastrointestinal bleeding by ranitidine in critically ill patients. In: Misiewicz J, Wormsley K, eds. The clinical use of ranitidine. Oxford, 1982:263–267.

55. Hummer-Siegal M, Jacquier A, Gerard A, et al. The effect of ranitidine is compared to that of placebo in 22 patients who are treated in intensive care for severe cerebral injuries [in French]. Ann Med Nancy L'est 1986;25:101–103.

56. Albin M, Freidl SJ, Hillman K. Continuous intragastric pH measurement in the critically ill and treatment with parenteral ranitidine. Intens Care Med 1985;11:295–299.

57. Bohrer H, Krier C, Gunter J, et al. Ranitidine bolus or infusion prophylaxis for stress ulceration. Crit Care Med 1989;17:381–382.

58. Rigaud D, Chastre J, Accary JP, et al. Intragastric pH profile during acute respiratory failure in patients with chronic obstructive pulmonary disease: effect of ranitidine and enteral feeding. Chest 1986;90:58–63.

59. Barth HO, Damman L, Wiser P, et al. Ranitidine versus cimetidine in preventing acute gastroduodenal bleeding: a randomized trial in 193 critically ill patients—a multicentre study in Germany. Intensivmedizin 1984;21:15–18.

60. Siepler J, Prindiville T, Nistikawa R, et al. Prophylaxis of stress ulceration in the ICU: a comparison of cimetidine and ranitidine constant infusion [Abstract]. Gastroenterology 1987;92:1639.

61. Ketterl R, Holscher A, Wiser H. Control of intragastric pH in patients with sepsis or peritonitis by ranitidine versus cimetidine: a double blind study [in German]. Z Gastroenterol 1984;22:602–608.

62. Reid SR, Bayliff CD. The comparative efficacy of cimetidine and ranitidine in controlling gastric pH in critically ill patients. Can Anaesth Soc J 1986;33:287–293.

63. More DG, Raper RF, Munroe IA, et al. Randomized, prospective trial of cimetidine and ranitidine for control of intragastric pH in the critically ill. Surgery 1985;97:215–224.

64. Naumann C, Listyosuputro R, Casty E, et al. Stress ulcer prevention in critically ill patients: famotidine versus ranitidine [Abstract]. Dig Dis Sci 1986;31:A166.

65. Friedl W, Krier E, Dammann H, et al. Intragastric pH profiles in critically ill surgical patients [in German]. Z Gastroenterol 1985;23:603–607.

66. Tryba M, Zevounou F, Torok M, et al. Prevention of acute stress bleeding with sucralfate, antacids, or cimetidine: a controlled study with pirenzepine as a basic medication. Am J Med 1985;79(suppl 2C):55–61.

67. Driks MR, Craven DE, Celli BR, et al. Nosocomial pneumonia in intubated patients given sucralfate as compared with antacids or histamine type 2 blockers. N Engl J Med 1987;317:1376–1382.

68. Borrero E, Cierro J, Chang J. Antacid versus sucralfate in preventing acute gastrointestinal tract bleeding in abdominal aortic surgery. Arch Surg 1986;121:810–812.

69. Tryba M. Prevention of stress bleeding with ranitidine or pirenzepine and the risk of pneumonia. J Clin Anesth 1988;1:12–20.

69a. Cannon LA, Heiselman D, Gardner W, Jones J. Prophylaxis of upper gastrointestinal tract bleeding in mechanically ventilated patients: a randomized study comparing the efficacy of sucralfate, cimetidine, antacids. Arch Intern Med 1987;147:2101–2106.

70. Tryba M. Prophylaxis of stress ulcer bleeding. A meta analysis. J Clin Gastroenterol 1991;13(suppl 2):S44–S55.

71. Lacroix J, Infante-Rivard C, Jenicek M, et al. Prophylaxis of upper gastrointestinal bleeding in intensive care units: A meta-analysis. Crit Care Med 1989;17:862–869.

72. Karlstadt R, Palmer R, McCafferty J, et al. Meta-analysis of cimetidine (CIM)-placebo (PL) controlled trials in the intensive care unit (ICU) [Abstract]. Gastroenterology 1992;102(4 Part 2):1351.

73. Ballesteros MA, Hogan DL, Koss MA, Isenberg JI. Bolus or intravenous infusion of ranitidine: effects on gastric pH and acid secretion. Ann Intern Med 1990;112:334–339.

74. Sanders SW, Buchi KN, Moore JG, et al. Pharmacodynamics of intravenous ranitidine after bolus and continuous infusion in patients with healed duodenal ulcers. Clin Pharmacol Ther 1989;46:545–551.

75. Larson G, Brown J, Wilson T, et al. Comparison of ranitidine versus placebo on 24 hour gastric pH and upper gastrointestinal (UGI) bleeding in head injury patients [Abstract]. Am J Gastroenterol 1989;84:1165.

76. Vorder Bruegge WF, Peura DA. Stress-related mucosal damage: review of drug therapy. J Clin Gastroenterol 1990;12(suppl 2):S35–S40.

77. Schuster DP. Stress ulcer prophylaxis: in whom? With what? Crit Care Med 1993;21:4–6.

78. Feldman M, Burton ME. Histamine$_2$-receptor antagonists. Standard therapy for acid-peptic diseases. N Engl J Med 1990;323:1672–1680.

79. McCarthy DM. Sucralfate. N Engl J Med 1991;325:1017–1025.

80. Zinner MJ, Rypins E, Martin LF, et al. Misoprostol vs. antacid in the prevention of stress bleeding and lesions in ICU patients: a multicenter prospective double-blind trial. Gastroenterology 1987;92(5 Pt 2):1711.

81. Earnest DL. Controlling gastric pH: the impact of newer agents on the critically ill patient. Ann Pharmacother 1990;24(suppl):S31–S34.

82. Donnelly D, May JR. Enteral nutrition prophylaxis against stress ulcers. Drug Intell Clin Pharm 1987;21:791–792.

83. Armstrong D, Castiglione F, Emde C, et al. The effect of continuous enteral nutrition on gastric acidity in humans. Gastroenterology 1992;102: 1506–1515.

84. Solem LD, Strate RG, Fischer RP. Antacid therapy and nutritional supplementation in the prevention of Curling's ulcer. Surg Gynecol Obstet 1979;148:367–370.

85. Choctaw WT, Fujita C, Zawacki BE. Prevention of upper gastrointestinal bleeding in burn patients: a role for "elemental" diet. Arch Surg 1980; 115:1073–1076.

86. Elmore MF, Knoll DM, Wagner DR. The effect of enteral nutrition gastric acidity with and without infusion of cimetidine [Abstract]. Am J Gastroenterol 1992;87:1267.

87. Valentine RJ, Turner WW, Borman KR, et al. Does nasoenteral feeding afford adequate gastroduodenal stress prophylaxis? Crit Care Med 1986;14:599–601.

88. Product Information for Tagamet. Smith Kline & French. Physicians' desk reference. ed. 47. 1993.

89. Product Information for Pepcid. Merck Sharp & Dohme. Physicians' desk reference, ed. 47. 1993.

90. Product Information for Axid. Eli Lilly. Physicians' desk reference. ed. 47. 1993.

91. Product Information for Zantac. Glaxo. Physicians' desk reference. ed. 47. 1993.

92. Aymard J-P, Aymard B, Netter P. et al. Haematological adverse effects of histamine H$_2$-receptor antagonists. Med Toxicol 1988;3:430–448.

93. Hinrichsen H, Halabi A, Kirch W. Hemodynamic effects of H$_2$-receptor antagonists. Eur J Clin Invest 1992;22:9–18.

94. Iberti TJ. The hemodynamic effects of H$_2$ antagonists in intensive care unit patients. J Intens Care Med 1990;5(suppl):S40–S43.

95. Tanner LA, Arrowsmith JB. Bradycardia and H$_2$-antagonists. Ann Intern Med 1988;109:434–435.

96. Goelzer SL, Farin-Rush C, Coursin DB. Ranitidine produces minimal hemodynamic depression in stable intensive care unit patients: a double-blind, prospective study. Crit Care Med 1988;16:8–10.

97. Coursin DB, Farin-Rusk C, Springman SR, et al. The hemodynamic effects of intravenous cimetidine versus ranitidine in intensive care unit patients: a double-blind, prospective, cross-over study. Anesthesiology 1988;69:975–978.

98. Hinrichsen H, Halabi A, Kirch W. Hemodynamic effects of different H$_2$-receptor antagonists. Clin Pharmacol Ther 1990;48:302–308.

99. Kirch W, Halabi A. Nizatidine significantly decreases heart rate [Abstract]. Clin Pharmacol Ther 1990;47:202.

100. Kirch W, Halabi A, Linde M, et al. Negative effects of famotidine on cardiac performance assessed by non-invasive hemodynamic measurements. Gastroenterology 1989;96:1387–1392.

101. Kirch W, Halabi A, Hinrichsen H. Hemodynamic effects of quinidine and famotidine in patients with congestive heart failure. Clin Pharmacol Ther 1992;51:325–333.

102. Salmon P, Fitzgerald D, Kenny M. No effect of famotidine on cardiac performance by noninvasive hemodynamic measurements. Clin Pharmacol Ther 1991;49:589–595.

103. Borow KM, Ehler D, Berlin R, et al. Influence of histamine receptors on basal left ventricular contractile tone in humans: assessment using the H$_2$ receptor antagonist famotidine and the beta-adrenoceptor antagonist esmolol as pharmacologic probes. J Am Coll Cardiol 1992;19:1229–1236.

104. Berlin RG. Famotidine does not have a negative inotropic effect [Letter]. Lancet 1987;1:1468.

105. Omote K, Namiki S, Sumita T, et al. Comparative studies on hemodynamic effects of intravenous cimetidine, ranitidine and famotidine in intensive care unit patients. Jpn J Anesthesiol 1987;36:940–947.

106. Heiselman DE, Chapman J, Malik M, et al. Hemodynamic status during famotidine infusion. Drug Intell Clin Pharm 1990;24:1163–1165.

107. Omote K, Namiki A, Nishikawa T, et al. Haemodynamic effects of famotidine and cimetidine in critically ill patients. Acta Anaesthesiol Scand 1990;34:576–578.

108. Cantu T, Korek J. Central nervous system reactions to histamine-2 receptor blockers. Ann Intern Med 1991;114:1027–1034.

109. Cerra FB, Schentag JJ, McMillen M, et al. Mental status, the intensive care unit and cimetidine. Ann Surg 1982;196:565–570.

110. Barth HO, Damman L, Wiser P, et al. Ranitidine and cimetidine in stress ulcer prophylaxis: a comparative multicenter study [in German]. Langenbecks Arch Chir 1984;362:131–138.

111. Das A, Freston J, Jacobs J, et al. An evaluation of safety in 37,252 patients treated with cimetidine or ranitidine. Intern Med 1990;11:127–149.

112. Slugg PH, Haug MT, Pippenger CE. Ranitidine pharmacokinetics and adverse central nervous system reactions. Arch Intern Med 1992;152:2325–2329.

113. Vial T, Goubier C, Bergeret A, et al. Side effects of ranitidine. Drug Safety 1991;6:94–117.

114. Juergens JP, Smith IS. Central nervous system symptoms and H_2-receptor antagonist. Post Marketing Surveillance 1991;5:135–144.

115. Lewis JH. Hepatic effects of drugs used in the treatment of peptic ulcer disease. Am J Gastroenterol 1987;82:987–1003.

116. Lewis JH, Zimmerman HJ. Drug-induced liver disease. Med Clin North Am 1989;73:775–792.

117. Sabesin SM. Clinical experience with hepatic effects of H_2-blockers. Adv Ther 1987;4:309–316.

118. Dobbs JH, Muir JG, Smith RN. H_2-antagonists and hepatitis [Letter]. Ann Intern Med 1986;105:803.

119. Saigenji K, Fukutomi H, Nakazawa S. Famotidine: postmarketing clinical experience. Scand J Gastroenterol 1987;229(suppl 134):34–40.

120. Pennington JE. Nosocomial respiratory infection. In: Mandell GL, Douglas RG, Bennett JE, eds. Principles and practice of infectious diseases, ed. 3. New York: Churchill Livingstone, 1990:2199–2205.

121. Niederman MS, Craven DE, Fein AM, et al. Pneumonia in the critically ill hospitalized patient. Chest 1990;97:170–181.

122. Bamberger DM. Diagnosis of nosocomial pneumonia. Semin Respir Infect 1988;3:140–147.

123. Du Moulin GC, Patterson DG, Hedley-Whyte J, et al. Aspiration of gastric bacteria in antacid-treated patients: a frequent cause of postoperative colonization of the airway. Lancet 1982;1:242–245.

124. Kahn RJ, Serruys-Schouten SE, Brimioulle S, et al. Influence of antacid treatment on the tracheal flora in mechanically ventilated patients [Abstract]. Crit Care Med 1982;10:229.

125. Garvey BM, McCambley JA, Tuxen DV. Effects of gastric alkalization on bacterial colonization in critically ill patients. Crit Care Med 1989;17:211–216.

126. Reusser P, Zimmerli W, Scheidegger D, et al. Role of gastric colonization in nosocomial infections and endotoxemia: a prospective study in neurosurgical patients on mechanical ventilation. J Infect Dis 1989;160:414–421.

127. Tryba M. Sucralfate versus antacids or H_2-antagonists for stress ulcer prophylaxis: a meta-analysis on efficacy and pneumonia rate. Crit Care Med 1991;19:942–949.

128. Fiddian-Green RG, Baker S. Nosocomial pneumonia in the critically ill: Product of aspiration or translocation. Crit Care Med 1991;19:763–769.

129. Inglis TJJ, Sherratt MJ, Sproat LJ, et al. Gastroduodenal dysfunction and bacterial colonisation of the ventilated lung. Lancet 1993;1:911–913.

130. Palmer RH. Nosocomial pneumonia in intubated patients [Letter]. N Engl J Med 1988;318:1464–1465.

131. Gachot B, Jebrak G, Legras A, et al. Nosocomial pneumonia in intubated patients [Letter]. N Engl J Med 1988;318:1465.

132. Metz C, Smith S, Larson G, et al. Acute incidence of pneumonia in a placebo-controlled study of ranitidine prophylaxis of stress related upper gastrointestinal bleeding (SR-UGIB) in patients with severe head injury [Abstract]. Am J Gastroenterol 1992;87:1342.

133. Cook DJ, Laine LA, Guyatt GH, et al. Nosocomial pneumonia and the role of gastric pH. Chest 1991;100:7–13.

134. Laine L. Rolling review: upper gastrointestinal bleeding. Aliment Pharmacol Ther 1993;7:207–232.

135. Collins R, Langman M. Treatment with histamine H_2 antagonists in acute upper gastrointestinal hemorrhage. N Engl J Med 1985;313:660–666.

136. Brunner G, Chang J. Intravenous therapy with high doses of ranitidine and omeprazole in critically ill patients with bleeding peptic ulcerations of the upper intestinal tract: an open randomized controlled trial. Digestion 1990;45:217–219.

137. Gabbrielli M, Pennati P, Trallori G, et al. Use of intravenous omeprazole in emergency cases of gastroduodenal hemorrhage [Letter]. Am J Gastroenterol 1992;87:1229.

138. Barie PS, Hariri RJ. Therapeutic use of omeprazole for refractory stress-induced gastric mucosal hemorrhage. Crit Care Med 1992;20:899–901.

139. Walt RP, Cottrell J, Mann SG, et al. Continuous intravenous famotidine for haemorrhage from peptic ulcer. Lancet 1992;340:1058–1062.

140. Daneshmend TK, Hawkey CJ, Langman MJS, et al. Omeprazole versus placebo for acute upper gastrointestinal bleeding: randomised double blind controlled trial. Br Med J 1992;304:143–147.

141. Peterson WL. Pharmacotherapy of bleeding peptic ulcer: is it time to give up the search? Gastroenterology 1989;97:796–797.

142. Brown C, Rees WDW. Drug treatment for acute upper gastrointestinal bleeding: works in selected subgroups of patients. Br Med J 1992;304:135–136.

143. Martin LF, Larson GM, Fry DE. Bleeding from stress gastritis: has prophylactic pH control made a difference? Am Surg 1985;51:189–193.

144. Kirchendoerfer LJ, Metz CA. Pharmacoeconomic evaluation of continuous infusion ranitidine for the prevention of upper gastrointestinal hemorrhage in head injury patients. In: Abstracts of the American Society of Hospital Phamacists 50th Annual Meeting, Denver, CO, June 7, 1993.

5

Pharmacologic Approach to the Control of Acute Gastrointestinal Bleeding

GARY R. ZUCKERMAN and PAUL E. BUSE

Gastrointestinal bleeding can represent a significant complication of peptic ulcer disease, portal hypertension, and various uncommon vascular lesions of the intestinal tract. The physician is often confronted with massive or submassive bleeding that requires volume expansion with fluids and/or blood products. The first priority in such patients is resuscitation and stabilization of vital signs to be followed by diagnostic evaluation for the bleeding source. It is obvious that morbidity and mortality may be affected if bleeding can be controlled, with the goal of stopping ongoing bleeding and preventing rebleeding. Although the majority of patients will spontaneously stop bleeding, the remaining patients will have ongoing bleeding or rebleeding requiring intervention such as surgery or endoscopic therapy, and a small number of patients will die from gastrointestinal bleeding. In this chapter, we review the pharmacologic approach to the control of acute gastrointestinal bleeding of various etiologies such as portal hypertension with bleeding esophageal varices and acid-peptic disease complicated by bleeding ulcers.

PHARMACOLOGIC MANAGEMENT OF VARICEAL HEMORRHAGE

Portal Hypertension

Gastrointestinal hemorrhage is a common and frequently lethal complication of portal hypertension. Even if the patient survives the index bleed, early rebleeding is the norm and long-term survival the exception. The pathogenesis of portal hypertension secondary to cirrhosis is complex and poorly understood. One simplistic theory is that there is a progressive increase in resistance to portal blood flow within the liver, due to the intrinsic liver disease (backwards hypothesis). This resistance coupled with increased portal blood flow due to the hyperdynamic circulation that characterizes advanced liver disease (forward hypothesis) results in portal hypertension (1). The ability to impact on the natural history of a patient with portal hypertension is difficult because of the typically irreversible nature of the impedance to portal blood flow. Additionally, in Western cultures, the preponderance of alcoholic cirrhosis as the primary cause of portal hypertension further complicates management because of the frequently poor functional status and low hepatocellular reserve seen in this population.

The development of varices is a compensatory mechanism through which the body attempts to decompress the hypertensive portal system through venous collaterals, thus creating the portocollateral circulation. Factors that predispose these varices to rupture and hemorrhage (2) are not well understood, but several purported risk factors are listed in Table 5.1. Increasing amounts of data suggest that a prerequisite for variceal formation and subsequent hemorrhage is the development of portal pressures in excess of 12 mm Hg (2).

Table 5.1
Factors Potentially Associated with an Increased Risk of Variceal Hemorrhage

High portal pressures ($\geq$11–12 mm Hg)
Large varices
Endoscopic stigmata (e.g., red whale marking)
Increased plasma volume
Poor overall clinical status
Ascites
Erosions secondary to gastroesophageal reflux

For these reasons, pharmacologic manipulation of the portal hypertensive state has specifically entailed attempts to decrease portal pressures and portocollateral blood flow. The various pathophysiologic parameters that can be manipulated in hopes of achieving this aim and the mechanism by which a few drugs are purported to accomplish this are listed in Table 5.2.

There is a large and growing body of literature evaluating the efficacy of a number of different classes of vasoactive medications in management of variceal bleeding. These studies can be grouped into three different categories according to the specific aims of the therapy, that is, primary and secondary prophylaxis as well as the management of the acute variceal hemorrhage. Primary prevention implies the ability to prevent bleeding in patients with known varices and no antecedent history of bleeding. Secondary prevention directs efforts towards preventing recurrent bleeding in patients who have bled before and subsequently stopped. The tremendous interest and effort that has been directed to this specific area of gastroenterology is primarily due to the very high mortality associated with variceal bleeding and the hope that an agent that could effectively control or prevent bleeding could directly improve mortality.

β-BLOCKERS

β-Blockers have received increasing attention over the last decade for their ability to improve hemodynamics and control bleeding in the portal hypertensive state. However, since the first controlled study by Lebrec et al. was published in 1981 (3), a number of conflicting studies have become available regarding propranolol's efficacy in both the primary and secondary prevention of variceal bleeding. An equally confusing body of literature exists that attempts to explain this purported effect on a pathophysiologic basis. The mechanism by which propranolol exerts its beneficial effect was initially thought to be related to a decrease in hepatic venous pressure gradient, the difference between free hepatic vein pressure and wedged hepatic vein pressure (4). This hypothesis has been refuted by some investigators on the basis that patients treated with placebo appear to have spontaneous improvement in their hyperdynamic circulation and portal hemodynamics that is not statistically different from that induced by propranolol (5).

A recent study by Groszmann et al. (6) compared changes in hepatic vein pressure gradients in 102 patients admitted with an acute variceal hemorrhage who were randomized in a blinded fashion to receive either propranolol or placebo. Hepatic vein pressure gradients were measured prior to randomization, and subsequently at 3, 12, and 24 months. There was a significant decrease in portal pressures in comparison to baseline at 3 months in the propranolol-treated group that was not seen in the control group. At 12 and 24 months, both groups experienced further reductions in portal pressures that were significant in comparison to baseline but not different between placebo and propranolol. One hypothesis provided to help explain this spontaneous, albeit delayed, improvement in hepatic vein pressure gradient was through the continual attrition of patients due to bleeding and death that tended to selectively remove patients with the highest portal pressures. Other studies using techniques to directly measure portal pressures have shown no change in portal pressures in up to a third of patients treated with propranolol (7). At best, the response of portal pressures to propranolol is variable and does not appear to correlate with risk of rebleeding except in cases where pressures are reduced to <12 mm Hg (6).

Table 5.2
Pathophysiologic Goals of Pharmacologic Manipulation of the Portal Hypertensive State

Decrease portal pressure
  A. Decrease portal blood flow
    1. Improve hyperdynamic circulation
      a. Decrease cardiac output (β-blockers)
    2. Increase splanchnic arteriole resistance
      a. Selectively (β-blockers, somatostatin)
      b. Nonselectively (vasopressins)
  B. Decrease portal venous resistance
    1. Direct portal venodilation (nitrates)
    2. Decrease perisinusoidal resistance
Decrease variceal pressure
  A. Decrease portal pressure
  B. Selectively decrease portocollateral blood flow (propranolol, somatostatin, metoclopramide)

Note: Parentheses indicate specific agent and its purported pathophysiologic effect.

Table 5.3
Controlled Trials of β-Blockers in the Primary Prevention of Variceal Hemorrhage

Study Agent	No. of Patients	Large Varices/ ETOH/Childs Class C (%)	Duration of Follow-up	Incidence (%) (control:β-blocker) Bleeding	Death
Propranolol (11)	230	23/90/46	14	27:17	36:22
Nadolol (12)	79	100/52/24	24	30:6*	22:6
Nadolol (13)	106	100/73/0	12	20:17	22:20
Propranolol (14)	174	14/40/17	28	35:21	31:43
Propranolol (15)	84	12/79/27	24	39:6*	46:34
Propranolol (16)	102	46/78/8	16	22:4*	22:16
Propranolol (17)	140	13/83/NA	15	18:18	22:15

Abbreviations: ETOH, alcohol-induced liver disease; NA, data not available.
*$P < .05$.

It appears that any effect on portal pressures may be directly related to a combination of the β- 1-mediated effects of decreased heart rate and subsequent decreased cardiac output as well as β- 2-mediated effects of increased splanchnic arteriolar tone (4). An alternative pathophysiologic explanation of propranolol's beneficial effect on the portal hypertensive state is related to its direct effects on the portocollateral circulation. Propranolol has been documented to decrease azygous blood flow (an indirect measurement of variceal blood flow) to a significantly higher degree than hepatic vein pressure gradients, hepatic blood flow, or cardiac output (8, 9). Recently, a study directly quantitating left gastric and portal vein blood flow using doppler techniques revealed that cirrhotic patients receiving propranolol had a significantly greater reduction in blood flow in the collateral vein, suggesting a selective effect of β-blockade on the portocollateral circulation (10).

Primary Prevention of Variceal Hemorrhage

Clinical trials of β-blockers to prevent the first episode of variceal hemorrhage have produced conflicting results (Table 5.3). Of the seven randomized trials (11–17), the three smallest have shown statistically significant reductions in the incidence of bleeding in patients treated with β-blockers [nadolol in one (12) and propranolol in the other two (15, 16)], but none has shown a significant impact on mortality. The trial by Pascal and Cales (11) showed a significant decrease in bleeding and mortality only when analyzing the specific subset of patients who were observed for 2 years during therapy. A few investigators have suggested that there is a risk of precipitating variceal hemorrhage in patients who stop therapy acutely (11).

The study by Lebrec et al. (13) reinforces the issue of compliance in this patient population by noting a statistically significant decrease in frequency of bleeding only in those patients who appeared to be compliant with the medication. A possible explanation for the disparity of results between studies relates to the hetcrogeneity of populations studied not only on a center-to-center basis but even within individual studies. Conn et al. (16) noted no benefit to therapy in the nonalcoholic, small varix subpopulation, and a suggested benefit in those with more advanced stages of liver disease, although they had very few Childs class C patients. Pascal and Cales (11) noted a more profound benefit in those patients with more advanced liver disease (Pugh scores 9–13) but excluded those with Pugh scores >14. The Italian multicenter study realized benefit in terms of a significant reduction in bleeding only in the ascites free population (14). Five recent meta-analyses have attempted to sort out these conflicting results and all have shown a statistically significant reduction in bleeding with no significant heterogeneity (18–21). However, none of the studies derived statistically significant effects on overall mortality.

From these data it is difficult to draw firm conclusions or make strong recommendations regarding the use of β-blockers. Toxicity of this therapy is relatively low, but side effects that necessitated discontinuation of the drug occurred in 3–30% of patients (4). Serious side effects, such as precipitation of liver failure, were uncommon although patients with decompensated hepatic function were almost universally excluded. Interestingly, the two studies using nadolol had the lowest incidence of side effects, implying a benefit to a non-hepatically metabolized nonselective β-blocker (12, 13). At present, it appears reasonable to consider the use of β-blockers in patients with portal hypertension and varices

that have never bled, particularly in the subgroup that is compliant and have large varices. Nevertheless, the fact that there are no data to suggest an effect on overall mortality should temper our enthusiasm for the use of these agents while awaiting further well-designed controlled trials.

Secondary Prevention of Variceal Hemorrhage

The initial and most promising study evaluating the efficacy of β-blockers in the secondary prevention of variceal hemorrhage was published by Lebrec et al. (3, 22) in preliminary form in 1981 and in final form in 1984 (Table 5.4). Follow-up at 2 years revealed an incidence of rebleeding in the propranolol-treated patients that was one-third of that of the control population. Subsequent to these publications, two studies noted no statistical benefit to treatment with propranolol (23, 24). Differences in study design were thought to explain this discrepancy, because the study by Burroughs et al. (23) evaluated patients with a more diverse array of chronic liver disease than those in the study of Lebrec et al. (22) in which 88% of patients had alcohol-induced cirrhosis. The study by Villeneuve et al. (24) randomized patients with advanced liver disease only hours after their acute hemorrhage had been controlled which explains their very high incidence of rebleeding and the high overall mortality regardless of the form of therapy.

Five of the subsequent six randomized controlled trials published in manuscript form in the English language revealed a statistically significant benefit to therapy with β-blockers in terms of a reduction in the frequency of rebleeding (25–30). The study by Colombo et al. (26) compared patient's receiving both propranolol and atenolol to a control group and found benefit only with propranolol. A possible explanation of the lack of significant benefit from atenolol may be related to its β-1 selectivity. Nadolol, a nonselective β-blocker was found to be effective in one small study (25). Prior to the work by Garden et al. (29), the data indicated that only those patients

Table 5.4
Controlled Trials of β-Blockers in the Secondary Prevention of Variceal Hemorrhage

Study Agent	No. of Patients	Prev/ETOH/ Childs Class C (%)	Time (days) F/U (mo)	Incidence (%) (control:β-blocker)	
				Rebleeding	Death
Propranolol (22)	74	62/88/0	21/24	68:21*	43:10*
Propranolol (23)	48	NA/100/38	8/19	50:46	9:15
Propranolol (24)	79	NA/57/37	0.7/22	81:76	38:45
Nadolol (25)	24	NA/75/0	15/19	71:25*	25:8
Propranolol, atenolol (26)	94	67/82/0	32/11	47:25* 47:31	23:12 23:10
Propranolol (27)†	50	60/0/NA	2/NA	80:20*	20:4
Propranolol (28)	36	54/44/0	21/12	56:28*	NA
Propranolol (29)	81	37/70/47	6/24	77:47*	44:37
Propranolol (30)	53	NA/100/38	8/19	61:47	34:20

Abbreviations: Prev, percentage of patients with a history of previous variceal bleeding; ETOH, percentage of patients with alcohol-induced cirrhosis; Time, period from initial bleed to randomization; F/U, duration of follow-up; NA, data not available.
*$P \leq .05$.
†All patients with presinusoidal portal hypertension.

with preserved hepatocellular function (Childs class A and B) benefitted from therapy with β-blockers. This recent study is unique from a number of standpoints, most notably its double-blinded design and the fact that all patients underwent one course of sclerotherapy to control their initial hemorrhage (29). Indeed, the incidence of rebleeding in Childs class C patients (excluding those with severe encephalopathy and evidence of hepatorenal renal syndrome) who were treated with propranolol was only 39% in comparison to 90% rebleeding in the placebo group ($P = .005$).

Secondary prevention of variceal hemorrhage with β-blockers does not appear to have a significant effect on overall survival, with only the initial study by Lebrec et al. (3) suggesting otherwise. Meta-analyses have all indicated a significant reduction in rebleeding, although only one meta-analysis found benefit in mortality (18–21, 31). That analysis has been criticized for the loose criteria used to select appropriate studies (18, 31).

Role of Sclerotherapy

Sclerotherapy to the point of variceal obliteration is the most widely practiced therapy to prevent recurrent variceal hemorrhage. Sclerotherapy's ability to effectively control the acute bleed and to impact on the risk of recurrent hemorrhage is well documented although its effect on overall mortality is uncertain (32, 33). Controlled trials comparing propranolol to repeated injection sclerotherapy in the secondary prevention of variceal hemorrhages are few with relatively small sample sizes. Of the four studies published in manuscript form in the English language (30, 34–36), only the study by Westaby et al. (36) found a significant difference in rebleeding between the two groups, and this was in favor of sclerotherapy (Table 5.5). Likewise, a meta-analysis revealed no difference in benefit to either of the therapeutic options (18). Variations in methodology between studies, particularly the heterogeneous clinical populations, differences in adjunctive medical management, and the typically early time at which patients were randomized in relation to the acute hemorrhage, make direct comparison of data between studies difficult. The study by Rossi et al. (30) comparing propranolol, sclerotherapy, and a control group revealed no significant advantage to either form of therapy. The number of patients studied was small but nonetheless this study raises the issue of the true therapeutic benefit of either form of therapy in long-term secondary prevention of variceal hemorrhage.

Table 5.5
Controlled Trials Comparing Endoscopic Sclerotherapy to Propranolol in the Secondary Prevention of Variceal Hemorrhage

Reference	No. of Patients	Prev/ETOH/ Childs Class C (%)	Time (days) F/U (mo)	Incidence (%) (propranolol:sclero)	
				Rebleeding	Death
34	65	NA/70/0	19/30	75:33*	46:31
35	70	30/83/30	2/11	29:28	15:8
36	108	0/55/0	1/12–64	54:45	42:38
30	53	NA/100/38	8/19	41:50	26:23

Abbreviations: Prev, percentage of patients with history of previous variceal hemorrhage; ETOH, percentage of patients with alcohol-induced cirrhosis; Time, period from initial bleed to randomization; F/U, duration of follow-up; SCLERO, endoscopic sclerotherapy; NA, data not available.
*$P < .02$.

An additional three studies have evaluated propranolol's efficacy as an adjunctive therapy to endoscopic sclerotherapy for the secondary prevention of variceal hemorrhage (37–39). O'Connor et al. (37) randomized 97 patients with predominantly advanced alcoholic cirrhosis who presented with acute variceal hemorrhage to either propranolol, propranolol with endoscopic sclerotherapy, or propranolol with transhepatic sclerotherapy. At 2 years they noted a nonstatistically significant decrease in major rebleeding in the group receiving propranolol plus endoscopic sclerotherapy (45%) as compared to either the group receiving propranolol alone (65%) or those receiving propranolol plus transhepatic sclerotherapy (60%). Interestingly, overall mortality was significantly lower in those undergoing endoscopic sclerotherapy in combination with propranolol (55%) as compared with those receiving propranolol alone (81%) or in combination with transhepatic sclerotherapy (77%).

Jensen and Karup (38) undertook a double-blinded study comparing repeated endoscopic sclerotherapy with placebo or a short (6 month) course of propranolol. They noted a decrease in rebleeding during the course of sclerotherapy in the propranolol-treated group (22% vs. 80%; $P < .05$). After variceal obliteration, which took an average of 5 months, the incidence of variceal recurrence, typically manifesting as bleeding, was higher in the placebo group (70% vs. 14%; $P < .01$).

Mortality was unchanged, however. These findings are difficult to reconcile in view of the marked reduction in recurrent hemorrhage, both early and late, without any effect on overall mortality. The mechanism by which propranolol could exert such a sustained effect on variceal recurrence after a relatively short course of therapy is unclear. The final study by Westaby et al. (39) was of a similar nature. Patients were randomized to receive repeated endoscopic sclerotherapy alone or repeated sclerotherapy plus propranolol. The incidence of bleeding was not different between the two groups, but the period of observation was short, limited only to the course of sclerotherapy.

In summary, the data regarding the use of β-blockers in the secondary prevention of variceal hemorrhage are controversial and the variability in study designs makes comparisons between trials difficult. Six of the nine individual randomized controlled trials and all meta-analyses found statistically significant reductions in the incidence of recurrent hemorrhage in those patients treated with propranolol. Additionally, the currently accepted technique for preventing secondary hemorrhage (sclerotherapy) does not appear to be significantly better than propranolol. A combined approach of endoscopic eradication coupled with β-blockade may hold additional promise. Evidence that β-blockade improves survival in this population is scant, however.

VASOPRESSIN

Vasopressin is a hormone produced by the posterior pituitary, the main physiologic function of which is regulation of the renal collecting tubules' permeability to water. When plasma concentrations increase, either in response to shock or due to exogenous, parenteral administration, this peptide then functions as a potent vasoconstrictor (40). In animal studies, vasopressin has a more pronounced vasoconstricting effect on the mesenteric vascular supply and other "less essential" vascular distributions such as the skin and musculoskeletal system. Through increased portal vascular resistance, portal venous blood flow decreases on the order of 35–72%. This decrease in portal blood flow does not necessarily result in a proportional decrease in portal pressures (11–50%), possibly because of compensatory increases in hepatic artery blood flow as well as a direct vasoconstrictive effect of vasopressin on the portal venous system.

Studies in humans, though less extensive, have suggested similar physiologic effects with decrements in portal blood flow in excess of changes in portal pressures. The vascular response to vasopressin appears to be similar regardless of the route of administration (intermittent intravenous bolus vs. continuous intravenous infusion vs. selective intraarterial administration) (41). Some investigators hypothesized that these beneficial changes in portal hemodynamics in response to vasopressin were unique to nonbleeding portal hypertensive subjects (42). In a recent study by Ready and colleagues (43), changes in portal hemodynamics were measured in patients with active acute variceal hemorrhage who were treated with vasopressin and compared with a control group of patients in whom the acute bleed stopped spontaneously. There was a significant and sustained decrease in wedged hepatic vein pressure, hepatic vein pressure gradient, and heart rate in the vasopressin-treated patients, a phenomenon not observed in the control group. There was no tachyphylaxis to the hemodynamic effects of the drug over the 26-hour period of the study.

Clinical studies evaluating the efficacy of this vasoactive compound in controlling active variceal hemorrhage are limited. There are three randomized studies that attempt to compare vasopressin to placebo therapy. The initial study by Merigan et al. published in 1962 (44), compared hourly intravenous boluses of vasopressin to placebo in patients who appeared to be bleeding from upper variceal sources. This small study revealed that all 15 placebo-treated patients continued to bleed, whereas approximately 50% of those treated with vasopressin continued to hemorrhage acutely (44). Subsequently Conn et al. (45) reported a study evaluating the efficacy of intra-arterial vasopressin in controlling acute upper gastrointestinal hemorrhage regardless of the source. Retrospective analysis of the subgroup of patients who were presumed to have a variceal source of hemorrhage (as less than 50% of the vasopressin group were "proven") revealed a significant benefit to those receiving intra-arterial vasopressin (71% vs 25% stopped bleeding). One confounding issue in the study design was the fact that the control group was treated with "conservative therapy" in which was included systemic vasopressin. The most recent study, by Fogel et al. (46) evaluated patients who presented with acute upper gastrointestinal hemorrhage who were subsequently randomized according to the etiology of their hemorrhage to receive continuous intravenous vasopressin or placebo. Of the 14 patients with documented variceal bleeding who received vasopressin, 8 stopped bleeding, as compared with 13 of 19 in the placebo group (no significant difference).

Two additional studies, one comparing vasopressin to sclerotherapy and the other to balloon tamponade, showed significantly higher rates of hemostatic control with sclerotherapy and no difference in comparison to tamponade (47, 48). These five studies represent the very limited amount of controlled data available to support the use of this agent in the management of acute variceal hemorrhage. As such, it is not readily apparent how this form of therapy has achieved such universal clinical favor.

Table 5.6
Vasopressin Compared with Vasopressin Plus Nitroglycerin in the Management of Acute Variceal Hemorrhage

| | | Dosage | | Incidence Control of Bleeding (%) | | |
| | | | | | Vasopressin + | |
Reference	No. of Patients	Vasopressin (U/min)	Nitroglycerin	Vasopressin	Nitroglycerin	Probability
55	39	0.33–0.66 iv	0.6 mg q 30 min sl	21	45	.21
53	57	0.4 iv	40–100 µg/min iv	44	68	<.05
54	69	0.4–0.8 iv	10 mg over 24 hr td	18	42	.11

Abbreviations: iv, continuous intravenous infusion; sl, sublingual; td, transdermal; q, every.

Toxicity related to the parenteral administration of vasopressin is mediated primarily by its generalized systemic vasoconstrictive properties (41). Increases in systemic vascular resistance result in decreased cardiac output, elevation of mean arterial pressures, and reflex bradycardia. This can precipitate myocardial ischemia or infarction, arrhythmias, cerebrovascular events, as well as mesenteric and peripheral ischemia. Administration of lower doses of vasopressin via selective intra-arterial routes is plagued with similar toxicities, no improvement in clinical end points, and the additional risks of arterial catheter placement (49, 50).

Because of the toxicities associated with its use, investigators have sought to counteract the systemic side effects of vasopressin with peripheral vasodilators such as nitroprusside, nitroglycerin, and isosorbide dinitrate (41). Besides its beneficial effects on the peripheral and coronary circulation, nitroglycerin has additional intrinsic beneficial effects on the portal circulation. Iwao and colleagues (51) reported the effects of propranolol on portal hemodynamics in 14 patients with compensated cirrhosis who were randomized to receive transdermal nitroglycerin or placebo. Direct measurement of portal vein pressures, hepatic vein pressures, and hepatic blood flow (by indacyanine green clearance) revealed that propranolol caused a decrease in portal venous pressure gradient, hepatic venous pressure gradient, and mean arterial pressure

without any decrement in hepatic blood flow. The mechanism by which nitroglycerin induces such beneficial changes is unknown, but is hypothesized to have to do with either a reduction in portal vein blood flow related to reflex splanchnic vasoconstriction in response to the decrease in mean arterial pressure or to a direct effect on hepatic sinusoidal pressures. Additionally, the adjuvant use of nitroglycerin with vasopressin reverses all the systemic effects produced by vasopressin while preserving and possibly potentiating the beneficial effects on the splanchnic hemodynamics (52).

These beneficial changes in hemodynamics that have been observed with combined therapy have translated into lower rates of toxicity in all clinical trials comparing vasopressin and nitroglycerin to vasopressin alone (53–55). Evidence suggesting that the combination of vasopressin and nitroglycerin will improve vasopressin's ability to control an acute variceal hemorrhage is limited. The first controlled study evaluating this issue by Tsai and co-workers (55) showed no significant difference in the incidence of cessation of bleeding between the two groups although there was a trend in favor of combined therapy (Table 5.6). Results from a study by Gimson et al. (53) revealed a statistically significant increase in control of bleeding in those patients receiving combined therapy compared with those treated with vasopressin alone. The most recent study, by Bosch and colleagues (54), showed no difference in initial control of hemorrhage, although there was a significant decrease in transfusion requirements, total dose of vasopressin, and need for balloon tamponade. Interestingly, each of these three studies administered the nitroglycerin via different routes (Table 5.6). The greatest limitation of the studies evaluating the efficacy of vasopressin in combination with nitroglycerin is the absence of a control group receiving placebo. In spite of that, two of three studies indicated less toxicity with combination therapy and two indicated statistically significant improvement in control of hemorrhage or severity of hemorrhage as judged by transfusion requirements and need for balloon tamponade. For these reasons, combined therapy with vasopressin and nitroglycerin appeared to be an improvement over administration of vasopressin alone.

TERLIPRESSIN

Investigators have attempted to modify the chemical structure of vasopressin in hopes of enhancing the specificity of the compound for the splanchnic vasculature, thereby improving efficacy and decreasing toxicity. Triglycyl vasopressin (terlipressin) is a "hormonogen" that has little intrinsic activity until converted to vasopressin (56). High concentrations of vasopressin have been detected for hours after the administration of terlipressin (57) thus enabling the drug to be administered in intravenous boluses at set intervals. In addition to the theoretical advantage of mesenteric selectivity, terlipressin has not been noted to induce plasminogen activator, as does vasopressin, thus potentially improving the hemostatic milieu in patients with acute hemorrhage (41). The hemodynamic effects of vasopressin and terlipressin appear similar (58).

There have been three placebo-controlled studies evaluating terlipressin's ability to control active variceal hemorrhage. The first such study by Walker et al. (59) found terlipressin to be of a significant benefit in controlling active bleeding at 36 hours (100 vs. 80%). Limitations in study design, however, included the variable use of sclerotherapy and balloon tamponade. Freeman and colleagues (60) found

no benefit to terlipressin with regard to ability to control hemorrhage in the first 24 hours. The most recent study by Söderlund and co-workers (61) revealed that 90% of patients treated with terlipressin stopped bleeding within 24 hours as compared with 59% in the placebo group ($P < .01$). A significant flaw in study design was that approximately 50% of patients did not show endoscopic evidence of active variceal bleeding at the time of randomization. One additional study found terlipressin in combination with nitroglycerin to be comparable to balloon tamponade when evaluating the end point of cessation of bleeding at 12 hours (62). The only randomized study directly comparing terlipressin to vasopressin found that 70% of the terlipressin-treated patients stopped bleeding in comparison with only 9% of those treated with vasopressin (63). This large discrepancy in incidence of persistent hemorrhage did not translate into a change in mortality. In addition, the small sample size and the use of the definition of treatment failure as that requiring balloon tamponade to control bleeding makes interpretation of these data difficult. Thus, to date, the available data do not suggest any significant advantage to the use of terlipressin over vasopressin in the acute control of active variceal hemorrhage. The drug is not currently available in North America.

Intravenous vasopressin has gained wide clinical use in the primary or initial management of acute variceal bleeding, and yet the data to support such use are limited at best and include its intra-arterial use. Its combination with nitroglycerin appears to offer a clinical advantage over vasopressin alone, but no controlled studies of this regimen have been done.

SOMATOSTATIN

Somatostatin is a 14-amino acid polypeptide with a variety of effects on multiple end organs. In normal subjects somatostatin reliably decreases splanchnic blood flow (64, 65), likely via the inhibitory effects of this hormone on the release of other gastrointestinal peptides (66). Somatostatin's physiologic effects on splanchnic hemodynamics in patients with portal hypertension secondary to cirrhosis are somewhat more controversial. Bosch and co-workers (67) noted a significant decrease in hepatic blood flow and wedged hepatic vein pressures in patients with portal hypertension in response to administration of 450 µg/hour of intravenous somatostatin without the concomitant deleterious effects of decreased heart rate and increased arterial pressure noted with vasopressin. Conversely, another study documented no changes in hepatic blood flow or wedged hepatic vein pressure in 8 patients with cirrhosis given 250 µg/hour of intravenous somatostatin, whereas 18 normal subjects experienced a significant decrease in hepatic blood flow in response to identical dosages (65). Kleber and colleagues (68) actually documented an increase in intravariceal pressure in response to a 250 µg bolus of somatostatin followed by a continuous intravenous infusion at 250 µg/hour. When assessing the hemodynamic response to SMS 201–995, a longer acting and more potent somatostatin analog, Wahren and Eriksson (69) noted a significant decrease in hepatic blood flow and wedged hepatic vein pressure in 8 patients with cirrhosis.

Clinical data evaluating the efficacy of somatostatin in controlling acute variceal hemorrhage are available in the form of two randomized, double-blind, placebo-controlled trials (70, 71). The first study, by Valenzuela et al. (70), examined 83 patients (most of whom had advanced alcoholic cirrhosis) who were randomized to receive somatostatin 250–500 µg/hour or placebo as a continuous intravenous infusion. Over the 30-hour period of the study, 65% of the somatostatin-treated patients and 83% of the placebo-treated patients stopped bleeding. This unusually high rate of spontaneous cessation of variceal hemorrhage noted in the placebo group makes interpretation of the results difficult. Burroughs et al. (71) noted more encouraging results in 120 patients with a somewhat more diverse array of etiologies of cirrhosis (only 52% alcohol related). Over the 5-day period of the study, 64% of the somatostatin-treated patients stopped bleeding in comparison with

41% in the placebo group. Additionally, the number of units of blood administered and their rates of transfusion were both significantly higher in the placebo group.

Four randomized-controlled trials comparing somatostatin to vasopressin have been published (72–75). Three indicated improved rates of hemostasis (67–100%) with somatostatin in the setting of acute variceal hemorrhage (73–75). It is difficult to be confident that these encouraging findings are significant because of the dubious utility of vasopressin and the relatively small size of these studies. Two other randomized studies compared somatostatin to balloon tamponade and found the two forms of therapy to be equally efficacious in the acute control of hemorrhage (76, 77). In the study by Averginos et al. (77), the incidence of rebleeding and complications was significantly lower in those treated with somatostatin as compared with the group managed with balloon tamponade alone. Toxicity of somatostatin in this clinical setting is minimal.

In summary, because of the variable results observed with somatostatin, both in terms of physiologic effect and clinical end points, further clinical trials are needed before we can justify the routine use of this medication for control of variceal hemorrhage.

METOCLOPRAMIDE

Metoclopramide is a pharmacologic agent that causes an increase in lower esophageal pressure via unclear mechanisms (78). Blood flow in the portocollateral circulation travels through the submucosal vessels that traverse the lower esophageal sphincter. By increasing muscular tone in this region one could theoretically increase resistance in the vascular bed and subsequently decrease variceal blood flow. Studies have revealed both a decrease in azygous vein blood flow and variceal pressure in response to intravenous metoclopramide (79, 80).

There is only one controlled clinical trial published in manuscript form evaluating the efficacy of metoclopramide in the setting of acute variceal hemorrhage (81). Forty-nine patients were randomized in a blinded fashion to receive 20 mg of metoclopramide or placebo intravenously at the time of documentation of an active variceal hemorrhage at endoscopy. Repeat endoscopy 15 minutes later revealed cessation of bleeding in 20 of 25 metoclopramide-treated patients as compared with 5 of 24 patients in the placebo group ($P < .05$). Blood transfusion requirements were also significantly lower in the group receiving metoclopramide.

The data concerning metoclopramide's ability to impact on the course of an acute variceal hemorrhage are potentially promising but preliminary.

PHARMACOLOGIC APPROACH TO PATIENTS WITH ACUTE GASTROINTESTINAL BLEEDING COMPLICATING ACID-PEPTIC DISEASE

Acute gastrointestinal bleeding complicating peptic ulcer disease is a common clinical problem with a presenting spectrum that varies from massive hematemesis and shock to a transient black stool associated with a decreased hematocrit in a hemodynamically stable patient. Acid-peptic diseases (duodenal ulcer, gastric ulcer, erosive gastritis, and esophagitis) are the most common diagnostic sources in patients with upper gastrointestinal bleeding (82). Fortunately, most patients stop bleeding without specific treatment (83), but as many as 25% of patients will rebleed during the next 72 hours after the index bleed (83). Although peptic lesions are commonly the source of this type of bleeding, usually upper endoscopy is necessary to specify the anatomic site and source of the bleeding. Once the diagnosis is verified, if not before, it would be ideal if a simple, nontoxic medication could be administered that would "turn off" the bleeding. This quest for an effective pharmacologic approach to the treatment of gastrointestinal bleeding is still ongoing.

Histamine-2 Receptor Antagonists (H₂ Antagonists)

Many physicians consider the administration of an H_2 antagonist the most practical, if not ideal, approach to patients with upper gastrointestinal bleeding. One survey has noted their use in 89% of patients with acute upper gastrointestinal bleeding, and the drug was ordered prior to endoscopy in 86% of cases (84). These data imply that this therapeutic approach is being used with the hope of stopping bleeding rather than as treatment for the ulcer.

The rationale for such an approach has a logical basis related to the effects of pH on blood clotting, but has yet to attain clinical verification. In vitro studies have demonstrated the association of altered blood clotting at the low pH values commonly found in gastric juice. There is a progressive prolongation of coagulation factors, including prothrombin time and altered platelet aggregation times, as pH falls below 7.0 (85). The presence of pepsin appears additive to this phenomenon (85). Whether these phenomenon are more or less important in the cessation of ongoing bleeding compared with the prevention of rebleeding or other factors such as vascular contraction remains unanswered.

Clinical trials evaluating the use of H_2 antagonists to stop ongoing bleeding or to prevent rebleeding have not demonstrated any significant benefit for these end points (83, 86). Although one study suggested a decreased mortality in cimetidine-treated patients, the authors presented conflicting data within the same study, and improvement in mortality was associated with no difference in cessation of hemorrhage (86). Certainly, the largest U.S., multicentered, randomized, placebo-controlled trial did not show any benefit for histamine-2 antagonists in stopping ongoing bleeding or preventing inhospital rebleeding (83). One reason for the poor showing for this pharmacologic approach may be the inability of the dosage forms to maintain adequate or high gastric pH values. It has been shown that bolus intravenous doses of H_2 antagonists, as were commonly used in the above studies, do not consistently maintain gastric pH (even above 4.0) for sustained periods in patients with peptic ulcer bleeding (87). Continuous infusion of a histamine-2 antagonist appears to be more efficacious than repeated bolus doses in maintaining gastric pH above 6.0 (88). However, even a randomized, placebo controlled trial utilizing continuous intravenous infusion of a histamine-2 antagonist failed to show any significant difference in cessation of bleeding, operative rates, or mortality for either group (89). Although continuous infusion of a histamine-2 antagonist offers improved pH control on intravenous bolus dosing, other approaches may be necessary to achieve and maintain achlorhydria. One such approach involves combining continuous infusion of a histamine-2 antagonist (e.g. cimetidine 100 mg/hour intravenously) with a continuous antacid drip given via nasogastric tube (0.5 ml/minute) (90). This regimen resulted in a gastric pH of 7.0 in all patients. Nevertheless when these investigators studied the efficacy of this combination regimen in a clinical setting compared to patients who received only intravenous cimetidine, there was no statistical advantage seen with either regimen in preventing recurrent ulcer bleeding (90, 91). This lack of clinical efficacy occurred even though the gastric pH was significantly higher in the group receiving combination therapy (pH 7.4 vs. 5.0).

A more recent study, using a similar combination of a histamine-2 antagonist administered intravenously and a continuous drip of antacid into the stomach compared the effect of this regimen to that of intravenous ranitidine alone in 25 patients with bleeding peptic ulcers (92). They found that overall control of bleeding (combining the ongoing bleeding group with the rebleeding group) was achieved in only 29% of patients in the combination therapy group compared with 50% of the patients in the control group ($P < .05$). These results should be tempered by the knowledge that the study population was small and the effect of therapy on each separate bleeding type (ongoing bleeding and rebleeding) was not significant. It would appear that the use of a histamine-2 antagonist to stop ongoing bleeding or prevent rebleeding in patients with peptic ulcer disease has not been validated. The value of combination

therapy with a continuous antacid gastric drip in achieving pH 7.0 may need to be studied with larger patient populations.

Omeprazole

The quest for an agent that can produce gastric anacidity has moved closer to clinical reality with the availability of omeprazole. It is envisioned that this pharmacologic agent can truly test the hypothesis that gastrointestinal bleeding can be improved in the presence of achlorhydria. Omeprazole is a substituted benzimidazole that inhibits the enzyme $H^+/K^+/ATPase$ on the secretory surface of the parietal cell. This enzyme, or "proton pump," catalizes the final step in acid secretion. Thus, omeprazole appears to block the final common pathway for all stimulators of parietal cell acid secretion. The standard 20-mg oral morning dose of omeprazole will reduce 24-hour gastric acidity by about 90% in duodenal ulcer patients (93). This contrasts with a 37–68% reduction in gastric acidity with conventional doses of histamine-2 antagonists (94).

Several studies have evaluated the use of intravenous omeprazole (which is not available in the United States) for bleeding (94, 95). Although the initial study suggested that omeprazole showed "promising" results compared with ranitidine, the study was not blinded (95). A large double-blind placebo controlled trial of more than 1000 patients with upper gastrointestinal bleeding found that omeprazole failed to reduce overall mortality, rebleeding, or transfusion requirements (96). Patients who received omeprazole had lower rates of blood in the stomach, active bleeding, and stigmata of recent bleeding compared with control patients, and although these findings, when lumped together, show a significant reduction in the endoscopic signs of bleeding, the individual findings were not significantly different. The authors of this study concluded that their findings "do not justify the routine use of acid inhibiting drugs in the management of hematemesis and melaena" (96). This study was different in design from the previously mentioned studies in that the intravenous route was only utilized for the first 24 hours and then oral omeprazole in a dosage of 40 mg every 12 hours was given.

A preliminary report in abstract form evaluated oral omeprazole (40 mg once a day) vs. intravenous ranitidine in patients with acute upper gastrointestinal bleeding (97). The authors reported that the overall recurrence of bleeding during hospitalization was significantly more frequent in the ranitidine-treated patients (97). These preliminary findings, while interesting, require further evaluation. Certainly the largest study to date does not offer any promise for the use of a potent acid inhibitor in the management of acute gastrointestinal bleeding (96). Supporters for this form of therapy would say that we still have not attained achlorhydria in all patients and thus the hypothesis has yet to be fully tested.

Other Agents Studied for Effect on Gastrointestinal Bleeding

TRANEXAMIC ACID

Tranexamic acid has had considerable experimental evaluation in Europe, but is not clinically available and has not been studied in the United States. It is an antifibrinolytic agent that is postulated to be beneficial by inhibiting the binding of plasminogen and activated plasmin to fibrin. There have been six randomized studies that have recently been summarized involving a total of 1267 patients with upper gastrointestinal bleeding (98, 99). These studies evaluated various end points, including rates of rebleeding, transfusion requirements, operation rates, and mortality, although some parameters, such as death, may not be directly related to the gastrointestinal bleeding. Only one study showed a statistically significant effect on the rebleeding rate (100). When tranexamic acid-treated patients were found to have a significantly lower mortality rate (4%) than a placebo control group (11%), it was not associated with a decreased transfusion rate or rebleeding rate (101). Thus, the results of the effect of tranexamic acid on gastrointestinal bleeding are variable and do not offer any conclusive benefit for such patients.

PROSTAGLANDINS

Prostaglandins are derivatives of arachidonic acid and have been shown to offer some protection to the gastric mucosa subjected to various toxic insults (102). Although prostaglandins can decrease gastric acid secretion, their mucosal protective abilities may be related to other mechanisms (103). They have been shown to increase bicarbonate secretion from gastric and duodenal mucosa, and to stimulate mucus production and surfactant-like phospholipids in the gastric mucosa (102).

Four prospective controlled trials have evaluated the use of various prostaglandin analogs to contain gastrointestinal bleeding. Three of the studies utilized prostaglandin E_1 (misoprostol) or prostaglandin E_2 analogs for acute nonvariceal hemorrhage (104–106). These studies involving a total of 253 patients did not show any advantage of the prostaglandin compared with placebo or antacids for the control of bleeding. One preliminary report involving 150 patients bleeding from gastritis or peptic ulcer disease showed the benefit of misoprostal over placebo with a significant decrease in transfusion requirements (from 3 to 2 units, $P = .02$) and the need for surgery (15% to 4%, $P = .05$) to stop bleeding (107). However, there was no benefit shown for misoprostal in preventing rebleeding during the same hospitalization. The validity of this preliminary report will need confirmation with the final publication.

ESTROGENS

Conjugated estrogens have been evaluated mainly in patients with nasal bleeding from hereditary hemorrhagic telangiectasias (Osler-Weber-Rendu [OWR] syndrome). The number of patients who have been studied with gastrointestinal bleeding due to OWR syndrome or angiodysplasia has been small. In double-blind crossover study of 10 patients with bleeding angiodysplasia and OWR, it was noted that all patients receiving placebo bled while only two patients bled while receiving estrogen therapy (108). There was also a lower transfusion requirement in the estrogen-treated patients (1 unit) compared with those in the placebo group (11 units). The above differences were statistically significant in favor of estrogen therapy.

Estrogens have been shown to improve the bleeding time in patients with chronic renal failure, but the mechanism of action has not been elucidated. A double-blind placebo controlled crossover study utilizing intravenous estrogen in six patients noted a significant improvement in bleeding time in all patients (109). Bleeding times were significantly better at 6 hours, reached a maximum on day 5, and persisted for 14 days after stopping the intravenously administered estrogen. These findings may be important for those patients with chronic renal insufficiency and bleeding from intestinal angiodysplasia. However, despite the association of chronic renal failure to upper gastrointestinal angiodysplasia, the link to a prolonged bleeding time has not been documented (82). Randomized trials examining the use of estrogen in these bleeding patients has not been conducted. An uncontrolled study evaluated seven patients with renal insufficiency who were bleeding from gastrointestinal angiodysplasia (110). An estrogen-progesterone combination resulted in cessation of bleeding for all patients. Obviously, controlled studies will be needed to accurately define the role of estrogen-progesterone therapy in these patients. However, until such time, selected patients may benefit from this approach. Other factors, including the unknown potential for thromboembolic complications, will need to be factored into the therapeutic equation.

DDAVP

One deamino (8-D-arginine) vasopressin is a synthetic analog of posterior pituitary hormone. DDAVP has been shown in a randomized double-blind crossover study to decrease bleeding time in patients with prolonged bleeding times due to uremia (111). This effect, however, only decreases the bleeding time for 2–4 hours (111). The mechanism of action is unknown, but is possibly related to improvement in factor VIII-deficient uremia patients. Case reports have noted benefit in a patient with OWR syndrome and in a patient bleeding from uremic gastritis (112, 113). There are as yet no controlled trials to confirm the value of DDAVP in various bleeding situations.

REFERENCES

1. MacMathung P. The pathogenesis of varice rupture. In: Westaby D, ed. Gastrointestinal endoscopy clinics of North America. Philadelphia: WB Saunders, 1992;2:1–15.
2. Boyer TD. Portal hypertension and bleeding esophageal varices. In: Zakim D, Boyer TD, eds. Hepatology. Philadelphia: WB Saunders, 1990:572–616.
3. Lebrec D, Nouel O, Berneau J, et al. Propranolol in prevention of recurrent gastrointestinal bleeding in cirrhotic patients. Lancet 1981;1:920–921.
4. Burroughs AK, McCormick PA. Long-term pharmacologic therapy of portal hypertension. In: Rikkers LF, ed. Surgical clinics of North America. Philadelphia: WB Saunders, 1990;70:319–339.
5. Pomier-Layrargues G, Villeneuve JP, Willems B, et al. Systemic and hepatic hemodynamics after variceal hemorrhage: effects of propranolol and placebo. Gastroenterology 1987;93:1218–1224.
6. Groszmann RJ, Basch J, Grace ND, et al. Hemodynamic events in a prospective randomized trial of propranolol versus placebo in the prevention of a first variceal hemorrhage. Gastroenterology 1991;99:1401–1407.
7. Rector WG. Propranolol for portal hypertension: evaluation of therapeutic response by direct measurement of portal vein pressure. Arch Intern Med 1985;145:648–650.
8. Bosch J, Mastai R, Kravetz D, et al. Effects of propranolol on azygous venous blood blow and hepatic and systemic haemodynamics in cirrhosis. Hepatology 1984;4:1200–1205.
9. Bosch J, Mastai R, Kravetz D, et al. Measurement of azygous venous blood flow in the evaluation of portal hypertension in patients with cirrhosis. Clinical and haemodynamic correlations in 100 patients. J Hepatol 1985;1:125–139.
10. Gaiani S, Blondi L, Fenyves D, Zironi G, Rigamonti A, Barbara L. Effect of propranolol on portosystemic collateral circulation in patients with cirrhosis. Hepatology 1991;14:824–829.
11. Pascal JP, Cales P. Multicentre Study Group: Propranolol in the prevention of first upper gastrointestinal tract hemorrhage in patients with cirrhosis of the liver and esophageal varices. N Engl J Med 1987;317:856–861.
12. Ideo G, Bellati G, Fesce E, et al. Nadolol can prevent the first gastrointestinal bleeding in cirrhotics: a prospective, randomized study. Hepatology 1988;8:6–9.
13. Lebrec D, Poynard T, Capron JP, et al. Nadolol for prophylaxis of gastrointestinal bleeding in patients

with cirrhosis: a randomized trial. J Hepatol 1988;7:118–125.

14. Italian Multicentre Project for Propranolol in Prevention of Bleeding: Propranolol prevents first gastrointestinal bleeding in nonascitic cirrhotic patients: final report of a multicentre randomized trial. J Hepatol 1989;9:75–83.

15. Andreani T, Poupon RE, Balkau B. et al. Preventive therapy of first gastrointestinal bleeding in patients with cirrhosis: results of a controlled trial comparing propranolol, endoscopic sclerotherapy and placebo. Hepatology 1991;12:1413–1419.

16. Conn HO, Grace ND, Bosch J, et al. Propranolol in the prevention of first hemorrhage from esophagogastric varices: a multicenter, randomized clinical trial. Hepatology 1991;13:902–912.

17. PROVA Study Group. Prophylaxis of first hemorrhage from esophageal varices by sclerotherapy, propranolol or both in cirrhotic patients: a randomized multicenter trial. Hepatology 1991;14:1016–1024.

18. Pagliaro L, Burroughs AK, Sorensen TIA, et al. Therapeutic controversies and randomized controlled trials (RCTs): prevention of bleeding and rebleeding in cirrhosis. Gastroenterol Int 1989;2:71–84.

19. Hayes PC, Davis JM, Lewis JA, Bouchier IAD. Meta-analysis of value of propranolol in prevention of variceal haemorrhage. Lancet 1990;336:153–156.

20. Pagliaro L, Burroughs AK, Sorensen TIA, et al. Beta-blockers for preventing variceal bleeding. Lancet 1990; :1001–1002.

21. Poynard T, Cales P, Pasta L, et al. Beta-adrenergic-antagonist drugs in the prevention of gastrointestinal bleeding in patients with cirrhosis and esophageal varices. N Engl J Med 1991;324:1532–1538.

22. Lebrec D, Poynard T, Bernuau J, et al. A randomized controlled study of propranolol for prevention of recurrent gastrointestinal bleeding in patients with cirrhosis: a final report. Hepatology 1984;4:355–358.

23. Burroughs AK, Jenkins WJ, Sherlock S, et al. Controlled trial of propranolol for the prevention of recurrent variceal haemorrhage in patients with cirrhosis. N Engl J Med 1983;309:1539–1542.

24. Villeneuve JP, Pomier-Layragues G, Infante-Rivard C, et al. Propranolol for the prevention of recurrent variceal haemorrhage: a controlled trial. Hepatology 1986;6:1239–1243.

25. Gatta A, Merkel C, Sarcedoti D, et al. Nadolol for prevention of variceal rebleeding in cirrhosis: a controlled clinical trial. Digestion 1987;37:22–28.

26. Columbo M, De Frachis R, Tommasini M, et al. Beta-blockade prevents recurrent gastrointestinal bleeding in well compensated patients with alcoholic cirrhosis: a multicentre randomized controlled trial. Hepatology 1989;9:433–438.

27. Kiire CF. Controlled trial of propranolol to prevent recurrent variceal bleeding in patients with non-cir-

rhotic portal fibrosis. Br Med J 1989;298:1363–1365.

28. Sheen IS, Chen TY, Liaw YF. Randomized controlled study of propranolol for prevention of recurrent esophageal varices bleeding in patients with cirrhosis. Liver 1989;9:1–5.

29. Garden OJ, Mills PR, Birnie GG, Murray GD, Carter DC. Propranolol in the prevention of recurrent variceal haemorrhage in cirrhotic patients. Gastroenterology 1990;98:185–190.

30. Rossi V, Cales P, Burtin P, et al. Prevention of recurrent variceal bleeding in alcoholic cirrhotic patients: prospective controlled trial of propranolol and sclerotherapy. J Hepatol 1991;12:283–289.

31. Rosellini SR, Miglio F. Beta-blockers and varices hemorrhage [Letter]. Lancet 1990;336:1503–1504.

32. Van Stiegmann G, Yamamoto M. Endoscopic techniques for the management of active variceal bleeding. In: Sivak M, Westaby D, eds. Gastrointestinal endoscopy clinics of North America. Philadelphia: WB Saunders, 1992;2:59–75.

33. Terblanche J, Burroughs AK, Hobbs KEF. Controversies in the management of bleeding esophageal varices. N Engl J Med 1989;320:1469–1475.

34. Alexandrino P, Martins Alves M, Pinto-Correla J. Propranolol or endoscopic sclerotherapy in the prevention of recurrence of variceal bleeding: a prospective, randomized controlled trial. J Hepatol 1988;7:175–185.

35. Fleig WE, Stange EF, Hunecke R, et al. Prevention of recurrent bleeding in cirrhotics with recent variceal hemorrhage: prospective, randomized comparison of propranolol and sclerotherapy. Hepatology 1987;7:355–361.

36. Westaby D, Poison RJ, Gimson AES, Hayes PC, Hayllar K, Williams R. A controlled trial of oral propranolol compared with injection sclerotherapy for the long-term management of variceal bleeding. Hepatology 1990;11:353–359.

37. O'Connor KW, Lehman G, Yune H, et al. Comparison of three nonsurgical treatments for bleeding esophageal varices. Gastroenterology 1989;96:899–906.

38. Jensen LS, Karup N. Propranolol in prevention of rebleeding from oesophageal varices during the course of endoscopic sclerotherapy. Scand J Gastroenterol 1989;24:339–345.

39. Westaby D, Melia W, Hegarty J, et al. Use of propranolol to reduce the rebleeding rate during injection sclerotherapy prior to variceal obliteration. Hepatology 1986;6:673–675.

40. Stump DL, Hardin TC. The use of vasopressin in the treatment of upper gastrointestinal hemorrhage. Drugs 1990;39:38–53.

41. Rector WG. Review: drug therapy for portal hypertension. Ann Intern Med 1986;105:96–107.

42. Valla D, Girod C, Lee SS, Braillon A, Lebrec D. Lack of vasopressin action on splanchnic hemody-

namics during bleeding: a study in concious, portal hypertensive rats. Hepatology 1988;8:10–15.

43. Ready JB, Robertson AD, Rector WG. Effects of vasopressin on portal pressure during hemorrhage from esophageal varices. Gastroenterology 1991;100:1411–1416.

44. Merigen TC, Plotkin GR, Davidson CS. Effect of intravenously administered posterior pituitary extract on hemorrhage from bleeding esophageal varices. N Engl J Med 1962;266:134–135.

45. Conn HO, Ramsby GR, Storer EH, Mutchnick IG, Joshi PH, et al. Intra-arterial vasopressin in the treatment of upper gastrointestinal hemorrhage: a prospective, controlled clinical trial. Gastroenterology 1975;68:211–221.

46. Fogel MR, Krauer CM, Andres LL, Mahal AS, Stein DET, et al. Continuous intravenous vasopressin in active upper gastrointestinal bleeding: a placebo-controlled trial. Ann Intern Med 1982;96:565–569.

47. Westaby D, Hayes PC, Gimson AES, Poison RJ, Williams R. Controlled clinical trial of injection sclerotherapy for active variceal bleeding. Hepatology 1989;9:274–277.

48. Correia JP, Alves MM, Alexandrino P, Silvera J. Controlled trial of vasopressin and balloon tamponade in bleeding esophageal varices. Hepatology 1984;5:885–888.

49. Choijkier M, Groszman RJ, Atterbury CE, Bos-Meir S, Blei AT, et al. A controlled comparison of continuous intra-arterial and intravenous infusions of vasopressin in hemorrhage from esophageal varices. Gastroenterology 1979;77:540–546.

50. Johnson WC, Widrich WC, Ansell JE, Robbins AH, Nabseth DC. Control of bleeding varices by vasopressin: a prospective randomized study. Ann Surg 1977;186:369–376.

51. Iwao T, Toyonaga A, Sumino M, et al. Hemodynamic study during transdermal application of nitroglycerin tape in patients with cirrhosis. Hepatology 1991;13:124–128.

52. Groszman RJ, Kravetz D, Bosch J, Glickman M, Bruix J, et al. Nitroglycerin improves the hemodynamic response to vasopressin in portal hypertension. Hepatology 1982;2:757–762.

53. Gimson AES, Westaby D, Hegarty J, Watson A, Williams R. A randomized trial of vasopressin and vasopressin plus nitroglycerin in the control of acute variceal hemorrhage. Hepatology 1986;6:410–413.

54. Bosch J, Groszman R, Garcia-Pagan JC Jr., et al. Association of transdermal nitroglycerin to vasopressin infusion in the treatment of variceal hemorrhage: a placebo-controlled clinical trial. Hepatology 1989;10:962–968.

55. Tsai Y-T, Lay C-S, Lai K-H, Ng W-W, Yeh Y-S, et al. Controlled trial of vasopressin plus nitroglycerin vs vasopressin alone in the treatment of bleeding esophageal varices. Hepatology 1986;6:406–409.

56. Prowse CV, Douglas JG, Forrest JAH, Forsling MF. Hemostatic effects of lysine vasopressin and triglycyl lysine vasopressin infusion in patients with cirrhosis. Eur J Clin Invest 1980;10:49–54.

57. Forsling ML, Aziz LA, Miller M, Davies R, Dohovan B. Conversion of triglycyl vasopressin to lysine-vasopressin in man. J Endocrinol 1980;85:237–244.

58. Rabol A, Juhl E, Schmidt A, Winkler K. The effect of vasopressin and triglycyl lysine vasopressin (glypressin) on the splanchnic circulation in cirrhotic patients with portal hypertension. Digestion 1976;14:285–289.

59. Walker S, Stiehl A, Raedsch R, Kommerell B. Teripressin in bleeding esophageal varices: a placebo-controlled double-blind study. Hepatology 1986;6:112–115.

60. Freeman JG, Cobden I, Record CO. Placebo-controlled trial of terlipressin (Glypressin) in the management of acute variceal bleeding. J Clin Gastroenterol 1989;11:58–60.

61. Söderlund C, Magnusson I, Torngren S, Lundell L. Terlipressin (triglycyl lysine vasopressin) controls acute bleeding esophageal varices: a double-blind, randomized, placebo-controlled trial. Scand J Gastroenterol 1990;25:622–630.

62. Fort E, Sautereau D, Silvain C, Ingrand P, Pillegand B, Beauchant M. A randomized trial of terlipressin plus nitroglycerin vs balloon tamponade in the control of acute variceal hemorrhage. Hepatology 1990;11:678–681.

63. Freeman JG, Lishman AH, Cobden I, Record CO. Controlled trial of terlipressin (glypressin vs vasopressin in the early treatment of esophageal varices. Lancet 1982;2:66–68.

64. Wahren J, Felig P. Influence of somatostatin on carbohydrate disposal and absorption in diabetes mellitus. Lancet 1976;2:1213.

65. Sonnenberg GE, Keller U, Perruchoud A, et al. Effect of somatostatin on splanchnic hemodynamics in patients with cirrhosis of the liver and in normal subjects. Gastroenterology 1981;80:526.

66. Rodriguez-Perez F, Groszman RJ. Pharmacologic treatment of portal hypertension. In: Groszman RJ, Grace ND, eds. Gastroenterology clinics of North America. Philadelphia: WB Saunders, 1992;21:15–40.

67. Bosch J, Kravetz D, Rodes J. Effects of somatostatin on hepatic and systemic hemodynamics in patients with cirrhosis of the liver: comparison with vasopressin. Gastroenterology 1981;80:518.

68. Kleber G, Sauerbruch T, Fischer G, et al. Somatostatin does not reduce oesophageal variceal pressure in liver cirrhosis. Gut 1988;29:153–156.

69. Wahren J, Eriksson LS. The influence of long-acting somatostatin analogue on splanchnic haemodynamics and metabolism in healthy subjects and patients with liver cirrhosis. Scand J Gastroenterol 1986;21(suppl 119):103–108.

70. Valenzuela JE, Schubert T, Fogel MR, et al. A multicenter, randomized, double-blind trial of somatostatin in the management of acute hemorrhage from esophageal varices. Hepatology 1989;10:958.

71. Burroughs AK, McCormick PA, Hughes MD, et al. Randomized, double-blind, placebo-controlled trial of somatostatin for variceal bleeding. Gastroenterology 1990;99:1388.

72. Kravetz D, Bosch J, Teres J, et al. Comparison of continuous somatostatin and vasopressin infusions in the treatment of acute variceal hemorrhage. Hepatology 1984;4:442–446.

73. Saari A, Livilaakso E, Inberg M, et al. Comparison of somatostatin and vasopressin in bleeding esophageal varices. Am J Gastroenterol 1990;85:804–807.

74. Jenkins SA, Baxter JN, Corbet W, Devitt P, Ware J, Shields R. A prospective randomized, controlled, clinical trial comparing somatostatin and vasopressin in controlling acute variceal hemorrhage. Br Med J 1985;290:275–278.

75. Bagarini M, Albertini M, Anza M, et al. Effect of somatostatin in controlling bleeding from esophageal varices. Ital J Surg Sci 1987;17:21–26.

76. Jamarillo JL, Mata M, Miño G, Costan G, Gómez-Camacho F. Somatostatin vs Sengstaben balloon tamponade for primary hemostasia of bleeding esophageal varices: a randomized pilot study. J Hepatol 1991;12:100–105.

77. Avgerinos A, Klonis C, Rekoumis G, Gouma P, Papadimitriou N, Raptis S. A prospective randomized trial comparing somatostatin, ballon tamponade, and the combination of both methods in the management of acute variceal hemorrhage. J Hepatol 1991;13:78–81.

78. Cohen S, Morris DW, Schoen HJ, DiMarino AJ. The effect of oral and intravenous metoclopramide on human lower oesophageal sphincter pressure. Gastroenterology 1976;70:484–487.

79. Mastai R, Grand L, Bosch J, et al. Effects of metoclopramide and domperidone on azgos venous blood flow in patients with cirrhosis and portal hypertension. Hepatology 1986;6:1244–1247.

80. Kleber G, Sauerbruch T, Fischer G, Geigenberger G, Paumgartner G. Reduction of transmoral esophageal variceal pressure by metoclopramide. J Hepatol 1991;12:362–366.

81. Gupta IP, Sharma MP. Control of variceal bleed with metoclopramide. Indian J Gastroenterol 1991;10:10–11.

82. Zuckerman GR, Cornette GL, Clouse RE, et al. Upper gastrointestinal bleeding in patients with chronic renal failure. Ann Intern Med 1985;102:588.

83. Zuckerman G, Welch R, Douglas A, et al. Controlled trial of medical therapy for active upper gastrointestinal bleeding and prevention of rebleeding. Am J Med 1984;76:361.

84. Bhatt BD, Meriano FV, Phipps TL, Ho H, Zuckerman MJ. Survey of H_2 antagonist usage in acute upper gastrointestinal hemorrhage. J Clin Gastroenterol 1990;12:14–16.

85. Green FW, Kaplan MM, Curtis LE, et al. Effects of acid and pepsin on blood coagulation and platelet aggregation. Gastroenterology 1978;74:38.

86. Barer D, Ogilvie A, Henry D, et al. Cimetidine and tranexamic acid in the treatment of acute upper-gastrointestinal tract bleeding. N Engl J Med 1983;308:1571.

87. Reynolds JR, Walt RP, Clark AG, Hardcastle JD, Langman MJ. Intragastric pH monitoring in acute upper gastrointestinal bleeding and the effect of intravenous climetidine and ranitidine. Aliment Pharmacol Ther 1987;1:23–30.

88. Fiorucci S, Clausi GC, Farinelli M, Santuce L, Pelli MA, Morelli A. Intragastric pH monitoring during antisecretory therapy in patient with gastrointestinal bleeding. Am J Gastroenterol 1987;84:1416–1420.

89. Basso N, Bagarani M, Brocci F, et al. Ranitidine and somatostatin: their effects on bleeding from the upper gastrointestinal tract. Arch Surg 1986;121:833.

90. Peterson WL, Richard CT: Sustained fasting achlorhydria: a comparison of medical regimens. Gastroenterology 1985;88:666.

91. Peterson WL, Hartless K, Meadows T. Prevention of recurrent ulcer bleeding: double-blind, randomized trial of a regimen designed to produce sustained achlorhydria. Gastroenterology 1990;98:A106.

92. Arora A, Tandon RK, Acharya SK, Tandon BN. The role of sustained achlorhydria in bleeding peptic ulcer. J Clin Gastroenterol 1991;13:147–153.

93. Holt S, Howden CW. Omeprazole: overview and opinion. Dig Dis Sci 1991;36:385–393.

94. Jones DB, Howden CW, Burget DW, Kerr GD, Hunt RH. Acid suppression in duodenal ulcer: a meta-analysis to define optimal dosing with antisecretory drugs. Gut 1987;28:1120–1127.

95. Brunner G, Chang J. Intravenous therapy with high doses of ranitidine and omeprazole in critically ill patients with bleeding peptic ulcerations of the upper intestinal tract: an open, randomized, controlled trial. Digestion 1990;45:217.

96. Daneshmel TK, Hawkey CJ, Langman MJS, Logan RFA, Long RG, Walt RP. Omeprazole vs placebo for acute upper gastrointestinal bleeding: randomized, double-blind, controlled trial. Br Med J 1992;304:143–147.

97. Rocca G, Fasseas P, Ricci E, Oliveri F, Franceschi M, Garetto G. A randomized clinical trial of oral omeprazole vs ranitidine I.V. in the medical treatment of acute gastrointestinal bleeding. Gastroenterology 1992;102:A153.

98. Henry DA, O'Connell DL. Effects of fibrinolytic inhibitors on mortality from upper gastrointestinal hemorrhage. Br Med J 1989;298:1142.

99. Zuckerman GR, Buse PE. Current medical and surgical management of nonvariceal upper gastrointes-

tinal bleeding. Gastrointest Endosc Clin N Amer 1991;1:263–289.

100. Bigg SJC, Hugh TB, Dodds AJ. Tranexamic acid and upper gastrointestinal hemorrhage: a double-blind trial. Gut 1976;17:729.

101. Barer D, Ogilvie A, Henry D, et al. Cimetidine and tranexamic acid in the treatment of acute upper gastrointestinal tract bleeding. N Engl J Med 1983;308:1571.

102. Aly A. Prostaglandins in clinical treatment of gastroduodenal mucosal lesions: a review. Scand J Gastroenterology 1987;22(suppl 137):43.

103. Buchanan N, Laferla G, Hearns D, et al. Effect of a single oral dose of enprostil on gastric secretion and gastrin release. Am J Med 1986;81(suppl 2A):40.

104. Levine BA, Sirinek KR, Gaski HV. Topical prostaglandin E_2 in the treatment of acute gastrointestinal hemorrhage. Arch Surg 1985;120:600.

105. Raskin JB, Camara DS, Levin BA, et al. Effect of 15(R)-15-methyl prostaglandin E_2 on acute upper gastrointestinal hemorrhage. Gastroenterology 1985;88:1550.

106. Bright-Asare P, Giannikopoulos I, Blackstone M, et al. Double-blind, controlled trial of misoprostol (cytotec) compared with antacids in subjects with acute GI bleeding. Gastroenterology 1986;90:1357.

107. Birnie GG, Akbar FE, Shroff ME, et al. A double-blind comparative study of misoprostol with placebo in acute upper gastrointestinal bleeding. Gastroenterol Int 1988;1(suppl):110.

108. Van Cutsem E, Rutgeerts P, Vantrappen G. Treatment of bleeding gastrointestinal vascular malformations with estrogen-progesterone. Lancet 1990;335:953.

109. Livio M, Mannucci PM, Vigano G, et al. Conjugated estrogens for the management of bleeding associated with renal failure. N Engl J Med 1986;315:731.

110. Bronner MH, Pate MB, Cunningham JT, et al. Estrogen-progesterone therapy for bleeding gastrointestinal telangiectasias in chronic renal failure. Ann Intern Med 1986;105:371.

111. Mannucci PM, Remuzzi G, Persineri F, et al. Deamino-8-D-arginine vasopressin shortens the bleeding time in uremia. N Engl J Med 1983;308:8.

112. Quitt M, Froom P, Veisler A. The effect of desmopressin on massive gastrointestinal bleeding in hereditary telangiectasia unresponsive to treatment with cryoprecipitate. Arch Intern Med 1990;150:1744.

113. Juhl A, Jorgensen F. DDAVP and life-threatening diffuse gastric bleeding in uremia. Acta Chir Scand 1987;153:75.

6

Helicobacter pylori and Ulcer Disease: Treatment Considerations

WALTER L. PETERSON

INTRODUCTION

Helicobacter pylori was "discovered" in 1983 when Warren and Marshall, two Australian investigators, reported spiral organisms in mucosal biopsies of patients with chronic active gastritis (1, 2). First named *Campylobacter* ("curved rod") *pylori*, its name was changed to *Helicobacter pylori* when biochemical and genetic characterization of the organism showed that it was not a member of the *Campylobacter* genus. The organism is a slow-growing, microaerophilic, Gram-negative rod, the most striking biochemical characteristic of which is abundant production of urease. *H. pylori* is very sensitive to low pH. However, if the organism is able to escape the effects of acidic gastric juice, it burrows through the mucus layer and colonizes the surface epithelium of gastric mucosa where the pH is near neutrality. It is found only on gastric epithelium (i.e., stomach and areas of gastric metaplasia) and virtually never penetrates the cell. It nevertheless elicits robust inflammatory and antibody responses that persist throughout life unless the organism is eradicated. *H. pylori* gastritis is associated with several important disease states, including peptic ulcer disease and gastric adenocarcinoma.

DIAGNOSIS

Diagnostic tests for *H. pylori* may be divided into those which do (invasive) or do not (noninvasive) require endoscopically obtained mucosal biopsies.

Noninvasive Tests

Detection of serum antibodies to H. pylori by an enzyme-linked immunosorbent assay (ELISA) is the most convenient and, when more widely available, will probably be the least expensive diagnostic test (3). It has virtually 100% positive and negative predictive values, being unreliable only after successful eradication of the organism with antimicrobial therapy. In this situation, serum antibody titers may remain elevated for a year or more even though the organism is no longer present in the stomach. Thus, in patients who have not received regimens effective against *H. pylori* a positive serology is evidence of active infection, whereas a negative serology strongly suggests that the organism is not present. It will primarily be used as a screening test for the presence of *H. pylori*, perhaps to determine the necessity of endoscopy. It should *not* be used to assess success of eradication therapy.

Another noninvasive means of detecting *H. pylori* are the *urea breath tests* (UBT), which are just now becoming available. Here, urea labeled with either ^{13}C or ^{14}C is ingested with a liquid meal (4). If urease is present, labeled carbon dioxide will be split off and absorbed into the circulation where its presence can be determined by analysis of expired breath. This test has virtually 100% positive predictive value and about 95% negative predictive value. Small numbers of organisms that can

93

be detected by direct examination of gastric tissue may not produce enough urease to be detected by the UBT. ^{13}C-labeled urea has the advantage of not being radioactive but requires a mass spectrometer for analysis; ^{14}C can be measured with a simple γ-counter but subjects an individual to a small dose of radioactivity. The UBT is especially valuable before and after antimicrobial therapy to determine whether eradication has been achieved. If the test is positive before therapy and remains positive 4–6 weeks after cessation of such therapy, therapy has failed. It the test becomes negative, only a small proportion of patients will still be infected. A decision to obtain gastric tissue to confirm eradication depends on the clinical situation and how important it is to ensure successful eradication.

Invasive Tests

Tissue obtained at endoscopy may be examined several ways for the presence of *H. pylori*. The presence of *H. pylori* urease can be determined by placing mucosal biopsies onto a *urea slide test* (e.g., CLO Test). If urease is present in the mucosal biopsy, it will split the urea into ammonia and carbon dioxide. The ammonia will raise the pH of the medium, which will change the color of a pH-sensitive indicator (phenol red) from yellow to red. This test may require several hours to become positive.

The most sensitive test for detecting *H. pylori* is *histologic examination* of mucosal biopsies. Pathologists with reasonable experience can readily detect even small numbers of organisms using routine hematoxylin and eosin or Giemsa stains (5).

The most specific test for the presence of *H. pylori* is *culture* of the organism from gastric mucosal biopsies, although sensitivity is diminished if the number of organisms is small, the patient has recently taken omeprazole or bismuth compounds, or if the culture technique is improper. Cultures should be kept for at least 7 days before being declared negative and discarded.

Strategy

The choice of a diagnostic test depends upon the clinical indication. If one wishes to screen patients with dyspepsia to decide if endoscopy is necessary, a serum antibody test is an excellent choice. In a younger individual in whom malignancy is not a concern and in whom there is no evidence of nonsteroidal anti-inflammatory drug usage, a negative serologic test for *H. pylori* virtually excludes the possibility of a peptic ulcer. Endoscopy in such patients could legitimately be postponed (6). The serum antibody test is also an excellent screening test for patients in whom diagnostic endoscopy has been performed in the past, but tissue was not obtained at the time for *H. pylori* testing.

Endoscopy is expensive and should rarely, if ever, be performed solely to diagnose *H. pylori*. On the other hand, if there is a valid clinical indication for diagnostic endoscopy, and *if* treatment of *H. pylori* is a reasonable therapeutic option, two mucosal biopsies should be obtained. One should be placed on the inexpensive urea slide test and the other placed in a bottle for histology. If the slide test is positive, the second biopsy may be discarded. If the slide test is negative the second biopsy can be sent for the more expensive histologic examination.

Because it will probably be more expensive and time consuming than serology, the urea breath test is less desirable as a screening test. However, for patients with known *H. pylori* infection who are to be treated with antimicrobial agents, a urea breath test performed before and 4–6 weeks after therapy is the preferred means to evaluate the success of eradication therapy. Such tests may be more widely available within the year.

EPIDEMIOLOGY

Refinement and standardization of nonendoscopic means of detecting *H. pylori* has been of major benefit in studies of the epidemiology of the infection. Large groups of subjects can be evaluated quickly and noninvasively.

Prevalence in Healthy Volunteers

The prevalence of *H. pylori* in healthy volunteers varies enormously depending upon ethnicity, country of origin, and age. In devel-

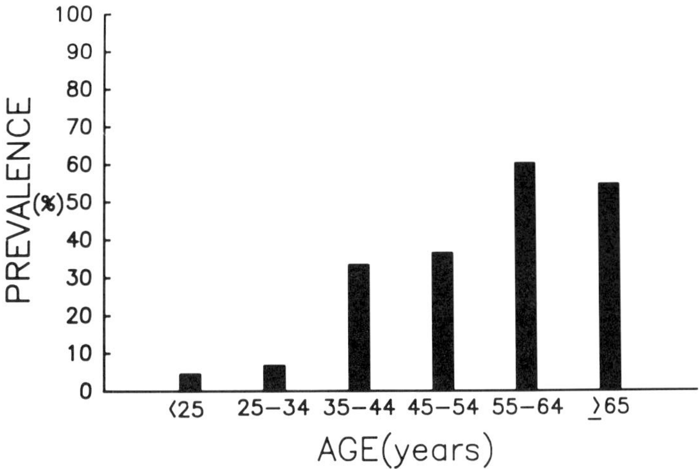

FIGURE 6.1. Age-related prevalence of *H. pylori* in healthy volunteers as determined by mucosal histology and culture. From Podolsky I, Lee E, Cohen R, Peterson WL. Prevalence of *C. pylori* (CP) in healthy subjects and patients with peptic diseases [Abstract]. Gastroenterology 1989;96:A394.

oped countries, there is a clear age-related increase in prevalence (7–9) (Fig. 6.1). Current evidence suggests this phenomenon may be due to a combination of age-related risk factors (as yet undefined) plus a generational cohort effect (10). A cohort effect is the result of overall differences in the risk of exposure depending upon year of birth. For example, today's cohort of 65 year olds, who have a high prevalence of *H. pylori*, would have had a prevalence when they were 30 years old higher than the prevalence in today's cohort of 30 year olds. Said another way, the prevalence in today's cohort of 30 year olds will be less when they reach 65 years of age than it is in today's cohort of 65 year olds. One explanation for the decrease in prevalence may be the rise in socioeconomic status from one generational cohort to another. In the United States, the age-related prevalence curves for Hispanic and black populations are higher than that for white populations (11) (Fig. 6.2).

While genetic differences in risk cannot be ruled out, this observation most likely represents a delay in generational improvements in socioeconomic status. If all this is true, one might predict that in several more generations, *H. pylori* infection will become uncommon in developed countries.

Generational differences in prevalence are much less obvious in healthy volunteers from developing countries. In such locations, there is a high prevalence regardless of age. This is not surprising given the lack of generational improvements in socioeconomic status in these countries.

Transmission of Infection

H. pylori has never been cultured, or even found, outside the human body. It is therefore unlikely that the bacterium is transmitted through environmental sources or traditional animal vectors such as insects, pets, or farm animals. Rather, it appears that the organism is transmitted from person to person. Support for this theory comes from studies in which family members, especially mothers, of an infected child are more likely to be infected than family members of an uninfected child (12, 13) (Table 6.1). Furthermore, the frequency of infection is higher in institutions of custodial care, where person-to-person transmission of disease is well known. On the other hand, there is no concordance of infection in sexually active couples without children (14). Whether transmission is oral-oral or fecal-oral is not known. *H. pylori* has been isolated from dental plaque (15, 16) and from stool (17). The fact that couples with children exhibit concordance of infection, while childless couples do not, and that children in institutions of custodial care have increased prevalence suggests that the fecal-oral route is more likely than the oral-oral one.

Risk Factors for Infection

Situations of economic deprivation and habitational crowding enhance the spread of *H. pylori* during childhood (18, 19) (Table 6.2). Indeed, it is likely that most adults who harbor the organism became infected during childhood, although young parents who were not infected as children may be infected by their children who are infected outside the home (e.g., child care centers) (Table 6.2). Interestingly, endoscopists have been reported to have a higher than expected prevalence of infection (20), presumably by handling endoscopes contaminated by patients with *H. pylori*. There is no apparent increase in rates of infection in immunocompromised subjects (21) and, although in theory they should, patients taking drugs that suppress gastric acidity have not been shown to be at increased risk.

HISTOLOGIC MANIFESTATIONS OF *H. PYLORI* INFECTION

Antral biopsies from adults who harbor *H. pylori* show focal epithelial cell damage as well as an inflammatory response in the lamina propria consisting of both polymorphonuclear leucocytes and mononuclear cells. The latter include B and T lymphocytes, monocytes, plasma cells, and eosinophils. The plasma cells secrete both IgG and IgA antibodies which may prevent invasion of the epithelial cells (22). Biopsies from the body of the stomach also usually demonstrate gastritis but may at times be normal. These histologic abnormalities are associated with reduced surface hydrophobicity of gastric mucosa, a phenomenon associated with impaired mucosal defense (23).

H. pylori is not merely a commensal that inhabits inflamed tissue, it causes the gastritis. Inoculation of *H. pylori* into experimental an-

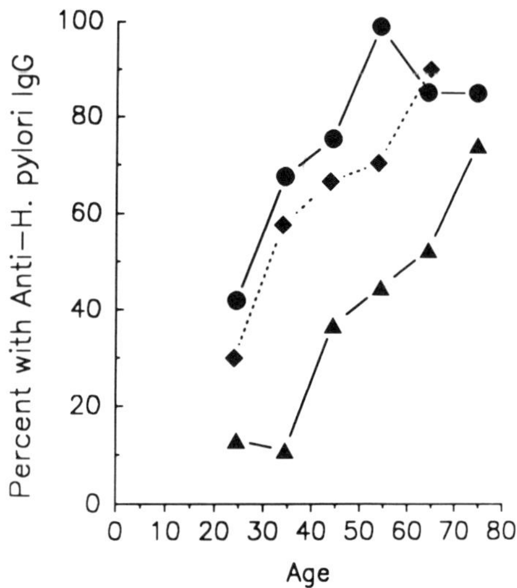

FIGURE 6.2. Age-related seroprevalence of *H. pylori* in healthy volunteers of different ethnicity. Closed circles = blacks; closed diamonds = hispanics; closed triangles = whites. From Malaty HM, Evans DG, Evans DJ, Jr, Graham D. *Helicobacter pylori* in hispanics: comparison with blacks and whites of similar age and socioeconomic class. Gastroenterology 1992;103:813–816.

Table 6.1
Seroprevalence of *H. pylori* in Family Members of Children with and without *H. pylori* [a]

	Children with H. pylori		Children without H. pylori	
	No.	%	No.	%
Siblings	18/22	82	5/37	14
Mothers	15/18	83	2/17	12
Fathers	10/16	62	6/16	38

[a]From Drumm B, Perez-Perez GI, Blaser MJ, Sherman PM. Intrafamilial clustering of *Helicobacter pylori* infection. N Engl J Med 1990;322:359–363.

imals has led to colonization in neonatal gnotobiotic piglets (24) and beagles and 2-month-old barrier-born pigs, although the histologic response is less granulocytic than in the human infection. The histologic response in the chimpanzee is reported to mimic more closely the response seen in humans (25). Germ-free mice inoculated with *Helicobacter felis*, a related organism found in cats, also develop a pro-

**Table 6.2
Living Conditions and *H. pylori* Seropositivity in Adult Life[a]**

		Odds Ratio
No. of children now	0	1.0
	1	1.85
	≥2	5.53
Persons/room in childhood	<0.7	1.0
	0.7–0.99	1.36
	1.0–1.29	4.04
	≥1.3	6.15

[a]From Mendall MA, Goggin PM, Molineaux N, et al. Childhood living conditions and *Helicobacter pylori* seropositivity in adult life. Lancet 1992;339:896–897.

nounced polymorphonuclear response and may prove to be a more convenient animal model (26). Two human subjects who intentionally ingested *H. pylori* developed an intense, neutrophilic inflammatory response, first in the antrum and then the body (27, 28). There was spontaneous resolution of infection and inflammation in one. In the second subject, infection was associated with hypochlorhydria, and while acid secretion ultimately returned, he was left with chronic active gastritis that ultimately resolved only with administration of triple antibiotic therapy (29).

Further evidence that *H. pylori* causes gastritis is found in studies in which the organism is eradicated by antimicrobial therapy. In virtually every instance where there is clear evidence of eradication of the organism, there is accompanying resolution of at least the active component of gastritis.

VIRULENCE FACTORS

A number of candidate virulence factors have been suggested to permit *H. pylori* to escape the bactericidal properties of gastric acid, colonize gastric epithelium, damage epithelial cells, and induce an inflammatory reaction. With the possible exception of immunocompromised hosts, invasion of human epithelial cells by *H. pylori* has not been documented.

Motility

Studies in gnotobiotic piglets have demonstrated that less motile strains of *H. pylori* are less virulent (30). This may be related to the need for the organism to penetrate the mucus layer to avoid the acid milieu of the gastric lumen.

Adherence

It is now clear that *H. pylori* possesses lectins that bind to glycolipids and/or glycoproteins on gastric epithelial cells. An *N*-acetylneuraminyllactose-binding fibrillar hemagglutinin has been described as has a specific gastric glycerolipid receptor (31, 32). Tight attachment of this fibrillar adhesin to the carbohydrate results in the formation of an attachment pedestal which in turn leads to actin polymerization and epithelial cell disruption (33). Failure of adherence, while having no effect on the inflammatory response, results in less epithelial cell injury (34).

Urease

Urease appears to be necessary for *H. pylori* to successfully colonize gastric epithelium. It was recently reported that a mutant strain of *H. pylori* without urease was unable to colonize gnotobiotic piglets (35). The reasons why urease may be necessary for colonization are unclear, but include protection of *H. pylori* from the bactericidal effect of acidic gastric juice (by surrounding the organisms with a cloud of ammonia) (36) or the enhancement of bacterial adherence (37). Urease, primarily through production of ammonia, is also cytotoxic and may be at least partially responsible for epithelial cell damage associated with *H. pylori* (38, 39).

Mediators of Inflammation

H. pylori elaborates proteins with chemotactic properties to recruit monocytes and neutrophils to the lamina propria (40) and both lipopolysaccharide (LPS)-dependent and LPS-independent soluble surface proteins that activate these inflammatory cells (41). Activation of inflammatory cells results in release of other inflammatory cytokines as well as reactive oxygen metabolites (42).

Cytotoxins

A vacuolating cytotoxin elaborated by *H. pylori* has been found by several laboratories (43–45). This putative toxin is believed to be an important factor in cellular injury associated with the organism.

PHYSIOLOGIC RESPONSE TO *H. PYLORI* INFECTION

Acid Secretion

Healthy subjects infected with *H. pylori* have significantly lower basal, but not peak or meal-stimulated, acid outputs when compared to uninfected subjects (46). The reason (or reasons) for the lower basal acid output is not clear but may involve a protein that inhibits acid secretion somewhere late in the enzymatic cascade of the parietal cell (47). Of interest, patients with duodenal ulcer who are infected with *H. pylori* have *high* basal and peak acid outputs (46). The discrepancy in acid secretion between healthy subjects and duodenal ulcer patients, each infected with *H. pylori*, is not known. One possibility is that duodenal ulcer patients have a less intense inflammatory response in the acid-secreting portion of the stomach than do healthy subjects (48), thereby permitting higher levels of basal acid secretion.

Serum Gastrin Concentrations

Both *H. pylori*-positive, healthy subjects and patients with duodenal ulcer exhibit fasting and meal-stimulated serum gastrin levels significantly higher than those of uninfected healthy subjects (46). Recent evidence suggests that hypergastrinemia is related to a relative deficiency of D cells, which secrete somatostatin. A deficiency of this natural inhibitor of gastrin release would explain higher levels of gastrin (49–51). Whether *H. pylori*-associated hypergastrinemia has any clinical relevance is unknown. However, it is possible that in *H. pylori*-infected individuals with no or only mild involvement of the body of the stomach, prolonged hypergastrinemia could lead to parietal cell hyperplasia and acid hypersecretion. Such individuals might be predisposed to the development of duodenal ulcer.

Gastric Emptying

There is no evidence that *H. pylori* infection has any effect on gastric motility.

ROLE OF *H. PYLORI* IN DISEASE STATES

Duodenal Ulcer Disease

The association between *H. pylori* gastritis and duodenal ulcer disease is now well-accepted, with more than 90% of all duodenal ulcer patients being infected. In fact, if nonsteroidal anti-inflammatory drug (NSAID) use is excluded, the prevalence of *H. pylori* in duodenal ulcer is virtually 100% (52). Association, however, does not prove causation. The strongest evidence to support a causal role for *H. pylori* in the pathogenesis of duodenal ulcer comes from controlled trials in which eradication of the organism is associated with a significant and substantial reduction in the rate of ulcer recurrence (53–56) (Table 6.3). The mechanism(s) by which *H. pylori* predisposes to duodenal ulcer remains unclear, although it is speculated that duodenal ulcers occur in areas of gastric metaplasia infected with *H. pylori*.

As plausible as this scenario is, several factors prompt caution concerning its acceptance. First, the randomized, controlled eradication trials to date all suffer from methodologic flaws, not the least of which is that none has a double-blind structure. Bismuth darkens the stools, a phenomenon that surely does not go unnoticed by the patients. Recognition by the patient that he or she is receiving active medication may bias the results. For example, the patient may communicate the observation of dark stools to the individual responsible for determining whether ulcer recurrence has or has not occurred. As another example, knowledge that he or she is receiving active medication may trigger psychologic factors favorable to reduction in the rate of recurrence. Second, patients in randomized controlled trials have been followed for ≤12 months. Thus, the true long-

Table 6.3

Recurrence of Duodenal Ulcer during 12 Months after Healing with Various Bismuth-containing Regimens or H$_2$ Receptor Antagonists[a]

Author	Regimens[b]	Time after Completion of Therapy Clearance of *H. pylori* Assessed (wk)	Clearance of *H. pylori* (%)	No. of Ulcers Recurring after Healing		Total	
				H. pylori Still Present	*H. pylori* Eradicated	No.	%
Coghlan	Cim	Immediately	17	11/14	1/4	12/18	67
	CBS		52	8/10	3/11	11/21	52
Marshall	Cim ± T		2	30/34	0/1	30/35	86
	CBS	2	32	7/8	1/7	8/15	53
	CBS + T		74	0/2	5/18	5/20	25
Rauws	CBS	4	10	16/19	0/2	16/21	76
	CBS + A + M		88	1/2	0/15	1/17	6
Graham	Ran	≥4	0			95[c]	
	Ran + BSS + M + TC′		96			12[c]	

[a]Adapted from Peterson WL. N Engl J Med 1991; 324:1043–1048.
[b]Cim = cimetidine 400 mg twice daily for 6 weeks; CBS = colloidal bismuth subcitrate 120 mg four times daily for 6 weeks; Cim ± 1 cimetidine 400 mg twice daily for 8 weeks; T = tinidazole 500 mg twice daily for 10 days; A = amoxicillin 375 mg three times daily for 4 weeks; M = metronidazole 500 mg three times daily for 10 days; Ran = ranitidine 300 mg at bedtime for 2–16 weeks; BSS = bismuth subsalicylate 5–8 tablets/day × 14 days; M = metronidazole 250 mg three times daily for 14 days; TC = tetracycline 500 mg four times daily for 14 days.
[c]Life table method.

term efficacy of eradication of *H. pylori* remains unknown. Third, both *H. pylori* infection and gastric metaplasia are common findings in healthy controls. If *H. pylori* is so important in duodenal ulcer disease, why do so few individuals infected with the organism ever develop an ulcer?

At least the first reservation may now be dismissed. In a recent double-blind study from Vienna, patients with acute duodenal ulcer were treated with either ranitidine alone (300 mg at bedtime) for 6–10 weeks or ranitidine plus amoxicillin (750 mg three times daily) and metronidazole (500 mg three times daily) for the first 12 days (57). Not only was ulcer healing significantly faster with the combination regimen, but 12-month recurrence was significantly reduced.

Thus, the role of *H. pylori* in duodenal ulcer disease, at least chronic recurrent ulcer disease, seems real, even if the mechanism is not well-understood. Said another way, *H. pylori* is a necessary, but not by itself sufficient, pathogenetic factor in a majority of patients with duodenal ulcer. In this regard, it is like gastric acid. Each is necessary for the formation of an ulcer, even to-gether they are not sufficient to produce an ulcer, the means by which each predisposes to ulceration is unknown, and suppression or eradication of either sharply reduces the rate of ulcer recurrence. Further work is needed to determine why some individuals with *H. pylori* develop duodenal ulcers, but most do not.

Gastric Ulcer Disease

Fewer studies are available assessing the role of *H. pylori* in gastric ulcer, but it seems likely that it is an important factor in many patients (56). Approximately 65% of patients with gastric ulcer will be infected with *H. pylori*, NSAID use is present in another 25% of patients, and in about 10% neither *H. pylori* nor NSAID use is present. If NSAIDs are excluded, approximately 80% of gastric ulcer patients are *H. pylori* positive. One trial with small numbers of patients reported a 1-year recurrence rate of 13% in gastric ulcer patients whose ulcer was healed with ranitidine plus H. pyloricidal therapy compared with 74% recurrence in patients healed with ranitidine alone (56). Further eradication studies are needed in patients with gastric ulcer.

Table 6.4
**Seroprevalence of *H. pylori* 13–14 Years before Diagnosis in Patients
with Gastric Adenocarcinoma and Matched Controls[a]**

	Parsonnet et al. (68)	Nomura et al. (69)
Cohort size (N)	128,992	5,908
Follow-up (yr)	14.2	13
No. (%) of patients with cancer (N)	246 (0.2%)	137 (2.3%)
No. of patients selected as cases	136	109
H. pylori		
Cases	80	94
Controls	60	76
Odds ratio		
All AC	3.6	6.0
Intest type	3.1	4.5
Diffuse type	8.0	
GEJ cancer	0.8	

[a]Nested case control studies from References 68 and 69. Key to abbreviations: AC = adenocarcinoma; GEJ = gastroesophageal junction.

Functional Dyspepsia

The syndrome of epigastric distress especially related to meals, in patients with no evidence of peptic ulcer, reflux esophagitis, pancreatitis, or gallbladder disease has been termed non-ulcer or, more recently, functional dyspepsia. The notion that symptoms in such patients might be related to *H. pylori* gastritis met with a burst of enthusiasm, and a number of studies were conducted to see if eradication of the organism would improve symptoms (58–64). Although several reported success, all of these early studies were fatally flawed, with uninterpretable results. There were no long-term measurements of symptoms, follow-up diagnostic tests were performed too early to ensure that eradication had occurred, and the regimens used are now known to be poorly effective against *H. pylori*. Recent studies in which more effective regimens have been used and in which eradication has been properly assessed suggest that symptoms are improved in patients regardless of whether *H. pylori* has been eradicated (65–67). Even these studies evaluate short-term symptom response only. Well-designed studies with large numbers of patients followed for a minimum of 1 year after treatment are not available. Until such studies prove the benefit of eradication of *H. pylori*, antimicrobial therapy in patients with functional dyspepsia should be avoided.

Gastric Adenocarcinoma

It has long been known that the sequence of mucosal histologic events leading to the intestinal type of gastric adenocarcinoma is as follows: chronic superficial gastritis, atrophic gastritis, intestinal metaplasia, dysplasia, adenocarcinoma. It is now generally accepted that *H. pylori* is by far the most common cause of chronic superficial gastritis, that in some patients *H. pylori* gastritis progresses to atrophic gastritis, and that there is an epidemiologic association between *H. pylori* and gastric adenocarcinoma (68–69) (Table 6.4). On the other hand, there are problems with this scenario. First, as shown in Table 6.4, patients with the diffuse type of gastric adenocarcinoma are also linked epidemiologically with *H. pylori*. Since this type of cancer is not related to chronic gastritis, it is possible that *H. pylori* is merely a marker for other pre-neoplastic conditions. Second, even if *H. pylori* is important, other factors must also play a role. The prevalence of *H. pylori* is very high, and yet only a small proportion of patients will progress to atrophic gastritis, much less intestinal metaplasia, dysplasia, and cancer. As with peptic ulcer, *H. pylori* may be in many individuals a necessary but far from sufficient factor in the pathogenesis of gastric adenocarcinoma.

It has been suggested that eradication of *H. pylori* might dramatically reduce the incidence of gastric adenocarcinoma, the second most common cause of death from cancer worldwide. On the other hand, the lack of proof that this would actually happen, as well as the staggering costs and logistical difficulties of treating millions of people with antimicrobial therapy, realistically preclude such thoughts.

TREATMENT OF *H. PYLORI*
Definition of Eradication

It has become clear that failure to detect *H. pylori* immediately after a course of antimicrobial therapy does not mean that the organism is truly eradicated. In many instances the organism has only been suppressed, with follow-up studies performed several weeks later readily disclosing its presence. Somehow, *H. pylori* finds "sanctuary sites," which temporarily preclude its detection but from which it ultimately emerges to regain its foothold. Thus, eradication is now defined as absence of the organism by tests performed no sooner than 4 weeks after cessation of therapy.

Antimicrobial Agents

A remarkable assortment of agents, alone and in combination, has been utilized to eradicate *H. pylori* (70–74). It is clear that none of the standard therapeutic agents for ulcer has any meaningful effect on the organism, although early reports suggested that bismuth or omeprazole might. However, these represented instances in which the organism was suppressed rather than truly eradicated. Bismuth or omeprazole alone eradicate *H. pylori* in less than 20% of cases (73, 75, 76). Monotherapy with amoxicillin, the fluoroquinolones, or the nitroimidazoles is also ineffective (76, 77). With the latter, rapid emergence of resistance to *H. pylori* occurs when metronidazole or tinidazole is given alone. In one series, 70% of *H. pylori* became resistant when treated with tinidazole alone (77). The most effective agent to date given as monotherapy is clarithromycin. In a dosage of 500 mg four times daily, clarithromycin eradicated *H. pylori* in 54% of infected healthy volunteers (78).

Because of the poor results with monotherapy and with the emergence of resistance when single antibiotic agents were used, combination regimens have been designed and tested. A recent meta-analysis of the best available *H. pylori* eradication trials suggested that double therapy with combinations of a nitroimidazole (metronidazole, tinidazole) with either amoxicillin or a bismuth compound resulted in an eradication rate of 55–60% (77). Studies using triple therapy for 1 to 4 weeks with bismuth (primarily colloidal bismuth subcitrate in a dosage of 120 mg four times daily) plus metronidazole (800–1500 mg/day) plus either amoxicillin (375–500 mg three times daily) or tetracycline (500 mg four times daily) have reported eradication rates of 70–90% (77). Results are highly dependent on patient compliance. In one study, success was achieved in 96% of patients who took at least 60% of their prescribed medication compared with 69% in patients who took less (79). Reasons for poor compliance include the complexity of the regimens and side effects. In one study, complications occurred in >50% of patients taking triple therapy, with 20% discontinuing therapy (80).

The cornerstone of double and triple therapy regimens appears to be metronidazole. Combinations that do not include metronidazole are not as effective. Although combining other antimicrobial agents with metronidazole has markedly reduced the acquisition of new resistance, it has not solved the problem of preexisting resistance to metronidazole. Several studies have reported substantially lower eradication rates with triple therapy in patients whose organism was resistant to metronidazole prior to therapy (80, 81). In some areas of the world the proportion of isolates resistant to metronidazole approaches 80% (82). In another report from the United Kingdom, 19% of primary isolates were resistant, with the rate significantly higher (72%) in women <40 years of age (83). The differences in rates of resistance are most likely related to differences in the previous use of metronidazole for other purposes (e.g., amebiasis, gynecologic diseases).

Because of side effects to triple antimicrobial therapy and metronidazole resistance, agents to replace metronidazole as well as newer combinations are being tested. Clarithromycin appears to be the best candidate to replace metronidazole in triple therapy, although results are still preliminary. Because they are effective against metronidazole-resistant organisms and appear to have fewer side effects, the most promising regimens are combinations of omeprazole and either amoxicillin or clarithromycin. Omeprazole in a dose of 40 mg/day plus either amoxicillin (2 g/day) or clarithromycin (500 mg three times daily) has been reported to eradicate *H. pylori* in up to 80% of cases (84, 85). Further data, however, are needed to confirm these preliminary results.

It is my opinion that, based on evidence currently available, a trial of *H. pylori*cidal therapy is reasonable for most patients who are *H. pylori* positive and have recurrent peptic ulcer disease. Such individuals might otherwise be candidates for long-term maintenance therapy with H_2-receptor antagonists or surgery, courses of action that are expensive and, with the latter, associated with some morbidity and mortality. Therefore, a course of antimicrobial therapy directed against *H. pylori* is a reasonable, relatively safe, and inexpensive alternative.

There are, however, several groups of ulcer patients whom I would not treat for *H. pylori*. These include patients with very mild disease, patients with Zollinger-Ellison syndrome, and patients who are old and infirm who might not tolerate the antimicrobial regimens. Because maintenance therapy with H_2-receptor antagonists is so effective, and until controlled trials are performed in these patients, I also do not advocate treatment of *H. pylori* in patients with a history of ulcer bleeding or perforation. Said another way, I would be unwilling at this time to stop maintenance H_2-receptor antagonist therapy in such patients even if eradication were successful. Since eradication will not change management, it serves no purpose. The only exception might be patients for whom maintenance H_2-receptor antagonist therapy has failed and who are not candidates for surgery.

The current gold standard in the United States is a 2-week course of triple therapy with Pepto bismol (2 tablets four times daily), metronidazole (250 mg three times daily), and tetracycline (500 mg four times daily) or amoxicillin (500 mg three times daily). Confirmation of *H. pylori* infection prior to therapy is essential (see diagnosis above) and, if at all possible, pre- and 4–6-week post-therapy breath tests should be obtained. If the post-therapy breath test is positive, therapy has failed and alternative measures are indicated.

It has been suggested that the family members of peptic ulcer patients in whom eradication has been achieved should also be treated to prevent reinfection. In my opinion, the rate of reinfection (probably no more than 0.5%/year) appears to be too low to justify such a practice at present.

Finally, until evidence of efficacy is available, treatment of patients with functional dyspepsia should be avoided.

THE FUTURE

During the 10 years since *H. pylori* was detected, an enormous amount of information has unfolded. During the next ten years, research will likely continue in several areas. One will certainly deal with the organism itself—how it is transmitted, how it produces gastritis. A more thorough understanding of its virulence factors will surely develop. A second area will explore the reasons why some infected individuals develop peptic ulcers or gastric adenocarcinoma, but most do not. A third will undoubtedly deal with new ways to eradicate *H. pylori* with less complicated, safer antimicrobial regimens or through novel means that attack the organism through its virulence factors (86, 87). Finally vaccine development *may* occur. Although this may pose difficult technical problems, early work in experimental animals suggests it can be accomplished (88). If successful, vaccination represents the most effective means of reducing the incidence of gastric adenocarcinoma in those parts of the world where it remains a major problem. Unfortunately, the very people at greatest need for such a vaccine reside in the countries with the least resources for purchase and distribution. This reality plus the ever-present risks of litigation inherent with vaccines, must be overcome before the enormous sums required to develop and test vaccines can be justified.

REFERENCES

1. Warren JR. Unidentified curved bacilli on gastric epithelium in active chronic gastritis [Letter]. Lancet 1983;1:1273.
2. Marshall B. Unidentified curved bacilli on gastric epithelium in active chronic gastritis [Letter]. Lancet 1983;1:1273–1274.
3. Evans DJ, Jr, Evans DG, Graham DY, Klein PD. A sensitive and specific serologic test for detection of *Campylobacter pylori* infection. Gastroenterology 1989;96:1004–1008.
4. Graham DY, Evans DJ, Alpert LC, et al. *Campylobacter pylori* detected noninvasively by the ^{13}C-urea breath test. Lancet 1987;29:1174–1177.
5. Peterson WL, Lee E, Feldman M. Relationship between *Campylobacter pylori* and gastritis in healthy humans after administration of placebo or indomethacin. Gastroenterology 1988;95:1185–1197.
6. Sobala GM, Crabtree JE, Pentith JA, et al. Screening dyspepsia by serology to *Helicobacter pylori*. Lancet 1991;338:94–96.
7. Podolsky I, Lee E, Cohen R, Peterson WL. Prevalence of *C. pylori* (CP) in healthy subjects and patients with peptic diseases [Abstract]. Gastroenterology 1989;96:A394.
8. Dooley CP, Cohen H, Fitzgibbons PL, et al. Prevalence of *Helicobacter pylori* infection and histologic gastritis in asymptomatic persons. N Engl J Med 1989;321:1562–1566.
9. Graham DY, Malaty HM, Evans DG, Evans DJ, Jr, Klein PD, Adam E. Epidemiology of *Helicobacter pylori* in an asymptomatic population in the United States. Gastroenterology 1991;100:1495–1501.
10. Parsonnet J, Blaser MJ, Perez-Perez GI, Hargrett-Bean N, Tauxe RV. Symptoms and risk factors of *Helicobacter pylori* infection in a cohort of epidemiologists. Gastroenterology 1992;102:41–46.
11. Malaty HM, Evans DG, Evans DJ, Jr, Graham D. *Helicobacter pylori* in hispanics: comparison with blacks and whites of similar age and socioeconomic class. Gastroenterology 1992;103:813–816.
12. Drumm B, Perez-Perez GI, Blaser MJ, Sherman PM. Intrafamilial clustering of *Helicobacter pylori* infection. N Engl J Med 1990;322:359–363.
13. Malaty HM, Graham DY, Evans DG, Adams E, Evans DJ. Transmission of *Helicobacter pylori* infec-
tion: studies in families of healthy individuals. Scand J Gastroenterol 1991;26:927–932.
14. Perez-Perez GI, Witkin SS, Decker MD, Blaser MJ. Seroprevalence of *Helicobacter pylori* infection in couples. J Clin Microbiol 1991;29:642–644.
15. Krajden S, Fuksa M, Anderson J, et al. Examination of human stomach biopsies, saliva and dental plaque for *Campylobacter pylori*. J Clin Microbiol 1989;27:1397–1398.
16. Shames B, Krajden S, Fuksa M, Babida C, Penner JL. Evidence for the occurrence of the same strain of Campylobacter pylori in the stomach and dental plaque. J Clin Microbiol 1989;27:2849–2850.
17. Thomas JE, Gibson GR, Darboe MK, Dale A, Weaver LT. Isolation of *Helicobacter pylori* from human faeces. Lancet 1992;340:1194–1195.
18. Sitas F, Forman D, Yarnell JWG, et al. *Helicobacter pylori* infection rates in relation to age and social class in a population of Welsh men. Gut 1991;32:25–28.
19. Mendall MA, Goggin PM, Molineaux N, et al. Childhood living conditions and *Helicobacter pylori* seropositivity in adult life. Lancet 1992;339:896–897.
20. Mitchell HM, Lee A, Carrick J. Increased incidence of *Campylobacter pylori* infection in gastroenterologists: further evidence to support person-to-person transmission of *C. pylori*. Scand J Gastroenterol 1989;24:396–400.
21. Edwards PD, Carrick J, Turner J, et al. *Helicobacter pylori*-associated gastritis is rare in AIDS: antibiotic effect or a consequence of immunodeficiency? Am J Gastroenterol 1991;86:1761–1764.
22. Blaser MJ. Hypotheses on the pathogenesis and natural history of *Helicobacter pylori*-induced inflammation. Gastroenterology 1992;102:720–727.
23. Goggin PM, Marrero JM, Spychal RT, et al. Surface hydrophobicity of gastric mucosa in *Helicobacter pylori* infection: effect of clearance and eradication. Gastroenterology 1992;103:1486–1490.
24. Krakowka S, Morgan DR, Kraft WG, Leunk RD. Establishment of gastric Campylobacter pylori infection in the neonatal gnotobiotic piglet. Infect Immun 1987;55:2789–2796.
25. Hazell SL, Eichberg JW, Lee DR, et al. Selection of the chimpanzee over the baboon as a model for *Helicobacter pylori* infection. Gastroenterology 1992;103:848–854.
26. Lee A, Fox JG, Otto G, Murphy J. A small animal model of human *Helicobacter pylori* active chronic gastritis. Gastroenterology 1990;99:1315–1323.
27. Marshall BJ, Armstrong JA, McGechie DB, Glancy RJ. Attempt to fulfill Koch's postulates for pyloric *Campylobacter*. Med J Aust 1985;142:436–439.
28. Morris A, Nicholson G. Ingestion of *Campylobacter pyloridis* causes gastritis and raised fasting gastric pH. Am J Gastroenterol 1987;82:192–199.
29. Morris AJ, Ali MR, Nicholson GI, Perez-Perez GI, Blaser MJ. Long-term follow-up of voluntary ingestion of *Helicobacter pylori*. Ann Intern Med 1991;114:662–663.

30. Eaton KA, Morgan DR, Krakowka S. *Campylobacter pylori* virulence factors in gnotobiotic piglets. Infect Immunol 1989;57:1119–1125.

31. Evans DG, Evans DJ, Moulds JJ, Graham DY. N-acetylneuraminyllactose-binding fibrillar hemagglutinin of *Campylobacter pylori*: a putative colonization factor antigen. Infect Immun 1988;56:2896–2906.

32. Lingwood CA, Pellizzari A, Law H, Sherman P, Drumm B. Gastric glycerolipid as a receptor for *Campylobacter pylori*. Lancet 1989;2:238–241.

33. Smoot DT, Mobley HLT, Gilliam T, Phelps P, Resau JH. Pedestal formation of *Helicobacter (Campylobacter) pylori* with gastric epithelial cells in vitro may require actin polymerization [Abstract]. Gastroenterology 1990;98:A127.

34. Hessey SJ, Spencer J, Wyatt JI, et al. Bacterial adhesion and disease activity in *Helicobacter*-associated chronic gastritis. Gut 1990;31:134–138.

35. Eaton KA, Morgan DR, Brooks C, Krakowka S. Essential role of urease in the pathogenesis of gastritis induced by *Helicobacter pylori* in gnotobiotic piglets. Infect Immun 1989;59:2470–2475.

36. Marshall BJ, Barrett LJ, Prakash C, McCallum RW, Guerrant RL. Urea protects *Helicobacter (Campylobacter) pylori* from the bactericidal effect of acid. Gastroenterology 1990;99:697–702.

37. Parsons CL, Stauffer C, Mulholland CS, Griffith DP. Effect of ammonium on bacterial adherence to bladder transitional epithelium. J Urol 1984;132:365–366.

38. Smoot DT, Bobley HLT, Chippendale GR, Lewison JF, Resau JH. *Helicobacter pylori* urease activity is toxic in human gastric epithelial cells. Infect Immun 1990;58:1992–1994.

39. Xu J, Goodwin CS, Cooper M, Robinson J. Intracellular vacuolization caused by the urease of *Helicobacter pylori*. J Infect Dis 1990;161:1302–1304.

40. Craig PM, Karnes WE, Territo MC, Walsh JH. *Helicobacter pylori* secretes a chemotactic factor for monocytes and neutrophils. Gut 1992;33:1020–1023.

41. Mai UEH, Perez-Perez GI, Wahl LM, et al. Soluble surface proteins from *Helicobacter pylori* activate monocytes/macrophages by lipopolysaccharide-independent mechanism. J Clin Invest 1991;87:894–900.

42. Mooney C, Keenan J, Munster D, et al. Neutrophil activation by *Helicobacter pylori*. Gut 1991;32:853–857.

43. Leunk RD, Ferguson MA, Morgan DR, Low DE, Simar AE. Antibody to cytotoxin infection by *Helicobacter pylori*. J Clin Microbiol 1990;28:1181–1184.

44. Hupertz V, Czinn S. Demonstration of a cytoxin from *Campylobacter pylori*. Eur J Clin Microbiol Infect Dis 1988;7:576–578.

45. Cover TL, Blaser MJ. Purification and characterization of the vacuolating toxin from *Helicobacter pylori*. J Biol Chem 1992;267:10570–10575.

46. Peterson W, Barnett C, Evans DJ, et al. Role of *H. pylori* in gastric acid secretion and serum gastrin concentrations in health subjects and patients with duodenal ulcer [Abstract]. Gastroenterology 1991;100:A140.

47. Cave DR, Vargas M. Effect of a *Campylobacter pylori* protein on acid secretion by parietal cells. Lancet 1989;2:187–189.

48. Dooley CP, Akriviadis E, El-Newihi HM, Dehesa M, Cohen H, Fitzgibbons PL. Distinctive features of *Helicobacter pylori* infection and gastroduodenal histology in duodenal ulcer [Abstract]. Gastroenterology 1990;98:A37.

49. Murthy UK, Linscheer R, Cho C. The hypergastrinemia in *Helicobacter pylori* (HP)-gastritis is due to a decrease in antral D cell density and D:G cell ratio [Abstract]. Gastroenterology 1992;102:A130.

50. Kaneko H, Nakada K, Mitsuma T, et al. *Helicobacter pylori* infection induces a decrease in immunoreactive-somatostatin concentrations of human stomach. Dig Dis Sci 1992;37:409–416.

51. Moss SF, Legon S, Bishop AE, Polak JM, Calam J. Effect of *Helicobacter pylori* on gastric somatostatin in duodenal ulcer disease. Lancet 1992;340:930–932.

52. Graham DY. *Campylobacter pylori* and peptic ulcer disease. Gastroenterology 1989;96:615–625.

53. Coghlan JG, Humphries H, Dooley C, et al. *Campylobacter pylori* and recurrence of duodenal ulcers: a 12-month follow-up study. Lancet 1987;2:1109–1111.

54. Marshall BJ, Goodwin CS, Warren JR, et al. Prospective double-blind trial of duodenal ulcer relapse after eradication of *Campylobacter pylori*. Lancet 1988;2:1437–1442.

55. Rauws EAJ, Tytgat GNJ. Cure of duodenal ulcer associated with eradication of *Helicobacter pylori*. Lancet 1990;335:1233–1235.

56. Graham DY, Lew GM, Klein PD, et al. Effect of treatment of *Helicobacter pylori* infection on the long-term recurrence of gastric or duodenal ulcer: a randomized, controlled study. Ann Intern Med 1992;116:705–708.

57. Hentschel E, Brandstatter G, Dragosics B, et al. Effect of ranitidine and amoxicillin plus metronidazole on the eradication of *Helicobacter pylori* and the recurrence of duodenal ulcer. N Engl J Med 1993;328:308–312.

58. Morgan D, Kraft W, Bender M, Pearson A. Nitrofurans in the treatment of gastritis associated with *Campylobacter pylori*. Gastroenterology 1988;95:1178–1184.

59. Glupczynski Y, Burette A, Labbe M, Deprez C, De Reuck M, Deltenre M. *Campylobacter pylori*-associated gastritis: a double-blind placebo-controlled trial with amoxycillin. Am J Gastroenterol 1988;83:365–372.

60. Rokkas T, Pursey C, Uzoechina E, et al. Non-ulcer dyspepsia and short term De-Nol therapy: a placebo controlled trial with particular reference to the role of *Campylobacter pylori*. Gut 1988;29:1386–1391.

61. Lambert JR, Dunn K, Borromeo M, Korman MG, Hansky J. *Campylobacter pylori*: a role in non-ulcer dyspepsia? Scand J Gastroenterol 1988;24(suppl 160):7–13.

62. Loffeld R, Potters H, Stobberingh E, Flendrig J, Van Spreeuwel J, Arends J. *Campylobacter*-associated gastritis in patients with non-ulcer dyspepsia: a double blind placebo controlled trial with colloidal bismuth subcitrate. Gut 1989;30:1206–1212.

63. Kang JY, Tay HH, Wee A, Guan R, Math MV, Yap I. Effect of colloidal bismuth subcitrate on symptoms and gastric histology in non-ulcer dyspepsia: a double blind placebo controlled study. Gut 1990;31:476–480.

64. Marshall BJ, Valenzuela JE, McCallum RW, et al. A placebo controlled clinical trial of bismuth subsalicylate for the treatment of *Helicobacter pylori*-associated gastritis [Abstract]. Gastroenterology 1990;98:A83.

65. Patchett S, Beattie S, Leen E, et al. *Helicobacter pylori* and non-ulcer dyspepsia. Gastroenterology 1992;103:340–347.

66. Elta G, Barnett J, Scheiman J, et al. The effect of treatment for *Helicobacter pylori* on non-ulcer dyspepsia symptoms [Abstract]. Gastroenterology 1992;102:A63.

67. Holcombe C, Thom C, Kaluba J, Lucas SB. *Helicobacter pylori* clearance in the treatment of non-ulcer dyspepsia. Aliment Pharmacol Ther 1992;6:119–123.

68. Parsonnet J, Friedman GD, Vandersteen DP, Chang Y, et al. *Helicobacter pylori* infection and the risk of gastric carcinoma. N Engl J Med 1991;325:1127–1131.

69. Nomura A, Stemmermann GN, Chyou P, Kato I, et al. *Helicobacter pylori* infection and gastric carcinoma among Japanese Americans in Hawaii. N Engl J Med 1991;325:1132–1136.

70. Graham DY, Borsch GMA. The who's and when's of therapy for *Helicobacter pylori*. Am J Gastroenterol 1990;85:1552–1555.

71. Glupczynski Y, Burette A. Drug therapy for *Helicobacter pylori* infection: problems and pitfalls. Am J Gastroenterol 1990;85:1545–1551.

72. Axon ATR. *Helicobacter pylori* therapy: effect on peptic ulcer disease. J Gastroenterol Hepatol 1991;6:131–137.

73. Chiba N, Rao BV, Rademaker JW, Hunt RH. Meta-analysis of the efficacy of antibiotic therapy in eradicating *H. pylori*. Am J Gastroenterol 1992;87:1716–1727.

74. Heatley RV. The treatment of *Helicobacter pylori* infection. Aliment Pharmacol Ther 1992;6:291–303.

75. Weil J, Bell GD, Powell K, et al. Omeprazole and *Helicobacter pylori*: temporary suppression rather than true eradication. Aliment Pharmacol Ther 1991;5:309–313.

76. Daw MA, Deegan P, Leen E, Omorain C. The effect of omeprazole on *Helicobacter pylori* and associated gastritis. Aliment Pharmacol Ther 1991;5:435–439.

77. Goodwin CS, Marshall BJ, Blincow ED, Wilson DH, Blackbourn S, Phillips M. Prevention of nitroimidazole resistance in *Campylobacter pylori* by coadministration of colloidal bismuth subcitrate: clinical and in vitro studies. J Clin Pathol 1988;41:207–210.

78. Peterson WL and members of the Clarithromycin/*H. pylori* Study Group. Clarithromycin as monotherapy for eradication of *Helicobacter pylori* [Abstract]. Am J Gastroenterol 1992;87:1274.

79. Graham DY, Lew GM, Malaty HM, et al. Factors influencing the eradication of *Helicobacter pylori* with triple therapy. Gastroenterology 1992;102:493–496.

80. Bell GD, Powell K, Burridge SM, et al. Experience with 'triple' anti-*Helicobacter pylori* eradication therapy: side effects and the importance of testing the pre-treatment bacterial isolate for metronidazole resistance. Aliment Pharmacol Ther 1992;6:427–435.

81. Weil J, Bell GD, Powell K, et al. *Helicobacter pylori* infection treated with a tripotassium dicitrato bismuthate and metronidazole combination. Aliment Pharmacol Ther 1990;4:651–657.

82. Glupczynski Y, Burette A, De Koster E, et al. Metronidazole resistance in *Helicobacter pylori* [Letter]. Lancet 1990;335:976–977.

83. Weil J, Bell GD, Powell D, et al. *Helicobacter pylori* and metronidazole resistance [Letter]. Lancet 1990;336:1445.

84. Bayerdorffer E, Mannes GA, Sommer A, et al. High dose omeprazole treatment combined with amoxicillin eradicates *Helicobacter pylori* [Abstract]. Gastroenterology 1992;102:A38.

85. Logan RPH, Gummett PA, Hegarty BT, Walker MM, Baron JH, Misiewicz JJ. Clarithromycin and omeprazole for *Helicobacter pylori* [Letter]. Lancet 1992;340:239.

86. Graham DY. Treatment of peptic ulcers caused by *Helicobacter pylori* [Editorial]. N Engl J Med 1993;328:349–350.

87. Goldschmiedt M, Peterson WL. The role of *H. pylori* in peptic ulcer disease. Semin Gastrointest Dis 1993;4:13–20.

88. Eaton KA, Krakowka S. Chronic active gastritis due to *Helicobacter pylori* in immunized gnotobiotic piglets. Gastroenterology 1992;103:1580–1586.

SECTION

II

DISORDERS OF GASTROINTESTINAL MOTILITY

7

A Pharmacologic Approach
to Noncardiac Chest Pain

SCOTT R. BRAZER and JOEL E. RICHTER

INTRODUCTION

Chest pain is a common symptom complaint; 12% of all adult members of a Seattle Health Maintenance Organization (HMO) complained of chest pain in a 6-month period (1). Chest pain is often an alarming symptom to both the patient and the physician because of its association with potentially life-threatening conditions such as ischemic heart disease. Of the Seattle HMO members who experienced chest pain, 35% sought medical care. Many of these patients underwent cardiac catheterization as part of their evaluation. In 1986, 775,000 cardiac catheterizations were performed in the United States (2); it is likely this figure has now eclipsed one million annually. Approximately 20% of patients with chest pain who undergo cardiac catheterization will have normal or insignificantly diseased coronary arteries (3, 4) and are grouped as "noncardiac chest pain."

A more accurate term is chest pain of undetermined etiology (CPUE) and such patients face a "good news/bad news" situation. The good news is that mortality is very low in this subgroup. In a study of 1977 consecutive patients seen at Duke University Medical Center with normal or insignificantly diseased coronary arteries, survival without a fatal cardiac event exceeded 98% at 10 years (4). The bad news is that the quality of life of these patients is markedly diminished. In the same study, 70% of 1631 patients had persistent chest pain, and the frequency did not decrease with time. Furthermore, the functional status of these patients was compromised; 50% could not perform moderate to heavy exercise without chest pain and 20% took a less demanding job because of their "heart problem." These patients also overutilized health care resources: in a single year 14% had a cardiac-related hospitalization, 31% took antianginal medication, 10% took antidepressants, and 17% took tranquilizers. It is estimated that the yearly medical cost for a single patient with CPUE is $3500 (5).

The complexity of CPUE has confounded researchers for over 100 years (6). CPUE is a heterogeneous disorder with similar symptoms occurring in patients with multiple disorders including gastrointestinal (e.g., esophageal motility disorders and gastroesophageal reflux), psychiatric (e.g., panic disorder and depression), cardiac (e.g., mitral valve prolapse and microvascular angina), or musculoskeletal (e.g., chest wall pain and fibromylagia) disorders. Unfortunately, association does not equate with causation. Many of the suggested causes of CPUE do not stand up to careful scrutiny (7). Furthermore, the history of CPUE brings to mind the story of the blind men and the elephant. In this story, six blind men touch different parts of an elephant so that they might "see" him. Each man sees the elephant from a distinct perspective and is convinced that the elephant is: a wall (the elephant's side); a spear (a tusk); a snake (the trunk); a tree (a leg); a fan (an ear); and a rope

109

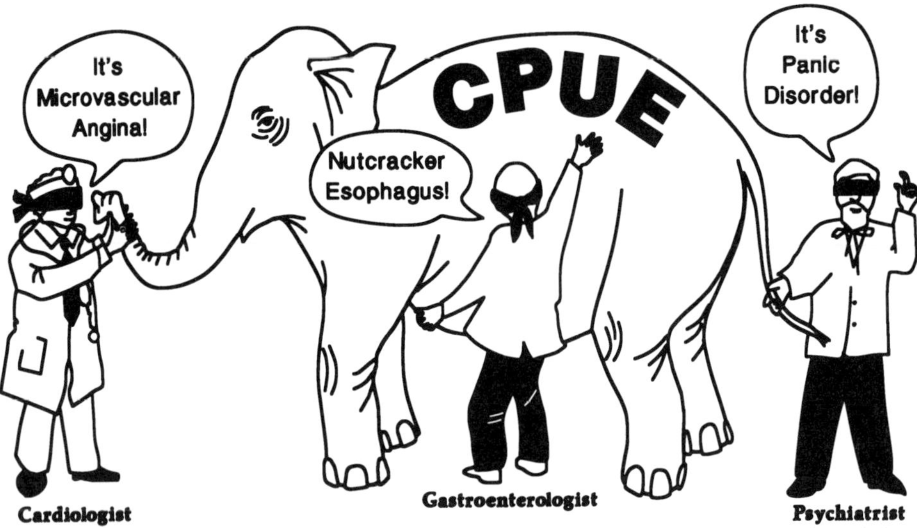

Figure 7.1. Specialists often "see" only their own areas of expertise when evaluating the patient with chest pain of undetermined etiology (CPUE).

(the tail). Using this analogy, gastroenterologists have ascribed CPUE to being an esophageal motility disorder or gastroesophageal reflux, cardiologists believe mitral valve prolapse or microvascular angina is the cause, and psychiatrists believe CPUE reflects an underlying panic disorder (Fig. 7.1). An overall view of CPUE has been provided by investigators whose studies look beyond their individual subspeciality (8–11). For example, Clouse and Lustman (8) found that 84% of patients with an esophageal motility disorder also carried a psychiatric diagnosis such as depression, somatization, and anxiety disorders; this contrasts with a 31% figure for patients with normal esophageal motility.

In this chapter, we will review the differential diagnosis of chest pain and then examine the treatment of these challenging patients.

DIFFERENTIAL DIAGNOSIS

Exclusion of significant coronary artery disease is essential in the workup of patients with chest pain. Although history remains the cornerstone of the evaluation, it does not always differentiate ischemic heart disease from other causes of chest pain (12–14). Even the experts occasionally miss significant coronary artery disease in patients with atypical pain (15, 16). Once coronary artery disease has been excluded, the differential can be narrowed to disorders of the esophageal, psychiatric, cardiovascular (other than epicardial coronary artery disease), and musculoskeletal systems. A nomogram, developed to predict the likelihood of esophageal chest pain (14), uses age and four historical features of esophageal chest pain: background chest discomfort, retrosternal pain without lateral radiation, regurgitation, and provocation with eating. Unfortunately, this model was developed in an extremely small patient sample (18 patients with esophageal chest pain) and is therefore unlikely to perform well in independent patient populations (17).

Esophageal Disorders

GASTROESOPHAGEAL REFLUX

The discovery that gastroesophageal reflux (GER) causes chest pain in some individuals is one of the most important clinical breakthroughs in the past decade. This advance followed the technological development of compact computerized systems with miniature pH probes that allow continuous ambulatory pH monitoring. Not only does ambulatory pH monitoring quantitate esophageal acid contact, but one can witness spontaneous episodes of chest pain and determine their temporal correlation with reflux episodes (Fig. 7.2).

DeMeester et al. were among the first to study patients with typical angina pectoris and normal coronary arteries with ambulatory pH monitoring (18). Abnormal acid contact times were observed in 23 of 50 (46%) of these patients. Subsequent studies have confirmed the findings of DeMeester et al. suggesting that gastroesophageal reflux is found in approximately one-fourth to one-half of all patients with CPUE (19, 20). Gastroesophageal reflux may also contribute to chest pain in patients with significant coronary artery disease (CAD). For example, 20 of 30 (67%) patients with CAD and refractory chest pain despite maximum medical therapy had evidence of gastroesophageal reflux-induced pain on ambulatory pH testing (21). The diagnosis of GER is extremely important in that it provides the potential for effective treatment.

The majority of patients with GER-induced chest pain give a history of typical reflux symptoms, such as heartburn, regurgitation, waterbrash, or dysphagia. The pain may be more frequent or severe after ingestion of a meal or assumption of the supine position, and may ameliorate with antacids. However, GER cannot be ruled out in the patient lacking heartburn. Ten to twenty per cent of patients with chest pain and GER do not have typical reflux symptoms (18, 22).

Exercise may provoke gastroesophageal reflux, producing a pattern of chest pain that has features similar to typical angina pectoris. Normal volunteers have four times more acid reflux during running than when at rest (23). Schofield and coworkers studied exercise induced GER in 52 patients with typical angina pectoris and normal coronary arteries using combined treadmill and ambulatory pH testing (24). While 11 patients exhibited increased acid contact time by 24 hour pH monitoring, an additional 13 patients had reflux and chest pain brought on only by exercise.

Treatment may be initiated in patients with CPUE and typical reflux symptoms on the basis of symptoms alone. However, the diagnosis of GERD should be established in patients who do not respond to empiric treatment, in patients in whom long-term treatment is proposed, or in patients who lack typical reflux symptoms. Several tests have been used to diagnose GERD (Table 7.1) including barium swallow, upper gastrointestinal (GI) endoscopy with or without biopsy, and ambulatory pH monitoring (22).

ESOPHAGEAL MOTILITY DISORDERS

Esophageal spasm was suggested as a cause of chest pain by Soranus of Ephesus in the 2nd century *A.D.* Osler believed hysterical or hypochondriacal patients suffered from "oesophagismus" (25). More recently, abnormal esophageal contractions and distention have been proposed to cause chest pain by stimulating mechanical nociceptors or inducing esophageal ischemia (26–28).

The advent of low-compliance, pneumohydraulic esophageal manometry in the late 1960s provided the opportunity to examine the relationship between abnormal esophageal motility and chest pain. Significant advances in our understanding of normal and abnormal esophageal motility followed the careful examination of normal volunteers and patients with chest pain (29, 30). New motility disorders were defined on the basis of abnormal esophageal peristalsis, and the amplitude or duration of contractions (Table 7.2).

Motility disorders can be delineated in 20–56% of patients with CPUE (19, 30–32). In the largest series to date, 910 patients with CPUE were studied at the Bowman Gray School of Medicine (30). Of the total, 13% had the nutcracker esophagus, 10% had nonspecific esophageal motility disorder, 3% had diffuse esophageal spasm, and 1% had hypertensive lower esophageal sphincter. Only 0.5% had achalasia.

Esophageal motility disorders may be suggested by a barium esophagram, but are best diagnosed with esophageal manometry. The

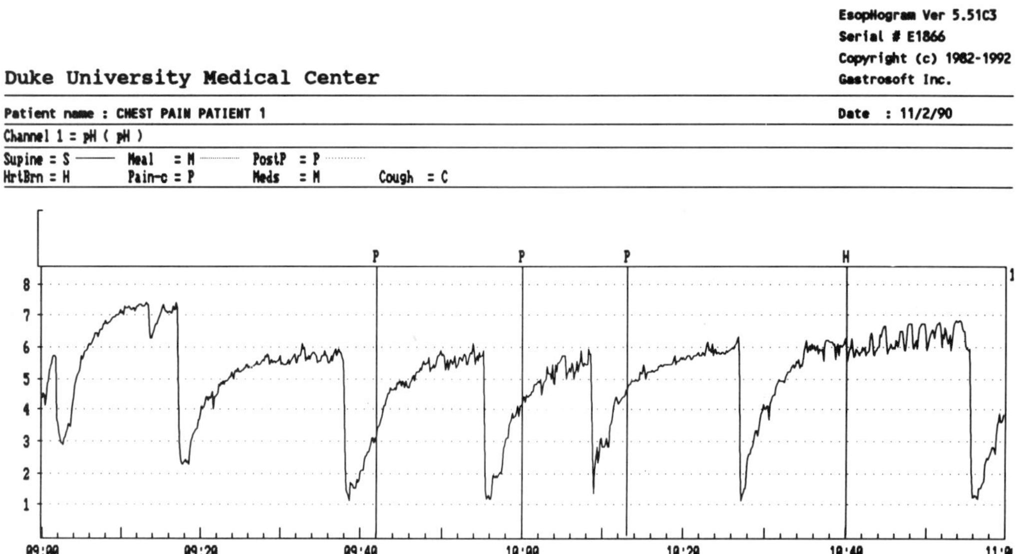

Figure 7.2. Temporal association of acid reflux and chest pain. A 2-hour segment of an ambulatory pH tracing from 9–11 *AM* in a patient with chest pain of undetermined etiology (CPUE) demonstrates an excellent correlation of chest pain episodes (*P*) with reflux episodes (defined as pH < 4).

nomenclature established by Castell and Richter are the most widely used (Table 7.2).

Only the well-recognized disorder of achalasia is a convincing cause of esophageal chest pain. It is a true disease with typical symptoms and characteristic anatomic findings. Patients with achalasia may complain of chest pain early in the course of their disease, before the symptoms of dysphagia predominate. Young patients with achalasia may complain of chest pain more often than the elderly (33). While dysphagia may occur in any patient with an esophageal motility disorder, patients with achalasia typically have progressive dysphagia for solids and liquids.

Unfortunately, the bulk of the evidence supporting motility disorders as a cause of chest pain is not convincing (7). First, the severity of manometric abnormalities does not correlate with the severity of the patient's chest pain. For example, the amplitude of esophageal contractions does not mirror chest pain severity in patients with the "nutcracker" esophagus. Second, the temporal relationship between abnormal esophageal contractions and chest pain is imperfect. Ambulatory mo-

tility monitoring may show a high amplitude or long duration contraction wave before an episode of chest pain, but these contraction abnormalities are as likely to occur after the episode of pain (Fig. 7.3) (31). Thus the esophageal motility disorder may be *due* to the pain rather than be its cause.

Although some of these new motility disorders may evolve to achalasia (34), many result from gastroesophageal reflux (35, 36), stress (37–39), a myopathy, a neuropathy, or an unidentified disorder that is related to both the chest pain and the motility disorder. Furthermore, some subjects are normal individuals who happen to fall in the extreme right tail of the distribution curve (i.e., false positive diagnosis of a motility disorder).

Psychiatric Disorders

ANXIETY DISORDERS

Panic disorder is the most common anxiety-related disease found in CPUE patients, occurring in one-third to one-half of these individuals undergoing psychiatric evaluation (40–43). The evidence that panic disorder

Table 7.1
Diagnostic Tests for Gastroesophageal Reflux Disease[a]

	Sensitivity	Specificity
	%	
Tests that indicate reflux potential		
Hypotensive lower esophageal sphincter (<10 mm Hg)	58	84
Tests that indicate esophageal damage		
Endoscopy ($>$ grade I esophagitis)	68	96
Mucosal biopsy	77	91
Double-contrast barium esophagram	60	93
Tests that show reflux		
Barium esophagram	40	85
Standard Acid Reflux Test		
Basal	40	99
Loading	84	83
Gastroesophageal scintigraphy	61	95
Ambulatory pH monitoring	88	98

[a]From Richter JE, Castell DO. Gastroesophageal reflux: pathogenesis, diagnosis, and therapy. Ann Intern Med 1982;97:93–103.

Table 7.2
Manometric Criteria for Diagnosis of Esophageal Motility Disorders

Diagnosis	Required Manometric Criteria
Achalasia	Aperistalsis of esophageal body
Nutcracker	Mean distal esophageal contraction >180 mm Hg; normal peristalsis
Diffuse esophageal spasm	Simultaneous contractions $>10\%$; intermittent normal peristalsis
Hypertensive lower esophageal sphincter	Lower esophageal sphincter pressure >45 mm Hg
Nonspecific esophageal motility disorder	Abnormal motility not described above

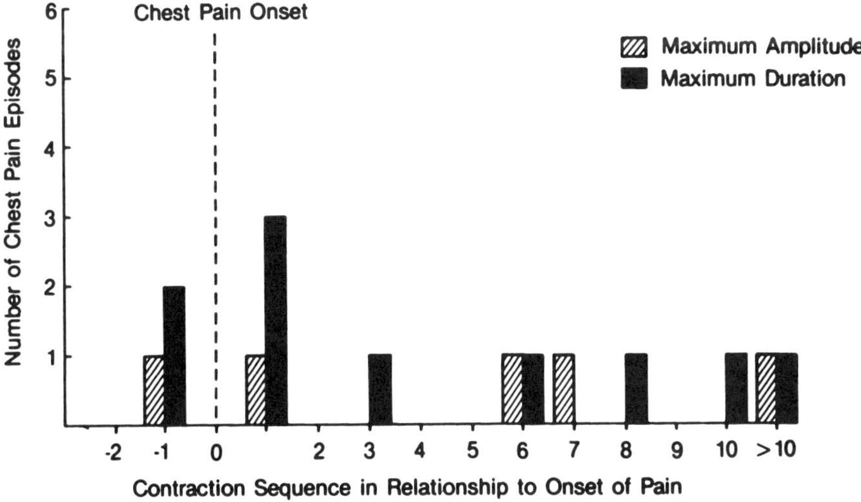

Figure 7.3. Temporal relation of abnormal esophageal contractions with chest pain by ambulatory motility testing. Abnormal esophageal contractions were as likely to occur after the onset of chest pain. From Peters L, Maas L, Petty D, et al. Spontaneous noncardiac chest pain: evaluation by 24-hour ambulatory esophageal motility and pH monitoring. Gastroenterology 1988;94:878–886.

causes chest pain is strong. First, 60% of patients with panic disorder complain of chest pain (44). Second, Katon found panic in 40% of patients with chest pain and normal coronary arteries vs. a prevalence of only 5% in patients with chest pain and coronary artery disease (43). Third, successful treatment of panic disorder improves chest pain (15, 45).

Although the cause of panic disorder is unknown, there are two primary hypotheses: a biologic hypothesis and a behavioral-cognitive hypothesis. The biological hypothesis attributes the disorder to a primary abnormality of the CNS, for example, lack of CNS control of the locus ceruleus. The locus ceruleus, a region near the fourth ventricle that is loaded with adrenergic neurons, may be stimulated by electric or pharmacologic means. This stimulation produces anxiety in humans and experimental animals. The behavioral-cognitive hypothesis suggests that panic attacks result from a phobic response to minor physical sensations. Gorman and colleagues have proposed a neuroantomical model that encorporates both hypotheses (46). Hyperventilation may play an important role in the genesis of chest pain in panic disorder (41, 47–49). Patients with chest pain and anxiety frequently have resting hypocapnia (41).

Panic disorder should be looked for in all patients with disabling chest pain, in patients with a past history of depression, and in those patients with social phobias. Panic disorder is diagnosed by history on the basis of DSM-IIIR criteria (Table 7.3). The Hospital Anxiety and Depression Scale is a brief, patient-administered questionnaire that has been validated against formal psychiatric interview (50). It has been used as a screen for anxiety and depression in patients with chest pain who are undergoing exercise tolerance testing (51). This diagnosis is extremely important because, like gastroesophageal reflux, panic disorder is treatable.

DEPRESSION

In one-half of cases, depressed patients present with a somatic symptom as chief complaint (52, 53), and chest pain is a frequent symptom. Depression is found in approximately one-third of patients with CPUE (43, 54) and may antedate or coexist with a panic disorder. In a series of 48 patients with CPUE, Carney and colleagues found major depression in 38%, panic disorder in 10%, and both conditions in 6% (54). Beitman et al. found that 44% of the patients with CPUE and panic disorder have either a current (21%) or past (23%) history of depression (55).

SOMATIZATION DISORDER

Somatization disorder is marked by multiple somatic complaints dating from childhood or early adulthood that defy medical explanation. Chest pain is often a symptom of somatization disorder (56, 57). It occurs primarily in women and is usually diagnosed in the fifth or sixth decades of life. A history of panic attacks is often present.

Cardiovascular Disorders

MICROVASCULAR ANGINA

Chest pain may result from myocardial ischemia despite anatomically normal coronary arteries. This condition is referred to as "syndrome X" or microvascular angina (58). Although it is very difficult to accurately quantitate myocardial blood flow in humans (59), several studies provide evidence of inadequate coronary perfusion reserve in these patients. First, increased myocardial lactate production, reflecting anaerobic metabolism, can be demonstrated in up to 100% of patients examined (60–62). Second, sustained coronary sinus oxygen desaturation (which is a response typical of obstructive coronary artery disease) has been demonstrated in two patients after atrial pacing (63). Third, coronary blood flow does not rise appropriately in these patients with pacing (61) or dipyridamole treatment (62). Fourth, exercise-induced wall motion abnormalities (64) or a fall in ejection fraction (65) are frequently seen in these patients. Fifth, Cannon and coworkers have demonstrated a relative increase in coronary vascular resistance in patients with CPUE in whom chest pain develops following intravenous er-

Table 7.3
DSM-IIIR Criteria for Diagnosis of Panic Disorder[a]

At least 4 attacks of intense fear or discomfort[b] in a 4-week period or one or more attacks followed by a period of at least 1 month of persistent fear of another attack in association with at least four of the following:

1. Dyspnea or smothering sensation
2. Dizziness, lightheadedness, or unsteady feelings
3. Palpitations or tachycardia
4. Trembling or shaking
5. Diaphoresis
6. Choking
7. Nausea or abdominal discomfort
8. Depersonalization or feelings of unreality
9. Paresthesias
10. Hot flashes or chills
11. Chest pain or discomfort
12. Fear of dying
13. Fear of going crazy or doing something uncontrolled

[a]From Anonymous. Diagnostic and statistical manual of mental disorders. 3rd ed rev. Washington DC: American Psychiatric Association, 1987.
[b]Symptoms not due to a medical illness.

gonovine and atrial pacing compared with patients in whom chest pain does not develop (66). These findings all support an underlying abnormality of the coronary microcirculation.

Although there is evidence for ischemia in these patients, the severity of chest pain is out of proportion to the degree of demonstrable ischemia. This may reflect heightened visceral nociception. In one study, 10 of 11 patients with CPUE, had their typical chest pain provoked by manipulation of a catheter in the right heart (67). No patient with valvular or coronary artery disease had chest pain with these maneuvers. Right heart catheter manipulation, right atrial pacing, and intracoronary injection of contrast caused chest pain in 29 of 36 patients with CPUE tested at the National Institutes of Health (NIH) (68). Only 2 of 33 patients with coronary artery disease and 0 of 10 patients with valvular heart disease experienced chest pain during these maneuvers.

The diagnosis of microvascular angina should be considered in patients with typical angina and normal coronary arteries. The diagnosis may be confirmed in clinical practice by demonstrating a functional abnormality (e.g., a fall in left ventricular ejection fraction with exercise) in patients with otherwise normal coronary angiography.

MITRAL VALVE PROLAPSE

Mitral valve prolapse is found in 7–56% of patients with CPUE in selected series (69, 70). The diagnosis of mitral valve prolapse can be made either by the typical auscultory findings of midsystolic click(s) and/or late systolic murmur or with echocardiography (71). However, the evidence supporting a causal association of mitral valve prolapse and chest pain is very weak (72); 80% of patients with chest pain and mitral valve prolapse also have an esophageal motility disorder (73) or a psychiatric disorder (54). The mere association of mitral valve prolapse with chest pain and panic disorder may be due to ascertainment bias. In an elegant study, Devereux et al. examined the first-degree relatives of symptomatic patients with mitral valve prolapse (74). Those relatives with mitral valve prolapse who did not present to medical attention were compared with two control groups without mitral valve prolapse. The study concluded that chest pain and panic attacks were not associated with mitral valve prolapse. Most investigators agree that mitral valve prolapse does not cause chest pain or panic disorder (75–77). Mayou (78) in his review on atypical chest pain stated, "It is likely that anxious patients find this incidental finding less than reassuring and that it may be

Table 7.4
Criteria for Diagnosis of Musculoskeletal Chest Pain[a]

Diagnosis requires the following major criteria plus at least two of the seven minor criteria.

Major Criterion

Palpation tenderness of the chest wall that is similar in quality and location to the spontaneously occurring pain

Minor Criteria

1. Pain accentuated by movement
2. Pain improved by local heat, cold, or analgesic
3. Dull, aching, or nagging pain with variable intensity and/or duration
4. Nocturnal attacks of pain are rare and, if present, clearly relate to position
5. Pain upon arising in the morning
6. At least one provocative test positive for exacerbation or onset of pain similar in quality and location to spontaneously occurring pain:
    a. Horizontal flexion of the arm
    b. "Crowing rooster" maneuver
7. Diffuse poorly defined musculoskeletal pain in locations beyond the chest

[a]From Brazer S, Schmitt C, Varia I, et al. Chest pain of undetermined etiology (CPUE): multiple MDs + tests = multiple diagnoses [Abstract]. Am J Gastroenterol 1992;87:1244.

a perpetuating factor for chest pain having quite a different etiology" (p. 399).

Musculoskeletal Disorders

Chest pain may result from musculoskeletal disorders including musculoskeletal (chest wall) chest pain, ankylosing spondylitis, fibromyalgia, Tietze's syndrome, rheumatoid arthritis, thoracic outlet syndrome, and slipping rib syndrome (79). Semble and Wise prospectively evaluated 101 patients with CPUE and found a definite musculoskeletal cause of chest pain in 16% (80). Levine and Maschette used a systematic musculoskeletal examination to determine the prevalence of musculoskeletal chest pain in a prospective study of 62 patients referred for cardiac catheterization (81). Of 25 patients with normal or insignificantly diseased coronary arteries, 5 (20%) met their criteria for musculoskeletal chest pain. Using published criteria (81, 82) modified by McCallum (Table 4.4), we have found musculoskeletal chest pain in 7 of 24 (29%) patients prospectively evaluated at Duke University Medical Center (83).

Patients with ankylosing spondylitis (84) or fibromyalgia (85) may present with chest pain. The diagnosis of ankylosing spondylitis is made by demonstrating reduced chest expansion with inspiration (≤3 cm) and observing the characteristic findings on thoracic spine

and pelvic X-ray. The diagnosis of fibromyalgia is based on the presence of >3 month history of widespread pain with >10 of 18 tender-point sites on digital palpation (86). Patients with fibromyalgia have significantly more obscure somatic complaints than do patients with rheumatoid arthritis (87).

Tietze's syndrome is a rare disorder marked by chest pain and swelling, usually of the left second or third costochondral cartilage (80). Rheumatoid arthritis may produce chest pain by affecting the manubriosternal or sternoclavicular joints. Patients with thoracic outlet syndrome may complain of chest pain and arm paresthesias due to compression of the brachial plexus and subclavian vessels (88).

Heightened Visceral Nociception

The coexistence of multiple disorders in a single patient (8–11) has led to the suggestion that an underlying abnormality could be linking these conditions. However, specific disturbances have not been identified. Leading candidates include a diffuse disorder affecting smooth muscle or, conversely, a neurosensory disturbance leading to abnormal visceral nociception (pain perception).

Heightened visceral nociception refers to the increased sensitivity to visceral stimuli that is found frequently in patients with CPUE (67–89). These patients develop chest pain in response to physiologic events that would cause no symptoms in normal individuals.

Provocative tests are directed toward delineation of heightened visceral nociception in that they use stimuli which characteristically cause chest pain in patients but not in healthy volunteers. These include tests used by gastroenterologists (e.g., the edrophonium test, acid perfusion test, or balloon distension test); psychiatrists (e.g., sodium lactate challenge or voluntary hyperventilation); cardiologists (e.g., rapid atrial pacing, adenosine or ergonovine administration); and rheumatologists (e.g., chest wall palpation).

Although these tests were initially designed to be markers of specific disorders, their specificity has been questioned. For example, it was traditionally taught that the acid perfusion test and edrophonium test were specific markers for gastroesophageal reflux disease and esophageal motility disorders, respectively. However, ambulatory pH and motility testing reveal that these provocative tests are equally likely to be abnormal in patients with either condition (90, 91). The overlap of positive edrophonium and acid perfusion tests in the same patient (92) suggests a more global abnormality of visceral nociception.

The abnormalities causing heightened visceral nociception are unknown. The disorder may result from malfunction of any component of the nociceptive pathway including the nociceptor itself, the ascending nociceptive pathway, the central nervous system, the descending antinociceptive pathway, or neurotransmitter release (93). Several neurotransmitters have been identified that play a role in pain perception and transmission including substance P, calcitonin gene-related peptide, and serotonin (94). Specific antagonists of the 5HT-3 receptor, for example, ondansetron and granisetron, may block visceral pain perception, as will be discussed.

TREATMENT
General Considerations
RANDOMIZED CONTROLLED TRIAL
Forty years ago, Hill argued that treatment efficacy must be established by using the ran-

domized controlled trial (95). Unfortunately, there are few randomized controlled trials examining treatment of patients with CPUE. The uncontrolled trials of patients with CPUE are particularly difficult to interpret because many patients are known to improve while receiving placebo. For example, Richter et al. found that the mean chest pain index improved nearly 25% with placebo in patients with the nutcracker esophagus (96). Dager and colleagues noted that 30–50% of patients with panic disorder improve when treated with placebo in controlled trials (97). Similarly, Clouse and coworkers found that chest pain intensity decreased by >50% with placebo treatment in patients with esophageal motility disorders (98).

PROBLEM OF INADEQUATE SAMPLE SIZE
Randomized controlled trials may miss a clinically important difference between treatments when in fact it exists because of an inadequate sample size (99). This is referred to as a type II error. Studies of CPUE patients are particularly prone to this problem because there is an extreme variation in the frequency and severity of chest pain within and among individual subjects. Sample sizes must be large in such instances. For example, a study having an 80% chance of finding a 50% drop in chest pain severity or frequency would require over 200 patients (mean and variance data from [96]).

Crossover studies, which use subjects as their own controls, seem to be an attractive way to reduce the required sample size. Unfortunately, crossover studies are appropriate only when the investigator can exclude a carryover effect. A carryover effect exists when the difference in efficacy varies with the order of treatment. For example, placebo may appear to be effective if it follows a therapeutic agent with a sustained effect. With rare exceptions, it is impossible to rule out a carryover effect without employing formal statistical tests. These tests require more patients than would be needed to do a parallel-design, randomized controlled trial.

PROBLEM OF PSYCHIATRIC DIAGNOSES IN "MEDICAL" PATIENTS

Physicians must be careful to explain that a psychiatric illness (e.g., panic disorder) is a real disorder like hypertension or diabetes (100). Patients with psychiatric disorders presenting for medical attention with somatic complaints are often reluctant to accept a psychiatric diagnosis, referral, or treatment. They may believe their physician considers their pain to be imaginary or "all in their head." Overcoming the stigma associated with the diagnosis of panic disorder is a difficult process for the patient. Patients may become angry, confused, and refuse further evaluation and treatment.

For all of these reasons, the results of published efficacy trials in the literature may not be generalizable to patients with CPUE as a whole. For example, patients who enroll in studies of panic disorder have sufficient insight to answer television or newspaper advertisements for study entry (101). These patients are likely to be much different than those patients with panic disorder and chest pain who believe they have heart disease. It is up to the skillful clinician to overcome the patient's anger and distrust of physicians in order to provide effective therapy. In a study of CPUE and panic disorder, one of the reasons that 75% of patients screened were not enrolled was the patient belief that pain was due to a medical rather than a psychiatric cause (102).

PATIENT-PHYSICIAN RELATIONSHIP

In some patients, a caring and compassionate physician may be all that is necessary to relieve chest pain (103). Patients who remembered being informed of an esophageal disorder required less medical care and suffered less disability and limitation of activities than did patients who did not recall being told or who did not have an esophageal disorder (104).

Effective treatment awaits the patient with CPUE whose physician is aware of these potential problems.

SPECIFIC DRUG THERAPY

Gastroesophageal Reflux Disease

A detailed treatment of gastroesophageal reflux disease is covered in Chapter 2. However, it is important to emphasize that there have been no randomized controlled trials specifically examining patients with gastroesophageal reflux presenting with the primary complaint of chest pain.

Three uncontrolled reports suggest that high-dose H_2-receptor antagonists or omeprazole are effective treatment. In the first, DeMeester et al. noted 7 of 12 patients with CPUE and evidence of GER improved on medical therapy (18). In the second study, 13 patients with CPUE and evidence of GER were treated in an open study with high-dose ranitidine (150 mg three times daily to 300 mg four times daily) (105). The mean symptom score improved from 2.87 to 0.68 after 8 weeks of therapy, and seven patients had complete resolution of their chest pain. In the third study, 13 of 20 patients (65%) with significant coronary artery disease and refractory chest pain (despite maximum medical therapy) had marked improvement of their chest pain after vigorous acid suppression with high dose H_2-blockers or omeprazole for 8 weeks (21).

Two uncontrolled series suggest that Nissen fundoplication surgery provides relief of chest pain in patients with CPUE and evidence of GER. DeMeester et al. noted improvement of chest pain in 10 of 11 patients following fundoplication (18). Similarly, in a series of 24 patients with CPUE and evidence of GER treated with Nissen fundoplication by Bancewicz et al. (106), 23 of 24 had resolution of their chest pain over a follow-up period of 3 to 6 years. Although these studies suggest that patients with chest pain and evidence of GER respond to medical or surgical antireflux treatment, they are uncontrolled, unblinded, and subject to investigator bias.

Richter and colleagues treated 16 patients with CPUE and abnormal ambulatory pH testing with omeprazole 20 mg daily for 8 weeks followed by placebo treatment for 8 weeks (107). Although patients knew they were initially treated with omeprazole, they were unaware of the replacement of active treatment with placebo during the second half of the trial. Twelve patients (75%) treated with omeprazole improved, but 7 of these had worsening of their chest pain when switched to placebo. While this study was not double-blinded and lacked concurrent controls, it provides the best evidence to date that aggressive acid suppressive therapy is superior to placebo in the treatment of these patients.

On occasion, a randomized controlled trial of GERD has included the frequency of chest pain in the patients studied. For example, Bremner et al. studied 125 patients with reflux esophagitis in a randomized, double-blind trial of ranitidine 150 mg twice daily vs. sucralfate 6 g daily (108). Chest pain was relieved in 63% of patients receiving ranitidine vs. 86% of those receiving sucralfate. In another study, ranitidine was more effective than placebo in decreasing chest pain (109).

TREATMENT RECOMMENDATIONS FOR GERD-RELATED CHEST PAIN

Patients with typical reflux symptoms and chest pain may be treated empirically with life-style modifications and usual doses of an H_2-blocker (e.g., ranitidine 150 mg or famotidine 20 mg twice daily, every day, and every evening 30 minutes after meals). However, atypical symptoms of gastroesophageal reflux, including chest pain, may be refractory to standard medical treatment. Patients who have failed an empiric trial of life-style modifications and H_2-blocker or those patients with chest pain alone should have the diagnosis of GER confirmed.

There are three treatment options for those patients with confirmed GER and refractory chest pain. First, they may respond to higher doses of an H_2-blocker. We suggest ranitidine 150 mg four times daily, 300 mg twice daily, or famotidine 40 mg twice daily. A second option is treatment with the proton pump inhibitor, omeprazole. We usually start treatment with 20 mg daily for 1 month. Those patients whose chest pain is not controlled may respond to higher doses, for example, 20 mg twice daily. High-dose omeprazole should be given two or three times daily before meals to improve absorption. Antireflux surgery should be considered for those patients with severe pain, proven gastroesophageal reflux, and strong evidence of a temporal association on ambulatory pH testing between reflux episodes and chest pain. We recommend this infrequently and only for patients in whom aggressive acid suppression has relieved their chest pain. The age of the patient, the expense of chronic medication, and the potential long-term risk of medical treatment (i.e., with omeprazole) are other factors to consider when recommending surgery.

Esophageal Motility Disorders

SMOOTH MUSCLE RELAXANTS

If esophageal motility disorders cause chest pain via abnormal smooth muscle contractions, it would be logical to presume that drugs relaxing smooth muscle would improve chest pain. Unfortunately, the experience with smooth muscle relaxants has been disappointing (110). To paraphrase Chalmers, investigations can be divided into two groups: those with enthusiasm and no controls vs. those with controls but no enthusiasm (111). Anticholinergic drugs (112, 113), hydralazine (114), nitrates (115), and calcium channel blockers (116, 117) can all decrease esophageal contraction amplitudes. Moreover, hydralazine (114), nitrates (114, 115), and calcium channel blockers (116–118) are all reported to be effective in the treatment of chest pain in patients with esophageal motility disorders when studied in an uncontrolled, unblinded fashion.

The five placebo-controlled trials examining the use of calcium channel blockers in patients with CPUE and esophageal motility disorders produce a different picture. Two studies concluded that calcium channel blockers relieve chest pain, while three studies concluded they were ineffective. In the first positive study, 15 patients with chest pain and an esophageal motility disorder (8 with hypertensive lower esophageal sphincter, 2 with diffuse esophageal spasm, 4 with achalasia, and 1 with nutcracker esophagus) were treated with nifedipine in a placebo-controlled, crossover trial (119). Of the 15 patients, 12 favored nifedipine over placebo, 1 preferred placebo, and 2 had no preference. In the second positive study, 22 patients with the nutcracker esophagus received diltiazem in a 16-week placebo-controlled, double-blind crossover trial (16). The mean chest pain index (severity × frequency) was lowered by approximately 50% during treatment with diltiazem 60–90 mg orally four times a day. Unfortunately, the dropout rate was excessive; only 14 of the original 22 patients completed the study. Furthermore, only 9 of those 14 patients would meet 1992 diagnostic criteria for nutcracker esophagus.

Three studies could show no treatment effect. In the first, 10 patients with esophageal spasm received nifedipine 10–40 mg orally three times per day for 4 weeks followed by placebo for at least 4 weeks (120). There were no differences in chest pain frequency or severity. In a second study, 14 patients with an esophageal motility disorder and chest pain or dysphagia completed an 8-week double-blind, placebo-controlled crossover trial comparing diltiazem 90 mg four times daily with placebo (121). Again, there was no improvement in chest pain while patients received diltiazem. Finally, Richter and coworkers studied the effects of nifedipine in 20 patients with the nutcracker esophagus in a 14-week, placebo-controlled double-blind crossover study (96). Although the distal esophageal contraction amplitude was decreased with active therapy (123 mm Hg vs. 198 mm Hg, $P < .005$), multiple parameters of chest pain (frequency, severity, and their product) were unaffected by nifedipine therapy.

The most obvious explanation for the discrepancy is that the negative studies are simply examples of a type II error. The largest study to date, that of Richter et al. with 20 patients (96), has nearly an 80% chance of missing a difference as large as 50% between active therapy and placebo. However, other factors are likely to be important because these drugs are not predictably effective in clinical practice.

OTHER TREATMENTS

In a well-designed study, Clouse and coworkers examined the effect of an antidepressant, trazodone, in the treatment of 35 patients with esophageal symptoms, about half of whom complained of chest pain and esophageal motility disorders (98). Twenty-nine patients completed the 6-week placebo-controlled, double-blind parallel trial of trazodone in a dosage of 100–150 mg orally every day. Although there were no differences in chest pain frequency or intensity, patients treated with trazodone had less distress from esophageal symptoms, including chest pain. Furthermore, patients treated with trazodone reported a greater overall global improvement. Thus, trazodone decreased chest pain distress without affecting esophageal motility.

Anecdotal reports suggest that esophageal bougienage may be effective treatment for patients with chest pain and esophageal motility disorders. However, Winters and coworkers found that placebo bougienage with a 24-F was as effective as therapeutic bougienage with a 54-F in patients with nutcracker esophagus (122).

Although uncontrolled series suggest that surgical myotomy is effective treatment of patients with chest pain and motility disorders (123), Stein and DeMeester believe that chest pain alone should never be an indication for myotomy (124).

TREATMENT RECOMMENDATIONS FOR ESOPHAGEAL MOTILITY DISORDER-ASSOCIATED CHEST PAIN

Esophageal motility disorders, other than achalasia, are very difficult to treat. It is important to remember that two treatable conditions may coexist in patients with an esophageal motility disorder, i.e., gastroesophageal reflux and panic disorder. Both should be excluded before embarking on long-term treatment or more extensive investigation.

Some patients with CPUE and an esophageal motility disorder will respond to calcium channel blockers. We recommend starting with nifedipine 10–20 mg orally four times daily 30 minutes before meals and every night.

The long-acting preparations may be used for long-term treatment. Nitrates and diltiazem may be tried in individual patient trials. Although trazodone 100–150 mg every day may work for some patients with esophageal motility disorders, the side effect of priapism limits its usefulness in men.

We do not recommend surgical myotomy for the treatment of any esophageal motility disorder, with the obvious exception of achalasia.

Psychiatric Disorders

PANIC DISORDER

The first step in treating a patient with panic disorder is patient education. Patients should be told about the disorder, its prevalence, possible etiology, and available treatments (125). Although there are no controlled treatment trials of panic disorder in CPUE patients, several randomized controlled trials have demonstrated the efficacy of several psychotropic drugs in patients with panic disorder diagnosed in a psychiatric setting.

Tricyclic Antidepressants

There are at least 14 double-blind, placebo-controlled studies of the use of imipramine (130–300 mg daily) in panic disorder (126, 127). Eleven show imipramine to be beneficial over placebo. The three negative studies suffer significant methodologic problems (126). A recent meta-analysis concluded that the average patient had a 25% improvement with imipramine over placebo (128); the mean time of response was 6 weeks. Approximately one-fourth of patients treated with imipramine in controlled trials drop out (126), many from troublesome side effects such as xerostomia, tachycardia, sexual dysfunction, or overstimulation. Clorimpramine also is effective based on a double-blind, placebo-controlled trial (129).

Benzodiazepines

Alprazolam, clonazepam (130), and diazepam (131) are effective drugs for the treatment of panic disorder based on placebo-controlled trials. Alprazolam was more effective than placebo in all 12 double-blind, placebo-controlled trials published to date (126, 127, 132). For example, in the largest series to date, alprazolam was proven effective in the treatment of panic attacks in an 8-week, placebo-controlled trial of 526 patients (101). At week 4, 50% of treated patients vs. 28% of controls receiving placebo were free of panic attacks. Although these patients did not present with CPUE, an uncontrolled trial suggests that alprazolam works in that group as well (102). In the meta-analysis by Wilkinson and colleagues (128), benzodiazepines were equal in efficacy to imipramine with an average improvement in patient symptoms of 25% and a mean response time of 7 weeks. Their advantage of rapid onset must be weighed against the risk of abuse, dependence, and withdrawal symptoms (126). Abuse seems limited primarily to patients with a personal or family history of drug or alcohol abuse. Therefore, these patients should receive an alternative therapy. Alprazolam should be slowly weaned by 0.25 mg every week after 6 months of therapy. Despite this slow tapering, symptoms of withdrawal may still occur. Alprazolam is better tolerated than imipramine; the drop out rate in randomized, controlled trials is approximately one-half that of imipramine-treated patients (13% vs. 27% [126]).

Serotonin Reuptake Inhibitors

Fluoxetine shows promise in the treatment of panic disorder in early, uncontrolled trials (133, 134). However, up to 50% of treated patients will experience overstimulation when treatment is begun with the standard 20 mg daily dose (133).

Monoamine Oxidase Inhibitors

Despite evidence of efficacy in a double-blind, placebo-controlled trial (135), this class of medications is not widely used in the United States because of fear of inducing hypertensive crisis.

β-Blockers

Although propranolol has been effective in the control of certain autonomic symptoms associated with anxiety such as diaphoresis, trembling, and palpitations (136), the effectiveness of propranolol in the treatment of panic disorder is controversial. In the only placebo-controlled trial, propranolol was no more effective than placebo in decreasing the frequency or severity of panic attacks after 5 weeks of therapy (137). Propranolol was shown to be equivalent to imipramine (138) and diazepam (139) in crossover studies. Neither study excluded the possibility of a carryover effect. In the most recent study (140), 15 patients receiving a mean daily dose of 182 mg of propranolol had improvement similar to that of 14 patients receiving a mean daily dose of 5 mg of alprazolam.

Cognitive/Behavioral Therapy

It is important that the CPUE patient learn to control stress and improve coping strategies. Klimes and coworkers randomized 31 patients with CPUE to either immediate or delayed cognitive-behavioral therapy (15). The cognitive-behavioral treatment focused on training patients to deal with pain, associated autonomic symptoms, and concerns about illness. Patients receiving cognitive-behavioral treatment had fewer days of pain, decreased total pain episodes, less activity avoidance, disruption, psychologic stress, and depressed mood.

DEPRESSION AND SOMATOFORM DISORDER

The treatment of depression and somatoform disorder is beyond the scope of this chapter. The reader is referred to standard texts or recent reviews by Calabrese and Markovitz (141), Smith (142), and Morrison (143).

TREATMENT RECOMMENDATIONS FOR PSYCHIATRIC DISORDER-RELATED CHEST PAIN

In those patients with panic disorder without severe anxiety, antidepressants are recommended as first-line therapy. We suggest that imipramine be used, beginning with a low dose, 10 mg every night, to minimize side effects. The dose should be increased slowly by 10 mg every 2–4 days to a dose of 50 mg. Thereafter, the dose may be increased by 25 mg every 2–4 days to a target of 150–200 mg every night (2.5 mg/kg/day). Eliciting a response may take 6–24 weeks (144) and patients may continue to improve for the first year of therapy. Patients should be maintained on treatment for at least 6 months or as long as there is continued improvement. Imipramine should be gradually tapered by 25 mg every 3 days. Despite the gradual tapering of the drug, fully 15–30% of patients will relapse within 2 years.

Those patients with severe anxiety may benefit from the more rapid effects of an anxiolytic. Alprazolam, begun in doses of 0.25–0.5 mg four times daily, will improve anxiety within 1–2 weeks.

Cardiovascular Disorders

MICROVASCULAR ANGINA

Cannon and coworkers treated 26 microvascular angina patients with either verapamil or nifedipine in a 1-month double-blind, placebo-controlled crossover study (145). The patient population was skewed because all subjects had responded to either verapamil or nifedipine in an unblinded lead-in phase. Not surprisingly, the 22 patients who completed the study suffered fewer episodes of chest pain while on the calcium channel blocker (21 in 28 days) than while on placebo (35 in 28 days). Twenty-two patients felt better overall on active treatment compared to placebo vs. just one patient who favored placebo (3 had no preference).

MITRAL VALVE PROLAPSE

In an uncontrolled study, propranolol improved chest pain in only 2 of 8 patients with mitral valve prolapse (146).

TREATMENT RECOMMENDATIONS FOR MICROVASCULAR ANGINA

Patients with typical exertional angina, normal coronary anatomy and an abnormal functional study (e.g., exercise tolerance test or radionuclide angiogram) may respond to

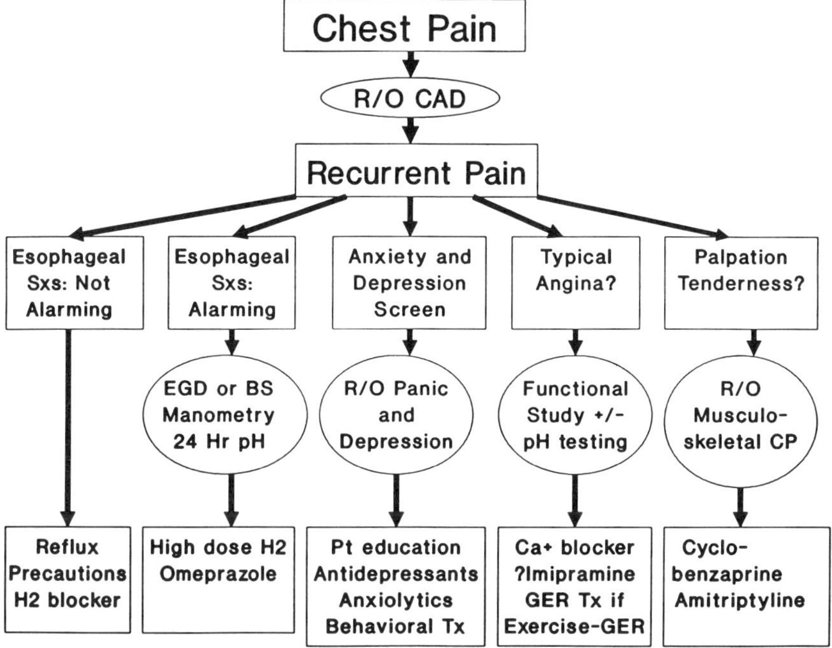

Figure 7.4. Algorithm for the evaluation and treatment of patients with chest pain.

treatment with a calcium channel blocker, i.e., verapamil 80 mg orally four times daily or nifedipine 10 mg four times daily.

Musculoskeletal Disorders

While patients with musculoskeletal chest pain alone may respond to nonsteroidal anti-inflammatory drugs (NSAIDs), fibromyalgia patients do not respond to NSAIDs alone (147). Cyclobenzaprine, 10–40 mg daily was studied in patients with fibromyalgia in a double-blind, placebo-controlled trial of 120 patients over a 12-week period (148). Cyclobenzaprine-treated patients had a nearly 30% decrease in pain severity of all types vs. <10% improvement in placebo-treated patients. In another randomized controlled trial of 42 patients with fibromyalgia, a cardiovascular training program decreased pain threshold scores and improved patient and physician global assessment scores (149). Finally, amitriptyline has been shown to be effective in the treatment of fibromyalgia (150, 151).

TREATMENT RECOMMENDATIONS FOR MUSCULOSKELETAL-RELATED CHEST PAIN

Patients with musculoskeletal chest pain may be treated with reassurance, local heat, NSAIDs, and, in certain cases, corticosteroid-lidocaine injection (152). Patients with CPUE overlapping with fibromyalgia may benefit from cyclobenzaprine (2.5–10 mg four times daily) or amitriptyline (10–50 mg at bedtime).

Heightened Visceral Nociception

Pain perception may be modified by serotonin antagonists or imipramine. Because heightened visceral nociception might result from a serotonergic hypersensitivity, Stark and coworkers studied the effects of ondansetron, a 5 HT_3 antagonist, in patients with abnormal esophageal balloon distension tests (153). Chest pain developed in these patients during inflation of an intraesophageal latex balloon at volumes that did not produce pain in normal control subjects. An intravenous injection of ondansetron prior to repeat balloon distension normalized the patients' response. In another study by the same investigators (154), 30 patients with CPUE were randomized to one of three treatment arms: placebo for 2 months; placebo for 1 month followed by clonidine 0.1 mg orally twice daily; and placebo for 1 month followed by imipramine 50 mg every night for 1 month. Chest pain decreased significantly in patients receiving imipramine only.

TREATMENT RECOMMENDATIONS FOR ABNORMAL VISCERAL NOCICEPTION

Patients with heightened visceral nociception may be identified on the basis of positive provocative tests. Potential treatments include trazodone 100–150 mg every day or imipramine 50 mg orally every night. The serotonin and cholecystokihin antagonists may prove effective treatments in the future. Research is underway to examine the role of these agents in the treatment of heightened visceral nociception.

SUMMARY

Patients with CPUE are often difficult to diagnose and manage effectively (Fig. 7.4). The initial step in the evaluation of these patients is to rule out coronary artery disease. Thereafter, physicians should not view CPUE as a single disorder, but must be aware of its multidimensional nature and complexity. Panic disorder and gastroesophageal reflux should be excluded in all CPUE patients with refractory pain; both are common and potentially most treatable.

REFERENCES

1. Von Korff M, Dworkin SF, Le Resche L, Kruger A. An epidemiologic comparison of pain complaints. Pain 1988;32:173–183.
2. Feinleib M, Havlik RJ, Gillum RF, Pokras R, McCarthy E, Moien M. Coronary heart disease and related procedures. National Hospital Discharge Survey Data. Circulation 1989;79(suppl 1):I13–I18.
3. Ockene IS, Shay MJ, Alpert JS, Weiner BH, Dalen JE. Unexplained chest pain in patients with normal coronary arteriograms: a follow-up study of functional status. N Engl J Med 1980;303:1249–1252.
4. Papanicolaou MN, Califf RM, Hlatky MA, et al. Prognostic implications of angiographically normal and insignificantly narrowed coronary arteries. Am J Cardiol 1986;58:1181–1187.
5. Richter JE, Bradley LA, Castell DO. Esophageal chest pain: current controversies in pathogenesis, diagnosis, and therapy. Ann Intern Med 1989;110:66–78.
6. DaCosta JM. On irritable heart: a clinical study of a form of functional cardiac disorder and its consequences. Am J Med Sci 1871;61:17–52.
7. Brazer SR. Chest pain of esophageal origin. Semin Gastrointest Dis 1992;3:166–175.
8. Clouse RE, Lustman PJ. Psychiatric illness and contraction abnormalities of the esophagus. N Engl J Med 1983;309:1337–1342.
9. Richter JE, Obrecht WF, Bradley LA, Young LD, Anderson KO. Psychological comparison of patients with nutcracker esophagus and irritable bowel syndrome. Dig Dis Sci 1986;31:131–138.
10. Schofield PM, Brooks NH, Colgan S, et al. Left ventricular function and oesophageal function in patients with angina pectoris and normal coronary arteriograms. Br Heart J 1987;58:218–224.
11. Cannon RO III, Cattau EL Jr, Yakshe PN, et al. Coronary flow reserve, esophageal motility, and chest pain in patients with angiographically normal coronary arteries. Am J Med 1990;88:217–220.
12. Schofield PM, Whorwell PJ, Jones PE, Brooks NH, Bennett DH. Differentiation of "esophageal" and "cardiac" chest pain. Am J Cardiol 1988;62:315–316.
13. McCroskery JH, Schell RE, Sprafkin RP, Lantinga LJ, Warner RA, Hill N. Differentiating anginal patients with coronary artery disease from those with normal coronary arteries using psychological measures. Am J Cardiol 1991;67:645–646.
14. Alban Davies H. Anginal pain of esophageal origin: clinical presentation, prevalence, and prognosis. Am J Med 1992;92(suppl 5A):5S–10S.
15. Klimes I, Mayou RA, Pearce MJ, Coles L, Fagg JR. Psychological treatment for atypical non-cardiac chest pain: a controlled evaluation. Psychol Med 1990;20:605–611.
16. Cattau EL Jr, Castell DO, Johnson DA, et al. Diltiazem therapy for symptoms associated with nutcracker esophagus. Am J Gastroenterol 1991;86:272–276.
17. Harrell FE, Lee KL, Califf RM, Pryor DB, Rosati RA. Regression modelling strategies for improved prognostic prediction. Stat Med 1984;3:143–153.
18. DeMeester TR, O'Sullivan GC, Bermudez G, Midell AI, Cimochowski GE, O'Drobinak J. Esophageal function in patients with anginal-like chest pain and normal coronary arteriograms. Ann Surg 1982;196:488–498.
19. Janssens J, Vantrappen G, Ghillebert G. 24-Hour recording of esophageal pressure and pH in patients with noncardiac chest pain. Gastroenterology 1986;90:1978–1984.
20. Hewson EG, Sinclair JW, Dalton CB, Richter JE. Twenty-four-hour esophageal pH monitoring: the

most useful test for evaluating noncardiac chest pain. Am J Med 1991;90:576–583.

21. Singh S, Richter JE, Hewson EG, Sinclair JW, Hacksaw BT. The contribution of gastroesophageal reflux to chest pain in patients with coronary artery disease. Ann Intern Med 1992;117:824–830.

22. Mattox HE III, Richter JE. Prolonged ambulatory esophageal pH monitoring in the evaluation of gastroesophageal reflux disease. Am J Med 1990;89:345–356.

23. Kraus BB, Sinclair JW, Castell DO. Gastroesophageal reflux in runners: characteristics and treatment. Ann Intern Med 1990;112:429–433.

24. Schofield PM, Bennett DH, Whorwell PJ, et al. Exertional gastro-oesophageal reflux: a mechanism for symptoms in patients with angina pectoris and normal coronary angiograms. Br Med J 1987;294:1459–1461.

25. Osler W. Principles and practice of medicine. New York: D. Appleton, 1892:340–341.

26. Meyer GW, Castell DO. Human esophageal response during chest pain induced by swallowing cold liquids. JAMA 1981;246:2057–2059.

27. Kahrilas PJ, Dodds WJ, Hogan WJ. Dysfunction of the belch reflex: a cause of incapacitating chest pain. Gastroenterology 1987;93:818–822.

28. MacKenzie J, Belch J, Land D, Park R, McKillop J. Oesophageal ischaemia in motility disorders associated with chest pain. Lancet 1988;2:592–595.

29. Richter JE, Wu WC, Johns DN, et al. Esophageal manometry in 95 healthy adult volunteers: variability of pressures with age and frequency of "abnormal" contractions. Dig Dis Sci 1987;32:583–592.

30. Katz PO, Dalton CB, Richter JE, Wu WC, Castell DO. Esophageal testing of patients with noncardiac chest pain or dysphagia. Results of three years' experience with 1161 patients. Ann Intern Med 1987;106:593–597.

31. Peters L, Maas L, Petty D, et al. Spontaneous noncardiac chest pain: evaluation by 24-hour ambulatory esophageal motility and pH monitoring. Gastroenterology 1988;94:878–886.

32. Ghillebert G, Janssens J, Vantrappen G, Nevens F, Piessens J. Ambulatory 24 hour intraoesophageal pH and pressure recordings v provocation tests in the diagnosis of chest pain of esophageal origin. Gut 1990;31:738–744.

33. Clouse RE, Abramson BK, Todorczjuk JR. Achalasia in the elderly. Effects of aging on clinical presentation and outcome. Dig Dis Sci 1991;36:225–228.

34. Vantrappen G, Janssens J, Hellemans J, Coremans G. Achalasia, diffuse esophageal spasm, and related motility disorders. Gastroenterology 1979;76:450–457.

35. Kahrilas PJ, Dodds WJ, Hogan WJ, Kern M, Arndorfer RC, Reece A. Esophageal peristaltic dysfunction in peptic esophagitis. Gastroenterology 1986;91:897–904.

36. Crozier RE, Glick ME, Gibb SP, Ellis FH, Veerman JM. Acid-provoked esophageal spasm as a cause of noncardiac chest pain. Am J Gastroenterol 1991;86:1576–1580.

37. Stacher G, Schmeierer G, Landgraf M. Tertiary esophageal contractions evoked by acoustic stimuli. Gastroenterology 1979;77:49–54.

38. Young LD, Richter JE, Anderson KO, et al. The effects of psychological and environmental stressors on peristaltic esophageal contractions in healthy volunteers. Psychophysiology 1987;24:132–141.

39. Anderson KO, Dalton CB, Bradley LA, Richter JE. Stress induces alteration of esophageal pressures in healthy volunteers and non-cardiac chest pain patients. Dig Dis Sci 1989;34:83–91.

40. Beitman BD, Basha I, Flaker G, et al. Atypical or non-anginal chest pain: panic disorder or coronary artery disease. Arch Intern Med 1987;147:1548–1552.

41. Bass C, Chambers JB, Kiff P, Cooper D, Gardner WN. Panic anxiety and hyperventilation in patients with chest pain: a controlled study. Q J Med 1988;69:949–959.

42. Ayuso Mateos JL, Bayon Perez C, Santo-Domingo Carrasco J, Olivares D. Atypical chest pain and panic disorder. Psychother Psychosom 1989;52:92–95.

43. Katon W, Hall ML, Russo J, et al. Chest pain: relationship of psychiatric illness to coronary arteriographic results. Am J Med 1988;84:1–8.

44. Beitman BD. Panic disorder in patients with angiographically normal coronary arteries. Am J Med 1992;92(suppl 5A):33S–40S.

45. Beitman BD, Basha IM, Trombka LH, et al. Pharmacotherapeutic treatment of panic disorder in patients presenting with chest pain. J Fam Pract 1989;28:177–180.

46. Gorman JM, Liebowitz MR, Fyer AJ, Stein J. A neuroanatomical hypothesis for panic disorder. Am J Psychiatry 1989;146:148–161.

47. Bass C, Kartsounis L, Lelliot P. Hyperventilation and its relation to anxiety and panic. Integr Psychiatry 1987;5:274–291.

48. Cowley DS, Roy-Byrne PP. Hyperventilation and panic disorder. Am J Med 1987;83:929–937.

49. Beck JG, Berisford MA, Taegtmeyer H. The effects of voluntary hyperventilation on patients with chest pain without coronary artery disease. Behav Res Ther 1991;29:611–621.

50. Zigmond AS, Snaith RP. The hospital anxiety and depression scale. Acta Psychiatr Scand 1983;67:361–370.

51. Channer KS, Papouchado M, James MA, Rees JR. Anxiety and depression in patients with chest pain referred for exercise testing. Lancet 1985;2:820–822.

52. Katon W, Kleinman A, Rosen G. Depression and somatization: a review: part 1. Am J Med 1982;72:127–135.

53. Katon W. Depression: somatic symptoms and medical disorders in primary care. Compr Psychiatry 1982;23:274–287.
54. Carney RM, Freedland KE, Ludbrook PA, Saunders RD, Jaffe AS. Major depression, panic disorder, and mitral valve prolapse in patients who complain of chest pain. Am J Med 1990;89:757–760.
55. Beitman BD, Basha I, Flaker G, DeRosear L, Mukerji V, Lamberti JW. Major depression in cardiology chest pain patients without coronary artery disease and with panic disorder. J Affect Disord 1987;13:51–59.
56. Monson RA, Smith GR Jr. Current concepts in psychiatry. Somatization disorder in primary care. N Engl J Med 1983;308:1464–1465.
57. Smith GR Jr, Monson RA, Ray DC. Patients with multiple unexplained symptoms: their characteristics, functional health, and health care utilisation. Arch Intern Med 1986;146:69–72.
58. Cannon RO III, Epstein SE. "Microvascular angina" as a cause of chest pain with angiographically normal coronary arteries. Am J Cardiol 1988;61:1338–1343.
59. Marcus ML, Wilson RF, White CW. Methods of measurement of myocardial blood flow in patients: a critical review. Circulation 1987;76:245–253.
60. Mammohansingh P, Parker JO. Angina pectoris with normal coronary arteriograms: hemodynamic and metabolic response to atrial pacing. Am Heart J 1975;90:555–561.
61. Greenberg MA, Grose RM, Neuburger N, Silverman R, Strain JE, Cohen MV. Impaired coronary vasodilator responsiveness as a cause of lactate production during pacing induced ischemia in patients with angina pectoris and normal coronary arteries. J Am Coll Cardiol 1987;9:743–751.
62. Opherk D, Zebe H, Weihe E, et al. Reduced coronary dilatory capacity and ultrastructural changes of the myocardium in patients with angina pectoris but normal coronary angiograms. Circulation 1987;63:817–825.
63. Crake T, Canepa-Anson R, Shapiro L, Poole-Wilson PA. Continuous recording of coronary sinus oxygen saturation during atrial pacing in patients with coronary artery disease or with syndrome X. Br Heart J 1988;59:31–38.
64. Cannon RO III, Banow RO, Bacharach SL, et al. Left ventricular dysfunction in patients with angina pectoris, normal epicardial coronary arteries, and abnormal vasodilator reserve. Circulation 1985;71:218–226.
65. Legrand V, Hodgson J, Bates E, et al. Abnormal coronary flow reserve and abnormal radionuclide exercise test results in patients with normal coronary angiograms. J Am Coll Cardiol 1985;6:1245–1253.
66. Cannon RO III, Watson RM, Rosing DR, Epstein SE. Angina caused by reduced vasodilator reserve of the small coronary arteries. J Am Coll Cardiol 1983;1:1359–1373.
67. Shapiro LM, Crake T. Poole-Wilson PA. Is altered cardiac sensation responsible for chest pain in patients with normal coronary arteries? Clinical observations during cardiac catheterisation. Br Med J 1988;296:170–171.
68. Cannon RO III, Quyyumi AA, Schenke WH, et al. Abnormal cardiac sensitivity in patients with chest pain and normal coronary arteries. J Am Coll Cardiol 1990;16:1359–1366.
69. Pasternak RC, Thibault GE, Savoia M, DeSanctis RW, Hutter AM Jr. Chest pain with angiographically insignificant coronary arterial obstruction: clinical presentation and long-term follow-up. Am J Med 1980;68:813–817.
70. Nakhjavan FK, Natarajan G, Seshachary P, Goldberg H. The relationship between prolapsing mitral leaflet syndrome and angina and normal coronary arteriograms. Chest 1976;70:706–710.
71. Devereux RB, Kramer-Fox R, Kligfield P. Mitral valve prolapse: causes, clinical manifestations, and management. Ann Intern Med 1989;111:305–317.
72. Alpert MA, Mukerji V, Sabeti M, Russell JL, Beitman BD. Mitral valve prolapse, panic disorder, and chest pain. Med Clin North Am 1991;75:1119–1133.
73. Koch KL, Davidson WR, Day FP, Spears PF, Voss SR. Esophageal dysfunction and chest pain in patients with mitral valve prolapse: a prospective study using provocative testing during esophageal manometry. Am J Med 1989;86:32–38.
74. Devereux RB, Kramer-Fox R, Brown WT, et al. Relationship between clinical features of the mitral valve prolapse syndrome and echocardiographically documented mitral valve prolapse. J Am Coll Cardiol 1986;8:763–772.
75. Savage DD, Devereux RB, Garrison RJ, et al. Mitral valve prolapse in the general population. 2. Clinical features: the Framingham study. Am Heart J 1983;106:577–581.
76. Dager SR, Comess KA, Saal AK, Dunner DL. Mitral valve prolapse in psychiatric settings: diagnostic assessment, research and clinical implications. Integr Psychiatry 1986;4:211–223.
77. Margraf J, Ehlers A, Roth WT. Mitral valve prolapse and panic disorder: a review of their relationship. Psychosom Med 1988;50:93–113.
78. Mayou R. Invited review: atypical chest pain. J Psychosom Res 1989;33:393–406.
79. Wright JT. Slipping-rib syndrome. Lancet 1980;2:632–634.
80. Semble EL, Wise CM. Chest pain: a rheumatologist's perspective. South Med J 1988;81:64–68.
81. Levine PR, Mascette AM. Musculoskeletal chest pain in patients with "angina": a prospective study. South Med J 1989;82:580–591.
82. Epstein SE, Gerber LH, Borer JS. Chest wall syndrome: a common cause of unexplained chest pain. JAMA 1979;241:2793–2797.

83. Brazer S, Schmitt C, Varia I, et al. Chest pain of undetermined etiology (CPUE): multiple MDs + tests = multiple diagnoses [Abstract]. Am J Gastroenterol 1992;87:1244.

84. Dawes PT, Sheeran TP, Hothersall TE. Chest pain: a common feature of ankylosing spondylitis. Postgrad Med J 1988;64:27–29.

85. Pellegrino MJ. Atypical chest pain as an initial presentation of primary fibromyalgia. Arch Phys Med Rehabil 1990;71:526–528.

86. Wolfe F, Smythe HA, Yunus MB, et al. The American College of Rheumatology 1990 criteria for the classification of fibromyalgia. Report of the Multicenter Criteria Committee. Arthritis Rheum 1990;33:160–172.

87. Kirmayer LJ, Robbins JM, Kapusta MA. Somatization and depression in fibromyalgia syndrome. Am J Psychiatry 1988;145:950–954.

88. Urschel HC Jr, Razzuk MA. Management of the thoracic-outlet syndrome. N Engl J Med 1972;286:1140–1143.

89. Richter JE, Barish CF, Castell DO. Abnormal sensory perception in patients with esophageal chest pain. Gastroenterology 1986;91:845–852.

90. Hewson EG, Dalton CB, Richter JE. Comparison of esophageal manometry, provocative testing, and ambulatory monitoring in patients with unexplained chest pain. Dig Dis Sci 1990;35:302–309.

91. Dalton CB, Hewson EG, Castell DO, Richter JE. Edrophonium provocative test in noncardiac chest pain: evaluation and testing techniques. Dig Dis Sci 1990;35:1445–1451.

92. de Caestecker JS, Pryde A, Heading RC. Comparison of intravenous edrophonium and oesophageal acid perfusion during oesophageal manometry in patients with non-cardiac chest pain. Gut 1988;29:1029–1034.

93. Lynn RB. Mechanisms of esophageal pain. Am J Med 1992;92(suppl 5A):11S–19S.

94. Tally NJ. Review article: 5-hydroxytryptamine agonists and antagonists in the modulation of gastrointestinal motility and sensation: clinical implications. Aliment Pharmacol Ther 1992;6:273–289.

95. Hill AB. The clinical trial. N Engl J Med 1952;247:113–119.

96. Richter JE, Dalton CB, Bradley LA, Castell DO. Oral nifedipine in the treatment of noncardiac chest pain in patients with the nutcracker esophagus. Gastroenterology 1987;93:21–28.

97. Dager SR, Kham A, Cowley DS, et al. Characteristics of placebo-response during long-term treatment of panic disorder. Psychopharmacol Bull 1990;26:273–278.

98. Clouse RE, Lustman PJ, Eckert TC, Ferney DM, Griffith LS. Low-dose trazodone for symptomatic patients with esophageal contraction abnormalities: a double-blind, placebo-controlled trial. Gastroenterology 1987;92:1027–1036.

99. Freiman JA, Chalmers TC, Smith H Jr, Kuebler RR. The importance of beta, the type II error and sample size in the design and interpretation of the randomized control trial: survey of 71 "negative" trials. N Engl J Med 1978;299:690–694.

100. Roy-Byrne PP. Integrated treatment of panic disorder. Am J Med 1992;92(suppl 1A):49S–54S.

101. Ballenger JC, Burrows GD, DuPont RL Jr, et al. Alprazolam in panic disorder and agoraphobia: results from a multicenter trial, I: efficacy in short-term treatment. Arch Gen Psychiatry 1988;45:413–422.

102. Beitman BD, Basha IM, Trombka LH, Jayaratna MA, Russell BD, Tarr SK. Alprazolam in the treatment of cardiology patients with atypical chest pain and panic disorder. J Clin Psychopharmacol 1988;8:127–130.

103. Sontag SJ. A piece of her heart. JAMA 1988;259:1071–1072.

104. Ward BW, Wu WC, Richter JE, Hacksaw BT, Castell DO. Long-term follow-up of symptomatic status of patients with noncardiac chest pain: is diagnosis of esophageal etiology helpful? Am J Gastroenterol 1987;82:215–218.

105. Stahl WG, Beton RR, Johnson CS, Brown CL, Waring JP. High-dose ranitidine in the treatment of patients with non-cardiac chest pain and evidence of gastroesophageal reflux [Abstract]. Gastroenterology 1992;102:168.

106. Bancewicz J, Osugi H, Marples M. Clinical implications of abnormal oesophageal motility. Br J Surg 1987;74:416–419.

107. Richter JE, Schan C, Burgard S, Bradley L. Placebo controlled trial of omeprazole in the treatment of acid-related non-cardiac chest pain (NCCP) [Abstract]. Am J Gastroenterol 1992;87:1255.

108. Bremner CG, Marks IN, Segal I, Simjee A. Reflux esophagitis therapy: sucralfate versus ranitidine in a double-blind multicenter trial. Am J Med 1991;91(suppl 2a):119S–122S.

109. Johannson K-E, Boeryd B, Johannson K, Tibbling L. Double-blind crossover study of ranitidine versus placebo in gastro-oesophageal reflux disease. Scand J Gastroenterol 1986;21:769–778.

110. Achem SR, Kolts BE. Current medical therapy for esophageal motility disorders. Am J Med 1992;92(suppl 5A):98S–105S.

111. Chalmers TC. A shortage of reliable data. N Engl J Med 1976;294:721–722.

112. Dodds WJ, Dent J, Hogan WJ, Arndorfer RC. Effect of atropine on esophageal motor function in humans. Am J Physiol 1981;240:G290–G296.

113. Allen M, Mellow M, Robinson MG, Orr WC. Comparison of calcium channel blocking agents and an anticholinergic agent on esophageal function. Aliment Pharmacol Therapeut 1987;1:153–159.

114. Mellow MH. Effect of isosorbide and hydralazine in painful primary esophageal motility disorders. Gastroenterology 1982;83:364–370.

115. Orlando RC, Bozymski EM. Clinical and manometric effects of nitroglycerin in diffuse esophageal spasm. N Engl J Med 1973;289:23–25.

116. Richter JE, Spurling TJ, Cordova CM, Castell DO. Effects of oral calcium channel blocker, diltiazem, on esophageal contractions: studies in volunteers and patients with nutcracker esophagus. Dig Dis Sci 1984;29:649–656.

117. Richter JE, Dalton CB, Biuce RG, Castell DO. Nifedipine: a potent inhibitor of contractions in the body of the human esophagus. Studies in healthy volunteers and patients with the nutcracker esophagus. Gastroenterology 1985;89:549–554.

118. Nasrallah SM. Nifedipine in the treatment of diffuse oesophageal spasm. Lancet 1982;2:1285.

119. Nasrallah SM, Tommaso CL, Singleton RT, Backhaus EA. Primary esophageal motor disorders: clinical response to nifedipine. South Med J 1985;78:312–315.

120. Alban Davies H, Lewis M, Rhodes J, Henderson A. Nifedipine for relief of esophageal chest pain? N Engl J Med 1982;307:1274.

121. Frachtman RL, Botoman VA, Pope CE II. A double-blind crossover trial of diltiazem shows no benefit in patients with dysphagia and/or chest pain of esophageal origin [Abstract]. Gastroenterology 1986;90:1420.

122. Winters C, Artnak EJ, Benjamin SB, Castell DO. Esophageal bougienage in symptomatic patients with the nutcracker esophagus: a primary esophageal motility disorder. JAMA 1984;252:363–366.

123. Traube M, Tummala V, Baue AE, McCallum RW. Surgical myotomy in patients with high-amplitude peristaltic esophageal contractions: manometric and clinical effects. Dig Dis Sci 1987;32:16–21.

124. Stein HJ, DeMeester TR. Therapy of noncardiac chest pain: is there a role for surgery? Am J Med 1992;92(suppl 5A):122S–128S.

125. Noyes R Jr, Chaudry DR, Domingo DV. Pharmacologic treatment of phobic disorders. J Clin Psychiatry 1986;47:445–452.

126. Matuzas W, Jack E. The drug treatment of panic disorder. Psychiatr Med 1991;9:215–243.

127. Anonymous. Drug treatment of panic disorder: comparative efficacy of alprazolam, imipramine, and placebo. Br J Psychiatry 1992;160:191–202.

128. Wilkinson G, Balestrieri M, Ruggeri M, Bellantuono C. Meta-analysis of double-blind placebo-controlled trials of antidepressants and benzodiazepines for patients with panic disorders. Psychol Med 1991;21:991–998.

129. Johnstone DG, Troyer IE, Whitsett SF. Clomipramine treatment of agorophobic women: an eight-week controlled trial. Arch Gen Psychiatry 1988;45:453–459.

130. Tesar GE, Rosenbaum JF, Pollack MH, et al. Clonazepam versus alprazolam in the treatment of panic disorder: interim analysis of data from a prospective, double-blind, placebo-controlled trial. J Clin Psychiatry 1987;48(suppl):16–19.

131. Dunner DL, Ishiki D, Avery DH, Wilson LG, Hyde TS. Effect of alprazolam and diazepam on anxiety and panic attacks in panic disorder: a controlled study. J Clin Psychiatry 1986;47:458–460.

132. Lydiard RB, Lesser IM, Ballenger JC, Rubin RT, Laraia M, DuPont R. A fixed-dose study of alprazolam 2 mg, alprazolam 6 mg, and placebo in panic disorder. J Clin Psychopharmacol 1992;12:96–103.

133. Gorman JM, Liebowitz MR, Fyer AJ, et al. An open trial of fluoxetine in the treatment of panic attacks. J Clin Psychopharmacol 1987;7:329–332.

134. Schneier FR, Liebowitz MR, Davies SO, et al. Fluoxetine in panic disorder. J Clin Psychopharmacol 1990;10:119–121.

135. Sheehan DV, Ballenger J, Jacobsen G. Treatment of endogenous anxiety with phobic, hysterical, and hypochondriacal symptoms. Arch Gen Psychiatry 1980;37:51–59.

136. Bass C. Chest pain and breathlessness: relationship to psychiatric illness. Am J Med 1992;92(suppl 1A):12S–17S.

137. Munjack DJ, Crocker B, Cabe D, et al. Alprazolam, propranolol, and placebo in the treatment of panic disorder and agorophobia with panic attacks. J Clin Psychopharmacol 1989;9:22–27.

138. Munjack DJ, Rebal R, Shaner R, et al. Imipramine versus propranolol for the treatment of panic attacks: a pilot study. Compr Psychiatr 1985;26:80–89.

139. Noyes R Jr, Anderson DJ, Clancy J, et al. Diazepam and propranolol in panic disorder and agorophobia. Arch Gen Psychiatry 1984;41:287–292.

140. Ravaris CL, Friedman MJ, Hauri PJ, McHugo GJ. A controlled study of alprazolam and propranolol in panic-disordered and agorophobic outpatients. J Clin Psychopharmacol 1991;11:344–350.

141. Calabrese JR, Markovitz PJ. Treatment of depression: new pharmacologic approaches. Primary Care 1991;18:421–433.

142. Smith GR Jr. Effectiveness of treatment for somatoform disorder patients. Psychiatr Med 1991;9:545–558.

143. Morrison J. Managing somatization disorder. DM 1990;36:542–591.

144. Ballenger JC. Pharmacotherapy of the panic disorders. J Clin Psychiatry 1986;47(6 suppl):27–32.

145. Cannon RO III, Watson RM, Rosing DR, Epstein SE. Efficacy of calcium channel blocker therapy for angina pectoris resulting from small-vessel coronary artery disease and abnormal vasodilator reserve. Am J Cardiol 1985;56:242–246.

146. Winkle RA, Lopes MG, Goodman DL, Fitzgerald JW, Schroeder JS, Harrison DC. Propranolol for

patients with mitral valve prolapse. Am Heart J 1977;93:422–427.

147. Yunus MB, Masi AT, Aldag JC. Short term effects of ibuprofen in primary fibromyalgia syndrome: a double blind, placebo controlled trial. J Rheumatol 1989;16:527–532.

148. Bennett RM, Gatter RA, Campbell SM, Andrews RP, Clark SR, Scarola JA. A comparison of cyclobenzaprine and placebo in the management of fibrositis: a double-blind controlled study. Arthritis Rheum 1988;31:1535–1542.

149. McCain GA, Bell DA, Mai FM, Halliday PD. A controlled study of the effects of a supervised cardiovascular fitness program on the manifestations of primary fibromyalgia. Arthritis Rheum 1988; 31:1135–1141.

150. Carette S, McCain GA, Bell DA, Fam AG. Evaluation of amitriptyline in primary fibrositis: a double-blind, placebo-controlled study. Arthritis Rheum 1986;29:655–659.

151. Goldenberg DL, Felson DT, Dinerman H. A randomized, controlled trial of amitriptyline and naproxen in the treatment of patients with fibromyalgia. Arthritis Rheum 1986;29:1371–1377.

152. Fam AG. Approach to musculoskeletal chest wall pain. Primary Care 1988;15:767–782.

153. Stark M Jr, Maher K, Gupta P, et al. Visceral afferent blockade with ondansetron (Zofran®) increases nociceptive thresholds in patients with chest pain of undetermined etiology [Abstract]. Am J Gastroenterol 1991;86:1305.

154. Gupta PK, Stark MT, Maher KA, Cannon RO, Quyymi A, Benjamin SB. Imipramine is superior to clonidine and placebo for amelioration of chest pain symptoms in patients enrolled in a double-blinded, two-drug, placebo-controlled study in chest pain of undetermined etiology (CPUE) [Abstract]. Am J Gastroenterol 1992;87:1248.

8

Gastroparesis, Nausea, and Vomiting[a]

ANDRE DUBOIS

Before describing the medications that are available to treat nausea, vomiting, and disorders affecting gastric emptying, it is important to understand the teleologic significance of these symptoms.

All living organisms have to absorb and digest a portion of the outside world to grow and survive, yet they have to defend themselves against potentially toxic substances that should not be allowed to enter into their bodies or cells. Some species (e.g., rodents) are unable to vomit, possibly because they have developed an exquisite sense of smell and taste that allows them to avoid most naturally occurring poisons. In contrast, some mammals (e.g., dogs) rely on vomiting to repel substances that should not be absorbed by their intestines. Primates combine both modes of defense, experiencing nausea and anorexia when presented with food or drink that has previously led to unpleasant experiences, while being able to vomit if this first line of defense is insufficient or suppressed because of more powerful motivations. In most species, a third line of defense is provided by the stomach, which may slow or suppress emptying of potential toxins and denature or dilute them before allowing them to reach the intestinal mucosa. If this latter mechanism fails, gastric distension and/or irritation of mucosal cells will initiate vomiting.

Nausea, vomiting, and gastric stasis may also occur in various conditions where there is no apparent benefit to be gained from these otherwise useful reflexes. For example, these symptoms may be induced by oral or parenteral administration of various medications, e.g., during chemotherapy. Nausea, vomiting, and gastric stasis may also occur following the production of toxins by bacteria, by viruses, or by the patients themselves in response to a noxious stimuli (e.g., allergy to food or radiotherapy). Finally, various diseases may disrupt the balance between excitatory and inhibitory mechanisms that normally regulate the functioning of the stomach and/or its regulation by the brain-gut axis. In all these conditions, nausea, vomiting, and gastric stasis may lead to significant morbidity, and the availability of powerful antiemetic and gastrokinetic agents represents a valuable addition to our therapeutic armamentarium.

In this chapter, the normal regulation of gastric motility and the mechanism of emesis production will first be reviewed. Diseases in which these medications may be of benefit will then be discussed. Finally, the medications available for the treatment of vomiting and gastric stasis will be described.

REGULATION OF GASTRIC MOTILITY

The functioning of the stomach is controlled by impulses that can be triggered by external (e.g., visual, olfactory, auditory, or motion) or internal (e.g., gastric distension, or presence of nutrients in the small intestine) stimuli perceived by the central and/or peripheral ner-

[a]The opinions and assertions contained herein are the private ones of the authors and are not to be construed as official or reflecting the views of the Department of Defense or the Uniformed Services University of the Health Sciences.

131

Table 8.1
Classes of Antiemetic and/or Prokinetic Agents

Anticholinergic and cholinomimetic agents
  Atropine
  Bethanechol
Histamine receptor antagonists
  Histamine H_1-receptor antagonists (e.g., Antivert)
  Histamine H_2-receptor antagonists (e.g., cimetidine)
Neuroleptic drugs
  Chlorpromazine (e.g., Thorazine)
  Prochlorperazine (e.g., Compazine)
Adrenergic-blocking drugs
  Bretylium
Substituted benzamides acting at multiple receptor
  sites
  Metoclopramide (Reglan)
  Renzapride (BRL-24924)
Dopamine antagonists
  Domperidone (R-33812, Motilium)
  Clebopride
$5-HT_3$-receptor antagonists
  Ondansetron (GR-38032F, Zofran, Glaxo)[a]
  Granisetron (BRL-43694, Kytril, SKB)[b]
  Tropisetron (ICS-205930, Novathan, Sandoz)[b]
  Batanopride (BMY-25801, Bristol Myers)[b]
  Evsatron (RG-12915, Rhone Poulenc Rorer)[b]
  Zacopride (AHR-11190B, AH Robbins)[b]
  Dolaselon (Anemet, Marion Merreli Dow)[b]
  Benzimidazolone derivatives
Specific $5-HT_4$-receptor agonists
  Cisapride (R-51619, Propulsid)
  Benzimidazolone derivatives
  Substituted pyrrolizidine 1
Opioid agonists and antagonists
  Naloxone
  Trimebutine
  Bremazocine
Motilin analogues
  Erythromycin
  Macrolide derivatives without antibiotic activity (e.g.,
  EM-523)

[a]Approved for chemotherapy-induced emesis and for postoperative nausea and vomiting.
[b]Investigational for chemotherapy-induced emesis and for postoperative nausea and vomiting.

vous system and conveyed to the stomach through nervous or humoral mechanisms. For example, gastric emptying is delayed when the acidity and caloric concentration of the gastroduodenal contents increase, and this effect is mediated by neurohumoral vectors released following stimulation of chemoreceptors located in the wall of the stomach and duodenum (1). Similarly, gastroduodenal mechanoreceptors mediate the stimulation of gastric motility induced by distension of the stomach,

as well as the inhibition produced by overdistension. Some hormones and neurotransmitters that regulate gastric motility may stimulate the contractility of the gastric antrum while inhibiting the tone of the proximal stomach, including the lower esophageal sphincter. In addition, the net effect on the movements of the gastric contents within and outside the stomach results from the complex integration of each of these actions. Therefore, only in vivo studies of gastric emptying allow the complete definition of the pathophysiologic role of various transmitters, whereas only in vivo and in vitro studies of mechanical and electrical activity of the stomach will permit the analysis and the interpretation of these effects.

Nervous Factors

The nervous control of the stomach relies on extrinsic nerves, which connect the central nervous system to the stomach, as well as on myenteric plexus and intramural descending and ascending nerves (2). In general, cholinergic nerves stimulate, while noradrenergic nerves inhibit gastric contractions. In addition, many other neurotransmitters are present within the afferent and efferent neurones of the intramural plexus, which thus play an important role in the sensation of nausea as well as in the regulation of gastric motility (3). In turn, these events may lead to emesis and/or increase or decrease gastric emptying.

The role of serotonin (5-hydroxytryptamine [5-HT]) in neurotransmission within the myenteric plexus is extremely complex. Clarification of these effects through the pharmacological characterization of responses and ligand-binding sites in various tissues led to the recognition of the four main serotonin receptors, and the development of specific antagonists for each of these receptors has renewed the interest in this field. In fact, several of these antagonists are effective in the treatment of nausea, vomiting, and gastric stasis, and some of them are already approved for use in the United States (Table 8.1). Their development started in 1957 when Gaddum and Pi-

Table 8.2
Serotonin (5-HT)-Receptor Family[a]

Family	Subtypes	Location and Function
5-HT$_1$	1A	CNS-primarily inhibitory effect on neuronal tissue
	1B	Periphery—primarily causes contraction of cranial vascular smooth muscle
	1C	(vasoconstriction)
	1D	
	1P	
	1-like	
5-HT$_2$		Generally excitatory effect on neuronal and muscle tissues leading to vasoconstriction, bronchoconstriction, contraction of GI smooth muscle, platelet aggregation
5-HT$_3$		CNS—chemotreceptor trigger zone (stimulates emesis)
		Peripheral nervous system—excitatory response to 5-HT (stimulates ACH release leading to contraction of ileum)
		Mediates vagally mediated reflex bradycardia (Bezold-Jarisch reflex)
		Activates pain from sensory nerve endings
5-HT$_4$		Modulation of GI motility
5-HT$_5$		?

[a]CNS, central nervous system; GI, gastrointestinal, ACH, acetylcholine.

carelli demonstrated that 5-HT contracts the guinea pig ileum by two different mechanisms: (a) direct action on the smooth muscle which is blocked by dibenzyline; and (b) indirect action through the release of acetylcholine by nerve endings, which is blocked by morphine (4). Based on these findings we postulated the existence of two 5-HT-receptor subtypes: (a) a D-receptor explaining the former action; and (b) an M-receptor mediating the latter action. However, neither dibenzyline nor morphine were specific or potent in their actions, and it is only recently that 5-HT receptors have been precisely classified and characterized because of the availability of specific antagonists. (Table 8.2). For example, the M-receptor was recently demonstrated to be the 5-HT$_3$-receptor (5). This latter receptor, along with the 5-HT$_{1A}$- and 5-HT$_{1P}$-receptors (6), appears to play an important role in the production and prevention of nausea, vomiting, and gastric stasis. In addition, a 5-HT$_4$-receptor with pharmacologic characteristics different than those of the 5-HT$_1$-, 5-HT$_2$-, and 5-HT$_3$-receptors has been described (7). This receptor may be responsible for some of the so far unexplained actions of the 4-amino-5-chloro-2-methoxy-substituted benzamide derivatives, such as metoclopramide, cisapride, zacopride, and renzapride. All

these compounds have the common property of being potent stimulants of gastrointestinal motility, while some of them are also 5-HT$_3$-receptor antagonists. The rank order of potency of these substituted benzamide derivatives in stimulating cyclic adenosine monophosphate (cAMP) formation in vitro was found to be: cisapride greater than renzapride greater than 5-HT greater than zacopride greater than metoclopramide (7). The nonadditivity of benzamide and 5-HT activities suggests that 5-HT and the substituted benzamide derivatives act on the same receptor. Only tropisetron, a 5-HT$_3$-receptor antagonist, competitively antagonized the stimulatory effect of cisapride, zacopride, and BRL 24924. However, the pK$_i$ (6–6.3) of tropisetron for the 5-HT$_4$-receptor was very different from its pK$_i$ for 5-HT$_3$-receptors (pK$_i$ = 8–10). In addition, other selective 5-HT$_3$-receptor antagonists with an carbazole group (ondansetron), with an indazole (granisetron), with a benzoate group (cocaine, MDL-72222), or with a piperazine group (quipazine) were ineffective in reversing the stimulatory effect of cisapride, zacopride, renzapride, and metoclopramide. Based and these and other observations, Tonini et al. (8) have proposed a hypothetical distribution of 5-HT-receptors on the neurones of the myenteric plexus that would explain these observations (Fig. 8.1). The role of serotonin in the regulation of gastric motility is further complicated by the fact that its release by enterochromaffin cells is autoregulated, being stimulated by activation of its 5-HT$_3$-receptors and inhibited by activation of its 5-HT$_4$-receptors (9).

The presence of opioid peptides has been demonstrated in the central nervous system as well as in neurones of the myenteric plexus (10), and studies on the effect of specific opioid antagonists on binding of [³H]naloxone and [³H]U69593 provided evidence for κ and μ sites, but not for δ sites, on dispersed gastric smooth muscle cells (11). Opioid peptides may cause vomiting, and they have been shown to play an important role in the regulation of gastric emptying, possibly by modulating pyloric motility (12). The regulation of the endogenous opiate system is not well understood, but recent evidence has suggested that it is regulated by endogenous antiopiate peptides which are able to stimulate gastric emptying in rodents (13). In dogs, κ-opioid agonists given intravenously have been shown to reduce the amplitude of the gastric relaxation induced by a standard meal whereas μ-agonists given intravenously increased markedly the feeding-induced relaxation (14). Orally administered κ-agonists at doses not exceeding 1 mg/kg enhanced gastric emptying of a solid meal, but slowed emptying of liquids, whereas doses greater than 1 mg/kg of μ-agonists slowed gastric emptying of both liquids and solids (15, 16). In primates, both μ- and κ-agonists decreased gastric emptying (17, 18). Finally, κ- but not μ-opioid agonists appear to act selectively on peripheral κ-receptors located in the wall of the proximal gut to inhibit the acoustic stress-induced stimulation of the hypothalamo-pituitary-adrenocortical axis (19).

In addition, all the peptides listed below under Hormonal Factors have been observed in neurones, and they may be involved as neurotransmitters in the myenteric plexus. Finally, the recent observation that nitric oxide (NO) may mediate the relaxation of the stomach to accommodate food or fluids (20) may

open new avenues in our understanding of nonadrenergic, noncholinergic neurotransmission in the gut, and possibly lead to the development of novel medications.

Hormonal Factors

Many hormones have been found to modify gastric motor activity, but their physiologic role or their involvement in gastric pathology is often difficult to establish.

Secretin. This hormone, which was the first to be described, is known to delay gastric emptying of liquids (21) and of solids (22). Since secretin is released by infusion of physiologic amounts of acid into the duodenum, it could play a role in the normal regulation of gastric emptying. Generally, secretin relaxes fundic and antral smooth muscle and contracts the pylorus, which may occur because secretin decreases the responsiveness of gastric smooth muscle to other neural and hormonal stimuli.

Cholecystokinin (CCK). Like secretin, CCK at low doses suppresses both gastric emptying and gastric secretion, which indicates that this peptide plays a physiologic role in the regulation of gastric emptying and secretion (21, 23). The physiologic role of CCK has been further demonstrated by the observation that the specific CCK-A antagonist L-364,718 (MK-329) abolishes the slowing effect of fat on gastric emptying both in monkeys (24) and in humans (25).

Gastrin. The gastrins and their analog pentagastrin may delay gastric emptying through two mechanisms: first, by stimulating gastric acid, which indirectly inhibits gastric emptying, and secondly, by directly relaxing the fundus and contracting the antrum (26). However, these latter direct actions occur only when high doses are administered, suggesting that gastrin may play only an indirect physiologic role in the regulation of gastric motility.

Motilin. Motilin is the only gastrointestinal peptide that has been found to stimulate gastric emptying of liquids in dogs (27) and of solids in humans (28), although emptying of fat was not increased by infusion of the pep-

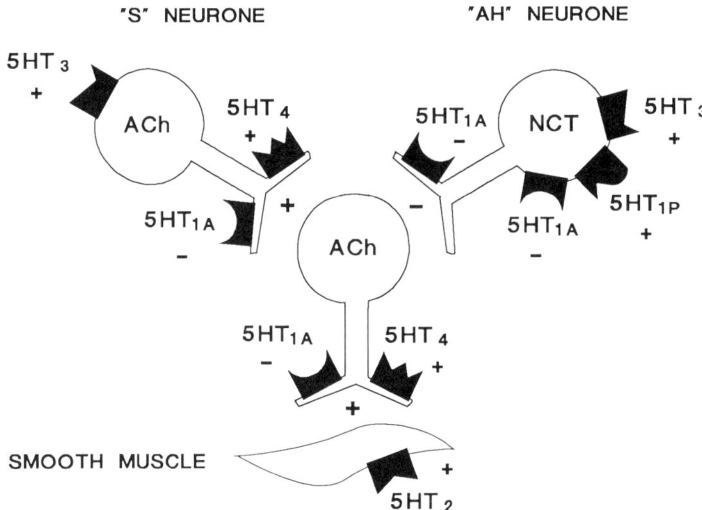

Figure 8.1. Schematic representation of the 5-HT receptors at the level of the myenteric plexus. The "S"-type neurones receive fast nicotinic synaptic input, whereas the "AH"-type neurones represent those noncholinergic inhibitory interneurones that show a long-acting afterpolarization following a single action potential (after Tonini et al. [3]).

tide (29). Motilin also stimulates phase III of the migrating myoelectric complex (MMC) (30), as well as postprandial gastric contractions (31). In fact, motilin may *be responsible* for the initiation of these MMCs (32), although the peptide may be released as a *consequence* of contractile activity (33). Early studies demonstrated that motilin was acting on specific myogenic receptors, as its action in vitro was independent of cholinergic or adrenergic neurones (34). However, subsequent studies have shown that the in vivo effect of natural motilin depends on the activation of cholinergic nerves, because the effect of exogenous motilin is abolished by vagotomy (27) and by atropine (35). The clinical importance of this peptide is likely to rise sharply with the recent discovery of the motilin-like activity of the antibiotic erythromycin, which allows the current development of potent and relatively inexpensive motilin analogs, called motilides or motilin-like macrolides (31).

Other Hormones. Vasoactive intestinal polypeptide, gastric inhibitory polypeptide, pancreatic polypeptide, and glucagon have been found to alter gastric smooth muscle activity, but their physiologic role in the regulation of gastric motility and emptying is unknown. More studies will be needed before such a role can be established.

Paracrine Mechanisms

Little is known about the effect of the release of local agents on gastric emptying. Prostaglandins of the E, F, and I classes have been found in significant amounts in the stomach wall and in the gastric juice. Because prostaglandins have a major effect on gastric emptying and secretion of acid, they could play a role in the regulation of gastric motility in health and diseases (36, 37). However, the current unavailability of specific antagonists makes the study of these effects difficult, and it has been precluding the development of medications that are devoid of unacceptable side effects.

MECHANISM OF EMESIS

Expulsion of the gastric contents during vomiting is a respiratory response integrated in a complex sequence of events that involves gastrointestinal reflexes. Multiple stimuli are

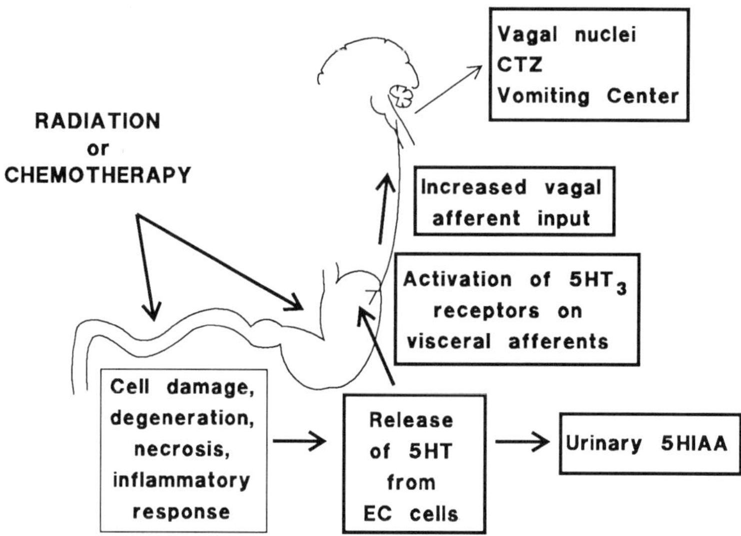

Figure 8.2. Putative mechanisms of serotonin involvement in the initiation of chemotherapy and radiation-induced emesis and gastric stasis. CTZ, chemoreceptor trigger zone; EC, enterochromaffin cell; 5HIAA, 5-hydroxy indole acetic acid.

probably involved concurrently when nausea and emesis are initiated. For example, radiation-induced vomiting may be reduced by limiting the movements of the patients during exposure to whole body radiation (38). Brain lesion studies have indicated that vomiting may be primarily coordinated by the chemoreceptor trigger zone (CTZ), also called the area postrema (39). The CTZ has been shown to contain dopamine, opiate, and serotonin receptors, and activation of one of these may lead to vomiting. In addition, receptors located in the gastrointestinal wall may convey stimuli to the central nervous system through afferent vagal pathways (40), and this may explain why changes in gastrointestinal motility may lower or elevate the threshold for a given emetogenic stimulus to produce vomiting. For example, postprandial antral hypomotility has been identified as a major abnormality in patients with unexplained nausea and vomiting (41).

The unique role of the CTZ in the production of emesis has been challenged by careful neuroanatomic studies that demonstrated that lesions believed to be specifically restricted to the CTZ had, in fact, extended into the vagal nuclei (42). Therefore, some of the concepts regarding the role of the area postrema in emesis and the associated suppression of gastric emptying may have to be re-evaluated. This task will be facilitated by the recent development of specific 5-HT-receptor agonists and antagonists, as illustrated by the current interpretation of 5-HT involvement in chemotherapy and radiotherapy-induced emesis (Fig. 8.2). However, as is often the case in medical research, a treatment for this symptom may be available before the pathophysiology is fully understood.

PATHOPHYSIOLOGY OF GASTRIC STASIS

Gastric emptying is suppressed when gastric motility is inhibited, but it is also suppressed in the presence of gastric hypermotility if peristalsis is uncoordinated. One difficulty in sorting out the cause of gastric retention is that most studies have used intraluminal manometry (43, 44), which is insensitive if the stomach is distended by gas, fluid, or food. Thus, a given contraction of the stomach wall will be recorded to a lesser extent if the stomach is distended because the distance between the gastric wall and the pressure sensor is greater than in an undistended stomach. Furthermore, a number of agents that increase gastric contractility may be ineffective in producing "normal" gastric emptying if their administration results in a greater increase of motility in the pyloroduodenal area than in the proximal stomach, or if they induce retropropagation of gastric waves.

Gastric retention may be diagnosed clinically in patients who complain of bloating if they vomit undigested food eaten more than 6 hours earlier, and this diagnosis can be confirmed by using the qualitative tests usually available. Milder cases of gastric retention also produce symptoms, but these can be detected only by more sensitive techniques such as scintigraphic measurement of gastric emptying. Furthermore, symptoms of gastric distension without retention of food may be observed in the presence of normal gastric emptying if there is gastric hypersecretion. This association may be observed in atypical cases of the Zollinger-Ellison syndrome, in which symptoms of gastric distension completely disappear after treatment with a Histamine H_2-antagonist (45), whereas most patients with the Zollinger-Ellison syndrome have normal intragastric volumes because they have enhanced gastric fractional emptying rates (46). Similarly, gastric retention in patients with duodenal ulcer may be more or less severe, depending on the degree of gastric hypersecretion (47). Thus, the diagnosis of gastric retention should not be based solely on an increased gastric volume either during fasting or after a saline load test, and additional investigations should be made in the presence of gastric hypersecretion. Specific diagnosis of gastric retention can be provided by intragastric (46) or intraduodenal (48) marker dilution techniques as well as by Technetium-tagged solid meals (49). A fractional emptying rate of <10%/minute (half-life of 6 minutes) after water or saline meals strongly suggests gastric retention. For solid meals, fractional emptying rates of <0.5%/minute after chicken liver

meals (49) suggest the diagnosis of gastric retention. If these sophisticated tests are not available, the steak and barium meal test (50, 51) may provide qualitative evidence of gastric retention if some barium is still present in the stomach 5 hours after ingestion of the meal.

DISEASES IN WHICH GASTRIC STASIS AND/OR EMESIS MAY BE OBSERVED

Peptic Ulcer Disease. Gastric retention is usually caused by pyloric stenosis due to scarring from a duodenal or pyloric channel ulcer or, more rarely, in the presence of gastric cancer. If the pylorus is patent, it will be difficult to determine whether gastric retention is brought about by an inhibition of gastric motility, or by a decrease in the grinding of food, or by an alteration of the gastric sieving process. Again, gastric hypersecretion will aggravate these symptoms (47). Gastric emptying was found to be delayed in gastric ulcer patients after a liquid meal (52), although this finding was not confirmed by others (53). The discrepancy may be related to differences in ulcer location in the two studies, because delayed emptying was found in patients with antral ulcers, but not in those with more proximal ulcers (54).

Diabetes. Diabetic gastroparesis is only one manifestation of a widespread gastrointestinal neuropathy observed in patients with long-standing insulin-dependent diabetes. Gastric emptying is delayed in 20–30% of diabetics (55), a phenomenon that appears to be related to insufficient control of glycemia, diabetic ketoacidosis, electrolyte imbalance, or associated autonomic neuropathy (56, 57). Thus, scintigraphic studies have demonstrated retarded gastric emptying in only 3 of 29 well-controlled patients with diabetes (58) and in 3 of 6 diabetics patients with autonomic neuropathy (56). Delayed gastric emptying is associated with low acid output (58) and a lower than expected incidence of duodenal ulcer but not of gastric ulcer. Since acid, which is known to inhibit gastric emptying, is often decreased in diabetes, the fact that emptying is normal in many diabetic patients could be related to their decreased acid secretion, but no information is available regarding this possibility. The mild gastric stasis that is often present in diabetes does not usually produce clinical symptoms, although it could play a role in the nausea and vomiting that is frequently reported. Moreover, the difficulty in controlling the blood sugar levels of some diabetic patients could be related to the slow rate at which food enters the intestines. In a series of 137 patients, 29% patients had nausea and vomiting, which is the most characteristic symptom of diabetic gastroparesis (59). In addition, 34% had abdominal pain, 27% had dysphagia, 22% had diarrhea, and 60% had constipation (59). In diabetic patients complaining of nausea and vomiting, as well as in some asymptomatic patients, gastric emptying of liquids is usually within the normal range, whereas emptying of solids is delayed (60, 61). This suppression of gastric emptying appears to be related to disturbances of coordinated antral motility (62), because this region is responsible for the emptying of both digestible and indigestible solids (63), and because there was no mechanical gastric outlet obstruction. In addition, the phase III of the interdigestive motor complex may be lacking (62).

The treatment of this condition is difficult. Administration of gastrokinetic agents such as metoclopramide may improve gastric emptying, but the side effects of this medication often necessitate its discontinuation (64). Therefore, there is a need for safer and more effective gastrokinetic agents. Some that show promise are domperidone (65), cisapride, erythromycin (66), or one of the nonantibiotic analog macrolides (31).

Collagen Diseases. Involvement of the stomach by collagen diseases produces atrophy of gastric smooth muscle cells, which are replaced by connective tissue. Radiologic methods have demonstrated that gastric emptying is decreased in patients with scleroderma (67). The early phase of gastric emptying appears normal or rapid, but small amounts of barium are often retained for many hours. Similar symptoms are often found in patients with other collagen diseases such as dermatomyos-

itis (68) and systemic lupus erythematosus (69).

Anorexia Nervosa. In primary anorexia nervosa, both gastric secretion and fractional emptying are decreased, which usually results in normal fasting gastric volumes (70). After liquid meals, however, the decrease of gastric fluid output is insufficient to compensate for the decrease of emptying, and postprandial gastric volumes are therefore greater than normal. Gastric emptying of solids is also delayed (71). Thus, the postprandial epigastric fullness often observed in anorexia nervosa could be related to a treatable gastric dysfunction and may not be related to a psychiatric disease. The cause of these disturbances is unknown, however.

Postoperative Ileus. Postoperative gastric atony and stasis result from neural reflexes causing norepinephrine release by sympathetic neurons in the wall of the stomach (72, 73). The result is atony of the stomach, slow emptying of liquids and solids, and absence of interdigestive contractions, which explains the clinical picture of gastric distension, bloating, and intragastric accumulation of secretions. Fortunately, the condition usually subsides spontaneously within a few days. Antiadrenergic agents have been shown to shorten or completely prevent the syndrome (72, 74), but the cardiovascular side effects of this therapy prevent its widespread use.

Tachygastria. In 1980, a new gastric motility disorder characterized by nausea and vomiting was described (75). In this syndrome, ectopic antral pacemakers, firing at rapid rates of 4–10 cycles/minute (tachygastria), suppressed the natural 3 cycles/minute gastric pacemaker, captured the gastric smooth muscle, and destroyed the usual orderly patterns of aborally directed gastric peristalsis. The ectopic pacemaker may also occur at irregular intervals (tachyarrhythmia). The pacesetter potentials generated by the ectopic pacemaker are retropropagated from the antrum orally to the body of the stomach. Action potentials and contractions phased by such orally moving cycles also have an oral direction. Therefore, normal gastric propulsion is impaired, and gastric stasis, distension, nausea, and vomiting result. The cause of the syndrome is unknown, but ectopic pacemakers have occurred in patients with autonomic dysfunction, gastric cancer, or following injection of prostaglandins (37). This diagnosis requires intragastric manometry or recording of the cutaneous electrogastrogram, and it cannot be made by conventional diagnostic methods. It is often confused with psychosomatic illness.

Short Bowel Syndrome. Patients with extended resection of the small intestine have a decreased gastric fractional emptying rate, in addition to acid hypersecretion (76). Both abnormalities are independent of parenteral hyperalimentation and they tend to subside after 3–6 months. The exact mechanism of these abnormalities is unknown, but they could be caused by the loss of inhibitory and excitatory intestinal peptide(s).

Pernicious Anemia. Since these patients have decreased gastric fluid secretion, fasting *gastric emptying rate* is decreased. However, the *fractional emptying rate* is normal (77). Thus, although gastric musculature is atrophied and serum gastrin is extremely high, no abnormality of stomach motility has been detected.

ANTIEMETIC AND GASTROKINETIC AGENTS

Most classical gastrokinetic agents have originated from the substituted benzamide class of compounds and, as such, have antiemetic properties related to their dopamine receptor antagonist properties. In addition, the antiemetic effects of prokinetic agents may be due in part to a reduction of the intragastric volume available for vomiting. On the other hand, motilin agonists may cause vomiting, possibly because they act at multiple receptor sites. Finally, anticholinergic agents with antiemetic properties may inhibit gastric emptying, and clinical benefits may be found without correlation to changes in gastric function. The complexity of this field may benefit from the ongoing discovery and development of specific antagonists of receptor subclasses. Although any current classification by receptor class may soon be obsolete and inaccurate, subsections of these chapters have been classified according to the receptor that is believed to mediate the main effect of families of drugs, and antiemetic and gastrokinetic properties have been discussed jointly for each drug (Table 8.1).

Anticholinergic and Cholinomimetic Agents

Anticholinergic drugs are effective in reducing motion sickness. For example, hyoscine significantly increased tolerance to cross-coupled stimulation and produced a significant though small reduction in eye velocity gain during pursuit eye movement (78). However, the efficacy of these agents is variable, and they have significant side effects (79). In addition, all anticholinergic agents inhibit gastric emptying to some extent.

On the other hand, muscarinic M_2-receptor agonists stimulate gastric motility, but their effect on gastric emptying is variable, and their clinical use is restricted by their cardiac and urinary side effects. Interestingly, the pharmacologic definition of a muscarinic M_3-receptor present only in glandular and smooth muscles of the gastrointestinal tract (80) may open new avenues for the development of novel gastrokinetic agents devoid of side effects.

Histamine Receptor Antagonists

Histamine H_1-receptor antagonists have been used to treat motion sickness, and some of these agents also suppress vertigo (e.g., Antivert). However, they cause drowsiness, and their effect on gastric emptying is unknown.

Histamine H_2-receptor antagonists potently inhibit acid and fluid secretion. Therefore, they reduce the risk of vomiting, especially during induction of anesthesia and immediately after surgery. In addition, histamine H_2-receptors appear to be involved in the regulation of gastric emptying (81), which could modify the effect of antiemetic agents.

Neuroleptic Drugs

Chlorpromazine (e.g., Thorazine) is a phenothiazine that has been used as an antiemetic, but its efficacy is relatively low, and its side effects are much greater than those of more recently developed agents. For example, only 49% of patients treated with chlorpromazine remained free from vomiting and had no, or only mild, nausea in the first 24 hours following administration of cytostatic drugs (82). Chlorpromazine reduces extrapyramidal manifestations associated with metoclopramide in cancer patients receiving chemotherapy (83).

Prochlorperazine (Compazine) has been one of the most widely used antiemetics. Although low doses are not effective in postoperative nausea and vomiting (10 mg intravenously intraoperatively) (83) or in cisplatin-induced emesis (10 mg orally four times daily) (85), the association of high doses of prochlorperazine with dexamethasone has been found to be as effective as high doses of metoclopramide plus dexamethasone (86). However, prochlorperazine may cause somnolence, dizziness, confusion, and parkinsonism, this latter syndrome being found in 8 of 2811 subjects (0.3%), 7 of those being over 60 years of age (87). In addition, dystonic reactions have been reported (88), and these effects are dose-related, being observed in all subjects given 1.2 mg/kg intravenously (89). Finally, at least one case of neuroleptic malignant syndrome has been reported following prochlorperazine (90). Its effect on gastric emptying is unknown.

Adrenergic Blocking Drugs

Blockade of the inhibitory effect of neuronal or circulating catecholamines stimulates gastric emptying (72–74). However, the cardiovascular side effects of the available medications have precluded their use in patients with gastric stasis.

Substituted Benzamides Acting at Multiple Receptor Sites

METOCLOPRAMIDE (REGLAN)

Metoclopramide was the first substituted benzamide derivative with potent gastrokinetic and antiemetic properties (91, 92). At the time of this writing, it remains the only such agent currently approved in the United States.

Mechanism of Action

The gastrokinetic and antiemetic effects of metoclopramide were initially attributed to its antidopaminergic properties (93). In rats, metoclopramide showed the profile of a centrally active dopamine D_2-antagonist, and it also displayed a stimulant effect on spontaneous gastric emptying, this latter effect being unrelated to dopamine D_2-antagonism (94). In addition, although it was later recognized that the antiemetic action of high doses of metoclopramide (4–10 mg/kg) is related to its 5-HT_3-receptor antagonist properties (95), the mechanism of its gastrokinetic effect remained unclear for a long time. In man, metoclopramide has no direct effect on gastric smooth muscle contractility in vitro, but it sensitizes the tissue to acetylcholine (96), and its gastrokinetic effect is dependent on tissue acetylcholine stores (97). Its ability to antagonize the action of 5-HT at neuronal receptor sites was recognized in 1970 (98), but it is only recently that its selective affinity for, and its agonist effect on, 5-HT_4-receptors (see below) has been fully studied (99).

Clinical Studies

Metoclopramide increased gastric emptying of water in patients with peptic ulcer disease (99), whereas gastric emptying of solids was increased in postvagotomy patients only in the presence of gastric stasis (101, 102). This effect could be related in part to the ability of metoclopramide to increase duodenojejunal motility during phase II without inducing a premature phase III (103). In a double-blind randomized study, 10 mg of metoclopramide four times daily was found to be superior to placebo in improving symptoms attributed to delayed gastric emptying as assessed by a "barium burger" test (104). Radionuclide measurement of gastric emptying has demonstrated objective improvement of diabetic gastroparesis after metoclopramide in some studies (56, 105–107). However, another study showed no significant change of emptying despite a symptomatic improvement (108). Although these observations indicate that both local and centrally mediated effects of the drug may be important, it is worth noting that most of these studies examined only the effect of acute administration of metoclopramide (56, 105, 106, 108). Finally, administration of metoclopramide for 3 weeks resulted in an improvement in both symptoms and gastric emptying of liquid in diabetics, but the symptomatic improvement was poorly correlated with enhancement of gastric emptying (107).

Higher doses of metoclopramide (2 mg/kg i.v., repeated 5 times) were shown to prevent cisplatin-induced emesis in humans, whereas lower doses were ineffective (109). This observation, in conjunction with the known weak 5-HT_3-antagonist properties of metoclopramide, led to the hypothesis that this effect was due to 5-HT_3 antagonism. In turn, this concept prompted the development of specific and potent antagonists that selectively inhibit the 5-HT_3-receptors located both in the central nervous system and in afferent nerve terminals located in the gut (see below) (110).

OTHER SUBSTITUTED BENZAMIDES

Other compounds of this family have been developed in an effort to isolate the gastrokinetic properties from the antidopaminergic effects of metoclopramide. Renzapride (BRL-24924, SmithKline Beecham) was shown to antagonize responses of myenteric neurons mediated by both 5-HT_{1F}- and 5-HT_3-receptors (111). In dogs, renzapride mitigated gastroparesis induced by an α_2-adrenergic agonist, while stimulating antroduodenal motility (112). In diabetic gastroparesis and autonomic neuropathy, renzapride also accelerated gastric emptying of both solids and liquids, an effect related to its potent 5-HT_4-agonist properties (see below) (113). It is not available in the United States.

Dopamine Antagonists

DOMPERIDONE (R-33812, MOTILIUM, JANSSEN PHARMACEUTICA)

Mechanism of Action

Domperidone is a dopamine antagonist with high potency and selectivity for binding to dopamine D_2-receptor sites in vitro (114). However, in vivo experiments have indicated that domperidone does not reach dopaminergic receptors in the central nervous system (115). This may explain why, unlike metoclopramide, domperidone is rarely associated with extrapyramidal side effects when given at therapeutic doses and why, contrary to neuroleptic agents, it does not modify the state of vigilance (116). However, like metoclopramide, it produces elevations of plasma prolactin via the inhibition of dopaminergic receptors in the pituitary gland (117).

Domperidone appears to stimulate propulsive gastric motor activity and gastroduodenal coordination by acting directly on an unknown smooth muscle receptor (118). Dopamine receptors have been demonstrated in the stomach; dopamine inhibits gastric motility and it increases the adaptive relaxation of the proximal stomach in response to ingestion of a meal (119, 120). Acute administration of domperidone decreased adaptive relaxation (121) and accelerated gastric emptying of liquid meals in normal subjects (122–124), although it may be less effective in increasing gastric emptying of solids (125, 126). Domperidone prevented radiation-induced vomiting in dogs (127), but not in monkeys (128), while the concurrent radiation-induced suppression of gastric emptying was not mitigated in either species. In addition, domperidone did not prevent cisplatin- or irradiation-induced emesis in ferrets (129).

Clinical Studies

Domperidone inhibited nausea following chemotherapy (130) or surgery (131). Domperidone also increased gastric emptying and concurrently improved symptoms in patients idiopathic gastroparesis (132), diabetes (65), and gastroesophageal reflux disease (126). In patients with the symptom complex of nausea and/or vomiting, epigastric discomfort or pain, abdominal bloating/distension and early satiety, 6 weeks of double-blind treatment with domperidone (20 mg four times daily) was significantly superior to placebo in ameliorating symptoms, but gastric emptying and/or gastric motility were not significantly improved in all series (133–135).

Side Effects

The main side effect of domperidone is an elevation of serum prolactin and the concomitant breast tenderness or enlargement, galactorrhea, and amenorrhea. In addition, a case of neuroleptic malignant syndrome was recently observed in a patient with severe insulin-dependent diabetes (134). It has not been approved for use in the United States.

CLEBOPRIDE

Receptor binding assay has shown that clebopride binds to the dopamine D_2-receptor with a high affinity, and to the α_2-adrenergic and 5-HT_2-receptor with relatively lower affinity (137). Clebopride showed no affinity for dopamine D_1, α_1-adrenergic, muscarinic acetylcholine, histamine H_1, or opioid receptors. In gastric strips, 10^{-8}–10^{-5} M clebopride enhanced the release of acetylcholine as well as the contractions evoked by electrical transmural stimulation. Three findings suggest that this enhancement is caused by the blockade of both the dopamine D_2-receptor and the α_2-adrenergic receptor. First, maximum responses obtained with the specific dopamine D_2-receptor antagonist domperidone and with the specific α_2-adrenergic receptor antagonist yohimbine were smaller than that with clebopride. Second, the sum of the effects of these two specific receptor antagonists was approximately equal to the effect of clebopride. Third, the facilitatory effect of clebopride was partially eliminated by pretreatment of the gastric strips with domperidone or yohimbine, and the facilitatory effect of clebopride was not observed in preparations treated with the combination of domperidone and yohimbine. Clebopride also antagonized

the inhibitory effects of dopamine and clonidine on the responses evoked by electrical transmural stimulation. Thus, clebopride appears to act on postganglionic cholinergic neurons at dopamine D_2- and α_2-adrenergic receptors in gastric strips to enhance the increased motility induced by stimulation of the enteric nervous system.

In patients with nonulcer-related dyspepsia, only one study has shown that clebopride increases gastric emptying and that this effect was correlated with subjective improvement (138). It remains investigational in the United States.

5-HT_3-Receptor Antagonists

Since the discovery in 1986 that a $5HT_3$-receptor antagonist could block cisplatin-induced emesis (110), a number of drugs specifically antagonizing this receptor have been developed, and the list is constantly growing (Item 7 in Table 8.1). Preclinical studies have shown that these medications modify a variety of physiologic functions, indicating that they may become clinically useful in a variety of diseases (139). The mechanism through which $5HT_3$-receptor antagonists prevent cisplatin-induced emesis has been suggested by a study performed in isolated and vascularly perfused segments of the guinea pig small intestine (140). In this preparation, cisplatin at 3 μM caused longitudinal muscle contractions that were abolished by scopolamine as well as a 90% increase of the release of 5HT and 5-hydroxyindoleacetic acid (5-HIAA) into the portal venous effluent. Interestingly, 30 and 100 μM cisplatin decreased the outflow of 5-HT and of its metabolite by 40–50%. The stimulatory effect of cisplatin was abolished in the absence of extracellular calcium or in the presence of tetrodotoxin, hexamethonium, or scopolamine. Several $5HT_3$-receptor antagonists also abolished the stimulatory effect of cisplatin but they did not significantly alter the outflow of 5-HT and 5-HIAA. Thus, cisplatin, at concentrations that occur during anticancer therapy in humans and induce emesis, increases the release of 5-HT from the small intestine of the guinea pig.

In addition, 5-HT$_3$-receptors appear to be located on vagal afferent fibers, since cisplatin-induced emesis is abolished by vagotomy but not by injection of tropisetron into the fourth ventricle (141). Furthermore, 5-HT$_3$-receptors located on vagal afferents may modify endogenous release of acetylcholine and thereby control the regulation of gastric interdigestive phase III activity by motilin (142). When given during phase III contractions, intravenous injections of granisetron and ondansetron instantly and dose-dependently inhibited the spontaneous and motilin-induced phase III contractions in the *innervated*, intact stomach of conscious dogs. At the same time, the duodenal phase III contractions were changed to a pattern of continuous contractions, the contractile force of which was 65% of the spontaneous phase III duodenal contractions, and these contractions immediately migrated aborally along the small intestine. However, spontaneous and motilin-induced phase III-like contractions in *denervated* Heidenhain pouches were not affected by 5-HT$_3$-receptor antagonists. When antagonists were given during phase I, they did not stimulate gastrointestinal contractions. The cyclic fluctuation of plasma motilin concentration with phase III activity in the stomach was also not influenced by 5-HT$_3$-receptor antagonists, but the next phase III gastric contractions were inhibited. However, 5-HT$_3$-receptor antagonists did not influence postprandial motility in either the innervated stomach or in the vagally denervated fundic pouch. Because 5-HT$_3$-receptors appear to be present in peripheral neurones of vagal afferents and in the enteric nervous system, these results suggest that motilin acts on 5-HT$_3$-receptors located on vagal afferents. Therefore, although most 5-HT$_3$-receptor antagonists do not increase gastric emptying, additional studies are necessary to determine whether the constipation and/or diarrhea occasionally observed during treatment are related to 5HT$_3$-receptor antagonist mediated to modifications of gastrointestinal motility.

Both clinical and comparative studies have shown that 5-HT$_3$-receptor antagonists are potent antiemetic agents during cisplatin and noncisplatin chemotherapy as well as during radiotherapy. In comparative studies, the antiemetic efficacy of 5-HT$_3$-receptor antagonists has been superior to conventional antiemetic drugs with regard to the acute chemotherapy-related symptoms, whereas further investigations are needed regarding their role as antiemetics in delayed chemotherapy-induced emesis and in other types of nausea and vomiting, such as that during the postoperative period. The affinity of these compounds for 5HT$_3$ and other receptors varies, and comparative efficacy of each of these compounds may show advantages and disadvantages for some of these agents. Side effects have been minor, consisting mainly of slight headaches, but possible increases in liver enzyme levels associated with the administration of some compounds need further evaluation. In addition, one of these compounds was shown to *cause* emesis (143), and some doses of 5HT$_3$-receptor antagonists may have weak agonistic activity on this receptor (144). Finally, potential clinical use in migraine and psychiatric disorders has been suggested. It is notable that only one case of extrapyramidal reactions was found in the literature (145). At this time, only ondansetron is approved for use in the United States.

ONDANSETRON
(GR-38032F, ZOFRAN, GLAXO)

Pharmacologic Properties and Mode of Action

Ondansetron is a carbazole that binds to 5-HT$_3$-receptors and, to a lesser extent, to 5-HT$_{1B}$, 5-HT$_{10}$ α_1-adrenergic and μ-opioid sites (146). It is a 5-HT$_3$-receptor antagonist that behaves as a reversible competitive antagonist of 5-HT-induced depolarization on both the rabbit and the rat isolated vagus nerve and on the rat superior cervical ganglion (147). Ondansetron was also shown to cause concentration-dependent parallel rightward displacement of the 2-methyl-5-HT concentration-contraction response curve on the longitudinal smooth muscle of the guinea pig ileum, whereas a portion of the response to 5-HT appeared resistant to ondansetron (147). At micromolar concentrations, this compound had negligible agonist or antagonist activity on other 5-HT or non-5-HT receptor-containing tissues on which it was tested (147). In vivo studies in the anesthetized rat showed that the ED_{50} for GR-38032F against the bradycardic response induced by 2-methyl-5-HT (von Bezold-Jarisch reflex) was 0.4 and 7.0 µg/kg for intravenous and oral administration, respectively, and a similar efficacy was observed in the anesthetized cat (147). In the ferret, it has been shown to inhibit vomiting induced by cisplatin, cyclophosphamide, or X-radiation (148), but the dose-response curve was highly nonlinear, suggesting that certain doses of the compound recruit some other pharmacologic action of the compound that interferes with the primary antiemetic action mediated by 5-HT_3-receptor antagonism (144). The inhibitory effectiveness of ondansetron on the Bezold-Jarisch reflex persisted for <3 hours after oral administration and for less than 15 minutes after intravenous administration (149). Because cisplatin selectively increases the levels of 5-HT and 5-HIAA in the intestinal mucosa, a possible site of the antiemetic action of ondansetron may be on 5-HT_3-receptors located on vagal afferents in the gastrointestinal tract (150).

Pharmacokinetics and Tolerance

Ondansetron is eliminated almost entirely by hepatic metabolism, and <5% of an intravenously administered dose is recovered intact in urine (151). The half-life of ondansetron is approximately 3.5 hours, it is slightly less in children and it is prolonged in the elderly. Neither clinical efficacy nor adverse effects have correlated with serum concentrations. Ondansetron is generally well-tolerated. Clinically relevant adverse effects include headache, diarrhea or constipation, sedation, and transient minor elevations of liver function tests.

Clinical Trials

Numerous studies have shown that ondansetron is an effective and safe agent for controlling cisplatin-induced nausea and vomiting (152). In one study that included 28 patients with cancer, nausea and vomiting were significantly decreased by administration of intravenous ondansetron (0.15 mg/kg, three times daily) given at 4-hour intervals beginning 30 minutes before administration of cisplatin compared with placebo (153). The median time to the first episode of emesis was 2.8 hours in the placebo group and 11.6 hours in the ondansetron group ($P < .001$); the median number of episodes in 24 hours was 5.5 in the placebo group and 1.5 in the ondansetron group ($P < .001$); the mean ($\pm$ standard error of the mean) number of regurgitations or dry heaves per episode was 3.2 ± 0.5 in the placebo group and 1.17 ± 0.1 in the ondansetron group ($P < .001$). Treatment with antiemetic rescue agents was required for the control of nausea and vomiting in 12 of 14 patients given placebo, but in none of the 14 patients given ondansetron. There were no adverse effects attributable to ondansetron. The urinary excretion of 5-hydroxyindoleacetic acid, the main metabolite of serotonin, was increased in all patients 2–6 hours after cisplatin chemotherapy, and the increases paralleled the episodes of emesis. Thus, cisplatin increases serotonin release from enterochromaffin cells, and ondansetron appears to act by blocking 5HT_3-receptors.

Ondansetron also was compared with metoclopramide for antiemetic efficacy in a randomized double-blind trial in 122 patients with advanced breast cancer (154). All patients were treated with epirubicin (>50 mg/m²) and cyclophosphamide (>500 mg/m²). Complete plus major control of vomiting and nausea tended to be greater with ondansetron than with metoclopramide (59–85% vs. 48–74% on day 1; $P = .230$ and 67–91% vs. 53–78% on days 2–3 after chemotherapy; $P = .122$). Over the 3-day study period, nausea was absent or mild in 60% of the patients treated with ondansetron compared with 45% of the patients given metoclopramide ($P = .064$).

The only drug-related side effects were gastrointestinal disturbance and headache in 1 patient receiving ondansetron and episodes of diarrhea, fever, hyperkinetic syndrome, fatigue, restlessness, and migraine with vomiting in 5 patients treated with metoclopramide. None of the changes in the biochemical or hematologic parameters was attributed to the antiemetic treatments.

In addition, a randomized double-blind crossover trial demonstrated that dexamethasone significantly improved the efficacy of ondansetron in the control of acute cisplatinum induced emesis (155). In this study, complete or major control was obtained in 49 of 71 (69%) patients after receiving ondansetron plus dexamethasone vs. 40 of 71 (56%) after receiving ondansetron alone ($P = .01$). This effect was most pronounced in the first 12 hours after chemotherapy. Patients receiving the combination also had significantly less nausea. Of the 53 patients who expressed a preference, 38 (72%) preferred the combination treatment ($P = .01$) to ondansetron alone. The effect of ondansetron on delayed emesis was less pronounced.

The efficacy of ondansetron against radiation-induced emesis was demonstrated in a study comparing oral ondansetron (8 mg three times daily) and metoclopramide (10 mg three times daily) in a group of 82 evaluable patients (156). One day after single-exposure radiotherapy treatments of 8–10 Gy to the upper abdomen, vomiting or retching was completely prevented in 97% of patients receiving ondansetron and in 46% of subjects receiving metoclopramide ($P < .01$), and nausea was also significantly better controlled by ondansetron ($P < .01$). During the 5 days of the study period, complete or major control of vomiting or retching was maintained in 92–100% of patients on ondansetron and in 70–95% of subjects in the metoclopramide group.

Ondansetron had no significant effect on motion-induced nausea or saccadic eye movement, although it produced a significant ($P < .05$) though small reduction in eye velocity gain during pursuit eye movement (78). These findings suggest that the 5-HT_3-receptor is not involved in the neural pathways that mediate motion sickness, but that it may have a role in the control of ocular pursuit.

GRANISETRON (BRL-43694, KYTRIL, SMITHKLINE BEECHAM)

Pharmacologic Properties and Mode of Action

Granisetron is an indazole which has been shown by radioligand binding studies to label potently 5-HT_3 recognition sites in rat cortical membranes, although the number of binding sites is very low (157). Granisetron is more potent and longer acting than ondansetron against cisplatin- and radiation-induced emesis in the ferret, and its dose-response curve is linear (144).

Pharmacokinetics and Side Effects

In volunteers, granisetron was widely distributed and also rapidly eliminated, largely through nonrenal mechanisms (158). Granisetron exhibited essentially linear kinetics over the dosage range studied (30–300 μg/kg). There was considerable intersubject variability in terminal phase half-life and total plasma clearance. Biologic activity of granisetron, as evidenced by significant inhibition of cutaneous 5-HT-induced, axon-reflex flare, was still apparent 24 hours after a single dose of 40 μg/kg. Single intravenous doses of 2.5–300 μg/kg of granisetron over a period of 30 minutes, and of 40–160 μg/kg administered over a 3-minute period, were well-tolerated and there were no serious adverse events. There were no consistent or clinically important effects on cardiovascular parameters (pulse rate, blood pressure, electrocardiogram). Single doses of 40–200 μg/kg (30-minute infusion) or 160 μg/kg (3-minute infusion) did not influence subjective state, psychomotor performance, or electroencephalogram results. The only adverse event reported consistently more frequently with granisetron than with placebo was constipation; this generally subsided spontaneously after 24–72 hours. Repeated intravenous doses of granisetron (up to 160 μg/kg twice daily for 7 days) were also well-tolerated. As in the single dose studies, constipation was the only adverse event reported consistently more frequently with active treatment than with placebo, but in no case did this necessitate withdrawal from the study or administration of a laxative.

Clinical Studies

Three double-blind, dose-ranging studies involving 996 chemotherapy-naive patients were conducted to determine the optimal prophylactic dose of intravenous granisetron for prevention of cytotoxic-induced emesis (160). The antiemetic efficacy of prophylactic intravenous granisetron doses ranging from 2–40 μg/kg (study 1) and 40–160 μg/kg (study 2) were examined in patients receiving high-dose cisplatin regimens. In study 3, intravenous of 40 and 160 μg/kg were compared in patients receiving other emetogenic cytotoxic therapies. In study 1, 67.9% (36 of 53) of patients were complete responders at 24 hours following the 40 μg/kg dose compared with 61.5% (32/52) and 30.8% (16/52) in the 10 and 2 μg/kg groups, respectively (40 vs. 2 μg/kg; P < .001). There were no significant differences between doses of 40 and 160 μg/kg in any efficacy parameter in studies 2 and 3. Granisetron was well-tolerated across the dose range examined and no dose-related toxicity was observed. In conclusion, a single 10–40 μg/kg prophylactic dose is effective in controlling cytotoxic-induced nausea and vomiting, and a single 3-mg intravenous dose may be given for the prevention of cytotoxic-induced emesis.

The antiemetic efficacy of granisetron was further demonstrated in a single-center, double-blind, placebo-controlled study conducted of 28 patients with malignant disease, naive to chemotherapy, receiving >80 mg/m² of cisplatin (161). Patients randomly received either granisetron (40 μg/kg) or placebo. Patients in both groups who experienced symptoms of vomiting and nausea were given as many as three 40-μg/kg doses of granisetron on an open-label basis, allowing the assessment of granisetron as an intervention antiemetic in the placebo group. Following gran-

isetron administration, 13 patients (93%) had no vomiting or nausea during the first 24 hours vs. 1 patient (1%) in the placebo group (P < .001).

Granisetron was also effective and safe in a series of twenty-four 3–15-year-old children given moderately or highly emetogenic chemotherapy for malignant disease (162). Single doses of 10, 20, and 40 μg/kg were given intravenously 1 hour before chemotherapy. After 40 μg/kg, 5 of 8 patients experienced no nausea or vomiting in the 24 hours after granisetron treatment. With 20 μg/kg, a similar response was seen, but with 10 μg/kg only 2 of 8 patients experienced complete antiemetic protection despite additional prophylactic chlorpromazine in this group. Granisetron was well-tolerated, and there were no clinically important changes in pulse rate, blood pressure, or electrocardiogram results. Thus, granisetron is well-tolerated by pediatric patients, and its antiemetic action lasted at least 24 hours after a single intravenous dose of 20 or 40 μg/kg.

Recently, a 7- or 14-day randomized, double-blind study was carried out in 930 chemotherapy patients to examine the efficacy and safety of oral granisetron at 0.25, 0.5, 1.0 or 2.0 mg twice daily (163). The number of patients enrolled into this study was able to detect a difference of 15% between groups (80% power). The preliminary results at 7 days showed that efficacy was significantly greater for the group receiving 1.0 mg twice daily (58.5%) than for the group receiving 0.25 mg twice daily (43.7%), thus indicating that the 1.0 mg twice daily dose was optimal in patients receiving moderately emetogenic chemotherapy. This conclusion was supported by the finding that there were more withdrawals from the 0.25- and 0.5-mg groups due to lack of efficacy. The adverse events most frequently reported (>5% of patients) were abdominal pain, constipation, headache, fever, leucopenia, and asthenia. The latter three are recognized side effects of the primary disease and of chemotherapy. Thus, oral granisetron at 1.0 mg twice daily is an effective antiemetic, offering a convenient dosing regimen without significant adverse events. It is currently awaiting FDA approval.

TROPISETRON (ICS-205930, SANDOZ)

Tropisetron showed higher affinity than ondansetron for 5-HT_3-receptors in the guinea pig ileum, although intravenous administration of either compound to anesthetized rats resulted in similar inhibition of the Bezold-Jarisch reflex (149). After oral administration to anesthetized rats, tropisetron was approximately twice as potent as ondansetron as an inhibitor of serotonin-induced bradycardia, and its effect lasted for >3 hours, with heart rate returning to control values 6 hours after oral administration. In dogs, intravenous tropisetron was equipotent compared with ondansetron in inhibiting cisplatin-induced emesis (149). It remains investigational at this time.

Human Studies

Given as a single dose prior to chemotherapeutic agents, tropisetron inhibited emesis and nausea for at least 24 hours, and no extrapyramidal side-effects have been reported to date (164). In addition, 10 and 20 mg tropisetron dose-dependently accelerated gastric emptying of a solid meal in 12 healthy subjects (165). However, a crossover, double-blind, placebo-controlled study showed that 0.15–0.18 mg/kg of intravenous tropisetron did not significantly modify gastric emptying and antral contractility in 13 patients with primary anorexia nervosa (166).

ZACOPRIDE (AHR-11190B, ROBBINS)

In the guinea pig ileum, the affinity of zacopride for 5-HT_3-receptors was similar to that of tropisetron, and greater than that of ondansetron. After intravenous administration to anesthetized rats, zacopride was approximately 10-fold more potent than either tropisetron or ondansetron in the inhibition of serotonin-induced bradycardia. After oral administration to anesthetized rats, zacopride remained approximately 10-fold more potent than tropisetron, and approximately 20-fold more potent than ondansetron as an inhibitor

of serotonin-induced bradycardia. Zacopride had a longer duration of inhibitory effectiveness than either ondansetron or tropisetron in urethane-anesthetized rats with maximal inhibition still apparent 6 hours after oral administration. Similarly, intravenous zacopride was 10-fold more potent than either compound as an inhibitor of cisplatin-induced emesis in animals (167, 168) and in human patients (169). However, emesis was *caused* by 0.3 mg/kg of oral zacopride in ferrets (170), an effect present only for the S-, but not for the R-enantiomer (169). In addition, a study of the ferret showed that emesis induced by 0.2 mg/kg of zacopride can be blocked by 1 mg/kg of tropisetron but not by 0.1–1 mg/kg of granisetron (171). Because tropisetron at high doses is reported to be a 5-HT_4-receptor antagonist, these findings suggest that activation of 5-HT_4-receptors could be responsible for zacopride-induced emesis. In addition, tropisetron at 1 mg/kg, but not granisetron or ondansetron, can also block the vagally mediated emesis induced by oral $CuSO_4$, suggesting that 5-HT_4-receptors involved in emesis are closely associated with abdominal vagal afferents. In monkeys, 0.3 mg/kg of zacopride caused no vomiting in healthy unirradiated animals, and the same dose prevented emesis induced by radiation (168). In patients receiving chemotherapy, intravenous doses <0.007 mg/kg were antiemetic against cisplatin, whereas intravenous doses >0.015 mg/kg *produced* vomiting in 50% of the subjects before they received cisplatin (143).

BENZIMIDAZOLONE DERIVATIVES (SEE ALSO UNDER SPECIFIC 5-HT_4-AGONISTS BELOW)

This novel class of 5-HT_3-receptor antagonists includes six ester or amide derivatives of benzimidazolone-1-carboxyl acid with a basic azabicycloalkyl moiety (compounds 1–3) and their respective ethyl derivatives (compounds 4–6) (172). In isolated preparations of the rabbit heart and of the guinea pig ileum, all compounds antagonized the 5-HT_3-receptor-mediated effects of serotonin, with potencies comparable with those of tropisetron and ondansetron. In the anesthetised rat, all agents potently inhibited the Bezold-Jarisch reflex whether given intravenously or intradermally, and intravenous administration of these compounds prevented cisplatin-induced emesis in dogs. All agents also accelerated gastric emptying of solids in rats, and compounds 4 and 5 were able to stimulate 5-HT_4-receptors in the isolated guinea pig ileum, as well as to enhance contractile activity in the Heidenhain gastric pouch of dogs, showing clear-cut prokinetic properties. Finally, one of these agents, DAU 6215 behaved as a competitive 5-HT_4-antagonist in the rat esophagus, showing an affinity equivalent to that of tropisetron for this receptor (173).

The antiemetic activity of DAU 6215 was investigated in animal models of cytotoxic treatment-evoked emesis and compared with the antiemetic activity of ondansetron and metoclopramide (174). In dogs, vomiting was induced by administration of intravenous cisplatin; in ferrets, the emetic response was elicited by administration of intravenous doxorubicin or X-ray exposure. Pretreatment with 0.1–1 mg/kg of DAU 6215 given intravenously or orally prevented the vomiting response to the different emetic agents. In the dog, the antiemetic potency of metoclopramide was 30 times lower than that of DAU 6215. Ondansetron was less potent than DAU 6215 against cisplatin and doxorubicin but was equally effective in the radiotherapy protocol. In this model, lengthening of the pretreatment time to 2 hours did not affect the antiemetic efficacy of DAU 6215, whereas it decreased that of ondansetron. The results demonstrate that DAU 6215 is a highly effective and long-lasting inhibitor of cytotoxic treatment-induced emesis in different animal species. This effect may be mediated in part by an inhibitory action on dopaminergic neurones of the ventral tegmental area (175).

Specific 5-HT_4-Receptor Agonists

As discussed above, the gastrokinetic properties of metoclopramide, of renzapride, and of some of the 5-HT_3-receptor antagonists could not be completely explained by its agonist or antagonist activity at any known receptor. This observation led to the concept of a 5-HT_4-receptor and to the subsequent demonstration that the prokinetic action of metoclopramide was correlated with its agonist activity at this receptor, which could also explain the effect of cisapride (7). In addition to the 5-substituted indole such as 5-HT, three other chemical classes of 5-HT_4-receptor agonists have been identified so far: the substituted benzamides such as cisapride and renzapride, the benzimidazolones such as BIMU-8, and the substituted pyrrolizidine. Interestingly, the 5-HT_3-receptor antagonist tropisetron also is a 5-HT_4-receptor antagonist, and the recent development of specific 5-HT_4-antagonists such as SB204070 will permit further clarification of the role of this receptor in the regulation of gastric motility. Since 5-HT_4-agonists produce tachycardia in a pig model (176), one will have to evaluate the possible risk that such a side effect could entail when the 5-HT_4-agonists are used as gastrokinetic agents.

CISAPRIDE (R-51619, PROPULSID, JANSSEN)

Receptor Binding Profile

Cisapride is a substituted piperidinyl benzamide that has been shown to stimulate gastrointestinal motility (177). In rat brain homogenates, cisapride showed binding affinity for 5-HT_2, dopamine D_2, and α_1-adrenergic receptors (178, 179). However, the affinity for 5-HT_3-receptor sites was three orders of magnitude weaker than that of zacopride (178), and there was virtually no affinity for 5-HT_4-receptors or for other neurotransmitter binding sites such as dopamine D_2, α_2-adrenergic, β-adrenergic, histamine H_1 and H_2 muscarinic M_1, cholinergic, opiate (μ), benzodiazepine, substance P, neurotensin, or Ca^{2+}-channel sites (181, 182). In addition, cisapride showed only weak or no interaction with the uptake of ^3H-norepinephrine, ^3H-serotonin, ^3H-dopamine, and ^3H-γ-aminobutyric acid (GABA) in synaptosomes. Finally, cisapride

Table 8.3
Effect of Cisapride and Metoclopramide on Mean EC_{50} of Several Gastrointestinal Preparations of Guinea Pig[a]

		EC_{50}	
	Effect	Cisapride	Metoclopramide
Gastroduodenal preparation: antroduodenal coordination	Increase	1.9×10^{-7} M[b] (1.4–2.7)	2.2×10^{-5} M (1.7–2.7)
Stomach: relaxation induced by dopamine	Decrease	1.0×10^{-6} M[b] (0.7–1.5)	1.7×10^{-5} M (1.0–2.9)
Ileum: contractile response to electrical stimulation	Increase	9.2×10^{-9} M[b] (4.4–20)	3.3×10^{-6} M (2.0–5.4)
Colon: tone	Increase	3.5×10^{-8} M[b] (2.5–5.0)	3.5×10^{-6} M (2.4–5.2)

[a]Values in parentheses represent the means $\pm$ confidence limits (after Schuurkes et al. [179]).
[a]EC, effective concentration.
[b]$P < .05$ compared with metoclopramide (covariance analysis).

displaced porcine motilin from its binding sites on rabbit duodenum (183, 184).

Mechanism of the Prokinetic Effect of Cisapride

The primary mechanism of action of cisapride appears to be an enhancement of the release of acetylcholine by the myenteric nerves of the plexus of Auerbach (180, 185). In vivo, this effect does not appears to involve the central nervous system, since the effect remains present in vagotomized dogs (186). The importance of acetylcholine release in the action of cisapride is illustrated by the observation that the majority of the gastrointestinal motor-stimulating effects of cisapride can be prevented or blocked by atropine in isolated tissues (180, 187, 188), in anesthetized dogs (186, 187), and in fasted and fed conscious dogs (186, 189). Thus, although cisapride itself is not a direct cholinergic agonist (187, 189, 190–192), the motor-stimulating effects of cisapride are observed only in the presence of a functional cholinergic tone. In addition, cisapride does not shift the dose-response curve to methacholine to the left as observed with neostigmine (180), thus indicating that cisapride does not act via blockade of acetyl-cholinesterase activity. Furthermore, experiments performed on the guinea pig ileum demonstrate that cisapride does not sensitize postjunctional smooth muscle muscarinic re-

ceptors (Table 8.3) (180). Finally, comparison of the effects of cisapride with those of the M_1-agonist McN-A-343 and the M_1-antagonist pirenzepine demonstrate that the enhanced release of acetylcholine produced by cisapride is not caused by inhibition of prejunctional muscarinic M_1-receptors (193). Similarly, opiate receptors do not appear to play a role as naloxone does not modify the response to cisapride either in vitro (194) or in vivo (195).

As expected from the weak affinity binding of cisapride for dopaminergic receptors, 2.5 mg/kg cisapride given orally to rats did not affect prolactin levels, suggesting a lack of antidopaminergic properties. However, 10 mg/kg oral cisapride enhanced prolactin levels by about 50% of the amount released by metoclopramide, and both compounds were equipotent at 40 and 160 mg/kg (194). Similarly, high doses of cisapride were needed to antagonize apomorphine agitation via central dopamine receptors (ED_{50} = 19.0 mg/kg subcutaneously) or to antagonize apomorphine-induced vomiting (ED_{50} = 3.3 mg/kg subcutaneously) (178). A comparison of doses needed to interact with dopaminergic receptors and doses that cause gastrointestinal prokinetic effects demonstrated that the dopamine-blocking properties are not involved in the motility-stimulating effects of cisapride (178). Motility-stimulating effects occurred at lower concentrations in vitro (twitch enhancement on ileum vs. binding affinity for dopamine receptors) and in vivo (gastric emptying rat vs. central apomorphine-induced agitation or gastric emptying in dogs vs. antagonism of apomorphine-induced vomiting) (178). The potential of cisapride to antagonize dopamine-induced gastric relaxation of the guinea pig in vitro may be due to functional antagonism.

Recent evidence suggests that the stimulatory effect of cisapride on the release of acetylcholine by the guinea pig ileum may involve both inhibitory and stimulatory 5-HT-receptors. However, 5-HT is more potent on the inhibitory receptor, whereas cisapride is more potent on the receptor that stimulates the release of acetylcholine (185). Thus, classical serotonergic receptors do not appear to be involved in the stimulatory effect of cisapride, as more potent and different 5-HT antagonists failed to enhance the contractile response of the guinea pig ileum to electrical stimulation (180). Furthermore, occupation of serotonergic receptors by these antagonists did not interfere with the stimulating effect of cisapride, suggesting that the classical antiserotonergic properties of cisapride, including those at 5-HT$_3$ sites, do not contribute to its motor-stimulating properties (180, 197–199). In both fetal mouse colliculi neurons and in adult guinea pig hippocampal membranes (200), cisapride is an agonist of the 5-HT$_4$-receptors positively coupled with adenylate cyclase, and pretreatment with serotonin prevents the direct effects of cisapride on the guinea pig ileum (7, 183, 188, 199). In the electrically stimulated longitudinal muscle myenteric plexus preparation from the guinea-pig ileum, cisapride (3.10^{-7} M), 5-HT, and a 5-HT$_4$-receptor agonist 5-MeOT ($3.10^{-10} - 10^{-6}$ M) induced similar effects, that is, enhancement of the twitch responses (202). In addition, the same study demonstrated that cisapride desensitized the response induced by 5-HT or 5-MeOT and 5-MeOT or 5-HT desensitized the effect induced by cisapride. Finally, preincubation of the preparations with 5-HT$_4$-receptor antag-

onists abolished the effects induced by cisapride, 5-HT, and 5-MeOT. Thus, 5-HT$_4$-receptors appear to mediate the effects of cisapride on guinea pig and cat tissues, as well as on human stomach strips (203), but the role of serotonergic mechanisms in the effects of cisapride in vivo remains to be determined.

However, all the stimulatory effects of cisapride could not be blocked by atropine, especially in the colon (180, 187, 188, 204), which indicates that part of the stimulatory effects of cisapride at some gastrointestinal sites may be independent of acetylcholine release. Although motilin could be involved, this effect does not seem to be important since the in vivo effect of motilin itself is inhibited by atropine (35).

Pharmacokinetics and Bioavailability

Oral cisapride is rapidly absorbed, oral bioavailability is 30–40%, and peak serum concentrations are reached after 1–2 hours (205). However, peak serum concentrations are higher if cisapride is taken with food.

Effects on Gastrointestinal Motility

In Vitro Studies (Fig. 8.3). Cisapride (10^{-9} to 10^{-6} M) enhanced motility in isolated preparations of the esophagus (206), stomach (178, 204), duodenum (184, 207), small intestine (186, 187, 195, 208), and large intestine (209, 210). Its motility-stimulating effects were demonstrated on strips of tissue from rat, rabbit, opossum, cat, dog, and human preparations. Concentrations $>10^{-6}$ M produced a less pronounced stimulatory effect or even caused inhibition, suggesting a bell-shaped dose-response curve. Interestingly, cisapride did not inhibit gastric relaxation induced by vagal nerve stimulation in the presence of atropine.

In Vivo Studies. Cisapride enhanced motility in various regions of the gastrointestinal tract in different animal species, both in the fed and fasted state, resulting in an accelerated transit through the alimentary canal.

Studies in Rats. Cisapride accelerated gastric emptying of acaloric liquid test meals in conscious rats with a minimum effective subcutaneous dose of 0.31 mg/kg (211). The maximal effects were observed from 0.63 to 5 mg/kg subcutaneously administered, whereas similar effects were observed with metoclopramide with higher doses, ranging from 1.25–20 mg/kg subcutaneous (211).

Studies in Dogs. In the fasting dog, cisapride-induced contractions of the stomach and small intestine were similar to those observed during the phase III of the migrating motor complexes (212). In contrast, bursts of motor activity induced by carbachol were observed only in the small intestine, and not in the stomach (212). Individual gastric and intestinal contractions induced by intravenous administration of 0.16–0.63 mg/kg of cisapride were propagated in an aboral direction, but, in contrast to naturally occurring motor complexes, the entire burst of activity did not migrate (31, 185, 188). However, administration of small doses of intravenous cisapride (0.02–0.03 mg/kg) induced premature phase III-like activity that migrated along the gut (190).

In conscious, fed dogs, cisapride enhanced the amplitude of postprandial contractions on the canine antrum, duodenum, jejunum, and colon after both intravenous (190, 212, 213) and oral (212) administration. Interestingly, the patterns of antral and duodenal contractions induced by cisapride after a small test meal resembled those observed in untreated animals after a normal meal (212). The characteristic pattern of antroduodenal motility after a normal meal consists of antral contractions linked to groups of one to three sequential duodenal contractions separated by periods of relative quiescence (antroduodenal coordination). When small meals are administered, coordination is incomplete. Administration of cisapride (1.25 mg/kg orally) in these circumstances doubled antroduodenal coordination, and this effect was abolished by administration of isopropamide (0.04 mg/kg intravenously) (212). The minimum effective oral dose for this effect was 0.31 mg/kg (212). In this pattern, the ratio of duodenal over antral slow wave frequency approximated 4.0, providing the electrical basis for optimal me-

chanical coordination (214). Cisapride was more potent than metoclopramide in enhancing antroduodenal amplitude and coordination (212). Intravenous cisapride increased the incidence of propagating duodenal contractions (215). In conscious dogs, gastric emptying of liquid, semisolid, and solid test meals was increased after intravenous (212, 216) and oral (217) administration. Finally, cisapride (0.3 mg/kg intravenously) stimulated motility in the duodenum and proximal jejunum after two-thirds resection of the stomach with Roux-en-Y reconstruction in dogs (218).

Human Studies. In 7 healthy volunteers, cisapride (10 mg intravenously) markedly increased the number of spike bursts during the interdigestive state (219). During the first 5-minute period, a nonmigrating phase III-like activity (stationary phase III) occurred, which lasted for 2.6 ± 0.4 minutes. This initial pattern was followed by an intense phase II activity, characterized by a 10-fold increase in the number of groups of repetitive spike bursts and a 6-fold increase in the number of ultrarapid single propagated spike bursts (ultrarapid peristaltic rushes). In addition, the delaying effect of a fat preload on gastric emptying was abolished by cisapride (220).

The effects of cisapride on morphine-induced delay of gastric emptying were compared to those of metoclopramide in 40 patients before surgery (221). Cisapride 10 mg reversed the delay in gastric emptying induced by morphine 10 mg, and this effect was significantly greater than after metoclopramide 10 mg.

Double-blind placebo-controlled trials have shown that cisapride improves gastric emptying in patients with gastric stasis of idiopathic (222) and diabetic origin (205, 222, 224), as well as in gastroparesis related to dystrophia myotonica (223) and progressive systemic sclerosis (226). In nonulcer-related dyspepsia, long-term oral cisapride significantly improved the symptoms and increased fasting antroduodenal motility (10 mg four times daily) (227) and gastric emptying (10 mg three times daily) (228). Finally, cisapride (10 mg four times daily for 6–12 weeks) was significantly superior to placebo in reducing symptoms of gastroesophageal reflux disease and in healing endoscopic esophagitis (229), the only indication to date for which it has received FDA approval.

BENZIMIDAZOLONES

In longitudinal muscle myenteric plexus preparations, nanomolar concentrations of the three azabicycloalkyl benzimidazolone derivatives DAU 6236, BIMU 1, and BIMU 8 caused a concentration-dependent enhancement of the amplitude of nerve-mediated cholinergic submaximal contractions to electrical stimulation (228). The potency of these compounds was equivalent or greater than that of the reference 5-HT_4-receptor *agonist* 5-methoxytryptamine. In whole ileal segments, 0.1–3 μM of DAU 6236, BIMU 1, and BIMU 8 increased markedly the number of peristaltic waves. Micromolar concentrations of tropisetron, a low-affinity *antagonist* of 5-HT_4-receptors, were able to antagonize the facilitatory effect on cholinergic transmission caused by benzimidazolone derivatives and 5-methoxytryptamine, and to reverse the increase in the number of peristalsic waves induced by DAU 6236, BIMU 1, and BIMU 8. In contrast, no effect was observed with micromolar concentrations of the potent and specific 5-HT_3-receptor antagonist ondansetron (230). Thus, benzimidazolone derivatives appear to act as 5-HT_4-receptor agonists in the guinea pig ileum, causing enhancement of acetylcholine release and peristaltic activity, and this action is similar to that of indoleamines and substituted benzamide derivatives with prokinetic properties. In the rat esophagus, BIMU 1 and BIMU 8 behaved as potent synthetic 5-HT_4-agonists (173). Additional experiments will determine whether these agents will be useful in the treatment of gastric stasis.

SUBSTITUTED PYRROLIZIDINE 1

One of these 5-HT_4-receptor agonists was similar to cisapride and renzapride in that it (1) stimulated fasting antral motility in dogs; (2) partially reversed gastroparesis induced by an α_2-adrenergic agonist; and (3) prevented cisplatin-induced emesis (230). Recently, more potent and more selective derivatives have been characterized (232), and this series of compounds may open new avenues for the development of more effective gastrokinetic agents that have fewer side effects. A more recent member of this family is AS-4370, which has no affinity for dopamine D_2, 5-HT_1, 5-HT_2, α_1-, and α_2-adrenergic binding sites (233). In dogs, this agent stimulated antro-duodenal activity without affecting colonic motility; this effect was abolished by atropine, but not by vagotomy (234), and its effect was enhanced by neostigmine. Thus, this compound appears to act by increasing the release of acetylcholine by nerve endings, possibly by stimulating 5-HT_4-receptors.

Opioid Agonists and Antagonists

Although the role of opioid receptors in the physiologic regulation of gastric emptying in man remains to be fully established, opioid agonists and antagonists may prove useful in the treatment of gastric stasis (235).

Naloxone increased gastric emptying in patients with functional dyspepsia and chronic idiopathic gastric stasis only if it was associated with duodenal dyskinesia, whereas no effect was observed if there was antral hypomotility (236). Therefore, opioid antagonists may have a place in the treatment of some types of gastroparesis, but the exact indications for such a treatment are at present unclear.

Trimebutine is an agent with both stimulatory and inhibitory effects on gastric motility, and it has been shown to increase gastric emptying (237) and to alleviate the symptoms of dyspepsia that is non-ulcer related (238). In guinea pig whole brain membranes and ileum myenteric plexus synaptosomes membranes, trimebutine possesses both agonistic and antagonistic properties without true specificity for μ-, δ-, and κ-opioid subtypes, thus suggesting that activation of any of these receptors may mediate its gastrointestinal motility effect (239). Trimebutine given at 5 mg/kg intravenously for 10 minutes initiated migrating phase III-like activity and, like morphine, caused a significant rise in plasma motilin that preceded the beginning of the premature phase III. Both effects were abolished by naloxone (240). In dogs, trimebutine induced gastric contractions (195) and antagonized acoustic stress-induced gastric motor disturbances, thus suggesting that it acts on peripheral κ-receptors located in the wall of the proximal gut (241).

Other opioid agents such as bremazocine also modify gastrointestinal motility (242), but as is the case for trimebutine, further studies will be necessary to evaluate whether this medication may be useful in the treatment of gastric stasis.

Motilin Analogs

The discovery that the antibiotic *erythromycin* has powerful prokinetic properties may allow the development of nonantibiotic macrolides that would be applicable for the treatment of gastroparesis. In the dog, intravenous administration of erythromycin induced bursts of strong contractions in the stomach and the duodenum that migrate along the small intestine to the terminal ileum. This effect may explain the fact that abdominal pain is a frequently observed side effect of this antibiotic. The frequency, contractile force, duration of contractions, and migrating velocity of erythromycin-induced contractions are similar to the contractions occurring spontaneously during interdigestive migrating motor complexes, as well as to those induced by the peptide motilin (243).

Also, in dogs, intravenous or intraduodenal administration of 3 μg/kg of an erythromycin derivative without antibiotic activity, EM-523, induced gastric contractions that subsequently migrated along the small intestine and were inhibited by atropine but not by naloxone (31).

In man, the effect of Erythrocin Lactobionate on intragastric pressure was studied in 13 normal subjects and in 8 patients with severe diabetic gastroparesis. A slow intravenous infusion of 40, 200, or 350 mg was given over a 20-minute period starting 10 minutes after the passage of phase III or after 180 minutes if

phase III was lacking. A 350-mg dose of erythromycin had no significant effect in normal subjects. At a 200-mg dose, an MMC was not elicited but a prolonged period of strong antral peristaltic contractions was observed in both groups. Erythromycin at 40 mg induced phase III of MMC in the antrum and upper small intestine in patients with diabetic gastroparesis, as well as in normal subjects (244).

In another study, 10 patients with diabetic gastroparesis were given either erythromycin (200 mg intravenously) or placebo over a 15-minute period following a standardized meal. Erythromycin normalized gastric emptying of both liquids and solids with a disappearance of the differences between emptying of liquids and of solids in the 10 subjects. Gastric emptying also improved in the 10 patients after 4 weeks of treatment with oral erythromycin (250 mg three times a day) but to a lesser degree (66).

Based on the above studies, erythromycin appears to be a potent gastrokinetic agent that accelerates gastric emptying and intestinal transit by stimulating normal gastrointestinal motility. However, oral bioavailability is known to be a problem with erythromycin, and the relation between its plasma levels and its gastrokinetic effects has not been evaluated. Furthermore, the development of nonantibiotic macrolides will be necessary before this type of agent can be applied on a wide scale in the treatment of gastric stasis.

CONCLUSIONS

In recent years, the treatment of nausea, vomiting, and gastric stasis has benefitted greatly from the rapid development of novel therapeutic agents, and many other medications will become available for both basic and clinical research in the near future. Except for the motilin analogs, the peptide antagonists and agonists currently under investigation have not been considered in this review, but the specific cholecystokinin A and B antagonists may represent a fruitful area of research (23, 24). However, many factors have to be weighed before these compounds become widely used in patients, such as their pharmacokinetics, duration of action, and side effects, and only many years of postmarketing surveillance will demonstrate which agents are most useful and effective.

REFERENCES

1. Hunt JN. Regulation of gastric emptying by neurohumoral factors and by gastric and duodenal receptors. In: Dubois A, Castell DO, eds. Esophageal and gastric emptying. Boca Raton FL: CRC Press, 1984:65–71.
2. Treacy PJ, Jamieson GG, Dent J, Devitt PG, Heddle R. Duodenal intramural nerves in control of pyloric motility and gastric emptying. Am J Physiol 1992;263:G1–G5.
3. Davison JS. Innervation of the gastrointestinal tract. In: Wingate DL, Christensen J, eds. A guide to gastrointestinal motility. London: John Wright and Sons, 1983:1–47.
4. Gaddum JH, Picarelli ZP. Two kinds of tryptamine receptors. Br J Pharmacol Chemother 1957;12:323–328.
5. Peroutka SJ. 5-Hydroxytryptamine receptor subtypes. Annu Rev Neurosci 1988;11:45–60.
6. Gershon MD, Altman RF. An analysis of the uptake of 5-hydroxytryptamine by the myenteric plexus of the small intestine of the guinea pig. J Pharmacol Exp Ther 1971;179:29–41.
7. Dumuis A, Sebben M, Bockaert J. The gastrointestinal prokinetic benzamide derivatives are agonists at the non-classical 5-HT receptor (5-HT$_4$) positively coupled to adenylate cyclase in neurons. Naunyn Schmied Arch Pharmacol 1989;340:403–410.
8. Tonini M, Rizzi CA, Manzo L, Onori L. Novel enteric 5HT$_4$ receptors and gastrointestinal prokinetic action. Pharmacol Res 1991;24:5–14.
9. Gebauer A, Merger M, Kilbinger H. Modulation by 5-HT$_3$ and 5-HT$_4$-receptors of the release of 5-hydroxytryptamine from guinea pig small intestine. Naunyn-Schmiedeberg Arch Pharmacol 1993;347:137–140.
10. Creese I, Snyder SH. Receptor binding and pharmacological activity of opiates in the guinea pig intestine J Pharmacol Exp Ther 1975;194:205–219.
11. Zhang L, Gu ZF, Pradhan T, Jensen RT, Maton PN. Characterization of opioid receptors on smooth muscle cells from guinea pig stomach. Am J Physiol 1992;262:G461–G469.
12. Reynolds JC, Ouyang A, Cohen S. Opiate nerves mediate feline pyloric responses to intraduadenal amino acids. Am J Physiol 1984;284 (Gastrointest Liver Physiol 11):G307–312.
13. Million M, Fioramonti J, Bueno L. Oral administration of Tyr-MIF-1 stimulates gastric emptying and gastrointestinal motility in rodents. Peptides 1992;13:469–474.
14. Gue M, Junien JL, Bueno L. Central and peripheral opioid modulation of gastric relaxation induced by feeding in dogs. J Pharmacol Exp Ther 1989;250:1006–1010.
15. Gue M, Fioramonti J, Junien JL, Bueno L. Orally administered kappa but not mu opiate agonists enhance gastric emptying of a solid canned food meal in dogs. J Pharm Pharmacol 1988;40:873–875.
16. Gue M, Fioramonti J, Honde C, Pascaud X, Junien JL, Bueno L. Opposite effects of kappa-opioid agonists on gastric emptying of liquids and solids in dogs. Gastroenterology 1988;95:927–931.
17. Shea-Donohue, PT, Adams N, Arnold J, Dubois A. Effects of met-enkephalin and naloxone on gastric emptying and secretion in rhesus monkeys. Am J Physiol 1983;245:G196–G200.
18. Touzeau PL, Shea-Donohue PT. Kappa agonists inhibit gastric emptying but not acid secretion in rhesus monkeys. J Pharmacol Exp Ther 1990;253:1010–1016.
19. Bueno L, Gue M, Fargeas MJ, Alvinerie M, Junien JL, Fioramonti J. Vagally mediated inhibition of acoustic stress-induced cortisol release by orally administered kappa-opioid substances in dogs. Endocrinology 1989;124:1788–1793.
20. Desai KM, Sessa WC, Vane JR. Involvement of nitric oxide in the reflex relaxation of the stomach to accommodate food or fluid. Nature 1991;351:477–479.
21. Chey MJ, Hitanant S, Hendricks J, et al. Effect of secretin and cholecystokinin on gastric emptying and gastric secretion in man. Gastroenterology 1970;58:820–827.
22. Kleibeuker JH, Beekhuis H, Piers DA, Schaffalitzky de Muckadell OB. Retardation of gastric emptying of solid food by secretin. Gastroenterology 1988;94:122–126.
23. Debas HT, Farooq O, Grossman MI. Inhibition of gastric emptying is a physiological action of cholecystokinin. Gastroenterology 1975;68:1211–1217.
24. Dubois A, Bruley S, Mizrahi M, Fiala N, Solomon T, Turkelson C. Role of cholecystokinin in the regulation of gastric function after caloric meals [Abstract]. Gastroenterology 1991;100:A439.
25. Liddle RA, Gertz BJ, Kanayama S, et al. Effect of a novel CCK receptor antagonist MK-329 on gall bladder contraction and gastric emptying in humans: implications for the physiology of CCK. J Clin Invest 1989;84:1220–1225.
26. Hunt JN, Ramsbottom N. Effect of gastrin II on gastric emptying and secretion during a test meal. Br Med J 1967;4:386–390.
27. Debas HT, Yamagishi Y, Dryburgh JR. Motilin enhances gastric emptying of liquids in dogs. Gastroenterology 1977;73:777–780.
28. Christofides ND, Modlin IM, Fitzpatrick ML, Bloom SR. Effect of motilin on the rate of gastric emptying and gut hormone release during breakfast. Gastroenterology 1979;76:903–907.
29. Christofides ND, Long RG, Fitzpatrick ML, MacGregor GP, Bloom SR. Effect of motilin on the

gastric emptying of glucose and fat in humans. Gastroenterology 1981;80:456–460.

30. Vantrappen G, Janssens J, Peeters, Bloom SR, Christofides N, Hellemans J. Motilin and the interdigestive migrating motor complexes. Am J Dig Dis 1979;24:497–500.

31. Inatomi N, Satoh H, Maki Y, Hashimoto N, Itoh Z, Omura S. An erythromycin derivative, EM-523, induces motilin-like gastrointestinal motility in dogs. J Pharmacol Exp Ther 1989;251:707–712.

32. Sarna S. Cyclic motor activity: migrating motor complex. Gastroenterology 1985;89:894–913.

33. Vantrappen G, Peeters TL. Motlin. In: Makhlouf GM, ed. Handbook of physiology. sect 6. Bethesda MD: American Physiological Society, 1989:545–558.

34. Strunz U, Domschke W, Mitzinegg P, Domschke S, Schubert F, Wunch E, Jageer E, Demling L. Analysis of motor effect of 13-norleucine motilin on the rabbit, guinea-pig, rat and human alimentary tract. Gastroenterology 1975;68:1485–1491.

35. Fox JE, Daniel EE, Jury J, Fox AE, Collins SM. Sites and mechanisms of action of neuropeptides on canine gastric motility differ *in vivo* and *in vitro*. Life Sci 1983;33:817–825.

36. Sanders KM, Bauer AJ, Publicover NG. Regulation of antral gastric slow wave frequency by prostaglandins. In: Roman C, ed. Gastrointestinal motility. Lancaster, United Kingdom: MTP Press, 1984:77–85.

37. Kim CH, Zinsmeister AR, Malagelada J.-R. Effect of gastric dysrhythmia on postcibal motor activity of the stomach. Dig Dis Sci 1988;33:193–199.

38. Westbrook C, Glaholm J, Barrett A. Vomiting associated with whole body irradiation. Clin Radiol 1987;38:263–266.

39. Borison HL, Wang SC. Physiology and pharmacology of vomiting. Pharmacol Rev 1953;5:193–230.

40. Borison HL, McCarthy LE. Neuropharmacology of chemotherapy-induced emesis. Drugs 1983;25:8–17.

41. Kerlin P. Postprandial antral hypomotility in patients with idiopathic nausea and vomiting. Gut 1989;30:54–59.

42. Borison HL, McCarthy LE, Douple EB, Johnson J, Borison R. Acute radiation-induced vomiting in area postrema-ablated cats. Radiat Res 1987;109:430–439.

43. Malagelada JR, Rees WDW, Mazzotta LJ, Go VLW. Gastric motor abnormalities in diabetic and postvagotomy gastroparesis: effect of metoclopramide and bethanechol. Gastroenterology 1980; 78:286–293.

44. Fox S, Behar J. Pathogenesis of diabetic gastroparesis: a pharmacological study. Gastroenterology 1980;78:757–763.

45. Mignon M, Bonnefond AN, Gratton J, Bonfils S. Repeated vomiting of gastric juice in a patient with Zollinger-Ellison syndrome: modifying influence upon clinical features. Dig Dis Sci 1981;26:752–754.

46. Dubois A, Van Eerdewegh P, Gardner JD. Gastric emptying and secretion in Zollinger-Ellison syndrome. J Clin Invest 1977;59:255–263.

47. Dubois A, Price SF, Castell DO. Gastric retention in duodenal ulcer disease: a reappraisal. Am J Dig Dis 1978;23:993–997.

48. Malagelada JR, Longstreth GF, Summerskill WHJ, Go VLW. Measurement of gastric functions during digestion of ordinary solid meals in man. Gastroenterology 1976;70:203–210.

49. Meyer JH, MacGregor IL, Gueller R, Martin P, Cavalieri R. ^{99m}Tc-tagged chicken liver as a marker of solid food in the human stomach. Am J Dig Dis 1976;21:293–304.

50. Stordy SN, Greig JH, Bogoch A. The steak and barium meal. Am J Dig Dis 1969;14:463–469.

51. Raskin H. Barium-burger roentgen study for unrecognized, clinically significant, gastric retention. South Med J 1971;64:1227–1235.

52. Bromster D. Gastric emptying rate in gastric and duodenal ulceration. Scand J Gastroenterol 1969;4:193–201.

53. George JD. New clinical method for measuring the rate of gastric emptying: the double sampling test meal. Gut 1968;9:237–242.

54. Griffith GH, Owen GM, Campbell H. Gastric emptying in health and gastroduodenal disease. Gastroenterology 1968;54:1–7.

55. Kassander P. Asymptomatic gastric retention in diabetes. Ann Intern Med 1958;48:797–812.

56. Campbell IW, Heading RC, Tothill P, Buist TAS, Ewing DJ, Clark FB. Gastric emptying in diabetic autonomic neuropathy. Gut 1977;18:462–467.

57. Feldman M, Corbett DB, Ramsey EJ, Walsh JH, Richardson CT. Abnormal gastric function in long-standing, insulin-dependent diabetic patients. Gastroenterology 1979;77:12–17.

58. Scarpello JHB, Barber DC, Hague RV, Cullen DR, Sladen GE. Gastric emptying of solid meals in diabetics. Br Med J 1976;2:671–673.

59. Feldman M, Schiller LR. Disorders of gastrointestinal motility associated with diabetes mellitus. Ann Intern Med 1983;98:378–384.

60. Wright RA, Clemente R, Wathen R. Diabetic gastroparesis: an abnormality of gastric emptying of solids. Am J Med Sci 1985;289:240–242.

61. Keshavarzian A, Iber FL, Vaeth J. Gastric emptying with insulin-requiring diabetes mellitus. Am J Gastroenterol 1987;82:29–35.

62. Camilleri M, Malagelada JR. Abnormal intestinal motility in diabetics with gastroparesis syndrome. Eur J Clin Invest 1984;14:420–427.

63. Meyer JH. Motility of the stomach and gastroduodenal junction. In: Johnson LR, Christensen J, Jackson MJ, Jacobson ED, Walsh JH, eds. Physiology

of the gastrointestinal tract. New York: Raven Press, 1987:613–629.

64. Schulze-Delrieu K. Metoclopramide. Gastroenterology 1979;77:768–779.

65. Horowitz M, Harding PE, Chatterton BE, Collins PJ, Shearman DJC. Acute and chronic effects of domperidone on gastric emptying in diabetic autonomic neuropathy. Dig Dis Sci 1985;30:1–9.

66. Janssens J, Vantrappen G, Peeters T, et al. Improvement of gastric emptying in diabetic gastroparesis with erythromycin. N Engl J Med 1990;322:1028–1031.

67. Peachy RDG, Creamer B, Pierce JW. Sclerodermatous involvement of the stomach and the small and large bowel. Gut 1969;10:285–292.

68. Feldman F, Marshak RH. Dermatomyositis with significant involvement of the gastrointestinal tract. Am J Roentgenol 1963;90:746–752.

69. Brown CH, Shirey EK, Haserick JR. Gastrointestinal manifestations of systemic lupus erythematosus. Gastroenterology 1956;31:649–655.

70. Dubois A, Gross HA, Ebert MH, Castell DO. Altered gastric emptying and secretion in primary anorexia nervosa. Gastroenterology 1979;77:319–323.

71. Holt S, Ford MJ, Grant S, Heading RC. Abnormal gastric emptying in primary anorexia nervosa. Br J Psychiat 1981;139:550–552.

72. Dubois A, Weise VK, Kopin IJ. Postoperative ileus in the rat: physiopathology, etiology and treatment. Ann Surg 1973;178:781–786.

73. Dubois A, Kopin IJ, Pettigrew K, Jacobowitz DM. Chemical and histochemical studies of postoperative sympathetic activity in the digestive tract. Gastroenterology 1974;66:403–407.

74. Catchpole BN. Ileus: use of sympathetic blocking agents in its treatment. Surgery 1969;66:811–820.

75. You CH, Lee KY, Chey WY, Menguy R. Electrogastrographic study of patients with unexplained nausea, bloating, and vomiting. Gastroenterology 1980;79:311–314.

76. Murphy JP, King DR, Dubois A. Treatment of gastric hypersecretion with cimetidine in the short bowel syndrome. N Engl J Med 1979;300:80–81.

77. Dubois A, Castell DO. Gastric emptying in pernicious anemia, a model for the study of secretagogues in the absence of acid. In: J Christensen, ed. Gastrointestinal motility. New York: Raven Press, 1980:233–237.

78. Stott JR, Barnes GR, Wright RJ, Ruddock CJ. The effect on motion sickness and oculomotor function of GR 38032F, a 5-HT$_3$-receptor antagonist with anti-emetic properties. Br J Clin Pharmacol 1989;27:147–57.

79. Homick JL, Kohl RL, Reschke MF, Degioanni J, Cintron-Trevina N. Transdermal scopolamine in the prevention of motion sickness: evaluation of the time course efficacy. Aviat Space Environ Med 1983;54:994–1000.

80. Hanack C, Pfeiffer A. Upper gastrointestinal porcine smooth muscle expresses M$_2$- and M$_3$-receptors. Digestion 1990;45:196–201.

81. Dubois A, Nompleggi D, Castell DO. Histamine H$_2$ receptor stimulation increases gastric emptying in monkeys. Am J Physiol 1988;255:G767–G771.

82. Marty M. A comparative study of the use of granisetron, a selective 5-HT3 antagonist, versus a standard anti-emetic regimen of chlorpromazine plus dexamethasone in the treatment of cytostatic-induced emesis. The Granisetron Study Group. Eur J Cancer 1990;26 (suppl 1):S28–S32.

83. Tsavaris NB, Papaioannou D, Beldecos D, et al. Comparison of antiemetic activity of chlorpromazine and high doses of metoclopramide in cisplatin-based chemotherapy. Acta Oncol 1990;29:1005–1009.

84. Cramb R, Fargas-Babjak A, Hirano G. Intraoperative prochlorperazine for prevention of post-operative nausea and vomiting. Can J Anaesth 1989;36:565–567.

85. Lane M, Smith FE, Sullivan REA, Plasse TF. Dronabinol and prochlorperazine alone and in combination as antiemetic agents for cancer chemotherapy. Am J Clin Oncol 1990;13:480–484.

86. Akhtar SS, Bano ZA, Bhat GM, Bhat MA. A double blind randomized cross-over comparison of high dose prochlorperazine with high dose metoclopramide for cisplatin-induced emesis. Oncology 1991;48:226–229.

87. Bateman DN, Darling WM, Boys R, Rawlins MD. Extrapyramidal reactions to metoclopramide and prochlorperazine. Q J Med 1989;71:307–311.

88. Schumock GT, Martinez E. Acute oculogyric crisis after administration of prochlorperazine. South Med J 1991;84:407–408.

89. Olver IN, Webster LK, Bishop JF, Clarke J, Hillcoat BL. A dose finding study of prochlorperazine as an antiemetic for cancer chemotherapy. Eur J Cancer Clin Oncol 1989;25:1457–1461.

90. Manser TJ, Warner JF. Neuroleptic malignant syndrome associated with prochlorperazine. South Med J 1990;83:73–74.

91. Justin-Besancon L, Laville C, Thominet M. Le métoclopramide et ses homologues: introduction à leur étude biologique. C R Acad Sci Paris 1964;258:4384–4386.

92. Pinder RM, Brogden RN, Sawyer PR, Speight TM, Avery GS. Metoclopramide: a review of its pharmacological properties and clinical use. Drugs 1976;12:81–131.

93. Peringer E, Jenner P, Donaldson IM, Marsden CD. Metoclopramide and dopamine receptor blockade. Neuropharmacology 1976;15:463–469.

94. Megens AA, Awouters FH, Niemegeers CJ. General pharmacology of the four gastrointestinal motility stimulants bethanechol, metoclopramide, trimebutine, and cisapride. Arzneimittelforschung 1991;41:631–634.

95. Miner WD, Sanger GJ, Turner DH. Evidence that 5-hydroxytryptamine₃ receptors mediate cytotoxic drugs and radiation-evoked emesis. Br J Cancer 1987;56:159–162.

96. Eisner M. Gastrointestinal effects of metoclopramide in man: in vitro experiments with human smooth muscle preparations. Br Med J 1968;4:679–680.

97. Hay AM, Man WK. Effect of metoclopramide on guinea pig stomach: critical dependence on intrinsic stores of acetylcholine. Gastroenterology 1979;76:492–496.

98. Bianchi C, Beani L, Crema C. Effect of metoclopramide on isolated guinea pig colon: 2. Interference with ganglionic stimulant drugs. Eur J Pharmacol 1970;12:332–341.

99. Bockaert J, Sebben M, Dumuis A. Pharmacological characterization of 5-hydroxytryptamine4 (5-HT₄) receptors positively coupled to adenylate cyclase in adult guinea pig hippocampal membranes: effect of substituted benzamide derivatives. Mol Pharmacol 1990;37:408–411.

100. Connell AM, George JD. Effect of metoclopramide on gastric function in man. Gut 1969;10:678–680.

101. Hancock BD, Bowen-Jones E, Dixon R, Dymock IW, Cowley DJ. The effect of metoclopramide on gastric emptying of solid meals. Gut 1974;15:562–467.

102. Metzger WH, Cano R, Sturdevant RAL. Effect of metoclopramide in chronic gastric retention after gastric surgery. Gastroenterology 1976;71:30–32.

103. Grandjouan S, Chaussade S, Couturier D, Thierman-Duffaud D, Henry JF. A comparison of metoclopramide and trimebutine on small bowel motility in humans. Aliment Pharmacol Ther 1989;3:387–393.

104. Perkel MS, Moore C, Hersh T, Davidson ED. Metoclopramide therapy in patients with delayed gastric emptying: a randomized double-blind study. Dig Dis Sci 1979;24:662–666.

105. Domstad PA, Kin EE, Coupal JJ, et al. Biologic gastric emptying time in diabetic patients using Tc⁹⁹ᵐ-labeled resin-oatmeal with and without metoclopramide. J Nucl Med 1980;22:1098.

106. Kim EE, Choy YC, Domstad PA, et al. Biologic gastric emptying time using Tc⁹⁹ᵐ-TETA polystyrene resin in various clinical situations. Eur J Nucl Med 1981;6:155–158.

107. Snape WJ, Nattle WM, Schwartz SS, Braunstein SN, Goldstein HA, Alavi A. Metoclopramide to treat gastroparesis due to diabetes mellitus: a double-blind, controlled trial. Ann Intern Med 1982;96:444–446.

108. Soergel KH, Palmer DP, Loo FD, Wood CM. Abnormal gastric emptying in diabetics and the effect of metoclopramide [Abstract]. Gastroenterology 1980;78:1265A.

109. Gralla RJ, Itri LM, Pisko SE, et al. Antiemetic efficacy of high dose metoclopramide: randomized trials with placebo and prochlorperazine in patients with chemotherapy-induced nausea and vomiting. N Engl J Med 1981;305:905–909.

110. Miner WD, Sanger GJ. Inhibition of cisplatin-induced vomiting by selective M-receptor antagonism. Br J Pharmacol 1986;88:497–499.

111. Mawe GM, Branchek TA, Gershon MD. Blockade of 5-HT-mediated enteric slow EPSP by BRL-24924: gastrokinetic effects. Am J Physiol 1989;257:G386–G396.

112. Gullikson GW, Virina MA, Loeffler R, Erwin WD. Alpha 2-adrenergic model of gastroparesis: validation with renzapride, a stimulator of motility. Am J Physiol 1991;261:G426–G432.

113. Mackie AD, Ferrington C, Cowan S, Merrick MV, Baird JD, Palmer KR. The effects of renzapride, a novel prokinetic agent, in diabetic gastroparesis. Aliment Pharmacol Ther 1991;5:135–142.

114. Leysen JE, Gommeren W. In vitro receptor binding profile of drugs in migraine. In: WK Amery, JM Van Nueten, A Wauquier eds. The Pharmacological Basis of Migraine Therapy. London: Pitman, 1984:255–266.

115. Laduron PM, Leysen JE. Domperidone, a specific in vitro dopamine antagonist devoid of in vivo central dopaminergic activity. Biochem Pharmacol 1979;28:2161–2165.

116. Costall B, Fortune DH, Naylor RJ. Neuropharmacological studies on the neuroleptic potential of domperidone (R 33,812). J Pharm Pharmacol 1979;31:344–347.

117. Cocchi D, Gil-Ad I, Parenti M, Stefanini E, Locatelli V, Muller EE. Prolactin-releasing effect of a novel antidopaminergic drug, domperidone, in the rat. Neuroendocrinology 1980;30:65–69.

118. Schuurkes JAJ, Helsen LFM, Ghoos ECR, Eelen JGMG, Van Nueten JM. Stimulation of gastroduodenal motor activity: dopaminergic and cholinergic modulation. Drug Dev Res 1986;8:233–241.

119. Schuurkes JAJ, Van Nueten JM. Is dopamine an inhibitory modulator of gastrointestinal motility? Scand J Gastroenterol 1981;16(suppl 67):33–36.

120. Valenzuela JE. Dopamine as a possible nerve transmitter in gastric relaxation. Gastroenterology 1976;71:1019–1022.

121. Bateman DN, Gooptu D, Whittingham TA. The effects of domperidone on gastric emptying of liquid in man. Br J Clin Pharmacol 1982;13:675–678.

122. Baeyens R, Van de Velde D, De Schepper A, Wollaert R, Reyntjens A. Effect of intravenous and oral domperidone on the motor function of the stomach and small intestine. Postgrad Med J 1979;55(suppl 1):19–23.

123. Broekaert A. Effect of domperidone on gastric emptying and secretion. Postgrad Med J 1979;55(suppl 1):11–14.

124. De Schepper A, Wollaert F, Reyntjens A. Effects of oral domperidone on gastric emptying and motility: a double-blind comparison with placebo and

metoclopramide. Arzneimittelforschung 1978;28: 1196–1199.

125. Akkermans LMA, Jacobs F, Dei HY, Wittebol P. Gastric emptying function of proximal and distal stomach and the effect of peripheral dopamine blockade [Abstract]. Gastroenterology 1983; 84:1087A.

126. Valenzuela JE, Miranda M, Ansari AN, Lim BR. Delayed gastric emptying in patients with reflux esophagitis [Abstract]. Gastroenterology 1981; 80:1307A.

127. Dubois A, Jacobus JP, Grissom MP, Eng RR, Conklin JJ. Altered gastric emptying and prevention of radiation induced vomiting in dogs. Gastroenterology 1984;86:444–448.

128. Dorval ED, Mueller GP, Eng RR, Durakovic A, Conklin JJ, Dubois A. Effect of ionizing radiation on gastric secretion and gastric motility in monkeys. Gastroenterology 1985;89:374–380.

129. Miner WD, Sanger GJ, Turner DH. Evidence that 5-hydroxytryptamine³-receptors mediate cytotoxic drug and radiation-evoked emesis. Br J Cancer 1987;56:159–162.

130. Hamers J. Cytostatic therapy-induced vomiting inhibited by domperidone. A double-blind cross-over study. Biomedicine 1978;29:242.

131. Fragen RJ, Caldwell N. A new benzimidazole antiemetic, domperidone, for the treatment of postoperative nausea and vomiting. Anesthesiology 1978;49:289–292.

132. McCallum RW. Review of the current status of prokinetic agents in gastroenterology. Am J Gastroenterol 1985;80:1008–1016.

133. Chey WY, You CH, Ange DA. Open and double-blind clinical trials of domperidone in patients with unexplained nausea and vomiting, abdominal bloating and early satiety [Abstract]. Gastroenterology 1982;82:1033A.

134. Corinaldesi R, Stanghellini V, Zarabini GE, et al. The effect of domperidone on the gastric emptying of solid liquid phases of a mixed meal in patients with dyspepsia. Curr Ther Res 1983;34:982–986.

135. Davis RH, Clench MH, Mathias JR. Effects of domperidone in patients with chronic unexplained upper gastrointestinal symptoms: a double-blind, placebo-controlled study. Dig Dis Sci 1988;33:1505–1511.

136. Spirt MJ, Cahn W, Thieberg M, Sachar DB. Neuroleptic malignant syndrome induced by domperidone. Dig Dis Sci 1992;37:946–948.

137. Takeda K, Taniyama K, Kuno T, et al. Clebopride enhances contractility of the guinea pig stomach by blocking peripheral D_2 dopamine receptor and alpha-2 adrenoceptor. J Pharmacol Exp Ther 1991;257:806–811.

138. Corinaldesi R, Stanghellini V, Raiti C, et al. Effect of chronic oral administration of clebopride and metoclopramide on gastric emptying of solids in patients with functional dyspepsia. Curr Ther Res 1985;38:790–797.

139. Fozard JR. Pharmacological relevance of 5-HT₃ receptors. In: Langer SZ, Brunello N, Racagni G, Mendlewicz J, eds. International Academy of Biomedical Drug Research. Vol 1: Serotonin receptor subtypes: pharmacological significance and clinical implications. Basel: Karger, 1992:44–55.

140. Schworer H, Racke K, Kilbinger H. Cisplatin increases the release of 5-hydroxytryptamine (5-HT) from the isolated vascularly perfused small intestine of the guinea-pig: involvement of 5-HT₃ receptors. Naunyn Schmiedebergs Arch Pharmacol 1991;344:143–149.

141. Fukui H, Yamamoto M, Sato S. Vagal afferent fibers and peripheral 5-HT₃ receptors mediate cisplatin-induced emesis in dogs. Jpn J Pharmacol 1992;59:221–226.

142. Itoh Z, Mizumoto A, Iwanaga Y, Yoshida N, Torii K, Wakabayashi K. Involvement of 5-hydroxytryptamine 3 receptors in regulation of interdigestive gastric contractions by motilin in the dog. Gastroenterology 1991;100:901–908.

143. Pisters KMW, Kris MG, Tyson LB, Clarck RA, Gralla RJ. Dose-ranging trial of zacopride: the emetic antiemetic. J Natl Cancer Inst 1992;84:717–718.

144. Andrews PLR, Bhandari P, Davey PT, Bingham S, Marr HE, Blower PR. Are all 5-HT₃ antagonists the same? Eur J Cancer 1992;28A(suppl 1):52–56.

145. Dobrow RB, Coppock MA, Hosenpud JR. Extrapyramidal reaction caused by ondansetron. J Clin Oncol 1991;9:1921.

146. Van Wijngaarden I, Tulp MTM, Soudijn W. The concept of selectivity in 5HT receptor research. Eur J Pharmacol 1990;188:301–312.

147. Butler A, Hill JM, Ireland SJ, Jordan CC, Tyers MB. Pharmacological properties of GR38032F, a novel antagonist at 5-HT₃ receptors. Br J Pharmacol 1988;94:397–412.

148. Tyers MB. Pharmacology and preclinical antiemetic properties of ondansetron. Semin Oncol 1992;19(suppl 10):1–18.

149. Cohen ML, Bloomquist W, Gidda JS, Lacefield W. Comparison of the 5-HT₃ receptor antagonist properties of ICS 205-930, GR38032F and zacopride. J Pharmacol Exp Ther 1989;248:197–201.

150. Stables R, Andrews PL, Bailey HE, et al. Antiemetic properties of the 5-HT₃-receptor antagonist, GR38032F. Cancer Treat Rev 1987;14:333–336.

151. Kohler DR, Goldspiel BR. Ondansetron: a serotonin receptor (5-HT₃) antagonist for antineoplastic chemotherapy-induced nausea and vomiting. DICP 1991;25:367–380.

152. Milne RJ, Heel RC. Ondansetron: therapeutic use as an antiemetic. Drugs 1991;41:574–595.

153. Cubeddu LX, Hoffmann IS, Fuenmayor NT, Finn AL. Efficacy of ondansetron (GR 38032F) and the

role of serotonin in cisplatin-induced nausea and vomiting. N Engl J Med 1990;322:810–816.

154. Marschner NW, Adler M, Nagel GA, Christmann D, Fenzl E, Upadhyaya B. Double-blind randomized trial of the antiemetic efficacy and safety of ondansetron and metoclopramide in advanced breast cancer patients treated with epirubicin and cyclophosphamide. Eur J Cancer 1991;27:1137–1140.

155. Smyth JF, Coleman RE, Nicolson M, et al. Does dexamethasone enhance control of acute cisplatin induced emesis by ondansetron? Br Med J 1991;303:1423–1426.

156. Priestman TJ, Roberts JT, Lucraft H, et al. Results of a randomized, double-blind comparative study of ondansetron and metoclopramide in the prevention of nausea and vomiting following high-dose upper abdominal irradiation. Clin Oncol 1990;2:71–75.

157. Nelson DR, Thomas DR. ^{3}H-BRL-43694 (Granisetron), a specific ligand for 5-HT$_3$ binding sites in rat brain cortical membranes. Biochem Pharmacol 1989;38:1693–1695.

158. Chugh Y, Saha N, Sankaranarayanan A, Sharma PL. Memory enhancing effects of granisetron (BRL 43694) in a passive avoidance task. Eur J Pharmacol 1991;203:121–123.

159. Upward JW, Arnold BD, Link C, Pierce DM, Allen A, Tasker TC. The clinical pharmacology of granisetron (BRL 43694), a novel specific 5-HT$_3$ antagonist. Eur J Cancer Clin Oncol 1990;26(suppl 1):S125–15.

160. Kamanabrou D. Intravenous granisetron-establishing the optimal dose. The Granisetron Study Group. Eur J Cancer Clin Oncol 1992;28A(suppl 1):S6–11.

161. Cupissol DR, Serrou B, Caubel M. The efficacy of granisetron as a prophylactic anti-emetic and intervention agent in high-dose cisplatin-induced emesis. Eur J Cancer Clin Oncol 1990;26(suppl 1):S23–27.

162. Lemerle J, Amaral D, Southall DP, Upward J, Murdoch RD. Efficacy and safety of granisetron in the prevention of chemotherapy-induced emesis in paediatric patients. Eur J Cancer Clin Oncol 1991;27:1081–1083.

163. Hacking A. Oral granisetron; simple and effective: a preliminary report. The Granisetron Study Group. Eur J Cancer Clin Oncol 1992;28A(suppl 1):S28–32.

164. Gamse R. Antiemetic action of 5-HT$_3$ receptor antagonists; review of preclinical and clinical results with ICS 205-930. Cancer Treat Rev 1990;17:301–305.

165. Akkermans LMA, Vos A, Hoekstra A, Roelofs JMM, Horowitz M. Effect of ICS-205930 (a specific 5-HT$_3$ receptor antagonist) on gastric emptying of a solid meal in normals subjects. Gut 1988;29:1249–1252.

166. Stacher G, Bergmann H, Granser-Vacariu GV, et al. Lack of systematic effects of the 5-hydroxytrypt-amine 3 receptor antagonist ICS-205930 on gastric emptying and antral motor activity in patients with primary anorexia nervosa. Br J Clin Pharmacol 1991;32:685–689.

167. Smith WL, Sancillo LF, Owera-Atepo JB, Naylor RJ, Lambert L. Zacopride, a potent 5-HT$_3$ antagonist. J Pharm Pharmacol 1988;40:301–302.

168. Dubois A, Fiala N, Bogo V. Prevention and treatment of the gastric symptoms of radiation sickness. Radiat Res 1988;115:595–604.

169. Sancilio LF, Pinkus LM, Jackson CB, et al. Studies on the emetic and antiemetic properties of zacopride and its enantiomers. Eur J Pharmacol 1991;192:365–369.

170. King GL. Emesis and defecations induced by the 5-hydroxytryptamine (5-HT$_3$) receptor antagonist zacopride in the ferret. J Pharmacol Exp Ther 1990;253:1034–1041.

171. Bhandari P, Andrews PL. Preliminary evidence for the involvement of the putative 5-HT$_4$ receptor in zacopride- and copper sulphate-induced vomiting in the ferret. Eur J Pharmacol 1991;204:273–80.

172. Turconi M, Donetti A, Schiavone A, et al. Pharmacological properties of a novel class of 5HT3 receptor antagonists. Eur J Pharmacol 1991;203:203–211.

173. Baxter GS, Clarke DE. Benzimidazolone derivatives act as 5-HT$_4$ receptor ligands in rat oesophagus. Eur J Pharmacol 1992;212:225–229.

174. Sagrada A, Turconi M, Bonali P, et al. Antiemetic activity of the new 5-HT$_3$ antagonist. DAU 6215 in animal models of cancer chemotherapy and radiation. Cancer Chemother Pharmacol 1991;28:470–474.

175. Prisco S, Pessia M, Ceci A, Borsini F, Esposito E. Chronic treatment with DAU 6215, a new 5-HT$_3$ receptor antagonist, causes a selective decrease in the number of spontaneously active dopaminergic neurons in the rat ventral tegmental area. Eur J Pharmacol 1992;214:13–19.

176. Villalon CM, den Boer MO, Heiligers JP, Saxena PR. Further characterization, by use of tryptamine and benzamide derivatives, of the putative 5-HT$_4$ receptor mediating tachycardia in the pig. Br J Pharmacol 1991;102:107–112.

177. Van Daele GHP, DeBruyn MFL, Sommen FM, et al. Synthesis of cisapride, a gastrointestinal stimulant derived from cis-4-amino-3-methoxypiperidine. Drug Dev Res 1986;8:225–232.

178. Schuurkes JAJ, Megens AAHP, Niemegeers CJE, Leysen JE, Van Nueten JM. A comparative study of the cholinergic vs the anti-dopaminergic properties of benzamides with gastrointestinal prokinetic activity. In: Szurzewski JH, ed. Cellular physiology and clinical studies of gastrointestinal smooth muscle. Excerpta Medica International Congress Series 725. Amsterdam: Excerpta Medica, 1987:231–247.

179. Karasawa T, Yoshida N, Furukawa K, Omoya H, Ito T. Comparison of gastrokinetic effect of AS-

4370, cisapride and BRL-24924. Eur J Pharmacol 1990;183:2181–2183.

180. Nelson DR, Thomas DR. [³H]-BRL 43694 (granisetron), a specific ligand for 5-HT₃ binding sites in rat brain cortical membranes. Biochem Pharmacol 1989;38:1693–1695.

181. Schuurkes JAJ, Van Nueten JM, Van Daele PGH, Reyntjens AJ, Janssen PAJ. Motor-stimulating properties of cisapride on isolated gastrointestinal preparations of the guinea pig. J Pharmacol Exp Ther 1985;234:775–783.

182. Horton RW, Lowther S, Chivers J, Jenner P, Marsden CD, Testa B. The interaction of substituted benzamides with brain benzodiazepine binding sites in vitro. Br J Pharmacol 1988;94:1234–1240.

183. Peeters TL, Bormans V, Matthijs G, Vantrappen G. Characterization of motilin receptors [Abstract]. Gastroenterology 1988;94:A347.

184. Gaion RM, Armani P, Grion AM, Dorigo P. Effects of cisapride on rat duodenum. Pharmacol Res Commun 1988;20(suppl 2):166.

185. Pfeuffer-Friederich I, Kilbinger H. Facilitation and inhibition by 5-hydroxytryptamine and R 51619 of acetylcholine release from guinea pig myenteric neurons. In: Roman C, ed. Gastrointestinal motility. United Kingdom: MTP Press, 1983:527–534.

186. Fujii K, Okajima M, Kawahori K. Effect of cisapride on the cholinergic control mechanisms of gastrointestinal motility in dogs. Jpn J Smooth Muscle Res 1988;24:1–12.

187. Nakayama S, Neya T, Yamasato T, Takaki M, Itano N. Effects of cisapride on the motility of digestive tract in dogs and guinea pigs. Jpn J Smooth Muscle Res 1985;21:1–9.

188. Snape WJ, Clarke DD, Ristow E. Effect of cisapride on colonic smooth muscle in vivo and in vitro [Abstract]. Gastroenterology 1985;88:1592A.

189. Suzuki T, Nakaya M, Nakamura T Itoh Z. Effect of cisapride on contractile activity of the gastrointestinal tract. Jpn Smooth Muscle Res 1985;21:139–149.

190. Neya T, Itano N, Mizutani M, Yamasato T, Takaki M, Nakayama S. The effect of cisapride on neural 5-HT receptors in guinea pig isolated ileum. Eur J Pharmacol 1985;106:221–222.

191. Summers RW, Flatt AJ. A comparative study of the effects of four motor-stimulating agents on canine jejunal spike bursts. Scand J Gastroenterol 1988;23:1173–1181.

192. Van Nueten JM, Van Daele PGH, Reyntjens AJ, Janssen PAJ, Schuurkes JAJ. Gastrointestinal motility stimulating properties of cisapride, a non-antidopaminergic non-cholinergic compound. In: Roman C, ed. Gastrointestinal motility. Lancaster, United Kingdom: MTP Press, 1983:513–520.

193. Schuurkes JAJ, Van Bergen PJE, Van Nueten JM. Prejunctional muscarinic (M₁)-receptor interactions on guinea-pig ileum: lack of effect of cisapride. Br J Pharmacol 1988;94:228–234.

194. Chen HT, Pan S. Mechanism of the acetylcholine-release effect of cisapride on guinea pig gastrointestinal tract. Chin Med J 1988;41:263–270.

195. Van Nueten JM, Schuurkes JAJ. Cisapride and trimebutine both induce strong contractions in the fasted state in conscious dogs, but via different mechanisms [Abstract]. Gastroenterology 1987;92:1680A.

196. De Coster R, Van Cauteren H, Wouters L. Effect of a single administration of cisapride and metoclopramide on serum prolactin in female rats. Janssen Research Foundation, Preclinical report R 51 619/64, Sept. 1988.

197. Tonini M, Galligan JJ, North RA. Effects of cisapride on cholinergic neurotransmission and propulsive motility in the guinea pig ileum. Gastroenterology 1989;96:1257–1264.

198. Nemeth PR, Gullikson GW. Gastrointestinal motility stimulating drugs and 5-HT receptors on myenteric neurons. Eur J Pharmacol 1989;166:387–391.

199. Hill JM, Bunce KT, Humphrey PPA. Investigation of the neuronal "non-5-HT," receptor mediating contraction of guinea pig ileum. Br J Pharmacol 1990;97:26.

200. Bockaert J, Sebben M, Dumuis A. Pharmacological characterization of 5-hydroxytryptamine₄ (5-HT₄) receptors positively coupled to adenylate cyclase in adult guinea pig hippocampal membranes: effect of substituted benzamide derivatives. Mol Pharmacol 1990;37:408–411.

201. Craig DA, Clarke DE. Pharmacological characterization of a neuronal receptor for 5-hydroxytryptamine in guinea pig ileum with properties similar to the 5-hydroxytryptamine₄ receptor. J Pharmacol Exp Ther 1990;252:1378–1386.

202. Meulemans AL, Schuurkes JA. Is the action of cisapride on the guinea-pig ileum mediated via 5-HT₄ receptors? Eur J Pharmacol 1992;212:51–59.

203. Schuurkes JAJ, Meulemans AM, Obertop H, Akkermans LMA. 5-HT₄-receptors on the human stomach [Abstract]. J Gastrointest Motil 1991;3:199A.

204. Syed M, Tokuno H, Tomita T. Effects of cisapride on isolated guinea pig colon. Jpn J Pharmacol 1989;51:47–56.

205. Brown CK, Khanderia U. Use of metoclopramide, domperidone, and cisapride in the management of diabetic gastroparesis. Clin Pharm 1990;9:357–365.

206. McKirdy HC, McKirdy ML, Marshall RW. Effects of cisapride on isolated muscle strips from human digestive tract. J Physiol 1990;422:88P.

207. Matthijs G, Peeters TL, Bormans V, Vantrappen G. In vitro relaxation of rabbit duodenum induced by high concentrations of cisapride. Gastroenterology 1987;92:1523A.

208. VandenBrink HW, Schuurkes JAJ, VanNueten JM, VanRossum JM. R 50595, a selective non-competitive antagonist of cisapride, BRL 24924 and 5-hy-

droxytryptamine on the guinea pig ileum. Eur J Pharmacol 1990;181:119–125.

209. Syed M, Tokuno H, Tomita T. Effects of cisapride on isolated guinea-pig colon. Jpn J Pharmacol 1989;51:47–56.

210. Den Hertog A, Van den Akker J. The effect of cisapride on smooth muscle cells of guinea-pig taenia caeci. Eur J Pharmacol 1986;126:31–35.

211. Megens AAHP, Canters LU, Artois KSK, Smeyers F, Keersmaekers RCA, Awouters F. Non-antidopaminergic, non-cholinergic stimulation of gastric emptying with cisapride (R 51619) in rats. Drug Dev Res 1986;8:243–250.

212. Schuurkes JAJ, Akkermans LMA Van Nueten JM. Stimulating effects of cisapride on antroduodenal motility in the conscious dog. In: Roman C, ed. Gastrointestinal motility. Lancaster, United Kingdom: MTP Press, 1983:95–102.

213. Schemann M, Ehrlein HJ. 5-Hydroxytryptophan and cisapride stimulate propulsive jejunal motility and transit of chyme in dogs. Digestion 1986;34:229–235.

214. Akkermans LMA, Roelofs JMM, Breedijk M, et al. Cisapride-induced temporal relationship between antral and duodenal electrical control activity (ECA) [Abstract]. Gastroenterology 1986;90:1323A.

215. Wülschke S, Ehrlein HJ, Tsiamitas C. The control mechanisms of gastric emptying are not overridden by motor stimulants. Am J Physiol 1986;251:G744–G751.

216. Thies P, Janisch HD, Wolff KU, Hampel KE. Gastric emptying and plasma VIP in response to oil in the stomach and the influence of cisapride. Ital J Gastroenterol 1987;19(suppl 3):54S.

217. Gué M, Fioramonti J, Bueno L. A simple double radiolabeled technique to evaluate gastric emptying of canned food meal in dogs: application to pharmacological tests. Gastroenterol Clin Biol 1988;12:425–430.

218. Schippers E, Hölscher A, Bollschweiler E, Siewert JR. Altered intestinal motility patterns after Roux-en-Y reconstruction [Abstract]. Gastroenterology 1989;96:A449.

219. Coremans G, Janssens J, Vantrappen G, Chaussade S, Ceccatelli P. Cisapride stimulates propulsive motility patterns in human jejunum. Dig Dis Sci 1988;33:1512–1519.

220. Stacher G, Bergmann H, Gaupmann G, et al. Fat preload delays gastric emptying: reversal by cisapride. Br J Clin Pharmacol 1990;30:839–845.

221. Rowbotham DJ, Bamber PA, Nimmo WS. Comparison of the effect of cisapride and metoclopramide on morphine-induced delay in gastric emptying. Br J Clin Pharmacol 1988;26:741–746.

222. Jian R, Ducrot F, Ruskone A, et al. Symptomatic, radionuclide and therapeutic assessment of chronic idiopathic dyspepsia. A double-blind placebo-controlled evaluation of cisapride. Dig Dis Sci 1989;34:657–664.

223. Horowitz M, Maddox A, Harding P, et al. Effect of cisapride on gastric and esophageal emptying in insulin-dependent diabetes mellitus. Gastroenterology 1987;92:1899–1907.

224. Feldman M, Smith HJ. Effect of cisapride on gastric emptying of indigestible solids in patients with gastroparesis diabeticorum: a comparison with metoclopramide and placebo. Gastroenterology 1987;92:171–174.

225. Horowitz M, Maddox A, Wishart J, Collins P, Shearman D. The effects of cisapride on gastric and oesophageal emptying in dystrophia myotonica. J Gastroenterol Hepatol 1987;2:285–293.

226. Horowitz M, Maddern G, Maddox A, Wishart J, Chatterton B, Shearman D. Effects of cisapride on gastric and esophageal emptying in progressive systemic sclerosis. Gastroenterology 1987;93:311–315.

227. Testoni PA, Bagnolo F, Fanti L, Passaretti S, Titobello A. Long-term oral cisapride improves interdigestive antroduodenal motility in dyspeptic patients. Gut 1990;31:286–290.

228. Corinaldesi R, Stanghellini V, Raiti C, Salgemini R, Barbara L. Effect of chronic administration of cisapride on gastric emptying of a solid meal and on dyspeptic symptoms in patients with idiopathic gastroparesis. Gut 1987;28:300–305.

229. Baldi F, Bianchi Porro G, Dobrilla G, et al. Cisapride versus placebo in reflux esophagitis: a multicenter double-blind trial. J Clin Gastroenterol 1988;10:614–8.

230. Rizzi CA, Coccini T, Onori L, Manzo L, Tonini M. Benzimidazolone derivatives: a new class of 5-hydroxytryptamine$_4$ receptor agonists with prokinetic and acetylcholine-releasing properties in the guinea pig ileum. J Pharmacol Exp Ther 1992;261:412–419.

231. Gullikson GW, Virina MA, Loeffler RF, et al. SC-49518 enhances gastric emptying of solids and liquid meals and stimulates gastrointestinal motility in dogs by a 5-hydroxytryptamine$_4$ receptor mechanism. J Pharmacol Exp Ther 1993;264:240–248.

232. Flynn DL, Zabrowski DL, Becker DP, et al. SC-53116: the first selective agonist at the newly identified serotonin 5-HT$_4$ receptor subtype. J Med Chem 1992;35:1486–1489.

233. Yoshida N, Omoya H, Oka M, Furukawa K, Ito T, Karasawa T. AS-4370, a novel gastrokinetic agent free of dopamine D$_2$ receptor antagonist properties. Arch Int Pharmacol Ther 1989;300:51–67.

234. Yoshida N, Ito T, Karasawa T, Itoh Z. AS-4370, a new gastrokinetic agent enhances gastrointestinal motor activity in conscious dogs. J Pharmacol Exp Ther 1991;257:781–787.

235. Dubois A. Endogenous opioids, gastric motility and gastric emptying. Gastroenterol Clin Biol 1987;11:B56–B60.

236. Narducci F, Bassotti G, Granata MT, et al. Functional dyspepsia and chronic idiopathic gastric stasis: role of endogenous opiates. Arch Intern Med 1986;146:716–720.
237. Tatsumi H. The effects of various gastrokinetic drugs on gastric emptying. Nippon Heikatsukin Gakkai Zasshi 1990;26:31–49.
238. Walters JM, Crean P, McCarthy CF. Trimebutine, a new antispasmodic in the treatment of dyspepsia. Ir Med J 1980;73:380–381.
239. Pascaud X, Petoux F, Roman F, Vauche D, Junien JL. Mode of action of trimebutine: involvement if opioid receptors. Presse Med 1989;18:298–302.
240. Poitras P, Boivin M, Lahaie RG, Trudel L. Regulation of plasma motilin by opioids in the dog. Am J Physiol 1989;257:G41–G45.
241. Gue M, Pascaud X, Honde C, Junien JL, Bueno L. Peripheral antagonistic action of trimebutine and kappa opioid substances on acoustic stress-induced gastric motor inhibition in dogs. Eur J Pharmacol 1988;146:57–63.
242. Romer D, Buscher H, Hill RC, et al. Bremazocine: a potent long-acting opiate kappa agonist. Life Sci 1980;27:971–978.
243. Itoh Z, Nakaya M, Suzuki T, Arai H, Wakabayashi K. Erythromycin mimics exogenous motilin in gastrointestinal contractile activity in the dog. Am J Physiol 1984;247:G688–G694.
244. Vantrappen G, Janssens J, Tack J, Muls E, Bouillon R, Peeters T. Erythromycin is a potent gastrokinetic in diabetic gastroparesis [Abstract]. Gastroenterology 1989;96:A525.

9

The Pharmacotherapy of the Irritable Bowel Syndrome

GERALD FRIEDMAN

The irritable bowel syndrome (IBS) is a functional disorder of the gastrointestinal tract for which there is no known anatomical or biochemical cause. IBS is, without doubt, the most commonest gastrointestinal disorder seen by gastroenterologists in office practice. The variability of the presenting complaints and the lack of confirmatory diagnostic tests make the diagnosis more difficult. Following the exclusion of organic disease, therapy is directed toward amelioration of symptoms by the selective introduction of dietary, psychologic, and pharmacologic techniques designed to reduce the factors triggering symptoms and suppressing existing symptoms.

Recent investigations suggest that the entire hollow tract may be involved in the irritable bowel syndrome, thus creating symptom complexes with both upper and lower gastrointestinal components (1). This chapter will concentrate mainly on the treatment of symptoms involving the small bowel and colon, since these anatomic areas evoke the majority of presenting complaints.

CLINICAL AND PATHOPHYSIOLOGIC PERSPECTIVES

Patients with IBS present with intermittent and recurrent symptoms that include abdominal pain and altered bowel habits, diarrhea, constipation, or alternating diarrhea and constipation. Following an analysis of patients with functional and organic diseases, Manning et al. (2) have suggested certain leading indicators that imply a positive diagnosis of IBS (Table 9.1). Symptoms found in patients with pain dominating IBS include: (a) pain relieved by defecation, (b) more frequent stools with the onset of pain, (c) looser stools with the onset of pain, (d) abdominal distension, (e) mucus in the stool, and (f) a feeling of incomplete evacuation after defecation. It is important to note that confounding factors clouding the diagnosis may include those related to autonomic lability, mood or behavioral disturbances, and hyperirritability of contiguous organs. As a result, many of these patients may have autonomic vasomotor dysfunction such as sweating, faintness, labile blood pressure and pulse, clammy hands, feet, and axillae, palpitations and precordial discomfort. Anxiety, depression, nervousness, lassitude, sleep disturbances, and difficulty in concentration may be present. Additionally, urinary frequency, dysmenorrhea, and dyspareunia may be noted. Symptoms may occur as a reaction to psychosocial stress, the ingestion of food, or in response to hormones or drugs. Clearly, there appears to be a hypersensitivity of the smooth muscle of the hollow tract in many instances sustained or triggered by psychologic input: in brief, a hypersensitivity of mind and muscle.

Demographic Considerations

In Western populations approximately 20–30% of individuals in all age groups have

163

symptoms consistent with the irritable bowel syndrome (3). It is estimated that one-fourth of these individuals will seek medical care and become patients. Why these individuals become patients involves a complex of health-seeking behavior based upon familial factors, individual psychologic features, cultural factors, early childhood experiences, and hyper-reactivity to life stresses. Obtaining essential background data in the patient's history is a primary step in laying the groundwork for diagnosis and therapy. In Western countries 65–75% of patients seen by physicians are females, whereas in countries such as India, male patients predominate.

Pathophysiologic Features

THE MIND

The psyche is intimately involved in the complex interplay of factors affecting the irritable bowel syndrome. In the realm of psychosocial features, the psyche is involved in health-seeking behavior. Early childhood experiences, familial influences, and psychologic trauma modify health-seeking patterns and determine how the illness is experienced (4) (Table 9.2).

As a group, IBS patients appear to be more neurotic, anxious, or depressed than the normal population. Their coping skills are limited, and they appear to be physiologically more sensitive to life stresses (5). Additionally, there is a higher frequency of psychiatric diagnoses, specifically anxiety, depression, and somatization. The altered "mind set," acting through neural and hormonal influences, appear to sensitize the gut, thus influencing gastrointestinal function.

The physician's ability to evaluate the patient's psychologic profile, distinguish stressful lifestyle features, and diagnose serious psychiatric illness is of prime importance in dealing with IBS patients. A review of the relationship of psychiatric disorders and gastrointestinal illness emphasizes the need for specific criteria for the diagnosis of psychiatric illness. Creade and Guthrie (5) analyzed controlled studies of the relationship of psychiatric illness and IBS. Their analysis allowed the conclusion that the prevalence of psychi-

Table 9.1
Symptoms in Pain-Dominating IBS[a]

1. Pain relieved by defecation
2. Frequent stools with onset of pain
3. Looser stools with onset of pain
4. Abdominal distension
5. Mucous in stool
6. Incomplete evacuation

[a]After Manning et al. (2)

Table 9.2
Psychologic Considerations in IBS

1. Influences of childhood experiences
2. Familial influences
3. Limited coping skills
4. Increased sensitivity to life stresses
5. Depression, anxiety, somatization

atric disorder in the populations of IBS patients studied was 40–50%. Self-administered interview tests may be helpful in the estimation of psychiatric disorder among IBS patients (6).

THE MUSCLE

Motor dysfunction of the entire hollow gastrointestinal (GI) tract may be involved in the symptomatic expression of the irritable bowel syndrome. Thus, esophageal motor dysfunction, gastric emptying disorders, aberrant small bowel motility, and colonic motor abnormalities have been reported in IBS patients (7–9).

The colon remains the major symptomatic focus of patients with IBS. The diagnostic emphasis of the positive features of IBS previously noted imply that colonic motor dysfunction frequently is a major presenting area of complaint. The availability of the rectum and left colon for intraluminal pressure studies has allowed ready investigation of these areas. The pathophysiologic markers of colonic motor dysfunction in IBS include the following:

1. Increased phasic contractions of high amplitude associated with spastic constipation
2. Decreased phasic contractions in patients with painless diarrhea

3. Postprandial abdominal pain and distension associated with exaggerated sigmoid responses
4. An increased sensitivity to inflated rectally-placed balloons in IBS patients
5. An increased frequency of 3 cycle/minute basic electrical rhythm (BER) activity in the rectum and sigmoid in IBS patients as compared with normal subjects
6. Short spike bursts from circular muscle in the colon correlated with abdominal pain in IBS patients more frequently than in normal subjects.

The inference in most cases is a hyperreactivity of colonic smooth muscle to intraluminal distending factors, neural, endocrine and psychologic factors, or combinations of these and other factors.

The ingestion of foods containing significant amounts of fat has been shown to increase the myoelectric activity and motility of the sigmoid colon. The same holds true for meals of high caloric content. Fatty food intake causes a delayed peak of sigmoid motor activity that is inhibited by a concomitant increase in protein or amino acids (9).

Recent experimental data have demonstrated small bowel motor abnormalities in IBS patients (10). Abnormalities of small bowel motility include:

1. Shorter daytime migrating motor complex periodicities
2. Increased jejunal discrete clustered contractions
3. Increased ileal propagating propulsive contractions
4. Increased motor activity in response to fatty meals, hormonal stimulation, and ileal balloon distension
5. Shorter duration of postprandial (fed) pattern
6. Altered ileocecal transit
7. Increased pain sensitivity to discrete clustered contractions and propagating propulsive contractions.

In summary, smooth muscle hyperreactivity appears to be a hallmark of both colonic and small bowel motor function in the IBS patient (11).

FOOD INTAKE AND IBS SYMPTOMS

The nutrient content, caloric density, frequency of feeding, psychologic state of the subject at the time of eating, physical state of the food, and other dietary factors all have a profound effect on the reactivity of the hollow tract at mealtime. The ingestion of food is a major triggering factor inducing symptoms in the IBS patient.

A prospective dietary history is an important consideration in the interpretation of symptoms. A detailed dietary history taken over a period of 7 days should include the quality and quantity of food consumed. The patient should record the nature and chronologic sequence of symptoms occurring following meals, as well as a description of the frequency and consistency of bowel movements. By utilizing this information, the physician may detect the relationship of symptom occurrence associated with the ingestion of lactose-containing foods, sorbitol intake, or fructose-sorbitol combinations. In addition, the frequency of ingestion of "gas-forming foods" such as cabbage, brussel sprouts, baked beans, apples, grapes, apple juice, etc., may be ascertained. Total caloric intake and dietary fat intake should be noted, since caloric density and fat intake may alter gastric, small bowel, and colonic motor function (Table 9.3).

Lactose intolerance may produce symptoms that are indistinguishable from those of IBS (12). Relatively reduced concentrations of lactase in the small intestinal mucosa allow passage of poorly digested lactose-containing foods into the colon. Colonic bacterial fermentation produces gaseousness, bloating, and an osmotic diarrhea. Thus, elimination or

Table 9.3
Dietary Factors Altering Motor Function in IBS

1. Caloric density of diet
2. Total fat intake
3. Amounts of cruciferous vegetables
4. Lactose containing foods
5. Foods containing fructose or sorbitol
6. Soluble and insoluble fiber content

reduction of lactose-containing foods in the diet may aid in the reduction of IBS symptoms. Sorbitol, a straight-chain hexahydric alcohol, is found naturally in foods such as peaches, apple juice, pears, and plums. It is an artificial sweetener frequently added to sugarless gums, dietetic jams, and chocolate. Sorbitol in doses >10 g produces abdominal pain, bloating, and diarrhea. Reduced ingestion of selected foods may be helpful in these patients. Fructose, alone or in combination with sorbitol, may produce abdominal distress presumably related to the fermentative effect of colonic bacteria on malabsorbed carbohydrates. Fructose is a common constituent of fruits, berries, and plants.

In summary, the elimination or reduction of lactose, sorbitol, and fructose-containing foods in selected patients may ameliorate or lessen symptoms of bloating, abdominal pain, and diarrhea.

GAS SYNDROMES

Excessive belching, postprandial abdominal distension, borborygmi, and the passage of excessive amounts of flatus are common complaints of the IBS patient. The volume, composition, and source of intestinal gas has been precisely investigated by Levitt and Bond (13). Their analyses provide a perspective in reducing the impact of gas-related symptoms in the IBS patient. The total volume of gas in the normal human GI tract varies between 100 and 200 ml, the same volume of gas being present in IBS patients. Thus, the symptomatic response of IBS patients is not volume related, but is rather a hypersensitivity of the smooth muscle of the hollow tract to the presence of gas and the aberrant aboral movement of intraluminal gas. The major intestinal gases are grouped according to their location in the hollow tract. The upper gastrointestinal tract contains oxygen, nitrogen, and carbon dioxide, whereas hydrogen, methane, and carbon dioxide are found in the colon. Oxygen and nitrogen are contributions from swallowed air, whereas carbon dioxide is produced by the interaction of acid and alkaline substances in the stomach. Much of the carbon dioxide generated is absorbed through the bloodstream. Avoidance of large meals of high caloric content, carbonated beverages, smoking, chewing gum, excessive fluid intake, and rapid eating may effectively reduce the amount of gas swallowed or generated in the stomach.

Gas generated in the lower gastrointestinal tract is the result of bacterial fermentation. Approximately 10–20% of ingested carbohydrates may be malabsorbed. Fermentation by the colonic flora results in the production of variable amounts of hydrogen, methane, carbon dioxide, and oxygen. Protein substrates, when fermented, may contribute to malodorous gaseous constituents. The elimination of known gas producers such as cabbage, beans, lentils, brussel sprouts, and legumes may reduce may reduce flatus production.

DIAGNOSTIC CONSIDERATIONS

An in-depth history remains the fundamental basis for diagnosis. A positive diagnosis of IBS requires fulfillment of the Manning criteria noted above as well as the following:

1. Patients with IBS usually have a multiyear history of intermittent and recurrent abdominal symptoms. The character of these symptoms remains constant.
2. An antecedent history of "infectious diarrhea" may result in later onset of IBS symptoms in the younger age group.
3. In the female population IBS symptoms are frequently exacerbated at the time of menses.
4. Due consideration should be accorded "confounding factors," particularly the use of over-the-counter drugs, which may alter bowel function.
5. Onset of IBS symptoms in patients >50 years of age requires attention to ruling out serious organic disease.
6. Deviation from the usual pattern of symptomatic presentation requires attention to further work-up to rule out organic disease.
7. Symptoms such as fever, weight loss, anorexia, persistent or progressive abdominal pain, intestinal bleeding, and symptoms awakening patients from sleep are rare in IBS patients and require analytic attention.

Following the history and dietary analysis, a basic evaluation requires a complete physical examination including a rectal and pelvic examination. A flexible sigmoidoscopic examination is necessary as well as a 72-hour stool collection for guaiac (hemoccult system). A complete blood analysis including a complete blood count (CBC), erythrocyte sedimentation rate and sequential multiple analyzer 18, and urinalysis is advisable as well as a thyroid profile. Patients presenting with diarrhea require a rectal smear for inflammatory cells, stools for ova and parasites, and a stool culture. These baseline studies are needed for diagnostic purposes and serve as a basis for future comparisons since IBS patients frequently have a lifetime of intermittent and recurrent symptoms.

TREATMENT OF IRRITABLE BOWEL SYNDROME

Effective treatment of patients with IBS requires a fundamentally secure patient-physician relationship. The physician must pursue historical information by using a nondirective, patient-centered interview. Warm, concerned physicians can engender the trust and confidence necessary to allay patients' fears and educate patients with respect to the origin of their symptoms. Such education and confidence will engage patients as partners in the ongoing therapeutic effort. It also establishes a foundation for a lifetime of continuing care required in a syndrome in which chronic recurrent symptoms is a hallmark.

Therapeutic Challenge

The ground rules for therapy in IBS require the following.

1. A cure, in most instances, is unlikely. Under the physician's guidance, the patient should understand that he or she does not have a disease, but rather a hypersensitive bowel. Further, the patient must understand that this hypersensitivity can be dulled or ameliorated by the introduction of life-style changes and the use of selected therapeutic agents on an ad hoc basis.

2. No single agent is available for the treatment of IBS patients. An analysis of controlled trials, using accepted trial designs, specific entry criteria, and precise efficacy measurements demonstrated that no single agent is effective in the treatment of IBS (14).

3. The absence of a universally accepted therapeutic agent for the treatment of patients with IBS does not negate the selection of rational therapies designed to ameliorate symptoms. Treatment is directed at reducing the frequency and intensity of triggering factors, as well as dampening the hypersensitive target smooth muscle.

Treatment Designs

The two major triggering factors associated with IBS symptoms are psychologic influences and the ingestion of food. Either alone or in combination, these factors set into motion the symptoms of abdominal pain, altered stool frequency, altered stool consistency, abdominal distension, and various gas syndromes.

Before discussing the pharmacologic agents used in the treatment of IBS, it should be noted that several psychologic techniques have been employed to modify symptoms and reduce the frequency of recurrent episodes.

PSYCHOTHERAPY, HYPNOTHERAPY, AND BEHAVIOR MODIFICATION

Patients who are seriously impaired psychologically should be referred for in-depth psychiatric assessment. However, even those patients with less serious psychologic impairment may benefit from psychotherapy. Whitehead and Crowell (15) reviewed the psychologic considerations in IBS and summarized the benefits of psychologic techniques. Their analysis of controlled studies of brief psychotherapy suggested that conversational psychotherapy focusing on current problems and applying coping techniques, produced beneficial effects. Both short- and long-term benefits were obtained showing greater reductions in dysphoric mood and in somatic symptoms of abdominal pain and diarrhea. Group psychotherapy appeared to be less valuable.

Several studies employing hypnotherapy directed efforts at inducing and practicing relaxation of mind and smooth muscle appear to be effective (16, 17). Patients >50 years of age and those with significant psychopathology were less likely to respond to this form of therapy.

Cognitive behavior therapy combines patient education regarding origins of bowel symptoms, progressive muscle relaxation training, and methods to reduce thoughts and attitudes that may contribute to stress. Several studies report beneficial results employing these techniques (18, 19).

Pharmacologic Interventions

Nowhere in gastroenterology is the art of medicine more important therapeutically than in the selection of appropriate therapeutic agents for the treatment of IBS. The patient's recording of dietary intake, chronologic sequence of symptoms, bowel activity, drug (including over-the-counter preparations) intake, unusual stressful incidents, and such confounding factors as the menstrual cycle should be recorded for a minimum of 7 days to obtain a baseline perspective of the predominant symptoms. The recording of these events and analysis by the physician immediately introduces a partnership status that builds confidence and cooperation into the therapeutic relationship. When such information is available, the predominant symptoms become apparent, allowing dietary adjustments and pharmacologic therapies to be thoughtfully introduced.

The predominant symptoms to be treated pharmacologically include *pain, diarrhea, constipation, abdominal distension and gas syndromes,* and *depression and anxiety.*

PAIN TREATMENT

The pain of IBS is chronic and recurrent. Pain may be noted anywhere in the abdomen, being commonest in the left and right lower quadrants (20–22). Pain is usually precipitated by the ingestion of food or stress and is frequently relieved by defecation or passing flatus. The relationship of pain and colonic or small bowel motor abnormalities is difficult to assess. IBS patients with severe postprandial abdominal pain have had demonstrable ab-

normalities in the gastrocolic response. The latter may be reproduced by intravenous cholecystokinin. Balloon distension at various sites in the colon may reproduce symptoms typical of pain in IBS (23). Similarly, balloon distension in the small bowel may elicit typical abdominal pain in some patients with IBS. Additionally, certain patterns of small bowel dysmotility are correlated with pain patterns (24). Symptoms of abdominal pain have been reported in association with propagating propulsive contractions (PPCs) and with some discrete clustered contractions (DCCs). Thus there appears to be a strong association between altered jejunal and ileal motility and symptoms of abdominal pain. Overall, motor function studies support the concept that IBS patients may have alterations in visceral pain perception, and that this altered neural input may be central to the abnormal motility disorders seen in IBS.

The mechanism of a lower pain threshold with GI tract distension in IBS appears to be a lower threshold for excitation of afferent terminals at the level of the mucosa and submucosa. It appears that mucosal compression from gut distension and mucosal/submucosal compression from gut wall contraction may more easily induce pain in patients with IBS. Visceral mechanoreceptors set at a lower threshold for excitation in IBS could explain these phenomena. In simpler terms, there appears to be a mucosal-submucosal and smooth muscle hyperreactivity evoking contractile activity that may be correlated with pain.

The presence of a variety of nongastrointestinal symptoms such as nocturia, urinary frequency and urgency, back pain, dyspareunia, and lethargy also support the concept of altered visceral pain perception, altered visceral pain discrimination, and a facilitation of mechanisms resulting in referred pain (25).

Patients with IBS may have altered visceral sensation and changes in afferent reflex mechanisms that modulate GI motility. These patients do not have a generalized increase in pain perception, but may have a distinct sensitivity to visceral afferent stimulation in both GI and other viscera. Whether the altered

Table 9.4
Anticholinergic Agents

Quarternary Ammonium Compounds

Methscapolamine bromide (Pamine)
Homatropine methyl bromide
Methantheline bromide (Banthine)
Propantheline bromide (Probanthine)
Anisotropine methyl bromide (Valpin)
Clidinium bromide (Quarzan)
Glycopyrrolate (Robinul)
Isopropamide iodide (Darbid)
Mepenzolate bromide (Cantil)
Trihexethyl chloride (Pathilon)

Tertiary Amine Compounds

Dicyclomine hydrochloride (Bentyl)

Newer Anticholinergic Agents

Cimetropium bromide
Hyoscyamine sulfate (Levsin)
Otilonium bromide
Pinaverium bromide
Prifinium bromide

"setpoint" to visceral afferent stimulation of IBS is intrinsic to the smooth muscle of viscera or secondary to central nervous system (CNS) and autonomic nervous system (ANS) modulation is not known. Many of the symptoms and abnormalities of small bowel and colonic motility in IBS probably result from these changes in afferent sensation and reflex mechanisms (26). These findings support the concept that IBS is an abnormality of intestinal motility in conjunction with a "sensitive" gut.

ANTICHOLINERGIC AGENTS

Anticholinergic medications (Table 9.4) are the most frequently used agents for treatment of IBS. These agents, which inhibit the actions of acetylcholine on autonomic effectors innervated by postganglionic cholinergic innervation, have little action at nicotinic receptor sites. The use of anticholinergics is based upon the pharmacologic property of reducing smooth muscle contractility, an implied antispasmodic effect. Depending upon the dose employed, these agents decrease the tone, amplitude, and frequency of peristaltic activity of the stomach, small bowel, and colon. Despite

their widespread use, no well-designed placebo-controlled study provides convincing evidence of their efficacy (27). There is evidence that anticholinergic agents may reduce the impact of neurohumoral-induced gastrocolic reflex upon sensitized colonic smooth muscle (28). Thus, postprandial pain of colonic origin may respond to the administration of small doses of anticholinergics administered 30 to 60 minutes before meals.

Efforts directed at obtaining greater selectivity at cholinergic neuroeffector sites resulted in the development of drugs with quarternary ammonium structure. These drugs are poorly absorbed from the GI tract and do not readily cross the blood-brain barrier. They have a prolonged action and have greater potency at nicotinic receptors. There is a clinical impression that the quarternary ammonium compounds have a relatively greater effect on GI activity, and that the doses necessary to treat GI disorders are more readily tolerated than are other agents of this type; this effect has been attributed to the additional element of ganglionic block (29).

Tertiary amine antimuscarinic compounds are purported to have greater antispasmodic properties. Dicyclomine hydrochloride (Bentyl) is representative of this group of agents.

Side effects of anticholinergic agents are essentially dose-related. Small doses depress salivary and bronchial secretions and sweating. Larger doses cause pupillary dilation, ocular accommodations, and tachycardia. Larger doses inhibit the parasympathetic control of the urinary bladder and gastrointestinal tract, inhibiting micturition and decreasing the tone and motility of the gut. From a practical point of view, it is prudent to start with small doses of anticholinergics (7.5 mg of *propantheline bromide* or 10 mg of *dicyclomine*). Titrating doses in this manner may help to minimize side effects.

Continued interest in the use of new anticholinergic agents has come from foreign investigators. *Pinaverium bromide* has been shown to have an inhibitory action on postprandial colonic motility (30, 31). A positive control study comparing *otilonium bromide* to pinaverium bromide in a limited 2-week study demonstrated a decrease in the frequency and intensity of pain episodes in IBS patients (32). In a multicenter, randomized controlled trial comparing otilonium to placebo, otilonium significantly reduced abdominal pain and bloating (33). *Cimetropium bromide* has been evaluated in studies ranging from 6 weeks to 6 months (34–36). In the longer term study, pain and anxiety were significantly decreased when compared with placebo. Constipation and diarrheal episodes did not differ significantly from placebo. Two open studies employing *prifinium bromide* suggest the possible value of this compound in reducing diarrhea and pain (37, 38).

There may be some theoretic advantage of combining sedative-anticholinergic drugs for the reduction of anxiety as well as inducing an antispasmodic effect (39). However, fixed dosage combinations are more difficult to assess and precise dosage adjustment in the individual patient cannot readily be accomplished.

In summary, anticholinergic agents appear to be effective in the reduction of postprandial sigmoidal motor dysfunction, reduction in "spastic pain," and in diminishing diarrheal episodes. These agents may be used judiciously in graded doses in an effort to reduce smooth muscle contractility or hyperreactivity on a short-term basis.

TREATMENT OF DEPRESSION AND ANXIETY

Depressive reactions are frequently reported among IBS patients who seek medical care (40). It should be noted that transient depressive reactions are often seen in medical practice, and are usually associated with situational factors such as grief, marital difficulties, vocational problems, and the like. Depression syndrome, however, is more pervasive and is associated with vegetative symptoms such as insomnia, decreased appetite, weight loss, diminished sexual interest, and inability to concentrate. These patients represent a major affective disorder and require psychiatric evaluations and appropriate therapy.

IBS patients experiencing depressive reactions in association with crampy abdominal pain may benefit from antidepressant medication in several ways:

1. Anticholinergic side effects of tri-cyclic antidepressants may be beneficial in reducing "spastic pain" (41).
2. An enhanced analgesic effect may be effected by antidepressants, particularly when pain and depression coexist (42).
3. Mood elevation induced by antidepressants may be a prime factor in the enhancement of coping mechanisms in the IBS patient.

THE SELECTION OF ANTIDEPRESSANT MEDICATION

When employed for an adequate period of time (6–8 weeks), most tricyclic antidepressants will produce a salutary response in 60–80% of depressed patients. The choice of an antidepressant medication is essentially based upon the response to and tolerance of prior treatment, the side effect profile, and potential drug interactions. In the treatment of IBS patients, the onset of action of anticholinergic and analgesic effects of tricyclic agents occurs much sooner than the antidepressant effect (24–48 hours). Thus, the full antidepressant dosage may not be needed to evoke a beneficial response.

Typical tricyclic antidepressants have three-ring molecular core and produce therapeutic responses in major depressions (43). The putative mechanism of action is the inhibition of the neuronal uptake of norepinephrine. The original antidepressant imipramine is the prototype of tricyclics and there are several analogues chemically related (Table 9.5) *Amitriptyline* (Elavil), *doxepin* (Sinequan), *trimipramine* (Surmontil), *maprotiline* (Ludiomil), and *amoxapine* (Asendin) are among those in popular use. Atypical antidepressants include *trazadone* (Desyrel) and *fluoxitine* (Prozac). Trazadone potentiates the action of 5-hydroxytryptamine, and fluoxetine is a potent selective inhibitor of the neuronal uptake of 5-hydroxytryptamine.

These drugs may affect sleep, resulting in a decrease in the number of awakenings and an increase in stage IV sleep. The impact of the tricyclics on the function of the autonomic

Table 9.5
Antidepressants

Typical Tricyclic Antidepressants

Imipramine (Tofranil)
Amitriptyline (Elavil)
Doxepin (Sinequan)
Amoxapine (Asendin)
Trimipramine (Ludiomil)

Atypical Antidepressants

Trazadone (Desyrel)
Fluoxitine (Prozac)

Table 9.6
Antianxiety Agents

Chlordiazepoxide (Librium)
Diazepam (Valium)
Lorazepam (Ativan)
Oxazepam (Serax)
Alprazolam (Xanax)
Buspirone (Buspar)

nervous system is believed to result from inhibition of norepinephrine transport into adrenergic nerve terminals and from antagonism of muscarinic cholinergic and α-1 adrenergic responses to autonomic transmitters. Major anticholinergic activity is noted with amitriptyline, doxepin, imipramine, protriptyline, and trimipramine. Minimal anticholinergic activity is noted with trazadone, fluoxetine, and bupropion. With the exception of fluoxetine (Prozac), antidepressants are started on a low dose which is then increased as tolerated into a therapeutic range. Several studies have implicated the relationship of inhibition of serotonin reuptake with chronic pain relief (44, 45). Doxepin is one of the most studied agents with respect to pain relief. This drug is often the tricyclic antidepressant of choice for pain relief because of its beneficial sedative effects on sleep disorders, its anxiolytic activity on the agitation accompanying chronic pain and depression, and its lesser impact on the cardiovascular system (46). Recent evidence suggests that enkephalins may also be involved in the mediation of pain reduction with antidepressants (47).

Tricyclics should be used with caution in patients with associated cardiovascular disorders and in the elderly. Particular attention should be accorded the impact on the cardiovascular system. Hypotension, sinus tachycardia, prolongation of conduction, and electrocardiographic EKG-evidence of flattening or inversion of T waves may occur. All tricyclics may produce these effects. A lesser effect on cardiac conduction has been noted with bupropion, fluoxetine and trazodone.

Recent interest in the role of antidepressants and IBS has resulted in several randomized, placebo-controlled studies suggesting the usefulness of the agents in depressed patients. Amineptine (48), desipramine (41), and trimipramine (49) induced clinical and psychologic improvement compared with placebo.

In summary, tricyclic antidepressants may be a valuable addition to the therapeutic regimen of depressed IBS patients. The selection of appropriate medication will, in large part, depend upon the degree and duration of depression, the presence of pain induced by spasticity, the chronicity of pain, the age of the patient, the presence of associated cardiovascular disease, interaction with other coincident medication, the need for appropriate monitoring, and the proposed duration of therapy.

ANTIANXIETY AGENTS

Episodic anxiety related to life experiences may trigger or exacerbate symptoms related to the irritable bowel syndrome. This type of anxiety is best treated with sympathetic understanding and guidance by the clinician. When the patient's ability to function requires the temporary assistance of antianxiety agents (Table 9.6), they should be given for brief periods for symptomatic relief. IBS is characteristically an intermittent and recurrent syndrome, thus habituation or addiction to these agents should be carefully avoided.

The selection of appropriate pharmacologic agents to ameliorate situational anxiety is based upon the patient's age, the presence of concomitant medication, the pharmacologic profile of the agent used, and the individual physician's familiarity with the drug.

The *benzodiazepines* are among the most commonly used antianxiety agents. When appropriately used, they are effective and have relatively low toxicity (50). The current view is that the actions of the benzodiazepines is a result of the neuronal inhibition mediated by γ-aminobutyric acid (51). There are differences to consider with respect to the pharmacokinetics and pharmacodynamics in the selection of these agents. For example, *chlordiazepoxide* (Librium) and *diazepam* (Valium) appear to be more slowly metabolized through the hepatic mono-oxygenase P-450 enzyme system in elderly persons. Caution should be exercised when other medications such as cimetidine, warfarin, and phenytoin are given, because they compete for metabolism through the same hepatic enzyme system. The usual adult dose of 10 mg of chlordiazepoxide three times daily should be modified in the elderly to 5 mg three times daily, while the usual dose of 5 mg of diazepam three times daily for anxiety should be reduced to 2.5 mg. Careful attention should be accorded to the cumulative effects of these drugs, and patients should be informed of possible alterations in judgment and performance while driving or performing tasks requiring intellectual and motor coordination. *Lorazepam* and *oxazepam* produce lesser pharmacokinetic impairment in the elderly patient because the latter agents are metabolized via the phase II conjugating hepatic enzyme system. Newer agents such as buspirone may prove effective as antianxiety agents in IBS, with a lesser potential for reduced intellectual or motor performance. This drug may be used in doses of 5–10 mg three times daily, with a possible delay in onset of action of 5–7 days.

In summary, anxiolytics may be used to ameliorate brief episodes of severe anxiety, thus avoiding habituation and dependence.

A special situation exists when IBS is associated with generalized anxiety disorder. Under these circumstances short term use of alprozolam has been utilized with dual benefit in reducing anxiety and IBS symptoms (52).

Other Agents of Potential Value for Painful IBS

PEPPERMINT OIL

Peppermint oil is a naturally occurring carminative oil that relaxes gastrointestinal muscle in vivo and in vitro (53). This agent has been demonstrated to be superior to placebo for relieving symptoms of IBS in a double-blind crossover trial (54). Additional support came from a limited study in which gelatin capsules containing peppermint oil (0.2 ml) coated with cellulose acetate phthalate (to ensure contents were only released in the distal intestine) were compared with placebo capsules (55). Subjectively, patients taking peppermint oil had statistically better results in reducing abdominal pain than patients receiving placebo. No effect on the number of bowel actions per day was noted. An opposite view point regarding the efficacy of peppermint oil employed a 4-week trial during which time gradations of pain severity, stool frequency, and distension were recorded (56). No statistical difference was noted between peppermint oil and placebo in this study. This drug is currently not available in the United States.

TRIMEBUTINE

Trimebutine (Jouveinal Laboratoires, Fresnes, France), a peripherally acting enkephalin analog, has been reported to reduce IBS symptoms in human (57, 58). Its stimulatory effects appear to be due to agonistic activity on μ and δ receptors of intramural, noncholinergic excitatory neurons, whereas its inhibitory effects are related to its action on κ enkephalinergic receptors of inhibitory neurons. A multicenter study comparing the safety and efficacy of trimebutine and mebeverine in the treatment of IBS demonstrated that both agents progressively relieved the pain of IBS over a 4-week period of time (59). However, no placebo arm was included in this study.

MEBEVERINE

Mebeverine hydrochloride (Duphar, Villeurbanne, France), a spasmolytic agent derived from papaverine, acts directly on smooth muscle. Published clinical trials have indicated its superiority over placebo in IBS patients (60, 61). Neither mebeverine nor trimebutine are available in the United States.

CALCIUM CHANNEL BLOCKERS

The exaggerated and prolonged motor response to eating in IBS patients may be a contributory cause of postprandial complaints. The effect of *nifedipine* (20 mg sublingually) on colonic myoelectric and contractile activity was recorded during fasting and after a mixed 1000-calorie meal. Nifedipine reduced the postprandial increase of both spike potential activity and motility index (62). A long-term trial of this agent may be of value in selected patients. *Nicardipine*, a dihydropyridine calcium antagonist administered intravenously, resulted in a decreased postprandial motility index, and diminished distension-induced rectal motor activity (63). Diltiazem, in a dosage of 60 mg three times daily had no greater benefit than placebo when tested in IBS patients (64).

TREATMENT OF DIARRHEA

Loperamide

Loperamide is a piperidine derivative that acts at opioid receptor sites in the intestine with resultant slowing of GI motility. Loperamide is poorly absorbed after oral administration and does not penetrate into the brain. Most of this agent is excreted in the feces. Loperamide is available as 2-mg capsules, the usual dose being 4–8 mg/day. Several double-blind, placebo controlled trials demonstrated the drug's efficacy in improving stool consistency, diminishing pain, and reducing urgency (65, 66). Self-titration of dose and administration in a single nightly dose proved to be safe and efficient.

Diphenoxylate

Diphenoxylate is a meperidine congener employed in the treatment of diarrhea. This drug is available only in combination with atropine sulfate (Lomotil) in tablets and liquid form. Each tablet contains 2.5 mg of diphenoxylate and 25 mcg. of atropine sulfate. The usual dosage is one to two tablets every 6–8 hours, as needed for diarrhea.

Other Agents

Oral *disodium cromoglycate* has been employed in an open study in an effort to reduce diarrhea in IBS patients selected because of possible food-induced loose bowel movements (67). The data suggest a possible protective role of disodium cromoglycate in food-dependent diarrheal type IBS with food allergy features.

TREATMENT OF CONSTIPATION

The constipation associated with the irritable bowel syndrome is physiologically treated with a dietary program supplemented with either insoluble (bran, whole wheat) or soluble fiber (psyllium, methylcellulose, calcium polycarbophil, fruits, and vegetables). An estimate of total dietary fiber content allows supplemental fiber to be added in small, graded amounts over a period of several weeks to avoid undue bloating and flatulence. Patience and persistence are necessary to produce salutary results and sustain these results on a long-term basis. Use of stimulant laxatives is to be discouraged.

The physical characteristics of fiber that contribute to their physiologic value include the following:

1. Water-holding capacity, which relates to the ability of fiber to hold and maintain water on hydrophilic sites on the fiber. The swell-volume of fiber contributes to the ability of fiber to distend the hollow tract and lubricate the stool. This fecal-bulking effect is more pronounced with soluble fibers, which hold more water than the insoluble fibers.
2. Viscosity or gel-forming capacity of fibers allow the formation of viscous gels, which delay gastric emptying and lubricate the stool.
3. Fermentation of fibers takes place in the colon by colonic bacteria. Soluble fibers are fermented to a much greater extent than insol-

uble fibers. The increased bacterial numbers resulting from fermentation contribute to colonic bulking. The end products of bacterial fermentation are short-chain fatty acids, gases, and water.

4. Bulking involves the increased volume of intraluminal contents. The indigestible fibers and water-adsorbing qualities, as well as the bacterial proliferation, all enhance total bulking actions.

5. Cation exchange and binding refers to the ability of fiber to adsorb cations. Fibers bind bile acids as well as certain minerals such as calcium, iron, and zinc. The cation exchange capacity may be associated with hydratability and ease of fermentation.

The actions of fiber noted here cause a feeling of satiety by delaying gastric emptying. Gastrointestinal transit time is affected by delayed gastric emptying (soluble fibers), slowed small bowel transit (soluble fibers form gels that also delay glucose absorption), and shortened colonic transit time (soluble fibers adsorb water, add to fecal bulking, increasing peristaltic activity; insoluble fibers increase colonic distension and thus peristalsis). Soluble fibers also bind bile acids in the distal small bowel. These bile acids are then excreted in the feces.

The uses of fiber in controlled IBS trials have been reviewed (68). Summarizing the evidence that dietary fiber has a beneficial effect on the symptoms of patients with IBS, the following conclusions may be drawn; (a) Constipated patients clearly derive a beneficial effect from dietary bulk. The dose of dietary fiber must be individually adjusted to each patient's response, allowing enough time to evaluate changes in stooling patterns and relief of pain. (b) The heterogeneity of symptoms makes it difficult to evaluate the benefits of dietary fiber on overall groups of IBS patients unless careful delineation of specific symptomatic responses are recorded. Colon-specific symptoms must be carefully defined and separated from those involving extracolonic hollow organ symptoms. (c) The high placebo response of IBS patients as well as the intermittent and recurrent frequency of symptoms demands the use of large numbers of patients studied over extended periods of time to obtain statistically valid results.

Prokinetic Agents

The clinical use of prokinetic agents has been expanding in the past several years. Metoclopramide, domperidone, cisapride, and erythromycin have all been utilized to enhance esophageal, gastric, small bowel, and colonic motor function. *Metoclopramide* increases the frequency and amplitude of gastric antral contractions. In the small intestine, metoclopramide induces increased peristaltic activity as an extension of the coordinated antroduodenal stimulatory activity. Metoclopramide's prokinetic effects are less pronounced in the distal small bowel and are minimal in the colon. *Domperidone*, an investigational benzimidazole derivative, is a specific dopamine antagonist that stimulates the proximal gastrointestinal tract and has antiemetic properties. This agent does not cross the blood-brain barrier, and rarely causes extrapyramidal side effects. Domperidone augments antral motility, improves antroduodenal coordinated propulsive activity, and accelerates small bowel transit. Milo (69), employing domperidone in a dosage of 10 mg four times daily in a double-blind placebo-controlled study suggested domperidone was effective in reducing postprandial flatulence and abdominal pain and in correcting abnormal bowel habits. Fielding's (70) placebo-controlled study failed to show the efficacy of domperidone when employed with a high fiber diet.

Cisapride, a benzamide derivative, is thought to facilitate acetylcholine release at the myenteric plexus. Cisapride stimulates digestive and interdigestive antroduodenal motility and improves gastric emptying. Colonic transit is significantly increased in humans, thus making this agent the first panprokinetic drug with effects ranging from esophagus to colon. In patients with constipation-predominant IBS, a randomized, double-blind placebo-controlled study over a 12-week period increased the frequency of stooling, reduced abdominal pain, and diminished flatulence (71). Further studies in constipa-

Symptom assessment
  7-day diary
  Food intake, bowel activity, symptoms
  Analysis of record
Predominant symptom:
PAIN
  Anticholinergics
  Antidepressants
  Calcium channel blockers
  Peppermint oil
  Mebeverine
  Trimebutine
Predominant symptoms
Psychologic

Anxiety	Depression
Anxiolytics	Antidepressants
	Hypnotherapy
	Psychotherapy

Predominant symptom
Dysmotility

Diarrhea	Constipation
Antidiarrheals	Fiber, prokinetics

Gas-bloated sensation

Dietary	Other
Eliminate lactose,	Lactaid, beano, charcoal
fructose, sorbitol,	
cruciferous vegetables	

Figure 9.1. Flow chart showing symptomatic therapies irritable bowel syndrome.

tion-predominant IBS patients will be valuable. The usual dose of cisapride is 10–20 mg three times daily. *Erythromycin* is a motilin receptor agonist with profound effects on gastric and small bowel motility as well as possible increased colonic motility (72). No studies of erythromycin in IBS patients are currently available. McCallum (73) provides an in-depth review of prokinetic agents in gastroenterology, many of which may have efficacy in IBS.

SUMMARY

The challenge that the IBS patient presents to the practicing physician is daunting. Organic disease must be ruled out. Effective treatment presupposes an in-depth history with special emphasis on the patient's leading symptoms(s), the severity of the symptom(s), the duration of the symptom(s), possible precipitating factors, and why the patient is now coming for medical care. Two areas of partic-

ular importance are the psychologic status of the patient and a careful dietary history. Modification or elimination of confounding factors such as over-the-counter drug intake, prior surgery, disease of contiguous organs, menstrual cycle, and concomitant other therapeutic agents is necessary. The pre-set goal of therapy is modification or reduction of the intensity of the major presenting symptoms. The overall measurement of success is patient satisfaction. Finally, follow-up surveillance is extremely important for follow-up purposes and to rule out intercurrent serious illness.

When used appropriately, the agents discussed in this section may be useful as pharmacologic aids to reduce the symptoms of IBS (Fig. 9.1). Their optimal use is as a temporary supportive measure during which time the patient learns to reduce triggering factors, improve coping techniques, gain an understanding of the origins of symptoms, and alter inappropriate dietary and life-style elements.

REFERENCES

1. Lennard-Jones JE. Functional gastrointestinal disorders. N Engl J Med 1983;308:431–435.
2. Manning AP, Thompson WG, Heaton KW, Morris AF. Towards a positive diagnosis of the irritable bowel. Br Med J 1975;2:653–654.
3. Thompson WC, Heaton W. Functional bowel disorders in apparently healthy people. Gastroenterology. 1980;79:283–288.
4. Drossman DA, Thompson WG. The irritable bowel syndrome: review and a graduated, multicomponent treatment approach. Ann Intern Med 1992;116(12 pt 1):1009–1016.
5. Creade F, Guthrie E. Psychologic factors in the irritable bowel syndrome. Gut 1987;28:1307–1318.
6. Dergatis R, Lipman RS, Rickles K, et al. The Hopkins Symptom Check List (HSCL): a self-report symptom inventory. Behav Sci 1974;19:1–15.
7. Whorwell PJ, Kloutur C, Smith CC. Esophageal motility in irritable bowel syndrome. Br Med J 1981;282:1101–1108.
8. Malageleda R, Stanghellini V. Manometric evaluation of functional upper gut symptoms. Gastroenterology 1985;88:1223–1231.
9. Snape WJ, Mataruzzo SA, Cohen S. Effect of eating and gastrointestinal hormones as human colonic myoelectrical and motor activity. Gastroenterology 1978;75:373–378.
10. Lind D. Motility disorders in the irritable bowel syndrome. Gastroenterol Clin North Am 1991; 20:279–296.

11. Friedman G. Nutritional therapy of irritable bowel syndrome. Gastroenterol Clin North Am 1989; 18:513–524.

12. Friedman G. Diet and the irritable bowel syndrome. Gastroenterol Clin North Am 1991;20:313–324.

13. Levitt D, Bond JH. Volume, composition and source of intestinal gas. Gastroenterology 1970;59:921–929.

14. Klein B. Controlled treatment trials in the irritable bowel syndrome: a critique. Gastroenterology 1988;95:232–241.

15. Whitehead E, Crowell MD. Psychologic considerations in the irritable bowel syndrome. Gastroenterol Clin North Am 1991;20:249–268.

16. Whorwell PJ. Hypnotherapy in irritable bowel syndrome. Lancet 1989;1:622.

17. Whorwell PJ, Prior A, Faragher EB. Controlled trial of hypnotherapy in the treatment of severe refractory irritable bowel syndrome. Lancet 1984;106:1232–1234.

18. Blanchard ED, Schwartz SP. Adaptation of a multicomponent treatment for irritable bowel syndrome to a small group format. Biofeedback Self-Regul 1987;12:63–69.

19. Neff DF, Blanchard ED. A multicomponent treatment for irritable bowel syndrome. Behav Ther 1987;18:70–83.

20. Kingham JGC, Dawson AM. Origin of right upper quadrant pain. Gut 1985;29:738–788.

21. Moriarity KF, Dawson AM. Functional abdominal pain: further evidence that the whole gut is affected. Br Med J 1982;1:1607–1612.

22. Ritchie J. Pain from distention of the pelvic colon by inflating a balloon in the irritable bowel syndrome. Gut 1973;14:125–132.

23. Sworbrick E, Batt L, Williams CB, et al. Site of pain from the irritable bowel syndrome. Lancet 1980;1:443–446.

24. Kellow E, Phillips SF. Altered small bowel motility in irritable bowel syndrome is correlated with symptoms. Gastroenterology 1987;92:1885–1893.

25. Whorwell PJ, McCallum M, Creed FH, et al. Noncolonic features of irritable bowel syndrome. Gut 1986;27:37–40.

26. Mayer EA, Raybould HE. Role of visceral afferent mechanisms in functional bowel disorders. Gastroenterology 1990;99:1688–1704.

27. Frey KJ. Are anticholinergics of use in the irritable colon syndrome. Gastroenterology 1975;68:1300–1307.

28. Sullivan WA, Cohen S, Snape WJ Jr. Colonic myoelectric activity in irritable bowel syndrome. N Engl J Med 1978;298:878–883.

29. Brown JH. Atropine, scopolamine and related antimuscarinic drugs. In: Bull TW, Nies AS, Taylor P, eds. *Goodman and Gilman's* The pharmacological basis of therapeutics. 8th ed. New York: Pergamon Press, 1990;158–160.

30. Fioramonti J, Frezimos J, Straumont G, Bueno L. Inhibition of the colonic motor response to eating by pinaverium bromide in irritable bowel syndrome patients. Fund Clin Pharmacol 1988;2:19–27.

31. Passaretti S, Sorghi M, Colombo E, Mazzotti G, Tittobello A, Gushendi M. Motor effects of locally administered pinaverium bromide in the sigmoid tract of patients with irritable bowel syndrome. Int J Clin Pharmacol Ther Toxicol 1989;27:47–50.

32. Defrance P, Cosini A. A comparison of the action of otilonium bromide and pinaverium bromide: study conducted under clinical control. Ital J Gastroenterol 1991;23(8 suppl):64–66.

33. Baldi F, Longonesi A, Blasi A, et al. Clinical and functional evaluation of the efficacy of otilonium bromide: a multicenter study in Italy. Ital J Gastroenterol 1991;23(8 suppl):60–63.

34. Ferrari A, Cavallero M, Spandre M, Gemme C, Rossini FP, Imbimbo BP. Six week double blind study of octylonium bromide vs. cimetnopium bromide. Clin Ther 1986;8:320–328.

35. Centonza V, Imbimbo BP, Campanozzi F, Attolini E, Daniotti S, Albano O. Oral cimetropium bromide, a new anti-muscarinic drug, for long-term treatment of irritable bowel syndrome. Am J Gastroenterol 1988;83:1262–1266.

36. Dobrilla G, Imbimbo BP, Piazzi L, Bensi G. Longterm treatment of irritable bowel syndrome with cimetropium bromide. Gut 1990;31:355–358.

37. Sasaki T, Takekashi T, Okoda T. Results of prifinium therapy in irritable bowel syndrome. Clin Ther 1985;7:512–521.

38. Sasaki D, Suzuki A, Yoshida Y, Okamoto K, Ohmi T, Talcahoshi S, et al. Treatment of irritable bowel syndrome with prifinium bromide. Clin Ther 1985;7:190–198.

39. Rhodes JB, Abrams JH, Manning RT. Controlled clinical trial of sedative-anticholinergic drugs in patients with the irritable bowel syndrome. J Clin Pharmacol 1978;18:340–345.

40. Hislap IG. Psychological significance of the irritable colon syndrome. Gut 1971;12:452–457.

41. Greenbaum RB, Mayle JE, Vanegeren LE, et al. The effects of desipramine on irritable bowel syndrome compared with atropine and placebo. Dig Dis Sci 1987;32:257–66.

42. Ward NG, Bloom VL, Friedel RO. The effectiveness of tricyclic antidepressants in the treatment of coexisting pain and depression. Pain 1979;7:331–41.

43. Baldessarini RJ. Drugs and the treatment of psychiatric disorders. In: Rall TW, Nies AS, and Taylor P, eds. *Goodman and Gilman's* The pharmacologic basis of therapeutics. 8th ed. New York: Pergamon Press, 1990;405–414.

44. Tura B, Tura SM. The analgesic effect of tricyclic antidepressants. Brain Res 1990;518:19–22.

45. Feinmann C. Pain relief by antidepressants: possible modes of action. Pain 1985;23:1–8.

46. Aronoff GM, Wagner JM, Spangler AS Jr. Chemical interventions for pain. J Consult Clin Psychol 1986;54:769–775.

47. Hameroff SR, Cork RC, Scherer K, et al. Doxepin effects on chronic pain, depression and plasma opioids. J Clin Psychiatry 1982;43:22–26.
48. Alevizos B, Christodoulou GN, Ioannidis C, et al. The efficacy of amineptine in the treatment of depressive patients with irritable bowel syndrome. Clin Neuropharmacol 1989;12(suppl 2):66–76.
49. Myren J, Loveland B, Larsen SE, Larsen S. A double-blind study of the effect of trimipramine in patients with the irritable bowel syndrome. Scand J Gastroenterol 1984;19:835–43.
50. Meyer R. Benzodiazepines in the elderly. Med Clin North Am 1982;66:1017–1035.
51. Mackler A, Schweizer E. Benzodiazepines as anxiolytic agents: The risks of long term treatment. Hosp Proct 1992;27:109–116.
52. Tollefson GD, Lexenberg M, Valentine R, Dunsmore G, Tollefson SL. An open label trial of alprosolam in comorbid irritable bowel syndrome and generalized anxiety disorder. J Clin Psychiatry 1991;52:502–508.
53. Hills JM, Aaronson PI. The mechanism of action of peppermint oil on gastrointestinal smooth muscle. Gastroenterology 1991;101:55–65.
54. Rees WDW, Evans BK, Rhodes J. Treating irritable bowel syndrome with peppermint oil. Br Med J 1979;2:835–836.
55. Dew MJ, Evans BK, Rhodes J. Peppermint oil for the irritable bowel: a multicenter trial. Br J Clin Pract 1984;38:397–398.
56. Nash P, Gould R, Barnardo DE. Peppermint oil does not relieve the pain of irritable bowel syndrome. Br J Clin Pract 1986;40:292–293.
57. Luttecke K. A trial of trimebutine in spastic colon. J Int Med Res 1978;6:86–88.
58. Moshal G. A clinical trial of trimebutine (mebutine) in spastic colon. J Int Med Res 1979;7:231–234.
59. Schaffstein W, Panijel M, Lutteche K. Comparative safety and efficacy of trimebutine versus mebeverine in the treatment of irritable bowel syndrome. Curr Ther Res 1990;47:136–145.
60. Tasman Jones C. A double blind cross over trial with mebeverine (Duspatalin) in irritable colon syndrome: results of 12 patients. NZ Med J 1973;77:232–235.
61. Lindner A, Selzer H, Cloosen V, et al. Pharmacological properties of mebeverine, a smooth muscle relaxant. Arch Int Pharmacodyn 1963;145:378–395.
62. Narducci F, Bassotti G, Gaburri M, Farroni F, Morelli A. Nifedipine reduces the colonic motor response to eating in patients with the irritable bowel colon syndrome. Am J Gastroenterol 1985;80:317–319.
63. Prior A, Harris SR, Whorwell PJ. Reduction of colonic motility by intravenous nicardipine in irritable bowel syndrome. Gut 1987;28:1609–1612.
64. Perez-Meteo M, Sillero C, Cuesta A, Vazquez N, Berbergal J. Diltiazem in the treatment of irritable bowel syndrome. Int J Clin Pharmacol Res 1986;6:425–427.
65. Lavo B, Stemstam M, Nielsen AL. Loperamide in treatment of irritable bowel syndrome: a double-blind, placebo-controlled study. Scand J Gastroenterol 1987;130(suppl):77–80.
66. Hovdenak N. Loperamide treatment of irritable bowel syndrome. Scand J Gastroenterol 1987;130(suppl):81–84.
67. Stefanini GF, Prati E, Albini MC, et al. Oral disodium cromoglycate treatment on irritable bowel syndrome: an open study on 101 subjects with diarrheic type. Am J Gastroenterol 1992;87:55–57.
68. Friedman G. Nutritional therapy of irritable bowel syndrome. Gastroenterol Clin Am 1989;18:513–524.
69. Milo R. Use of the peripheral dopamine antagonist, domperidone in the management of gastrointestinal symptoms in patients with irritable bowel syndrome. Curr Med Res Opin 1980;6:577–583.
70. Fielding JF. Domperidone treatment in the irritable bowel syndrome. Digestion 1983;23:125–127.
71. Van Outryve M, Milo R, Toussaint J, Van Eegham P. "Prokinetic" treatment of constipation-predominant irritable syndrome: a placebo-controlled study of cisapride. J Clin Gastroenterol 1991;13:49–57.
72. Hasler W, Heldinger A, Soudak H, et al. Erythromycin promotes colonic transit in humans: mediation via motilin receptors. Gastroenterology 1990;98:A358.
73. McCallum RW. Review of the current status of prokinetic agents in gastroenterology. Am J Gastroenterol 1985;80:1008.

10

Constipation Syndromes

MARY JEANNE KREEK and JOAN A. CULPEPPER-MORGAN

Constipation is a symptom complex that includes, but is not limited to, decreased frequency of defecation, hard consistency of stool, difficulty in stool passage, and the need for laxatives. It is estimated that approximately 2% of the population of the United States suffers from constipation. It is more common in women, nonwhites, persons over 65 years of age, and in lower socioeconomic groups (1, 2). In 1989, Johanson et al. estimated that cathartics were prescribed for more than 3 million people per year and that over 200 million dollars per year was spent on over-the-counter laxatives in the United States (2). Although constipation is a common complaint, it is an infrequent cause of hospitalization, loss of days of work, or death when compared with other gastrointestinal disorders such as gall bladder disease or peptic ulcer disease. Nevertheless, constipation is a prevalent medical problem and accounts for about 1% of physician visits in the United States annually.

The morbidity associated with the syndrome and its treatment is clinically significant. Prolonged constipation may cause megacolon, obstruction/obstipation, perforation, and even death, especially in the elderly (3). Improper treatment of constipation can result in imbalances of fluids and electrolytes, damage to bowel epithelium, damage to the enteric nervous system, and the syndrome of cathartic colon.

Etiology

The etiology of constipation is multifactorial. Reversible causes may be superimposed on irreversible disorders of the structure or function of the bowel (Table 10.1) (4). For example, lack of dietary fiber, ingestion of constipating medications, and mechanical obstruction are all potentially reversible causes of the syndrome of constipation. Conversely, constipation may be caused by diseases of the nerves or muscles involved with bowel motility. Disorders of electrolytes, acid-base balance, and endocrine function can cause constipation. These factors should be identified and corrected when possible.

In addition to these identifiable causes of bowel pathology, behavioral problems associated with toileting, especially in children, may exacerbate constipation. Specifically, straining, ignoring the urge to defecate, eating a low-fiber diet, and abusing laxatives may all worsen this symptom complex. The two most potent stimulants of bowel motility are the increase in physical activity after sleep and the colonic emptying stimulated by a meal (5). Bowel retraining programs encourage defecation at these times.

Most patients with constipation do not have an identifiable cause of constipation, as noted in Table 10.1. Clinically this description includes several diverse groups of patients. These groups include the constipated elderly, the patient with constipation in the setting of irritable bowel, and the young woman with life-long constipation. These patients also can be classified by some objective physiologic measures, which can then be used to quantify the efficacy of the various laxative agents.

Table 10.1
Etiology of Constipation

Potentially reversible causes of constipation
  Mechanical obstruction
    Neoplasm
    Adhesion
    Hernia
    Volvulus
  Metabolic abnormalities
    Diabetes
    Hypothyroidism
    Panhypopituitarism
    Porphyria
    Uremia
    Hypokalemia
    Hypercalcemia
  Drug induced
    Opioid analgesics
    Anticholinergics
    Psychotherapeutic agents
    Heavy metal intoxication (lead, mercury, etc.)
    Laxative abuse
Usually irreversible causes of constipation
  Neurogenic
    Peripheral
      Agangliosis (Hirschsprung disease)
      Ganglioneuromatoses (Von Recklinghausen,
        tuberous sclerosis, etc.)
      Autonomic neuropathy
      Chagas disease
    Central
      Spinal cord injury
      Multiple sclerosis
      Organic mental syndromes
  Myopathic
    Scleroderma
    Amyloidosis
    Familial visceral myopathy

Most forms of constipation, despite their etiology, will cause a measurable decrease in stool passage combined with a less measurable decrease in ease of stool passage. Stool passage may be quantified by determining stool frequency or stool weight. Having a bowel movement less than three times a week is considered consistent with constipation (4). Stool wet weight within a range of 35–400 g/24 hours is considered normal (6). A range this large makes it difficult to document significant changes in stool passage in clinical studies. Most patients with chronic constipation pass stools that are on average 100 g/day, but there is significant overlap with non-constipated controls. The ease of stool passage may be as-sessed by questionnaire or quantified by determining the ratio of stool wet to dry weight.

Beyond these general measures of stool passage, constipation may be quantified and categorized by its effect on colonic transit time (Table 10.2). Patients who have delayed transit of radio-opaque markers throughout the colon that results in less than 80% of the markers passed within 5 days have colonic inertia (6–8). In some patients with colonic inertia this delay is limited to the distal rectosigmoid, and is termed hindgut dysfunction (9). Other patients with idiopathic chronic constipation have normal colonic transit, but their ability to initiate and complete the complex neuromuscular event of defecation is impaired by some dysfunction of their pelvic musculature (9–11). This may be acquired as in women who have had multiple or traumatic parturitions, or due to a congenital anatomic defect such an abnormal defecatory angle (12, 13).

There is still another group of patients who have normal transit and are able to defecate but seem not to sense the presence of stool in the rectum. This sensory deficit may be due to local nerve damage, spinal cord damage, or lack of cortical awareness and processing as in some cases of organic brain syndrome (12, 13). Patients in this last group may present with fecal impaction or overflow incontinence.

Pathophysiology

In addition to transit studies, electromyographic studies are also used to determine the efficacy of laxatives in the treatment of all

Table 10.2
Idiopathic Chronic Constipation

Slow transit constipation (colonic inertia)
  Total colonic inertia
  Hindgut dysfunction
Normal transit constipation (defecatory disorders)
  Acquired-pelvic trauma
  Abnormal defecatory angle
  Impaired rectoanal sensation
    Local nerve damage
    Central decreased cortical awareness

types of chronic constipation. Small bowel motility has been characterized to a greater degree than large bowel motility. A full description of the complex electrophysiology of small and large bowel motility is beyond the scope of this chapter and has been reviewed elsewhere. Still, several points should be highlighted (14, 15). Normal small bowel motility may be divided into fasting and fed motility patterns. The fasting pattern, also sometimes called the interdigestive migrating motor complex (MMC), has four distinct phases. Phase III of the MMC is a peristaltic wave that is important in emptying residual food and bacteria from the small bowel between meals. The absence of this motility pattern is associated with bacterial overgrowth but not with constipation (15, 16). The fed motility pattern of the small bowel is associated with mixing contractions and seems designed to maximize contact time between food and the absorptive surface of the intestine. Some constipated patients have normal orocecal transit times. Other forms of chronic idiopathic constipation may be part of a disease entity that slows the small as well as the large bowel (17–19).

The normal colon has two distinct types of myoelectric activity. Long spike bursts (LSBs) of high-frequency electrical activity, associated with long duration contractions, are propulsive in nature. On the other hand, the colon also demonstrates short duration contractions that are associated short spike bursts (SSBs) of electrical activity and are nonpropulsive contractions. Most patients with constipation have more short spike burst activity than propulsive myoelectrical activity. Increases in SSBs associated with mixing contractions have been correlated with prolongation of the intestinal transit time. The SSBs and the LSBs are phasic contractions, which occur periodically in normal human and canine colon (16).

The small bowel and the colon also exhibit giant migrating contractions or peristaltic rushes. In the small bowel, these are two to three times larger in amplitude and 4–5 times longer in duration than the phasic contractions mentioned above (16, 20). They are initiated in the mid-small bowel and migrate rapidly to proximal colon. This contractile pattern is associated with cramps and diarrhea, and may be the motility pattern designed for toxin removal as it is seen in cases of infectious diarrhea or after radiation therapy. In the colon of the dog these giant migrating contractions are associated with the mass movement of the colon that precedes defecation (16, 20). In nonpathologic states in humans and dogs, they occur approximately once or twice per day. Yet, in colitis and other diarrheal states their frequency of occurrence is greatly increased (21–23).

Defecation finally occurs when the bolus of stool that has been delivered to the distal rectosigmoid colon is expelled by the integrated activity of the neuromuscular structures of the anus and rectum. The internal and external anal sphincters are in a state of tonic contraction. Rectal distension produces relaxation of the internal sphincter and contraction of the external sphincter. The external sphincter provides volitional control of rectal emptying. It responds to voluntary effort, increased intra-abdominal pressure dilation, perianal stretching, and rectal distension (14). The stretching of the anus and rectum not only leads to defecation, but also increases propulsion in more proximal colonic segments (24). Thus rectal stimulation from enemas and suppositories can lead to defecation.

The preceding brief overview of the pathophysiology of constipation is important to understand the mechanisms of action of the many available laxatives and cathartics. The better we can characterize normal motility and the ways in which it can be modified, the more successful we will be in the rational development of drugs to treat specific forms of constipation.

Indications for Laxatives

In defining laxative drug actions, it is important to distinguish laxation from catharsis. Laxation is the evacuation of formed fecal material from the rectum, and is the desired result from the treatment of constipation with laxatives. Catharsis is the evacuation of un-

Table 10.3
Classification of Laxatives by Time of Onset and Effect on Stool Consistency[a]

Softening of Stool 1–3 days	Soft or Semifluid Stool 6–8 hours	Watery Evacuation 1–3 hours
Dietary fiber Docusates Lactulose	Diphenylmethanes Anthraquinones	Nonabsorbable salts Castor oil

[a]Modified from Brunton (26).

Table 10.4
Indications for Use of Laxatives and Cathartics

Laxation
  Constipation
  Avoid spontaneous valsalva
    Anorectal surgery
    Postmyocardial infarction
    Postpartum

Catharsis
  Bowel retraining
  Fecal impaction
  Preparation for surgery
  Preparation for endoscopy
  Preparation for radiologic procedure
  Clean-out after barium procedure
  Helminth elimination
  Removal of poisons after toxic ingestion

formed usually watery fecal material from the entire colon. Catharsis is total bowel cleansing or purgation (25). This type of effect may be desired prior to diagnostic or therapeutic endoscopic procedures. It also would be needed prior to surgical or radiologic procedures. Catharsis not only causes abrupt laxation, but results in a loss of fecal flora. While this may be desirable before a surgical procedure, the loss of bacterial flora decreases the ability of the colon to salvage malabsorbed carbohydrate, leading to a prolonged diarrheal state after the initiating agent has been discontinued (23).

Although most of the agents described below promote laxation, some are actually cathartics that, at low doses, are used as laxatives. Cathartics may be roughly distinguished from laxatives by the time to onset of action, as has been suggested by some (26) (Table 10.3). However, as will be described more fully later in the chapter, cathartics promote giant migrating contractions of the colon and are strongly prosecretory, thus initiating diarrheal mechanisms. Laxatives decrease mixing contractions and thus favor the gradual aboral progression of bowel contents. Their secretory effects are minimal.

It should be noted that constipation is just one of several acceptable indications for the use of laxatives (Table 10.4). As described above, most patients with idiopathic chronic constipation probably have an underlying motility disorder. Nevertheless there are several situations in which laxation may need to be induced in individuals who probably have normal bowel motility (Table 10.4). For example, after anorectal surgery or immediately post partum, one may want to decrease straining at stool. After radiologic procedures using barium, rapid drug-aided evacuation may be required. Before many surgical or diagnostic procedures, total bowel catharsis is desired. These situations involve giving laxative drugs to individuals with essentially normal bowel motility. In these settings, the drug response is brisk and predictable. However, the efficacy of laxative drugs in the treatment of chronic constipation is rarely as predictable because the underlying bowel motility of the patients is abnormal.

Until recently, surprisingly little was known or proven about the mechanism of action and/or efficacy of most of the agents used to treat constipation. This was especially true of the anthraquinones and the diphenylmethanes. Misconceptions regarding drug actions and toxicities have remained unchanged for over 50 years. Although much progress has been made recently in clarifying the mechanisms of

Table 10.5
Types of Fiber

Nonpolysaccharides
   Lignin
Polysaccharides
   Nonstarch polysaccharides
      Celluloses
      Noncelluloses
         Hemicelluloses
         Mucilages
         Gums
         Pectins

drug action, often modern clinical trials to judge drug efficacy are lacking. Many trials have appeared in the endoscopic and surgical literature regarding the cathartic efficacy of these drugs, but, these studies cannot be extrapolated to provide data on their use in chronic constipation.

Despite these limitations, we have attempted to group these laxative agents mechanistically. The major classes include the luminal agents that modify the stool content and indirectly affect bowel motility and secretion. The second major class comprises the specific prokinetic agents that work by binding to specific gut receptors and thereby affect motility and sometimes secretion. Finally, we will discuss the many commonly used nonspecific prokinetic agents that affect motility and secretion, but not through specific receptors. These nonspecific agents mediate their response primarily by releasing proinflammatory messengers.

LUMINAL AGENTS

Luminal laxative agents are those that act primarily by changing the composition of the luminal contents of the bowel without directly affecting its neuromuscular structures. They indirectly affect the motility of the gut by increasing luminal residue and/or luminal water. The bowel responds to mechanical stretch caused by a bolus by contracting proximally and relaxing distally to propel the bolus forward. Thus, luminal stretch promotes peristalsis (27). The goal of treatment with these agents is try to produce a stool that contains more residue and more water. Residue includes undigested food particles as well as bacterial mass. Some of these agents increase stool water by filling the lumen with osmotically active substances, others increase the bacterial content of the stool, and some agents do both. A stool that contains more water will be easier to pass. Simply adding bulk without increasing water intake can lead to bowel obstruction (28). Finally, it should be noted that some of the ionic agents thought simply to be osmotic agents may directly stimulate the neuromuscular and neurosecretory apparatus of the gut.

Dietary Fiber

Dietary fiber is the part of food that is resistant to digestion by gastrointestinal enzymes. Crude fiber is an older term that defines fiber as what is left after sequential chemical digestion with acid, alkali, water, ethanol, and ether (29, 30). The first definition is more physiologic and is currently preferred. Most fiber consists of nonstarch polysaccharides (Table 10.5). Lignin, which is the only nonpolysaccharide fiber, is a polymer of phenolic alcohol and is insoluble in water. The remaining nonstarch polysaccharides can be further subdivided into cellulose and noncellulose fibers. Cellulose fibers are not soluble in water. Noncellulose polysaccharides include hemicelluloses, mucilages, gums, and pectins. The water solubility of noncellulose polysaccharides is variable and is an important factor in determining their metabolic activity (31, 32).

The fermentation of fiber by colonic bacteria produces short-chain fatty acids (SCFAs) and increases the mass of colonic bacteria. SCFAs can be used by the colonic epithelium as a source of fuel (33). Dietary fibers differ significantly with respect to their ability to be fermented (Table 10.6), which is determined by the chemistry of the fiber, the degree of water solubility, and the form in which the fiber is ingested (32). Lignin and cellulose fibers are poorly fermented by colonic bacteria, whereas hemicelluloses, gums, and pectins are almost totally fermented. Although any form of wheat bran contains a combination of in-

Table 10.6
Fermentation of Dietary Fibers (31)

Fiber Type	% of Fermentation
Lignin	0
Cellulose	15
Hemicellulose	56–87
Mucilages	85–95
Pectins	90–95

soluble lignins and moderately fermentable hemicelluloses, fine bran is more readily fermented than coarse bran and has less effect on gastrointestinal (GI) transit (34). The metabolic process of fermentation can decrease stool water. Therefore the use of highly fermentable fibers like pectins and mucilages has been suggested for the treatment of diarrhea. Still, the water holding capacity of dietary fiber is not sufficient to overcome a secretory diarrhea (31). Conversely, fiber that is not digested in the small bowel or by the colonic bacteria can osmotically attract water into the colon, increase stool bulk, and improve transit times (35).

Foods vary considerably with respect to the type of fiber they contain. Cereals and grains generally contain negligible amounts of pectins and contain the greatest amounts of lignin and pentose-containing polysaccharides, the hemicelluloses. Thus they are poorly digested, poorly fermented, insoluble fibers. However, they are the best at increasing stool bulk and do so in a dose-dependent fashion (36). They also shorten transit times in normal control subjects to a greater degree than does cabbage or apple fiber (37). Vegetables and fruits contain more pectins and hemicelluloses. They are more water soluble and produce stool that is moister and thus easier to pass, without having a great effect on transit time (34). Legumes contain more mucilages and gums. These water-soluble fibers are almost entirely fermented. Some authors have suggested that water soluble fibers that produce gas during fermentation are less effective at increasing bacterial cell mass and thus have a negligible effect on either the rate or the ease of stool

passage (38). However, these types of fibers may be the most important in the lipid-lowering and glucose-controlling effect of dietary fiber (33).

It should be noted that SCFAs may be prokinetic agents, as one recent study demonstrated a decrease in bowel transit time in rats given SCFAs directly into the terminal ileum (39). In dogs this effect is blocked by lidocaine, prostacyclin, naloxone, and calcium channel antagonists but not by muscarinic, adrenergic, or cholinergic blockade (40). This implies that the natural fermentation of fiber by the cecal bacteria with the physiologic reflux of cecal contents into the terminal ileum could accelerate intestinal transit time. This effect seems to be mediated by the enteric nervous system.

Dietary fiber may be increased by attempting to increase a person's intake of whole grains, fruits, and vegetables (32). It also may be increased by taking any one of several commercially available fiber supplements, such as psyllium husk derivatives, purified methylcellulose, and calcium polycarbophil (Table 10.7). These products increase stool weight and decrease transit time in a dose-dependent fashion. They are fermented only moderately but are water soluble, which is an important property for palatability. Still, it should be noted that wheat bran produces a greater decrease in intestinal transit time than do psyllium laxatives (41). Therefore, wheat bran is the most effective fiber laxative.

Dietary fiber is perhaps the most well-studied category of laxative agents. Epidemiologic and pathophysiologic studies suggest that increasing dietary fiber is the best way to improve all causes of constipation (42). However, results of controlled studies do not strongly support this hypothesis. Current Western diets include approximately 15–20 g/day of dietary fiber, which is estimated to be half what it was over a century ago (29, 43). It is also estimated to be one-third of the diet of rural Africans (42). Studies of normal volunteers have shown that increasing dietary fiber by 12–20 g/day will increase stool wet weight and result in faster transit times (44). Several

Table 10.7
Luminal Agents: Dose and Onset of Action (60, 222, 239)

Class	Drug Name	Dose Range	Onset of Action (hr)
Dietary fiber	Wheat bran	20–30 g	12–72
	Psyllium seed	3–30 g	12–72
	Methlycellulose	4–6 g	12–72
	Sterculia	5–10 g	12–72
	Calcium polycarbophil	1–6 g	12–72
	Malt soup extract	12 g	12–72
Nonabsorbable salts	Magnesium sulfate	10–30	0.5–3
	Magnesium citrate	18 g/12 oz	0.5–3
	Magnesium hydroxide	2.4–4.8	0.5–3
	Sodium phosphate	10 g	0.5–3
	Polyethylene glycol-3350	4 l	1.0–3
Nonabsorbable sugars	Glycerin	3 g (rectally)	0.5
	Sorbitol	120 ml	0.5
	Lactulose		24–48
Lubricants	Mineral oil	15–45 ml	6–8

studies evaluating the efficacy of wheat bran in elderly patients in chronic care facilities have demonstrated a decrease in laxative use and an improved stool function (45–47). In this group of chronically constipated adults who may or may not have underlying disordered motility, wheat bran supplementation may be efficacious (48–50).

Although constipated patients will increase stool weight and transit time when treated with dietary fiber, it is important to note that a meta-analysis of studies evaluating the effect of wheat bran on constipation concluded that constipated patients will still have lower stool weights and slower transit times than normal subjects, whether or not they consume bran (51, 52). In addition, patients with severe idiopathic chronic constipation do not consume less fiber than nonconstipated control subjects and are not helped by the addition of fiber to their diets (53). Therefore, in many patients with chronic constipation, there is still an underlying motility disorder of the bowel that should be treated by using prokinetic agents.

Finally, fiber therapy is not totally benign. When given without sufficient water, large doses of fiber can result in bowel obstruction (28). Prolonged administration of 10–20 g of wheat bran daily can sometimes decrease calcium and iron levels in the elderly (54, 55). Psyllium products also have been reported rarely to cause allergic reactions, occasionally with anaphylaxis (56, 57). Although white fiber may be important in maintaining optimal bowel function in normal persons or in improving lipid or glucose metabolism, its role in the treatment of severe chronic constipation is probably adjunctive.

Nonabsorbable Salts

The nonabsorbable salts include magnesium, sulfate, phosphate, and citrate. These are also called the saline laxatives; all were thought originally to act by a simple osmotic mechanism, drawing water into the lumen. However, Harvey and Read have proposed that magnesium causes the release of CCK, that in turn stimulates active intestinal secretion, pancreatic secretion, and intestinal motility (58). Magnesium citrate increases the number of colonic motor complexes and increases the number of giant migrating complexes associated with defecation. Oral magnesium sulfate increases sigmoid motor activity as measured by the motility index (59). The CCK mediator theory is provocative, yet remains unproven.

The rapid (1–6 hour) onset of action of these agents favors a humoral mechanism primarily affecting the large bowel. Nevertheless, it is likely that both mechanisms contribute to the total effect of these drugs.

The effects of the saline laxatives are rapid and difficult to titrate. The order of potency of the different salts is reported to be sulfate > magnesium > phosphate > tartrate (60). These agents are more appropriately termed cathartics than laxatives. They do not promote normal motility, but they rapidly empty the bowel of its contents. They are most appropriate as pre-endoscopic or preradiologic examination preparation for treatment of poisoning or for parasitic elimination.

Although these agents are considered "nonabsorbable," about 20% is absorbed and this is the mechanism by which they produce toxicity (60). Clinically significant hypermagnesemia (>5.0 mg/dl) is uncommon in adults treated with magnesium citrate even when they are given 960 ml for the treatment of overdose (61). Still, significant electrolyte disturbances do occur in children, especially neonates receiving saline laxatives (62, 63). Cardiac patients have occasionally developed congestive failure because of saline laxatives. Electrolyte imbalances can occur in renal patients, especially with those laxatives that contain large amounts of phosphate. Hypocalcemia, tetany, onetetany, hypernatremia, and hyperphosphatemia have all been reported to occur.

Polyethylene glycol (PEG)-based balanced electrolyte solutions have been developed for total bowel cleansing before diagnostic procedures (64). There are several brands currently available. These solutions are true cathartics, allowing approximately 1 gallon of fluid to be flushed through the bowel with minimal absorption. Although these saline laxatives are used primarily for the purpose of cleaning out, they may be useful in the obstipated patient for a one-time catharsis before the patient attempts establishment of a new bowel routine. In addition, PEG-based solutions have been used with efficacy in some cases of chronic constipation (65). They are an option to consider for a patient with severe debilitating symptoms. Side effects are minimal and include nausea and vomiting. The effects of long-term therapy with PEG solutions in patients with idiopathic chronic constipation are unknown.

Nonabsorbable Sugars

The nonabsorbable sugars include lactulose, glycerin, sorbitol, mannitol, and other sugar alcohols (Table 10.7). The enzymes of the small intestine do not digest these substances. Lactulose is the prototypical substance in this group. It is a disaccharide that is not hydrolyzed until it reaches the cecum. There, cecal bacteria metabolize it first to fructose and galactose and further to lactic acid, acetic acid, formic acid, carbon dioxide, and hydrogen gas. These acids have an osmotic effect and draw water into the lumen of the colon. The low luminal pH produced by the acids also may stimulate colonic propulsive motility (66). Lactulose has shown efficacy against vincristine-induced constipation, opioid-induced constipation, and constipation in the elderly. It was shown in one multicenter study to be more effective than anthraquinone and diphenylmethane-type stimulant laxatives in the treatment of chronic constipation (67). Another study reports lactulose to be as effective and better tolerated than bran in the treatment of chronic constipation (68). Yet it should be noted that the less expensive sugar alcohol, sorbitol, was shown to be as effective as lactulose for elderly patients with constipation (69). In that study the two drugs also had similar side effect profiles. The doses required are 20–40 grams daily in divided doses. Side effects include flatulence and cramps. Diarrhea and electrolyte disturbances may occur if large doses are used or if therapy is given for a long time. However, damage to the myoelectric structures of the bowel with chronic use has not been reported.

Lubricants

Mineral oil is commonly used simply to lubricate the bowel wall and reduce intraluminal sticking of the stool, thus easing its passage.

The oral administration of this agent is occasionally associated with the aspiration of lipoid droplets into the lungs (70). This is especially true for elderly individuals who may be edentulous. In these individuals, droplets of oil may become trapped in the interstices of the mouth and then aspirated into the lungs during sleep. A decrease in absorption of fat-soluble vitamins A, D, K, and E also may occur with prolonged mineral oil therapy (71).

Enemas and Suppositories

Despite their chemical diversity, enemas and suppositories (except those containing mineral oil) are luminally active agents that stimulate the defecatory reflex by very similar mechanisms. They all stretch the anus and rectum by increasing the luminal content of gas or liquid. This increases the rectal volume and the stretching initiates the defecatory reflex (72). Phosphate enemas release carbon dioxide; glycerin suppositories are osmotically active and attract water; simple tap water enemas also are effective because they stimulate rectal emptying and colonic motility by stretching the rectum.

Enemas and suppositories are generally used as adjuncts to orally administered laxatives in the treatment of chronic constipation or for the relief of fecal impaction. They may be most useful in patients with hindgut dysfunction. The effect of clearing the rectum with enemas is important in re-establishing a normal bowel routine, but, the effect of these agents is not sustained (73). In addition, enemas containing nonspecific prokinetic agents like bisacodyl should not be used chronically (see below).

SPECIFIC PROKINETIC AGENTS

Specific prokinetic agents are those laxatives that increase intestinal motility by binding directly to specific neuromuscular receptors within the bowel wall. Their actions mimic (agonist) or inhibit (antagonist) the actions of known specific neurotransmitters. The binding of endogenous or exogenous ligands to specific receptors in the gastrointestinal tract can affect motility, secretion, or both. Table 10.7 lists the activity of a select group of gastrointestinal neurotransmitters on motility. It is important to distinguish motility effects from transit effects. Several drugs, especially the opioids, increase bowel motility but actually delay transit. That is because the pattern of motility produced by opioids is one of increased mixing or nonpropulsive contractions. In addition, some cases of diarrhea are associated with decreased motility and increased secretion, leading to rapid movement of intestinal contents through a flaccid bowel (16). Therefore hypermotility does not always translate into increased transit speed.

Table 10.8 lists the putative actions that result from the specific binding of clinically relevant classes of ligands. Clinically significant prokinetic agents in this group include bethanechol, metoclopramide, domperidone, cisapride, naloxone, and erythromycin. Although each of these agents exhibits specific binding to certain receptor types in vitro, their in vivo activity may not correlate exactly to their in vitro binding.

Cholinomimetics

Cholinomimetic agents mimic the action of acetylcholine by either binding to muscarinic receptors or by increasing the concentration of endogenous acetylcholine at the receptor site as with acetylcholinesterase inhibitors.

BETHANECHOL

Bethanechol is a cholinomimetic used as a promotility agent that binds directly to muscarinic receptors (74). It nonspecifically stimulates all bowel motility and secretion. Its use is associated with many unpleasant side effects, including cramps, diarrhea, flushing, bradycardia, and blurred vision. While it has little efficacy in increasing either gastric, small bowel, or colonic transit (74), it has been used successfully in some cases of postoperative ileus (75). Also, it may be useful in maintaining cholinergic balance in patients receiving drugs such as tricyclic antidepressants with prominent anticholinergic side effects. In these limited settings it may have efficacy in the treatment of constipation (76).

Table 10.8
Actions of Gut Receptor Activation by Agonists (75)[a]

Ligand Class	Receptor Subtype	Receptor Location	Colonic Action
Muscarinic	M2	Smooth muscle	↑ Motility
Adrenergic	α-1	Postsynaptic smooth muscle	↓ Motility
	α-2	Presynaptic adrenergic neurons	↓ Motility
	β-2	Presynaptic smooth muscle	↓ Motility
	β-1	Ganglionic plexus?	↓ Motility
Dopaminergic	D2	CNS only	↓ Motility
Serotonergic	5HT3	"Enteric"	↑ Motility
			↑ Secretion
Opioid	μ2, κ	Myenteric plexus smooth muscle	↑ Motility (mixing)
	μ1, δ	Submucosal plexus	↑ Secretion
Motilin	?		↑ Motility
Calcium channels	?		↓ Motility
Dihydropyridine			↓ Secretion

[a] ↑ = increased, ↓ = decreased, ? no data available, CNS = central nervous system.

Monoaminergics

Included in this category are drugs that are thought to bind to catecholamine receptors such as the adrenergic or dopaminergic receptors and drugs that may interact with serotonin receptors. The drugs in this category are classified by their in vitro binding activity in brain tissue. However, it should be noted that little work has been done that correlates this in vitro activity with prokinetic activity or lack of prokinetic activity in human intestinal motility. In fact, several of these agents have cross-reactivity with monoaminergic systems other than the ones predicted by their binding in brain tissue.

The stimulation of adrenergic receptors, including pre- and postsynaptic α and β receptors in the gut generally decreases gastrointestinal motility and secretion. Clonidine, an α-2 agonist, was shown to prolong GI transit time in normal male volunteers (77) and has been shown to have antidiarrheal efficacy (78). Another study showed that the bowel-slowing effect of clonidine was reversible by idazoxan, an α-2 antagonist, and that idazoxan had no effect on gastric or orocecal transit when given alone (79). The prominent cardiovascular effects of these agents hinder their clinical usefulness in the treatment of intestinal hypomotility. However, as will be discussed, some other monoaminergic agents may exert their effects by weak stimulation of the adrenergic system.

Although it had been theorized that several prokinetic agents acted via dopamine receptors, it had not been shown conclusively that dopamine receptors played a role in controlling intestinal motility. Neither dopamine nor its synthesizing enzyme tyrosine hydroxylase has been demonstrated in the enteric nervous system (75). Metoclopramide is not a specific dopamine antagonist (80). It has significant cross-reactivity with α-2 adrenergic receptors and causes the release of acetylcholine. It also may work through serotonergic receptors. Domperidone, which is more specific for D2-receptors than metoclopramide, has less effect on intestinal motility. Finally, it should be noted that dopamine itself can interact with adrenergic receptors. Thus evidence for a significant role for dopamine as a gastrointestinal neurotransmitter is lacking.

Serotonin is abundant in the enterochromaffin cells of the normal gastrointestinal tract (81). It probably mediates the diarrhea that is so prominent in the carcinoid syndrome. It has recently been shown that a combination of serotonin (5-hydroxytryptamine [5-HT]) antagonists—5HT-2 and 5HT-3 will totally abolish the secretion produced by cholera toxin without affecting the increase in cyclic adenosine monophosphate (cAMP) produced by cholera toxin. In that same experiment, using rat jejunum, researchers found that those serotonin antagonists lacked efficacy against the diarrhea produced by prostaglandin E2 (PGE-2) or bisacodyl. Therefore, serotonin ligands appear to modulate bowel secretion by a mechanism that is independent of prostaglandins and cAMP (82).

Serotonin is increased in the colonic mucosa of some patients with idiopathic chronic constipation (83). Serotonin agonists have been shown to convert fed-mixing small bowel motility in dogs to propulsive-fasting type motility patterns and to increase the numbers of giant migrating complexes (84). Recall that in dogs these giant migrating complexes usually precede defecation. In humans, serotonin increases small bowel and proximal colon propulsive motility while simultaneously causing decreased distal colonic motility (85, 86). Ondansetron, a 5HT-3 antagonist used for the treatment of chemotherapy-induced and postoperative nausea and vomiting increases colonic transit time in a dose-dependent fashion in normal men (87). Still, Murrell et al. were unable to show any difference in bowel motility response to intravenous serotonin in patients with constipation or diarrhea (86). Moreover, Hendrix et al. noted that intraluminal serotonin did not produce the same motility effects in the same subjects as intravenous serotonin (88). Therefore, although the role of the serotonergic system in the regulation of bowel motility and secretion has yet to be defined, the role is probably a very significant one.

METOCLOPRAMIDE

Metoclopramide is a nonspecific dopamine (D2) antagonist. It binds to these receptors in the area postrema to reduce nausea and vomiting, especially after chemotherapy (89). However, it is unclear what receptors metoclopramide acts on in the gut (80). It is more effective in accelerating upper gastrointestinal transit than colonic transit. Numerous studies have demonstrated its ability to increase gastric emptying and small intestinal transit

times. Metoclopramide has been effective in some cases of vincristine-induced ileus (90). It increases colonic spike activity and binds in vitro to colonic tissue (74). However, it has no efficacy in the syndromes of constipation or intestinal pseudo-obstruction (91).

Metoclopramide is known to facilitate the release of acetylcholine, but this may be mediated by serotonin receptors instead of dopamine receptors (91, 92). Metoclopramide blocks α-2 adrenergic receptors in the guinea pig ileum, but not enough to account for its acetylcholine release. Parkinsonian-like symptoms such as tremor, restlessness, akathisia, and tardive dyskinesias that occur with high doses of this drug limit its general use (74). These central antidopaminergic effects may be compounded by peripheral antidopaminergic side effects like gynecomastia. Diarrhea and abdominal cramps are rare.

DOMPERIDONE

Domperidone is also a dopamine (D2) antagonist with some adrenergic cross-reactivity. However, unlike metoclopramide it does not cross the blood-brain barrier and does not promote acetylcholine release (93). It is poorly absorbed and undergoes extensive first pass biotransformation. Nevertheless, it is an effective antiemetic and accelerates gastric emptying with none of the parkinsonian side effects associated with metoclopramide when given orally. It can increase prolactin release like metoclopramide, and may cause galactorrhea in women and rarely gynecomastia in men (93). Domperidone is probably a weak α-2 adrenergic antagonist in the gut like metoclopramide. It does not affect serotonin receptors (91). Unlike metoclopramide it has no effect on colonic spike activity, and thus no efficacy in diseases of delayed colonic transit.

CISAPRIDE

Cisapride is a prokinetic agent that is structurally related to metoclopramide, yet it is not a dopamine antagonist. The exact mechanism and location of its action are still unknown. Like metoclopramide, it promotes the release of acetylcholine. Again, like metoclopramide, there is some evidence that cisapride may act via serotonin (5HT-3) receptors (92). In the upper gut, it induces an MMC-like activity front followed by a prolonged phase II. In the colon, it caused colonic MMC-like activity that was followed by defecation in two dogs that were tested (94).

Although its site of action is not known, cisapride has demonstrated broad efficacy in both upper and lower gastrointestinal hypomotility disorders. It effectively treats gastroparesis in diabetics (95). It increased stool frequency, decreased transit time, and decreased laxative use in children with chronic constipation (96). Cisapride was effective in a randomized control trial in adults with irritable bowel syndrome-related constipation. These patients demonstrated increased stool frequency, improved stool consistency, and decreased abdominal pain (97). Improved laxation also was shown in a randomized controlled trial and a blinded crossover trial of patients with idiopathic chronic constipation (98). There have been case reports of cisapride improving bowel action in paraplegics with total gut slowing (99). It has also been effective in decreasing transit time in patients with pseudo-obstruction (100).

It is interesting that in 12 normal men, cisapride prolonged colonic transit time while decreasing gastric emptying time and small bowel transit time (101). In another study of 10 normal men, cisapride had no effect on gastric emptying, accelerated orocecal transit time, and accelerated colonic transit time (102). The reason for the discordance between the drug action in normal control subjects and those with organic disease is not known. No treatment limiting side effects have been noted with cisapride use in most studies; however, small but significant increases in heart rate and blood pressure have been reported (103).

Motilin Agonists

Motilin stimulates premature MMCs in the small intestine (104). Morphine has the same effect, but motilin does not work via opioid receptors because as the effects of opioids and motilin are not identical. Motilin can induce isolated cecal giant migrating complexes (GMCs) but morphine does not (20). Stimulation of motilin receptors in the upper gastrointestinal tract is associated with accelerated gastric emptying in normal and diabetic subjects (105).

ERYTHROMYCIN

At low doses erythromycin is a motilin agonist. Erythromycin shortens orocecal transit time in normal adults, as measured by the lactulose breath hydrogen test (106). It has also been shown to accelerate gastric emptying in patients with diabetic gastroparesis (107). Studies are currently under way to develop a motilin agonist that does not have any antimicrobial action.

Opioid Antagonists

Opioid agonists have a profound effect on gastrointestinal motility that has been recognized for thousands of years (108). Constipation is a well-known side effect of treatment with exogenous opioid drugs such as morphine, meperidine, and methadone (109, 110). Opioid drugs acutely increase bowel motility and decrease transit time in the opioid, naive patient (111, 112). Most patients who are treated with opioid drugs for more than an hour develop bowel slowing (113).

Opioids slow intestinal transit by several mechanisms. They decrease propulsive intestinal contractions (LSBs), increase mixing intestinal contractions (SSBs), and decrease intestinal secretion (114, 115). Opioids may do this by relaxing longitudinal smooth muscle while contracting circular muscle (116, 117). Transit time studies of the human gastrointestinal tract have documented that opioid drugs delay gastric emptying, delay small intestinal transit, and delay colonic transit (113, 118). The net result is a decrease in stool wet and dry weight, stool volume, and the number of defecations (118, 119), leading to the development of constipation.

Exogenous opioids administered acutely to the opioid naive human or dog have induced premature phase III migrating motor complexes (MMCs) in the small intestine (112, 120). This effect has been noted with opioid alkaloids as well as peptides (112). In opioid-naive humans, intravenous morphine changed the pattern of large bowel myoelectrical activity from a predominance of propagating contractions to nonpropagating contractions (115). In opioid-naive dogs, naloxone infusion may decrease the frequency of the MMC or abolish its appearance altogether (121). In opioid-naive humans, intravenous naloxone reversed the delay of transit induced by the ileal infusion of lipid (122, 123). Intravenous naloxone also has been shown to increase transit selectively in the transverse colon and the rectosigmoid of opioid-naive humans without affecting the number of defecations (118). These effects imply that the normal physiologic function of endogenous opioids in the bowel is to promote the transition from a fasting to a fed bowel motility pattern.

In rodents, opioids potently inhibit toxin-induced diarrhea. In isolated rabbit ileal loops, opioids inhibit secretion (124, 125). In humans, however, the increase in net absorption produced by opioids is due to an increase in contact time produced by an increase in colonic capacitance caused by opioid agonists (126, 127). Therefore the antisecretory effect of opioids in humans is due to their effect on bowel motility.

It has only recently been appreciated that opioid drugs act on specific opioid receptors in the enteric nervous system (128). There are currently three accepted types of opioid receptor (129). These receptors were originally classified by the in vitro bioassay system in which they were the most plentiful and, alternatively, by prototypic agonists. The μ type opioid receptor was originally described in the guinea pig ileum. Morphine was its prototypic agonist. The mouse vas deferens is believed felt to have a predominance of δ type opioid

receptors. The endogenous enkephalin opioids are the prototypic agonists for this receptor. Finally, the rabbit vas deferens is considered to be a pure preparation of κ type opioid receptors for which the endogenous dynorphin opioids are the prototypic agonists (129).

Since the original descriptions of these opioid receptor types, opioid receptors have been subclassified. Pasternak postulated the existence of a μ-1 receptor subtype that is a shared high affinity site between μ and δ agonists (130, 131). It is so far only discernible by treatment with the irreversible antagonist naloxonazine. Pasternak has shown that the effect of opioids on bowel motility is mediated by μ-2 receptor subtypes in rodents. Early studies by Binder implicated the δ preferring enkephalins in the antisecretory effects of opiates in rodents (132). However, recent studies in rodents showing this effect to be more potent than the antitransit effect and occurring with high potency with either δ or μ agonists, suggests a μ-1 or naloxonazine-sensitive mechanism (130, 133, 134).

Besides the existence of opioid receptors there are also three generally accepted classes of endogenous opioid peptides (129). The pro-opiomelanocortin (POMC) derivatives, particularly β-endorphin, bind predominantly to μ and δ type opioid receptors. The proenkephalin-A derivatives bind to δ opioid receptors slightly more than μ and have minimal κ type receptor activity. Finally, there are the prodynorphin derivatives, including a large family of actively processed dynorphin peptides that generally have a ten-fold higher affinity for κ receptor agonists than any of the other endogenous opioids (129).

Endogenous opioid peptides have been demonstrated in the myenteric plexus of the guinea pig, rat, mouse, cat, and pig by immunohistochemical and radioimmunologic techniques (114, 135, 136). We have presented preliminary studies showing the presence of preproenkephalin mRNA throughout the gastrointestinal tract of the guinea pig (137). Biosynthesis of enkephalins has been shown in the guinea pig myenteric plexus by the incorporation of radio-labeled amino acids (138). Opioid peptides have been localized in the neuronal cell bodies and nerve fibers of the myenteric and submucosal plexus (139). They have been found in nerve processes that project into the circular muscle layer of rat (135). In 1977, Polak et al. showed enkephalin peptides throughout the human intestinal tract (140).

The presence of specific opioid receptor binding has been demonstrated in the longitudinal muscle and myenteric plexus tissue homogenates of the guinea pig and rat small intestine (128, 141). We showed preliminary evidence of the existence of μ, δ, and κ opioid receptor binding in the guinea pig colon (142). There has also been preliminary localization of μ and δ opioid receptors in the circular muscle, submucosal plexus, and myenteric plexus of the guinea pig and rat by autoradiographic techniques (143, 144). These results would have to be considered preliminary because the relatively nonspecific ligands used in these studies could not distinguish δ from μ opioid receptors (145). Opioid receptors have also been found in isolated circular smooth muscle preparations from guinea pigs and humans (146).

NALOXONE

Naloxone is uniquely suited to treat problems of gastrointestinal motility because, unlike naltrexone or nalmefene, its bioavailability is limited, for the most part, to the gastrointestinal tract. Opioids may affect gastrointestinal transit by interacting with opioid receptors in either the brain, the spinal cord, or the enteric nervous system (114, 147). Many studies have shown that the intracerebroventricular administration of opioids will produce gastrointestinal slowing (148). Yet, this effect can be abolished in most species by truncal vagotomy (149). Selective administration of opioids to the spine also slows gastrointestinal transit in humans and some rodent species (131, 150). However, we hypothesized that it is the interaction of exogenous opioids with the enteric nervous system that is the most crucial aspect

of understanding the effect that chronic administration of opioids has on the gut.

Several lines of evidence led to the above conclusions. In 1973, Kreek noted that methadone-maintained patients who received naloxone administered by the oral route underwent a withdrawal syndrome that was limited, in most cases, to the gastrointestinal tract (151). This effect was probably localized to the gut, because naloxone undergoes extensive first pass biotransformation when absorbed through the intestine (152–154). Thus, naloxone, when administered orally, reverses opioid effects at the gut level while having minimal effect on the central nervous system.

In 1986, this observation was furthered by oral administration of naloxone to individuals who were receiving opioids chronically for the treatment of pain and who were suffering from chronic constipation (152). It was demonstrated that the amelioration of constipation occurred, although most of the naloxone that was present in the circulation was the inactive biotransformed naloxone-6-glucuronide (154). It was also demonstrated that the mild signs of systemic withdrawal that occurred with this treatment occurred when higher levels of active naloxone were present in the circulation (154).

Others have confirmed and expanded upon these observations. In opioid-naive humans, it has been shown that loperamide, an opioid agonist that acts only on gut opioid receptors, causes intestinal slowing that can be reversed by administration of naloxone (16 mg of oral as well as 8 mg intravenous) (155, 156). Sykes used oral naloxone to treat constipation in patients receiving opioids chronically for pain (157). Just as our own study, they also demonstrated amelioration of constipation without recrudescence of pain or precipitation of withdrawal. Another group did not show any benefit from oral naloxone therapy in opioid-tolerant individuals (158). But, the dose of oral naloxone that they used was admittedly low, ranging from 0.4–4 mg orally. Schang et al. examined the effect of parenteral naloxone on colonic SSBs and LSBs and found no effect (115). However, the dose of naloxone was only

1.6 mg intramuscular, far below that which had been effective in other gastrointestinal studies.

In studies of rodents, Manara et al. showed that gut levels of opioids correlated better with the gut effects of opioids than either blood levels or central nervous system levels (159). Additionally, in this study they showed that the two best methods of administration to achieve these levels were the oral route and the intraperitoneal route. Thollander et al. (160) recently studied the difference between the withdrawal syndrome caused by intravenous naloxone, which crosses the blood-brain barrier, and intravenous methylbromide naloxone, which does not enter the central nervous system, in morphine-dependent rats. The rats that received intravenous naloxone exhibited classical signs of rodent withdrawal, including ptosis, chattering teeth, wet dog shakes, and escape behavior, as well as profuse diarrhea. Morphine-tolerant rats that received intravenous methylbromide naloxone experienced diarrhea only. These findings were similar to those of Kreek who administered naloxone orally with methadone in a combination preparation to methadone-maintained patients (151). Therefore, we conclude that the enteric nervous system mediates the most important effects of exogenous and endogenous opioids on gastrointestinal transit.

Although rodent studies are invaluable in providing detailed data regarding the location of opioid receptors and endogenous opioid peptides and the expression of DNA, one must use caution when extrapolating these data to humans because of the species differences in the gastrointestinal response to exogenous opioids. In 1984, Tavani et al. reported that the κ-agonist U-50, 488H did not slow gastrointestinal transit in the rat, and concluded that κ-receptors were not involved in the pathogenesis of opioid-induced constipation in humans (161). Yet, in 1988, we showed that despite a lack of efficacy in the rat, κ-agonist U-50,488H was equipotent with morphine in producing delay of orocecal transit in the guinea pig when given orally (162). Other investigators have demonstrated

transit delay with the same κ-agonist administered intraperitoneally in the mouse (163). In later studies, we showed that the μ-preferring antagonist, nalmefene, which has more potency at the κ-receptor site than the μ-preferring antagonist naloxone given at similar doses, was more potent than naloxone in reversing the orocecal transit delay produced by κ-agonist U-50,488H (164). These results were not surprising in that Unterwald et al., in an autoradiographic study of guinea pig and rat brain, have documented the paucity of high-affinity κ-opioid receptors in the central nervous system of the rat (165). At this time it is not known whether humans are like guinea pigs, rats, or mice. A recent study by Bansinath et al. showed differential responses to κ-agonists between different strains within the same species mouse (166). Thus the gastrointestinal response to opioid agonists and antagonists depends on the species studied, the opioid receptor density of the tissue, the receptor type specificity of the opioid drug, and the route of administration.

We have hypothesized that the endogenous opioid system not only plays a role in the pathophysiology of opioid-induced constipation, but also plays a role in the pathogenesis of other disorders of gastrointestinal motility. Specifically, some forms of idiopathic chronic constipation and constipation in the elderly may be due to an enhanced relative or absolute activity of the endogenous opioid system. In 1983, Kreek et al. reported the amelioration of constipation in two patients with idiopathic chronic constipation using oral naloxone (167). Later Schang et al. reported in detail on one patient with intestinal pseudo-obstruction who continued to manifest bowel slowing despite having a colectomy (168). The administration of subcutaneous naloxone in this patient improved gastric emptying and normalized intestinal transit. These positive effects reversed when naloxone was withdrawn.

Kreek et al. showed an association between advancing age and increasing levels of circulating β-endorphin (169). Kaiko et al. reported that the requirement for pain medica-

Table 10.9
Nonspecific Agents: Dose and Onset of Action (60, 222, 239)

Class	Drug Name	Dosage Range (mg)	Onset of Action (hr)
Anthraquinones	Standardized senna	374–748	6–12
	Cascara sagrada fluid extract	200–400	6–12
	Danthron	75	6–12
	Aloe	250	6–12
Diphenyl methanes	Bisacodyl	10–30	6–12
	Phenolphthalein	30–270	6–12
	Oxyphenasitin[a]		
Surfactants	Sodium docusate	50–360	24–48
	Calcium docusate	50–360	24–48
	Potassium docusate	50–300	24–48
	Castor oil	15–60 ml	3
	Bile salts[b]		

[a]No longer available.
[b]No longer used for this indication.

tion decreases with advancing age (170). We have reported preliminary evidence that older guinea pigs (33 months vs. 6 months) seem to have more μ-type opioid receptors in their colons than their young counterparts (171). These observations implied an increase in endogenous opioid system activity with age. To test the hypothesis that this increase in endogenous opioid activity may contribute to the increased prevalence of constipation in advancing age, Kreek et al. administered 8 mg of oral naloxone three times daily in a double-blind random cross-over design to 12 nursing home residents whose mean age was 82 years. Fecal wet weight increased significantly. These results implied that the decrease in stool output seen in advancing age may be due to an excess activity of endogenous opioids (152).

Finally, acute stress produces motility effects that mimic the acute administration of opioids in humans and inhibits gastrointestinal transit in animals (112, 172, 173). No model of chronic human stress has been identified or studied with respect to bowel motility, however. It was recently shown that individuals with chronic spinal cord injury, that is, injury of >1 year's duration, have chronically low levels of circulating β-endorphins (174). Chronically stressed an-

imals also have low levels of circulating endorphins, while the endorphin content of the anterior pituitary may be high (175, 176). Low levels of circulating β-endorphins have also been described in humans actively abusing short-acting opioid agonists and in morphine-tolerant rats (177, 178). In the stressed rat, low levels of circulating β-endorphin may be associated with higher anterior pituitary levels of POMC peptides and POMC mRNA (179). In the opioid-dependent animal, low levels of circulating β-endorphin are associated with low levels of pituitary POMC peptides and mRNA (180). Therefore in constipation that is associated with chronic stress, gut levels of endogenous opioids may be high, causing hypomotility.

Chronic constipation is a prevalent problem for individuals with spinal cord injury of several years' duration (181). There is one case report of constipation in a quadriplegic treated with oral naloxone (182). A patient who was 21 years status post–spinal cord injury who suffered from acute pseudo-obstruction was treated with intravenous followed by oral naloxone (personal observation). The patient responded well and was eventually able to have spontaneous bowel movements without the drug.

NONSPECIFIC PROKINETIC AGENTS

These are the laxative agents that historically have been called stimulant or irritant laxatives (Table 10.9). They are the most commonly consumed laxative compounds (183), although despite their widespread use, clinical trials demonstrating their safety and efficacy in the long-term treatment of chronic constipation are lacking. This group of drugs includes the anthraquinone derivatives, the diphenylmethane derivatives, and the surfactants. These agents increase fluid and electrolyte secretion and also increase intestinal motility. We have termed these agents nonspecific prokinetic agents because, although they all produce direct neuromuscular stimulation of the intestines, these effects are not mediated by specific endogenous neurohormonal receptors.

There is much evidence that their effects may be partially mediated by increasing prostaglandin synthesis and/or increasing intracellular cAMP. This may represent a low-grade inflammatory response due to epithelial and/or myenteric tissue destruction produced by these agents since the bowel also releases prostaglandins when exposed to endotoxin, radiation, and some allergens (184). In these conditions, a motility pattern develops that is identical to the one seen with nonspecific prokinetic laxatives (23). Therefore, although these agents are not irritants in the sense that they produce gross mucosal edema and erythema, they are irritant in that they activate proinflammatory mechanisms in the gut.

Anthraquinones

This group includes danthron, senna, aloe, and cascara derivatives. Most of the laxatives in this category are vegetable derivatives that have been used for centuries (185). The ring substitutions at C^3 and at C^4 determine the final active compound. None of these compounds except danthron are active in the upper bowel because they have to be biotransformed by the colonic bacteria. Danthron and the other monoanthrones tend to be irritating to the oral mucosa because they are ingested in their active form. Thus, nature has allowed

for the formation of less toxic forms of the active moiety by drying or aging the plant source. This results in the formation of either a dianthrone in which two monoanthrone moieties are joined at the C-10 location or a glycoside with a glucose at the same C-10 site. Rhein anthrone is the active moiety of the senna plant. It forms a dianthrone or sennoside when dried for purposes of ingestion. Barbaloin is the monoanthrone glycoside active component of aloe. Cascara contains the glycosides barbaloin and chrysaloin. The inactivation of the native anthraquinone by drying is reversed by the action of the colonic bacteria, which can split the dianthrone and remove any glucose moieties present to leave the active compound (185). Thus the delay in onset of action of oral sennosides of between 6 and 12 hours occurs because compound must reach the colon and be metabolized by the bacterial flora.

Orally administered sennosides produce giant migrating contractions and diarrhea in the dog (186). They inhibit the postprandial increase in colonic spiking activity, which is probably mediated by endogenous opioids, while simultaneously emptying the entire colon (123, 187). In rats they induce mass movements that empty the colon (188). Sennosides produce migrating LSBs and high amplitude contractions associated with the urge to defecate in normal and constipated subjects (189). Although sennosides do produce net water and electrolyte secretion, it has been shown that the promotility effect occurs before enough fluid can build up in the intestine to promote diarrhea (190, 191). In normal men, Senokot accelerates transit times, increases stool wet weight, and increases stool dry weight (119). In these experiments the fiber content of the diet was kept constant. Bacterial mass was measured and found to account for most of the increase in stool dry weight caused by Senokot.

The motility pattern produced by sennosides and its active moiety rhein anthrone has been induced by colonic instillation of fatty acids, bile acids, indigestible particles, and infection. Sennosides increase the production of

PGE-2 in rodents. In humans prostaglandins can produce diarrhea. The induction of mucous secretion caused by rhein anthrone can be mimicked by PGE-2 and blocked by indomethacin (192). However, it has not yet been proven that anthraquinones work entirely by this mechanism. This is especially true since pretreatment with indomethacin did not completely reverse the net fluid secretion caused by rhein anthrone (193). Rhein anthrone also releases histamine in rodent colon (194). This is another potential mechanism of senna action.

A 1953 report on the efficacy of standardized senna stated that it produced a "good response" in 93 of 101 patients. The seven patients who did not respond had chronic constipation (195). It has also been reported that senna is more effective than a magnesium hydroxide and mineral oil combination (94% vs. 36%) in treating patients with drug-induced constipation (196). However, there are few studies in the current medical literature that demonstrate the clinical safety and efficacy of anthraquinone laxatives in chronic constipation. One study of elderly nursing home patients revealed the anthraquinone to be equally as effective as lactulose. This study also concluded that both agents were better than placebo in increasing the number of bowel movements per week as well as the number of markers (73). Another study of constipated adults (average age 26.1 years) who were treated with psyllium alone or psyllium plus senna has demonstrated an added benefit of the addition of senna. Only those patients treated with psyllium and senna increased stool wet as well as stool dry weight (197). A recent randomized controlled study examining an aloe-psyllium mixture concluded that this combination was more effective than placebo in increasing the frequency of bowel movements and decreasing the use of laxatives (198).

The toxicity of anthraquinones to the bowel is presently a subject of controversy. Although the syndrome of cathartic colon is acknowledged to exist (consisting of laxative abuse associated with an ahaustral colon, melanosis coli, and histologic evidence of myenteric plexus damage), it is not clear which laxatives alone or in combination are responsible for the damage. Many of the original descriptions of cathartic colon were of necessity retrospective and could not fully explore the chemical nature of all drugs taken by particular patients over their lifetimes (199).

Acute and subacute studies evaluating senna toxicity in humans and in animals have been conflicting. Most agree that *Melanosis coli* is a harmless reversible side effect due to anthracene laxative use (200). An early, much quoted, retrospective comparison of the colons of human laxative abusers with the colons of mice treated with a senna mixture postulated that the similar damage seen in the myenteric plexus in these two situations was due to anthraquinone ingestion (46). Still, other studies of dogs and rodents state that even after months of therapy damage due to pure anthraquinones cannot be demonstrated by light or electron microscopy (201–203). It has been postulated that the myenteric plexus damage reported in earlier studies and case reports was due to contamination with free monoanthrones such as danthron. However, evidence of colonic damage by danthron has been difficult to establish (201). From the available evidence we conclude that anthraquinones are probably not neurotoxic when used alone in the recommended dosages.

Diphenylmethanes

The diphenylmethane derivatives include the commonly prescribed drugs bisacodyl and phenolphthalein (Table 10.9). Also included in this group is oxyphenasitin, which is no longer commercially available because of its hepatotoxicity (183). When given in combination with sodium docusate, it produced a chronic active hepatitis. It is possible that the surfactant increased its absorption and consequently its hepatotoxicity. *Bisacodyl* is a prodrug that is absorbed by the small intestine, conjugated, and re-excreted in the bile. It is then deconjugated in the colon to picosulfate and exerts most of its effect there (204). However, it should be noted that bisacodyl can be activated in an alkalinized stomach. Activation in the upper gut can cause abdominal cramping, nausea, and vomiting (60).

At low doses, bisacodyl increases mucus and potassium secretion in rodent colon. Bisacodyl increases net sodium and water excretion in the jejunum of humans and in the colon of rodents (72, 205, 206). It is a potent inhibitor of intestinal absorption and thus produces a net increase in delivery of water to the colon in rodents and humans (207). The increase in flow produced by bisacodyl is linearly related to the decrease in transit time in humans (205). In addition, unlike opioids, which increase absorption by increasing colonic capacitance, bisacodyl does not decrease total gut volume (126, 127, 205). Bisacodyl is more potent at causing net fluid secretion than is senna (208). Bisacodyl induces the release‘ of PGE-2 after colonic administration (209, 210). The release of prostaglandins may secondarily increase cAMP, but that is not considered to be the primary mechanism of action of bisacodyl itself (206, 211). Besides prostaglandin release, there is some evidence that diphenylmethanes increase the transfer of larger molecular weight substances by increasing the leakiness of intercellular tight junctions. Chronic administration of bisacodyl decreases the effects of acute administration of bisacodyl on fluid and electrolyte flux in rodents (212).

Diphenylmethanes affect motility as well as secretion. Oxyphenasitin induced mass peristalsis in the colon of humans that is indistinguishable from the naturally occurring mass peristalsis. Bisacodyl and oxyphenasitin cause colonic giant migrating contractions (213). Higher doses of the compounds produced even more mass movements and were associated with diarrhea. Schang et al. showed that bisacodyl abolishes short spike bursts and increases the number of propagating spike bursts along with producing abdominal cramps and urgency (214, 215).

Bisacodyl will produce peristalsis in the distal colon of some, but not all, patients with slow transit constipation (54). It seemed no better or worse than lactulose in the treatment of patients with chronic constipation (67). In 1959 Dreiling et al. administered bisacodyl for 6 months to 32 patients with chronic constipation and reported that approximately 84% continued to respond well without side effects (216). There are other anecdotal reports that chronic treatment with bisacodyl is safe in cases of neurogenic bowel syndrome (217). Because of its toxicity, however, bisacodyl is not recommended for the chronic treatment of constipation. Unlike the anthraquinones, the diphenylmethanes definitely cause damage to enterocytes (218). When instilled rectally, they cause sloughing of the surface epithelium and a neutrophilic infiltration that resembles early inflammatory bowel disease (219). Bisacodyl also damages small bowel epithelium (207). It should be noted that when used as a cathartic and added to balanced PEG solutions, bisacodyl seems to result in more patients having total removal of fecal material (53% vs. 82%) (220).

Phenolphthalein is activated after absorption by the small bowel and secretion in the large bowel in a manner similar to bisacodyl. White and yellow phenolphthalein are widely available in several over-the-counter laxative preparations. Yellow phenolphthalein is approximately three times more potent than white phenolphthalein (221). Chronic use has been reported to cause malabsorption of vitamin D and calcium, resulting in rickets. Chronic use or abuse can cause a hyperaldosterone hyperkalemic syndrome that mimics Bartter syndrome. Skin hypersensitivity reactions, toxic epidermal necrolysis, and bullous reaction in sun light have also been reported (222, 223).

Surfactants

Dioctyl sodium and *calcium sulfosuccinate* (the docusates), *bile acids*, and *castor oil* are all anionic surfactants. The docusates are marketed primarily as stool-wetting agents. They are surfactants in vitro and thus could soften the stool by promoting the miscibility of oil and water (71). However, it has been shown that these agents do not simply allow for better

Table 10.10
Summary of Current Knowledge Regarding the Effect of Laxatives on Bowel Motility and Secretion[a]

| | Small Bowel | | Colonic | | | |
Agent	Transit Time	Mixing Contractions (SSBs)	Propulsive Contractions (LSBs)	Mass Movements	Stool Water	Stool Solids
Dietary fiber	↓	?	↑	?	↑	↑
Magnesium	↓	–	↑	↑	↑↑	
Lactulose	↓	?	?	?	↑↑	
Metoclopramide	↓	?	↑	?	–	–
Cisapride	↓	?	↑	?	↑	↑
Erythromycin	↓	?	?	?	?	?
Naloxone	↓	↓	–	–	↑	↑
Anthroquinones	↓	↓	↑	↑	↑↑	↑
Diphenylmethanes	↓	↓	↑	↑	↑↑	?
Docusates	–	?	?	?	–	–
Castor oil	↓	↓↓	↓↓	↓	↑↑	?
Mineral oil	?	?	?	?	↑?	?

[a] ↑ = increased, ↓ = decreased, ? = no data available, – = no effect on this parameter.

mixing of the stool, they actually promote the net intestinal secretion of water (190, 224). Docusate sodium is a competitive inhibitor of phosphodiesterase and thus increases intracellular cAMP (225). It abolishes glucose transport in the jejunum and ileum (226). This may be due to the toxic effect that these agents have on the epithelial cells (227).

Controlled studies documenting the efficacy of these agents are few. One study of chronically ill and geriatric constipated patients showed that docusate calcium may be significantly better than dioctyl sodium sulfosuccinate and that the docusate sodium may be no better than placebo (228). Another study of constipated elderly individuals showed no advantage of docusate calcium over placebo (229). These studies were done of individuals who probably had abnormal colonic motility. Earlier studies have reported efficacy of the docusates in postpartum constipation and postoperative stool softening, that is, in individuals who have normal underlying bowel motility (60). However, a recent study of docusate sodium in normal subjects revealed no change in stool solids or water (230). Use of surfactants with other potentially hepatotoxic laxatives and drugs may increase the hepatocellular damage of these other drugs by increasing their absorption. This is especially

true of drugs like quinidine or danthron. Therefore the overall efficacy of the docusates is minimal and they may have significant toxicity. Their use is not recommended in cases of severe colonic inertia. When bowel motility is normal they may be helpful.

Castor oil is converted in the small bowel to its active form, ricinoleic acid, which is also an anionic surfactant. Unlike the anthraquinones and the diphenylmethanes, the small bowel is the primary site of action of castor oil. Therefore the onset of action for this agent is usually 1–3 hours. Ricinoleic acid induces significant water and electrolyte secretion. It increases membrane permeability to macromolecules greater than 4 \ (71). It stimulates cAMP but by a nonphosphodiesterase-related method (225). The increase in cAMP produced by ricinoleic acid is probably an indirect effect mediated by prostaglandins. Ricinoleic acid does not increase intestinal motility. In fact, it inhibits small bowel motility while it increases net fluid secretion, leading to the rapid flow of contents through the small bowel (231, 232). Castor oil is clearly toxic to the bowel. It causes the destruction of the epithelium. Ricinoleate will decrease the number of ganglion cells in the submucosal plexus of rat jejunum when administered chronically (233). This drug is best suited for occasional use such as for preprocedure catharsis.

SUMMARY

A comprehensive approach to the treatment of constipation with laxatives would involve first eliminating or minimizing any reversible causes of constipation (Table 10.1). Certain causes of constipation may be amenable to very specific therapy. For example, constipation due to treatment with anticholinergic agents may be amenable to treatment with bethanechol and opioid-induced constipation may benefit from treatment with orally administered naloxone. (Table 10.10) Irreversible causes of neuromuscular damage also should be identified because they will not respond to the treatment approach described below.

Improvement of bowel habit behaviors should always be attempted. Fluid and fiber intake should be maximized, while the use of nonspecific stimulant laxatives should be minimized. Patients should be encouraged to attempt bowel action at times when colonic activity is naturally known to increase—that is, in the morning when increased physical activity increases colonic motility and after meals when the gastrocolic reflex attempts to empty the colon to prepare it to accept the coming small bowel contents. Gentle stimulation of the defecatory reflex by glycerin or even bisacodyl suppositories at the time of increased bowel motility may be all that is needed to promote regular bowel activity. Prolonged constipation leads to a distended overstretched bowel that must be decompressed before normal reflexes resume. This is especially true in children in whom bowel retraining programs that include the short-term use of laxatives and cathartics can produce a sustained improvement in bowel habit and bowel motility (67, 234).

If these procedures are unsuccessful, then a motility disorder should be suspected and colonic transit time should be evaluated. If the delivery of colonic contents to the distal rectosigmoid is globally delayed, then a specific prokinetic agent with colonic efficacy like cis-apride, oral naloxone, or erythromycin should be tried (Table 10.10). At the current time, none of these agents is approved for the treatment of constipation, but studies are ongoing.

Finally, constipation syndromes that have resulted primarily from hindgut disorders should be evaluated by anorectal manometry and defecography. The latter test involves lateral X-rays taken of the patient attempting to reproduce the act of defecation. Occasionally, surgically correctable lesions will be discovered. These include obstructed defecation due to pelvic floor spasm or adult Hirshsprung disease. Anorectal myotomy may be indicated in these rare cases. These examinations may also reveal incomplete defecation due to a lax pelvic floor caused by perineal descent. Such patients may benefit from pelvic strengthening exercises and/or biofeedback (6, 13).

PERSPECTIVES FOR THE FUTURE

It should be noted that attempts to define idiopathic chronic constipation by consistent changes in the histopathology of the enteric nervous system have been unsuccessful. Nevertheless, there have been a few provocative studies evaluating the changes in enteric plexus hormones that occur in these patients. The myenteric plexus is rich in peptide hormones whose functions are incompletely understood (235).

Excess secretion of vasoactive intestinal peptide (VIP) in the gastrointestinal tract is associated with profound watery diarrhea characterized by increased secretion and muscular relaxation of the bowel wall. Opioids, on the other hand, decrease bowel transit by increasing nonpropulsive contractions. Opioids also decrease secretion. Koch et al. determined that four patients with idiopathic chronic constipation had decreased VIP peptides and normal levels of metenkephalins (236). If VIP normally opposes endogenous opioid activity, then decreased VIP activity would lead to constipation secondary to unopposed opioid activity. These patients might respond to oral naloxone.

In another study motilin release was impaired in 12 patients with chronic constipa-

Table 10.11
Mechanism of Laxative Action and Toxicity[a]

Agent	Mechanism/Mediator	Toxicity
Fiber	Bowel wall stretch	Obstruction
	Osmotic action	Loss of divalent cations
	SCFAs prokinetic?	Anaphylaxis
Magnesium	Cholecystokinin release	Hypermagnesemia
	Osmotic action	Congestive heart failure
Lactulose	Osmotic action	Bloating, gas
PEG	Osmotic action	Bloating, gas, nausea, vomiting
Cisapride	Serotonin agonist or antagonist	(Unknown)
Erythromycin	Motilin agonist	Antimicrobial
Naloxone	Opioid antagonist	May precipitate abstinence in tolerant individuals
Anthraquinones	Prostaglandin release	*Melanosis coli*
	Histamine release	Enteric plexus damage??
Diphenylmethanes	Increased cAMP	Enteric plexus damage
	Prostaglandin release?	Light-sensitive bullous rashes
		Cathartic colon
		Pseudo-Bartter syndrome
Surfactants	Increased cAMP	Epithelial damage
		Enteric plexus damage

[a]SCFAs, short-chain fatty acids; cAMP, cyclic adenosine monophosphate.

tion. Motilin is prokinetic and its decrease could lead to constipation. Therefore, these patients might respond well to erythromycin.

An increase in mucosal serotonin has been demonstrated in six of eight patients with idiopathic constipation. In man, serotonin affects the proximal motility of the colon differently than the distal colon. It is conceivable that excess serotonin could lead to hindgut hypomotility, and decreased serotonin could lead to foregut hypomotility. Cisapride might be working on one of these systems.

In the preceding review of laxative agents, we have attempted to classify these agents by their predominant mechanism of action and to highlight the effects of these agents on bowel motility. As more is known regarding normal bowel motility with its fasting and fed patterns and bowel motility that functions to rid the gut of some unwanted toxin, we may be able to choose laxative agents by the particular motility patterns that they produce. The traditional "irritant laxatives" or nonspecific laxatives seem to produce a prostaglandin-mediated motility pattern consistent with bowel irritation or inflammation and characterized by frequent mass movements or peristaltic rushes and increased secretion;—the motility pattern of diarrhea or inflammation (Table 10.11) (22, 23, 237, 238). On the other hand, fiber and the specific prokinetic laxatives affect the normal or nonirritated fasting and fed motility pattern of the large and small bowel. Those agents that are most effective at reducing the mixing/fed motility patterns and promoting the propulsive/fasting motility patterns will have the greatest efficacy in diseases characterized by bowel inertia. They will have little direct effect on bowel secretion. Although activation of prodiarrheal mechanisms is desirable for catharsis, it is not necessary or desirable for the prokinetic laxatives of the future. The more we understand normal human physiology, the more we can specifically target opioid, motilin, or serotonin receptors and avoid the nonspecific activation of prostaglandin-mediated mechanisms.

ACKNOWLEDGMENTS

We acknowledge the assistance of Charles J. Morgan, M.D., and Robert A. Schaefer, M.D., in the preparation of this chapter. I also thank Peter R. Holt and Martin H. Floch for their training and guidance in the field of gastroenterology (J.A.C.-M.).

REFERENCES

1. Everhart JE, Go VL, Johannes RS, Fitzsimmons SC, Roth HP, White LR. A longitudinal survey of self-reported bowel habits in the United States. Dig Dis Sci 1989;34:1153–1162.

2. Johanson JF, Sonnenberg A, Koch TR. Clinical epidemiology of chronic constipation. J Clin Gastroenterol 1989;11:525–536.

3. Alessi CA, Henderson CT. Constipation and fecal impaction in the long-term care patient. Clin Geriatr Med 1988;4:571–588.

4. Devroede G. Constipation. In: Sleisenger MH, Fordtran JS, eds. Gastrointestinal disease: pathophysiology, diagnosis, management. Philadelphia: Saunders, 1989;331–368.

5. Mountjoy CQ, Haward LRC, Godding EW. Some determinants of defaecation. Lancet 1971;2:319.

6. Read NW, Timms JM. Defecation and the pathophysiology of constipation. Clin Gastroenterol 1986;15:937–965.

7. Shouler P, Keighley MR. Changes in colorectal function in severe idiopathic chronic constipation. Gastroenterology 1986;90:414–420.

8. Frieri G, Parisi F, Corazziari E, Caprilli R. Colonic electromyography in chronic constipation. Gastroenterology 1983;84:737–740.

9. Martelli H, Devroede G, Arhan P, Duguay C. Mechanisms of idiopathic constipation: outlet obstruction. Gastroenterology 1978;75:623–631.

10. Read NW, Timms JM, Barfield LJ, Donnelly TC, Bannister JJ. Impairment of defecation in young women with severe constipation. Gastroenterology 1986;90:53–60.

11. Barnes PR, Hawley PR, Preston DM, Lennard-Jones JE. Experience of posterior division of the puborectalis muscle in the management of chronic constipation. Br J Surg 1985;72:475–477.

12. Devroede G, Arhan P, Duguay C, Tetreault L, Akoury H, Perey B. Traumatic constipation. Gastroenterology 1979;77:1258–1267.

13. Miller R, Mortensen NJ: Anorectal physiology. Surg Annu 1989;21:303–326.

14. Cohen S, Snape WJ Jr. Movement of the small and large intestine. In: Sleisenger MH, Fordtran JS, eds. Gastrointestinal disease: pathophysiology, diagnosis and management. Philadelphia: Saunders, 1989;1088–1105.

15. Sarna SK: Cyclic motor activity: migrating motor complex: 1985. Gastroenterology 1985;89:894–913.

16. Bueno L, Frexinos J, Fioramonti J. Role of motility in pathogenesis of constipation and diarrhea. Pharmacology 1988;36:15–22.

17. Waller SL. Differential measurement of small and large bowel transit times in constipation and diarrhoea: A new approach. Gut 1975;16:372–378.

18. Camboni G, Basilisco G, Bozzani A, Bianchi PA. Repeatability of lactulose hydrogen breath test in subjects with normal or prolonged orocecal transit. Dig Dis Sci 1988;33:1525–1527.

19. Marzio L, Del Bianco R, Donne MD, Pieramico O, Cuccurullo F. Mouth-to-cecum transit time in patients affected by chronic constipation: effect of glucomannan. Am J Gastroenterol 1989;84:888–891.

20. Sarna SK, Prasad KR, Lang IM. Giant migrating contractions of the canine cecum. Am J Physiol 1988;254:G595–G601.

21. Sethi AK, Sarna SK. Colonic motor response to a meal in acute colitis. Gastroenterology 1991;101:1537–1546.

22. Sethi AK, Sarna SK. Colonic motor activity in acute colitis in conscious dogs. Gastroenterology 1991;100:954–963.

23. Read NW. Colon: relationship between epithelial transport and motility. Pharmacology 1988;36:120–125.

24. Hyland CM, Foran JD. Dioctyl sodium sulphosuccinate as a laxative in the elderly. Practitioner 1968;200:698–699.

25. Panton ON, Atkinson KG, Crichton EP, Schulzer M, Beaufoy A, Germann E. Mechanical preparation of the large bowel for elective surgery comparison of whole-gut lavage with the conventional enema and purgative technique. Am J Surg 1985;149:615–619.

26. Brunton LL. Agents affecting gastrointestinal water flux and motility, digestants, and bile acids. In: Gilman AG, Rall TW, Nies AS, Taylor P, eds. Goodman and Gilmans the pharmacological basis of therapeutics. ed. 8. New York: Pergamon Press, 1990;914–932.

27. Hirst GD. Mechanisms of peristalsis. Br Med Bull 1979;35:263–268.

28. Miller DL, Miller PF, Dekker JJ. Small-bowel obstruction from bran cereal [Letter]. JAMA 1990;263:813–814.

29. Cummings JH. Dietary fibre. Gut 1973;14:69–81.

30. Mendeloff AI. Dietary fiber and human health. N Engl J Med 1977;297:811–814.

31. Frankenfield DC, Beyer PL. Dietary fiber and bowel function in tube-fed patients. J Am Diet Assoc 1991;91:590–596, 599.

32. Council on Scientific Affairs. Dietary fiber and health. JAMA 1989;262:542–546.

33. Royall D, Wolever TM, Jeejeebhoy KN. Clinical significance of colonic fermentation. Am J Gastroenterol 1990;85:1307–1312.

34. Wrick KL, Robertson JB, Van Soest PJ, et al. The influence of dietary fiber source on human intestinal transit and stool output. J Nutr 1983;113:1464–1479.

35. Hillman L, Peters S, Fisher A, Pomare EW. Differing effects of pectin, cellulose and lignin on stool pH, transit time and weight. Br J Nutr 1983;50:189–195.

36. Jenkins DJ, Peterson RD, Thorne MJ, Ferguson PW. Wheat fiber and laxation: dose response and equilibration time. Am J Gastroenterol 1987;82:1259–1263.

37. Cummings JH, Branch W, Jenkins DJ, Southgate DA, Houston H, James WP. Colonic response to dietary fibre from carrot, cabbage, apple, bran. Lancet 1978;1:5–9.

38. Tomlin J, Read NW. Comparison of the effects on colonic function caused by feeding rice bran and wheat bran. Eur J Clin Nutr 1988;42:857–861.

39. Richardson A, Delbridge AT, Brown NJ, Rumsey RD, Read NW. Short chain fatty acids in the terminal ileum accelerate stomach to caecum transit time in the rat. Gut 1991;32:266–269.

40. Kamath PS, Phillips SF. Initiation of motility in canine ileum by short chain fatty acids and inhibition by pharmacological agents. Gut 1988;29:941–948.

41. Andersson H, Bosaeus I, Falkheden T, Melkersson M. Transit time in constipated geriatric patients during treatment with a bulk laxative and bran: a comparison. Scand J Gastroenterol 1979;14:821–826.

42. Burkitt DP, Walker AR, Painter NS. Effect of dietary fibre on stools and the transit-times, and its role in the causation of disease. Lancet 1972;2:1408–1412.

43. Taylor R. Management of constipation: 1. High fibre diets at work. Br Med J 1990;300:1063–1064.

44. Calcium polycarbophil (Mitrolan). Med Lett Drugs Ther 1981;23:52.

45. Sandman PO, Adolfsson R, Hallmans G, Nygren C, Nystrom L, Winblad B. Treatment of constipation with high-bran bread in long-term care of severely demented elderly patients. J Am Geriatr Soc 1983;31:289–293.

46. Smith B. Effect of irritant purgatives on the myenteric plexus in man and the mouse. Gut 1968;9:139–143.

47. Hull C, Greco RS, Brooks DL. Alleviation of constipation in the elderly by dietary fiber supplementation. J Am Geriatr Soc 1980;28:410–414.

48. Donald IP, Smith RG, Cruikshank JG, Elton RA, Stoddart ME. A study of constipation in the elderly living at home. Gerontology 1985;31:112–118.

49. Bannister JJ, Abouzekry L, Read NW. Effect of aging on anorectal function. Gut 1987;28:353–357.

50. Whitehead WE, Drinkwater D, Cheskin LJ, Heller BR, Schuster MM. Constipation in the elderly living at home: definition, prevalence, and relationship to lifestyle and health status. J Am Geriatr Soc 1989;37:423–429.

51. Hamilton JW, Wagner J, Burdick BB, Bass P. Clinical evaluation of methylcellulose as a bulk laxative. Dig Dis Sci 1988;33:993–998.

52. Muller-Lissner SA. Effect of wheat bran on weight of stool and gastrointestinal transit time: a meta-analysis. Br Med J (Clin Res Ed) 1988;296:615–617.

53. Preston DM, Lennard-Jones JE. Severe chronic constipation of young women: 'idiopathic slow transit constipation.' Gut 1986;27:41–48.

54. Persson I, Raby K, Fonss-Bech P, Jensen E. Effect of prolonged bran administration on serum levels of cholesterol, ionized calcium and iron in the elderly. J Am Geriatr Soc 1976;24:334–335.

55. Kinnunen O, Salokannel J. Comparison of the effects of magnesium hydroxide and a bulk laxative on lipids, carbohydrates, vitamins A and E, and minerals in geriatric hospital patients in the treatment of constipation. J Int Med Res 1989;17:442–454.

56. Sussman GL, Dorian W. Psyllium anaphylaxis. Allergy Proc 1990;11:241–242.

57. Busse WW, Schoenwetter WF. Asthma from psyllium in laxative manufacture. Ann Intern Med 1975;83:361–362.

58. Harvey RF, Read AE. Mode of action of the saline purgatives. Am Heart J 1975;89:810–812.

59. Harvey RF, Read AE. Effects of oral magnesium sulphate on colonic motility. Gut 1973;14:425–425.

60. Pietrusko RG. Use and abuse of laxatives. Am J Hosp Pharm 1977;34:291–300.

61. Woodard JA, Shannon M, Lacouture PG, Woolf A. Serum magnesium concentrations after repetitive magnesium cathartic administration. Am J Emerg Med 1990;8:297–300.

62. Mofenson HC, Caraccio TR. Magnesium intoxication in a neonate from oral magnesium hydroxide laxative. J Toxicol Clin Toxicol 1991;29:215–222.

63. Schindler AM. Isolated neonatal hypomagnesaemia associated with maternal overuse of stool softener [Letter]. Lancet 1984;2:822.

64. Davis GR, Santa Ana CA, Morawski SG, Fordtran JS. Development of a lavage solution associated with minimal water and electrolyte absorption or secretion. Gastroenterology 1980;78:991–995.

65. Krevsky B, Malmud LS, D'Ercole F, Maurer AH, Fisher RS. Colonic transit scintigraphy: a physiologic approach to the quantitative measurement of colonic transit in humans. Gastroenterology 1986;91:1102–1112.

66. Bond JH, Levitt MD. Effect of dietary fiber on intestinal gas production and small bowel transit time in man. Am J Clin Nutr 1978;31:S169–S174.

67. Connolly P, Hughes IW, Ryan G. Comparison of "Duphalac" and "irritant" laxatives during and after treatment of chronic constipation: a preliminary study. Curr Med Res Opin 1974;2:620–625.

68. Rouse M, Chapman N, Mahapatra M, Grillage M, Atkinson SN, Prescott P. An open, randomised, parallel group study of lactulose versus ispaghula in the treatment of chronic constipation in adults. Br J Clin Pract 1991;45:28–30.

69. Lederle FA, Busch DL, Mattox KM, West MJ, Aske DM. Cost-effective treatment of constipation in the elderly: a randomized double-blind comparison of sorbitol and lactulose. Am J Med 1990;89:597–601.

70. Rosenow EC 3d. The spectrum of drug-induced pulmonary disease. Ann Intern Med 1972;77:977–991.

71. Fingl E, Freston JW. Antidiarrhoeal agents and laxatives: Changing concepts. Clin Gastroenterol 1979;8:161–185.

72. Ewe K. The physiological basis of laxative action. Pharmacology 1980;20:2–20.

73. Brocklehurst JC, Kirkland JL, Martin J, Ashford J. Constipation in long-stay elderly patients: its treatment and prevention by lactulose, poloxalkol-dihydroxyanthroquinolone and phosphate enemas. Gerontology 1983;29:181–184.

74. Reynolds JC. Prokinetic agents: a key in the future of gastroenterology. Gastroenterol Clin North Am 1989;18:437–457.

75. Ruoff HJ, Fladung B, Demol P, Weihrauch TR. Gastrointestinal receptors and drugs in motility disorders. Digestion 1991;48:1–17.

76. Everett HC. The use of bethanechol chloride with tricyclic antidepressants. Am J Psychiatry 1975;132:1202–1204.

77. Rubinoff MJ, Piccione PR, Holt PR. Clonidine prolongs human small intestine transit time: use of the lactulose-breath hydrogen test. Am J Gastroenterol 1989;84:372–374.

78. Ooms LA, Degryse AD, Janssen PA. Mechanisms of action of loperamide. Scand J Gastroenterol Suppl 1984;96:145–155.

79. Baxter AJ, Edwards CA, Holden S, Cunningham KM, Welch IM, Read NW. The effect of two alpha 2-adrenoreceptor agonists and an antagonist on gastric emptying and mouth-to-caecum transit time in humans. Aliment Pharmacol Ther 1987;1:649–655.

80. Willems JL, Buylaert WA, Lefebvre RA, Bogaert MG. Neuronal dopamine receptors on autonomic ganglia and sympathetic nerves and dopamine receptors in the gastrointestinal system. Pharmacol Rev 1985;37:165–216.

81. Penttila A, Lempinen M. Enterochromaffin cells and 5-hydroxytryptamine in the human intestinal tract. Gastroenterology 1968;54:375–381.

82. Beubler E, Horina G. 5-HT2 and 5-HT3 receptor subtypes mediate cholera toxin-induced intestinal fluid secretion in the rat. Gastroenterology 1990;99:83–89.

83. Lincoln J, Crowe R, Kamm MA, Burnstock G, Lennard-Jones JE. Serotonin and 5-hydroxyindoleacetic acid are increased in the sigmoid colon in severe idiopathic constipation. Gastroenterology 1990;98:1219–1225.

84. Siegle ML, Ehrlein HJ. Effects of various agents on ileal postprandial motor patterns and transit of chyme in dogs. Am J Physiol 1989;257:G698–G703.

85. Fink S, Friedman G. The differential effect of drugs on the proximal and distal colon. Am J Med 1960;28:534–540.

86. Murrell TGC, Wangel AG, Deller DJ. Intestinal motility in man, IV: effect of serotonin in subjects with diarrhea and constipation. Gastroenterology 1966;51:656–663.

87. Gore S, Gilmore IT, Haigh CG, Brownless SM, Stockdale H, Morris AI. Colonic transit in man is slowed by ondansetron (GR38032F), a selective 5-hydroxytryptamine receptor (type 3) antagonist. Aliment Pharmacol Ther 1990;4:139–144.

88. Hendrix TR, Atkinson M, Clifton JA, Ingelfinger FJ. The effect of 5-hydroxytryptamine on intestinal motor function in man. Am J Med 1957;23:886–893.

89. Albibi R, McCallum RW. Metoclopramide: pharmacology and clinical application. Ann Intern Med 1983;98:86–95.

90. Garewal HS, Dalton WS. Metoclopramide in vincristine-induced ileus. Cancer Treat Rep 1985;69:1309–1311.

91. Kilbinger H, Weihrauch TR. Drugs increasing gastrointestinal motility. Pharmacology 1982;25:61–72.

92. Nemeth PR, Gullikson GW. Gastrointestinal motility stimulating drugs and 5-HT receptors on myenteric neurons. Eur J Pharmacol 1989;166:387–391.

93. Brogden RN, Carmine AA, Heel RC, Speight TM, Avery GS. Domperidone: A review of its pharmacological activity, pharmacokinetics and therapeutic efficacy in the symptomatic treatment of chronic dyspepsia and as an antiemetic. Drugs 1982;24:360–400.

94. Lee KY, Chey WY, You CH, Shah AN, Hamilton D. Effect of cisapride on the motility of gut in dogs and colonic transit time in dogs and humans [Abstract]. Gastroenterology 1984;86:1157.

95. Camilleri M, Malagelada JR, Abell TL, Brown ML, Hench V, Zinsmeister AR. Effect of six weeks of treatment with cisapride in gastroparesis and intestinal pseudoobstruction. Gastroenterology 1989;96:704–712.

96. Staiano A, Cucchiara S, Andreotti MR, Minella R, Manzi G. Effect of cisapride on chronic idiopathic constipation in children. Dig Dis Sci 1991;36:733–736.

97. Van Outryve M, Milo R, Toussaint J, Van Eeghem P. "Prokinetic" treatment of constipation-predominant irritable bowel syndrome: a placebo-controlled study of cisapride. J Clin Gastroenterol 1991;13:49–57.

98. Muller-Lissner SA. Treatment of chronic constipation with cisapride and placebo. Gut 1987;28:1033–1038.

99. Hellstrom PM, Aly A, Johansson C. Cisapride stimulates small intestinal motility and relieves constipation in myelopathy due to cervical spinal stenosis: case report. Paraplegia 1990;28:261–264.

100. Camilleri M, Brown ML, Malagelada JR. Impaired transit of chyme in chronic intestinal pseudoobstruction Correction by cisapride. Gastroenterology 1986;91:619–626.

101. Madsen JL. Effects of cisapride on gastrointestinal transit in healthy humans. Dig Dis Sci 1990;35:1500–1504.

102. Edwards CA, Holden S, Brown C, Read NW. Effect of cisapride on the gastrointestinal transit of a solid

meal in normal human subjects. Gut 1987;28:13–16.

103. Stacher G, Gaupmann G, Mittlebach G, Schneider C, Steinringer H, Langer B. Effects of oral cisapride on interdigestive motor activity, psychomotor function and side effect profile in healthy man. Dig Dis Sci 1987;32:1223–1230.

104. Sarna S, Condon RE, Cowles V. Morphine versus motilin in the initiation of migrating myoelectric complexes. Am J Physiol 1983;245:G217–G220.

105. Schmid R, Schusdziarra V, Allescher HD, Bofilias I, Buttermann G, Classen M. Effect of motilin on gastric emptying in patients with diabetic gastroparesis. Diabetes Care 1991;14:65–68.

106. Lehtola J, Jauhonen P, Kesaniemi A, Wikberg R, Gordin A. Effect of erythromycin on the oro-caecal transit time in man. Eur J Clin Pharmacol 1990;39:555–558.

107. Janssens J, Peeters TL, Vantrappen G, et al. Improvement of gastric emptying in diabetic gastroparesis by erythromycin: preliminary studies. N Engl J Med 1990;322:1028–1031.

108. Jaffe JH, Martin WR. Opioid analgesics and antagonists. In: Gilman AG, Rall TW, Nies AS, Taylor P, eds. Goodman and Gilman's The pharmacological basis of therapeutics. ed. 8. New York: Pergamon Press, 1990:485–521.

109. Rogers M, Cerda JJ. The narcotic bowel syndrome. J Clin Gastroenterol 1989;11:132–135.

110. Fetterman LE. Colonic fecal impaction in a young drug addict [Letter]. JAMA 1967;202:144.

111. Ingram DM, Catchpole BN. Effect of opiates on gastroduodenal motility following surgical operation. Dig Dis Sci 1981;26:989–992.

112. Camilleri M, Malagelada JR, Stanghellini V, Zinsmeister AR, Kao PC, Li CH. Dose-related effects of synthetic human beta-endorphin and naloxone on fed gastrointestinal motility. Am J Physiol 1986;251:G147–G154.

113. Adler HF, Atkinson AJ, Ivy AC. Effect of morphine and dilaudid on the ileum and of morphine, dilaudid, and atropine on the colon of man. Arch Intern Med 1942;69:974–985.

114. Kromer W. Endogenous and exogenous opioids in the control of gastrointestinal motility and secretion. Pharmacol Rev 1988;40:121–162.

115. Schang JC, Hemond M, Hebert M, Pilote M. How does morphine work on colonic motility? An electromyographic study in the human left and sigmoid colon. Life Sci 1986;38:671–676.

116. Tonini M, Onori L, Perucća E, Manzo L, De Ponti F, Crema A. Depression by morphine of the excitability of intrinsic inhibitory neurons in the guinea-pig colon. Eur J Pharmacol 1985;115:317–320.

117. Grider JR, Makhlouf GM. Role of opioid neurons in the regulation of intestinal peristalsis. Am J Physiol 1987;253:G226–G231.

118. Kaufman PN, Krevsky B, Malmud LS, et al. Role of opiate receptors in the regulation of colonic transit. Gastroenterology 1988;94:1351–1356.

119. Stephen AM, Wiggins HS, Cummings JH. Effect of changing transit time on colonic microbial metabolism in man. Gut 1987;28:601–609.

120. Sarna S, Northcott P, Belbeck L. Mechanism of cycling of migrating myoelectric complexes: effect of morphine. Am J Physiol 1982;242:G588–G595.

121. Poitras P, Boivin M, Lahaie RG, Trudel L. Regulation of plasma motilin by opioids in the dog. Am J Physiol 1989;257:G41–G45.

122. Kinsman RI, Read NW. Effect of naloxone on feedback regulation of small bowel transit by fat. Gastroenterology 1984;87:335–337.

123. Sun EA, Snape WJ Jr, Cohen S, Renny A. The role of opiate receptors and cholinergic neurons in the gastrocolonic response. Gastroenterology 1982; 82:689–693.

124. McKay JS, Linaker BD, Higgs NB, Turnberg LA. Studies of the antisecretory activity of morphine in rabbit ileum in vitro. Gastroenterology 1982; 82:243–247.

125. McKay JS, Linaker BD, Turnberg LA. Influence of opiates on ion transport across rabbit ileal mucosa. Gastroenterology 1981;80:279–284.

126. Schiller LR, Santa Ana CA, Morawski SG, Fordtran JS. Mechanism of the antidiarrheal effect of loperamide. Gastroenterology 1984;86:1475–1480.

127. Schiller LR, Davis GR, Santa Ana CA, Morawski SG, Fordtran JS. Studies of the mechanism of the antidiarrheal effect of codeine. J Clin Invest 1982;70:999–1008.

128. Pert CB, Snyder SH. Opiate receptor: demonstration in nervous tissue. Science 1973;179:1011–1014.

129. Leslie FM. Methods used for the study of opioid receptors. Pharmacol Rev 1987;39:197–249.

130. Pasternak GW, Wood PJ. Multiple mu opiate receptors. Life Sci 1986;38:1889–1898.

131. Porreca F, Mosberg HI, Hurst R, Hruby VJ, Burks TF. Roles of mu, delta and kappa opioid receptors in spinal and supraspinal mediation of gastrointestinal transit effects and hot-plate analgesia in the mouse. J Pharmacol Exp Ther 1984;230:341–348.

132. Binder HJ, Laurenson JP, Dobbins JW. Role of opiate receptors in regulation of enkephalin stimulation of active sodium and chloride absorption. Am J Physiol 1984;247:G432–G436.

133. Shook JE, Lemcke PK, Gehrig CA, Hruby VJ, Burks TF. Antidiarrheal properties of supraspinal mu and delta and peripheral mu, delta and kappa opioid receptors: Inhibition of diarrhea without constipation. J Pharmacol Exp Ther 1989;249:83–90.

134. Megens AA, Canters LL, Awouters FH, Niemegeers CJ. Is in vivo dissociation between the antipropulsive and antidiarrheal properties of opioids in rats related to gut selectivity. Arch Int Pharmacodyn Ther 1989;298:220–229.

135. Wang YN, Lindberg I. Distribution and characterization of the opioid octapeptide met5-enkephalin-

arg6-gly7-leu8 in the gastrointestinal tract of the rat. Cell Tissue Res 1986;244:77–85.

136. Nishimura E, Kwok YN, McIntosh HS. Characterization of opioid peptides in the rat stomach. Biochem Cell Biol 1986;64:733–742.

137. Zhang J, Albeck H, Culpepper-Morgan J, Friedman J, Kreek MJ. Distribution of preproenkephalin mRNA in the gastrointestinal tract of the guinea pig [Abstract]. Clin Res 1988;36:402A.

138. Sosa RP, McKnight AT, Hughes J, Kosterlitz HW. Incorporation of labelled amino acids into the enkephalins. FEBS Lett 1977;84:195–198.

139. Steele PA, Costa M. Opioid-like immunoreactive neurons in secretomotor pathways of the guinea-pig ileum. Neuroscience 1990;38:771–786.

140. Polak JM, Bloom SR, Sullivan SN, Facer P, Pearse AG. Enkephalin-like immunoreactivity in the human gastrointestinal tract. Lancet 1977;1:972–974.

141. Monferini E, Strada D, Manara L. Evidence for opiate receptor binding in rat small intestine. Life Sci 1981;29:595–602.

142. Culpepper-Morgan JA, Holt PR, Kreek MJ. Measurement of relative mu, kappa, and delta opioid receptor subtype densities in guinea pig colon [Abstract]. Clin Res 1987;35:407A–407A.

143. Nishimura E, Buchan AM, McIntosh CH. Autoradiographic localization of mu- and delta-type opioid receptors in the gastrointestinal tract of the rat and guinea pig. Gastroenterology 1986;91:1084–1094.

144. Dashwood MR, Debnam ES, Bagnall J, Thompson CS. Autoradiographic localisation of opiate receptors in rat small intestine. Eur J Pharmacol 1985;107:267–269.

145. Hargreaves M, Briggs CA. Effect of carbohydrate ingestion on exercise metabolism. J Appl Physiol 1988;65:1553–1555.

146. Bitar KN, Makhlouf GM. Selective presence of opiate receptors on intestinal circular muscle cells. Life Sci 1985;37:1545–1550.

147. Thoren T, Tanghoj H, Mattwil M, Jarnerot G. Epidural morphine delays gastric emptying and small intestinal transit in volunteers. Acta Anaesthesiol Scand 1989;33:174–180.

148. Gmerek DE, Cowan A, Woods JH. Independent central and peripheral mediation of morphine-induced inhibition of gastrointestinal transit in rats. J Pharmacol Exp Ther 1986;236:8–13.

149. Tache Y, Garrick T, Raybould H. Central nervous system action of peptides to influence gastrointestinal motor function. Gastroenterology 1990; 98:517–528.

150. Wattwil M. Postoperative pain relief and gastrointestinal motility. Acta Chir Scand Suppl 1988; 550:140–145.

151. Kreek MJ. Plasma and urine levels of methadone. Comparison following four medication forms used in chronic maintenance treatment. NY State J Med 1973;73:2773–2777.

152. Kreek MJ, Marsh F, Albeck H, et al. Effects of opioid antagonist naloxone on fecal evacuation in patients with idiopathic chronic constipation, irritable bowel syndrome, and narcotic induced constipation [Abstract]. Alcohol Drug Res 1986;6:168.

153. Culpepper-Morgan JA, Inturissi C, Portnoy R, Kreek MJ. Oral naloxone treatment of narcotic induced constipation: dose response. NIDA Res Monogr 1989;95:399–400.

154. Culpepper-Morgan JA, Inturrisi CE, Portenoy RK, et al. Treatment of opioid induced constipation with oral naloxone: A pilot study. Clin Pharmacol Ther 1992;52:90–95.

155. Basilisco G, Camboni G, Bozzani A, Paravicini M, Bianchi PA. Oral naloxone antagonizes loperamide-induced delay of orocecal transit. Dig Dis Sci 1987;32:829–832.

156. Basilisco G, Bozzani A, Camboni G, et al. Effect of loperamide and naloxone on mouth-to-caecum transit time evaluated by lactulose hydrogen breath test. Gut 1985;26:700–703.

157. Sykes NP. Oral naloxone in opioid-associated constipation [Letter]. Lancet 1991;337:1475.

158. Robinson BA, Johansson L, Shaw J. Oral naloxone in opioid-associated constipation [Letter]. Lancet 1991;338:581–582.

159. Manara L, Bianchi G, Ferretti P, Tavani A. Inhibition of gastrointestinal transit by morphine in rats results primarily from direct drug action on gut opioid sites. J Pharmacol Exp Ther 1986;237:945–949.

160. Thollander M, Hellstrom PM, Svensson TH. Suppression of small intestinal motility and morphine withdrawal diarrhoea by clonidine: peripheral site of action. Acta Physiol Scand 1989;137:385–392.

161. Tavani A, Gambino MC, Petrillo P. The opioid kappa-selective compound U-50, 488H does not inhibit intestinal propulsion in rats. J Pharm Pharmacol 1984;36:343–344.

162. Culpepper-Morgan J, Kreek MJ, Holt PR, LaRoche D, Zhang J, O'Bryan L. Orally administered kappa as well as mu opiate agonists delay gastrointestinal transit time in the guinea pig. Life Sci 1988;42:2073–2077.

163. Ramabadran K, Bansinath M, Turndorf H, Puig MM. Stereo-specific inhibition of gastrointestinal transit by kappa opioid agonists in mice. Eur J Pharmacol 1988;155:329–331.

164. Culpepper-Morgan J, LaRoche D, Nguyen J, Lewis V, Kreek MJ. Orally administered opioid antagonists reverse both mu and kappa opioid agonist delay of oro-cecal transit in the guinea pig [Abstract]. Clin Res 1989;37:366A.

165. Unterwald EM, Knapp C, Zukin RS. Neuroanatomical localization of kappa-1 and kappa-2 opioid receptors in rat and guinea pig brain. Brain Res 1991;562:57–65.

166. Bansinath M, Ramabadran K, Turndorf H, Puig MM. Kappa-opiate agonist-induced inhibition of gastrointestinal transit in different strains of mice. Pharmacology 1991;42:97–102.

167. Kreek MJ, Schaefer RA, Hahn EF, Fishman J. Naloxone, a specific opioid antagonist, reverses chronic idiopathic constipation. Lancet 1983;1:261–262.

168. Schang JC, Devroede G. Beneficial effects of naloxone in a patient with intestinal pseudoobstruction. Am J Gastroenterol 1985;80:407–411.

169. Kreek MJ, Raghunath J, Spagnoli D, Mueller D, Stubbs V, Paris P. Possible age-related changes in levels of beta-endorphin in humans. Alcohol Drug Res 1986;6:117.

170. Kaiko RF. Age and morphine analgesia in cancer patients with postoperative pain. Clin Pharmacol Ther 1980;28:823–826.

171. Culpepper-Morgan JA, Holt PR, Kreek MJ. Colonic opiate receptors change with age: Preliminary data [Abstract]. NIDA Res Monogr 1989;81:276.

172. Stanghellini V, Malagelada JR, Zinsmeister AR, Go VL, Kao PC. Stress-induced gastroduodenal motor disturbances in humans: possible humoral mechanisms. Gastroenterology 1983;85:83–91.

173. Joris JL, Dubner R, Hargreaves KM. Opioid analgesia at peripheral sites: A target for opioids released during stress and inflammation. Anesth Analg 1987;66:1277–1281.

174. Culpepper-Morgan JA, Twist DJ, Petrillo CR, Soda KM, Kreek MJ. Beta-endorphin and cortisol abnormalities in spinal cord injured individuals. Metabolism 1992;41:578–581.

175. Young EA, Akil H. Cortioctropin-releasing factor stimulation of adrenocorticotropin and beta-endorphin release: Effects of acute and chronic stress. Endocrinology 1985;117:23–30.

176. Shiomi H, Watson SJ, Kelsey JE, Akil H. Pretranslational and posttranslational mechanisms for regulating beta-endorphin-adrenocorticotropin of the anterior pituitary lobe. Endocrinology 1986;119:1793–1799.

177. Ho WK, Wen HL, Ling N. Beta-endorphin-like immunoactivity in the plasma of heroin addicts and normal subjects. Neuropharmacology 1980;19:117–120.

178. Martinez JA, Vargas ML, Fuente T, Garcia JDR, Milanes MV. Plasma beta-endorphin and cortisol levels in morphine-tolerant rats and in naloxone-induced withdrawal. Eur J Pharmacol 1990;182:117–123.

179. Hollt V, Przewlocki R, Haarmann I, et al. Stress-induced alterations in the levels of messenger RNA coding for proopiomelanocortin and prolactin in rat pituitary. Neuroendocrinology 1986;43:277–282.

180. Hollt V, Haarmann I, Herz A. Long-term treatment of rats with morphine reduces the activity of messenger ribonucleic acid coding for the beta-endorphin/ACTH precursor in the intermediate pituitary. J Neurochem 1981;37:619–626.

181. Glick ME, Meshkinpour H, Haldeman S, Hoehler F, Downey N, Bradley WE. Colonic dysfunction in patients with thoracic spinal cord injury. Gastroenterology 1984;86:287–294.

182. Bhansali LD, Moccia RM. Naloxone for the treatment of pseudo-obstruction of colon in a spinal cord injury [Abstract]. Arch Phys Med Rehabil 1989;70:A52.

183. Corazziari E, Materia E, Bausano G, et al. Laxative consumption in chronic nonorganic constipation. J Clin Gastroenterol 1987;9:427–430.

184. Herman AG, Vane JR: Endotoxin and production of prostaglandins by the isolated rabbit jejunum. Influence of indomethacin. Arch Int Pharmacodyn Ther 1975;213:328–329.

185. de Witte P, Lemli L: The metabolism of anthranoid laxatives. Hepatogastroenterology 1990;37:601–605.

186. Staumont G, Fioramonti J, Frexinos J, Bueno L. Changes in colonic motility induced by sennosides in dogs: evidence of a prostaglandin mediation. Gut 1988;29:1180–1187.

187. Fioramonti J, Staumont G, Garcia-Villar R, Bueno L. Effect of sennosides on colon motility in dogs. Pharmacology 1988;36:23–30.

188. Spiessens C, Ceuterick L, Ponette E, Janssens J, Lemli J. Combined manometric and radiological study of the changes in colonic motility induced by sennosides in rats. Pharmacology 1988;36:66–72.

189. Frexinos J, Staumont G, Fioramonti J, Bueno L. Effects of sennosides on colonic myoelectrical activity in man. Dig Dis Sci 1989;34:214–219.

190. Binder HJ, Donowitz M. A new look at laxative action. Gastroenterology 1975;69:1001–1005.

191. Leng-Peschlow E. Dual effect of orally administered sennosides on large intestine transit and fluid absorption in the rat. J Pharm Pharmacol 1986;38:606–610.

192. Yagi T, Miyawaki Y, Nishikawa A, Horiyama S, Yamauchi K, Kuwano S. Prostaglandin E2-mediated stimulation of mucus synthesis and secretion by rhein anthrone, the active metabolite of sennosides A and B, in the mouse colon. J Pharm Pharmacol 1990;42:542–545.

193. Yagi T, Miyawaki Y, Nishikawa A, Yamauchi K, Kuwano S. Suppression of the purgative action of rhein anthrone, the active metabolite of sennosides A and B, by indomethacin in rats. J Pharm Pharmacol 1991;43:307–310.

194. Autore G, Caliendo G, Pepe A, Capasso F. Perfusion of rat colon with sennosides, rhein and rhein-anthrone concentration-related histamine release. Eur J Pharmacol 1990;191:97–99.

195. Flintan P, Weeden GD. Standardised senna. Lancet 1953;1:497.

196. Izard MW, Ellison FS. Treatment of drug-induced constipation with a purified senna derivative. Conn Med 1962;26:589–592.

197. Marlett JA, Li BU, Patrow CJ, Bass P. Comparative laxation of psyllium with and without senna in an ambulatory constipated population. Am J Gastroenterol 1987;82:333–337.

198. Odes HS, Madar Z. A double-blind trial of a celandin, aloe vera and psyllium laxative preparation in adult patients with constipation. Digestion 1991;49:65–71.

199. Smith B. Disorders of the myenteric plexus. Gut 1970;11:271–274.

200. Oster JR, Materson BJ, Rogers AI. Laxative abuse syndrome. Am J Gastroenterol 1980;74:451–458.

201. Case MT, Smith JK, Nelson RA. Acute mouse and chronic dog toxicity studies of danthron, dioctyl sodium sulfosuccinate, poloxalkol and combinations. Drug Chem Toxicol 1977;1:89–101.

202. Kiernan JA, Heinicke EA. Sennosides do not kill myenteric neurons in the colon of the rat or mouse. Neuroscience 1989;30:837–842.

203. Rudolph RL, Mengs U. Electron microscopical studies on rat intestine after long-term treatment with sennosides. Pharmacology 1988;36:188–193.

204. Sund RB, Songedal K, Harestad T, Salvesen B, Kristiansen S. Enterohepatic circulation, urinary excretion and laxative action of some bisacodyl derivatives after intragastric administration in the rat. Acta Pharmacol Toxicol (Copenh) 1981;48:73–80.

205. Ewe K. Effect of bisacodyl on intestinal electrolyte and water net transport and transit: Perfusion studies in men. Digestion 1987;37:247–253.

206. Farack UM, Gruber E, Loeschke K. The influence of bisacodyl and deacetylbisacodyl on mucus secretion, mucus synthesis and electrolyte movements in the rat colon in vivo. Eur J Pharmacol 1985;117:215–222.

207. Saunders DR, Sillery J, Rachmilewitz D, Rubin CE, Tytgat GN. Effect of bisacodyl on the structure and function of rodent and human intestine. Gastroenterology 1977;72:849–856.

208. Leng-Peschlow E. Effects of sennosides A + B and bisacodyl on rat large intestine. Pharmacology 1989;38:310–318.

209. Smith GS, Warhurst G, Tonge A, Turnberg LA. Prostaglandins are not mediators of the intestinal response to cholera toxin. Gut 1985;26:680–682.

210. Beubler E, Juan H. Is the effect of diphenolic laxatives mediated via release of prostaglandin E. Experientia 1978;34:386–387.

211. Rachmilewitz D, Karmeli F. Laxatives and the cAMP system [Letter]. Dig Dis Sci 1981;26:94–95.

212. Beubler E. Influence of chronic bisacodyl treatment on the effect of acute bisacodyl on water and electrolyte transport in the rat colon. J Pharm Pharmacol 1985;37:131–133.

213. Hardcastle JD, Mann CV. Physical factors in the stimulation of colonic peristalsis. Gut 1970;11:41–46.

214. Schang JC, Hemond M, Hebert M, Pilote M. Changes in colonic myoelectric spiking activity during stimulation by bisacodyl. Can J Physiol Pharmacol 1986;64:39–43.

215. Schang JC. Effects of bisacodyl on the myoelectric spiking activity of the human sigmoid colon [Abstract]. Gastroenterology 1985;88:1573.

216. Dreiling DA, Fischl RA, Fernandez O. The therapeutic usefulness of Dulcolax (bisacodyl), a new nonpurgative laxative. Am J Dig Dis 1959;4:311–320.

217. Jones RF, Hall GJ. Management of the neurogenic bowel using durolax solution. Med J Aust 1979;1:309.

218. Saunders DR, Haggitt RC, Kimmey MB, Silverstein FE. Morphological consequences of bisacodyl on normal human rectal mucosa: effect of a prostaglandin E1 analog on mucosal injury. Gastrointest Endosc 1990;36:101–104.

219. Meisel JL, Bergman D, Graney D, Saunders DR, Rubin CE. Human rectal mucosa: proctoscopic and morphological changes caused by laxatives. Gastroenterology 1977;72:1274–1279.

220. Girard CM, Rugh KS, DiPalma JA, Brady CE III, Pierson WP. Comparison of Golytely lavage with standard diet/cathartic preparation for double-contrast barium enema. Am J Roentgenol 1984;142:1147–1149.

221. McGuigan HA, Steigmann F, Dyniewicz JM. Evaluation of the laxative effect of some commonly used laxative substances: With particular reference to dosage. Am J Dig Dis 1944;11:284–289.

222. Laxatives and cathartics. In: AMA drug evaluations annual 1992. Chicago: American Medical Association, 1991:863–877.

223. Walker NI, Bennett RE, Axelsen RA. *Melanosis coli*: A consequence of anthraquinone-induced apoptosis of colonic epithelial cells. Am J Pathol 1988;131:465–476.

224. Moriarty KJ, Kelly MJ, Beetham R, Clark ML. Studies on the mechanism of action of dioctyl sodium sulphosuccinate in the human jejunum. Gut 1985;26:1008–1013.

225. Simon B, Kather H. Interaction of laxatives with enzymes of cyclic AMP metabolism from human colonic mucosa. Eur J Clin Invest 1980;10:231–234.

226. Sund RB, Matheson I. Glucose and cation transport in rat jejunum, ileum and colon in vivo: effects of anionic and nonionic surfactants, and of desoxycholate. Acta Pharmacol Toxicol (Copenh) 1978;42:253–258.

227. Bretagne JF, Vidon N, L'Hirondel C, Bernier JJ. Increased cell loss in the human jejunum induced by laxatives (ricinoleic acid, dioctyl sodium sulphosuccinate, magnesium sulphate, bile salts). Gut 1981;22:264–269.

228. Fain AM, Susat R, Herring M, Dorton K. Treatment of constipation in geriatric and chronically ill

patients: a comparison. South Med J 1978;71:677–680.

229. Castle SC, Cantrell M, Israel DS, Samuelson MJ. Constipation prevention: empiric use of stool softeners questioned. Geriatrics 1991;46:84–86.

230. Chapman RW, Sillery J, Fontana DD, Matthys C, Saunders DR. Effect of oral dioctyl sodium sulfosuccinate on intake-output studies of human small and large intestine. Gastroenterology 1985;89:489–493.

231. Stewart JJ, Bass P. Effects of ricinoleic and oleic acids on the digestive contractile activity of the canine small and large bowel. Gastroenterology 1976;70:371–376.

232. Gaginella TS, Stewart JJ, Gullikson GW, Olsen WA, Bass P. Inhibition of small intestinal mucosal and smooth muscle cell function by ricinoleic acid and other surfactants. Life Sci 1975;16:1595–1605.

233. Fox DA, Epstein ML, Bass P. Surfactants selectively ablate enteric neurons of the rat jejunum. J Pharmacol Exp Ther 1983;227:538–544.

234. Loening-Baucke VA, Younoszai MK. Effect of treatment on rectal and sigmoid motility in chronically constipated children. Pediatrics 1984;73:199–205.

235. Fox JA. Control of gastrointestinal motility by peptides: old peptides, new tricks—new peptides, old tricks. Gastroenterol Clin North Am 1989;18:163–177.

236. Koch TR, Carney JA, Go L, Go VL. Idiopathic chronic constipation is associated with decreased colonic vasoactive intestinal peptide. Gastroenterology 1988;94:300–310.

237. Otterson MF, Sarna SK, Moulder JE. Effects of fractionated doses of ionizing radiation on small intestinal motor activity. Gastroenterology 1988;95:1249–1257.

238. Karaus M, Sarna SK, Ammon HV, Wienbeck M. Effects of oral laxatives on colonic motor complexes in dogs. Gut 1987;28:1112–1119.

239. Tedesco FJ, DiPiro JT. Laxative use in constipation. American College of Gastroenterology's Committee on FDA-Related Matters. Am J Gastroenterol 1985;80:303–309.

11

Hiccups: Reasons and Remedies

JAMES H. LEWIS

The term "hiccup" refers to the sudden contraction of the inspiratory muscles terminated by abrupt closure of the glottis to produce the characteristic sound. Indeed, the origin of the word "hiccup" appears to represent the onomatopoietic attempt to vocalize the sound that is made while hiccuping. Similarities in the spelling and pronunciation of hiccup in other languages (e.g., "hicka" in Swedish, "hikke" in Norwegian and Danish, "hipo" in Spanish, and "hoquet" in French) suggest that this is probably the case (1). The term "hiccough" has been used as an alternative spelling of hiccup, but more likely represents the previously held (but mistaken) notion that hiccups occur as a result of a respiratory reflex (2). The origin of the word "singultus," the medical term for hiccups, is lost in antiquity, but may have been derived from the Latin root "singult," meaning a sob or speech broken by sobs, or the act of catching the breath in sobbing. Alternatively, it may have been related to the Latin term meaning "the convulsive catching of breath" or "a rattling in the throat" of a dying person (1).

Nearly everyone has had a bout of hiccups at one time or another, and they have been the subject of medical curiosity throughout the centuries. Most hiccups occur as brief, self-limited episodes lasting only a few seconds or minutes. Hiccups that last more than 48 hours or recur at frequent intervals are referred to as "persistent" and often imply a serious underlying physical or metabolic disorder. Occasionally, hiccups are intractable, occurring continuously for months or years, and may result in significant morbidity and even death (1).

While favorite hiccup cures abound, the phenomenon remains incompletely understood. As a result, the treatment of hiccups can be quite difficult and is often very frustrating. Hiccup cures date from the time of Hippocrates, prompting the following remark by Charles Mayo in a discussion 60 years ago: "The amount of knowledge on any subject such as this can be considered as being in inverse proportion to the number of different treatments suggested and tried for it. Perhaps one is justified in saying that there is no disease which has had more forms of treatment and fewer results from treatment than has persistent hiccup" (3).

This chapter will review what is known of the pathophysiology of hiccups and summarize the various treatment modalities that have been tried in order to present a rational approach to the management of this curious disorder. Since most individuals attempt a physical or mechanical maneuver to stop a bout of hiccups prior to initiating any form of drug therapy, these nonpharmacologic treatments will be discussed first, followed by a review of drug therapy for hiccups.

PATHOPHYSIOLOGY

The precise pathophysiologic mechanisms responsible for hiccuping continue to elude anatomists, physiologists, and neurologists. In his *Aphorisms*, Hippocrates (4) mentioned several conditions associated with hiccups: "In inflammation of the liver, hiccough is bad";

**Table 11.1
Conditions Associated with
Self-Limited Hiccups[a]**

Gastric distension
  Overeating, eating too fast
  Drinking carbonated beverages
  Aerophagia
  Air insufflation during gastroscopy

Sudden change in temperature
  Ingesting very hot or cold food or beverages
  Taking a cold shower
  Entering or leaving a hot or cold room

Alcohol ingestion

Excess smoking

Psychogenic
  Sudden excitement
  Emotional stress

[a]References provided in Lewis (1).

and "hiccough supervening on excessive purging [or on copious flux of blood] is a bad sign." The Greek physician, Galen, believed that hiccups were caused by "arousing the stomach to violent emotions," an etiology also eluded to by Paulus Aegineta, who discussed "fullness of stomach," the presence of "acrid or pungent humors in the stomach," and "rigors" among the causes of hiccups in his writings in the Middle Ages (3). Inflammation of the stomach (due to spoiled food) was also the agreed upon cause of hiccups by the early Arabian and Methodist schools of medicine. Fernelius, another medieval medical authority, wrote that "singultus is a convulsive motion of the stomach in an attempt to dislodge what is impacted in the body of it. Very frequently it repeats, like a cough, and deadens what is irritating" (5).

Unlike reflexes such as coughing, sneezing, vomiting, gagging, and withdrawal from heat or pain, hiccups does not appear to serve any known useful or protective function (6). However, it has been observed that other mammals can hiccup (7) and it is well known that hiccups occur during fetal and neonatal life (8–10). Hiccups thus may represent a vestigial remnant of a primitive reflex whose functional

or behavioral significance is now lost (6), although Fuller suggests that they be reclassified as an essential intrauterine reflex that allows exercise of the inspiratory muscles without inhalation of liquid (11). Despite the commonplace occurrence of fetal hiccups, their exact purpose remains a mystery.

Early clinical observation suggested that hiccups were the result of diaphragmatic contractions. Not until 1833, however, when an Edinburgh physician, T. Shortt, recommended blistering the skin over the origin and course of the phrenic nerves as a means of treating the condition, was a relationship between hiccups and the phrenic nerve recognized (12). While the knowledge that hiccuping was due to central as well as peripheral causes was shared by several individuals in the first half of this century, it was not until 1943 that Bailey reported that the hiccup "reflux" had its own center in the upper cervical segments of the spinal cord (13). Bailey is also credited with being one of the first to suggest that afferent impulses were conveyed over vagal sympathetic as well as sensory fibers of the phrenic nerve.

Bailey's observations were confirmed and extended by subsequent investigators who expanded the concept that a hiccup results from stimulation of one or more limbs of its reflex arc. In current theory, as described by Salem et al. (14), the afferent limb of the reflex is comprised of the vagus and phrenic nerves and by the sympathetic chain arising from the sixth to the twelfth thoracic segments, with the "hiccup center" being located in the spinal cord between the third and fifth cervical segments. The efferent limb remains primarily the phrenic nerve, although efferents to the glottis and accessory muscles of respiration are also thought to be involved in hiccuping. The contribution of these accessory muscle groups has been emphasized by reports of patients who continue to hiccup even after transection of both phrenic nerves (15).

Early researchers believed that the inspiratory muscle contractions involved in hiccuping were the result of an involuntary respiratory reflex (16). However, electrophysiologic studies of three subjects with persistent hiccups demonstrated that hiccups are not the end result of a respiratory reflex, nor is the diaphragm the only muscle involved (6). Hiccups have been shown to have only a negligible effect on ventilation, despite the glottis closing approximately 35 msec after the onset of the diaphragmatic discharge. In addition, expiration is inhibited during the entire time of the inspiratory muscle discharge, making it exceedingly unlikely that hiccups can be mediated by any known reflex activity of the respiratory center (6). Newsom Davis concluded that the hiccup "discharge" consists of single or repeated bursts of activity generated by a supraspinal mechanism independent of the pathways controlling rhythmic breathing. This theory has been supported by the observations of Nathan et al. (17) that bilateral hemidiaphragm involvement is associated with the simultaneous discharge of the intercostal muscles of the anterior scalene muscles.

HICCUP FREQUENCY

Hiccups usually occur with a frequency of 4–60/minute, and the instantaneous frequency of hiccups remains relatively constant for the same individual (18). If more than a few hiccups occur together, they often become "established," producing a hiccup bout that does not stop until a certain minimum number of hiccups has occurred. The number of hiccups in any given bout is characteristically either <7 or >63, according to observations of >75 patients (19). The frequency and amplitude of hiccups appear to be controlled independently, as no significant correlation between the two was evident when hiccups were studied during quiet breathing, breath holding, coughing, and other ventilator maneuvers (6). While not linked to the respiratory center, the frequency of hiccups increases with a fall in arterial $_pCO_2$ and decreases with a rise in arterial $_pCO_2$ (20).

A number of fluoroscopic studies have demonstrated that hiccups are often unilateral and confined to the left hemidiaphragm (13, 14, 18). However, bilateral involvement probably occurs with an equal frequency, although the contractions on one side may be dominant (1, 17, 21).

Persistent hiccups occur much more frequently in men than in women. For example, among 220 patients seen at the Mayo Clinic between 1935 and 1963, 181 (82%) were men and only 39 (18%) were women (22). Others also have observed hiccups to be predominantly a male malady (23). Mayo thought this male predominance was attributable to hiccups being caused by a bacterial infection arising in the prostate gland (3). The true reason for this apparent male predisposition remains unknown.

CONDITIONS ASSOCIATED WITH HICCUPS

Inflammation of the liver, inanition, excessive bloodletting, or purging and distension or irritation of the stomach were among the first recorded causes of hiccups (1). Since then, scores of additional disorders have been added to the list (Tables 11.1 and 11.2).

Benign, Self-Limited Causes

Overdistension of the stomach (due to overeating, aerophagia, or drinking carbonated beverages) is one of the most frequent causes of self-limited hiccups (Table 11.1). Insufflation of air into the stomach during endoscopy may also induce transient hiccups. The mechanism by which gastric distension causes hiccups appears to be stimulation (stretching?) of the gastric branches of the vagus nerve or possible direct irritation of the diaphragm by the overinflated stomach. Other causes of transient benign hiccups include a sudden change in body or environmental temperature (such as eating or drinking very hot or cold foods or beverages, taking a cold shower, and entering or leaving a warm or cold room). The pathophysiologic explanation for hiccups induced by temperature change is unknown, although Roth has suggested "hypersensitivity" of the hiccup reflex arc (24).

Overindulgence in alcohol has long been recognized as a cause of hiccups. The mechanism of alcohol-induced hiccups is unclear, but may relate to the ingestion of large quan-

Table 11.2
Causes of Persistent and Intractable Hiccups[a]

Central nervous system
 Structural lesions
  Intracranial neoplasms
  Hydrocephalus
  Multiple sclerosis
  Brainstem tumors
  Syringomyelia
  Ventriculi-peritoneal shunt
  Glaucoma
  Parkinson disease
 Vascular lesions
  Vascular insufficiency
  Arteriovenous malformation
  Intracranial hemorrhage
  Temporal arteritis
 Trauma
  Skull fracture
  Epilepsy
 Infectious causes
  Meningitis
  Encephalitis
  Neurosyphilis
  Brain abscess

Toxic-metabolic causes
 Uremia
 Diabetes mellitus
 Alcohol
 Gout
 Hyponatremia
 Hypokalemia
 Hypocalcemia
 Hypocarbia (hyperventilation)
 Fever
 Insulin shock therapy

Diaphragmatic irritation
 Diaphragmatic tumors
 Eventration
 Myocardial infarction
 Pericarditis
 Hiatus hemia
 Splenomegaly (various causes)
 Hepatomegaly (various causes)
 Subphrenic abscess
 Perihepatitis
 Esophageal cancer
 Aberrant cardiac pacemaker electrode

Irritation of the vagus nerve
 Meningeal branches
  Meningitis
 Pharyngeal branches
  Pharyngitis
  Laryngitis
 Auricular branches
  Hair, insect, or foreign body irritating tympanic
   membrane
 Recurrent laryngeal nerve
  Goiter
  Neck cysts, tumors
  Scrofula

 Thoracic branches
  Pneumonia
  Empyema
  Bronchitis
  Asthma
  Pleuritis
  Achalasia
  Sarcoidosis
  Esophageal obstruction
  Esophagitis
  Thoracic aortic aneurysm
  Tuberculosis
  Myocardial infarction
  Pericarditis
  Mediastinitis
  Cor pulmonale
  Herpes zoster
  Lung cancer
  Mediastinal himatoma
 Abdominal branches
  Gastric atony (distention)
  Gastric cancer
  Gastritis
  Peptic ulcer
  Gastric ulcer
  Pancreatic cancer
  Pancreatitis
  Pseudocyst
  Intraabdominal abscess
  Bowel obstruction
  Cholelithiasis
  Cholecystitis
  Abdominal aortic aneurysm
  Ulcerative colitis
  Crohn's disease
  Gastrointestinal hemorrhage
  Hydronephrosis
  Prostatic disorders
  Parasitic infestation
  Appendicitis
  Hepatitis

Drugs
 α-Methyldopa
 Short-acting barbiturates
 Dexamethasone
 Methylprednisolone
 Diazepam
 Chlordiazepoxide

General anesthesia
 Inadequate ventilation
 Suppression of normal inhibitory influences
 Intubation (stimulation of glottis)
 Recovery period
 Traction or viscera
 Hyperextension of the neck (stretching of phrenic
  nerve roots)
 Gastric distension or ileus

Table 11.2—*continued*
Causes of Persistent and Intractable Hiccups[a]

Postoperative causes	*Psychogenic causes*
Manipulation of diaphragm or adjacent organs	Hysterical neurosis (worry, anxiety, fear)
Prostatic and urinary tract surgery	Conversion reaction
Craniotomy (various operations)	Sudden shock
Thoracotomy (various operations)	Grief reaction
Laparotomy (cholecystectomy, gastrectomy,	Malingering
colectomy, sympathectomy)	Personality disorders
	Anorexia nervosa
Infectious causes	Enuresis
Meningitis	
Encephalitis (epidemic and nonepidemic)	*Familial*
Typhoid fever	
Cholera	*Idiopathic*
Candida esophagitis	
Malaria	
Herpes zoster	
Acute rheumatic fever	
Influenza	
Tuberculosis	

[a]References provided in Lewis (1) and in the text.

tities of alcoholic beverages causing gastric distension, or possibly to the effects of alcohol on the cerebral cortex that remove inhibitions normally serving to inhibit the hiccup reflex (2). Sudden excitement or emotional stress may also lead to transient hiccuping, possibly by an effect on the hiccuping center. Excessive smoking is also listed as a cause of hiccups, but without any satisfactory pathogenic explanation (16).

Causes of Persistent Hiccups

Over 100 causes of persistent or intractable hiccups have been described (1). Several additional causes of hiccups have been reported since I reviewed this subject in 1985. These include achalasia (25), trimethoprim-sulfamethoxazole-induced esophageal ulcer (26), methylprednisolone therapy (27), Parkinson disease (28), sarcoidosis (29), Addison disease (30), hyponatremia due to psychogenic polydipsia (31), glaucoma (32), hyperventilation and respiratory alkalosis in a tracheostomy patient (33), as a complication of internal jugular vein cannulation resulting in a hematoma compressing the right phrenic nerve (34), and familial hiccups (35). These new hiccup causes have been incorporated into the list given in

Table 11.2. Hiccups in this category are often the result of underlying structural, metabolic, inflammatory, or infectious disorders that stimulate one or more limbs of the hiccup reflex arc. In men, organic causes were found to be responsible for 93% of hiccups (vs. 7% attributed to psychogenic causes) in large series from the Mayo Clinic. The opposite was observed in women, in whom organic causes accounted for only 8% of cases, while psychogenic factors were thought to be causative in 92%. In many patients the cause of hiccups cannot be ascertained, although this obviously depends on the extent of the work-up, including psychologic evaluation.

According to the latest *Guinness Book of World Records* (36), the dubious honor for hiccuping the longest continues to belong to Charles Osborne of Anthon, Iowa, who has been listed for most of the past decade as having hiccuped since the 1920s without any known cause. It is estimated that he has hiccuped nearly 380 million times, based on more than 17,000 times per day, or 12 hiccups per minute. His ailment has not prevented him from leading a normal life or fathering eight children in the process, although he is quoted as complaining that his false teeth keep falling out!

Intractable hiccups are not always so benign. They have resulted in the inability to eat and debilitating weight loss, exhaustion, insomnia, cardiac arrhythmias, electrocardiogram (ECG) artifacts, wound dehiscence, and occasionally have been implicated in the deaths of some patients (1). In preterm infants, hiccups may interfere with normal ventilation, as airway closure may persist after the hiccups stop, and in infants with endotracheal tubes in place, hiccups may increase minute ventilation, leading to respiratory alkalosis, as the presence of the tube prevents glottic closure (8). Interestingly, in many patients persistent hiccups sometimes stop completely during sleep, only to recur again when the patient awakens (17).

Hiccups Due to Anesthesia and Surgery

One of the most commonly encountered clinical scenarios during which hiccups occur is general anesthesia. Several possible predisposing factors include hyperextension of the neck resulting in stretching of the roots of the phrenic nerve, traction on the diaphragm or viscera during surgery, the use of short-acting barbiturates, inadequate ventilation, and gastric distension or ileus in the recovery period. In addition, too light a plane of anesthesia may suppress inhibitory influences that normally function to prevent hiccups. Similarly, as the neuromuscular blocking action of certain muscle relaxants starts to wear off, return of diaphragmatic activity may be associated with hiccups (14, 37).

Postoperative hiccups accounted for 25% of the hiccups in men with an established organic basis for their hiccups in a Mayo Clinic series (22). More than half of these hiccup episodes followed intra-abdominal operations, with the remainder due to urinary tract, central nervous system, and chest operations. Postoperative hiccups usually appeared within 4 days of surgery and often interfered with sleeping and eating.

Hiccup Epidemics

Among the more curious causes of hiccups is that related to epidemic encephalitis or influenza. Hiccup epidemics were recorded during the 1919, 1922, and 1924 influenza-encephalitis outbreaks in Winnipeg, Canada, and during similar outbreaks in other parts of the world (7, 38). Bouts of hiccups during these epidemics lasted between 45 minutes and 1 hour, and occurred every 2–3 hours, with recovery after a few days. Rosenow isolated a neurogenic strain of *streptococcus* (*Streptococcus singultus*) from throat and urine cultures of affected patients that was alleged to have produced diaphragmatic contractions when inoculated into experimental animals (7).

Gastrointestinal Causes of Hiccups

Of particular interest to gastroenterologists, hiccups are reported as being due to a variety of gastrointestinal (GI) and hepatic conditions. These include gastroesophageal reflux (39–43), infectious (e.g., *Candida*) esophagitis; esophageal obstruction from rings, webs, or carcinoma (44); achalasia (25); extrinsic compression of the esophagus from mediastinal structures (1); and a variety of inflammatory, ulcerative, and obstructive gastric, hepatobiliary, pancreatic, and intestinal lesions (see Table 11.2). Patients with diffuse abdominal carcinomatosis or widespread surgical adhesions may develop intractable hiccups for which little or no therapy is effective. For many of the other more specific disease entities, treatment may in fact lead to a complete cessation and remission of the hiccups (see section below on Specific Hiccup Cures).

HICCUP TREATMENTS

Historical Cures

There have been almost as many treatments suggested for curing hiccups as there have been causes identified. One patient who hiccuped for more than 8 years reportedly received over 60,000 letters containing possible cures. Ironically, only his prayers to St. Jude, the patron saint for lost causes, were ultimately said to be successful (45).

The origins of many of the better known hiccup cures can be traced back hundreds and even thousands of years. Hippocrates (46) wrote in the fourth century *B.C.* that "In the case of a person afflicted with hiccough, sneezing coming on removes the hiccough." Celsus (47) also wrote that "sneezing puts an end to hiccough," as did Galen (3). Plato is credited with being the first to recommend a sudden thump on the back as means of "scaring away" hiccups (48). Unexpected fright was also listed as a cure by believers in natural magic 2,000 years later (3), and excitement, anxiety, and pain are still recognized as a means to end a bout of hiccups. Eryxmachus the Physician is quoted in Plato's "Symposium" as telling Aristophanes to hold his breath, gargle with water, and, if need be, tickle his nose to induce a sneeze, after which "even the most violent hiccough is sure to go" (49).

Pliny the Elder suggested 15 to 16 hiccup cures (3), but it was not until the fifth century *A.D.* that a treatment for hiccups was based on a specific cause when Aetius recommended that cupping instruments be applied to the chest, abdomen, and back for hiccups thought to be due to inflammation of the stomach and adjacent organs (3). Paulus Aegineta advocated emetics (assisted by sneezing) to empty the stomach if it was distended or contained "spoiled food." Noting that sneezing alone would not cure hiccups when the stomach was empty, the same author also recommended giving "rue with wine or nitre in honeyed water or hartwort or carrot, or cumin, or ginger, or calamint or celtic nard" (3). Similar herbal remedies were prescribed by a number of other medical authorities in the Middle Ages (5). Plugging the ears with the fingers (in combination with breath holding) was advocated by Lupton in 1627 (3). For many generations grandmothers have apparently known about the usefulness of swallowing granulated sugar and holding one's breath (50, 51).

Physical and Mechanical Means of Treating Hiccups

The "modern era" of hiccup treatment may be considered to have begun 150 years ago when Shortt described blistering of the skin over the course of the phrenic nerves in the neck (12). Since then, a number of therapies designed to disrupt the transmission of impulses along the phrenic nerves have been described (1), including galvanic (electric) stimulation, Novocaine injections, digital compression, crushing, avulsing, traction, and transection. Others have sprayed vapocoolants or applied ice to the skin overlying the phrenic nerves at the root of the neck. Rhythmic tapping over the fifth cervical vertebra at the level of the origin of the phrenic nerves has also been successful (Table 11.3).

Measures aimed at counterstimulating the diaphragmatic contractions that occur during hiccuping have included pulling the knees up to the chest or leaning forward to compress the diaphragm, applying ice or a mustard plaster to the epigastrium, or applying external pressure to the points of diaphragmatic insertion (1). Continuous positive airway pressure or other means to hyperinflate the lungs is thought to act by stimulating the Hering-Breuer inflation reflex, which inhibits not only the normal respiratory pattern but the abnormal hiccup pattern as well (52). Other acts that may disrupt the respiratory rhythm and reduce hiccup frequency to below a critical threshold level include sneezing, performing a Valsalva maneuver, breath holding, hyperventilation, and involuntary gasping induced by the inhalation of smelling salts or the result of being surprised by sudden fright or pain (1). Inhaling 5% carbon dioxide or breathing into a paper bag have also been used as a means of ending hiccups (53). Kappis suggested compressing the upper part of the thyroid cartilage physically to prevent the patient from hiccuping, with the caveat that the airway not be choked off (54). Since no relationship is believed to exist between hiccups and the respiratory center, why do these methods work? Such respiratory maneuvers may terminate hiccups through a direct inhibitory effect of acute respiratory acidosis on diaphragmatic contractility (55).

Relief of gastric distension by emetics, gastric lavage, or nasogastric aspiration has been effective when the stomach is overdistended by food, liquid, or air or is obstructed by me-

Table 11.3
Common Mechanical Methods Available for Treating Hiccups[a]

Stimulation of uvula or nasopharynx
  Forcible traction of the tongue
  Lifting the uvula with a spoon
  Catheter stimulation
  Gargling with water
  Sipping ice water
  Sucking on hard candy
  Swallowing dry granulated sugar
  Swallowing hard bread or crushed ice
  Drinking from the far side of a glass
  Swallowing agent with noxious taste
    (vinegar, angostura bitters)
  Instilling of noxious irritants (ammonia, ether)
	Relief of gastric distension
	  Emetic-induced vomiting
	  Nasogastric aspiration
	  Gastric lavage

Interruption of respiratory rhythm
  Valsalva maneuver
  Gasping (noxious odors or sudden fright)
  Sneezing
  Continuous positive airway pressure
  Breath holding
  Compression of the thyroid cartilage
	Disruption of the phrenic nerve
	  Novocaine injection (nerve block)
	  Percussion over C^5 vertebra
	  Vapocoolant sprays or ice
	  Electric stimulation
	  Phrenic crush
	  Transection

Respiratory center stimulants
  Breathing 5% of carbon dioxide
  Hyperventilation
  Breath holding
  Rebreathing into a paper bag or dead space tubing
	Counterirritation of the diaphragm
	  Supraorbital pressure
	  Carotid sinus massage
	  Removal of hair or foreign body irritating tympanic
	    membrane
	  Digital rectal massage

Counterirritation of the vagus nerve
  Pulling the knees up to the chest
  Leaning forward to compress the chest
  Mustard plaster to epigastrium
  Applying pressure at points of diaphragmatic
    insertion
	Psychiatric
	  Behavior modification
	  Hypnosis
	
	Miscellaneous
	  Cardioversion
	  Acuncture
	  Prayer

[a]References provided in (1).

chanical or functional disorders (1). Relief of esophageal obstruction secondary to a Schatzki lower esophageal ring or carcinoma has also ended persistent hiccups (44). In a patient of my own with *Candida* esophagitis, persistent hiccups were finally ended after successful antifungal therapy.

Travell has long believed that the "trigger point" for hiccups is located in the uvula (21), which may explain why measures that stimulate the soft palate and pharynx are often able to terminate a bout of hiccups. Forcible traction of the tongue (credited to William Osler [16]), lifting the uvula with a spoon (21), and stimulating the pharynx with a catheter or cotton-tipped swab (14, 56) have been used successfully. Intraoperative hiccups stopped

promptly in 64 of 65 patients when the pharynx was manipulated with a rubber or plastic catheter using a to-and-fro motion, inserted through a nostril to a depth of 3–4 1/2 inches (14). Although 10 of these patients had recurrence of hiccups during surgery, all responded to repeat catheter manipulation. These authors reported similar success for 20 conscious patients with hiccups of 3 hours' to 4 days' duration of various causes. The hiccups stopped immediately in all of these patients after the pharynx was stimulated; 8 had recurrent hiccups, which again stopped in 6 patients on retreatment. Goldsmith used a similar technique to stop hiccups in a "dozen or so persons" by massaging a cotton-tipped swab for 60 seconds at the junction of the hard and soft palates (56). The success of this method suggests that irritation of the soft palate of the pharynx inhibits afferent impulses transmitted via the vagus nerve, thereby interrupting the hiccup reflex. Laryngotracheal stimulation is thought to act by a similar mechanism, since coughing is known to decrease hiccup frequency and may end a bout of hiccups (6). Spiro mentioned that passing a rubber esophageal bougie into the stomach often stopped hiccups in his practice (1). Whether this technique works by stimulating the diaphragm or the pharynx, or both, is not clear.

Stimulation of vagal afferents may also account for the success of swallowing dry granulated sugar (50, 51, 57). Engleman et al. gave 1 teaspoon of dry granulated sugar to 12 patients with hiccups of short duration (<6 hours) and recorded prompt success in all 12. Seven of eight additional patients with more persistent hiccups (24 hours' to 6 weeks' duration) that were previously unresponsive to other treatments also responded quickly. Three patients in this group with recurrent hiccups responded to repeat therapy (57). Although granulated sugar has been given to countless numbers of persons with hiccups, as with most other "cures," few published reports on the method are available, and all have been anecdotal and uncontrolled.

Other methods that stimulate the pharynx include swallowing hard bread or crushed ice, sipping ice water, dripping noxious substances into the nasopharynx, spraying cocaine into the larynx, and administering vinegar or other noxious tastes orally (1). Moses et al. (58) instilled 11 of ether into the nostrils of 27 patients with hiccups during abdominal surgery and observed the hiccups stopped "immediately" in 26. Although no untoward effects were recorded, others consider the use of ether potentially dangerous and have substituted the instillation of ice water into the nostrils of intubated patients with equal efficacy (59). Neither ether nor ice water has been evaluated to any extent in unanesthetized patients with chronic hiccups. Herman and Nolan (60) reported that alcohol-related hiccups

were treated successfully with a lemon wedge soaked with angostura bitters. Of their 16 patients, 14 responded within 1 minute and remained hiccup-free for at least 2 hours.

Counterirritation or blockade of vagal impulses is also the proposed mechanism for the success of carotid sinus massage, digital compression over the eyeballs, rectal massage, and manipulation of an aberrant hair irritating the tympanic membrane (1). At least two patients have been successfully treated with digital rectal massage (61, 62). In the case described by Fester, rectal massage was performed following incomplete success from a Valsalva maneuver, carotid sinus massage, and digital eyeball compression. The increase in vagal tone (which is the probable underlying mechanism for the success of these other vagal maneuvers) also applies to digital massage, which has been used to successfully terminate paroxysmal supraventricular tachycardia (61). In a report by Goldenberg et al., a patient developed hiccups in the setting of ventricular tachycardia and responded only to the use of cardioversion. The authors recommended that this treatment modality be used only in patients with a specific indication such as a life-threatening arrhythmia (63). Hiccups as the initial presentation of glaucoma was recently described in a patient in whom digital eyeball compression was used as a vagal maneuver to terminate a bout of hiccups after several other physical maneuvers were unsuccessful (32). The physician noted elevated intraocular pressure during digital compression, which led to the diagnosis of glaucoma. The hiccups eventually stopped following the use of a spoonful of sugar followed by drinking a glass of water from the opposite rim.

Drinking from the far side of a glass has been proposed as a means of terminating hiccups through "cerebral concentration" (2), although it may act simply as a pharyngeal stimulant. Competition for "neural energy" as a means of curing hiccups has been reported by Kirkman (64). His approach was somewhat less conventional than others in that he offered a financial reward of ten dollars if the

Table 11.4
Pharmacotherapy of Hiccups[a]

Major tranquilizers	*Parasympathomimetics*
Chlorpromazine	Edrophonium
Haloperidol	
	Parasympatholytics
Anticonvulsants	Atropine
Diphenylhydantoin	Quinidine
Valproic acid	
Carbamazepine	*Antispasticity agents*
Magnesium sulfate	Baclofen
Central nervous system	*Calcium channel blockers*
stimulants	Nifedipine
Methylphenidate	
Benzedrine sulfate	*Antidepressants*
Amyl nitrate	Amitriptyline
Ephedrine	
Nikethamide	Serotonin antagonists
	Ondansetron
Anesthetic stimulants	
Ketamine	*Dopamine antagonists*
	Metoclopramide
Muscle relaxants	
Mephenesin	*Dopamine agonists*
Orphenadrine citrate	Amantadine
	Levodopa/carbidopa
Narcotic analgesics	
Pentazocine	*Antiarrhythmics*
Apomorphine	Lidocaine
Hyoscine	
Hydrobromide	

[a]Medications listed are those with reported success.

"hiccupper" could voluntarily continue to hiccup on demand. Kirkman states that this approach worked among his family, friends, and few patients, leading him to postulate that "the neural energy was suddenly drained from the [hiccup] pathway and the [patient] simply could not hiccup." In commenting on this "cure," Nathan (17) was skeptical that his or any other academician's salary would allow for a controlled study of Kirkman's method.

Miscellaneous Nondrug Hiccup Treatments

A number of clinicians have resorted to behavioral modification, hypnosis, and even acupuncture when treating patients with intractable hiccups. At least two authors have reported the successful use of negative reinforcement techniques in reducing the frequency of hiccups resistant to more conventional therapies (65, 66). Both employed a noxious stimulus (instillation of an ammonia solution into the pharynx in one case and use of verbal reprimands plus a rubber tube to induce gagging in the other, respectively, as a form of mild punishment in emotionally disturbed patients. Whether or not pharyngeal irritation alone would have been sufficient to end the hiccups without the use of operant conditioning in either patient is not known.

Successful use of hypnosis has been reported by several authors (67–71). Bendersky and Baren used hypnotic suggestion to treat a patient with prolonged hiccups secondary to a myocardial infarction (67). Kirkner and West described a patient with hiccups associated with metastatic adenocarcinoma of the colon unresponsive to phrenic nerve block whose attacks were controlled with hypnotherapy (69). Smedley and Barnes also used relaxation and countersuggestion techniques to terminate episodes of postoperative hiccups (70). Through the use of hypnosis, both Theohar and McKegney (68) and LeCron et al. (71) successfully uncovered deep-seated psychologic problems that were at the root of their patients' hiccups. In both instances, further hypnosis ultimately terminated the hiccup episodes.

Acupuncture has been used in Asia to treat hiccups for many years (72), and the technique has been reported to influence the course of intractable hiccups favorably in at least one Western study (73). Its major limitation as a hiccup cure appears to be only the availability of physicians skilled in its application.

DRUG THERAPY FOR HICCUPS

A variety of pharmacologic agents have been used in the treatment of intractable hiccups when mechanical or physical measures fail (Table 11.4). As is the case with most reports dealing with physical maneuvers to stop hiccups, the results of nearly all of these reports have been largely anecdotal (1, 74–76). Nevertheless, in many instances, they represent the only available data on the possible treatment efficacy of certain drugs for hiccups. Additionally, given the difficulty in collecting a large enough series of patients with intractable hiccups in order to perform controlled clinical trials, and the fact that no new studies on the pathophysiology of hiccups have appeared since the early 1970s, it is not surprising that breakthroughs in the pharmacologic treatment of this disorder are generally lacking. Moreover, as with many other disorders for which therapy is often not successful, most authors have published only their positive results. We know very little about how often specific drug treatments do *not* work from the available literature. Nevertheless, the following section reviews in detail the results of the published studies suggesting treatment efficacy for hiccups with a variety of centrally and peripherally acting agents.

Major Tranquilizers

Among the centrally active medications that have been the most effective in treating hiccups, *chlorpromazine* is the agent that has probably been most widely utilized. It gained most of its notoriety in the 1950s, when reports first appeared that cited cure rates in the range of 80% among patients with intractable hiccups of various etiologies (77, 78). For example, among the patients treated by Friedgood and Ripstein (77), 41 of 50 had a prompt response, with the hiccups stopping almost immediately. In the small number of refractory patients who received a second 50 mg intravenous dose 2–4 hours later, 5 of 9 decreased the severity of their hiccups, although they did not completely subside. Only 4 patients remained completely unresponsive to this treatment. For most patients, 25–50 mg given intravenously is considered to be more effective than either the oral or the intramuscular routes (75). The butyrophenone, *haloperidol*, has also been reported to be effective in "several" patients, perhaps relating to its dopamine antagonist effects. The effective dose appears to be between 2 and 12 mg/day, with some patients responding to a single 2 mg intramuscular dose (79–81).

Anticonvulsants

Diphenylhydantoin given as a 200 mg intravenous bolus followed by 100 mg four times

daily orally reportedly achieved success in a "number" of patients, although it is not always effective (82, 83). *Valproic acid* was said to be curative in four of five patients with chronic hiccups of diverse etiologies. A dose of 15 mg/kg/day orally or rectally (increased by increments of 250 mg in divided doses every 2 weeks as needed) controlled hiccups for periods of up to 1 year (84). While only two of five patients were able to taper the dose successfully, none developed hepatic dysfunction, which can be severe, especially in children (85). Valproic acid is postulated to act in the central nervous system by enhancing the inhibitory effects of γ-amino butyric acid (GABA). *Carbamazepine* 200 mg four times daily orally successfully stopped hiccups due to multiple sclerosis within 24 hours in one patient (86, 87). A patient with hiccups associated with pulmonary tuberculosis responded to 5 ml of a 25% *magnesium sulfate* solution given intramuscularly (88). Curiously, the benzodiazepines have not been useful in treating hiccups. *Diazepam* has been reported to worsen hiccuping episodes (89), a finding consistent with the observation that hiccups may be induced when the drug is given as premedication for the induction of anesthesia or endoscopy (90). *Chlordiazepoxide* has also been reported to cause hiccups (91).

Central Nervous System Stimulants

A number of central nervous system (CNS) stimulants have been used with variable success in treating anesthesia-related hiccups. Macris (92) and Vasiloff et al. (93) both reported that *methylphenidate* (20 mg intravenously administered) was rapidly effective in the anesthesia setting. Fry also reported success with 6–12 mg intravenous in "scores" of patients (94). Gregory and Way (95), however, were unable to demonstrate any benefit over placebo of a 10-mg dose of methylphenidate given to 51 unanesthetized patients in a controlled study. However, they admitted that the lower dose, as well as possible differences between anesthetized and unanesthetized patients, may have explained why their results differed from those of other investigators.

Ephedrine (5 mg intravenous bolus injections) was "rapidly effective" in 10 of 11 patients with hiccups that occurred during anesthesia in one study (96). *Benzedrine sulfate* (10–20 mg twice daily) arrested postoperative hiccups in 2 patients (97), possibly because of its smooth muscle relaxant effect. A single report of success with *nikethamide* (2–5 mg intravenous) has been recorded (98). *Ketamine*, an anesthetic stimulant, has been reported to terminate hiccups rapidly in several patients given 25–55 mg (0.4–0.5 mg/kg) given intravenously during anesthesia or postoperatively (99–101). This dose represents only about one-fifth of the normal anesthetic dose. In animals, ketamine has caused seizures due to its pronounced central nervous system stimulant effect. In humans, it is postulated that the drug blocks the hiccup center by increasing efferent impulses and decreasing afferent stimuli (99).

Sedative/Hypnotics

Among the various sedative-hypnotic agents, *pentobarbital* (25–50 mg intravenous) was effective in four patients who developed hiccups after transurethral prostatectomy (37). *Phenobarbital* is listed as being unreliable in controlling hiccups (102), perhaps because it has also been implicated as a cause of hiccups (37). As mentioned under "anticonvulsants," the *benzodiazepines* have not been useful as a class in the control of hiccups.

Muscle Relaxants/Antispasticity Agents

The muscle relaxants *mephenesin* and *orphenadrine* have both been reported to be effective for short periods of time in a small number of patients (103–105). These centrally acting skeletal muscle relaxants have been used in doses of 2500 mg orally and 60 mg intravenously, respectively.

Baclofen (lioresal) is a derivative of the inhibitory neurotransmitter γ-amino butyric acid (GABA) that was first proposed for use in treating hiccups in 1988 (106). Subsequently, it has received additional notoriety with its anecdotal success (35, 107, 108) and more recently was shown to be useful in a randomized controlled clinical trial (109). The drug was initially developed for reducing the frequency and severity of spasticity caused by multiple sclerosis and other diseases of the spinal cord, particularly following traumatic injury (110). When given orally in a dosage of 5–20 mg every 6–12 hours, success has been reported in hiccups unresponsive to most other agents (109), including hiccups due to renal failure in patients receiving chronic peritoneal dialysis or hemodialysis (107), and an interesting entity referred to as "familial hiccups" (35). Baclofen is rapidly absorbed after oral administration with a half-life of 3 to 4 hours and is excreted largely unchanged by the kidneys. Side effects include drowsiness, insomnia, dizziness, weakness, ataxia, and confusion. It is said to be poorly tolerated by elderly patients and sudden withdrawal after long-term use may cause auditory and visual hallucinations, anxiety, and tachycardia. Respiratory depression, seizures, and coma have been reported following significant overdose. Treatment is usually initiated with 5 mg twice daily with the dosage escalated at 3-day intervals until a maximum of 20 mg four times daily has been reached. Abrupt withdrawal should be avoided and it should be administered cautiously in patients with impaired renal function. It is not recommended for use in patients with spasticity due to stroke or other cerebral lesions (110).

Narcotic Analgesics

A number of narcotic agents have been successfully used to treat hiccups, including *pentazocine, apomorphine*, and *hyoscine hydrobromide* (92, 111). *Morphine* by itself is said to be rarely effective (18). *Amyl nitrate* inhalation has been reported to terminate hiccups temporarily (112), possibly by its irritative action on the nasal mucosa, but its success is reported as variable (111).

Tricyclic Antidepressants

Amitriptyline is known to synchronize electroencephalogram (EEG) activity and to act on brain amines (113), although its exact mechanism of action in the treatment of hiccups remains unclear. Nevertheless, anecdotal success is reported using 30 mg given in three divided doses (114). In one case, an attempt at dose reduction was unsuccessful in maintaining a remission and the full dose had to be reinstituted (113).

Calcium Channel Blocking Agents

Several patients have been treated successfully with *nifedipine* in an initial dosage of 10 mg twice daily, escalated to 20 mg three times a day as needed (115, 116). Nonresponders, however, have also been described. As nifedipine does not readily enter the central nervous system, its actions are thought to be peripheral.

Dopamine Antagonists

Agents in this class act on the autonomic nervous system, and are regularly tried in patients with chronic hiccups. In addition to chlorpromazine, haloperidol, and apomorphine (all described above), *metoclopramide* has been used successfully in several patients (117–119). Madanagopolan reported that 10 mg given orally every 6 hours or 5–10 mg given intramuscularly or intravenously every 8 hours terminated hiccups of diverse etiologies (including gastric dilatation due to diabetic gastroparesis) in 14 patients. While relief from hiccups lasted up to 8 hours, maintenance therapy for an additional 10 days was advised (119). Unpleasant neuropsychiatric side effects are common and represent a limiting factor to its use.

Dopamine Agonists

Amantadine is a dopaminergic agonist that has been described anecdotally as having been successful for a patient with Parkinson's disease (28). In that case, 100 mg daily produced complete control of hiccups during the one year of treatment that was described. The combination of *levodopa/carbidopa* also was effective with this patient.

Parasympathomimetics/ Parasympatholytics

Edrophonium chloride (5 mg intravenous) has been effective in terminating hiccups, possibly by disrupting cholinergic impulse transmission (37). *Atropine* is said to be beneficial in protecting against hiccups during anesthesia, with a 1 mg intravenous bolus reported to be effective (37). In addition, *quinidine sulfate* (10 grains orally or intramuscularly every 3–4 hours) was helpful in eight of nine patients with chronic hiccups, perhaps by prolonging the refractory period of striated muscle (110).

Serotonin Antagonists

Ondansetron (Zofran) a specific 5HT-3 antagonist, is currently used in the management of chemotherapy-induced emesis and postoperative nausea and vomiting (120). A recent report describes its successful control of hiccups in a patient with metastatic gastric adenocarcinoma, whose symptomatology also included uncontrolled vomiting (121). Although the mechanism by which ondansetron stops hiccups is unclear, it may relate to the drug's effects on blocking the serotonin neurotransmitter 5-hydroxytryptamine (5HT-1) at its receptors in the central and peripheral nervous systems (120). As such, it warrants further study, especially in patients in whom hiccups is associated with emesis.

Lidocaine

Pretreatment with lidocaine in a dose of 1 mg/kg body weight intravenously has been reported to reduce the risk of hiccups associated with induction of anesthesia with methohexital (122) and more recently was successful in alleviating hiccups associated with pneumonitis when given as a 1 mg/kg iv loading dose followed by a 2- to 4-mg/min continuous infusion for 24 hr (123). These authors caution that close monitoring for lidocaine toxicity should be performed during such an infusion.

SPECIFIC HICCUP CURES

Table 11.5 lists a number of causes of hiccups that have been successfully treated by physical maneuvers or drug therapy directed specifically at the cause. While most of these treatments seem self-evident, there are relatively few reports chronicling the success of a spe-

Table 11.5
Specific Hiccup Therapies

Hiccup Cause	Successful Physical Maneuver or Drug Treatment[a]
Parkinson disease	Amantadine
	Levodopa/carbidopa
Alcohol	Angostura bitters-soaked lemon wedge
Addison disease	Steroid replacement
Candida esophagitis	Antifungal treatment
Herpetic esophagitis	Acyclovir
Hyponatremia	Correct electrolyte imbalance
Carcinomatosis with vomiting	Ondansetron
Renal failure requiring dialysis	Baclofen
Reflux esophagitis	H_2-blocker or antireflux surgery
Cardiac arrhythmia (ventricular tachycardia)	Cardioversion
Seizure disorder	Amitriptyline
Coronary or valvular heart artery disease	Nifedipine
Foreign body in ear canal	Removal
Esophageal obstruction or achalasia	Esophageal dilation
Intraoperative	Catheter stimulation of pharynx; ether instillation into nostrils; ephedrine, benzedrine, ketamine
Postoperative	Splanchnicectomy

[a]As reported in the literature.

cific therapy directed against a specific cause of hiccups in the literature. In addition, a number of caveats remain. One, in particular, relates to reflux esophagitis. While some investigators have used antireflux surgery successfully to relieve hiccups associated with severe reflux esophagitis (40), there are several reports suggesting that hiccups may be the cause of reflux rather than its consequence (39, 41–43). As a result, antireflux surgery in some patients has relieved only the heartburn, but not hiccups (39, 42, 43). It has been suggested, therefore, that antireflux surgery is most likely to be beneficial in treating intractable hiccups if medical therapy for reflux is initially helpful, and if acid perfusion consistently provokes the hiccups (40, 43). It certainly seems reasonable that prior to considering a surgical approach to hiccups in the setting of reflux, these prior conditions be satisfied.

Other esophageal causes of hiccups that have been treated by specific therapy directed at the underlying esophageal condition include achalasia (25), esophageal rings, and some causes of obstructing carcinoma (44); all of which have been successfully treated with esophageal dilatation. Seeman and Traub re-

cently described their experience with 15 patients treated for achalasia, 9 of whom had hiccups (25). Hiccups were noted to have begun after dysphagia had been present for 6–108 months. Interestingly, in most patients, hiccups were present only following meals and ended when the dysphagia subsided (generally after ingestion of liquids or after forced regurgitation). Hiccups did not develop after dilation in patients in whom hiccups were absent at baseline. Of the 9 patients with achalasia-associated hiccups, 5 were women, which stands in contrast to the widely quoted report from the Mayo Clinic series in which the majority of individuals with an organic cause of hiccups were men (22). One case of hiccups caused by herpetic esophagitis successfully treated with acyclovir was recently reported (124).

GUIDELINES FOR TREATING TRANSIENT HICCUPS

Hiccup episodes that last only a few minutes may be annoying or sometimes socially embarrassing, but rarely require treatment other than simple physical maneuvers (1). Breath holding, breathing into a paper bag, pulling on the tongue, sneezing, swallowing a teaspoonful of granulated sugar, sucking on hard candy, drinking from the far side of the glass, or holding one's nose and ears closed while swallowing, or sudden fright, alone or in combination, are usually effective. In cases in which hiccups last longer than 30 or 60 minutes, manual stimulation of the nasopharynx with a finger, rubber catheter, or cotton-tipped applicator; lifting the uvula with a spoon or other device; or inducing a gasp with smelling salts or other noxious substances can be tried if simpler measures are ineffective. Not recommended as home measures are instilling ammonia or ether into the nasopharynx, performing carotid sinus massage, applying supraorbital pressure, digital compression to the root of the neck over the course of the phrenic nerve, compressing the thyroid cartilage, or massaging the rectum digitally. Nasogastric aspiration and manipulation or removal of an aberrant hair, insect, or other foreign object in the auditory canal should also not be employed without proper instruction or supervision.

Occasionally, women in their second or third trimester of pregnancy will note rhythmic fetal movements that can be attributed to fetal hiccuping. These hiccups can be routinely seen on sonography, and in many instances, such episodes can be terminated when the mother leans forward or turns onto her side to change position. Interestingly, fetal hiccups are said to recur in subsequent pregnancies, and often occur at the same time of the day, and may persist in the infant after birth.

GUIDELINES FOR TREATING PERSISTENT HICCUPS

A thorough search for an underlying cause usually reveals an organic etiology in over 90% of men with persistent hiccups. Women, however, are less likely to have an identifiable organic cause according to older reports in the literature (22), although this is not a hard and fast rule. Although there are no studies that have examined what percentage of hiccups can be expected to resolve when the underlying disorder is corrected, it is assumed that many,

if not most, hiccups will stop when the specific cause is successfully treated (Table 11.5). If hiccups persist despite specific therapy, physical manipulation such as pharyngeal stimulation or gastric aspiration can be tried. Hiccups that remain refractory to these measures will often require the use of pharmacologic agents as listed in Table 11.4. In the past, many authorities have recommended chlorpromazine in a dosage of 25–50 mg intravenously every 6 hours as initial drug therapy. If this proves successful in terminating the hiccups, then oral chlorpromazine (at the same dosage) can be maintained for a period of 7–10 days. If chlorpromazine fails to terminate the episode, a number of second-line drugs are available. These include intravenous metoclopramide (10 mg every 4 hours), although I personally now favor the use of one of the more recently described therapies such as baclofen, nifedipine, amitriptyline, or ondansetron as initial therapy. Should these agents fail, intravenous lidocaine can be tried as recently described (123).

For hiccups unresponsive to both physical maneuvers and drug therapy, disruption of the phrenic nerve can be considered, especially in patients in whom persistent hiccups are the cause of significant discomfort or serious morbidity. A temporary phrenic nerve block using a long-acting agent such as bupivacaine, should be attempted before a more permanent phrenic crush or transsection procedure is carried out. If a permanent nerve block or surgery is contemplated, it is recommended that fluoroscopic examination of the diaphragm be performed to determine which leaflet is contracting, or to determine if one leaflet is dominant in cases of bilateral involvement (125). It should be remembered that phrenic nerve block and phrenic crush procedures have not been uniformly successful in terminating bilateral hiccups, even when both sides have been treated (1). Moreover, impaired pulmonary function and frank respiratory failure have occurred as a result of bilateral diaphragmatic paralysis (126), and such an approach seems justified only in extreme cases and with ventilatory support services available. It is reasonable to first exhaust all conservative treatment approaches, including hypnosis, psychotherapy, and even acupuncture if it is available, before proceeding with a bilateral phrenic nerve crush or transsection. For hiccups that defy all of the treatment measures listed above, perhaps Dr. Kirkman still has money to spare—although I am sure that with inflation, the amount offered as a monetary reward to stop hiccuping is now significantly more than his original ten dollars.

REFERENCES

1. Lewis JH. Hiccups: causes and cures. J Clin Gastroenterol 1985;7:539–552.
2. Hulbert NG. Hiccoughing (hiccup or singultus). Practitioner 1951;167:286–289.
3. Mayo CW. Hiccup. Surg Gynecol Obstet 1932;55:700–708.
4. Hippocrates. Aphorisms. In: Jones WHS, trans. Hippocrates: Vol. 4. The Loeb Classical Library. Cambridge: Harvard University Press, 1962: lib. V:1viii, p. 173;lib. VII:xvii, p. 197.
5. Riddel WR. Hippocrates and hiccup. Med J Rec 1930;132:40–41.
6. Newsom Davis J. An experimental study of hiccup. Brain 1970;93:851–872.
7. Rosenow EC. Diaphragmatic spasms in animals produced with a streptococcus from epidemic hiccup: preliminary report. JAMA 1921;76:1745–1747.
8. Brouillette RT, Thach BT, Abu-Osba YK, Wilson SL. Hiccups in infants: characteristics and effects on ventilation. J Pediatr 1980;96:219–225.
9. Dunn AM. Fetal hiccups. Lancet 1977;2:505.
10. Miller FC, Gonzales F, Mueller E, et al. Fetal hiccups: an associated fetal heart rate pattern. Obstet Gynecol 1983;62:253–255.
11. Fuller GN. Hiccups and human purpose. Nature 1990;243:420.
12. Shortt T. Hiccup, its causes and cure. Edinburgh Med Surg J 1833;39:305.
13. Bailey H. Persistent hiccup. Practitioner 1943;150:173–177.
14. Salem MR, Baraka A, Rattenborg CC, Holaday DA. Treatment of hiccups by pharyngeal stimulation in anesthetized and conscious subjects. JAMA 1967;202:126–130.
15. Campbell MF. Malignant hiccup: with report of a case following transurethral prostatic resection and requiring bilateral phrenicectomy for cure. Am J Surg 1940;48:449–455.
16. Bellingham-Smith E. The significance and treatment of obstinate hiccough. Practitioner 1938;140:166–171.
17. Nathan MD, Leshner RT, Keller AP Jr. Intractable hiccups (singultus). Laryngoscope 1980;90:1612–1618.
18. Samuels L. Hiccup: a ten year review of anatomy, etiology, and treatment. Can Med Assoc J 1952;67:315–322.
19. Anthoney JR, Anthoney SL, Anthoney DJ. On temporal structure of human hiccups: ethology and chronobiology. Int J Chronobiol 1978;5:477–492.
20. Shim C. Motor disturbances of the diaphragm. Clin Chest Med 1980;1:128–129.
21. Travell JG. A trigger point for hiccup. J Am Osteopath Assoc 1977;77:308–312.
22. Souadjian JV, Cain JC. Intractable hiccup: etiologic factors in 220 cases. Postgrad Med 1968;43:72–77.
23. Fisher CM. Protracted hiccup—a male malady. Trans Am Neurol Assoc 1967;92:231–233.
24. Roth JLA. Hiccup. In: Bockus HL, ed. Gastroenterology. ed. 3. Philadelphia: WB Saunders, 1974;1:88–89.
25. Seeman H, Traub M. Hiccup and achalasia. Ann Intern Med 1991;115:711–712.
26. Seibert D, Al-Kawas F. Trimethoprim-sulfamethoxazole, hiccups, and esophageal ulcers. Ann Intern Med 1986;105:976.
27. Baethge BA, Lidsky MD. Intractable hiccups associated with high-dose intravenous methylprednisolone therapy. Ann Intern Med 1986;104:58–59.
28. Askenasy JJM, Boiangiu M, Davidovitch S. Persistent hiccup cured by amantadine. N Engl J Med 1988;318:711.
29. Connolly JP, Craig TJ, Sanchez RM, et al. Intractable hiccups as a presentation of central nervous system sarcoidosis. West J Med 1991;155:78–79.
30. Hardo PG. Intractable hiccups—an early feature of Addison's disease. Postgrad Med J 1989;65:918–919.
31. Cronin RE. Psychogenic polydipsia with hyponatremia: Report of 11 Cases. Am J of Kidney Dis 1987;9:410–416.
32. Carmichael C. Glaucoma presenting as Hiccups [Letter]. JAMA 1988;261:702.
33. Campbell LA, Schwartz SH. An unusual cause of respiratory alkalosis. Chest 1991;100:1159.
34. Topaz O, Sharon M, Rechavia E, et al. Traumatic internal jugular vein cannulation. Ann Emerg Med 1987;16:1394–1395.
35. Lance JW, Bassil JT. Familial intractable hiccup relieved by Baclofen. Lancet 1989;2:276–277.
36. McFarlan D, ed. Guinness book of world records, 1990–1991. New York: Bantam Books, 1991.
37. Butt HR Jr, Hamleberg W, Jacoby J. Hiccup: its possible cause and treatment in anesthesia. Anesth Analg 1961;40:182–185.

38. Rosenow EC. Further studies on the etiology of epidemic hiccup (singultus) and its relation to encephalitis. Arch Neurol Psychiatry 1926;15:712–734.
39. Shay SS, Myers RL, Johnson LF. Hiccups associated with reflux esophagitis. Gastroenterology 1984;87:204–207.
40. Gluck M, Pope CE II. Chronic hiccups and gastroesophageal reflux disease: the acid perfusion test as a provocative maneuver. Ann Intern Med 1986;105:219–220.
41. Triadafilopoulos G. Hiccups and esophageal dysfunction. Am J Gastroenterol 1989;84:164–169.
42. Fisher MJ, Mittal RK. Hiccups and esophageal reflux: cause and effect? Dig Dis Sci 1989;34:1277–1280.
43. Marshall JB, Landreneau RJ, Beyer KL. Hiccups: esophageal manometric features and relationship to gastroesophageal reflux. Am J Gastroenterol 1990;85:1172–1175.
44. Kaufman HJ. Hiccups: an occasional sign of esophageal obstruction. Gastroenterology 1982;82:1443–1445.
45. McWhirter R, ed. Guinness book of world records, ed. 13. New York: Sterling Publishing, 1974:41.
46. Hippocrates. Aphorisms. In: Jones WHS, trans. Hippocrates: Vol. 4. The Loeb classical library. Cambridge: Harvard University Press, 1962:lib, VI:xiii, p. 183.
47. Celsus C. De medicina. In: Spencer WG, trans. Celsus: DeMedicina: the Loeb classical library. Cambridge: Harvard University Press, 1962:bk. II, section 8:16, p. 139.
48. Obis P Jr. Remedies for hiccups. Nursing 1974;4:88.
49. Plato. The symposium. Quoted in Hulbert NG: Hiccoughing (hiccup or singultus). Practitioner 1951;167:288–289.
50. Schisel AD, Rhodes RH. Hiccup remedies [Letter]. N Engl J Med 1972;286:323.
51. Margolis GM. Hiccup remedies [Letter]. N Engl J Med 1972;286:323.
52. Baraka A. Inhibition of hiccup by pulmonary inflation. Anesthesiology 1970;32:271–273.
53. Gigot AF, Flynn PD. Treatment of hiccups. JAMA 1952;150:760–764.
54. Kappis M. Origin and treatment of hiccups. JAMA 1924;83:228.
55. Juan G, Calverly P, Talamo C, Schnader J, Roussos C. Effect of carbon dioxide on diaphragmatic function in human beings. N Engl J Med 1984;310:874–879.
56. Goldsmith S. A treatment for hiccups [Letter]. JAMA 1983;249:1566.
57. Engleman EG, Lankton J, Lankton B. Granulated sugar as treatment for hiccups in conscious patients [Letter]. N Engl J Med 1971;285:1489.
58. Moses JA, Ramachandran KP, Surendran D. Treatment of hiccups with instillation of ether into nasal cavity. Anesth Analg 1970;49:367–368.
59. Ravindran RS. A simple technique to stop hiccups during endotracheal anaesthesia [Letter]. Anesth Analg 1981;60:121.
60. Herman JH, Nolan DS. A bitter cure [Letter]. N Engl J Med 1981;305:1654.
61. Fester FM. Termination of intractable hiccups with digital rectal massage [Letter]. Ann Emerg Med 1988;17:872.
62. Odeah M, Bassan H, Oliven A. Termination of intractable hiccups with digital rectal message. J Intern Med 1990;227:145–146.
63. Goldenberg IF, Ochi RP, Almquist A, Benditt DG. Cardioversion for intractable hiccups: A frightening cure [Letter]. N Engl J Med 1987;316:883.
64. Kirkman B. Discussion. In: Nathan et al. Intractable hiccups (singultus). Laryngoscope 1980;90:1618.
65. Salkind MR. The treatment of intractable hiccup by operant conditioning with negative incentive. Practitioner 1971;206:535–537.
66. Van Heuven PF, Smeets PM. Behavioral control of chronic hiccuping associated with gastrointestinal bleeding in a retarded epileptic male. J Behav Ther Exp Psychiatry 1981;12:341–345.
67. Bendersky G, Baren M. Hypnosis in the termination of hiccups unresponsive to conventional treatment. Arch Intern Med 1959;104:417–420.
68. Theohar C, McKegney FP. Hiccups of psychogenic origin: a case report and review of the literature. Compr Psychiatry 1970;11:377–384.
69. Kirkner FJ, West PM. Hypnotic treatment of persistent hiccup: a case report. Br J Med Hypnotism 1950;1:22–24.
70. Smedley WP, Barnes WT. Postoperative use of hypnosis on a cardiovascular service: termination of persistent hiccups in a patient with an aortorenal graft. JAMA 1966;197:149–150.
71. LeCron M, Fields A, Levine B. Postoperative prolonged hiccups relieved through the uncovering by hypnosis of the psychological cause. Ann West Med Surg 1951;5:937–938.
72. Li X, Yi J, Qi B. Treatment of hiccough with auriculo-acupuncture and auriculo-pressure—a report of 85 Cases. J Trad Chin Med 1990;10:257–259.
73. Bondi N, Bettelli A. Treatment of hiccup by acupuncture in patients under anesthesia and in conscious patients. Minerva Med 1981;72:2231–2234.
74. Kaufmann HJ. Hiccups: causes, mechanisms, and treatment. Pract Gastroenterol 1983;7:28–32.
75. Williamson BWA, MacIntyre IMC. Management of intractable hiccup. Br Med J 1977;2:501–503.
76. Middleton RK, Hart LL. Drug therapy for hiccups. Drug Intell Clin Pharm 1987;21:259–261.
77. Friedgood CE, Ripstein CB. Chlorpromazine (Thorazine) in the treatment of intractable hiccups. JAMA 1955;157:309–310.
78. Davignon A, Laurieux G, Genest J. Chlorpromazine in the treatment of persistent hiccough. Union Med Can 1955;84:282.

79. Korczyn AD. Hiccup [Letter]. Br Med J 1971; 2:590–591.

80. Scarnati RA. Intractable hiccups (singultus): report of case. J Am Osteopath Assoc 1979;79:127–129.

81. Ives TJ, Fleming MF, Weart CW, et al. Treatment of intractable hiccups with intramuscular haloperidol. Am J Psychiatry 1985;142:1368–1369.

82. Petroski D, Patel AN. Diphenylhydantoin for intractable hiccups [Letter]. Lancet 1974;1:739.

83. Newsom Davis J. Diphenylhydantoin for hiccups [Letter]. Lancet 1974;1:997.

84. Jacobson PL, Messenheimer JA, Farmer TW. Treatment of intractable hiccups with valproic acid. Neurology 1981;31:1458–1460.

85. Zimmerman HJ, Ishak KG. Valproate-induced hepatic injury: analysis of 23 fatal cases. Hepatology 1982;2:591–597.

86. McFarling DA, Susac JO. Carbamazepine for hiccoughs [Letter]. JAMA 1974;230:962.

87. McFarling DA, Susac JO. Hoquet diabolique: intractable hiccups as a manifestation of multiple sclerosis. Neurology 1979;29:797–801.

88. MacKay-Dick J. Hiccup [Letter]. Br Med J 1971;1:591.

89. Fariello RG, Mutani R. Treatment of hiccup [Letter]. Lancet 1974;2:1201.

90. Greenblatt DJ, Shader RI. Benzodiazepines in clinical practice. New York: Raven Press, 1974: 203.

91. Winstead DK. Hiccups following ingestion of oral chlordiazepoxide. Am J Psychiatry 1976;136: 719.

92. Macris SG. Methylphenidate for hiccups [Letter]. Anesthesiology 1971;34:201.

93. Vasiloff N, Cohen DD, Dillon JB. Effective treatment of hiccup with intravenous methylphenidate. Can Anaesth Soc J 1965;12:306–310.

94. Fry ENS. Management of intractable hiccup [Letter]. Br Med J 1977;2:704.

95. Gregory GA, Way WL. Methylphenidate for the treatment of hiccups during anesthesia. Anesthesiology 1969;31:89–90.

96. Sohn YZ, Conrad LJ, Katz RL. Hiccup and ephedrine. Can Anaesth Soc J 1978;25:431–432.

97. Shaine MS. Benzedrine sulphate in persistent hiccough: a report of 2 cases. Am J Med Sci 1938;196:715–717.

98. Gilston A. Nikethamide for hiccough [Letter]. Anaesthesia 1979;34:1060.

99. Shantha TR. Ketamine for the treatment of hiccups during and following anesthesia: a preliminary report. Anesth Analg 1973;52:822–824.

100. Tavakoli M, Corssen G. Control of hiccups by ketamine: a preliminary report. Ala J Med Sci 1974;31:229–230.

101. Teodorowicz J, Zimny M. The effect of ketamine in patients with refractory hiccups in the postoperative period: preliminary report. Anasth Intensivther Not fallmed 1975;3:271–272.

102. Lamphier TA. Methods of management of persistent hiccup (singultus). Maryland State Med J Nov 1977;80–81.

103. Catalano R. Centrally acting skeletal muscle relaxants in persistent hiccup. Acta Neurolog (Napoli) 1973;28:466–470.

104. Gibbs AE. Two cases of persistent hiccups treated with orphenadrine citrate. Practitioner 1963; 191:646.

105. Finch JW. Rapid control of persistent hiccups by orphenadrine citrate. Med Times 1966;94:485–488.

106. Burke AM, White AB, Brill N. Baclofen for intractable hiccups. N Engl J Med 1988;318: 1354.

107. Yaqoob M, Prabhu P, Abmed R. Baclofen for intractable hiccups. Lancet 1989;2:562–563.

108. Bhalotra R. Baclofen therapy for intractable hiccoughs. J Clin Gastroenterol 1990;12:122.

109. Ramirez FC, Graham DY. Treatment of intractable hiccup with baclofen: results of a double-blind randomized, controlled, cross-over study. Am J Gastroenterol 1992;87:1789–1791.

110. Cedarbaum JM, Schleifer LS. Drugs for Parkinson disease, spasticity, and acute muscle spasms. In: Gilman AG, Rall TW, Nies AS, Taylor P. Goodman and Gilman's the pharmacological basis of therapeutics, ed. 8. New York: Pergamon Press, 1990:479–480.

111. Bellet S, Nadler CS. The use of quinidine sulfate in the treatment of hiccup, a preliminary report. Am J Med Sci 1948;216:680–686.

112. Nairn RC. Case of hiccups: revival of old remedy. Lancet 1947;1:829–830.

113. Longo VG. Effects of psychotropic drugs on the EEG of animals. In: Clark WG, delGuidice J, eds. Principals of psychopharmacology. ed. 2. New York: Academic Press, 1978:247–260.

114. Stalnikowicz R, Fich A, Troudart T. Amitriptyline for intractable hiccups. N Engl J Med 1986;315:64–65.

115. Mukhopadhyay P, Osman MR, Wajima T, Wallace TI. Nifedipine for intractable hiccups. N Engl J Med 1986;314:1256.

116. Lipps DC, Gabbari B, Mitchell MH, Daigh JD Jr. Nifedipine for intractable hiccups. Neurology 1990;40:531–532.

117. Douthwaite AH. Hiccup [Letter]. Lancet 1968; 1:144.

118. Middleton RSW. The use of metoclopramide in the elderly. Postgrad Med J 1973; July (suppl):90–93.

119. Madanagopolan N. Metoclopramide in hiccup. Curr Med Res Opin 1975;3:371–374.

120. Cubeddu LX, Hoffmann IS, Fuenmayor NT, Finn AL. Efficacy of ondansetron (GR38032F) and the role of serotonin in cisplatin-induced nausea and vomiting. N Engl J Med 1990;322: 810–816.

121. Mulvenna PM, Regnard CFB. Subcutaneous ondansetron. Lancet 1992;339:1059.
122. Weksler N, Stav A, Ovadia L, et al. Lidocaine pretreatment effectively decreases incidence of hiccups during methohexitrone administration for dilitation and currettage. Acta Anaesthesiol Scand 1992; 36:772–774.
123. Dunst MN, Margolin K, Horak D. Lidocaine for severe hiccups [Letter]. N Engl J Med 1993; 329:890–891.
124. Cain JS, Amend W. Herpetic esophagitis causing intractable hiccups [Letter]. Ann Intern Med 1993;119:249.
125. Benzon HJ, Prasad YS, Borthwell DA. The value of fluoroscopy before performing a phrenic nerve block. Anesthesiology 1981;55:469–470.
126. Eisele JH, Noble MIM, Katz J, et al. Bilateral phrenic nerve block in man. Technical problems and respiratory effects. Anesthesiology 1972; 37:64–69.

12

The Pharmacologic Approach to Intestinal Gas Syndromes

HARRIS R. CLEARFIELD

The passage of oral or rectal gas is often considered amusing and lends itself easily to jokes, epithets, and a variety of interesting literary uses. One might assume that it is abnormal to belch or pass flatus, yet witness the discomfort of those who cannot belch, such as those individuals with the gas-bloat syndrome that may follow fundoplication surgery for hiatal hernia, or the serious consequences of being unable to pass flatus. The humor probably results from the public display of gas passage rather than the physiologic need. Although gas passage is not only useful but required, symptoms of belching, flatulence, and "gas pains" are commonly encountered in an ambulatory practice. These discomforts may not have prompted medical consultation in the past, but almost any chronic, unexplained distress now tends to trigger cancer fears. The frequency of gas-related symptoms has resulted in a variety of dietary and pharmacologic therapies that have not generally been subjected to scientific scrutiny. Knowledge of the pathophysiology of the various disorders is required in order to plan a treatment program, recognizing the technical difficulties in confidently measuring the ingestion, internal generation, and interactions of the many major and trace gases.

BELCHING

Pathophysiology

Belching brings back atmospheric air that has been swallowed; thus the 80% nitrogen and 20% oxygen composition. Understanding of the sequence of events that lead to belching was aided by the observations of McNally et al. who introduced increasing quantities of air into the stomach and measured the intragastric pressure response (1). A pressure increase of 4–7 mm Hg occurred with instilled volumes of 200–600 ml of air, but no further increase was recorded despite the introduction of 1000 ml of air. This plateau effect requires receptive relaxation of gastric smooth muscle and the striated muscle of the abdominal cavity. The gastroesophageal junction widened when the plateau was reached, thus permitting gas reflux into the esophagus. The esophageal air was emptied back into the stomach by a secondary peristaltic wave.

More recent studies by Kahrilas et al. confirmed the relaxation of the lower esophageal sphincter (LES) prior to belching, thus creating a common gastroesophageal cavity (2). Belching results when the upper esophageal sphincter (UES) also relaxes. The initiating event for UES relaxation was found to relate to esophageal distension rather than LES relaxation. Voluntary belching appears to be initiated by an abrupt increase in intra-abdominal pressure, which leads to increased esophageal pressure and subsequent UES relaxation. It is likely that esophageal reflux of gas occurs frequently in response to normal gastric distension, but the gas is usually returned to the stomach by secondary peristalsis. Gas reflux into the esophagus is more common in the sitting than supine position, possibly because the gastroesophageal junction lies posteriorly and may be occluded by liquid or solid gastric contents when a person is supine.

Management

Occasional belching is a normal and perhaps satisfying event. Witness the patients with upper abdominal discomfort who somewhat wistfully say, "If I could only belch." Some patients believe they are belching excessively, a complaint that is difficult to quantify, while others present with pathologic belching characterized by an extremely loud event that is sure to attract attention.

The common denominator for these complaints is swallowed air. Some patients with organic upper abdominal disorders such as esophagitis, peptic ulcer, or neoplasm may instinctively swallow air with the hope that the belching process will provide relief. Unfortunately, voluntary air swallowing and forced belching leads, paradoxically, to increasing gastric gas accumulation. The new onset of significant belching in an adult should prompt consideration of diagnostic studies, particularly in patients who fail to respond to empiric management.

The approach to aerophagia should include an evaluation of swallowing patterns. Patients with a postnasal discharge or ill-fitting dentures may swallow excessively, accumulating small quantities of gastric air with each swallow. Tense individuals and those who suck on pipes or cigars may swallow more frequently. It is not uncommon to encounter patients who clearly swallow before each eructation but are unaware of the maneuver. Such patients should be counseled about their habit with explanations about the air swallowing/belching interaction, and asked to simply stop swallowing. The results of this approach are variable. Patients with pathologic (loud) belching are usually found to have an emotional disorder and should be treated appropriately.

Diet should be evaluated carefully, since ingestion of carbonated soft drinks or beer is an obvious explanation for gastric distension and belching. Sucking on hard candy and chewing gum lead to excess swallowing and increased gastric gas accumulation. Rapid eating can also result in excess air swallowing.

There are a number of simethicone-containing products advertised for the treatment of gaseousness. Simethicone is a defrothicant that has the capability of altering the surface tension of small air bubbles so that they coalesce into larger bubbles. Although this property of simethicone has been used during upper endoscopic procedures to reduce the frothing that results when air mixes with bile, it is difficult to translate this effect to human symptomatology. There have been few studies that confidently demonstrate any therapeutic effectiveness of simethicone, either alone or in combination with antacids, in patients with belching as a primary complaint.

After dinner mints were originally offered to aid digestion. More recent studies demonstrated that peppermint and other carminatives relax the LES. Any benefit attributable to mints is probably related to the induced postprandial relaxation of the LES, which may permit belching and relief of gastric distension, although the same mechanism might also lead to reflux.

Indigestion has been commonly treated with sodium bicarbonate. A unique complication of this therapy was described by Murdfield in 1926 (3). His patient consumed considerable quantities of beer (6–8 liters were found in his stomach) and then ingested sodium bicarbonate which promptly resulted in severe abdominal pain secondary to gastric perforation. Several additional cases have subsequently been described, prompting the recommendation that sodium bicarbonate not be used for the treatment of acid/peptic disorders (4). Fordtran et al. reported that 1/2 teaspoon of baking soda could result in the release of 475 ml of carbon dioxide as a result of acid neutralization (5). Acute gastric distension is most likely to occur when sodium bicarbonate is taken by an individual with considerable gastric distension and acid who is unable to belch the rapid gas accumulation. The rare but unfortunate sequellae of this therapy are illustrated by the following epitaph found on a gravestone in Burlington, Massachusetts (6):

> Here lies the body of Mary Ann Lowder,
> She burst while drinking a Seidlitz powder,
> Called from the world to her heavenly rest,
> She should have waited till it effervesced.

FLATULENCE

Pathophysiology

The principal gases in flatus are N_2, O_2, CO_2, CH_4, and H_2. Swallowed air provides the N_2 and O_2. The N_2 passes through the gastrointestinal tract, but the O_2 is absorbed and is also metabolized by aerobic colonic bacteria so that O_2 concentration in flatus is low. Fermentation of undigested carbohydrate is a major contributor to flatus volume (7). Carbon dioxide and hydrogen generation increase after meals. If flatulence is excessive and a high concentration of flatus N_2 is present, there is a high likelihood that air swallowing plays a dominant role. N_2 could diffuse from the blood to the gut lumen if the PN_2 was reduced to a point below that of blood because of increased production of other luminal gases.

Gastric acid is neutralized by duodenal and pancreatic bicarbonate, with the release of 22.4 ml of CO_2 for each mEq of acid neutralized. Rather large volumes of CO_2 can be formed in this manner, particularly after meals. The CO_2 is largely absorbed in the mid- to distal ileum, but the clinical implications of this proximal small bowel gas production are uncertain.

Bacterial fermentation of nonabsorbed carbohydrate, classically, beans, results in considerable generation of H_2 and CO_2. Lactase deficiency is another common cause of flatulence, since the unabsorbed lactose is metabolized by bacteria to short-chain fatty acids, CO_2, and H_2. Approximately 14% of H_2 production is absorbed from the small and large bowel and excreted in the breath. The measurement of breath hydrogen concentrations is easily performed and will provide information regarding the presence of small bowel bacterial overgrowth and the presence of lactase deficiency (high breath hydrogen levels after lactose ingestion) (8).

Carbon dioxide, hydrogen, nitrogen, and methane are odorless. Trace gases such as skatole and indole have been assigned the odor responsibility, although several methyl sulfides have also been incriminated (9). Hydrogen and methane are combustible, thus the need to cleanse the bowel thoroughly before endoscopic polypectomy in order to avoid a colonic explosion while passing an electric current through the base of a polyp (10).

Management

Patients may complain of excess gas passages and/or foul odor. Before an extensive investigation is launched, it is often helpful to quantify the number of gas passages per day, since patients have nothing with which to compare their experience. Levitt et al. reported that healthy young males have 13.6 ± 5.6 gas passages per day (11). The patient should be instructed to keep a diary for 3–4 days, listing the time and number of gas passages, the foods ingested, and any discomfort. If their tallies do not exceed the limits listed above, patients may be comforted by the knowledge that they are normal. Appropriate diagnostic studies should be considered if crampy distress or change in bowel habits accompany the gaseousness. Giardiasis, for example, may result in flatulence and diarrhea.

The initial approach to excess flatulence should be the elimination of foods likely to increase colonic gas elimination, such as drinking carbonated beverages, chewing gum, or sucking on hard candies. Foods containing poorly digestible carbohydrates such as brown or lima beans, cabbage, broccoli, and cauliflower may lead to excess colonic gas production. Lactase deficiency can be evaluated by breath hydrogen testing or elimination of milk, ice cream, and cottage cheese. Yogurt and other cheeses contain less lactose. Other sugars, such as sorbitol (found in diet products) and fructose may lead to gaseousness. Another strategy is to pursue an "addition" diet, starting with a small core of foods that produce no problems and gradually adding foods until symptoms occur, in order to identify offending substances.

Pharmacologic measures claiming to control flatus frequency or odor have been poorly documented. There is little convincing evidence to support the claims for simethicone and its ability to reduce the quantity of flatus production (12). Activated charcoal has also received mixed reviews in the few studies evaluating its efficacy (13, 14). The latter may conceivably have some value if odor is the primary complaint. Simethicone and activated charcoal have been combined in one product, but convincing evidence of its value is lacking. If milk-based products are identified as a risk factor but cannot be completely withdrawn, the use of milk and ice cream to which lactase has been added in manufacture or subsequently added by the patient has proven helpful.

ABDOMINAL DISTENSION

Abdominal distension is a common complaint that occurs more often in women, usually becomes more noticeable as the day progresses (most apparent after the evening meal), and is frequently attributed to gaseousness. Many patients, however, do not report increased belching or flatulence. Furthermore, there is no reliable correlation between the total quantity of bowel gas and symptoms of bloating and distension (15, 16). It is often helpful to examine the patient when the distension is noticeable (a late afternoon appointment) and to observe the abdomen with the patient erect. If distension is present, the abdomen should be inspected when the patient is recumbent. If the distension is no longer apparent and the rectus muscles are flaccid, the diagnosis is probably not related to excess intestinal gas. Women who have had one or more pregnancies and men with debilitating illnesses often experience thinning or atrophy of the rectus muscles and hence lack the ability to provide the necessary abdominal support. If the distension is present when the patient is recumbent, the clinician should search for organic disorders such as partial obstruction and ascites.

Management

Many patients who complain of abdominal distension are treated with a variety of anticholinergic and/or sedative medications with their predictable side effects. These medications will be of little assistance if the cause of distension is related to atrophy of the rectus muscles. The prominence of the complaint in the late afternoon and evening is probably due to reflex relaxation of the rectus muscles after meals, with gas ingestion or generation playing a less important role. There is no apparent increase in the total volume of intestinal gas measured in patients with bloating and other functional gastrointestinal symptoms. The patient should be advised to embark upon a strengthening program centering on rectus-tensing exercises, often variations of the standard "sit-up." Older patients and those not interested in a rigorous body-building effort are not likely to benefit from this approach and may have to settle for reassurance and the use of a support garment.

"GAS" PAINS

Crampy abdominal pain is a prominent feature of the irritable bowel syndrome (IBS). The discomfort is found more often in patients with constipation (spastic colon) than those with the diarrhea predominant form. Excess intestinal gas has been offered as the cause for the abdominal pain, but has not been documented (15, 16). Lasser et al. demonstrated that patients with irritable bowel respond to infusion of small amounts of infused air with considerably more discomfort than the same quantity infused into the upper small bowel of normal patients (17). This suggests that the IBS patients have an exaggerated motility response to small amounts of intestinal gas. The following examples of localized gas pain are probably the result of gas-induced bowel spasm.

If there is gas accumulation in the hepatic flexure, the discomfort will be experienced in the right upper quadrant: this has been labeled the hepatic flexure syndrome. The distress is occasionally described as "pressure" pain and may easily be confused with gallstone disease, but is distinguishable from that disorder by the frequency (often daily for months or years) and absence of liver function abnormalities, fever, back radiation, and other signs of inflammation. If the patient has gallstones it is unlikely that cholecystectomy will relieve the pain of the hepatic flexure syndrome, and the recurrence of pain after surgery has been erroneously described as the "postcholecystectomy syndrome."

If there is considerable gas accumulation in the stomach the patient may experience high midline pressure pain that could radiate to the low substernal region. This could simulate angina pectoris, although the frequent occurrence after meals, relief with belching, and lack of relationship to exertion should help to exclude a cardiac etiology.

Gas may accumulate in the splenic flexure and give rise to left upper quadrant discomfort that may radiate to the left chest and also simulate cardiac disease. Relief of symptoms with defecation or passage of flatus plus lack of relationship to exertion should help in distinguishing the distress from ischemic heart disease.

Management

The complaint of persistent abdominal discomfort should prompt appropriate studies to rule out organic disorders. If a functional etiology seems likely, efforts should be made to reduce air swallowing, sucking on hard candies, ingestion of carbonated beverages, eating of gas-forming foods (such as broccoli, cabbage, brown beans, and cauliflower), and ingestion of lactose. An anticholinergic preparation may be tried in an effort to reduce the exaggerated motility response, but sufficient dosage should be used to exert an effect. Anticholinergic therapy should be administered 45–60 minutes before meals in an effort to produce bowel relaxation prior to the food-induced motility and gas production. Unfortunately, older patients may not tolerate this approach and the side effects on the eyes, prostate, and bowel function may be unacceptable.

PNEUMATOSIS CYSTOIDES INTESTINALIS

Pneumatosis cystoides intestinalis is characterized by the presence of gas-filled blebs on the mucosal or serosal surfaces of the small or large bowel. Numerous explanations have been offered and include the possibility of air dissection from the rupture of emphysematous blebs along the aorta to the gut, peptic ulcer disease causing pyloric obstruction leading to the dissection of gastric air into the bowel wall, and mucosal ulcerative disease elsewhere in the intestinal track that permits gas dissection. Some patients are asymptomatic while others experience pneumoperitoneum from serosal bleb rupture or bowel obstruction secondary to compromise of the lumen by large gas-filled blebs.

Management

Asymptomatic blebs do not require specific therapy, although a search for mucosal disease may prove helpful. We have encountered a 23-year-old patient with cystic fibrosis in whom a sigmoid colon obstruction developed from *Pneumotosis coli*. One option was to decompress the blebs by needle aspiration during colonoscopy. We chose to administer 100% oxygen by mask for 4 hours followed by a 30-minute rest, with the cycle repeated for 48 hours. A repeat obstruction series showed complete disappearance of the gas. The pulmonary status worsened with this therapy, but, fortunately, no major decompensation occurred. This approach is predicated on the likelihood that the high concentration of venous oxygen would permit nitrogen in the blebs to diffuse back into the blood. Another option to consider is the use of metronidazole therapy, since anaerobic gas-forming bacteria may gain entrance to the mucosa and generate sufficient hydrogen gas to cause bleb formation (18).

Recently, a report of *P. coli* exacerbated during high-altitude air flight was reported (19). In this instance, lower abdominal cramping and rectal bleeding developed in a young man at cruising altitudes during midflight on a transatlantic crossing. Upon landing in London, the patient was given a barium enema that revealed multiple polypoid lesions involving the right colon which were subsequently identified as submucosal air-filled cysts, which was confirmed on colonoscopic examination. Areas of recent hemorrhage were observed overlying the mucosa of several cysts, which explained the patient's complaint of rectal bleeding. The patient remained entirely asymptomatic at sea level but continued to have recurrence of his symptoms during subsequent transatlantic flights. Although the Federal Aviation Administration mandates that cabin pressures be maintained at or below 10,000 feet, it was surmised that the volume of the colonic cysts varied with changes in cabin pressure, leading to capillary hemorrhage and abdominal pain. It was recommended that this individual avoid high-altitude flying in the future. This recommendation may also benefit other patients with this condition.

REFERENCES

1. McNally EF, Kelly JE, Ingelfinger FJ. Mechanism of belching: effects of gastric distention with air. Gastroenterology 1964;46:254–259.
2. Kahrilas PJ, Dodds WJ, Dent J, Wyman JB, Hogan WJ, Arndorfer RC. Upper esophageal sphincter function during belching. Gastroenterology 1986;91:133–140.
3. Murdfield P. Rupture of the stomach from sodium bicarbonate. JAMA 1926;87:692–693.
4. Mastrangelo MR, Moore EW. Spontaneous rupture of the stomach in a healthy adult man after sodium bicarbonate ingestion. Ann Intern Med 1984; 101:649–650.
5. Fordtran JS, Morawski SG, Santa Ana CA, Rector FC. Gas production after reaction of sodium bicarbonate and hydrochloric acid. Gastroenterology 1984;87:1014–1021.
6. Downs NM, Stonebridge PA. Gastric rupture due to excessive sodium bicarbonate ingestion. Scot Med J 1989;34:534–535.
7. Tomlin J, Lowis C, Read NW. Investigation of normal flatus production in healthy volunteers. Gut 1991;32:665–669.
8. Sciarretta G, Giacobazzi G, Verri A, Zanirato P, Garuti G, Malaguti P. Hydrogen breath test quantification and clinical correlation of lactose malabsorption in adult irritable bowel syndrome and ulcerative colitis. Dig Dis Sci 1984;1098–1104.
9. Levitt MD. Only the nose knows. Gastroenterology 1987;93:1437–1438.
10. Monahan DW, Peluse FE, Goldner F. Combustible colonic gas levels during flexible sigmoidoscopy and colonoscopy. Gastrointest Endosc 1992;38:40–43.
11. Levitt MD, Lasser RB, Schwartz JS, Bond JH. Studies of a flatulent patient. New Engl J Med 1976;295:260–262.
12. Lifschitz CH, Irving CS, Smith EO. Effect of simethicone-containing tablet on colonic gas elimination in breath. Dig Dis Sci 1985;30:426–430.
13. Potter T, Ellis C, Levitt M. Activated charcoal: in vivo and in vitro studies of effect on gas formation. Gastroenterology 1985;88:620–624.
14. Jain NK, Patel VP, Pitchumoni CS. Efficacy of activated charcoal in reducing intestinal gas: a double-blind clinical trial. Am J Gastroenterol 1986;81:532–535.
15. Chami TN, Schuster MM, Bohlman ME, Pulliam TJ, Kamal N, Whitehead WE. A simple radiologic method to estimate the quantity of bowel gas. Am J Gastroenterol 1991;86:599–602.
16. Maxton DG, Martin DF, Whorwell PJ, Godfrey M. Abdominal distension in female patients with irritable bowel syndrome: exploration of possible mechanisms. Gut 1991;32:662–664.
17. Lasser RB, Bond JH, Levitt MD. The role of intestinal gas in functional abdominal pain. New Engl J Med 1975;293:524–526.
18. Gillon J, Tadesse K, Logan RFA, Holt S, Sircus W. Breath hydrogen in pneumatosis cystoides intestinalis. Gut 1979;20:1008–1111.
19. Blosser RA, Esrick M, Lewis JH, Benjamin SB. Pneumatosis exacerbated during high altitude commercial flight [Abstract]. Am J Gastroenterol 1992;87:1352.

INFLAMMATORY, INFECTIOUS, AND OTHER DIARRHEAL SYNDROMES

13

Pharmacotherapy of Inflammatory Bowel Diseases

STEPHEN B. HANAUER and GEERT D'HAENS

Inflammatory bowel diseases (IBD) are generally divided into two defined clinical entities, Crohn's disease and ulcerative colitis, with overlapping epidemiologic, clinical, endoscopic, and pathologic features (1). Both conditions are chronic disorders with remissions and exacerbations. Their differential diagnosis is based upon radiographic, endoscopic, and pathologic criteria and the location of the intestinal inflammation. Crohn's disease can occur anywhere in the gastrointestinal tract, from the mouth to the anal canal, whereas ulcerative colitis is confined to the colon and occasionally associated with some backwash ileitis. Primary differences between the two diseases are the focality and the depth of inflammation: inflammation of Crohn's disease is focal and involves all layers of the intestinal wall, whereas ulcerative colitis is a continuous inflammation mainly limited to the colonic mucosa distal to a variable proximal extent in individual patients. While the present therapy for IBD has been based largely upon serendipitous empiricism and nonspecific approaches to inflammation, the impact of current therapeutic interventions has allowed insight into the mechanisms of the gut immune and inflammatory cascades which will no doubt permit therapies to emerge.

PATHOGENESIS

The pathogenesis of IBD is, in spite of extensive research, still unknown. Therefore, it also is unclear whether Crohn's disease and ulcerative colitis are caused by the same triggering agents or events, and whether both conditions each represent one single disease or a group of entities with similar clinical presentations. As with other organ systems, the gastrointestinal tract appears limited in its ability to react to various injuries.

Many epidemiologic studies have shown familial clustering of IBD (2, 3), suggesting inherited susceptibility, common antigenic exposure, or both. Linkages between histocompatibility antigens and other genetic markers for IBD are currently beginning to be revealed (4).

Increased permeability of the intestine to ethylenediamine tetracetic acid (EDTA) and polyethylene glycol (PEG) has been reported in patients with Crohn's disease and healthy family members (5), although this possible weakening of the tight junctions shown as significant structural abnormalities on electron microscopic examination (6, 7), has not been reproducibly confirmed (8).

The intestinal barrier in ulcerative colitis also appears aberrant because of the lack of colonic mucin species IV (9). Increased mucosal permeability could potentially facilitate intestinal entry of a variety of antigens, possibly primary triggers of the immune response.

Initiation

Although no coherent concept is yet available regarding the pathogenesis of IBD, it is commonly accepted that a variety of antigenic triggers in susceptible individuals may set off a complex, excessive (unbalanced) immune response leading to chronic intestinal inflammation. Exogenous antigens proposed over the years as possible triggers include *Mycobacterium paratuberculosis* (10, 11), endotoxins (12), enterobacterial common antigen (13), cell wall-defective *Pseudomonas*-like bacteria (14), small RNA viruses (15), peptidoglycans from the Gram-positive bacterial cell wall (16), and the bacterial chemotactic peptide formyl-methionyl-leucyl-phenylalanine (FMLP).

Besides exogenous antigens, autoantigenicity has been a postulated explanation for these chronic conditions (18). Recently, the intestinal vascular endothelium has been suggested to be the primary site of a primary vasculitic inflammation leading to secondary mucosal damage (19), possibly secondary to a measles-like virus (20).

Autoimmunity also could be initiated by an exogenous agent whose antigen(s) show molecular mimicry with substances of the intestine, thus causing an ongoing inflammatory response even after elimination of the primary offender. Antineutrophil cytoplasmic antibodies and anticolonic antibodies against Mr 40,000 protein (restricted to colon, biliary tree, and skin) both commonly found in ulcerative colitis, favor the autoimmunity hypothesis (21, 22).

A completely different scenario includes a fundamental deficiency of the immune response or its regulation to an otherwise harmless antigen. There is an increased number of total and activated T cells (measured by HLA-Dr expression) in IBD mucosa, but the ratio of helper to suppressor cells is normal (23). The interleukin 2-producing CD4+ T cell population, to the contrary, was found to be three to four times lower in IBD patients than in controls (24), and, although no abnormalities in T suppressor cells themselves have consistently been shown, suppressor-inducer cells (bearing Leu 3+ 8+ markers) were found to be functionally defective (25). Also, IBD epithelium in vitro failed to induce non-antigen-specific suppressor T cells, which may explain chronic unlimited inflammation (26). In addition, a distinct deficiency of nat-

ural killer cells and large granular lymphocytes in normal and diseased bowel segments was recently described in children with IBD (27).

Activation of the humoral immune system is most likely a secondary phenomenon, reflected by the increased number of plasma cells and B cells in the inflamed epithelium and by the elevated levels of total IgM and IgG, with predominantly IgG1 in ulcerative colitis and IgG2 in Crohn's disease (28, 29).

Psychologic factors, which are not likely to initiate inflammation, may interact with the enteric immune system via a functional relationship with the central nervous and neuroendocrine systems to affect the normal counteraction (homeostasis) in this organ system where (controlled) chronic inflammation is the norm (30).

Amplification

In recent years a large number of mediators that amplify and regulate the inflammatory reaction have been elucidated. These include arachidonic acid-derived molecules (prostaglandins, leucotrienes, and platelet-activating factor), cytokines such as interferons, interleukins, and tumor necrosis factor (TNF), complement-derived products (C3b, C5a, bradykinin), and neuropeptides (23). Although they have impact on many physiologic sequences (vasodilation, increased vascular permeability), studies with specific synthesis inhibitors and competitive receptor antagonists have revealed a significant redundancy and counter-regulation within most immune and inflammatory cascades. Despite the overlap, it is important to understand the contribution of the different pathways and their complex interactions to begin to optimize medical treatment while evolving new therapeutic strategies.

THE ARACHIDONIC ACID PATHWAY

Lipid extracts of colonic mucosa from IBD patients contain significantly more arachidonic acid than mucosal extracts from control subjects (31), and this presence of inflammatory cells correlates with the arachidonic acid composition of phospholipids in colonic mucosa (32). The arachidonic acid cascade consists of two major pathways, giving rise to two groups of inflammatory mediators: cycloxygenase (prostaglandins, thromboxanes) and lipoxygenase products (leucotrienes) (Figure 13.1).

During incubation in vitro, the release of cyclo-oxygenase-derived products by normal intestinal mucosa seems to be much greater than the release of leukotrienes (33). IBD-mucosa, on the contrary, releases large amounts of both cyclo-oxygenase and lipoxygenase products (34), suggesting the presence of endogenous stimuli for leucotriene synthesis or accumulation of cells with high lipoxygenase activity, such as macrophages and neutrophils (35). Increased formation of leukotrienes was confirmed in inflamed tissue from Crohn's disease patients, but not from uninvolved areas (36).

The major products of the lipoxygenase pathway are 5,12-dihydroxyeicosatetraenoic acid (LTB4) and 5-hydroxyeicosatetraenoic acid (5-HETE). LTB4 is the most potent chemotactic agent for neutrophils known in IBD, thus amplifying the inflammatory response. Its concentration in colonic IBD mucosa is up to 50 times higher than in normal mucosa (37). Anti-LTB4 antisera in vitro cause an almost complete blockage of the chemotactic response to IBD-mucosa (38). LTB4 also increases vascular permeability and induces neutrophil aggregation and degranulation (39). However, because it is mainly synthetized by the neutrophils themselves, LTB4 is unlikely to play a significant role in the initiation of the inflammatory response (40).

5-HETE is a less potent chemotactic agent and also induces neutrophil degranulation (40). In rabbit colonic mucosa it was shown to induce chloride secretion (41). The other leukotrienes are called "sulfidoleucotrienes" (LTC4, LTD4, LTE4). They increase the permeability of venules and induce smooth muscle contraction (42).

Whereas lipoxygenase is primarily present in neutrophils and mononuclear cells, cyclo-oxygenase has been identified in all mamma-lian cells (39). Cyclo-oxygenase produces a wide variety of prostaglandins. Their concentration is clearly increased in direct relationship with disease activity in inflamed tissue, feces, rectal dialysate, venous blood, and urine of IBD patients (43, 44). Administration of oral PGE1 and intravenous PGF2α causes watery diarrhea in humans because of increased mucosal secretion of water and electrolytes (45), and correlates with stimulation of adenylate cyclase activity and inhibition sodium-potassium-adenosine triphosphotase activity (46). Many prostanoids, particularly PGE2, produce increased vascular permeability, vasodilation, edema, and fever (47) and may also interfere in the release of toxic free radicals (48).

Nonsteroidal anti-inflammatory drugs (NSAIDs) inhibit cyclo-oxygenase and prostaglandin synthesis. IBD patients often experience deterioration in their symptoms when treated with NSAIDs (49, 50). A possible explanation for this phenomenon is diversion of the arachidonic acid cascade toward lipoxygenase products or an imbalance between prostanoids and leucotrienes (51). It may well be that certain molecules of the prostaglandin family exert a protective rather than harmful effect in the intestine (23, 47).

In Crohn's disease, imbalance of prostacyclin (measured by its stable breakdown product 6-keto PGF1α) and thromboxane, both cyclo-oxygenase products, was shown even in the absence of inflammation (52). F-series prostaglandins and TXA2 generally produce mesenteric vasoconstriction, while E-series and PGI2 (prostacyclin) evoke vasodilation. Thromboxane/prostacyclin imbalance may lead to an altered cytoprotective capacity or reduced suppressor cell activity in Crohn's disease (47), or participate in the chronicity of the inflammatory response (53).

Platelet-activating factor is another lipid inflammatory mediator released by endothelial and inflammatory cells (40). Its concentration is also increased in IBD mucosa (54), leading to direct damage, possibly by inducing ischemic necrosis. Platelet-activating factor enhances the inflammatory cascade via platelet

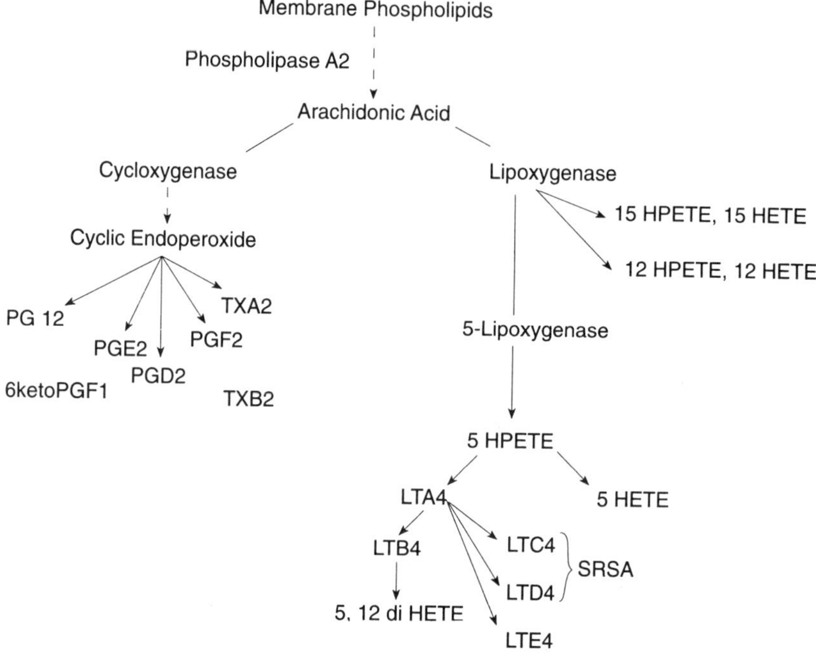

Figure 13.1. Arachidonic acid metabolism. PG, prostaglandin; TX, thromboxane; LT, leucotriene; HPETE, hydroxyperoxyeicosatetraenoic acid; HETE, hydroxy-eicosatetraenoic acid; SRSA, slow-releasing substance of anaphylaxis.

and neutrophil aggregation, degranulation, chemotaxis, and release of other arachidonic acid metabolites.

CYTOKINES

Cytokines are immunoregulatory molecules (polypeptides) produced by monocytes (monokines), lymphocytes (lymphokines), and mast cells. They each regulate specific cellular functions, sometimes acting upon the same cells from which they are secreted (55).

Interleukin-1 (IL-1) is a key molecule in the inflammatory response. It is produced by activated macrophages and colonic mucosa. Inflamed colonic mucosa produces significantly higher quantities of IL-1 than normal mucosa (56), and in Crohn's disease spontaneously enhanced IL-1 production by peripheral blood monocytes was observed (57). IL-1 is able to release neutrophils from the bone marrow, and prostanoids and platelet-activating factor from inflammatory cells

(58). It can cause fever and amplify the proliferative response of T cells via the induction of interleukin-2.

Interleukin-2 (IL-2), mostly produced by CD4+ helper cells, stimulates clonal expansion of effector T cells and proliferation of B cells with antibody synthesis. IL-2 activity was found to be decreased in IBD lamina propria, the concentration of IL-2 producing CD4+ cells being three to four times lower than in control cultures, suggesting that primary abnormalities of the intestinal CD4+ T cell function could play an important role in the immunopathogenesis of IBD (59). Soluble serum IL-2 receptor, exclusively expressed by activated T cells, is elevated in patients with Crohn's disease in accordance with disease activity (60).

Other lymphokines (IL-3, IL-4, IL-5, transforming growth factor β) also stimulate antibody synthesis and proliferation of effector T cells (61).

Interferons have both antiviral and antiproliferative properties and can decrease the number of suppressor T cells, reduce hyper-γ-globulinemia and enhance the defective natural killer activity detected in IBD (40). Interferon may generate its effect through the induction of the enzyme (2'-5')oligo-adenylate synthetase. However, no difference in adenylate cyclase activity could be determined in lamina propria mononuclear cells and epithelial cells from IBD and control tissue (62). Therefore, it appears unlikely that the inflammatory response in IBD is mediated by interferon.

Tumor necrosis factors and transforming growth factors also play an important role in modulating the immune response. In mice with severe graft-vs.-host disease, intestinal involvement and mortality were greatly reduced by the administration of antibodies to tumor necrosis factor (63).

COMPLEMENT ACTIVATION

Primary deficiencies in the complement cascade have never been detected in IBD. Increased catabolism of C3 with elevated levels of C3c has been reported in patients with Crohn's disease (64). C5a was found to be a major chemoattractant agent and, like C3b, also activates the kinin system. Complement factors may contribute to the formation of immune complexes in both the circulation and in inflamed tissue (65).

NEUROPEPTIDES

In colonic tissue from IBD patients, arterioles and venules in all layers express high levels of substance P receptor binding sites (66). The substance P concentrations in ulcerative colitis tissue is twice as high as in normal colonic mucosa (67). Substance P not only induces intestinal secretion of water and electrolytes but also acts as a vasodilator, enhances intestinal peristalsis, and plays an important role in both the efferent central transmission of information and regulation of inflammation (40, 68). Substance K and neuromedin K have a less well-defined function in the inflammatory regulation.

DIRECT IMMUNE-MEDIATED CYTOTOXICITY

Inflamed mucosa of IBD patients contains increased cytotoxic T cell activity (69). Many early experiments have shown this toxicity to be mediated by antibodies (70). Natural killer cytolytic effect is probably unimportant in IBD, since natural killer activity seems to be low in blood and intestinal tissue from IBD patients (71, 72) and natural killer activity induced by IL-2 is also significantly diminished (73). CD3-triggered peripheral blood lymphocytes, on the contrary, have greater cytotoxic activity in IBD patients than in control subjects (74, 75).

NEUTROPHIL-DERIVED OXIDANTS

Activated by a number of proinflammatory stimuli (LTB4, platelet-activating factor), neutrophils produce and release large quantities of reactive oxygen metabolites such as the superoxide anion radical $(O_{2\,-})$ and hydrogen peroxide (H_2O_2) (75). In the presence of certain metals, these will generate the highly cytotoxic hydroxyl radical OH*, which is capable of oxidizing and peroxidizing proteins, carbohydrates, and lipids, and also of altering enzymatic function and membrane permeability. Activated neutrophils and monocytes also secrete myeloperoxidase, catalyzing the oxidation of chloride ions to hypochlorous acid (HOCl), the most cytotoxic agent of the neutrophil.

In addition to injuring the intestinal epithelium, these oxidants also inactivate certain powerful protease inhibitors such as α-1-protease inhibitor and α-2-macroglobulin. The levels of antioxidant enzymes (superoxide dismutase, catalase, glutathion peroxidase) protecting tissues from oxidative aggression are generally lower in colonic mucosa than in other body tissues such as the liver (77).

ANTIINFLAMMATORY AGENTS

Corticosteroids

PHARMACOLOGY

Corticosteroids are the most potent and most widely used agents for the treatment of moderate to severe IBD. They bind with high affinity to an intracellular cytoplasmic steroid receptor that is uniformly present in all human cells (78). A structural change in the receptor steroid complex allows entry into the nucleus, where mRNA polymerase activity is induced for the synthesis of certain proteins (eg, β-receptors, GH, etc.) and suppressed for other proteins (eg, IL-1 and IL-2), finally resulting in an anti-inflammatory effect (79).

Phospholipase activity on arachidonic acid is inhibited (possibly by means of lipomodulin), thus reducing prostaglandin and leukotriene levels (80). The production of the vasoactive substance kinin is also suppressed. Probably the most important effect of steroids consists in a decreased adherence of neutrophils to the vessel wall (demargination) and migration into the site of inflammation (81). Only at very high doses do neutrophilic phagocytosis and intracellular destruction of bacteria seem to be impaired (82).

Lymphopenia is caused by a lymphocytic shift to the bone marrow. The T cells become functionally defective, possibly because of reduced IL-1 production by the monocytes, and the IgA and IgG secretion by B cells is lowered (83). Monocyte bactericidal function and chemotaxis are reduced, with steroid concentrations 30 times lower than those affecting neutrophils (84).

Pharmacokinetics

The oral bioavailability of the classic, nonsynthetic corticosteroids ranges from 50–80%. Once absorbed, 90% of plasma steroids are bound to albumin and, to a lesser degree, transcortin. The pharmacologic effect depends on the free plasma steroid concentration, which is increased in hypoalbuminemia (85). Prednisone and cortisone are converted in the liver to their active forms, prednisolone and hydrocortisone. Although the plasma half-life of steroids is only 1–3 hours, their biologic half-life extends up to 12–36 hours. The plasma half-life is prolonged with oral contraceptives, which raise transcortin levels (86). Elimination occurs by urinary excretion and various metabolic pathways and is increased in asso-

ciation with barbituates and other known stimulants of hepatic enzymes.

Systemic absorption of rectal corticosteroids is somewhat less than that of similar oral doses. Twenty-six percent of rectally administered hydrocortisone is absorbed by a healthy rectum (87). Colonic absorption of prednisolone and methylprednisolone is only 17% and 22% of their oral absorption rates (88, 89). If the colonic mucosa is inflamed, however, up to 50–80% may reach the blood stream (90).

Studies with radio-opaque enemas have shown that they may reach as high as the splenic flexure, especially if the colon is inflamed (91). Topical application of cortisone foam, however, was found only to reach as far as the midsigmoid and, again, higher in patients with active disease (92).

Newer conjugates or synthetic steroids continue to be developed to improve topical anti-inflammatory activity with limited systemic availability and impact on the hypothalamic-pituitary-adrenal axis (79). Topical prednisolone metasulphobenzoate (PMSB) is poorly absorbed compared with conventional steroids (93).

Tixocortol pivalate is a synthetic derivative of cortisol with a low bioavailability (10–20%) because of its high first pass effect in the liver (94). Intestinal absorption is limited, making this substance less suitable for development of oral preparations (95). The receptor affinity is similar to that of hydrocortisone, but much higher doses can be given topically without significant adverse effects.

The glucocorticosteroids with substitution in the 17-α position are beclomethasone diproprionate, budesonide, and fluticasone proprionate. Their glucocorticosteroid effect is at least 100 times higher than that of hydrocortisone, and, because of their high first-pass hepatic metabolism, the pituitary-adrenal axis is less suppressed (79, 95).

Beclomethasone diproprionate is converted by the liver to monoproprionate and further to beclomethasone (96). Budesonide's topical potency is 200 times higher than that of hydrocortisone and 2 times higher than that of

Table 13.1

Agent	Anti-inflammatory effect	Mineralocorticoid effect	Oral bioavailability (%)	Half-time plasma (min)	Half-time biol (hr)	Receptor affinity
Hydrocortisone	1	2+	50–60	90	8–12	1
Prednisolone	4	1+	80	200	12–36	13
Methylprednisolone	5	0	75	180	12–36	13
Dexamethasone	30	0	65–70	100–300	36–54	
Budesonide	200	0	10–15			1000

beclomethasone (97). It is 35% water soluble, which is 100 times more than beclomethasone and fluticasone. Its bioavailability is about 10–20% and the metabolites have 100 times less glucocorticosteroid activity than budesonide itself (79, 98).

Fluticasone proprionate is an α-proprionate with a fluorinated chain in the β-position. It is marked by poor intestinal absorption, low water solubility, and a glucocorticosteroid potency similar to that of budesonide (79, 99) (Table 13.1).

Clinical Use

ULCERATIVE COLITIS

Systemic Therapy. Although many uncontrolled trials reported the benefits of corticosteroids and corticotropin (ACTH) for the treatment of ulcerative colitis, it was not until 1955 that Truelove and Witts convincingly demonstrated the efficacy of these agents in a comparative trial. Cortisone 100 mg/day resulted in 70% vs. 40% success with placebo (100). An even greater benefit was shown with prednisone 40–60 mg/day, with remission rates of 89% vs. 33% in a control group (101).

In dose-ranging studies, 60 mg of prednisone was not more effective than 40 mg/day and produced more side effects. Both doses were superior to 20 mg in achieving clinical remission (102). Once daily oral administration of 40 mg of prednisone was equally as effective as 4 doses of 10 mg (103). This policy became standard for oral outpatient therapy, because it is believed to cause less adrenal suppression. Intensive intravenous corticosteroid treatment of severe colitis (prednisolone

60 mg/day) resulted in improvement or remission within 5 days in more than 60%, with 87% remaining in remission during the next 6 weeks. Remission was more frequently sustained in patients with a first colitis attack or with only distal colonic disease (104).

Despite the benefits of steroid therapy in acute attacks of ulcerative colitis, continuation of treatment has not been found effective in maintaining remission. Controlled trials showed an identical relapse rate with steroids and placebo (105, 106).

Corticotropin (ACTH) 80 U/day intramuscularly and oral cortisone 200 mg/day were found to be equally effective in ulcerative colitis. Patients with a first colitis attack responded somewhat better to ACTH but had a higher relapse rate in the following year (105). Two subsequent trials comparing ACTH with hydrocortisone have demonstrated comparable benefits although there is a suggestion that ACTH may be superior in patients without recent steroid exposure, but is clearly not as effective for patients on steroid therapy (107, 108). In addition, ACTH induces enhanced mineralocorticosteroid side effects and, possibly, adrenal hemorrhage (109).

Oral use of the semisynthetic corticosteroids such as budesonide and fluticasone proprionate is currently under investigation and appears very promising in terms of their lower systemic side effects of these agents (110).

Topical Therapy. Since enemas do not reach beyond the splenic flexure, their primary use in ulcerative colitis is confined to the treatment of left-sided colitis. Topical use of 100

mg hydrocortisone has been effective in 60% of patients after 1 week of treatment, with 72% of patients going into remission within 3 weeks (111). Similar benefits have been shown with prednisolone-21-phosphate enemas (112). In addition, corticosteroid suppositories and foam, which are often better tolerated than enemas, are also clearly more effective than placebo (113, 114), with the foam preparation being better tolerated for proctitis.

The presence of rectal involvement as a constant feature of ulcerative colitis has led to the investigation of novel steroid applications to minimize systemic effects. Prednisolone metasulphobenzoate in 20-mg enemas has been equally as effective as prednisone enemas, with diminished adrenal suppression (115). Tixocortol pivalate enemas, 250 mg, have been as effective as hydrocortisone enemas, 100 mg, over a 3-week period yet have no systemic side effects because of their fast hepatic and extrahepatic biodegradation (116). Higher doses (500–1000 mg) may even be more effective in more resistant colitis (117).

Beclomethasone diproprionate in dosages between 2 and 5 mg/day is as effective as conventional steroids with much lower adrenal suppression than its less lipophilic parent molecule, betamethasone (118).

Budesonide enemas, 2 mg/dl, have been found to be significantly better than prednisolone enemas at 2 weeks but not at 4 weeks. Serum cortisol levels were not influenced (119). No clear dose-response could be defined with 1, 2, and 4 mg.

CROHN'S DISEASE

Systemic Therapy. The National Cooperative Crohn's Disease Study (NCCDS) (120) was the first controlled clinical trial of corticosteroids in patients with Crohn's disease. Sixty per cent of patients with small bowel disease went into remission while receiving prednisone 0.25–0.75 mg/kg, compared with 30% receiving placebo. Colonic disease, perianal disease, and extraintestinal complications, however, were not significantly affected. The European Cooperative Crohn's Disease Study

(ECCDS) (121) for the most part confirmed these findings in 1984 (80% remission vs. 15% for those receiving placebo after 100 days), but showed efficacy of steroids regardless of the site of disease involvement. Neither of these trials was able to prove an additional benefit in combination with sulfasalazine.

Very few data are available on the intravenous use of steroids for active Crohn's disease. In a small series of 49 patients, 76% achieved immediate remission with a combination of intravenous steroids given as outlined by Truelove and Jewell for ulcerative colitis (122), together with antibiotics, parenteral nutrition, and cessation of oral intake (123).

Corticosteroids have not been effective in preventing recurrent disease after bowel resection or as maintenance therapy during remission (124). Although the ECCDS did show some benefit from low doses of 6-methylprednisolone (8 mg/d) in patients who initially responded to treatment of active disease, steroid use cannot be recommended as a maintenance regimen (121).

ACTH and beclomethasone have also been used for Crohn's disease, but were not found to be superior over the commonly used corticosteroids (125). An open trial of fluticasone diproprionate, 20 mg/day, showed a significant reduction in the Crohn's disease activity index (CDAI) from 193 ± 84 to 121 ± 50 and in the labeled leucocyte excretion from 28 ± 21% to 14 ± 7% (126), without changes in serum cortisol levels or response to ACTH. It was concluded that this synthetic corticosteroid was very promising for use with Crohn's disease; however, recent controlled trials have been less optimistic (127). On the other hand, preliminary data with an enteric-coated preparation of budesonide suggest the potential for efficacy without systemic toxicity (110).

Topical Therapy. The rationale for topical therapy for distal colonic Crohn's disease is similar to that for ulcerative colitis. There are no data regarding comparability, however. Nevertheless, the transmural nature of Crohn's disease probably limits efficacy compared with ulcerative colitis.

Adverse Effects

Side effects from corticosteroids depend on the dose and the duration of treatment and can affect almost all organ systems. Short-term side effects include emotional disturbances (euphoria, mania, mood swings, depression, and even psychosis), insomnia and "jitteriness," increased appetite, and fluid and sodium retention (128, 129). Metabolic alterations such as hyperglycemia, potassium depletion, and metabolic alkalosis can occur. Long-term side effects are clinically not as evident, but are often more dangerous and even irreversible. Prednisone dosages <10 mg/day are generally well tolerated, but as a rule no steroid dose should be considered safe in the long run.

Steroid-induced osteoporosis is related to lifetime steroid dose and is often more severe in postmenopausal females (130). Aseptic necrosis of the femoral head occurs in 1% of patients (131). On the other hand, steroid-induced myopathy does not depend on the dose or duration of treatment (132). Ocular side effects consist of cataract formation. Increased intraocular pressure and glaucoma have been reported as well (133, 134).

Metabolic complications include diabetes, hypertension, hypernatremia, and fluid retention. Controversy exists regarding the potential for steroid therapy to accelerate atherogenesis (135) or induce gastric mucosal injury (136). To a certain degree, the normal cellular immunity is inhibited and an increased rate of infections has been reported when high doses are used (137).

The most serious problem in children with IBD is growth retardation, which may be somewhat lessened by alternate-day treatment (138). Steroids seem to inhibit both bone growth and epiphyseal closure. Finally, the hypothalamic-hypophyseal axis can become suppressed after a long period of treatment, making abrupt cessation extremely hazardous (139). The "steroid withdrawal syndrome" includes fever, anorexia, arthralgias, and general weakness (133). Adrenal stimulation tests can be used to assess recovery of the adrenal glands after long-term suppression, but the diagnosis may remain complicated (140).

Steroids during Pregnancy

Corticosteroids cross the placenta by simple diffusion, but fetal adrenal suppression occurs rarely (141). The activity of the inflammatory disease seems to be the key determinant regarding fetal outcome (142). A national survey showed a lower incidence of fetal complications in IBD patients treated with medication, including corticosteroids, than in untreated patients (143). Prednisone is not transferred to the breast milk and complications in breast-fed infants whose mothers were treated with steroids have not been reported (144).

AMINOSALICYLATES

Pharmacology

Topical administration of sulfasalazine (SASP), 5-aminosalicylic acid (5-ASA, mesalamine), and sulfapyridine to patients with distal ulcerative colitis has shown improvement of disease activity with the first two molecules, but not with the last. This strongly suggests that 5-ASA is an active moiety of sulfasalazine (145). Based on the pharmacokinetic properties of SASP and 5-ASA, which include low systemic absorption, the effect appears to be local (146). Sulfapyridine has been shown to reduce bacterial colonization but does not affect inflammation (146, 147).

Numerous immunologic and anti-inflammatory effects of sulfasalazine and 5-ASA have been reported, and as the pathophysiology of IBD is slowly being unraveled, previously unrecognized properties are being detected (148).

In the arachidonic acid pathway, 5-ASA inhibits cyclo-oxygenase and thus lowers prostaglandin levels in IBD patients with active disease (149, 150). Indomethacin and other potent cyclo-oxygenase inhibitors, however, do not exert any beneficial effect at all (151), making it unlikely that mechanism of action is important. Whereas cyclo-oxygenase can be found in almost all mammalian cells, lipoxygenase is only present in inflammatory cells.

5-ASA and SASP inhibit lipoxygenase activity and the synthesis of LTB4 and 5-HETE in inflamed colonic mucosa in concentrations that are easily achieved in the colonic lumen and lower than those required for cyclo-oxygenase inhibition (inhibitory concentration for 50% of the enzyme (IC50) 6 mM vs. 10 mM) (152–154). This is now considered one of the most important ASA effects. In the same cascade, 5-ASA also appears to inhibit platelet-activating factor production in mucosal samples from ulcerative colitis patients (155).

A second possible mechanism is the inhibitory effect of 5-ASAS and SASP on human neutrophil function, including phagocytosis, chemotaxis, degranulation (156), and the binding of FMLP to its receptor on neutrophils (157). This last effect is the only one accomplished with sulfasalazine concentrations that are reached in the serum of treated patients. The same effects have been demonstrated with 5-ASA but higher serum levels seem to be required.

IL-1 production from colonic biopsies is reduced by 5-ASA (158). This may limit T cell proliferation and activation, as well as lymphocyte responsiveness and cytotoxicity (159, 160). In addition, it has recently been shown that 5-ASA inhibits mitogen-stimulated peripheral blood and intestinal mononuclear cell production of IgG, IgM, and IgA (161).

Possibly the most potent mechanism of action by 5-ASA is related to its antioxidant properties, which occur at lower concentrations (IC50: 10–1000 μM) than those required to affect cyclo-oxygenase (IC50: 10,000 μM), lipoxygenase (IC50: 6,000 μM), or neutrophil function (IC50: >5,000 μM) (76, 148). 5-ASA not only causes rapid conversion of superoxide to hydrogen peroxide (H_2O_2) or oxygen (O_2) (IC50: 10–20 μM) (162), but is also very effective in scavenging the hydroxyl radical (IC50: 400–1,000 μM). The latter equally occurs with sulfasalazine and *N*-acetyl-5-ASA (163).

Another effect unique to 5-ASA, which has not been demonstrated with sulfasalazine or *N*-acetyl-5-ASA, is the inhibition of lipid peroxidation because of the scavenging of peroxyl free radicals (IC50: 5–10 μM) (164) and hypochlorous acid (IC50: 25–400 μM). In addition, 5-ASA chelates iron (IC50: 300 μM), thus inhibiting the interaction with superoxide and hydrogen peroxide (165). 5-ASA seems to be selective in protecting α-1-protease inhibitor against this radical (163) and in scavenging hemoprotein-associated oxidants (166).

4-Aminosalicylic acid (PAS, with the amino group in the para instead of the meta position) has been used extensively in the treatment of tuberculosis in doses up to 10–12 g/day without nephrotoxicity (167). It shares some of the anti-inflammatory properties with 5-ASA such as the reduction of FMLP-induced permeability (168), but is a weaker free radical scavenger (169).

PHARMACOKINETICS

Sulfasalazine is composed of 5-aminosalicylic acid (5-ASA, mesalamine) linked to sulfapyridine by an azo bond. After oral ingestion, about 20–30% of the parent drug is absorbed from the upper gastrointestinal tract (170), bound to plasma proteins, and excreted unmetabolized in the bile. Only a small percentage is excreted in the urine (171). Most of the drug is delivered in the distal small bowel and the colon, where colonic bacteria cleave the azo bond to release 5-ASA and sulfapyridine (172, 173). The latter is absorbed from the colon, acetylated by the liver, and excreted in the urine as free sulphonamide or acetyl or glucuronide derivative. The genetically determined acetylator status will hereby affect serum sulfapyridine levels (174).

The 5-ASA fraction is partially absorbed (20–30%), also acetylated by the liver (in a nongenetically determined fashion), and excreted in the urine. Most of the drug, however, will be acetylated by colonic bacteria or within epithelial cells, and excreted in the feces (175).

If mesalamine (5-ASA) is orally administered, it is readily absorbed from the proximal small bowel, acetylated, and primarily excreted as *N*-acetyl-mesalamine in the urine

Table 13.2
Mesalazine (5-ASA) Preparations

Product	Type of release	Preparation	Urinary recovery (%)
Pentasa	Sustained (pH/time)	5-ASA encaptulated in ethylcellulose microgranules	30–55
Asacol	Delayed (pH > 7)	5-ASA coated with Eudragit-S	20–35
Claversal		5-ASA in Na-glycine buffer coated	
Salofalk	Delayed (pH > 6)	with Eudragit-L	25–45
Rowasa	Delayed (pH > 4.5)	5-ASA coated with coteric opadry	60

(146, 176). Once the drug is delivered to the colon, however, absorption is very poor and acetylation is triggered by colonic bacteria. Oral delivery systems therefore require either a carrier molecule like sulfapyridine or appropriate coating to prevent absorption in the proximal small bowel (146, 176).

Balsalazide is such an azo compound, linking mesalamine to the inert carrier aminobenzoyl-β-alanine. It has similar dissolution characteristics to olsalazine (including azoreductase activity) (177, 178).

Olsalazine is an azodisalicylate (Dipentum) composed of two mesalamine molecules linked by the same azo bond that is present in sulfasalazine. Almost no absorption occurs in the small bowel. Once the dimer arrives in the colon, it is broken down by bacteria, a process that can be impaired by accelerated colonic transit or alteration of the normal flora. One olsalazine molecule will thus release twice the molar quantity of 5-ASA (179–181).

Pentasa tablets or capsules are the only form of "sustained-release" 5-ASA, and are microencapsulated in ethylcellulose-coated microgranules (182). The size of the beads and the pH of the environment (>7.5) determine the release rate. Current formulations release approximately 50% of their 5-ASA in the small intestine and the remainder in the colon, unaffected by colonic transit time or resection (183, 184). Pharmacokinetic studies have confirmed greater small bowel delivery than the other 5-ASA preparations, but the absorption and urinary excretion appear to be similar (185).

Asacol is 5-ASA coated with an acrylic-based resin (Eudragit-S) that dissolves at pH 7 (186). Release studies have shown that asacol actually begins to break down in the terminal ileum, since the intestinal pH gradually increases toward the terminal ileum and slightly drops in the cecum because of bacterial fermentation. One 400-mg tablet delivers the same amount of 5-ASA as 1 gm of sulfasalazine. The urinary excretion of 5-ASA in asacol approaches 40% of the administered dose (185, 187).

Salofalk, Claversal, and Mesasal are 5-ASA preparations buffered by sodium carbonate and glycine and coated with Eudragit-L, dissolving at pH levels >6, which is generally in the distal small bowel. Urinary recovery of 5-ASA and acetyl-5-ASA falls within the upper range (35–45%) of that of the other oral 5-ASA preparations (185–188).

Rowasa is yet another pH-release preparation that is currently under investigation (189) (Table 13.2).

Because of its poor solubility and ease of oxidation, topically administered mesalamine requires a wax matrix (suppositories) or addition of antioxidants to enemas and foams (176). Absorption in the distal colon ranges from 20–40% depending on inflammation, retention time, and pH. Acidification of enemas significantly lowers 5-ASA absorption.

4-Aminosalicylic acid is considerably more stable in solution than 5-ASA. Clinical trials have therefore mostly focused on its topical use in ulcerative colitis (167, 190).

Therapeutic Use

ULCERATIVE COLITIS

Oral Use of Sulfasalazine. Since Svartz's 1941 report of 80–90% rate of improvement in patients with active ulcerative colitis, several controlled studies have confirmed the value of sulfasalazine in the first-line treatment of mild to moderate disease (191). Several trials have demonstrated a favorable response in 64–80% of patients treated with sulfasalazine vs. 35–40% in patients treated with placebo (192, 193). Some patients needed as many as 4 weeks of treatment before clinical improvement occurred. Success rates were higher with 6 g than with 4 g/day but the side effects also increased with higher doses. Sulfasalazine therapy is started in low doses, 500 mg twice daily, and gradually increased to 1 g four times daily with food.

For more *severe ulcerative colitis*, systemic steroids are clearly superior to sulfasalazine in success rate and speed of inducing remission (194). No data are available regarding possible additional benefits of sulfasalazine when combined with steroids. In this combination, allergic side effects from sulfasalazine may be masked.

The usefulness of sulfasalazine in the maintenance therapy of quiescent ulcerative colitis has been demonstrated extensively. In a dose of 2 g/day, 70% of treated patients were in remission at 1 year, as compared with 24% with placebo (195). A randomized dose-range study by Azad-Khan et al. in 1980 showed relapse rates of 9%, 14%, and 33% at 1 year with daily doses of 1, 2, and 4 g/day and a side effect frequency related to the dose (196). This has led to the common practice of using 2 gm/day to maintain a state of remission. In case of relapse, this dose can be increased to 4–6 gm/day. No important side effects have been reported with chronic, even lifelong, treatment with sulfasalazine.

Oral Use of Aminosalicylates. The oral 5-ASA formulations have been found to be more effective than placebo and equal to sulfasalazine for mild and moderate ulcerative colitis. Olsalazine (Dipentum) 2–3 g/day (197, 198)

in equivalent amounts of 5-ASA, has been as effective as sulfasalazine.

In comparative European studies, Asacol, at a dose of 800 mg/day, produced similar results to sulfasalazine 2 g/day (199). Subsequent placebo-controlled U.S. studies have suggested a somewhat different dose-response to Asacol in active ulcerative colitis requiring 2.4–4.8 g/day to achieve superiority over placebo (200, 201).

Discrepant results from comparisons with sulfasalazine vs. placebo also have been seen with Salofalk (Claversal and Mesasal) where 1.5 g/day demonstrated improvement comparable to that induced by sulfasalazine 3 g/day in active ulcerative colitis at 8 weeks (202). However, a double-blind trial with placebo 2 and 4 g/day of 5-ASA only showed significant improvement in disease activity with a 4-g dose (203).

Likewise, Pentasa, a sustained-release preparation, has been superior to placebo in inducing remission and clinical improvement in active ulcerative colitis with 2–4 g daily doses (204).

Preliminary studies have been conducted with a coated oral 4-ASA preparation showing promising results. A placebo-controlled trial reported 55% remission with 4 g of coated 4-ASA vs. 5% with placebo. Patients intolerant of sulfasalazine were more likely to respond to 4-ASA (205).

In maintenance therapy of quiescent ulcerative colitis, the aminosalicylates have demonstrated similar efficacy to sulfasalazine with improved tolerance. Olsalazine has been superior to placebo in preventing relapse (77% vs. 55%) at 6 months (206). Asacol 1.6–2.4 g/day is as effective as sulfasalazine 2–4 g/day (22 vs. 20%) (207). Salofalk 750 mg/day compared with sulfasalazine 1.5 g/day (208) and trials comparing equimolar amounts of 5-ASA from Pentasa (1.5 g/day) and sulfasalazine 1 g three times daily (209) showed that both mesalamine preparations provided similar benefit with fewer side effects, even in sulfasalazine-tolerant patients (208).

Mesalamine preparations are superior to placebo and equal to sulfasalazine in the treatment of both active ulcerative colitis and maintenance therapy. They also seem to cause fewer side effects than sulfasalazine, with approximately 80% of patients intolerant of sulfasalazine being able to tolerate an oral, non-linked 5-ASA or olsalazine (210). Although data are limited in comparing the various aminosalicylate formulations in different settings of ulcerative colitis, there may be situations that favor proximal vs. distal release preparations (211). Further comparative studies are necessary to assess the concept of targeted delivery for 5-ASA in ulcerative colitis.

Topical Therapy with Aminosalicylates. Topical mesalamine preparations appear superior to placebo and topical hydrocortisone in the treatment of distal ulcerative colitis (remission 57% with hydrocortisone vs. 93% with 5-ASA) (211, 212). Campieri et al. described 327 courses of treatment in 144 ulcerative colitis patients with 2–4 g of 5-ASA in 100-ml enemas and reported clinical benefit in 88% (213). Of the 44 subjects who did not tolerate sulfasalazine orally, only 5 were unable to tolerate the mesalamine enemas (214). In a subsequent placebo-controlled series, it was shown that the response to mesalamine enemas was not influenced by concurrent treatment with sulfasalazine, and that patients on low doses of steroids did not respond as well as those not treated with steroids (211). A large dose-ranging trial yielded equal efficacy of mesalamine enemas in doses of 1, 2, and 4 g (215). However, the higher dose (4-g) mesalamine enemas appear to be the most effective therapy for patients with "refractory" distal colitis, inducing improvement in up to 75% of patients with disease limited to the left colon, independent of prior therapeutic approaches (216).

In patients with ulcerative colitis limited to the rectum (proctitis), mesalamine suppositories, 200 mg twice daily, were found to be superior to 3 g/day of sulfasalazine at 4 weeks (217). An absent dose-response was also confirmed comparing 500 mg twice vs. three times daily in patients with active proctitis (218).

As with oral aminosalicylate therapy for ulcerative colitis patients with distal disease treated with topical mesalamine (219, 220), maintenance therapy is necessary to prevent relapse. It remains unclear whether oral sulfasalazine or oral aminosalicylate treatment can maintain remissions induced by topical mesalamine (216).

Although more limited than the experience with mesalamine enemas, results with topical 4-ASA appear similar in distal ulcerative colitis (205, 221, 222), although some patients who have not responded to mesalamine have noted clinical benefit on changing to 4-ASA (205).

CROHN'S DISEASE

The benefits of sulfasalazine in active Crohn's disease have been controversial because of discrepancies in dosing, site of disease, and definitions of response.

Oral Therapy with Sulfasalazine. In the National Cooperative Crohn's Disease Study, sulfasalazine (1 g/15 kg) was superior to placebo for a 17-week period in patients with colonic involvement, but ineffective if the disease was confined to the small bowel, and less effective if the patients had been taking corticosteroids before randomization. No additional benefit was obtained from the combination of sulfasalazine and corticosteroids over corticosteroids alone (120). Similarly, the European Cooperative Study confirmed the efficacy of sulfasalazine treatment, 3 g/day, in the presence of colonic disease (58% vs. 42% remission with placebo) (121).

However, smaller studies have reported some benefit in patients with small bowel Crohn's disease (223, 224) and the empiric observations of Goldstein et al. (225) are shared by many clinicians. In clinical trials, low doses of sulfasalazine were found to be ineffective in maintaining remission, regardless of the distribution of the disease (120, 121), and in preventing recurrence after surgical resection, although there may be some maintenance benefit with "high-dose" therapy (226).

Oral Therapy with Aminosalicylates. Several trials have begun to demonstrate benefits of oral mesalamine in Crohn's disease. Salofalk 1.5 g/day provided similar results to sulfasalazine 3 g/day in reducing the Crohn's disease activity index (CDAI) (227). In higher doses of 3 g/day, Salofalk was as effective as a standard prednisone regimen at 12 weeks. However, prednisone reduced the CDAI significantly more rapidly (228). A large multicenter study evaluating Pentasa also showed that higher doses, 4 g/day, were necessary to induce significant reduction in the CDAI, and that 1 g and 2 g/day were ineffective (229). In the prevention of Crohn's disease relapse, mesalamine 500 mg three times daily has been superior to placebo over a 1-year period (relapse rate 22% vs. 36%) (230). The lower relapse rates were especially favorable in patients with isolated ileal disease (8% vs. 31%) and prior bowel resection (14% vs. 47%). Alternative formulations have been beneficial at doses between 2.4 and 3 gm/day (231, 232). Additional studies are needed to determine the role of each mesalamine product, the optimal dose for the various disease patterns, and the use of these agents in maintaining clinical and endoscopic remission.

Topical Therapy with Aminosalicylates. Topical use of 5-ASA suppositories (500 mg three times daily) improved the CDAI in two of four patients with rectal disease (233). No further data on the usefulness of topical treatment are available.

Adverse Effects

The major problem with sulfasalazine treatment is the incidence of side effects, ranging from 10–45% in patients with ulcerative colitis and to 80% in healthy subjects (234, 235). Most of the side effects correlate with serum levels of sulfapyridine and depend on the hepatic acetylator status of the patient (234). Patients who are slow acetylators tend to experience more side effects, with effects gradually increasing to doses up to 4 g/day. Common symptoms are feelings of malaise, nausea, vomiting, headaches, epogastric discomfort, and diarrhea (235–237). The discomfort can sometimes be overcome by gradual titration or reduction of the dose (desensitization), the use of enteric-coated tablets, and administration of the drug with meals (235). The benefit of slowly increasing the dose might consist in the induction of hepatic enzymes for the metabolism of sulfapyridine (238).

Generalized allergic reactions include fever, skin rash, arthralgias, and lymphadenopathy. Megaloblastic anemia due to impaired folic acid absorption (239) and low-grade hemolysis (240) have been noted and are much more common than agranulocytosis, thrombocytopenia, and red cell aplasia (24). Many physicians now routinely add folic acid to sulfasalazine therapy. Other hypersensitivity phenomena may involve almost every organ system. Cutaneous reactions include a maculopapular rash, urticaria, a bluish discoloration of the skin, or most rarely, toxic epidermal necrolysis and Stevens-Johnson syndrome (235, 241). Hepatic manifestations include sulfa-induced cholestasis, allergic or granulomatous hepatitis and, rarely, massive hepatic necrosis (242). Pancreatitis has also been reported (243). Tracheolaryngitis with bronchospasm, eosinophilic pneumonia, and fatal subacute fibrosing alveolitis can occur (244, 245), as well as Raynaud phenomenon, drug-induced lupus, and transient neurotoxicity (246, 247).

Sulfasalazine often causes reduction in sperm counts and sperm motility, most likely because of its antifolate effect (248–250). A clear correlation was found with the patient's acetylation status, with more severe abnormalities occurring in patients who were slow acetylators (251). These effects commonly lead to infertility but are completely reversible within 3 months after withdrawal of the drug (248, 251).

Other complications of sulfasalazine treatment are the development of bloody diarrhea and worsening colitis (252–254). An undefined immunologic hypersensitivity seems to be involved, since this type of reaction can be masked by corticosteroids and, along with other inflammatory complications such as pancreatitis, allergic nephritis, and myocarditis are likely related to the salicylate moiety (210, 255–257).

The safety profile of the other aminosalicylates is still under intensive investigation. Only 20% of patients who do not tolerate sulfasalazine experience similar side effects with 5-ASA (headache, nausea, rash) (210). The major target organ of 5-ASA toxicity seems to be the kidney (256, 258). Interstitial nephritis in animal models, however, only occurred with serum levels ten times higher than the levels attained in humans at therapeutic doses (256). There have been single reports of allergic membranous nephropathy and nephrotic syndrome (257, 258). In patients receiving long-term treatment and high doses, the potential of salicylate-induced nephropathy exists but the frequency has not yet been demonstrated (259). Oligospermia with sulfasalazine is completely reversible when the patient is switched to any other 5-ASA preparation (260).

Diarrhea is a unique side effect of olsalazine and is due to small intestinal (mostly chloride) secretion (258, 261). A healthy colon can absorb the extra fluid, but with colitis, worsening diarrhea is common (206). The problem can generally be overcome by starting with low doses and slowly titrating them upward. Only 6% of patients in controlled trials had to discontinue olsalazine completely because of diarrhea (206, 262). The acute, worsening colitis reported with sulfasalazine has been seen virtually co-occurrently with 5-ASA (263, 264). Finally, single cases of pancreatitis, pneumonitis, and pericarditis have been noted (265–267).

Aminosalicylates Used during Pregnancy

Sulfasalazine and its metabolites cross the placenta but do not appear to exert any harmful effects on the fetus (143, 144). Extensive data about the safety of aminosalicylates during pregnancy are still lacking but, as with sulfasalazine, can also be safely continued during lactation (146, 258, 268, 269).

IMMUNOMODULATORS

6-Mercaptopurine and Azathioprine

PHARMACOLOGY/PHARMACOKINETICS

After a variable intestinal absorption, 50–55% of azathioprine is converted by the hepatocyte into 6-mercaptopurine (6-MP). Azathioprine is metabolized in the liver to mercaptopurine, which is then converted to thioinosinic acid by the enzyme hypoxanthineguanine phosphoribosyltransferase (HGPRT). The latter inhibits several reactions in the de novo purine ribonucleotide synthesis and in the DNA synthesis phase of the cell cycle (270). The most important effect of these drugs may be a depression of natural killer (NK) cell cytotoxicity (81), as it was originally shown in multiple sclerosis (271). This relationship also has been correlated with the clinical response in Crohn's disease (272). Suppressor T cell function also has been found to be affected in transplant patients treated with azathioprine (273).

CLINICAL USE

Ulcerative Colitis

The first therapeutic success with high doses of mercaptopurine (300 mg/day) was reported in 1962 (274). A later double-blind study adding azathioprine or placebo to corticosteroids did not find any different benefit at 1 month (275). However, Caprilli et al. in 1975 showed similar clinical and endoscopic improvement with sulfasalazine and azathioprine over a 3-month period first suggesting a prolonged interval prior to clinical benefit (276).

Subsequent trials have clarified the usefulness of azathioprine and 6-MP as steroid-sparing agents. A University of Chicago trial showed that adding azathioprine 1.5 mg/kg to a conventional steroid regimen permitted reduction of the steroid dose without significantly affecting the disease activity (277), while Kirk and Lennard-Jones, using doses between 2 and 2.5 mg/kg of azathioprine, also showed an additional anti-inflammatory effect with 69% vs. 16% endoscopic improvement (278). In one large, uncontrolled series evaluating the maintenance therapy of ulcerative colitis, 73% of patients responding to 6-MP were reported to remain in remission for ≥2 years, but 77% relapsed when the drug was discontinued after 1 year of remission (279). These results have now been confirmed by a large, controlled trial evaluating azathioprine maintenance therapy (280).

In summary, 6-MP and azathioprine seem to have an important steroid-sparing and, in higher doses, intrinsic anti-inflammatory effect (281). The onset of action for doses between 1 and 2.5 mg/kg is estimated between 3 and 6 months. Long-term maintenance therapy is beneficial to patients who respond.

Crohn's Disease

Neither early short-term trials (2–4 months) nor the NCCDS over a 4-month period showed a significant effect of 6-MP or azathioprine on Crohn's disease activity (120, 282, 283). A preliminary trial including nine patients treated with azathioprine alone for 8–16 months showed that all of them responded, with closure of fistulae and without relapses. These results demonstrated the slow response to the drug, which is now widely recognized (284). In a double-blind crossover study over a 1-year period in New York, 67% of patients who were unresponsive to corticosteroids or sulfasalazine responded to 6-MP, compared with 8% who responded to placebo (285). Of these, 55% had steroids discontinued and another 20% had steroids reduced in the 6-MP group. Improvement or closure of fistulae occurred in 50–86% of the patients (286). Ten per cent had to be withdrawn because of side effects and 32% of patients took 3 months or more to respond (285). These findings confirmed the steroid-sparing effect reported earlier with azathioprine (287).

The value of these drugs in maintaining remission was examined in two controlled trials, which showed 79–95% maintenance of remission at 1 and 3 years with 6-MP or azathioprine vs. 59% with placebo (285, 288). No studies have evaluated the use of azathioprine and 6-MP in the prevention of recurrent disease after surgery or compared the efficacy between the two agents. Because of the conversion of azathioprine to 6-MP, most clinicians have presumed the two are similar (81). It remains to be determined how to evaluate appropriate dosing or whether it is necessary to induce neutropenia in order to obtain maximal clinical benefit (289).

ADVERSE EFFECTS

The most common side effect is bone marrow suppression, which is related to dose and warrants close follow-up of leukocyte and platelet counts (every 2 weeks for the first 3 months, then every month) (290). The dose for initiation of treatment should not exceed 50 mg/day. A hypersensitivity-type pancreatitis occurs in about 3–15% of treated patients and resolves upon withdrawal of therapy (291). Other allergic reactions include fever, skin rash, and arthralgia (290). Nausea, hair loss, peripheral neuropathy, and dose-related hepatotoxicity (both cholestatic and hepatocellular) have been reported (292).

Two long-term complications that still seem to cause great reluctance in using these drugs are the presumed increased incidence of infections and the development of lymphomas. Frequently reported infections include shingles, cytomegalovirus, and pneumonia. In the nontransplant population, however, none of these associations have significantly been demonstrated (290). The single reports of lymphomas concurred with the same incidence observed in the general population (293), despite an increased risk of lymphoproliferative disorders in IBD independent of immunosuppressive therapy (294).

6-MERCAPTOPURINE AND AZATHIOPRINE USE DURING PREGNANCY

Azathioprine crosses the placenta rather poorly. More than 1000 pregnancies have been reported in renal transplant patients and patients with autoimmune diseases who are receiving immunesuppression, and the frequency of birth defects does not seem to exceed that of the general population (295). The same was noted in IBD patients (296, 297). Therefore, treatment with azathioprine or 6-MP, whether the patient is actually taking the drug or discontinued it before pregnancy, is not considered an indication for therapeutic abortion. In patients on a maintenance regimen, the risk of a disease flare-up during the pregnancy should be weighed against the unknown risk of immunomodulators.

Cyclosporine A

PHARMACOLOGY

Cyclosporine A (CyA) is a cyclic undecapeptide extracted from soil fungi and is being used widely in the prevention of transplant organ rejection. It has greatly improved the clinical outcome for transplant patients. Its mechanism of action is a reversible inhibition of the synthesis and/or release of interleukin-2 and interleukin-2 receptors from T helper cells. This results in depression of the helper T cell function and the entire cell-mediated immune response. CyA also lowers the production of B cell activating factors and interferon-γ by T helper cells (298–300).

PHARMACOKINETICS

Because oral CyA is a lipophilic agent stabilized in suspension with olive oil, its intestinal absorption is fairly unpredictable, ranging between 12% and 35%, with a maximum absorption at about 4 hours after ingestion (300). Inflammation as in regional enteritis or after radiotherapy, as well as a shortened bowel length can reduce absorption significantly (301, 302). The intravenous solution is stabilized with alcohol and castor oil. The drug is metabolized by the cytochrome P-450 system in the liver and its metabolites are mainly excreted via the bile. Biliary diversion can thus play a role in drug malabsorption (303, 304). CyA cannot be absorbed by normal or inflamed colon. On the other hand, CyA tissue concentrations in the colon are among the highest in the body (305).

CLINICAL USE

Ulcerative Colitis

In an early series, five patients with severe ulcerative colitis that was unresponsive to corticosteroids all responded to CyA in doses of 10 mg/kg/day after 4–6 weeks (306). In an uncontrolled trial of patients with severe ulcerative colitis, a continuous infusion of CyS A 4 mg/kg/day induced clinical improvement in the majority (307), results that have now been confirmed in a controlled trial of adjunctive CyS A with intravenous steroids (308), with 80% of steroid-unresponsive patients improving with intravenous CyS compared with none of the patients continuing on "intensive" intravenous steroid therapy alone. These data suggest that there may be a place for CyA in the therapy of severe, steroid-resistant ulcerative colitis, since the clinical effect can be seen within 1–2 weeks. However, the long-term benefits still remain to be proven (300).

Topical application of CyA with enemas has been tried for severe proctosigmoiditis, by analogy with the topical use of 5-ASA and steroids. Three uncontrolled studies reported a success rate of 50–75% at 2–4 weeks with maintenance of remission between 38% and 50% after discontinuing the enemas. The different dosages used (250 and 350 mg/day and 1.5 and 5 mg/kg/day) did not correlate with the results (309–311). Recent controlled trials have failed to confirm the uncontrolled experience, however (312).

Crohn's Disease

Of 15 patients with severe Crohn's ileitis and ileocolitis, 10 treated with 5–10 mg/kg of oral CyA for 16 weeks responded within 4 weeks. Of these, 3 remained in remission for more than 1 year (313). A second open-label study administered 4.5–10 mg/kg of oral CyA to 7 patients, of whom 6 responded within 2–4 weeks but 5 relapsed within 1 week of stopping the CyA (314).

In a placebo-controlled trial with 5–7.5 mg/kg of CyA twice a day, 59% of patients treated with CyA responded over a 3-month period compared with 32% who responded with placebo. Side effects did not necessitate withdrawal of treatment in any patient. The outcome did not differ between ileitis or ileocolitis patients. Six months after discontinuing CyA (at 1 year) there was no difference in sustained remission between the two groups (315). The rapid onset of clinical benefit emphasized the potential benefit of CyA over the other immunesuppressive agents, but the therapy may need to be continued in order to sustain remission (316).

CyA has recently also been shown to be useful in the treatment of actively draining fistulas, with an average of about two-thirds initial closure and about 50% sustained closure after discontinuation of cyclosporine (317). Oral doses for this indication are 8–10 mg/kg/day, in some reports preceded by continuous intravenous infusion of 4 mg/kg/day (307, 317).

ADVERSE EFFECTS

The side effects of CyA include neurologic symptoms in 20% (tremor, paresthesias, headaches, confusion, somnolence, depression, and seizures) and hypertrichosis in 50% (nausea and vomiting, hyperglycemia, gynecomastia, and impaired spermatogenesis) (299). Patients with low cholesterol are more susceptible to neurotoxic complications, including seizure (319). Hepatitis and cholestatic liver function abnormalities can be seen. Gingival hyperplasia has been noted in about 2% of patients. The most worrisome side effect is nephrotoxicity and the possibility of permanent kidney damage. The glomerular filtration rate appears to be lowered by about 20% in almost all treated patients, but generally the kidney function returns to baseline after therapy is stopped. Irreversible tubular atrophy and interstitial fibrosis have been found to develop in a few patients (300). Most of these side effects seem to be related to dose. A number of reports have been published on the increased incidence of infections (2%) and of malignant lymphoma (0.3%) (300). Topical applications of CyA, to date, have been very well tolerated without significant toxicity (300). Of note, a few patients have been reported to worsen or develop colitis while receiving CyA (320).

CyA DURING PREGNANCY

A considerable number of transplant patients receiving CyA have gone through successful pregnancies without an increased incidence of fetal abnormalities. At the present time there is insufficient experience, however, to evaluate CyA use during pregnancy in patients with IBD.

The Future

As our comprehension of the etiopathogenesis, immune, and inflammatory events occurring in IBD advances (321), so too will our ability to intervene with rationale medical therapy. Our current ability to observe and describe the multitude of mediators and immunoinflammatory cascades is beginning to open the door to an expanding armamentarium of new (322) and more specific medical approaches which we can expect to improve upon the plight of patients with, as yet, medically incurable IBD (322–325).

REFERENCES

1. Podolsky DK. Inflammatory bowel disease (first of two parts) [Review article]. New Engl J Med 1991; 325:928–937, 1008–1016.
2. Kirsner JB. Inflammatory bowel disease: clinical, etiological and genetic aspects. In: Rotter JI, Samloff I, eds. The genetics and heterogeneity of common gastrointestinal disorders. New York: Academic Press, 1980:261–280.
3. Ortholm M, Munkholm P, Langholz E, et al. Familial occurrence of inflammatory bowel disease. New Engl J Med 1991;324:84–88.
4. Toyoda H, Wang SJ, Yang HY, et al. Distinct associations of HLA Class II genes with inflammatory bowel disease. Gastroenterology 1993; 104:741–748.
5. Ainsworth M, Erikson J, Weever R, et al. Intestinal permeability of Cr-labelled ethylene diaminetetraacetic acid in patients with Crohn's disease and their healthy relatives. Scand J Gastroenterol 1989; 24:993–998.
6. Hollander D. Crohn's disease: a permeability disorder of the tight junction? Gut 1988;29:1621–1624.
7. Madara JL. Loosening tight junctions. J Clin Invest 1989;83:1089–1094.
8. Hollander D. The intestinal permeability barrier: a hypothesis as to its regulation and involvement in Crohn's disease. Scand J Gastroenterol 1992; 27:721–726.
9. Podolsky DK, Fournie DA. Emergence of antigenic glycoprotein structures in ulcerative colitis detected through monoclonal antibodies. Gastroenterology 1988;95:371–378.

10. Chiodini FJ. Crohn's disease and the mycobacter-ioses: a review of comparison of two disease entities. Clin Microb Rev 1990;2:90–117.

11. Kobayashi K, Blaser MJ, Brown WR. Immunohis-tochemical examination for mycobacteria in intestinal tissue from patients with Crohn's disease. Gastroenterology 1989;96:1009–1015.

12. Elson CO. Endotoxin and the mucosal immune response. In: Strober W, Hanson LA, Sell KW, eds. Recent advances in mucosal immunity. New York: Raven Press, 1982:73–80.

13. Bull DM, Ignaczk TF. Enterobacterial common antigen-induced lymphocyte reactivity in inflammatory bowel disease. Gastroenterology 1973;64:43–50.

14. Parent K, Mitchell PD. Bacterial variants: etiologic agent in Crohn's disease? Gastroenterology 1976; 71:365–368.

15. Whorwell PJ, Phillips CA, Beeken WL, et al. Isolation of reovirus-like agents from patients with Crohn's disease. Lancet 1977;1:1169–1171.

16. Sartor RB, Cromartie WJ, Powell DW, Schwab JH. Granulomatous enterocolitis induced in rats by purified bacterial cell wall fragments. Gastroenterology 1990;98:929–935.

17. LeDuc LE, Nast CC. Chemotactic peptide-induced acute colitis in rabbits. Gastroenterology 1990; 98:929–935.

18. Fiocchi C, Farmer RG. Autoimmunity in inflammatory bowel disease. Clin Asp Autoimmun 1987; 1:12–19.

19. Wakefield AJ, Sankey EA, Dhillon AP, et al. Granulomatous vasculitis in Crohn's disease. Gastroenterology 1991;100:1279–1287.

20. Wakefield AJ, Pittilo RM, Sim R, et al. Evidence of persistent measles virus infection in Crohn's disease. J Med Virol 1993;39:345–353.

21. Das KM, Vecchi M, Sakamaki S. A shared and unique epitope(s) on human colon, skin and biliary epithelium detected by a monoclonal antibody. Gastroenterology 1990;98:464–469.

22. Duerr RH, Targan SR, Landers CJ, Sutherland LR, Shanahan F. Anti-neutrophil cytoplasmic antibodies in ulcerative colitis. Gastroenterology 1991;100:1590–1596.

23. Schreiber S, Raedler A, Stenson WF, MacDermott. The role of the mucosal immune system in inflammatory bowel disease. Gastroenterol Clin N Am 1992;21:451–502.

24. Kusugami K, Matsuura T, West GA, Youngman KR, Rachmilewitz D, Fiocchi C. Loss of interleukin-2 producing intestinal CD4+ cells in inflammatory bowel disease. Gastroenterology 1991; 101:1594–1605.

25. Ming RH, Kekahbah EL, Strickland RG. Analysis of peripheral B cell helper and suppressor-inducer function of T cells in patients with Crohn's disease. Gastroenterology 1987;92:1536.

26. Mayer L, Eisenhardt L. Defect in immunoregulatory intestinal epithelial cells in inflammatory bowel disease, current status and future approach. In: MacDermott RP, ed. Excerpta Medica International Congress Series 1988;775:9–16.

27. Hadziselimovic F, Emmons LR, Schaub U. Natural killer cell and large granular lymphocyte deficiency in the gut of children with inflammatory bowel disease. Can J Gastroenterol 1990;4:303–308.

28. MacDermott RP, Nah GS, Bertovich MJ, et al. Alterations of IgM, IgG, and IgA synthesis and secretion by peripheral blood and intestinal mononuclear cells from patients with ulcerative colitis and Crohn's disease. Gastroenterology 1981;81:844–852.

29. MacDermott RP. Alterations in serum immunoglobulin G subclasses in patients with ulcerative colitis and Crohn's disease. Gastroenterology 1989; 96:164–168.

30. Sternberg EM, Chrousos GP, Wilder RL, Gold PW. The stress response and the regulation of inflammatory disease. Ann Intern Med 1992;117:854–866.

31. Pacheco S, Hillier K, Smith C. Increased arachidonic acid levels in phospholipids of human colonic mucosa in inflammatory bowel disease. Clin Sci 1987;73:361–364.

32. Nishida T, Miwa H, Shigematsu A, et al. Increased arachidonic acid composition of phospholipids in colonic mucosa from patients with acute ulcerative colitis. Gut 1987;28:1002–1007.

33. Dreyling KW, Hoppe U, Peskar BA, et al. Leucotriene synthesis by human gastrointestinal tissue. Biochim Biophys Acta 1986;878:184–193.

34. Peskar BM, Dreyling KW, Peskar BA, et al. Enhanced formation of sulfidopeptide-leucotrienes in ulcerative colitis and Crohn's disease: inhibition by sulfasalazine and 5-aminosalicylic acid. Agents Actions 1986;18:381–383.

35. Peskar BM. Inflammatory mediators in inflammatory bowel disease. Can J Gastroenterol 1990;4: 289–294.

36. Dreyling KW, Hoppe U, Peskar BA, et al. Leukotrienes in Crohn's disease: effect of sulfasalazine and 5-aminosalicylic acid. Adv Prostaglandin Thromboxane Leukotriene Res 1987;17:339–343.

37. Sharon P, Stenson WF. Enhanced synthesis of leukotriene B4 by colonic mucosa in inflammatory bowel disease. Gastroenterology 1984;86:453–460.

38. Lobos EA, Sharon P, Stenson WF. Chemotactic activity in inflammatory bowel disease: role of leucotriene B4. Dig Dis Sci 1987;32:1380–1388.

39. Stenson WF. Role of eicosanoids as mediators of inflammation in inflammatory bowel disease. Scand J Gastroenterol 1990;25 (suppl 172):13–18.

40. Rachmilewitz D. Mediators of inflammation and pathogenesis. In: Gitnick G, ed. Inflammatory bowel disease, diagnosis and treatment. New York: Igaku-Shoin, 1990:35–42.

41. Musch MW, et al. Bradykinin stimulated electrolyte secretion in rabbit and guinea pig intestine. J Clin Invest 1983;71:1073–1083.

42. Lewis RA, Austen KF. The biologically active leukotrienes: biosynthesis, metabolism, receptors, functions and pharmacology. J Clin Invest 1984; 73:889–897.

43. Gould SR. Assay of prostaglandin-like substances in faeces and their measurement in ulcerative colitis. Prostaglandins 1976;11:489–497.

44. Gould SR, Brash AR, Connolly ME. Increased prostaglandin production in ulcerative colitis. Lancet 1977;2:98.

45. Matuchansky C, Coutrot S. The role of prostaglandins in the study of intestinal water and electrolyte transport in man. Biomedicine 1978;28:143–148.

46. Rachmilewitz D. Prostaglandins and diarrhea. Gastroenterology 1980;78:1283–1285.

47. Lauritsen K, Laursen LS, Bukhave K, Rask-Madsen J. Inflammatory intermediaries in inflammatory bowel disease. Int J Colorectal Dis 1989;4:75–90.

48. Babbs CF. Oxygen radicals in ulcerative colitis. Free Rad Biol Med 1992;13:169–181.

49. Campieri M, Lanfranchi GA, Bazzochi G, et al. Prostaglandins, indomethacin and ulcerative colitis. Gastroenterology 1980;78:193.

50. Hawkey CJ, Rampton DS. Benaxoprofen in the treatment of active ulcerative colitis. Prostagland Leucotrienes Med 1983;10:405–410.

51. Wallace JL, Keenan CM, Gale D, Shoupe TS. Exacerbation of experimental colitis by nonsteroidal anti-inflammatory drugs is not related to elevated leukotriene B_4 synthesis. Gastroenterology 1992; 102:18–27.

52. Hawkey CJ, Karmeli F, Rachmilewitz D. Imbalance of prostacyclin and thomboxane synthesis in Crohn's disease. Gut 1983;24:881–885.

53. Palestine AG, Nussenblatt RB, Chan CC. Side effects of systemic cyclosporin in patients not undergoing transplantation. Am J Med 1984;77: 652–656.

54. Eliakim R, Karmeli F, Razin E, et al. Role of platelet activating factor in ulcerative colitis. Gastroenterology 1988;95:1167–1173.

55. Fiocchi C. Lymphokines and the intestinal immune response: role in inflammatory bowel disease. Immunol Invest 1989;18:91–102.

56. Cockburn ITR, Krupp P: The risk of neoplasms in patients treated with cyclosporin A. J Autoimmunity 1989;2:723–731.

56. Ligumski M, Simon PL, Karmeli F, et al. Interleukin-1: possible mediator of the inflammatory response in ulcerative colitis. Gastroenterology 1988;94:263.

57. Satsangi J, Wolstencroft RA, Caso J, et al. Interleukin-1 in Crohn's disease. Clin Exp Immunol 1987;67:594–605.

58. Dinarello CA. Interleukin-1. Dig Dis Sci 1988; 33:255–355.

59. Kusugami K, Matsuura T, West GA, et al. Loss of Interleukin-2-producing intestinal CD4+ T cells in inflammatory bowel disease. Gastroenterology 1991;101:1594–1605.

60. Mueller C, Knoflach P, Zielinski CC. T cell activation in Crohn's disease. Gastroenterology 1990; 98:639–646.

61. Grob V, Andus T, Leser HG, Roth M, Scholmerich J. Inflammatory mediators in chronic inflammatory bowel disease. Klin Wochenschr 1991;69:981–987.

62. Rachmilewitz D, Stalnikowitz R, Karmeli F, et al. Role of interferon in the pathogenesis of IBD. In: Rachmilewitz D, ed. Inflammatory bowel disease. The Hague: Martinus Nijhoff, 1987;87–94.

63. Piguet PF, Grau GE, Allet B, Vasailli P. Tumor necrosis factor-cachectin is an effector of skin and gut lesions of the acute phase of graft vs. host disease. J Exp Med 1987;166:1290–1299.

64. Elmgreen J, Berkowicz A, Sorensen H. Hypercatabolism of complement in Crohn's disease: assessment of circulating C3c. Acta Med Scand 1983; 214:403–407.

65. Hodgson HTT, Potter BJ, Jewell DP. Immune complexes in ulcerative colitis and Crohn's disease. Clin Exp Immunol 1977;29:187–196.

66. Mantyk CR, Gates TS, Zimmerman RP, et al. Receptor binding sites for substance P but not substance K or neuromedin K are expressed in high concentrations by arterioles, venules and lymph nodes in surgical specimens obtained from patients with ulcerative colitis and Crohn's disease. Proc Natl Acad Sci USA 1988;85:3235–3239.

67. Goldin E, Karmeli F, Selinger Z, et al. Colonic substance P levels are increased in ulcerative colitis and decreased in chronic severe constipation. Dig Dis Sci 1989;34:754–757.

68. Lembeck F, Holzer P. Substance P as neurogenic mediator of antidromic vasodilation and neurogenic plasma extravasation. Naunyn Schmiedebergs Arch Pharmacol 1979;310:175–183.

69. Shorter RG, Cardoza M, Huizinga KA, et al. Further studies of in vitro cytotoxicity of lymphocytes for colonic epithelial cells. Gastroenterology 1969; 57:30–35.

70. Shorter RG, McGill DB, Bahn RC. Cytotocicity of mononuclear cells for autologous colonic epithelial cells in colonic diseases. Gastroenterology 1984; 86:13–22.

71. Kett K, Rognum TO, Brandtzaeg P. Mucosal subclass distribution of immunoglobulin G-producing cells is different in ulcerative colitis and Crohn's disease of the colon. Gastroenterology 1987;83:919–924.

72. Gibson PR. NK cells, IBD and cancer. Gastroenterology 1986;90:1314–1315.

73. Fiocchi C, Hilfiker ML, Youngman KR, et al. Interleukin-2 activity of human intestinal mucosal mononuclear cells: decreased levels of inflammatory bowel disease. Gastroenterology 1984;86:734–742.

74. Shanahan F, Leman B, Deem R, et al. Enhanced peripheral blood T cell cytotoxicity in inflammatory bowel disease. Gastroenterology 1989;9:55–64.

75. Cantrell M, Prindiville T, Gershwin ME. Auto-antibodies to colonic cells and subcellular fractions in inflammatory bowel disease: do they exist? J Autoimmunity 1990;3:307–320.

76. Yamada T, Grisham MB. Role of neutrophil-derived oxidants in the pathogenesis of intestinal inflammation. Klin Wochenschr 1991;69:988–994.

77. Allgayer H. Clinical relevance of oxygen radicals in inflammatory bowel disease: facts and fashion. Klin Wochenschr 1991;69:1001–1003.

78. Baxter JD. The effects of glucocorticoid therapy. Hosp Prac 1992:111–134.

79. Brattsand RL. Steroid development: a case of enhanced selectivity for the bowel wall. Res Clin Forums 1993;15:17–33.

80. Hawkey CJ, Truelove SC. Effect of prednisolone on prostaglandin synthesis by rectal mucosa in ulcerative colitis, investigation by laminar flow bioassay and radioimmunoassay. Gut 1981;22:190–193.

81. Hawthorne AB, Hawkey CJ. Immunosuppressive drugs in inflammatory bowel disease. Drugs 1989;38:267–288.

82. Stossel TP, Mason RJ, Hartung J, Vaughan M. Quantitative studies of phagocytosis by polymorphonuclear leucocytes: use of emulsions to measure the initial rate of phagocytosis. J Clin Invest 1972; 51:615–624.

83. Cupps TR, Fauci AS: Corticosteroid-mediated immunoregulation in man. Immunol Rev 1982; 65:133–155.

84. Rinehart JJ, Balcerak SP, Sagone AL, Lobuglio AF. Effects of corticosteroids on human monocyte function. J Clin Invest 1974;54:1337–1343.

85. Meikle AW, Weed AJ, Tyler FH. Kinetics and interconversion of prednisolone and prednisone studied with new radioimmunassays. J Clin Endocrinol Metab 1975;41:717–721.

86. Boekenoogen SJ, Szefler SJ, Jusko WJ. Prednisolone disposition and protein binding in oral contraceptive users. J Clin Endocrinol Metab 1983; 56:702–709.

87. Cann PA, Holdsworth CD. Systemic absorption from hydrocortisone foam enema in ulcerative colitis. Lancet 1987;1:922–923.

88. Wood W, Walters G, Matts S. Urinary excretion of prednisolone after intrarectal steroid therapy. Br Med J 1963;2:24–26.

89. Sandbar S, West K. Rectal absorption of radio-active 6-alpha-methyl prednisolone in ulcerative colitis. J Med Liban 1961;4:380–386.

90. Halvoren S, Myren J, Aakvaag A. On the absorption of prednisone and prednisolone disodium phosphate after rectal administration. Scand J Gastroenterol 1969;4:851.

91. Matts S, Gaskell G. Retrograde colonic spread of enemata in ulcerative colitis. Br Med J 1961;2:614–616.

92. Farthing M, Rutland M, Clark M. Retrograde spread of hydrocortisone containing foam given intrarectally in ulcerative colitis. Br Med J 1979; 2:822–824.

93. Hamilton I, Pinder IF, Dickinson RJ, et al. A comparison of prednisolone enemas with low-dose oral prednisolone in the treatment of acute distal ulcerative colitis. Dis Colon Rect 1984;27:701–702.

94. Jumiem JL. Pharmacology of tixocortol pivalate, a glucocorticoid belonging to the 21-thiosteroid family. In: Henry JF, ed. 1st Meeting 21-thiosteroids. Mediators in inflammation: the local response. Montrouge, France: John Libbey Eurotext, 1988: 65–70.

95. Brattsand R. Overview of newer glucocorticosteroid preparations for inflammatory bowel disease. Can J Gastroenterol 1990;4:407–414.

96. Martin LE, Tanner RJN, Clark TJH, Cochrane MB. Absorption and metabolism of orally administered beclomethasone dipropionate. Clin Pharmacol Ther 1974;15:267–275.

97. Axelsson B, Brattsand R, Andersson PH, et al. Relationship between glucocorticosteroid effect of beclomethasone 17-alpha-21-dipropionate, beclomethasone 17-alpha-propionate and beclomethasone as studied in human, mouse and rat tissue. Respiration 1984;46(suppl 1):4.

98. Rutgeerts P. Budesonide enemas for topical therapy of ulcerative colitis. Can J Gastroenterol 1990; 4:415–419.

99. Harding S. Human pharmacology of fluticasone. XIVth congress of the European academy of allergology and clinical immunology. Berlin, Sept 17–22, 1989.

100. Truelove SC, Witts LJ. Cortisone in ulcerative colitis: final report on a therapeutic trial. Br Med J 1955;2:1041–1048.

101. Lennard-Jones JE, Longmore AJ, Newel AC, et al. An assessment of prednisone, salazopyrin and topical hydrocortisone hemisuccinate used as outpatient treatment of ulcerative colitis. Gut 1960;1:217–222.

102. Baron JH, Connell AM, Kanaghinis TG, et al. Outpatient treatment of ulcerative colitis. Br Med J 1967;2:441–443.

103. Powell-Tuck J, Brown RL, Lennard-Jones JE. A comparison of oral prednisolone given as single or multiple daily doses for active proctocolitis. Scand J Gastroenterol 1978;13:833–837.

104. Truelove SC, Lee EG, Willoughby CP, et al. Further experience in the treatment of severe attacks of ulcerative colitis. Lancet 1978;2:1086–1088.

105. Truelove SC, Witts LJ. Cortisone and corticotrophin in ulcerative colitis. Br Med J 1959;1:387–394.

106. Lennard-Jones JE, Misiewicz JJ, Connell AM, et al. Prednisone as maintenance treatment for ulcerative colitis in remission. Lancet 1965;1:188–189.

107. Powell-Tuck J, Buckell NA, Lennard-Jones JE. A controlled comparison of corticotropin and hydro-

cortisone in the treatment of severe proctocolitis. Scand J Gastroenterol 1977;12:971–975.

108. Meyers S, Sachar DB, Goldberg JD, Janowitz HD. Corticotropin versus hydrocortisone in the intravenous treatment of ulcerative colitis: a prospective, randomized, double-blind clinical trial. Gastroenterology 1983;85:351–357.

109. Dunlap SK, Meiselman MS, Breuer RI, Panella JS, Ficho TW, Reid SE Jr. Bilateral adrenal hemorrhage as a complication of intravenous ACTH infusion in two patients with inflammatory bowel disease. Am J Gastroenterol 1989;84:1310–1312.

110. Rutgeerts P, Lofberg R, Malchow H, et al. Budesonide vs. prednisolone for the treatment of active ileocecal Crohn's disease: a European multicenter trial [Abstract]. Gastroenterology 1993;104:A772.

111. Truelove SC. Treatment of ulcerative colitis with local hydrocortisone hemisuccinate sodium: report on a controlled therapeutic trial. Br Med J 1958;2:1072–1077.

112. Matts S. Local treatment of ulcerative colitis with prednisolone-21-phosphate enemata. Lancet 1960; 1:517–519.

113. Lennard-Jones JE, Baron JH, Connell AM, et al. A double-blind controlled trial of prednisolone-21-phosphate suppositories in the treatment of idiopathic proctitis. Gut 1962;3:207–210.

114. Ruddell WSJ, Dickonson RJ, Dixon MF, et al. Treatment of distal ulcerative colitis (proctosigmoiditis) in relapse: comparison of hydrocortisone enemas and rectal hydrocortisone foam. Gut 1980;21:885–889.

115. McIntyre PB, Macrae FA, Berghouse L, et al. Therapeutic benefits from a poorly absorbed prednisolone enema in distal colitis. Gut 1985;26:822–824.

116. Hanauer SB, Kirsner JB, Barrett WE. The treatment of left-sided ulcerative colitis with tixocortol pivalate [Abstract]. Gastroenterology 1986;90; A1449.

117. Mulder CJJ, Tytgat GNJ. Topical corticosteroids in inflammatory bowel disease [Review article]. Aliment Pharmacol Ther 1993;7:125–130.

118. Kumana CR, Meghi M, Seaton T, et al. Beclomethasone dipropionate enemas for treating inflammatory bowel disease without producing Cushing's syndrome or hypothalamic pituitary adrenal suppression. Lancet 1982;1:579–583.

119. Danielsson A, Hellers G, Lyrenas E. A controlled trial of budesonide versus prednisolone retention enemas in active distal ulcerative colitis. Scand J Gastroenterol 1987;22:987–992.

120. Summers RW, Switz DM, Sessions JT, et al. National Cooperative Crohn's Disease Study: results of drug treatment. Gastroenterology 1979;77:847–869.

121. Malchow H, Ewe K, Brandes JW, et al. European Cooperative Crohn's Disease Study (ECCDS): results of drug treatment. Gastroenterology 1984; 86:249–266.

122. Truelove S, Jewell D. Intensive intravenous regimen for severe attacks of ulcerative colitis. Lancet 1974;1:1067–1070.

123. Shepherd H, Barr G, Jewell D. Use of intravenous steroid regimen in the treatment of acute Crohn's disease. J Clin Gastroenterol 1986;8:154–159.

124. Jewell DP, Phil D. Corticosteroids for the management of ulcerative colitis and Crohn's disease. In: Ginsberg AL, ed. Gastroenterology clinics of North America. Philadelphia: Saunders, 1989;18:21–34.

125. Meyers S, Sachar DB. Medical therapy of Crohn's disease. In: Kirsner JB, Shorter R, eds. Inflammatory bowel disease. Ed. 3. Philadelphia: Lea and Febiger, 1988:477–503.

126. Carpani de Kaski M, Hodgson HJ. Fluticasone propionate in inflammatory bowel disease. Can J Gastroenterol 1990;4:417–419.

127. Hawthorne AB, Record CO, Holdsworth CD, et al. Double blind trial of oral fluticasone propionate versus prednisolone in the treatment of active ulcerative colitis. Gut 1993;34:125–128.

128. Dujorne CA, Azarnoff DL. Clinical complications of corticosteroid therapy. Med Clin North Am 1973;57:331–1342.

129. Meyers S. Oral and parenteral corticoids. In: Peppercorn MA, ed. Therapy of inflammatory bowel disease: new medical and surgical approaches. New York: Dekker, 1990:3–34.

130. Compston JE, Judd D, Crawley EO, et al. Osteoporosis in patients with inflammatory bowel disease. Gut 1987;28:410–415.

131. Varil N, Sparberg M. Steroid-related osteonecrosis in inflammatory bowel disease. Gastroenterology 1989;96:62–67.

132. Mandel S. Steroid myopathy: insidious cause of muscle weakness. Postgrad Med 1982;72:207–215.

133. Kusunoki M, Moeslein G, Shoji Y, et al. Steroid complications in patients with ulcerative colitis. Dis Colon Rectum 1992;35:1003–1009.

134. Tripathi RC, Kirschner BS, Kipp M, et al. Corticosteroid treatment for inflammatory bowel disease in pediatric patients increases intraocular pressure. Gastroenterology 1992;102:1957–1961.

135. Nashel DJ. Is atherosclerosis a complication of long-term corticosteroid treatment? Am J Med 1986;80:925–929.

136. Conn HO, Blitzer BL. Non-association of adrenocorticosteroid therapy and peptic ulcer. New Engl J Med 1976;294:473–479.

137. Stuck AE, Minder CE, Frey FJ. Risk of infectious complications in patients taking glucocorticosteroids. Rev Infect Dis 1989;6:954–963.

138. Sadeghi-Nejad A, Senior B. The treatment of ulcerative colitis in children with alternate-day corticosteroids. Pediatrics 1968;43:840–884.

139. Chamberlin P, Meyer WJ. Management of pituitary-adrenal suppression secondary to corticosteroid therapy. Pediatrics 1981;67:245–251.

140. Christy NP. Pituitary-adrenal function during corticosteroid therapy [Editorial]. New Engl J Med 1992;326:266.

141. Murphy BEP, Clark SJ, Donald IR, et al. Conversion of maternal cortisol to cortisone during placental transfer to the human fetus. Am J Obstet Gynecol 1974;118:538–541.

142. Barocco BJ, Korelitz BI. The influence of inflammatory bowel disease and its treatment on pregnancy and fetal outcome. J Clin Gastroenterol 1984;6:211.

143. Mogadam M, Dobbins WC, Korelitz BI, et al. Pregnancy in inflammatory bowel disease: effect of sulfasalazine and corticosteroids on fetal outcome. Gastroenterology 1981;80:72.

144. Darvasi RS. Pregnancy. In: Gitnick, ed. Inflammatory bowel disease, diagnosis and treatment. New York: Igaku-Shoin, 1990:517–522.

145. Azad Khan AK, Piris J, Truelove SC. An experiment to determine the active therapeutic moiety of sulphasalazine. Lancet 1977;2:892–895.

146. Klotz U. Clinical pharmacokinetics of sulfasalazine, its metabolites and other prodrugs of 5-aminosalicylic acid. Clin Pharmacokinet 1985;10:285–302.

147. West B, Lendrum R, Hill MJ, et al. Effects of sulfasalazine (Salazopyrin) on faecal flora in patients with inflammatory bowel disease. Gut 1974;15:960–965.

148. Gaginella TS, Walsh RE. Sulfasalazine: multiplicity of action. Dig Dis Sci 1992;37:801–812.

149. Hoult JRS, Moore PK. Effects of sulfasalazine and its metabolites on prostaglandin synthesis, inactivation and actions on smooth muscle. Br J Pharmacol 1980;68:719–730.

150. Hoult JRS. Pharmacological and biochemical actions of sulfasalazine; section 1: mode of action. Drugs 1986;32:18–26.

151. Rampton DS, Sladen GE. Prostaglandin synthesis inhibitors in ulcerative colitis: flurbiprofen compared with conventional treatment. Prostaglandins 1981;21:417–425.

152. Peskar BM, Dreyling KW, May B, et al. Possible mode of action of 5-aminosalicylic acid. Dig Dis Sci 1987;32:51S–56S.

153. Allgayer H, Stenson WF. A comparison of effects of sulfasalazine and its metabolites on the metabolism of endogenous versus exogenous arachidonic acid. Immunopharmacology 1988;15:39–46.

154. Lauritsen K, Laursen LS, Bukhave K, et al. Effects of topical 5-aminosalicylic acid and prednisolone on prostaglandin E2 and leukotriene B4 levels determined by equilibrium in vivo dialysis of rectum in relapsing ulcerative colitis. Gastroenterology 1986;91:837–844.

155. Eliakim R, Karmeli F, Razin E, et al. Role of platelet activating factor in ulcerative colitis: enhanced production during active disease and inhibition by sulfasalazine and prednisolone. Gastroenterology 1988;95:1167–1173.

156. Molin L, Standahl O. The effect of sulfasalazine and its active components on human polymorphonuclear leukocyte function in relation to ulcerative colitis. Acta Med Scand 1979;206:451–457.

157. Stenson WF, Mehta J, Spilberg J. Sulfasalazine inhibits the binding of formylmethionylleucylphenylalamine (FMLP) to its receptor on human neutrophils. Biochem Pharmacol 1984;33:407–412.

158. Lamming CED, Mahida YR, Hawkey CJ. 5-aminosalicylic acid inhibits interleukin-1-beta production by colonic biopsies in organ culture [Abstract]. Gastroenterology 1989;96:A285.

159. Holdstock G, Chastenay BF, Krawitt EL. Increased prostaglandin producing suppressor cells in inflammatory bowel disease not sensitive to sulfasalazine. Gastroenterology 1981;80:1177.

160. Gibson PR, Jewell DP. Sulphasalazine and derivatives, natural killer activity and ulcerative colitis. Clin Sci 1985;69:177–184.

161. MacDermott RP, Schloemann SR, Bertovich MJ, et al. Inhibition of antibody secretion by 5-aminosalicylic acid. Gastroenterology 1989;96:442–448.

162. Craven PA, Pfanstiel J, Saito R, et al. Actions of sulfasalazine and 5-aminosalicylic acid as reactive oxygen scavengers in the suppression of bile acid-induced increases in colonic epithelial cell loss and proliferative activity. Gastroenterology 1987;92:1998–2008.

163. Aruoma OI, Washil M, Halliwell B, et al. The scavenging of oxidants by sulfasalazine and its metabolites: a possible contribution to their anti-inflammatory effects? Biochem Pharmacol 1987;36:3739–3742.

164. Ahnfelt-Ronne I, Nielsen OH. The anti-inflammatory moiety of sulfasalazine, 5-aminosalicylic acid, is a radical scavenger. Agents Actions 1987;21:191–194.

165. Grisham MB. Effect of 5-aminosalicylic acid on ferrous sulfate-mediated damage to deoxyribose. Biochem Pharmacol 1990;39:2060–2063.

166. von Ritter C, Grisham MB, Granger DN. Sulfasalazine metabolites and dapsone attenuate formylmethionylleucyl-phenylalanine-induced mucosal injury in rat ileum. Gastroenterology 1989;96:811–816.

167. Ginsberg AL, Beck LS, McIntosh TM, et al. Treatment of left-sided ulcerative colitis with 4-aminosalicylic acid enemas. Ann Intern Med 1988;108:195–199.

168. Von Ritter C, Grisham MB, Granger DN. Effect of 5-aminosalicylic acid, 4-ASA, N-acetyl 5-ASA and sulfapyridine on FMET-LEU-PHE induced ileitis in rats [Abstract]. Gastroenterology 1988;94:A624.

169. Nielsen OH, Ahnfeldt-Ronne I. 4-aminosalicylic acid, in contrast to 5-aminosalicylic acid, has no effect on arachidonic acid metabolism in human neutrophils, or on the free radical 1,1-diphenyl-2-picrylhydrazyl. Pharmacol Toxicol 1988;62:223–226.

170. Schroder H, Campbell DES. Absorption, metabolism and excretion of salicylazosulfapyridine in man. Clin Pharmacol Ther 1972;13:539–551.

171. Das KM, Chowdhury JR, Zapp B, et al. Small bowel absorption of sulfasalazine and its hepatic metabolism in human beings, cats and rats. Gastroenterology 1979;77:280–284.

172. Das KM, Eastwood MA, McManus JPA, et al. The role of the colon in the metabolism of salicylazosulfapyridine. Scand J Gastroenterol 1974;9:137–141.

173. Peppercorn MA, Goldman P. The role of intestinal bacteria in the metabolism of salicylazosulfapyridine. J Pharmacol Exp Ther 1972;181:555–562.

174. Das KM, Eastwood MA. Acetylation polymorphism of sulfapyridine in patients with ulcerative colitis and Crohn's disease. Clin Pharmacol Ther 1975;18:514–520.

175. Ireland A, Jewell DP. Mechanism of action of 5-aminosalicylic acid and its derivatives. Clin Sci 1990;78:119–125.

176. Bondesen S, Rasmussen SN, Rask-Madsen J, et al. 5-aminosalicylic acid in the treatment of inflammatory bowel disease. Acta Med Scand 1987;221:227–242.

177. McIntyre PB, Rodrigues CA, Lennard-Jones JE, et al. Balsalazide in the maintenance treatment of patients with ulcerative colitis, a double blind comparison with sulfasalazine. Aliment Pharmacol Ther 1988;2:237–243.

178. Chan RP, Pope DJ, Gilbert AP, et al. Studies of two novel sulfasalazine analogs, ipsalazide and balsalazide. Dig Dis Sci 1093;28:609–615.

179. Van Hogezand RA, Van Hees PAM, Zwanenberg B, et al. Disposition of disodium azodisalicylate in healthy subjects: a possible new drug for inflammatory bowel disease. Gastroenterology 1985;88:717–722.

180. Willoughby CP, Aronson JR, Agback H, et al. Distribution and metabolism in healthy volunteers of disodium azodisalicylate, a possible new drug for ulcerative colitis. Gut 1982;23:1081–1087.

181. Lauritsen K, Hansen J, Ryde M, et al. Colonic azodisalicylate metabolism determined by in vivo dialysis in healthy volunteers and patients with ulcerative colitis. Gastroenterology 1984;86:1496–1500.

182. Rasmussen SN, Bondesen S, Hvidberg EF, et al. 5-aminosalicylic acid in a slow-release preparation: bioavailability, plasma level, and excretion in humans. Gastroenterology 1982;83:1062–1070.

183. Christensen LE, Slot O, Sanchez C, et al. Release of 5-aminosalicylic acid from Pentasa during normal and accelerated intestinal transit time. Br J Clin Pharmacol 1987;23:365–369.

184. Bondesen S, Tage-Jensen U, Jacobsen O, et al. 5-aminosalicylic acid in patients with ileo-rectal anastomosis: a comparison of the fate of sulfasalazine and Pentasa. Eur J Clin Pharmacol 1986;31:23–26.

185. Rijk MCM, van Schaik A, van Tongeren JHM. Disposition of 5-aminosalicylic acid by 5-aminosalicylic acid-delivering compounds. Scand J Gastroenterol 1988;23:107–112.

186. Dew MJ, Ebden P, Kidwai NS, et al. Comparison of the absorption and metabolism of sulfasalazine and acrylic-coated 5-aminosalicylic acid in normal subjects and patients with ulcerative colitis. Br J Clin Pharmacol 1984;17:474–476.

187. Dew MJ, Ryder REJ, Evans N, Evans BK, Rhodes J. Colonic release of 5-aminosalicylic acid from an oral preparation in active ulcreative colitis. Br J Clin Pharmacol 1983;16:185–187.

188. Klotz U, Maier KE, Fischer C, et al. A new slow-release form of 5-aminosalicylic acid for the oral treatment of inflammatory bowel disease: biopharmaceutic and clinical pharmacokinetic characteristics. Arzneimittel forschung 1985;53:636–639.

189. McLeod RS, Cohen Z, Vari BJ, et al. The release profile of a controlled release preparation of 5-aminosalicylic acid (Rowasa I) in humans. Dis Colon Rectum 1990;33:21–25.

190. O'Donnell LJD, Arvind AS, Hoang P, et al. Double blind, controlled trial of 4-aminosalicylic acid and prednisolone enemas in distal ulcerative colitis. Gut 1992;33:947–949.

191. Svartz N. Sulfasalazine II: some notes on the discovery and development of salazopyrin. Am J Gastroenterol 1988;83:497–503.

192. Moertel CG, Bargen JA. A critical analysis of the use of salicylazosulfapyridine in chronic ulcerative colitis. Ann Intern Med 1959;51:879.

193. Dick AP, Grayson MJ, Carpenter RG, et al. Controlled trial of sulphasalazine in the treatment of ulcerative colitis. Gut 1964;5:437.

194. Truelove SC, Watkinson G, Draper G. Comparison of corticosteroids and sulphasalazine treatment in ulcerative colitis. Br Med J 1062;2:1708–1711.

195. Misiewicz JJ, Lennard-Jones JE, Connell AM, et al. Controlled trial of sulphasalazine in maintenance therapy of ulcerative colitis. Lancet 1965;1:185–188.

196. Azad Khan AK, Howes DT, Peres J, et al. Optimum dose of sulphasalazine for maintenance treatment of ulcerative colitis. Gut 1980;21:232–240.

197. Selby WS, Barr GD, Ireland A, et al. Olsalazine in active ulcerative colitis. Br Med J 1985;291:1373–1375.

198. Meyers S, Sachar DB, Present DH, et al. Olsalazine sodium in the treatment of ulcerative colitis among patients intolerant of sulfasalazine. Gastroenterology 1987;93:1255–1262.

199. Riley SA, Mani V, Goodman MJ, et al. Comparison of delayed release 5-ASA (mesalazine) and sulfasalazine in the treatment of mild to moderate ulcerative colitis relapse. Gut 1988;29:669–674.

200. Schroeder KW, Tremaine WJ, Ilstrup DM. Coated oral 5-aminosalicylic acid therapy for mildly to

moderately active ulcerative colitis. New Engl J Med 1987;317:1625–1629.

201. Sninsky CA, Cort DH, Shanahan F, et al. Oral mesalamine (Asacol) for mildly to moderately active ulcerative colitis. Ann Intern Med 1991;115:350–355.

202. Rachmilewitz D. Coated mesalazine (5-aminosalicylic acid) versus sulfasalazine in the treatment of ulcerative colitis: a randomized trial. Br Med J 1989;298:82–86.

203. Sutherland LR, Robinson M, Onstad G, et al. A double-blind, placebo controlled, multicenter study of the efficacy and safety of 5-aminosalicylic acid tablets in the treatment of ulcerative colitis. Can J Gastroenterol 1990;4:463–467.

204. Hanauer SB, Schwartz J, Robinson M, et al. Mesalamine capsules for treatment of active ulcerative colitis: results of a controlled trial. Am J Gastroenterol 1993;88:1188–1197.

205. Ginsberg AL, Davis ND, Nochomovitz LE. Placebo-controlled trial of ulcerative colitis with oral 4-aminosalicylic acid. Gastroenterology 1992;102:448–452.

206. Sandberg-Gertzen H, Jarnerot G, Draaz W. Azodisal sodium in the treatment of ulcerative colitis. Gastroenterology 1986;90:1024–1030.

207. Dew MJ, Harries AD, Evans N, et al. Maintenance of remission in ulcerative colitis with 5-aminosalicylic acid in high doses by mouth. Br Med J 1983;287:23–24.

208. Rutgeerts P. Comparative efficacy of coated oral 5-aminosalicylic acid (Claversal) and sulfasalazine for maintaining remission in ulcerative colitis. Aliment Pharmacol Ther 1989;3:183–191.

209. Mulder CJJ, Tytgat GNJ, Weterman IT, et al. Double-blind comparison of slow-release 5-aminosalicylate and sulfasalazine in remission maintenance in ulcerative colitis. Gastroenterology 1988;95:1449–1453.

210. Rao SS, Cann PA, Holdsworth CD. Clinical experience of the tolerance of mesalazine and olsalazine in patients intolerant to sulphasalazine. Scand J Gastroenterol 1987;22:332–336.

211. Courtney MG, Nunes DP, Bergin CF, et al. Randomized comparison of olsalazine and mesalazine in prevention of relapses in ulcerative colitis. Lancet 1992;339:1279–1281.

212. Campieri M, Lanfranchi GA, Bazzocchi G, et al. Treatment of ulcerative colitis with high-dose 5-aminosalicylic acid enemas. Lancet 1981;2:270–271.

213. Lanfranchi GA, Campieri M, Brignola C, et al. Treatment of ulcerative colitis patients with high-dose 5-ASA enemas: report of 2 years in an outpatient clinic [Abstract]. Gastroenterology 1984;86:1151.

214. Campieri M, Lanfranchi GA, Brignola C, et al. 5-aminosalicylic acid as rectal enemas in ulcerative colitis in patients unable to take sulphasalazine. Lancet 1982;1:403.

215. Campieri M, Gionchetti P, Belluzzi A, et al. Optimum dosage of 5-aminosalicylic acid as rectal enemas in patients with active ulcerative colitis. Gut 1991;32:929–931.

216. Hanauer SB. 5-ASA therapy. Netherland J Med 1989;35(suppl):S11–S20.

217. Van Hees PA, Bakker JH, Van Tongeren JHM. Effect of sulphapyridine, 5-aminosalicylic acid and placebo in patients with idiopathic proctitis: a study to determine the active therapeutic moiety of sulphasalazine. Gut 1980;21:632.

218. Williams CN. Efficacy and tolerance of 5-aminosalicylic acid suppositories in the treatment of ulcerative proctitis: a review of two double-blind, placebo controlled trials. Can J Gastroenterol 1990;4:472–475.

219. Biddle WL, Greenberger NJ, Swan JT, et al. 5-aminosalicylic acid enemas: effective agent in maintaining remission in left-sided ulcerative colitis. Gastroenterology 1988;94:1075–1079.

220. Hanauer SB, Borgen L, Reiss L, Rowasa Study Group. Maintenance treatment of ulcerative proctitis with mesalamine suppositories: results of a multicenter two year controlled trial. Gastroenterology 1992;102:A634.

221. Selby WS, Bennett MK, Jewell DP. Topical treatment of distal ulcerative colitis with 4-aminosalicylic acid enemas. Digestion 1984;29:231–234.

222. Campieri M, Lanfranchi GA, Bertoni F, et al. A double-blind clinical trial to compare the effects of 4-aminosalicylic acid to 5-aminosalicylic acid in topical treatment of ulcerative colitis. Digestion 1984;29:204–208.

223. Van Hees PAM, Van Lier HJJ, Van Elteren PH, et al. Effects of sulphasalazine in patients with active Crohn's disease: a contolled double-blind study. Gut 1981;22:404–409.

224. Rijk MC, van Hogezand RA, van Lier HJ, van Tongeren JH. Sulphasalazine and prednisone compared with sulphasalazine for treating active Crohn's disease. Ann Intern Med 1991;114:445–450.

225. Goldstein F, Farquhar S, Thornton JJ, Abramson J. Favorable effects of sulfasalazine on small bowel Crohn's disease: a long-term study. Am J Gastroenterol 1987;82:848–853.

226. Ewe K, Herfarth C, Malchow H, Jesdinsky HJ. Postoperative recurrence of Crohn's disease in relation to radicality of operation and sulfasalazine prophylaxis: a multicenter trial. Digestion 1989;42:224–232.

227. Maier K, Fruhmorgen P, Bode JC, et al. Erfolgreiche akutbehandlung chronisch-entzundlicher Darmerkrankungen mit oraler 5-aminosalicylsaure. Dtsch Med Wochenschr 1985;10:363–368.

228. Martin F, Sutherland L, Beck IT, et al. Oral 5-ASA versus prednisone in short term treatment of Crohn's disease: a multicenter controlled trial. Can J Gastroenterol 1990;4:452–457.

229. Singleton JW, Hanauer SB, Gitnick GL, et al. Mesalamine capsules for the treatment of active Crohn's disease: results of a 16-week trial. Gastroenterology 1993;104:1293–1301.

230. Thomson ABR. Coated oral 5-aminosalicylic acid versus placebo in maintaining remission of inactive Crohn's disease. Aliment Pharmacol Ther 1990; 4:55–64.

231. Prantera C, Pallone F, Brunetti G, Cottone M, Miglioli M, the Italian IBD Study Group. Oral 5-aminosalicylic acid (Asacol) in the maintenance treatment of Crohn's disease. Gastroenterology 1992;103:363–368.

232. Gendre JP, Mary JY, Florent C, et al. Oral mesalamine (Pentasa) as maintenance treatment in Crohn's disease: a multicenter placebo-controlled study. Gastroenterology 1993;104:435–439.

233. Klotz U, Maier K, Fischer C, et al. Therapeutic efficacy of sulfasalazine and its metabolites in patients with ulcerative colitis and Crohn's disease. New Engl J Med 1980;303:1499–1502.

234. Schroder H, Price-Evans DA. Acetylator phenotype and adverse effects of sulphasalazine in healthy subjects. Gut 1972;13:278–284.

235. Taffet SL, Das KM. Sulfasalazine: adverse effects and desensitization. Dig Dis Sci 1983;28:833–842.

236. Nielsen OH. Sulfasalazine intolerance: a retrospective survey of the reasons for discontinuing treatment with sulfasalazine in patients with chronic inflammatory bowel disease. Scand J Gastroenterol 1982;17:389–393.

237. Das KM, Eastwood MA, McManus JPA, et al. Adverse reactions during salicylazosulfapyridine therapy and the relation with drug metabolism and acetylator phenotype. New Engl J Med 1973;289:491–495.

238. Korelitz BI, Present DH, Rubin PH, et al. Desensitization to sulfasalazine after hypersensitivity reactions in patients with inflammatory bowel disease. J Clin Gastroenterol 1984;6:27.

239. Franklin JL, Rosenberg IH. Impaired folic acid absorption in inflammatory bowel disease: effects of salicylazosulfapyridine (azulfidine). Gastroenterology 1973;64:517–525.

240. Van Hees PAM, Van Elferen LW, Van Rossum JM, et al. Hemolysis during salicylazosulfapyridine therapy. Am Gastroenterol 1978;70:501–505.

241. Davies GE, Palek J. Selective erythroid and megakaryocytic aplasia after sulfasalazine administration. Arch Intern Med 1980;140:1122.

242. Gulley RM, Mirza A, Kelley CE. Hepatotoxicity of salicylazosulfapyridine: a case report and review of the literature. Am J Gastroenterol 1979;72:561–564.

243. Block MB, Genant HK, Kirsner JB. Pancreatitis as an adverse reaction to salicylazosulfapyridine. New Engl J Med 1970;282:380–382.

244. Williams T, Eidus L, Thomas P. Fibrosing alveolitis, bronchiolitis obliterans, and sulfasalazine therapy. Chest 1982;81:766–768.

245. Averbuch M, Halpern Z, Hallak A, Topilsky M, Levo Y. Sulfasalazine pneumonitis. Am J Gastroenterol 1985,80.343–345.

246. Reid J, Holt S, Housley E, et al. Raynaud's phenomenon induced by sulphasalazine. Postgrad Med J 1980;56:106–107.

247. Wallace IW. Neurotoxicity associated with a reaction to sulphasalazine. Practitioner 1970;204:850–851.

248. Toth A. Reversible toxic effect of salicylazosulfapyridine on semen quality. Fertil Steril 1979;31:538.

249. Birnie GG, McLeod TF, Watkinson G. Incidence of sulfasalazine-induced male infertility. Gut 1982; 22:452.

250. Hudson E, Dore C, Sowter C, et al. Sperm size in patients with inflammatory bowel disease on sulfasalazine treatment. Fertil Steril 1982;38:77.

251. Toovey S, Hudson E, Hendrey WF, et al. Sulfasalazine and male infertility: reversibility and possible mechanism. Gut 1981;22:445.

252. Werlin SL, Grand RJ. Bloody diarrhea: a new complication of sulfasalazine. J Pediatr 1978;92:450.

253. Schwartz AG, Targan SR, Saxon A, Weinstein WM. Sulfasalazine-induced exacerbation of ulcerative colitis. New Engl J Med 1982;306:409.

254. Ruppin J, Domschke S. Acute ulcerative colitis: a rare complication of sulfasalazine therapy. Hepatogastroenterology 1984;31:192.

255. Calder IC, Funder CC, Green CR, et al. Nephrotoxic lesions from 5-aminosalicylic acid. Br Med J 1987;1:152–154.

256. Bilyard KG, Joseph EC, Metcalf R. Mesalazine: an overview of key preclinical studies. Scand J Gastroenterol 1990;25(suppl 172):52–55.

257. Novis BH, Korzets Z, Chen P, Bernheim J. Nephrotic syndrome after treatment with 5-aminosalicylic acid. Br Med J 1988;296:1442.

258. Jarnerot G. Newer 5-aminosalicylic based drugs in chronic inflammatory bowel disease. Drugs 1989; 37:73–86.

259. Riley SA, Lloyd DR, Mani V. Tests of renal function in patients with quiescent colitis: effects of drug treatment. Gut 1992;33:1348–1352.

260. Cann PA, Holdworth CD. Reversal of male infertility on changing treatment from sulfasalazine to 5-aminosalicylic acid. Lancet 1984;1:1119.

261. Pamukcu R, Hanauer SB, Chang EB. Effect of disodium azodisalicylate on electrolyte transport in rabbit ileum and colon in vitro: comparison with sulfasalazine and 5-aminosalicylic acid. Gastroenterology 1988;95:975–981.

262. Jewell DP, Ireland A. Controlled trial comparing olsalazine and sulfasalazine for maintenance treatment of ulcerative colitis. Scand J Gastroenterol 1988;23(suppl 148):45–47.

263. Austin CA, Cann PA, Jones TH, et al. Exacerbation of diarrhea and pain in patients treated with 5-aminosalicylic acid for ulcerative colitis. Lancet 1984;1:917–918.

264. Chakraborthy TK, Bhatia D, Heading RC, et al. Salicylate induced exacerbation of ulcerative colitis. Gut 1987;28:613–615.

265. Sachedina B, Saibil F, Cohen LB, Whitley J. Acute pancreatitis due to 5-aminosalicylate. Ann Intern Med 1989;110:490–492.

266. Kristensen KS, Hoegholm A, Bohr L, Friis S. Fatal myocarditis associated with mesalazine. Lancet 1990;1:605.

267. Reinoso MA, Schroeder KW, Pisani RJ. Lung disease associated with orally administered mesalamine for ulcerative colitis. Chest 1992;101:1469–1471.

268. Jarnerot G, Into-Malmberg MB. Sulfasalazine treatment during breast feeding. Scand J Gastroenterol 1979;14:869.

269. Lewis JH, Weingold AB. The use of gastrointestinal drugs during pregnancy and lactation. Am J Gastroenterol 1985;80:912.

270. Elion GB. Biochemistry and pharmacology of purine analogs. FASEB 1967;26:898–904.

271. Shih WWH, Ellison GW, Myers LW, Durkos-Smith D, Fahey JL. Locus of selective depression of human natural killer cells by azathioprine. Clin Immunol Immunopath 1982;23:672–681.

272. Brogan M, Hiserodt J, Olicer M, et al. The effect of 6-mercaptopurine on natural killer cell activities in Crohn's disease. J Clin Immunol 1985;5:204–211.

273. Duclos H, Maillot MC, Kreis H, Galanaud P. T-suppressor function impairment in peripheral blood lymphocytes from transplant patients under azathioprine and corticosteroids. Transplantation 1979;28:437–438.

274. Bean RHD. The treatment of chronic ulcerative colitis with 6-mercaptopurine. Med J Australia 1962;49:592–593.

275. Jewell DP, Truelove SC. Azathioprine in ulcerative colitis: final report on controlled therapeutic trial. Br Med J 1974;4:627–630.

276. Caprilli R, Carratu R, Babbini M. A double-blind comparison of the effectiveness of azathioprine and sulfasalazine in idiopathic proctitis. Am J Dig Dis 1975;20:115–120.

277. Rosenberg JL, Wall AJ, Levin B, Binder HJ, Kirsner JB. A controlled trial of azathioprine in the management of chronic ulcerative colitis. Gastroenterology 1975;69:96–99.

278. Kirk AP, Lennard-Jones JE. Controlled trial of azathioprine in chronic ulcerative colitis. Br Med J 1982;284:1291–1292.

279. Present DH, Chapman ML, Rubin PH. Efficacy of 6-mercaptopurine in refractory ulcerative colitis [Abstract]. Gastroenterology 1988;94:A359.

280. Hawthorne AB, Logan RFA, Hawkey CJ, et al. Randomized controlled trial of azathioprine withdrawal in ulcerative colitis. Br Med J 1992;305:20–22.

281. Hawthorne AB, Hawkey CJ. Immunosuppressive drugs in inflammatory bowel disease: a review of their mechanisms of efficacy and place in therapy. Drugs 1989;38:267–288.

282. Rhodes J, Beck P, Bainton D, Campbell H. Controlled trial of azathioprine in Crohn's disease. Lancet 1971;2:1273–1276.

283. Klein M, Binder HJ, Mitchell M, Aaronson R, Spiro H. Treatments of Crohn's disease with azathioprine: a controlled evaluation. Gastroenterology 1974;66:916–922.

284. Drucker WR, Jeejeeboy KN. Azathioprine: an adjunct to surgical therapy of granulomatous enteritis. Ann Surg 1970;172:618–625.

285. Present DH, Korelitz BI, Wisch N, et al. Treatment of Crohn's disease with 6-mercaptopurine: a long-term randomized double-blind study. New Engl J Med 1980;302:981–987.

286. Korelitz BI, Present DH. Favorable effect of 6-mercaptopurine in fistulas of Crohn's disease. Dig Dis Sci 1985;30:58–64.

287. Rosenberg JL, Levin B, Wall AJ, et al. A controlled trial of azathioprine in Crohn's disease. Am J Dig Dis 1975;20:721–726.

288. O'Donoghue VP, Dawson AM, Powelltuck J, et al. Double-blind withdrawal trial of azathioprine as maintenance treatment for Crohn's disease. Lancet 1978;2:955–957.

289. Korelitz BI. Immunosuppressives. In: Peppercorn MA ed. Therapy of inflammatory bowel disease: new medical and surgical approaches. New York: Dekker, 1990:103–133.

290. Present DH, Meltzer SJ, Krumholz MP, Wolke A, Korelitz BI. 6-mercaptopurine in the management of inflammatory bowel disease: short and long term toxicity. Ann Intern Med 1989;111:641–649.

291. Haber DJ, Meltzer SJ, Present DH, Korelitz BI. Nature and course of pancreatitis caused by 6-mercaptopurine in the treatment of inflammatory bowel disease. Gastroenterology 1986;91:982–986.

292. DePinho RA, Burke CS, Lefkowitch JH. Azathioprine and the liver: evidence favoring idiosyncratic, mixed cholestatic-hepatocellular injury in humans. Gastroenterology 1984;86:162–165.

293. Kinlen LJ. Incidence of cancer in rheumatoid arthritis and other disorders after immunesuppressive treatment. Am J Med 1985;78(suppl A):44–49.

294. Greenstein AJ, Sachar DB, Smith H, et al. A comparison of cancer risk in Crohn's disease and ulcerative colitis. Cancer 1981;48:2742–2745.

295. Hou S. Pregnancy in women with chronic renal disease. New Engl J Med 1985;312:836–839.

296. Goldstein F. Immunosuppressant therapy of inflammatory bowel disease. J Clin Gastroenterol 1987;9:654–658.

297. Alstead EM, Ritchie JK, Lennard-Jones JE, Farthing MJG, Clark ML. Safety of azathioprine in pregnancy in inflammatory bowel disease. Gastroenterology 1990;99:443–446.

298. Schreiber SL. Chemistry and biology of the immunophilins and their immunosuppressive ligands. Science 1991;251:283–287.

299. Kahan BD. Cyclosporin. New Engl J Med 1989; 321:1725–1738.

300. Sandborn WJ, Tremaine WJ. Cyclosporin treatment of inflammatory bowel disease. Mayo Clin Proc 1992;67:981–900.

301. Williams JD, Salaman JR, Griffin PJA, Hillis AN, Ross W, Williams GT. Malabsorption of cyclosporin in renal transplant recipient with Crohn's disease. Lancet 1987;1:914–915.

302. Atkinson K, Britton K, Paull P, et al. Detrimental effect of intestinal disease on absorption of orally administered cyclosporin. Transplant Proc 1983; 15(suppl 1):2446–2449.

303. Venkataramanan R, Burckart GJ, Ptachcinski RJ. Pharmacokinetics and monitoring of cyclosporin following orthotopic liver transplantation. Semin Liv Dis 1985;5:357–368.

304. Drewe J, Beglinger CH, Kissel T. The functional length of the small bowel determines the extent of peroral cyclosporin absorption in man [Abstract]. Gastroenterology 1991;100:A684.

305. Sandborn WJ, Strong RM, Forland SC, Chase RL, Cutler RE. The pharmacokinetics and colonic tissue concentrations of cyclosporin after IV, oral, and enema administration. J Clin Pharmacol 1991; 31:76–80.

306. Bianchi Porro G, Panza E, Petrillo M. Cyclosporin A in acute ulcerative colitis. Ital J Gastroenterol 1987;9:40–41.

307. Lichtiger S, Present DH. Cyclosporin A in the treatment of severe, refractory, ulcerative colitis. Lancet 1990;336:15–19.

308. Lichtiger S, Present DH, Kornbluth A, Hanauer S. Cyclosporin A in the treatment of severe, refractory ulcerative colitis: a double-blinded placebo controlled trial [Abstract]. Gastroenterology 1993; 104:A732.

309. Sandborn WJ, Tremaine WJ, Schroeder KW, Batts KP, Lawson GM. Cyclosporin (CYA) enemas for treatment of treatment-resistant, ulcerative proctosigmoiditis (UPS) [Abstract]. Gastroenterology 1992;102:A690.

310. Brynskov J, Freund L, Thomsen OO, Anderson CB, Rasmussen SN, Binder V. Treatment of refractory ulcerative colitis with cyclosporin enemas. Lancet 1989;1:721–722.

311. Ranzi T, Campanini MC, Velio P, Quarto di Paol F, Bianchi P. Treatment of chronic proctosigmoiditis with cyclosporin enemas [Letter]. Lancet 1989;2:97.

312. Sandborn WJ, Tremaine WJ, Batts KP, Pemberton JH, Phillips SF. Fecal short chain fatty acid (SCFA) concentrations are lower in patients with pouchitis and primary sclerosing cholangitis (PSC) [Abstract]. Gastroenterology 1993;104:A775.

313. Peltekian KM, Williams CN, McDonald AS, Roy PD, Czolpinska E. Open study of cyclosporin in patients with severe active Crohn's disease refractory to conventional therapy. Can J Gastroenterol 1988;2:5–11.

314. Bianchi PA, Mindelli M, Quarto di Palo F, Ranzi T. Cyclosporin for Crohn's disease. Lancet 1984;2:1242–1243.

316. Brynskov J, Freund L, Rasmussen N, et al. Final report on a placebo-controlled, double-blind, randomized, multicentered trial of cyclosporine treatment in active chronic Crohn's disease. Scand J Gastroenterol 1991;26:689–696.

317. Stange EF, Fleig WE, Rehklau E, Ditschuneit H. Cyclosporin A treatment in inflammatory bowel disease. Dig Dis Sci 1989;34:1387–1392.

318. Hanauer SB, Smith MB. Rapid closure of Crohn's disease fistulas with continuous intravenous cyclosporin A. Am J Gastroenterol 1993;88:646–649.

319. DeGroen PC, Aksamit AJ, et al. Central nervous system toxicity after liver transplantation. New Engl J Med 1987;317:861–866.

320. Passfall J, Distler A, Riecken EO, Zeitz M. Development of ulcerative colitis under the immunosuppressive effect of cyclosporine. Clin Invest 1992; 70:611–613.

321. Gibson PR, Pavli P. Pathogenic factors in inflammatory bowel disease, I; ulcerative colitis. Dig Dis 1992;10:17–28.

322. Thomson AW. The spectrum of action of new immunosuppressive drugs. Clin Exp Immunol 1992; 89:170–173.

323. Hodgson HJF. Immunological aspects of inflammatory bowel diseases of the human gut. Special Conference issue. Agents Actions 1992:C27–C31.

324. Hawkey CJ, Mahida YR, Hawthorne AB. Therapeutic interventions in gastrointestinal disease based on an understanding of inflammatory mediators. Special Conference Issue. Agents Actions 1992: C22–C26.

325. Hanauer SB, Stathopoulos G. Risk-benefit assessment of drugs used in the treatment of inflammatory bowel disease. Drug Safety 1991;6:192–219.

326. Hanauer SB. Inflammatory bowel disease revisited: newer drugs. Scand J Gastroenterol 1990;25(suppl 175):97–106.

14

Treatment of Intra-abdominal Infections

GARY L. SIMON and SHERWOOD L. GORBACH

The development of an intra-abdominal infection, secondary to perforation of the gastrointestinal tract, is a common problem in clinical medicine. The diagnosis is entertained in a patient with abdominal pain accompanied by peritoneal signs such as a board-like abdomen, rebound tenderness, and decreased bowel sounds. X-ray films often reveal free air under the diaphragm, although this may not be present in patients whose infections have been localized by the omentum or other structures. The clinical presentation usually does not vary substantially, whether perforation occurs in the stomach or in the colon, but significant differences in the microbiology and subsequent therapeutic approach relate to the site of perforation, as will be discussed below.

NORMAL FLORA OF THE GASTROINTESTINAL TRACT

The normal gastrointestinal microflora is made up of more than 400 different bacterial species (1, 2). These organisms are not randomly distributed throughout the gastrointestinal tract, but rather reside in specific ecologic niches. The flora of the stomach and proximal small intestine differs significantly from that found in the terminal ileum and colon.

Many bacteria are destroyed on contact with gastric acid. Microbiologic analysis of gastric fluid from individuals who produce normal amounts of gastric acid reveals that nearly 50% are sterile (1). Among the remaining subjects, the bacterial population is rather sparse, consisting of Gram-positive, facultative forms. The predominant organisms are *Streptococcus, Staphylococcus, Lactobacillus,* and *Candida.* In contrast, the bacterial population of the colon represents an enormously complex and well-populated ecosystem (1, 2). Bacterial concentrations in excess of 10^{12}/ml are encountered. Anaerobic bacteria outnumber aerobic/facultative bacteria by a ratio of more than 1000 to 1. The most frequently isolated anaerobic micro-organisms are *Bacteroides, Bifidobacterium* and *Eubacterium, Peptostreptococcus,* and *Clostridium.* Aerobic isolates include various species of *Enterobacteriaceae, Enterococcus,* and *Streptococcus.* Within the small intestine there is a gradual transition from the sparse Gram-positive microflora of the stomach to the more luxuriant Gram-negative populations of the colon. It is in the distal ileum that Gram-negative species begin to outnumber Gram-positive organisms.

Leakage of intraluminal contents into the intestinal cavity may be attributable to a traumatic injury, surgery, or other pathologic process. Traumatic injuries commonly involve knives, guns, and motor vehicles. Postoperative infections related to the surgeon's scalpel may occur, and the importance of antibiotic prophylaxis in this setting should not be overlooked (3, 4). Pathologic processes that lead to bowel perforation include cancer, diverticulitis, appendicitis, cholecystitis, ulcer disease, ischemic necrosis, and inflammatory bowel disease.

The microbiology of an intra-abdominal infection that results from a perforated viscus will depend upon the microflora of the involved segment of bowel. Thus, in patients who perforate a gastric ulcer an abscess may develop with predominantly facultative Gram-positive bacteria (5, 6). Since *Candida albicans* is frequently found in the stomach, it is not surprising that such patients may have intra-abdominal infection due to this microorganism (6). Anaerobic bacteria such as *Bacteroides fragilis* and facultative Gram-negative bacilli are more likely to be found in patients with intra-abdominal infection following a colonic perforation.

ANIMAL MODEL OF INTRA-ABDOMINAL SEPSIS

An animal model of intra-abdominal sepsis has been developed that mimics many aspects of the human disease (7, 8). Laboratory rats are surgically implanted with gelatin capsules containing pooled fecal contents in a slurry with 10% barium sulfate. The gelatin capsules dissolve and the animal is subjected to free-flowing feces within the peritoneal cavity reminiscent of a patient who undergoes a barium enema and suffers a perforation.

The animals develop a two-phase illness characterized by an early stage of peritonitis and sepsis with a 40% mortality rate, and a late phase associated with intraperitoneal abscess formation. Microbiologic analyses of these two phases have shown that the early stage is attributable to facultative coliform bacteria, whereas the latter stage is due to anaerobic bacteria, in particular *B. fragilis.*

The role of aerobic/facultative and anaerobic bacteria in this process has been further characterized by utilizing antimicrobial probes (9). Antibiotics that were effective against facultative coliforms prevented the early phase of peritonitis and septic shock, but, lacking activity against anaerobic species, they did not prevent abscess formation. Similarly, administration of drugs with good antimicrobial activity against anaerobic microorganisms could prevent intraperitoneal abscess formation, but did not affect the early mortality caused by sepsis.

HUMAN INFECTION

The microbiology of intra-abdominal infection resulting from leakage of intraluminal contents has been well defined (10–13). Like the animal model, it is a mixed infection with both aerobic/facultative and anaerobic microorganisms. Among the aerobic/facultative bacteria, *Escherichia coli* is the leading isolate. Other Gram-negative organisms such as *Klebsiella, Enterobacter, Proteus,* and *Pseudomonas* are frequently present. *Streptococcus, Enterococcus,* and *Staphylococcus* are also found. *B. fragilis* is the most frequently identified anaerobic component of these infections. Other anaerobic organisms include *Clostridium,* other *Bacteroides* species, *Fusobacterium,* and *Peptostreptococcus.*

TREATMENT OF INTRA-ABDOMINAL INFECTION: THE ROLE OF ANTIBIOTICS

The role of anaerobic bacteria in the development of human intraperitoneal infection was illustrated in a study published in 1973 in which a conventional antibiotic regimen (cephalothin and kanamycin) was compared with a regimen employing an antibiotic with activity against anaerobic bacteria (clindamycin) (14). Among patients who had undergone abdominal trauma with spillage of intraluminal contents, 52 received cephalothin and kanamycin, whereas 48 were treated with clindamycin and kanamycin. There were 14 failures in the cephalothin group; 11 of these were attributed to anaerobic bacteria. There were 5 failures in the clindamycin group, of which only 1 involved anaerobic bacteria. These results were statistically significant and demonstrated the necessity of treating patients with drugs that have activity against the anaerobic components of the intestinal microflora.

These findings have been confirmed in other studies in which treatment failures occurred when β-lactam antibiotics with limited activity against anaerobic bacteria were used in the treatment of intra-abdominal infections (Table 14.1). For example, cefamandole, cefotaxime, and cefoperazone are β-lactam antibiotics that have poor activity against many *Bacteroides* species. Neither cefamandole nor

Table 14.1
Treatment of Intra-abdominal Sepsis Comparison of Regimens with Good or Poor Antierobic Activity

Study	Drugs with poor antianaerobic activity	Failure rate (%)	Drugs with good antiaerobic activity	Failure rate (%)
Thadepalli et al. (14)	Cephalothin/kanamycin	27	Clindamycin/kanamycin	10
	Cefamandole	23		
Berne et al. (18)	Cefoperazone	14	Clindamycin/gentamicin	2.5
			Cefoxitin	6
Gentry et al. (16)	Cefamandole	20	Ticarcillin/tobramycin	10
			Clindamycin/tobramycin	20
Jones et al. (15)	Cefamandole	32	Cefoxitin	13
	Cefotaxime	18		
Lau et al. (20)	Cefoperazone	16	Moxalactam	6
	Cefamandole	20		
Baird (17)	Cefoperazone	10	Clindamycin/gentamicin	0

cefoperazone were effective in preventing abscess formation in the treatment of patients with bacterial peritonitis secondary to penetrating abdominal trauma (15, 16). Similarly, poor results were noted in patients with acute appendicitis who received cefamandole or cefoperazone alone (17–20).

Another study illustrating this point was published by Jones and coworkers, who compared the administration of cefamandole, cefoxitin, and the combination of clindamycin and tobramycin in a group of patients who had suffered penetrating intra-abdominal trauma (15). Considering only those patients who sustained colonic injuries, the infection rates for clindamycin/tobramycin were 33%; for cefamandole 62%; and for cefoxitin 19%. These differences were statistically significant. In an analogous study of patients with acute appendicitis, the infection rates were as follows: cefamandole 23%, cefoperazone 14%, and clindamycin/gentamicin 2.5% (17).

The gynecologic counterpart to intra-abdominal sepsis is postcesarean endomyometritis. The bacteriology is similar and the treatment regimens that are employed are often identical. A well-done study by diZerega and coworkers illustrates the necessity of utilizing antibiotics with good anaerobic activity (21). In this study of 200 patients comparing penicillin and gentamicin with clindamycin and gentamicin, there was a significantly higher failure rate among the penicillin-gen-

tamicin recipients (29%) compared with those receiving clindamycin-gentamicin (5%, $P <$ .001).

Similar findings were noted in a comparative study of cefazolin and clindamycin/gentamicin given as prophylactic regimens for patients undergoing cesarean section (22). There were eight infections noted among 51 patients receiving cefazolin (a drug with poor activity against many abdominal anaerobic bacteria), whereas no infections were seen in 54 patients receiving the combination regimen.

A microbiologic correlation with these clinical findings was noted by a Snydman et al. who found that postpartum women with endomyometritis that did not respond to administration of penicillin or ampicillin were often infected with *Prevotella* (formerly *Bacteroides*) *bivia* or *disiens*, organisms that contain a β-lactamase that renders them resistant to penacillins (23).

Antianaerobic Antibiotics

A number of antibiotics have activity against anaerobic pathogens. Clindamycin, metronidazole, and chloramphenicol are all quite active against most anaerobic pathogens, including *B. fragilis*. The excellent anaerobic activity profile of both clindamycin and metronidazole has been well-documented in numerous clinical trials (14, 17, 24–29). Indeed, the combination of clindamycin (or metronidazole) with an aminoglycoside represents a "gold standard" to which newer regimens are compared for efficacy.

Animal model studies have suggested that metronidazole is the most active agent in the treatment of anaerobic infections. In studies of experimental abscesses, metronidazole is associated with the greatest reduction in bacterial concentrations (30). However, clinical data do not suggest any material difference between these two agents (24, 27–29). For example, the Canadian Metronidazole-Clindamycin Study group compared clindamycin and metronidazole, each with gentamicin, in patients with serious intra-abdominal infections (27). There were four failures among 72 patients who received metronidazole and three failures in the clindamycin group.

A similar multicenter study was done by a European group led by Van der Auwera (28). In this study, a variety of other agents with poor antianaerobic activity were added to the treatment regimen if aerobic/facultative organisms were isolated. The rates for complete cure, clinical improvement, and failure were similar for both groups.

Another approach has been to combine an antianaerobe agent with a broad-spectrum β-lactam antibiotic that has excellent activity against aerobic/facultative organisms, but acts only marginally against anaerobic species. Burbrick et al. found that the combination of clindamycin and ceftazidime was as effective as the combination of clindamycin and tobramycin (31). Microbiologic efficacy, defined as eradication of the pathogenic organisms, was superior with the clindamycin-ceftazidime regimen.

Chloramphenicol has excellent activity against anaerobic pathogens and, unlike clindamycin or metronidazole, is also active against a variety of aerobic/facultative Gram-negative bacilli. Thus, chloramphenicol is potentially useful as a single agent in treating patients with intra-abdominal sepsis. Unfortunately, chloramphenicol was used most frequently in an earlier era, when controlled clinical trials were not the standard for determining efficacy. Recent studies have combined chloramphenicol with aminoglycosides in order to provide activity against *Pseudomonas aeruginosa*. These studies have shown that chloramphenicol/aminoglycoside is comparable to clindamycin/aminoglycoside (31, 32).

β-Lactam Antibiotics

A number of β-lactam antibiotics have been developed that have good activity against anaerobic pathogens. In general, penicillin is adequate to treat infections due to *Clostridium*, *Fusobacterium*, or *Peptostreptococcus*. However, *Bacteroides*, in particular those members of the *B. fragilis* group, contain a potent β-lactamase. Therefore, a basic requirement for β-lactam antibiotic used to treat the anaerobic component of intra-abdominal sepsis is that the drug be resistant to this β-lactamase activity.

One of the earliest agents to be successfully utilized in this capacity was cefoxitin. Cefoxitin, unlike many other cephalosporin antibiotics, contains a methoxyl group bound to C^7 on the R side chain. This methoxyl group confers resistance to *B. fragilis* β-lactamase (33).

Tally and coworkers compared cefoxitin with clindamycin and amikacin in patients with intra-abdominal infections (34). In this study, some patients were given cefoxitin and amikacin because of concern for resistant aerobic/facultative Gram-negative bacilli. A total of 37 patients received cefoxitin, 16 received cefoxitin alone, and an additional 7 initially received amikacin but had the aminoglycoside discontinued within 72 hours. This study found that cefoxitin with or without amikacin was equivalent in efficacy to clindamycin and amikacin.

Another study of cefoxitin with or without an aminoglycoside was conducted by a group at the University of Maryland (35). In this study 26 patients received cefoxitin alone and 5 received cefoxitin and an aminoglycoside. When compared with a clindamycin and tobramycin regimen, the cefoxitin-containing regimen was therapeutically equivalent. However, the microbiology in those patients in the cefoxitin group who were classified as clinical failures was characterized by the more frequent isolation of resistant Gram-negative bacilli.

Another study used a variation on this theme by comparing clindamycin and tobramycin with a regimen of cefoxitin and initially tobramycin (36). Tobramycin was discontinued after 72 hours in those patients (63%) in whom no cefoxitin-resistant Gram-negative bacilli were isolated. The two regimens were therapeutically equivalent. A more rigorous study was done by Nichols et al. comparing cefoxitin as a single agent with clindamycin and gentamicin in patients with penetrating abdominal trauma (37). The results of that study clearly demonstrated that cefoxitin is therapeutically equivalent to clindamycin and gentamicin in patients with community-acquired intra-abdominal infection.

These results were confirmed in a study by Malangoni et al. who found that cefoxitin when given in a dose of 3 g every 8 hours was as effective as a clindamycin/tobramycin regimen (38). There were 21 therapeutic failures among the 112 patients who were evaluated; 17 of these 21 failures were attributed to antibiotic-resistant organisms, including 16 clindamycin-resistant organisms and 10 cefoxitin-resistant organisms.

Cefoxitin is efficacious in the treatment of infections following cesarean section (39, 40). In a randomized study of 98 women in whom such infections developed, the cure rates were 75% for cefoxitin and 76% for clindamycin with gentamicin.

These studies have demonstrated the efficacy of cefoxitin in the treatment of intra-abdominal and pelvic infections. Given these findings, it is reasonable to consider cefoxitin as a useful single agent for the treatment of community-acquired intra-abdominal infections. It must be recognized, however, that cefoxitin has a limited spectrum of activity against aerobic/facultative Gram-negative bacilli. Nosocomial pathogens such as *Enterobacter* and *P. aeruginosa* are uniformly resistant. This suggests that cefoxitin may not be adequate for hospital-acquired intra-abdominal infections. In patients with such infections, a regimen with a broader spectrum of activity would be more effective.

Other β-lactam antibiotics also have been studied as single agents for the treatment of intra-abdominal sepsis. In the United States, moxalactam is a drug of historic interest only. This drug, in which the sulfur atom in the 6-membered ring is replaced by an oxygen atom, has good in vitro activity against aerobic/facultative Gram-negative bacilli as well as excellent activity against anaerobic micro-organisms (41). Indeed, the in vitro spectrum of activity of moxalactam is broad enough so that many hospital-acquired infections could be treated with this drug as a single agent. Comparative studies of moxalactam vs. either clindamycin and an aminoglycoside or cefoxitin demonstrated equivalent efficacy (41–44). However, use of moxalactam declined dramatically when it became associated with an increase in bleeding that was attributed, at least in part, to a methylthiotetrazole side chain that inhibits prothrombin synthesis (45, 46).

Cefotetan and cefmetazole are cephalosporin antibiotics that have activity comparable to cefoxitin (47–50). Cefotetan has been shown to be therapeutically equivalent to cefoxitin with the added advantage of requiring less frequent administration. Lewis and coworkers demonstrated equivalent efficacy with a 12 hourly regimen for cefotetan compared with a 6 hourly regimen for cefoxitin (47). There was, however, a 50% higher incidence of adverse effects noted in the cefotetan group. Most frequently, these adverse effects were gastrointestinal, including diarrhea, nausea, and vomiting.

Semisynthetic penicillins such as mezlocillin, ticarcillin, or piperacillin also show activity against anaerobic bacteria (32, 51–54). Harding and coworkers, in a well-controlled study, compared clindamycin, chloramphenicol, and ticarcillin in patients with intra-abdominal and pelvic sepsis (32). In addition, all patients received gentamicin. The results showed equal therapeutic activity.

Table 14.2
Comparative Studies with Imipenem in the Treatment of Intra-abdominal Sepsis

Study	Agent	Success rate (%)
	Imipenem	96
Scandinavian Study Group (66)	Clindamycin/Gentamicin	85
	Imipenem	94
Gonzenbach et al. (61)	Clindamycin/Gentamicin	89
	Imipenem	83
Solomkin et al. (62)	Clindamycin/Tobramycin	70
	Imipenem	79
	Clindamycin	
Poenaru et al. (65)	(or Metronidazole)/Tobramycin	67
	Imipenem	88
Hackford et al. (60)	Clindamycin/Tobramycin	80
	Imipenem	96
Eckhauser et al. (67)	Clindamycin/Aminoglycoside	92

Piperacillin has been used as a single agent in the treatment of intra-abdominal infections. A comparative study of cefoxitin and piperacillin demonstrated therapeutic equivalence between these two agents (53). In another study, no significant difference was evident when piperacillin was compared with the combination of cefuroximine and metronidazole (54).

Virtually every "third-generation" antibiotic has been used in patients with intra-abdominal infection. In general, there are few well-controlled clinical trials examining the relative efficacy of these agents. Ceftizoxime has been reputed to have good activity, (10, 55, 56) although careful in vitro studies demonstrate that the drug is inactivated when exposed to a high inoculum of *B. fragilis* (57).

Imipenem is the first carbapenem antibiotic to be approved by the FDA. It is a broad-spectrum antibiotic with activity against both aerobic/facultative and anaerobic micro-organisms (58). The drug is metabolized by renal dehydropeptidase, which results in the production of a nephrotoxic moiety. To prevent this nephrotoxicity, imipenem is administered in combination with an inactive agent, cilastatin, which preferentially binds to renal dehydropeptidase and prevents imipenem metabolism. Cilastatin not only prevents the nephrotoxicity, but serves to prolong the half-life and increase serum concentrations (59).

There have been a number of studies (60–67) examining the role of imipenem/cilastatin in the treatment of intra-abdominal sepsis (Table 14.2). For the most part these studies have shown that imipenem is equivalent to the traditional combination regimen of clindamycin and an aminoglycoside. A more striking result was noted in an early study by the Scandinavian Study Group suggesting that imipenem was superior to the clindamycin/gentamicin combination in patients with a wide variety of infections (66). There were nine failures in the clindamycin/gentamicin group as compared with only two failures among those patients receiving imipenem. However, patients who were randomized to receive the combination regimen may have received less than optimal dosages of gentamicin. Aminoglycoside dosages were adjusted to achieve peak serum concentrations of >4 µg/ml. More recent studies have shown that clinical response in patients with Gram-negative infections is correlated with higher aminoglycoside serum concentrations (68).

This issue was more clearly addressed in a study by Solomkin et al. in which clindamycin and tobramycin were compared with imipenem/cilastatin in 162 patients (62). Of 81 patients who received clindamycin, 24 failed, whereas only 14 of 81 imipenem patients failed ($P = .043$). This difference was primarily attributable to the persistence of aerobic/facultative Gram-negative bacteria in patients who received clindamycin and tobramycin. Although the aminoglycoside dose was adjusted to provide peak serum concentrations of >6 μg/ml, patients who failed took 4.58 days to reach this peak. This delay in achieving therapeutic aminoglycoside concentrations may account for the greater number of clinical failures in the clindamycin/tobramycin group.

The same drugs were studied by Poenaru and coworkers, who noted a 4% septic death rate among 52 patients with intra-abdominal infections who received imipenem compared with a 13% septic mortality in patients receiving clindamycin and tobramycin (65). This difference failed to reach statistical significance. A similar but also not statistically significant trend was noted in another study in which imipenem was compared with clindamycin and netilmicin (61). In that study, 81% of patients receiving imipenem were cured and 13% improved, whereas 67% of clindamycin/netilmicin recipients were cured and 22% improved.

A review of the imipenem/cilastatin experience suggests that this combination may be superior to the clindamycin/aminoglycoside combination. The basis for this superiority appears to lie with the relative efficacy of these drugs in treating the aerobic/facultative component of infections. In many patients the aminoglycoside dose produces subtherapeutic blood levels, which leads to clinical failure.

ROLE OF AMINOGLYCOSIDES

Aminoglycoside antibiotics such as gentamicin, tobramycin, netilmycin, and amikacin are active against a broad spectrum of aerobic/facultative Gram-negative bacteria. Because of their wide spectrum of in vitro activity, these antibiotics are frequently employed in the treatment of patients with intra-abdominal infections (69). However, because aminoglycosides are not active against anaerobic microorganisms, they must be used in combination with drugs that are active against anaerobes such as clindamycin, metronidazole, and chloramphenicol or with β-lactam antibiotics such as cefoxitin or piperacarcillin.

Aminoglycoside antibiotics are both ototoxic and nephrotoxic. These adverse affects are seen more commonly in debilitated patients. Advanced age, volume depletion, hypotension, and concomitant use of other nephrotoxic or ototoxic agents all increase the incidence of toxicity (70). Patients with intra-abdominal sepsis frequently have such complicating factors and are thus at increased risk for the development of aminoglycoside toxicity. This has been confirmed in comparative studies of patients with intra-abdominal sepsis, showing that patients who receive an aminoglycoside-containing regimen have a higher incidence of nephrotoxicity as measured by an increase in serum creatinine (35, 37, 41, 42, 62, 68, 69, 71). Aminoglycoside ototoxicity with cochlear and/or vestibular damage also has been documented (69, 72, 73).

The toxic/therapeutic ratio for aminoglycosides is quite small, so that the administration of these drugs must be accompanied by careful monitoring of serum concentrations. An adequate dose of aminoglycoside must be given to assure that peak values for gentamicin or tobramycin range from 4–12 μg/ml while trough values should be less than 2 μg/ml in order to minimize the risk of nephrotoxicity. As noted above, there are data to suggest that, at least in some trials, treatment failures may be more common in regimens in which an aminoglycoside antibiotic is employed. Because this appears to be attributable to inadequate serum concentrations, establishing proper dosage is an absolute requirement.

Aztreonam

Aztreonam is a β-lactam antibiotic that is active against aerobic/facultative Gram-negative bacteria and has been employed as an aminoglycoside substitute in combination regimens (71, 74, 75). Evaluating worldwide experience with aztreonam, Henry noted that the cure rates were 95% for patients receiving aztreonam compared with 81% for patients receiving tobramycin (74). However, this was based on a compilation of trials rather than a single, well-controlled study. When aztreonam has been compared directly with tobramycin and both groups were given clindamycin, Williams and Hotchkiss found virtually identical clinical response rates (71). Microbiologic response rates were slightly, but not significantly, higher in the aztreonam group.

The combination of a β-lactam with a β-lactamase inhibitor has been compared with a clindamycin-aminoglycoside regimen (76–79). The use of ticarcillin/clavulanate was therapeutically equivalent to clindamycin and tobramycin in patients with intra-abdominal infections and to the use of cefoxitin in patients with pelvic infections (76, 77). However, the clinical response to cefoperazone plus sulbactam was significantly better (93%) than that seen with the combination of clindamycin and tobramycin (74%) (78). A Swedish group found that pipercillin plus tazobactam produced a significantly higher cure rate than imipenem-cilastatin in treating intra-abdominal infections (91% vs. 69%, respectively) (79).

The results of these studies in patients with intra-abdominal sepsis indicate that successful therapy requires the administration of an agent(s) that has activity against both aerobic/facultative and anaerobic pathogens. In patients with community-acquired infections, it may be unnecessary to employ an aminoglycoside antibiotic since certain β-lactam antibiotics, such as cefoxitin, cefotetan, cefmetazole or piperacillin have shown efficacy when given as single agents.

The situation in patients with nosocomial infection is more complex by virtue of the presence of resistant aerobic/facultative Gram-negative organisms. In general, most patients require combination regimens that includes use of an antianaerobe agent in combination with an aminoglycoside or a broad-spectrum β-lactam antibiotic. Imipenem and the β-lactam/β-lactam inhibitor drugs are notable exceptions. These drugs can be employed as single agents in patients with nosocomial intra-abdominal infections.

TREATMENT OF SPECIFIC CAUSES OF INTRA-ABDOMINAL SEPSIS

In the discussion that follows, several representative causes of intra-abdominal infection are reviewed and their antibiotic treatment plans are summarized.

Acute Appendicitis

The microbiology of acute appendicitis is virtually identical with that seen in other types of intra-abdominal infections involving the distal small bowel and colon. Aerobic/facultative and anaerobic micro-organisms are present, and the predominant species are *B. fragilis* and *E. coli* (80–83).

A number of studies have now demonstrated that the incidence of postoperative wound infections can be reduced by the preoperative administration of antibiotics in patients undergoing appendectomy (17, 18, 84–92). In general, the agents employed in acute appendicitis are similar to those used in patients with penetrating injuries of the abdomen.

An early study by Leigh and coworkers demonstrated the efficacy of antibiotics for patients undergoing appendectomy (86). They found a 6% incidence of wound infection in patients receiving lincomycin compared to with a 17% incidence in untreated control patients (*P* < .02). Similar findings were noted by Donovan et al. who observed a 20% infection rate among patients undergoing appendectomy without antibiotics compared to with a 4% rate among patients receiving clindamycin and 6% for those receiving cefazolin (92). A placebo-controlled trial of clindamycin and gentamicin revealed a 10.2% infection rate for patients with nonperforating appendicitis who received a placebo, which was reduced to 5.3% among patients receiving antibiotics (87).

Two placebo-controlled studies of cefoxitin have been performed in patients with appendicitis. In one study, no infections were noted in 52 patients who received cefoxitin compared with 10 infections in 51 patients who received placebo (88). A much larger study by Bauer and coworkers revealed an 8.3% infection rate among control subjects receiving placebo compared with 2.5% among patients receiving cefoxitin (89). In this study a significantly lower infection rate was noted among cefoxitin-treated patients who had normal appendixes as well as among those with acute or gangrenous appendicitis (56).

The importance of the anaerobic flora in patients with acute appendicitis is evident from studies of β-lactam antibiotics with only marginal activity against anaerobic pathogens. A three-way comparative trial of cefoperazone vs. cefamandole vs. clindamycin/gentamicin demonstrated that the clindamycin/gentamicin regimen was superior, illustrating the need for using drugs with antianaerobic activity in treating appendicitis (19).

Another study involved 95 patients who were randomized to receive cefoxitin and 94 randomized to receive the combination of ampicillin and metronidazole (80). There were 10 wound infections in each group. However, intra-abdominal abscesses developed in only 2 patients who received cefoxitin compared with 12 patients who received ampicillin and metronidazole.

Metronidazole, a drug with excellent activity against anaerobes that is inactive against aerobic/facultative species, appears to be a poor choice as a single agent used for appendicitis patients. In a controlled study, metronidazole, alone or in combination with either cefazolin or tobramycin, was compared with a placebo (83). The incidence of infection in the four groups was 13%, 4%, 3%, and 17%, respectively, for patients receiving metronidazole, metronidazole plus cefazolin, metronidazole plus tobramycin, and placebo, respectively. The results of this study suggest that activity against aerobic/facultative pathogens is an important consideration in patients with appendicitis.

This point was further illustrated in another study in which metronidazole in combination with cefotetan was significantly better in treating appendicitis than metronidazole alone

(93). On the other hand, no difference was evident between metronidazole alone vs. metronidazole plus gentamicin (94). Similarly, three doses of metronidazole were as effective as the combination of metronidazole, ampicillin and gentamicin (95).

An interesting report from Los Angeles County Hospital described a high incidence of *P. aeruginosa* in primary cultures from patients with appendicitis (96). Despite the relatively frequent isolation of this organism (11% of patients), it appeared that clinical response was not related to its presence. Therapeutic failure was associated with in vitro resistance to *Bacteroides*. Furthermore, in patients who received combination antibiotic regimens, the serum concentrations of aminoglycoside did not correlate with outcome.

A number of other antibiotic regimens are efficacious in patients with appendicitis (20, 43, 81, 94). These include cefotaxime, moxalactam, imipenem, and the combination of clindamycin and aztreonam.

Patients undergoing surgery for acute appendicitis clearly benefit from antibiotic therapy. The results of these studies suggest that a regimen should include agents with activity against both aerobic/facultative and anaerobic micro-organisms. Short-course therapy (one to three doses) appears to be adequate for patients with acute nonperforated appendicitis,whereas longer treatment is needed for patients with gangrenous or perforated appendices.

Pancreatic Abscess

Pancreatic abscess usually occurs as a complication of pancreatitis. Enzymes released by the acutely inflamed pancreas result in tissue necrosis, establishing an environment conducive for bacterial growth. At the same time, edema of the common bile duct or pancreatic duct may impede drainage. The combination of obstruction and necrosis provides an excellent milieu for infection and abscess formation.

The bacteriology of pancreatic abscess reflects the flora of the biliary tract (97, 98). Enteric bacteria are frequently found, including

E. coli, Klebsiella sp., Enterococcus, and *Staphylococcus*. Other organisms identified in patients with pancreatic abscess include *Pseudomonas, Proteus*, and *Streptococcus*. Anaerobic bacterial isolates are less frequently found.

As with other visceral abscesses, the mainstay of therapy for patients with pancreatic abscesses is surgical drainage. Antibiotic choices are based on bacteriologic analysis of abscess fluid obtained at surgery or by percutaneous needle aspiration. The choice of antibiotics for empiric therapy should be similar to that used for patients with other biliary tract infections. Broad-spectrum β-lactam antibiotics active against Enterobacteriaceae are the agents of initial choice, pending microbiologic studies. In patients in whom the presence of *Enterococcus* is suspected, piperacillin plus an aminoglycoside is a useful regimen in that it provides activity against aerobic/facultative and anaerobic pathogens as well as *Enterococcus*. Timentin, the combination of ticarcillin and a β-lactamase inhibitor, clavulanic acid, may be substituted for piperacillin. Timentin has the added advantage of showing activity against *Staphylococcus aureus*.

Cholecystitis

The most frequently recognized complication of cholelithiasis is the development of acute cholecystitis, which is a mechanical disorder resulting from obstruction of the cystic duct. In some patients the gall bladder is sterile, and there is no need for antibiotic therapy of cholecystitis. However, in most individuals, cholecystitis is complicated by the presence of infection in the gall bladder. The source of the infecting bacteria is bile that is contaminated by retrograde spread of bacteria from the bowel. The incidence of bactobilia (bacteria in bile) is higher in patients who are elderly, have jaundice and/or common duct stones, have prolonged or severe symptoms, or have acute cholecystitis superimposed on chronic cholecystitis (99, 100).

The microbiology of infected bile is representative of the microflora of the upper intestine (99, 101, 102). *E. coli, Klebsiella*, and *Enterococcus* are frequently identified. *P. aeru-*

ginosa is occasionally found in elderly patients. Anaerobic bacteria such as *Bacteroides* and *Clostridium* may be present in polymicrobial infections, particularly in elderly patients or those with common duct stones.

Retrospective analyses of patients with acute cholecystitis suggest that antibiotics do not affect the course of the disease, perhaps because it is difficult to achieve adequate concentrations of antibiotics in the gallbladder and bile when obstruction is present (103). Nevertheless, in patients who are febrile and toxic, antibiotics should be administered. The combination of piperacillin with an aminoglycoside has the advantage of providing activity against *Enterobacteriaceae, Enterococcus*, and anaerobes.

There are convincing data to indicate that prophylactic antibiotics reduce the incidence of postoperative wound infection in patients who undergo cholecystectomy surgery (98, 103, 104). A variety of cephalosporin antibiotic agents has proven successful as a prophylactic agent.

Cholangitis

Although cholangitis is often clinically indistinguishable from cholecystitis, most patients have signs and symptoms of severe sepsis with high fever and chills. Obstruction of the common bile duct is more frequently complicated by bacteremia and septic shock than is obstruction of the cystic duct (103–107).

The bacteriology of cholangitis is similar to that seen in cholecystitis. Aerobic/facultative Gram-negative bacilli, enterococci, and anaerobic bacteria predominate. Empiric therapy should be directed against these organisms.

The regimen of ampicillin and gentamicin has been employed for the treatment of cholangitis because of the activity of this combination against aerobic/facultative Gram-negative bacilli and enterococci. Others have recommended the use of cephalosporins with activity against anaerobes or the combinations of an aminoglycoside with either clindamycin or metronidazole.

Mezlocillin is an acyl-ureidopenicillin with activity against the major pathogens found in patients with cholangitis. A randomized study comparing mezlocillin with the combination of ampicillin and gentamicin revealed that the mezlocillin had a superior response rate (83% vs. 41%, respectively) (108). This may be due to the higher biliary concentrations achieved by mezlocillin than by either ampicillin or gentamicin. Mezlocillin also has better activity against anaerobic pathogens than does the combination regimen. On the other hand, a comparative study of piperacillin, another antibiotic excreted in the bile, with ampicillin and gentamicin showed no significant difference between these regimens (109).

The combination of a penicillin and an aminoglycoside provides activity against *Enterococcus. Enterococcus faecalis* is isolated from the bile in 34–55% of patients with cholangitis. Because cholangitis is frequently complicated by bacteremia, patients with enterococcal bacteremia are at risk of seeding the heart valves and developing endocarditis.

In addition to mezlocillin and piperacillin, azlocillin, ceftriaxone, and cefoperazone are excreted in the bile. However, the relative importance of biliary antibiotic concentrations in the treatment of cholangitis is controversial. Studies have shown that gentamicin, an antibiotic that is not concentrated in the bile, can reduce the incidence of wound sepsis and bacteremia. In any event, these drugs, either alone or in combination with other agents, may be useful in the treatment of patients with cholangitis. It should be noted, however, that cefoperazone and ceftriaxone, unlike the ureidopenicillins, have relatively poor activity against anaerobic organisms, notably *B. fragilis*, so that a regimen employing these drugs should include either clindamycin or metronidazole. Finally, it should be recognized that patients with common duct obstruction and cholangitis require endoscopic or surgical intervention.

Liver Abscess

Pyogenic liver abscess may arise as a result of direct extension from a contiguous focus, biliary tract obstruction and cholangitis, or hematogenous spread of organisms via the portal venous system or the hepatic artery. Hepatic abscess may be single or multiple, depending upon the etiology and the source of the infecting organisms.

The bacteriology of hepatic abscess involves aerobic/facultative and anaerobic micro-organisms (110–116). More than two-thirds of all hepatic abscesses are polymicrobial. Aerobic/facultative species include *Enterobacteriaceae*, other aerobic Gram-negative bacilli, *S. aureus*, and *Streptococcus*. Anaerobic organisms include *Bacteroides*, *Fusobacterium*, *Clostridium*, and *Peptostreptococcus*.

The approach to treatment of hepatic abscess depends on a knowledge of the bacteriology and the characteristic features of the abscess (111, 117, 118). In patients with a large, single abscess, surgical or percutaneous drainage is both diagnostic and therapeutic. In patients with multiple small abscesses, therapeutic drainage may not be possible. Nevertheless, percutaneous aspiration may be useful in defining the microbial etiology, especially if blood cultures are sterile.

Empiric therapeutic regimens should incorporate antibiotics with activity against aerobic/facultative and anaerobic pathogens. Regimens that were listed for the treatment of intra-abdominal sepsis should be adequate for most patients, pending the results of cultures. Once culture results are available, antibiotics should be adjusted based on the microbiologic sensitivities. The duration of therapy may be quite prolonged. Patients who do not undergo surgical drainage may require treatment for several months.

REFERENCES

1. Simon GL, Gorbach SL. Intestinal flora in health and disease. Gastroenterology 1984;86:174–193.
2. Hentges DE. Anaerobes as normal flora. In: Finegold SM, George WL, eds. Anaerobic infections in humans. San Diego: Academic Press, 1989;37–53.
3. Clarke JS, Condon RE, Bartlett JG, et al. Preoperative oral antibiotics reduce septic complications of colon operations: results of prospective, randomized, double-blind clinical study. Ann Surg 1977; 186:251–259.
4. Washington JA II, Dearing WHH, Judd ES, et al. Effect of preoperative regimen on development of

infection after intestinal surgery: prospective, randomized, double-blind study. Ann Surg 1974; 180:567.

5. Boey J, Wong J, Ong GB. Bacteria and septic complication in patients with perforated duodenal ulcers. Am J Surg 1982;143:635–639.

6. Marsh PK, Tally FP, Kellum J, et al. Candida infections in surgical patients. Ann Surg 1983;198:42.

7. Weinstein WM, Onderdonk AB, Bartlett JG, Gorbach SL. Experimental intra-abdominal abscesses in rats: development of an experimental model. Infect Immunol 1974;10:1250–1255.

8. Onderdonk AB, Weinstein WM, Sullivan NM, Bartlett JG, Gorbach SL. Experimental intra-abdominal abscesses in rats: quantitative bacteriology of infected animals. Infect Immunol 1974;10:1256–1259.

9. Weinstein WM, Onderdonk AB, Bartlett JG, Louie TJ, Gorbach SL. Antimicrobial therapy of experimental intra-abdominal sepsis. J Infect Dis 1975; 132:282–286.

10. Bennion RS, Baron EJ, Thompson JE, et al. The bacteriology of gangrenous and perforated appendicitis-revisited. Ann Surg 1990;211:165.

11. Gorbach SL. Treatment of intra-abdominal sepsis. In: Finegold SM, Bartlet J, Chow AW, et al. Management of anaerobic infections. Ann Intern Med 1975;83:377.

12. Lorber B, Swenson RM. The bacteriology of intra-abdominal infections. Surg Clin North Am 1975; 55:1349.

13. Altemeier WA, Culbertson WR, Fullen WD, Shook CD. Intra-abdominal abscesses. Am J Surg 1973; 125:70–79.

14. Thadepalli H. Gorbach SL, Broido PW, et al. Abdominal trauma, anaerobes, and antibiotics. Surgery 1973;137:270.

15. Jones RC, Thal ER, Johnson NA, Gollihar LN. Evaluation of antibiotic therapy following penetrating abdominal trauma. Ann Surg 1985;201:576–585.

16. Gentry LO, Feliciano DV, Lea AS, et al. Perioperative antibiotic therapy for penetrating injuries of the abdomen. Ann Surg 1984;200:561–566.

17. Baird IM. Multicentered study of cefoperazone for treatment of intra-abdominal infections and comparison of cefoperazone with cefamandole and clindamycin plus gentamicin for treatment of appendicitis and peritonitis. Rev Infect Dis 1983;5(suppl):165.

18. Berne TV, Yellin AW, Appleman MD, Heseltine PNR. Antibiotic management of surgically treated gangrenous or perforated appendicitis. Am J Surg 1982;144:8–13.

19. Heseltine PNR, Yellin AE, Appleman MD, et al. Perforated and gangrenous appendicitis: an analysis of antibiotic failures. J Infect Dis 1983;148:322–329.

20. Lau W-Y, Fan S-T, Chu K-W, et al. Randomized prospective and double-blind trial of new beta-lactams in the treatment of appendicitis. Antimicrob Agents Chemother 1985;28:639–642.

21. deZerega G, Yonekura L, Subir R, Nakamura RM, Ledger WJ. A comparison of clindamycin-gentamicin and penicillin-gentamicin in the treatment of post-cesarean section endomyometritis. Am J Obstet Gynecol 1979;134:328.

22. Herman G, Cohen A, Talbot G, Coghlan R, Faidley-Mangen P, MacGregor RR. Cefoxitin versus clindamycin and gentamicin in the treatment of postcesarean section infections. Obstet Gynecol 1986;67:371–376.

23. Snydman DC, Tally FP, Knuppel R, et al. Bacteroides bivius and Bacteroides disiens in obstetrical patients: clinical findings and antimicrobial susceptibilities. J Antimicrob Chemother 1980;6:519–525.

24. Smith JA, Skidmore AG, Forward AD, et al. Prospective, randomized double-blind comparison of metronidazole and tobramycin with clindamycin and tobramycin in the treatment of intra-abdominal sepsis. Ann Surg 1980;192:213–220.

25. Lennard ES, Minshew BH, Dellinger P, et al. Stratified outcome comparison of clindamycin-gentamicin vs. chloramphenicol-gentamicin for treatment of intra-abdominal sepsis. Arch Surg 1985; 120:889–898.

26. Rowlands BJ, Ericsson CD. Comparative studies of antibiotic therapy after penetrating abdominal trauma. Am J Surg 1984;148:791–795.

27. Canadian Metronidazole-Clindamycin Study Group. Prospective, randomized comparison of metronidazole and clindamycin, each with gentamicin, for the treatment of serious intra-abdominal infection. Surgery 1983;93:221–229.

28. Van der Auwera P, Collier J, Goris RJA, et al. A comparison of metronidazole and clindamycin for the treatment of intra-abdominal anaerobic infection: a multicenter trial. J Antimicrob Chemother 1982;10:57–66.

29. Kirkpatrick JR, Anderson BJ, Louie JJ, et al. Double-blind comparison of metronidazole plus gentamicin and clindamycin plus gentamicin in intra-abdominal infection. Surgery 1983;93:215.

30. Joiner KA, Lowe B, Dzink J, et al. Comparative efficacy of 10 antimicrobial agents in experimental infections with Bacteroides fragilis. J Infect Dis 1982;145:561–568.

31. Bubrick MP, Heim-Duthoy KL, Yellin AE, et al. Ceftazidime/clindamycin versus tobramycin/clindamycin in the treatment of intra-abdominal infections. Am Surg 1990;56:613–617.

32. Harding GKM, Buckwold FJ, Ronald AR, et al. Prospective, randomized comparative study of clindamycin, chloramphenicol, and ticarcillin, each in combination with gentamicin, in therapy for intra-abdominal and female genital tract sepsis. J Infect Dis 1980;142:384–393.

33. Birnbaum J, Stapley EO, Miller AK, et al. Cefoxitin, a semisynthetic cephamycin: a microbiological overview. J Antimicrob Chemother 1978;4(suppl B):15–32.

34. Tally FP, McGowan K, Kellum JM, Gorbach SL, O'Donnell TF. A randomized comparison of cefoxitin with or without amikacin and clindamycin plus amikacin in surgical sepsis. Ann Surg 1981;193:318–323.

35. Drusano GL, Warren JW, Saah AJ, et al. A prospective randomized controlled trial of cefoxitin versus clindamycin-aminoglycoside in mixed anaerobic-aerobic infections. Surg Gynecol Obstet 1982;154:715.

36. Nicolle LE, Harding GKM, Louie TJ, et al. Cefoxitin plus tobramycin and clindamycin plus tobramycin. Arch Surg 1986;121:891–896.

37. Nichols RL, Smith JW, Lein DB, et al. Risk of infection after penetrating abdominal trauma. N Engl J Med 1984;311:1065.

38. Malangoni MA, Condon RE, Spiegle CA. Treatment of intraabdominal infections is appropriate with single-agent or combination antibiotic therapy. Surgery 1985;98:648–655.

39. Heseltine PNR, Berne TV, Yellin AE, et al. The efficacy of cefoxitin vs. clindamycin/gentamicin in surgically treated stab wounds of the bowel. J Trauma 1986;26:241–245.

40. Hofstetter SR, Pachter HL, Bailey AA. A prospective comparison of two regimens of prophylactic antibiotics in abdominal trauma: cefoxitin versus triple drug. J Trauma 1984;24:307–310.

41. Stone HH, Strom PR, Fabian TC, Dunlop WE, Third-Generation cephalosporins for polymicrobial surgical sepsis. Arch Surg 1983;118:193–200.

42. Tally FP, Kellum JM, Ho JL. Randomized prospective study comparing moxalacatam and cefoxitin with or without tobramycin for the treatment of serious surgical infections. Antimicrob Agents Chemother 1986;29:244–249.

43. Schentag JJ, Wels PB, Reitberg DP, et al. A randomized clinical trial of moxalactam alone versus tobramycin plus clindamycin in abdominal sepsis. Ann Surg 1982;198:35–41.

44. Stellato TA, Danzinger LH, Hau T, et al. Moxalactam vs. tobramycin-clindamycin: a randomized trial in secondary peritonitis. Arch Surg 1988;123:714.

45. Barza M, Furie B, Brown AE, et al. Defects in vitamin K-dependent carboxylation associated with moxalactam treatment. J Infect Dis 1986;153:1166–1169.

46. Agnelli G, Del Favavero A, Parise P, et al. Cephalosporin-induced hypoprothrombinemia: is the N-methylthiotetrazole side chain the culprit? Antimicrob Agents Chemother 1986;29:1108–1109.

47. Lewis RT, Duma RT, Echols RM, et al. Comparative study of cefotetan and cefoxitin in the treatment of intra-abdominal infections. Am J Obstet Gynecol 1988;158:728–735.

48. Souza Dias MB, Jacobus NV, Tally FP, Gorbach SL. Activity of cefotetan against anaerobic bacteria. Diagn Microbiol Infect Dis 1986;4:359–363.

49. Wilson SE, Boswick JA Jr, Duma RF, et al. Cephalosporin therapy in intraabdominal infections. Am J Surg 1988;155:61–66.

50. Cornick NA, Jacobus NV, Gorbach SL. Activity of Cefmetazole against anaerobic bacteria. Antimicrob Agents Chemother 1987;31:2010–2012.

51. O'Donnell V, Mandall AK, Lou MA Sr, et al. Evaluation of carbenicillin and a comparison of clindamycin and gentamicin combined therapy in penetrating abdominal trauma. Surg Gynecol Obstet 1978;147:525–529.

52. Fink MP, Helsmoortel CM, Arous EJ, et al. Comparison of safety and efficacy of parenteral ticarcillin/clavulanate and clindamycin/gentamicin in serious intra-abdominal infections. J Antimicrob Chemother 1989;24(suppl B):147–156.

53. Najem AZ, Kaminski AC, Spillert CR, Lazaro EJ. Comparative study of parenteral piperacillin and cefoxitin in the treatment of surgical infections of the abdomen. Surg Gynecol Obstet 1983;157:423–425.

54. Paakkonen M, Alhava EM, Huttunen R, et al. Piperacillin compared with cefuroxime plus metronidazole in diffuse peritonitis. Eur J Surg 1991;157:535.

55. Fu KP, Neu HC. Antibacterial activity of ceftizoxime, a beta-lactamase stable cephalosporing. Antimicrob Agents Chemother 1981;19:414–423.

56. Browder W, Smith JW, Vivoda LM. Nonperforative appendicitis: a continuing surgical dilemma. J Infect Dis 1989;159:1088–1094.

57. Eley A, Greenwood D. Activity of ceftizoxime against Bacteroides fragilis: comparison with benzylpenicillin, cephalothin and cefoxitin. Antimicrob Agents Chemother 1981;20:332–335.

58. Neu HC, Labthavikul P. Comparative in vitro activity of N-formimidoyl thienamycin against Gram-positive and Gram-negative aerobic and anaerobic species and its beta-lactamase stability. Antimicrob Agents Chemother 1982;21:180–187.

59. Drusano GL, Standiford HC, Ruslamante C, et al. Multiple dose kinetics of imipenem/cilastatin. Antimicrob Agents Chemother 1984;26:715–721.

60. Hackford AW, Tally FP, Reinhold RB, Barza M, Gorbach SL. Prospective study comparing imipenem/cilastatin with clindamycin and gentamicin for the treatment of serious surgical infections. Arch Surg 1988;123:322–326.

61. Gonzenbach HR, Simmen HP, Amgwerd R. Imipenem (N-F-thienamycin) versus netilmicin plus clindamycin. Ann Surg 1987;205:271–275.

62. Solomkin JS, Dellinger EP, Christou NV, et al. Results of a multicenter trial comparing-imipenem/cilastatin to tobramycin/clindamycin for intra-abdominal infections. Ann Surg 1990;212:581–591.

63. Kager L, Nord CE. Imipenem/cilastatin in the treatment of intraabdominal infections: a review of worldwide experience. Rev Infect Dis 1985;7(suppl 3):S518–S521.

64. Leaper DJ, Kennedy RH, Sutton A, et al. Treatment of acute bacterial peritonitis: a trial of imipenem/cilastatin against ampicillin-metronidazole-gentamicin. Scand J Infect Dis 1987;52(suppl):7.

65. Poenaru D, Santis MD, Christou NV. Iminpenem versus tobramycin antianaerobe antibiotic therapy in intra-abdominal infections. Can J Surg 1990;33:415–422.

66. Scandinavian Study Group. Imipenem/cilastatin versus gentamicin/clindamycin for treatment of serious bacterial infections. Lancet 1984;1:868–871.

67. Eckhauser FE, Knol JA, Raper SE, et al. Efficacy of two comparative antibiotic regimens in the treatment of serious intra-abdominal infections: results of a multicenter study. Clin Ther 1992;14:97–109.

68. Moore RD, Smith CR, Lietman PS. Association of aminoglycoside plasma levels with mortality in patients with Gram-negative bacteremia. J Infect Dis 1984:149–154.

69. Ho JL, Barza J. Role of aminoglycoside antibiotics in the treatment of intra-abdominal infection. Antimicrob Agents Chemother 1987;31:486–491.

70. Leitman PS, Smith CR. Aminoglycoside nephrotoxicity in humans. Rev Infect Dis 1983;5(suppl 2):284–293.

71. Williams RR, Hotchkiss D. Aztreonam plus clindamycin vs. tobramycin plus clindamycin in the treatment of intraabdominal infections. Rev Infect Dis 1991;13(suppl 7):S629–S633.

72. Fee WE. Gentamicin and tobramycin: Comparison of ototoxicity. Rev Infect Dis 1983;5(suppl 2):304–313.

73. Kahlmeta G, Dahlager J. Aminoglycoside toxicity: a review of clinical studies published between 1975 and 1982. J Antimicrob Chemother 1984;13(suppl A):9–22.

74. Henry SA. Overall clinical experience with aztreonam in the treatment of intra-abdominal infections. Rev Infect Dis 1985;7(suppl 1):S729–S733.

75. Birolini D, Moraes MF, de Souza OS. Aztreonam plus clindamycin versus tobramycin plus clindamycin for the treatment of intra-abdominal infections. Rev Infect Dis 1985;7(suppl 4):724–S728.

76. Fink MP, Helmoortel CM, Arous EJ, et al. Comparison of the safety and efficacy of parenteral ticarcillin/clavulanate and clindamycin/gentamicin in serious intra-abdominal infections. J Antimicrob Chemother 1989;24(suppl B):147–156.

77. Pastorek JG Jr, Aldridge KE, Cunningham GL, et al. Comparison of ticarcillin plus clavulanic acid with cefoxitin in the treatment of female pelvic infection. Am J Med 1985;79(5B):16–23.

78. Jauregui LE, Appelbaum PC, Fabian TC, et al. A randomized clinical study of cefoperazone and sulbactam versus gentamicin and clindamycin in the treatment of intra-abdominal infections. J Antimicrob Chemother 1990;25:423–433.

79. Brismar B, Malmborg AS, Tunevall G, et al. Piperacillin-tazobactam versus imipenem-cilastatin for treatment of intra-abdominal infections. Antimicrob Agents Chemother 1992;36:2766–2773.

80. The Danish Multicenter Study Group. A Danish multicenter study: cefoxitin versus ampicillin + metronidazole in perforated appendicitis. Br J Surg 1984;71:144–146.

81. Heseltine PNR, Yellin AE, Appleman, et al. Imipenem therapy for perforated and gangrenous appendicitis. Surg Gynecol Obstet 1986;162:43–48.

82. Pokorny WJ, Kaplan SL, Mason EO Jr. A preliminary report of ticarcillin and clavulanate versus triple antibiotic therapy in children with ruptured appendicitis. Surg Gynecol Obstet 1991;1729(suppl):54–56.

83. El-sefi TA, El-awadi HM, Shehata ML, et al. The place of antibiotics in the prevention of post-appendicectomy sepsis: a prospective study of 400 cases. Int Surg 1986;71:18–21.

84. Busuttil RW, Davidson RK, Fine M, Tompkins RK. Effect of prophylactic antibiotics in acute nonperforated appendicitis. Ann Surg 1981;194:502–509.

85. Everson NW, Fossard DP, Nash JR, McDonald RC. Wound an infection following appendectomy: the effect of extraperitoneal wound drainage and systemic antibiotic prophylaxis. Br J Surg 1977;64:236–238.

86. Leigh DA, Pease R, Henderson H, et al. Prophylactic lincomycin in the prevention of wound infection following appendicectomy: a double blind study. Br J Surg 1976;63:973–977.

87. Fine M, Busuttil RW. Acute appendicitis: efficacy of prophylactic preoperative antibiotics in the reduction of septic mortality. Am J Surg 1978;135:210–213.

88. Winslow RE, Dean RE, Harley JH. Acute nonperforating appendicitis. Arch Surg 1983;118:651–655.

89. Bauer T, Vennits B, Hol B, et al. Antibiotic prophylaxis in acute nonperforated appendicitis. Ann Surg 1989;209:307–311.

90. Krukowski ZH, Irwin ST, Denholm S, Matheson NA. Preventing wound infection after appendicectomy: a review. Br J Surg 1988;75:1023–1033.

91. Gorbach SL. Antimicrobial prophylaxis for appendectomy and colorectal surgery. Rev Infect Dis 1991;13(suppl 10):S815–S820.

92. Donovan IA, Ellis D, Gatehouse D, et al. One dose antibiotic prophylaxis against wound infection after appendectomy: a randomized trial of clindamycin, cefoxatin sodium and placebo. Br J Surg 1976;66–69.

93. Wilson RG, Taylor EW, Lindsay G, et al. A comparative study of cefotetan and metronidazole against metronidazole alone to prevent infection after appendectomy. Surg Gynecol Obstet 1987;164:447–451.

94. Flannigan GM, Clifford RP, Carver RA, et al. Antibiotic prophylaxis in acute appendicitis. Surg Gynecol Obstet 1983;156:209–211.

95. Grant C, Twum-Danso K, Al-Awami MS, et al. Prophylaxis against post-appendicectomy wound infection: a controlled clinical trial of intravenous (I.V.) metronidazole-ampicillin-gentamicin. Int Surg 1989;7:129–132.

96. Yellin AE, Heseltine PNR, Berne TV, et al. The role of *Pseudomonas* species in patients treated with ampicillin and sulbactam for gangrenous and perforated appendicitis. Surg Gynecol Obstet 1985;161:303–307.

97. Holden JL, Berne TV, Rosoff LSR. Pancreatic abscess following acute pancreatitis. Arch Surg 1976;111:858–861.

98. Miller TA, Lindenaue SM, Frey CF, et al. Pancreatic abscess. Arch Surg 1974;108:545–551.

99. Keighley MRB, Drysdale RB, Quoraiski AH, et al. Antibiotic treatment of biliary sepsis. Surg Clin North Am 1975;55:1370–1390.

100. Truedson H, Elmros T, Holm S. The incidence of bacteria in gallbladder bile at acute and elective cholecystectomy. Acta Chir Scand 1983;149:307–313.

101. Pitt HA, Postier RG, Cameron JC. Biliary bacteria: significance and alteration after antibiotic therapy. Arch Surg 1982;117:445–449.

102. Finegold S. Anaerobes in biliary tract infection. Arch Intern Med 1979;139:1338–1339.

103. Kune GA, Burdon JGW. Are antibiotics necessary in acute cholecystitis? Med J Aust 1975;2:627–630.

104. Hirschmann JV, Inui TS. Antimicrobial prophylaxis: a critique of recent trials. Rev Infect Dis 1980;2:1–23.

105. Lipsett PA, Pitt HA. Acute cholangitis. Surg Clin North Am 1990;70:1297–1312.

106. Muller EL, Pitt HA, Thompson JE Jr, et al. Antibiotics in infections of the biliary tract. Surg Gynecol Obstet 1987;165:285.

107. Keighley MR, Drysdale RB, Quoraishi AH. Antibiotic treatment of biliary sepsis. Surg Clin North Am 1975;55:1379.

108. Gerecht WB, Henry NK, Hoffman WW, et al. Prospective randomized comparison of mezlocillin therapy alone with combined ampicillin and gentamicin therapy for patients with cholangitis. Arch Intern Med 1989;149:1279.

109. Thompson JE Jr, Pitt HA, Doty JE, et al. Is a broad spectrum penicillin adequate therapy for cholangitis? Surg Gynecol Obstet 1990;171:275.

110. Frey CF, Zhu Y, Suzuki M, Isaji S. Liver abscesses. Surg Clin North Am 1989;69:259–271.

111. Gyorffy EJ, Frey CF, Silva J Jr, McGahan J. Pyogenic liver abscess: diagnostic and therapeutic strategies. Ann Surg 1990;206:699–705.

112. Branum GD, Tyson GS, Branum MA, Meyers WC. Hepatic abscess: changes in etiology, diagnosis, and management. Ann Surg 1990;212:655–662.

113. Stain SC, Yellin AE, Donovan AJ, Brien HW. Pyogenic liver abscess. Mod Treat Arch Surg 1991;126:991–996.

114. Barnes PF, DeLock KM, Reynolds TN, et al. A comparison of amebic and pyogenic abscess of the liver. Medicine 1987;66:472–483.

115. Rubin RH, Swartz MN, Malt R. Hepatic abscess: changes in clinical bacteriologic and therapeutic aspects. Am J Med 1974;57:601–610.

116. Sabbaj J. Anaerobes in liver abscess. Rev Infect Dis 1984;6(suppl):152–155.

117. Maler JA Jr, Reynolds TB, Yellin AE. Successful medical treatment of pyogenic liver abscess. Gastroenterology 1979;77:618–622.

118. Herbert DA, Fogel DA, Rothman J, et al. Pyogenic liver abscesses: successful nonsurgical therapy. Lancet 1982;1:134–136.

15

Secretory and Miscellaneous Noninfectious Diarrhea

LOUIS Y. KORMAN

Diarrheal diseases represent a major public health problem. Fortunately, in the United States deaths in adults secondary to diarrhea are uncommon. Over a 9-year period, 14,000 adults over age 75 died as an immediate or underlying result of a diarrheal illness (1). In contrast, in developing nations dehydration due to infectious diarrhea often represents an overwhelming public health problem (2–5).

Although diarrheal illness is not often lethal, it is a common and debilitating illness. Rotavirus infection accounts for 3.5 million cases of severe diarrhea in infants and young children. During the initial preparations for Operation Desert Shield in August 1990, outbreaks of diarrheal disease occurred at rates of 50–100/1,000 soldiers/week in some units (2).

It is common for the practitioner to encounter patients complaining of alterations in bowel function. The prevalence of this complaint and the disorders associated with it are difficult to quantify. Clearly, it is a common complaint given the numerous potions and nostrums found on the shelves of pharmacies and in the lore of families. It is the responsibility of the practitioner to approach the problem of diarrheal illness with the same sense of clarity of thought required of other disorders.

DEFINITIONS

Although it is beyond the scope of this chapter to undertake a detailed review of the pathophysiology and differential diagnosis of all diarrheal disorders, it is appropriate to emphasize fundamental principles that the practitioner should consider in the general management of diarrhea. The reader is directed to several excellent reviews of the subject of diarrheal illness in order to supplement the discussion in this chapter (6–12).

Diarrhea, from the Greek "to run," may be defined as an increase in the frequency and liquidity of stool. More specifically, diarrhea represents an increase in stool weight above 200 g/day for an average adult in the developed world. It should be evident that there is significant variation in stool weight and a broad range that can be considered normal. Because it is impractical to measure stool weight in all patients who present complaining of diarrhea, it is paramount to obtain as accurate an assessment of the degree of diarrhea as possible in order to appropriately classify the patient's condition.

CLASSIFICATION

Any approach to the treatment of diarrheal illness requires an understanding of the etiology and pathogenesis of the disorder. Diarrheal disorders have been classified according to a number of schemas which are necessary to provide an orientation to diagnosis and therapy (11–13). Classification can be based on both clinical and pathophysiologic views of the disease. Because the number of disorders that are associated with diarrhea are legion, simply listing the etiologies is of little practical use. It is necessary when making a decision regarding therapy to match therapy to both the clinical and pathophysiologic nature of the disorder.

Clinical Classification of Diarrheal Disorders

Clinically, diarrheal disorders may be classified as either acute or chronic. Acute diarrhea is self-limited, lasting <2 weeks. Chronic diarrhea is defined as diarrhea lasting >2 weeks. It is important to note that after an episode of acute diarrhea the patient may continue to have altered bowel habits. Although meeting the criteria for chronic diarrhea, this clinical picture represents the gradual recovery of function of the gastrointestinal tract after an episode of acute diarrhea, often of infectious etiology. The distinction between acute and chronic diarrhea is not entirely semantic. A diagnosis of chronic diarrhea implies a more extensive search for the etiologic basis of the disturbance. This search represents a significant degree of expense and inconvenience on the part of physician and patient.

Further clinical subdivision of diarrheal illness can be made on evidence of gastrointestinal inflammation. This subdivision is based on the presence of blood in the stool by history (hematochezia) or the finding of occult blood by a peroxidase reaction (Hemoccult). Additionally, a simple stool smear for white blood cells (methylene blue stain) documents the presence of mucosal inflammatory response. Direct visualization of the intestinal mucosa with either sigmoidoscopy or colonoscopy may be useful but is usually not necessary, except in cases of subacute or chronic inflammatory diarrhea.

Pathophysiologic Classification of Diarrhea

Any diarrheal illness associated with a substantial increase in fecal weight is the result of a perturbation of intestinal transport such that net flow of fluid and electrolytes into the lumen is increased.

Secretory diarrhea is defined as a net increase in water and electrolyte transport that occurs as a result of increased chloride secretion and/or decreased sodium absorption. Cholera is the prototypical secretory diarrhea. Cholera toxin binds to the enterocyte cell membrane and irreversibly increases the production of cyclic adenosine monophosphate (cAMP), which in turn increases the net secretion of fluid and electrolytes. The clinical result is a profuse isosomotic watery diarrhea without any substantial morphologic alteration in the epithelium.

Osmotic diarrhea is the result of the presence of osmotically active particles in the intestinal lumen which is accompanied by an increased flow into the lumen to reduce osmolarity. Magnesium-based and nondigestible carbohydrate (e.g., lactulose, sorbitol) laxatives act by increasing intraluminal osmolarity and intraluminal fluid. The result of the net flow into the lumen is an increase in stool weight and a therapeutic diarrhea.

Diarrhea caused by disturbances in motility or mucosal permeability are difficult to classify pathophysiologically. The diarrhea associated with disturbances in motility is often accompanied by increased secretion. Inflammatory diarrhea such as colitis associated with shigellosis represents a combination of altered secretion, increased permeability to osmotically active particles, and altered motility.

Specific Disorders

TUMOR-RELATED DIARRHEA

The diarrhea associated with tumors is usually the result of excessive production of hormones capable of altering the normal balance of absorption and secretion (14). The condition is rare and is manifested by persistent diarrhea even in the fasting state. The volume of the diarrhea is usually 1 liter/day and is secretory—that is, there is no osmotic gap when stool electrolytes are measured. When the tumor is examined immunohistochemically, multiple peptides are identified having a potential role in the diarrheal syndrome.

Verner and Morrison or Pancreatic Cholera Syndrome. This disorder is manifested by watery diarrhea, hypokalemia, hypochlorhydria or achlorhydria, and acidosis (WDHHA).

WDHHA is associated with excess secretion of VIP by islet cell, ganglioneuroblastoma, pheochromocytoma, neuroblastoma, small cell carcinoma of the lung or mast cell tumors (15, 16). There have been case reports of pancreatic cholera associated with islet cell tumors that do not contain vasoactive intestinal peptide (VIP). Furthermore, immunohistochemical staining of tumors demonstrates the presence of multiple peptides.

VIP is a neurotransmitter that causes secretory diarrhea by increasing cAMP in intestinal epithelial cells, resulting in increased secretion and decreased absorption. The diagnosis is usually made by a finding of elevated VIP levels in the serum. Treatment is directed toward resection of the tumor and reduction of circulating hormone levels. Even in patients with metastatic disease, reducing the amount of tumor can reduce the tumor load. Antitumor agents such as streptozotocin and 5-fluorouracil have been useful in treating advanced disease. Treatment may also be targeted to hormone release as well as to the intestine itself. Octreotide, a synthetic analog of somatostatin, caused significant improvement in diarrhea in most of the patients treated (17).

Zollinger-Ellison Syndrome. This disorder frequently presents with diarrhea (18). Hypergastrinemia produces excess acid secretion which produces malabsorption as well as anatomic injury to the proximal small intestinal mucosa. Pancreatic enzymes are inactive and bile salts precipitate at acid pH. Treatment is directed at tumor localization and resection and at reduction of acid secretion. Omeprazole rapidly and significantly reduces acid output and results in disappearance of the diarrhea and malabsorption (19).

Carcinoid Syndrome. Serotonin and substance P are elevated in carcinoid syndrome and are likely to be the agents responsible for the diarrhea (20). The diagnosis is made by the finding of elevated 5-hydroxyindoeacetic acid in the urine. Treatment includes tumor resection, chemotherapy with streptozotocin and 5-fluorouracil or cyclophosphamide, and tumor devascularization by angiographic em-

bolization. Octreotide will significantly reduce both the diarrhea and systemic manifestations of the disease.

Medullary Carcinoma of the Thyroid. Calcitonin, prostaglandins, somatostatin, serotonin, and VIP have all been found in this tumor. Approximately one-third of the patients will have diarrhea (21). The diagnosis is made by a finding of elevated calcitonin levels. Treatment is primarily directed at surgical resection. Chemotherapy may be warranted as well as treatment with octreotide for patients with severe diarrhea.

COLLAGENOUS COLITIS

Infiltration of the colonic mucosa by inflammatory cells and collagen deposition in the lamina propria are associated with diarrheal disorders (22–24). Microscopic colitis may be an early form of this disorder, because of the absence of collagen deposition. The therapy of this disorder is based on anecdotal reports. Symptomatic therapy with antidiarrheals and fiber should be considered initially. Trials of sulfasalazine and corticosteroids have been published and there is some evidence that corticosteroids reduce collagen deposition. The role of corticosteroids should be weighed against their long-term toxicity.

BACTERIAL OVERGROWTH

The role of increased bacterial content of the proximal small bowel in the pathogenesis of diarrhea is unclear. It is presumed that high bacterial counts either alter the metabolism of foodstuffs, resulting in osmotic catharsis, or bacterial toxins directly stimulate intestinal secretion (25). Diagnosis is difficult and practitioners often resort to a therapeutic trial of antibiotics to assess response. Agents with broad-spectrum activity against bacterial flora such as tetracycline, ampicillin, sulfamethoxazole/trimethoprim, and quinolones are used. The duration and need for recurrent courses is entirely dependent on the clinical response. It is important to establish some objective guidelines such as documentation of a decrease in stool frequency to assess response.

LACTOSE INTOLERANCE AND CARBOHYDRATE MALABSORPTION

The inability to metabolize carbohydrate is an important cause of diarrhea. Although the diarrhea may not be profuse, alteration in liquidity and frequency and gas production can be quite disturbing. Lactase deficiency is the most common problem, often developing later in life (26). The severity of symptoms is dependent on the quantity of lactose sugars consumed. When the capacity of the enzyme is exceeded, symptoms ensue. Treatment is based on elimination of lactose from the diet. Supplemental lactase is sometimes effective.

Fructose and sorbitol are sugars commonly encountered in the diet that are poorly absorbed. Stool analysis will demonstrate an osmotic gap because of the presence of osmotically active particles and the stool pH will be <6. Diagnosis can be made by careful dietary history and elimination diets. Treatment is based on elimination of the offending agent by careful attention to food labeling.

BILE ACID-INDUCED DIARRHEA

The role of bile salts in the diarrhea associated with ileal resection is clear (27, 28). In these patients colonic bile salt concentrations are high enough to alter transport. These patients respond to bile salt-binding materials such as cholestyramine. Bile acid malabsorption and its role in idiopathic chronic diarrhea, postvagotomy, and postcholecystectomy is less clear. Although, bile acid excretion may be elevated in some of these conditions, the response to cholestyramine is disappointing. In cases where a secretory diarrhea is present and bile acid malabsorption is considered, a therapeutic trial is warranted. Cholestyramine in large doses, 9 g four times daily to start, and then reduction if there is a therapeutic response.

CHRONIC IDIOPATHIC SECRETORY DIARRHEA

The diagnosis of this disorder is not straightforward because it is considered a diagnosis of exclusion (29, 30). Diagnostic studies should include examination of and biopsy of the small and large bowel, and a search for malabsorptive, infectious, and endocrinologic etiologies. Chronic idiopathic secretory diarrhea is characterized by fasting stool weight >500 g/24 hours and a secretory pattern on stool electrolytes. Symptom onset may occur after an acute diarrheal illness or may be insidious. A recent study suggests that this is a self-limited disease that may require many months to resolve. Treatment with opiate antidiarrheals in high doses and psyllium may be necessary to control symptoms. There are few data on the use of other antidiarrheal agents and their use should be weighed against risk and cost.

THERAPEUTIC PRINCIPLES

The danger of acute diarrheal illness is dehydration, and therapy should be directed at reducing stool output and maintaining adequate oral replacement. In contrast, chronic diarrhea can be debilitating without producing dehydration. With both acute and chronic diarrhea, therapy should be directed at the etiologic agent whenever the cause can be identified. However, in some instances, diagnosis is impractical or impossible and the practitioner must rely on symptomatic therapies. Symptomatic therapy carries the risk of missing an underlying treatable disorder and of exacerbating an underlying condition. Antidiarrheal agents have been reported to precipitate toxic megacolon when used in the setting of infectious or idiopathic inflammatory bowel disease.

THERAPEUTIC AGENTS

Oral Rehydration Therapy

Rehydration therapy represents a major advance in the treatment of diarrheal disease (31–34). The physiologic basis for this approach to therapy is the observation that transmucosal transport of sodium and water is increased when glucose is present in the lumen. This phenomenon is based on the finding of a solute-coupled transport process in the enterocyte. Glucose uptake by the enterocyte is accompanied by uptake of sodium followed by paracellular movement of chloride.

Table 15.1
Oral Rehydration Solutions for Treatment of Diarrhea[a]

Solution	Na	K	Cl	Citrate	Bicarbonate	Glucose
WHO solution	90	20	80	30		111
Pedialyte	45	20	35	10		140
Resol	50	20	50	11		111
Infalyte	50	25	45		30	111
Gatorade	23.5	<1	17			(40)
Coca-cola	1.6	<1			13	(100)
Apple juice	<1	25	30			(120)
Tea	0	0	0	0	0	0
Chicken soup	250	8	250	0	0	0

[a]All values are given as millimoles per liter except those in parentheses which are given as grams per liter.

The uptake of salt followed by water results in an increase in absorption that can substantially reduce the volume of fluid in the lumen. Oral rehydration may reduce fluid loss enough to avoid clinically significant dehydration.

Rehydration therapy can be effective independent of the etiology of the diarrhea because the nutrient-linked sodium cotransport mechanism remains intact (Table 15.1). The principle of therapy is to replenish fluid and electrolyte loss by frequent administration of an appropriate glucose and electrolyte solution in frequent, small volumes. Numerous mixtures derived from folklore and household practice have been used. Fortunately, the severity of most adult diarrheal illness in developed countries and normal renal function permit a variety of solutions to be effective. Soda, soup, and caffeinated beverages are often used, but are not properly balanced. Soda contains high concentrations of glucose, little sodium, and is hyperosmotic. Soup contains little glucose and is a hypertonic salt solution. Dilute tea is often used, but it has insufficient sodium and requires the addition of glucose to facilitate transport. Furthermore, caffeine is a phosphodiesterase inhibitor and may exacerbate an underlying secretory diarrhea by increasing cAMP.

Several rehydration solutions are commercially available (Table 15.1). It is important to recognize that oral rehydration therapy must begin soon after the diarrhea starts. The solution must be administered in small amounts at frequent intervals to avoid gastric distension and to minimize any stimulus to vomiting. The efficacy of rehydration therapy may be monitored by determining whether the patient produces a light tea-colored, i.e., dilute, urine every 4–6 hours. Adults may need to drink up to 1 liter/hour for rehydration and approximately 200 ml/hour for maintenance. There is some concern that oral rehydration solutions may produce hypernatremia (34).

Fiber Supplements

Psyllium hydrophilic mucilloid, calcium polycarbophil, and carboxymethylcellulose are often used to treat constipation. Although it is counterintuitive to use these agents in the setting of diarrheal illness, bulk laxatives are useful in selected circumstances. These agents are of little use in acute diarrheal illness, but appear to be useful alone or in combination with other agents in altering the frequency and consistency of stool (35–39).

Fiber supplements adsorb water and alter the viscosity of stool. Recent studies suggest equivalent doses of different fiber products have markedly different effects on fecal water output, stool viscosity, and the perception of stool fluidity. Psyllium appears to be most effective at producing a perception of increased stool solidity, in spite of an increase in stool water. Subjects with pharmacologically induced diarrhea eliminate more water with the addition of psyllium. Although psyllium increased stool water output and viscosity, the perceived effect was an improvement in stool fluidity.

Dosage

Dosage of fiber supplements is dependent on achieving the desired result. Thus, the dose should be titrated to achieve an improvement in the patients perception. Psyllium may be given in dosages of up to 30 g/day. Objective data on the effect of carboxymethylcellulose is unavailable. Calcium polycarbophil increased viscosity but did little to provide the sensation of increased stool form. In fact, more water was eliminated by patients receiving calcium polycarbophil than in control patients (38).

Opiates: Natural and Synthetic

Naturally occurring opiates are among the oldest medicinals, dating back to the Sumerians (ca. 4000 *BCE*). Modern formulations may be obtained that are based on extracts of opium that contain numerous alkaloids, including morphine and codeine as well as papaverine. The action of these agents is based on their interaction with intestinal opiate receptors (40–48). Several subtypes of the opiate receptor (μ, δ, κ, ϵ, and σ) have been identified on smooth muscle, neurons, and enterocytes. These opiate receptor subtypes have differential affinities for their naturally occurring ligands: the enkephalins and dynorphin. The effect of antidiarrheals which are not selective in their affinity may be on motility as well as transport. The ideal opiate would be an agent selective for receptors on the intestinal subsystem, for example, smooth muscle or enterocyte that is physiologically responsible for the diarrhea and does not cross the blood-brain barrier.

CODEINE AND OTHER NARCOTIC ANALGESICS

Meperidine, morphine, and hydromorphone hydrochloride (Dilaudid) are *not* indicated in the treatment of diarrheal diseases. However, the clinician should recognize that these agents can effectively potentiate the action of other agents used in the treatment of diarrhea. Codeine sulfate can be used in the treatment

of diarrhea, but it has some central nervous system side effects that may limit its use. Codeine also has a significant habituating potential.

Dosage

Codeine sulfate dosage should be titrated but 60 mg orally four times a day may be used.

PAREGORIC

This agent has often been used in functional gastrointestinal disorders associated with diarrhea. It is prepared as a camphorated tincture of opium and contains morphine 2 mg/5 ml. It is effective as an antidiarrheal but has sedating and addictive properties.

Dosage

The appropriate dosage is 5–10 ml orally as often as four times daily.

TINCTURE OF OPIUM, DEODORIZED

This agent may be used in the treatment of severe diarrhea. It should be remembered that opium is approximately 10% morphine. Tincture of opium is highly addictive and has sedating properties. It is currently in use in the treatment of AIDS-associated diarrhea.

Dosage

A dosage of 0.6 ml orally as often as four times per day is appropriate.

DIPHENOXYLATE HYDROCHLORIDE WITH ATROPINE SULFATE

This agent is a meperidine congener that has significant constipating effects. High doses (40–60 mg) will produce opium-like central nervous system effects, and for this reason this compound is formulated in combination with an anticholinergic to prevent abuse. Diphenoxylate has limited central nervous system permeability and appears to act predominantly at the μ-opiate receptor on smooth muscle. The effect is therefore a reduction in motility rather than alteration in transport. The anticholinergic component will produce dry mouth, blurred vision, and urinary retention. There may be some salutory effect of the anticholinergic effect in reducing motility and secretion, but this is not well-defined.

Dosage

A dosage of 2.5–5 mg orally four times per day is appropriate. Doses are often administered after each loose stool but should be individualized according to the severity of symptoms.

DIFENOXIN

This agent is also chemically related to meperidine and is combined with atropine sulfate to prevent abuse. Difenoxin is the principal active metabolite of diphenoxylate, and the dose required for therapeutic effect is significantly reduced. Both diphenoxylate and difenoxin should be used with caution because of their potential for central nervous system toxicity, including respiratory depression.

Dosage

A dosage of 1–2 mg should be given initially, and then 1 mg after each loose stool or every 3–4 hours. The total dose should not exceed 8 mg in 24 hours.

LOPERAMIDE

Loperamide is available over the counter and is frequently used in the treatment of diarrhea. The duration of action is approximately 4 hours and it can be used safely in high doses. The predominant effect of loperamide is on motility via the μ-receptor. In vitro studies suggest an effect on transport via the δ-receptor. Loperamide is used to control diarrhea in almost all diarrheal conditions, including adjunctive therapy for oral rehydration, acute traveler's diarrhea, dumping syndrome, high-output ileostomy, and irritable bowel syndrome.

Dosage

An initial dose of 4 mg followed by 2 mg after each loose stool until control is achieved is appropriate. The dose should then be individualized according to symptoms. The maximum daily dose is as much as 8 mg/day but higher doses have been used for AIDS-associated diarrhea.

Adrenergic Agonists

Adrenergic agents can stimulate absorption and inhibit secretion of fluid and electrolytes by interacting with specific receptors at multiple sites including enterocytes (49–56). Clonidine, lidamidine, and methoxy-tolazoline have similar properties in reducing diarrhea. Unfortunately, the utility of these agents is limited by their antihypertensive effect. Studies have been performed to dissociate the antidiarrheal effect from the central effects of hypotension, lightheadedness, depression, and fatiguability.

Clonidine, a selective α_2 adrenergic agonist, should be tried in patients with intractable diabetic diarrhea. The diabetic autonomic neuropathy appears to be associated with an increase in adrenergic tone and increased secretion and/or motility in these patients. The central hypotensive effect is less striking because of the autonomic neuropathy. Success is limited, and not all patients respond, but clonidine should be considered after simple measures such as fiber and low doses of opiates have been tried. In addition, clonidine may be useful in patients with diarrhea due to opiate withdrawal.

Dosage

The appropriate dosage is 1.0–1.5 mg/day. These doses are relatively high. The dose should be titrated and patients should be monitored carefully for side effects.

Hormones: Steroids and Somatostatin

Steroid hormones are ordinarily not considered to be antidiarrheal compounds but are included here because of their profound effect on inflamed mucosa. Steroids reduce the production of inflammatory mediators that stimulate secretion by enterocytes. They also increase absorption by the intestinal mucosa by acting directly on the epithelium to increase sodium absorption and decrease conductance.

The direct effect of steroids may be based on their action as a mineralocorticoid.

Dosage

Prednisone dosage is adjusted based on the severity of inflammatory disease. The maximum dose generally used is 60 mg orally each day.

Octreotide, a synthetic analog of somatostatin, has been used extensively in the treatment of diarrheal diseases (17, 57–65). Somatostatin and its analogs act on hormone release and on enterocytes to decrease ion transport. It is most effective in disorders that are the result of ectopic hormone secretion such as pancreatic cholera (VIP) and carcinoid syndrome. The effect of octreotide may be predominantly to reduce hormone release and less to decrease enterocyte secretion.

Octreotide has also been used in the treatment of diarrhea associated with short bowel syndrome, colostomies, ileostomies, and pancreatic fistulas. Octreotide must be injected subcutaneously and has a relatively short half-life. An acute side effect is hyperglycemia; long-term side effects include increased frequency of gallstones.

Octreotide also has been advocated as a treatment for AIDS-associated diarrhea. Several studies have suggested an improvement in some individuals; however, octreotide will result in a complete or partial response in less than 50% of patients. Most of the patients who do respond have no identifiable pathogens. Thus, octreotide should be used after conventional therapy with high doses of antidiarrheals and psyllium have failed.

Dosage

The dose should be titrated to achieve the desired effect. Starting dose is 50 μg subcutaneously every 8 hours, and may be increased to as much as 500 μg subcutaneously every 8 hours. In tumor-related diarrhea, doses should start at 150 μg subcutaneously every 8 hours.

Miscellaneous Agents

Bismuth Subsalicylate. This agent has been used in the treatment of traveler's diarrhea (66). It is likely to act by binding bacterial toxin. Bismuth subsalicylate does not appear to have activity in viral diarrhea or in other conditions associated with diarrhea.

Phenothiazines. These agents are not often used in the treatment of diarrheal disorders. They appear to have some effect on the intracellular signal transduction process. In addition, the phenothiazines often have anticholinergic effects that may contribute to some antidiarrheal action (67, 68). Phenothiazines have been used to reduce the volume requirement for oral rehydration therapy.

Calcium Channel Blockers. An important side effect of these agents is constipation, suggesting that calcium channel blockers alter motility and/or transport (69). These agents are not generally used in the treatment of diarrheal disorders.

Lithium Salts. Lithium chloride has been used in the treatment of a patient with a VIP-secreting tumor but has not been used in other conditions (70).

Indomethacin. The action of nonsteroidal anti-inflammatory drugs on the gastrointestinal tract is complex. Indomethacin inhibits cyclo-oxygenase and increases prostaglandin production. This should increase secretion but in vitro it appears to be proabsorptive. The drug may be tried for diarrhea caused by neuroendocrine tumors, villous adenomas, radiation enteritis, and irritable bowel syndrome (71–74). It should not be used in inflammatory bowel disease.

Cholestyramine. Cholestyramine is an ion exchange resin used in the treatment of pseudomembranous colitis due to *Clostridium difficile* infection (75, 76). The presumed mechanism of action is to bind toxin and reduce its effect on the epithelium. In addition, cholestyramine will bind bile salts and is used in the treatment of bile salt-induced diarrhea. The utility of cholestyramine in bile salt diarrhea associated with ileal resection will depend on the amount of small intestine resected. If >100 cm of ileum is removed, cholestyramine will result in bile salt depletion, worsen malabsorption, and increase the diarrhea. Cholestyramine may also be useful in the treatment of other causes of diarrhea, but the literature to support this approach is limited.

REFERENCES

1. Lew JF, Glass RI, Gangarosa RE, Cohen IP, Bern C, Moe CL. Diarrheal deaths in the United States, 1979–1987. JAMA 1991;265:3280–3285.
2. Hyams KD, Bourgeois AL, Merrell BR, et al. Diarrheal disease during Operation Desert Shield. N Engl J Med 1991;325:1423–1428.
3. Blacklow NR, Greenberg HB. Viral gastroenteritis. N Engl J Med 1991;325:252–264.
4. Snyder JD, Merson MH. The magnitude of the global problem of acute diarrheal disease: a review of active surveillance data. Bull WHO 1982;60:605–613.
5. Greenough WB III, Bennett RG. Diarrhea in the elderly. In: Hazzard WR, Andres R, Bierman EL, Blass JP, eds. Principles of geriatric medicine and gerontology. New York: McGraw Hill; 1990:1168–1176.
6. Cooke HJ. Neural and humoral regulation of small intestinal electrolyte transport. In: Johnson LR, ed. Physiology of the gastrointestinal tract. New York: Raven Press, 1987:1307–1350.
7. Powell DW. Approach to the patient with diarrhea. In: Yamada T, ed. Textbook of gastroenterology. Philadelphia: Lippincott, 1991:732–778.
8. Field M. Diarrheal diseases. New York: Elsevier, 1991.
9. Donowitz M, Welsh MJ. Regulation of mammalian small intestinal electrolyte secretion. In: Johnson LR, ed. Physiology of the gastrointestinal tract. New York: Raven Press, 1987:1351–1388.
10. Fine, KD, Krejs, GJ, Fordtran, JS. Diarrhea. In: Sleisenger MH, Fordtran JS, eds. Gastrointestinal disease, ed. 4. Philadelphia: WB Saunders, 1989:290–316.
11. Fedorak RN, Rubinoff MJ. Basic investigation of patient with diarrhea. In: Field M, ed. Diarrheal diseases. New York: Elsevier, 1991:191–218.
12. Schiller LR. Chronic diarrhea of obscure origin. In: Field M, ed. Diarrheal diseases. New York: Elsevier, 1991:219–238.
13. Binder HJ. Absorption and secretion of water and electrolytes by small and large intestine. In: Sleisenger MH, Fordtran JS, eds. Gastrointestinal disease, ed. 4. Philadelphia: WB Saunders, 1989:1022–1044.
14. Rood RP, Donowitz M. Endocrine tumor-associated diarrheal syndromes. In: Field M, ed. Diarrheal diseases. New York: Elsevier, 1991:397–411.
15. Verner JV, Morrison AB. Islet cell tumor and a syndrome of refractory diarrhea and hypokalemia. Am J Med 1958;25:374–380.
16. O'Dorisio TM, Mekhjian HS. VIPoma syndrome. In: Cohen S. Soloway RD, eds. Hormone-producing tumors of the gastrointestinal tract. New York: Churchill Livingston; 1985;101–116.
17. Maton PN, O'Dorisio TM, Howe BA, et al. Effects of a long-acting somatostatin analogue (SMS 201-995) in a patient with pancreatic cholera. N Engl J Med 1985;312:17–21.
18. Jensen RT, Foppman JL, Gardner JD. Gastrinoma. In: Go VLW et al., eds. The exocrine pancreas. New York: Raven Press; 1986:727–744.
19. Lamers CBHW, Lind T, Moberg S, et al. Omeprazole in Zollinger-Ellison syndrome. N Engl J Med 1984;310:900–902.
20. Vinik AI, Mcleod MK, Fig LM, Shapiro B, Lloyd RV, Cho K. Clinical features, diagnosis, and localization of carcinoid tumors and their management. Gastroenterol Clin North Am 1989;18:865–896.
21. Sizemore GW. Medullary carcinoma of the thyroid gland. Semin Oncol 1987;14:306–314.
22. Rams H, Rogers AI, Ghandur-Mnaymneh L. Collagenous colitis. Ann Intern Med 1987;106:108–113.
23. Rask-Madsen J, Grove O, Hansen MGJ, et al. Colonic transport of water and electrolytes in a patient with secretory diarrhea due to collagenous colitis. Dig Dis Sci 1983;28:1141–1146.
24. Jessurun J, Yaardley JH, Lee EL, et al. Microscopic and collagenous colitis: different names for the same condition? Gastroenterology 1986;91:1583–1584.
25. Moriarty KJ, Turnberg LA. Bacterial toxins and diarrhea. Clin Gastroenterol 1986;12:529–543.
26. Caspary WF. Diarrhea associated with carbohydrate malabsorption. Clin Gastroenterol 1986;15:631–655.
27. Arlow FL, Dekovich AA, Priest RJ, Beher WT. Bile-acid mediated postcholecystectomy diarrhea. Arch Intern Med 1987;147:1327–1329.
28. Fromm H, Malavolti M. Bile acid-induced diarrhea. Clin Gastroenterol 1986;15:567–582.
29. Read NW, Krejs GJ, Read MG, Santa Ana CA, Morawski SG, Fordtran JS. Chronic diarrhea of unknown origin. Gastroenterology 1980;78:264–270.
30. Afsalpurkar RG, Schiller LR, Little KH, Santangelo WC, Fordtran JS. The self-limited nature of chronic idiopathic diarrhea. N Engl J Med 1992;327:1849–1852.
31. Greenough WB III, Maung-U K. Oral rehydration therapy. In: Field M, ed. Diarrheal diseases. New York: Elsevier, 1991:485–499.
32. Pierce NF, Sack RB, Mitra RC, et al. Replacement of water and electrolyte losses in cholera by an oral glucose electrolyte solution. Ann Intern Med 1969;70:1173–1181.
33. Santosham M, Greenough WB III. Oral rehydration therapy: a global perspective. J Pediatr 1991;118:S44–S51.
34. Elliott EJ, Cunha-Ferreira R, Walker-Smith JA, Farthing MJG. Sodium content of oral rehydration solutions: a reappraisal. Gut 1989;2:719–723.
35. Smalley JR, Klish WJ, Campbell MA, Brown MR. Use of psyllium in the management of chronic nonspecific diarrhea of childhood. J Pediatr Gastroenterol Nutr 1982;1(3):361–363.
36. Longstretch GF, Fox D, Youkeles L, Forsythe AB, Wolochow DA. Psyllium therapy in irritable bowel syndrome. Ann Intern Med 1981;95:53–55.

37. Harvey RF, Heaton KW, Pomera EW. Effects of increased dietary fiber on intestinal transit. Lancet 1973;1:1278–1279.

38. Eherer AJ, Santa Ana CA, Porter J, Fordtran JS. Effect of psyllium, calcium polycarbophil and wheat bran on secretory diarrhea induced by phenolphthalein. Gastroenterology 1992;104:1007–1012.

39. Qvitzau S, Matzen P, Madsen P. Treatment of chronic diarrhea: loperamide versus ispaghula husk and calcium. Scand J Gastroenterol 1988;23:1237–1240.

40. Dobbins J, Racusen L, Binder HJ. Effect of d-alanine methionine enkephalin amide on ion transport in rabbit ileum. J Clin Invest 1980;66:19–28.

41. Kachur JF, Miller RJ, Field M. Control of guinea pig intestinal electrolyte secretion by a delta-opiate receptor. Proc Natl Acad Sci USA 1980;77:2753–2756.

42. Schiller LR, Davis GR, Santa Ana CA, Morawski SG, Fordtran JS. Studies of the mechanism of the antidiarrheal effect of codeine. J Clin Invest 1982;70:999–1008.

43. Schiller LR, Santa CA, Morawski SG, Fordtran JS. Mechanism of the antidiarrheal effect of loperamide. Gastroenterology 1984;86:1475–1480.

44. Sun EA, Snape WJ, Cohen S, Renny A. The role of opiate receptors and cholinergic neurons in the gastrocolonic response. Gastroenterology 1982;82:689–693.

45. Kaufman PN, Krevsky B, Malmud LS, et al. Opiate receptors in regulation of colonic transit. Gastroenterology 1988;94:1351–1356.

46. Telford GL, Condon RE, Szurszewski JH. Opioid receptors and the initiation of migrating myoelectric complexes in dogs. Am J Physiol 1989;256:G72–G77.

47. Shook JE, Lemcke PK, Gehrig CA, Hruby VJ, Burks TF. Antidiarrheal properties of supraspinal mu and delta and peripheral mu, delta and kappa opioid receptors: inhibition of diarrhea without constipation. J Pharmacol Exp Ther 1989;249:83–90.

48. Kramer W. Endogenous and exogenous opioids in the control of gastrointestinal motility and secretion. Pharmacol Rev 1988;40:121–162.

49. Carey HV, Cooke HJ. Neuromodulation of intestinal transport in the suckling mouse. Am J Physiol 1989;256:R481–R486.

50. Cooke HJ, Shannard K, Highison G, Wood JD. Effects of neurotransmitter release on mucosal transport in guinea pig ileum. Am J Physiol 1983;245:G745–G750.

51. Zimmerman TW, Dobbins JW, Binder HJ. Mechanism of cholinergic regulation of electrolyte transport in rat colon in vitro. Am J Physiol 1982;242:G116–G123.

52. Steadman CJ, Phillips SG, Camilleri M, Talley NJ, Haddad A, Hanson R. Control of muscle tone in the human colon. Gut 1992;33:541–546.

53. Field M, McColl. Ion transport in rabbit ileal mucosa: III. Effects of catecholamines. Am J Physiol 1973;225:852–857.

54. Chang EB, Field M, Miller RJ. Enterocyte α-2-Adrenergic receptors: yohimbine and p-amino clonidine binding relative to ion transport. Am J Physiol 1983;244:G76–G82.

55. Fedorak RN, Field M, Chang EB. Treatment of diabetic diarrhea with clonidine. Ann Intern Med 1985;102:197–199.

56. Dharmsathaphorn K. α-2-Adrenergic antagonists: a newer class of antidiarrheal drugs. Gastroenterology 1986;91:769–773.

57. Raijman I, Cragoe E, Sellin J. Hormonal and pharmacologic regulation of sodium absorption in rabbit cecum in vitro. Dig Dis Sci 1992;37:1874–1881.

58. Grubb BR, Bentley PJ. Effects of corticosteroids on short-circuit current across the cecum of the domestic fowl. J Comp Physiol 1992;162:690–695.

59. Lauritsen K, Laursen LS, Bukhave K, Rask-Madsen J. In vivo effects of orally administered prednisolone on prostaglandin and leucotriene production in ulcerative colitis. Gut 1987;28:1095–1101.

60. Sandle GI, McGlone F. Acute effects of dexamethasone on cation transport in colonic epithelium. Gut 1987;28:701–705.

61. Davis GR, Camp RC, Raskin P, Krejs GJ. Effect of somatostatin infusion on jejunal water and electrolyte transport in a patient with secretory diarrhea due to malignant carcinoid syndrome. Gastroenterology 1980;78:346–350.

62. Dharmasathaphorn K, Racusen I, Dobbins JW. Effect of somatostatin on ion transport in the rat colon. J Clin Invest 1980;66:813–820.

63. Barrett KE, Dharmasathaphorn K. Pharmacologic approaches to the therapy of diarrheal diseases. In: Field M, ed. Diarrheal diseases. New York: Elsevier, 1991:501–516.

64. Cello JP, Grendell JH, Basuk P, et al. Effect of octreotide on refractory AIDS-associated diarrhea: a prospective, multicenter clinical trial. Ann Intern Med 1991;115:705–710.

65. Catnach SM, Anderson JV, Fairclough PD, et al. Effect of octreotide on all stone prevalence and gall bladder motility in acromegaly. Gut 1993;34:270–273.

66. DuPont HL, Ericsson CD. Prevention and treatment of traveler's diarrhea. N Engl J Med 1993;328:1821–1827.

67. Holmgren J, Lange S, Lonnroth I. Reversal of cyclic AMP-mediated intestinal secretion in mice by chlorpromazine. Gastroenterology 1978;75:1103–1108.

68. Jennische E, Lonnroth I. Effects of chlorpromazine on fluid transport across the intestinal mucosa of the rat. Acta Pharmacol Toxicol (Copenh) 1982;50:305–309.

69. Donowitz M, Levin S, Powers G, Elta G, Cohen P, Cheng H. Ca2 + channel blockers stimulate ileal and colonic water absorption. Gastroenterology 1985;89:858–866.

70. Pandol SJ, Korman LY, McCarthy DM, Gardner JD. Beneficial effects of oral lithium carbonate in the treatment of pancreatic cholera syndrome. N Engl J Med 1980;302:1403–1404.

71. Davies GR, Wilkie ME, Rampton DS. Effects of metronidazole and misoprostol on indomethacin induced changes in intestinal permeability. Dig DIs Sci 1993;38:417–425.

72. Clarke LL, Argenzio RA. NaCl transport across equine proximal colon and the effect of endogenous prostanoids. Am J Physiol 1990;259:G62–G69.

73. Smith PL, Blumberg JB, Stoff JS, Field M. Antisecretory effects of indomethacin on rabbit ileal mucosa in vitro. Gastroenterology 1981;80:356–365.

74. Donowitz M, Cheng HY, Sharp GW. Effects of phobol esters on sodium and chloride transport in rat colon. Am J Physiol 1986;25:G509–517.

75. Rowe GG. Control of diarrhea by cholestyramine administration. Am J Med Sci 1968;255:84–88.

76. Allan JG, Russell RI. Double-blind controlled trial of cholestyramine in the treatment of post-vagotomy diarrhea. Gut 1975;10:830.

16

Pharmacotherapy of Gastrointestinal Tract Infections in Patients with Acquired Immunodeficiency Syndrome

DOUGLAS SIMON and LAWRENCE J. BRANDT

Gastrointestinal involvement is extremely common during the course of human immunodeficiency virus (HIV) infection. The gastrointestinal organs that are most frequently affected are the esophagus, small intestine, and colon. Esophageal involvement typically results in dysphagia, odynophagia, and occasionally substernal chest pain. Small intestinal involvement most often results in diarrhea and malabsorption, while colonic disease manifests with diarrhea or bloody diarrhea. This chapter will review the pharmacology and use of agents available to treat the pathogens that commonly affect the esophagus and intestine of patients with AIDS. The clinical characteristics of these infections have been reviewed elsewhere (1–3) and will not be discussed here.

AGENTS USED TO TREAT FUNGAL DISEASES

The most commonly encountered fungus in the gastrointestinal tract of HIV-infected individuals is *Candida albicans. C. albicans* results in thrush and esophagitis, both of which are extremely common in HIV-infected individuals; less common fungal species that may cause esophagitis include *Candida tropicalis, Candida krusei*, and *Torulopsis glabrata.*

Treatment options for fungal esophagitis can be divided into three categories: topical antifungal agents (clotrimazole and nystatin), oral absorbable antifungal agents (ketoconazole, fluconazole, and itraconazole), and intravenous antifungal agents (amphotericin).

Antifungal agents can be discussed according to their molecular structures and divided into the polyenes, imidazoles, and triazoles. Amphotericin and nystatin are polyene antifungal agents that function by binding to ergosterol. Polyene interaction with ergosterol results in the formation of pores or channels, with an increase in permeability of the fungal membrane and leakage of a variety of small molecules (4). The imidazole antifungal agents include ketoconazole, clotrimazole, and miconazole. Fluconazole and itraconazole are triazole agents. Both imidazole and triazole agents bind to the fungal cytochrome P-450 enzyme, lanosterol 14-α-demethylase, thus halting the conversion of lanosterol to ergosterol (4–6), a principal component of the fungal sterol membrane. This inhibition leads to accumulation of 14-α-methyl sterols which in turn interferes with the close packing of acyl chain phospholipids, impairs membrane bound enzyme systems, and inhibits fungal growth (4–6). The triazoles, fluconazole and itraconazole, have a minimal effect on mammalian cytochrome P-450 and, compared to ketoconazole, have less of an effect on human steroid hormone production (7). In theory, the effects of the imidazole and triazole antifungal agents should antagonize those of the polyenes because of decreased ergosterol synthesis, but clinically this has not been a problem in HIV-infected patients (8).

Ketoconazole (Nizoral) is a commonly prescribed oral antifungal agent and is well-absorbed after an oral dose. A 200-mg dose results in serum levels of 2.6–4 μg/ml, which is adequate to treat most fungal infections (9). Maksymiuk and colleagues (10) have reported that cancer patients receiving ketoconazole (200 mg four times daily for 2–3 weeks) have shown elevated ketoconazole blood levels. Espinel-Ingroff and colleagues (11) showed therapeutic blood levels in 40 patients receiving ketoconazole (600 mg daily for up to 6 months) for non-life-threatening fungal infections. Initial data indicated ketoconazole absorption could be increased by administration of the agent with food, but recent data has shown that higher serum levels of the drug result when it is taken fasting. This increased absorption results because the pH of the stomach is lower during fasting than during a meal, and ketoconazole, being a dibasic compound, requires hydrogen ions to render it neutral and thus permit its absorption across lipid membranes (12). A decrease in the functional parietal cell mass, referred to as "AIDS gastropathy," has been reported to occur in AIDS patients (13). AIDS gastropathy may result in reduced gastric acid secretion, thus reducing the absorption of ketoconazole and resulting in treatment failure. Similarly, antisecretory agents, such as H_2-receptor antagonists, by inhibiting gastric acid secretion, can also result in subtherapeutic serum ketoconazole levels and treatment failure (14). It has been suggested that taking the drug with a carbonated beverage or cranberry juice might enhance its absorption (15).

Data on distribution of ketoconazole in human tissues are limited and variable levels of the drug in the cerebrospinal fluid have been reported. Ketoconazole is 99% bound to plasma proteins, mainly albumin, and undergoes extensive hepatic metabolism with only 2–4% excreted unchanged in the urine (12). There are conflicting data on the half-life of ketoconazole, with a range of 2–8.1 hours reported after a single oral 200-mg dose (10, 12, 16). Ketoconazole metabolism can be accelerated when the agent is taken with either isoniazid or rifampin, resulting in subtherapeutic blood levels and possible treatment failure (17). Renal failure does not alter ketoconazole pharmacokinetics and dose adjustment is not required in patients with renal impairment (12). No data exist on ketoconazole pharmacokinetics in patients with hepatic dysfunction, but since hepatic metabolism is a major route of elimination, the drug probably should be used cautiously in patients with established hepatic dysfunction. Ketoconazole is extremely well-tolerated, with nausea, vomiting, abdominal pain, and pruritus being the most common reported side effects (12). Transient liver test abnormalities occur in approximately 10% of ketoconazole-treated patients (18), with a small number developing symptomatic liver dysfunction (19, 20). Gynecomastia has also been reported (21).

Fluconazole (Diflucan) has special pharmacokinetic properties of high metabolic stability and water solubility that contribute to its therapeutic activity. Ninety percent of an oral dose is detected in the circulation, with peak plasma concentrations occurring by 2 hours (7). Neither gastric pH or food influence fluconazole absorption (7). The volume of distribution is similar to that of the total body water, and approximately 11% of the drug is bound to plasma proteins (20, 22). Fluconazole has good penetration into the cerebrospinal fluid, as well as into tissues such as the liver, spleen, lung, kidney, muscle, and brain (23). Fluconazole is eliminated by the kidneys, with 80% of a dose recovered in the urine and an elimination half-life of 27–37 hours (7, 23, 24). These properties allow for once a day dosing, but dosage should be adjusted for renal function; for example, in patients with a glomerular filtration rate less than 20 ml/minute, the elimination half-life is increased to 98 hours (7). Three hours of hemodialysis lowers fluconazole plasma levels by 48%, but blood levels remain constant during the 2-day interdialysis period (7). The effect of fluconazole on the cytochrome P-450 enzyme complex has been reported possibly to alter the P-450 metabolism of several drugs, including phenytoin (25), coumadin (26), and oral hypoglycemic agents (7), with variable reports on blood cyclosporine levels (27, 28). Liver test abnormalities occur in approximately 1% of fluconazole-treated patients, which is significantly less than that occurring with ketoconazole (7). Rare cases of exfoliative skin reactions and hepatic necrosis also have been reported (7, 29).

Itraconazole (Sporanox) has pharmacokinetic properties of both ketoconazole and fluconazole. Itraconazole is available in Europe and is currently under consideration by the FDA for release in the United States. Itraconazole has poor bioavailability, with approximately 30% of an oral dose being absorbed when taken with a meal and wide interpatient variability in serum levels (30, 31). Like ketoconazole, itraconazole requires gastric acid for oral absorption, and, therefore, serum levels may be decreased in patients with AIDS gastropathy and those being treated with H_2-receptor antagonists (32, 33). Serum levels of itraconazole also can be decreased by coadministration of rifampin (34) and phenobarbital (35), and itraconazole has been reported to elevate serum digoxin levels (36). Also, like ketoconazole, itraconazole is highly protein bound and undergoes hepatic metabolism to inactive metabolites (30). At identical doses serum levels achieved with itraconazole are less than those with ketoconazole, but the volume of distribution of itraconazole is 20 times greater, giving it good penetration into skin, kidney, liver, lung, bone, and muscle (30, 32, 33). As with fluconazole, variable effects of itraconazole on blood cyclosporine levels have been reported (37, 38).

The half-life of itraconazole has been reported to range from 24–42 hours, similar to that of fluconazole, but it does not penetrate the cerebrospinal fluid as fluconazole does (30, 32). Itraconazole is eliminated by the liver, but only limited data are available on its use in patients with hepatic dysfunction; dose adjustments are not required in patients with renal insufficiency. Alteration of the dose, use

of a different antifungal agent, or monitoring blood levels carefully in cases of hepatic dysfunction seems reasonable, since itraconazole is metabolized in the liver. The safety profile of itraconazole is similar to that of fluconazole, with anorexia, rash, headache, nausea, and vomiting being the most frequently observed side effects (15, 30, 32, 39). At a dose of 400 mg/day itraconazole has no effect on serum levels of cortisol or testosterone (30), but Sharkey et al. (40) reported that at higher doses, itraconazole can cause reversible adrenal suppression. Transient abnormalities of serum transaminases occur in 1% of treated patients (30, 39), but to date, there have been no reports of drug-induced hepatitis.

Amphotericin B (fungizone and others) is reserved for patients with *Candida* esophagitis who are unable to swallow or for whom other antifungal agents have been ineffectual. Since absorption of amphotericin from the gastrointestinal tract is negligible, it is given intravenously. Amphotericin is insoluble at a neutral pH, and it is prepared with deoxycholate as a solubilizing agent (41). The amphotericin-deoxycholate complex is disrupted in the blood and the free amphotericin is then largely bound to β-lipoprotein (4, 41). Only 2–5% of the drug is recovered in the urine unchanged (4, 42) and animal studies indicate that hepatic and biliary disease have no effect on its metabolism (43). Autopsy studies indicate that one-third of the intravenous dose can be extracted from tissues, with the greatest amount found in the liver and spleen, followed by the kidney and lung (44, 45). The serum half-life of amphotericin is 10–18 hours in the serum, but it can be prolonged to 40 hours when the creatinine clearance is less than 5 ml/minute (4, 41, 42).

Side effects are common with amphotericin administration. Fever, chills, rigors, vomiting and headache can occur during intravenous infusion but may be attenuated by premedicating with aspirin or meperidine and hydrocortisone (15). Azotemia has been reported to occur in up to 80% of individuals receiving amphotericin for deep mycoses; the azotemia is dose-dependent, transient, and can be exacerbated by concomitant use of other nephrotoxic agents (i.e., aminoglycosides) (4, 41, 46). Renal tubular acidosis, with K+ and Mg2+ wasting and hypochromic and normocytic anemia secondary to diminished erythropoietin production, can also occur.

Topical agents include the imidazole, clotrimazole (Mycelex) troches and the polyene, nystatin (Mycostatin, Nilstatin) suspension. A dose of oral clotrimazole is almost 90% absorbed, but bioavailability is less than 5% because of its extensive first-pass metabolism (47). Nystatin, being a polyene antifungal like amphotericin, is not absorbed by the gastrointestinal tract (4). Topical agents are reasonable therapy for patients with mild to moderate oral thrush. Since they are neither absorbed, nor have an extensive first-pass metabolism, they have no drug interactions and lack side effects.

USE OF ANTIFUNGAL AGENTS IN THE TREATMENT OF CANDIDA ESOPHAGITIS

The treatment protocol that we use for *Candida* esophagitis begins with either topical agents or ketoconazole, depending on the severity of the patient's symptoms. Clotrimazole is usually given as 10-mg troches five times a day, and for nystatin 500,000–1.5 million units (5–15 ml) per day. The daily ketoconazole dose is 200–400 mg administered in two divided doses. Some patients dislike the taste of nystatin and the inconvenience of troches and prefer ketoconazole. In the rare patient who is unable to swallow, low dose amphotericin can be used as initial therapy until symptoms improve and the patient can be given an oral agent. There are limited data on the duration, dose, and effectiveness of amphotericin therapy in *Candida* esophagitis, but low doses (0.1–0.3 mg/kg/day) are recommended (4, 41), since this drug is extremely effective and produces rapid symptom resolution. If there is no symptomatic improvement by 1–2 weeks, the patient is then evaluated with esophagoscopy. Esophagoscopy is essential if empiric therapy for *Candida* esophagitis had been used initially. If *Candida* is the only pathogen identified by esophagoscopy,

then either fluconazole or low-dose amphotericin can be used. The usual fluconazole dose is 100–200 mg once daily. Gastric pH should be determined during endoscopy, and if it is alkaline, giving supplemental acid or raising the dose of ketoconazole should be considered before a different medication is tried. If symptomatic improvement does not follow fluconazole therapy within a few weeks, then the patient should undergo another esophagoscopy, and amphotericin should be given if *Candida* is again the only pathogen identified. During repeat esophagoscopy, culturing the yeast for species determination may also be helpful. Species such as *Torulopsis glabrata* or *Candida tropicalis* may be the cause of the esophagitis and both are resistant to certain antifungal agents.

There are limited data on the effectiveness of antifungal agents in treating *Candida* esophagitis. Laine and colleagues in an 8-week double-blind, randomized trial comparing fluconazole to ketoconazole showed fluconazole to be superior (48). Fluconazole resulted in a greater percentage of symptomatic improvement (66% vs. 55%), endoscopic resolution of disease, (87% vs. 53%) and a more rapid resolution of symptoms. Both drugs had minimal side effects. Cost is also an issue; fluconazole therapy at Montefiore Medical Center and Albert Einstein Medical Center costs five times more than does ketoconazole treatment ($10 vs. $2 per day). Smith and colleagues (49) compared itraconazole to ketoconazole in a 4-week double-blind, randomized protocol trial in 111 HIV-positive patients with oral and esophageal candidiasis. There were no differences in clinical and mycological response rates, with 93% success in each group after 8 weeks of therapy. One patient treated with itraconazole discontinued therapy because of a rash, and five ketoconazole patients discontinued therapy because of rash in one, hepatotoxicity in two, and nausea in two. The cost-effectiveness of itraconazole compared with that of fluconazole is unknown.

There are no controlled trials on the role of maintenance therapy for chronic or recurrent *Candida* esophagitis in patients with AIDS. Ketoconazole (100–200 mg/day) or topical agents can be used for such therapy in patients with frequent relapses. Another option is to instruct patients to initiate low-dose ketoconazole or a topical antifungal agent with the onset of thrush or esophageal symptoms. Prolonged use of fluconazole has led to resistant candidiasis (15).

AGENTS USED TO TREAT VIRAL DISEASES

The two most common viruses causing gastrointestinal disorders in HIV-infected individuals are cytomegalovirus and herpes simplex virus. Cytomegalovirus can infect any organ of the gastrointestinal tract, but the esophagus and colon are most commonly involved. Cytomegalovirus infection typically produces ulcerated lesions due to mucosal ischemia which results from viremia, endothelial deposition of virus, and subsequent vasculitis. Gastrointestinal tract infection with herpes simplex virus typically involves the esophagus and the rectum. The mechanism of esophagitis involves reactivation of latent virus in the trigeminal ganglia, with oropharyngeal viral shedding (symptomatic or asymptomatic) and finally swallowing of the virus into the esophagus. There have also been reports of reactivated herpes simplex virus causing esophageal infection directly from the vagus and celiac ganglia.

Three agents are available to treat gastrointestinal viral infections: acyclovir, ganciclovir, and foscarnet. Foscarnet is approved by the FDA for the treatment of cytomegalovirus retinitis that is refractory to ganciclovir therapy, but there are some data on its use in gastrointestinal viral infections.

Ganciclovir

Ganciclovir, (cytovene) 9-[(1,3-dihydroxy-2-propoxy)methyl] guanine (DHPG), is an acyclic nucleoside analog of 2′-deoxyguanosine that requires phosphorylation to a triphosphate derivative by cellular kinases in order for it to become active. Monophosphorylation is achieved via an induced host-encoded deoxyguanosine kinase (50) with subsequent phosphorylations by cellular guanylate kinase and phosphoglycerate kinase (50, 51). The ganciclovir triphosphate is a highly competitive inhibitor for the incorporation of deoxyguanosine triphosphate into viral DNA, and thereby inhibits viral DNA polymerase (52, 53). Ganciclovir triphosphate inhibition of DNA polymerase has much greater affinity for viral than for cellular DNA polymerase (53). The ganciclovir triphosphate is also incorporated into the growing viral DNA chain, which, in effect, reduces DNA chain elongation (52). The production of ganciclovir triphosphate is 100 times greater in cytomegalovirus-infected cells than in non-infected cells, which probably in some way relates to enhanced uptake by infected cells (54).

Ganciclovir demonstrates activity in vitro against cytomegalovirus, herpes simplex virus 1 and 2, Epstein-Barr virus, varicella-zoster virus, and adenovirus (52). It is more potent against cytomegalovirus than acyclovir is and appears to have a synergistic effect with interferons against cytomegalovirus (53).

Ganciclovir is not absorbed via the gastrointestinal tract and currently must be given intravenously (although an oral form is under investigation). The half-life of ganciclovir is 3–4 hours and plasma levels are linearly related to the infused drug within a dose range of 1–5 mg/kg (55, 56). The drug is 1–2% bound to plasma proteins (52) and is well-distributed throughout the body with good levels in the eye, cerebrospinal fluid, and tissues (52). Almost an entire intravenous dose of ganciclovir is excreted in the urine unchanged, indicating that both glomerular filtration and tubular secretion are involved in ganciclovir elimination (52, 56, 57). Plasma levels of ganciclovir increase in a linear fashion as creatinine clearance decreases (57). Weller and colleagues (56) have reported that its half-life is increased to 9–30 hours in patients with a creatinine clearance of 20–50 ml/min/1.73^2. Four hours of hemodialysis will lower plasma ganciclovir concentrations by almost 50% (52, 58).

The most frequent toxicity of ganciclovir therapy is hematologic, especially in patients with AIDS (59). Neutropenia and thrombocytopenia occur in up to 40% and 20%, respectively (52). Patients with platelet counts of <100,000/μl before therapy, are more likely to develop significant drug-related thrombocytopenia (52). Anemia has been reported in 2% of individuals (60). The hematologic toxicity of ganciclovir is reversible with discontinuation of therapy. Fever, rash, and liver test abnormalities have been reported in 2% of ganciclovir-treated patients (52). Ganciclovir should not be given to patients receiving imipenim/cilastatin (52) since there have been reports of generalized seizures during such combined therapy. Zidovudine and other drugs that can effect rapidly dividing cells should not be given with ganciclovir, since significant hematologic toxicity may result (52, 61).

Acyclovir

Acyclovir, (9-[(2-hydroxyethoxy)-methyl])-guanine, is an acyclic analog of $2'$-deoxyguanosine that also requires transformation to a triphosphate for it to inhibit viral DNA synthesis. The selectivity of acyclovir against herpes viruses and varicella zoster virus is due to the initial phosphorylation that is catalyzed by viral-encoded thymidine kinase (51, 62). The subsequent phosphorylations are performed by cellular guanylate kinase and other cellular enzymes (64). The acyclovir triphosphate is both a preferential inhibitor and a substrate for viral DNA polymerase. After binding to the viral DNA polymerase, the triphosphate acyclovir is incorporated into the DNA primer (64). This incorporation of triphosphate acyclovir prevents further chain elongation and has been termed a "suicide inactivator" (63). The effectiveness of acyclovir is enhanced both by viral DNA polymerase being more sensitive to its effect than is the host cellular DNA polymerase and the limited uptake of acyclovir into noninfected cells (65). Resistance of herpes simplex virus to acyclovir is well-known and is usually due to a viral lack or deficiency in thymidine kinase (64). Evidence of modified viral DNA polymerase has also been encountered recently (64).

Acyclovir also has in vitro activity, in decreasing order of effectiveness, against herpes type 1, herpes type 2, varicella-zoster virus, Epstein-Barr virus, and cytomegalovirus (62, 64). Currently, it is the most effective antiviral agent against herpes simplex virus 1 and 2.

Orally administered acyclovir (Zovirax) has only a 15–30% bioavailability due to its inconsistent and incomplete absorption (66). Peak plasma concentrations occur 1.5–2.5 hours after oral administration (66). Contradictory data exists on the effect of dosage on blood levels. Brigden and Whitman (67) reported that plasma acyclovir levels were similar after single 200- and 600-mg oral doses, suggesting that oral absorption of this drug is a saturable process. De Miranda and Blum (66) reported that steady-state peak and trough concentrations and area under the curve doubled when the dosage changed from 200–400 mg every 4 hours, indicating that absorption and plasma levels are dosage-dependent. Intravenous administration of acyclovir every 8 hours results in steady-state plasma levels that are directly proportional to the administered dose; there is no accumulation without significant renal dysfunction (63, 66, 68). Data on tissue and fluid distribution of the drug are limited, but because of its limited protein binding, tissue concentrations appear to be excellent (69). Penetration into the cerebrospinal fluid gives a concentration of acyclovir that is approximately 50% of the plasma levels and similar to that in the aqueous humor.

Acyclovir is eliminated by the kidneys with 45–79% of a dose recovered unchanged in the urine and the remainder consisting of acyclovir metabolites (62, 70). Acyclovir is eliminated not only by glomerular filtration but also by tubular secretion; probenecid has been shown to increase plasma levels. The half-life of acyclovir is 2–3 hours but increases to 20 hours with end-stage renal disease (64). Hemodialysis decreases plasma acyclovir levels by almost 60% and lowers the half-life to 5.7 hours (71). Peritoneal dialysis is less effective than hemodialysis in lowering plasma acyclovir levels and has been reported to lower the half-life to 14–18 hours (72).

The major toxicity of oral acyclovir when used in high doses for acute herpes infection is gastrointestinal, with nausea, vomiting, abdominal pain, and some lightheadedness (64). Studies of low-dose acyclovir used for long-term prophylaxis against herpes show no difference in side effects between acyclovir and placebo-treated patients (73). Isolated cases of rashes (lichenoid and maculopapular eruptions) (74, 75), neurotoxicity, and thrombocytopenia have been reported with oral acyclovir use (76). The most common adverse reaction of intravenous acyclovir is phlebitis and inflammation at the administration site (64). Renal dysfunction due to precipitation of intravenously administered acyclovir in the renal tubules has been reported, but can be minimized by adequate hydration, slow intravenous infusions, and adjustment of the dose in patients with renal dysfunction (64). Reversible neurologic (tremor) and psychiatric (confusion, hallucinations and delusions) manifestations have been reported with intravenous acyclovir administration and appear to be related to high plasma levels (62, 77). Finally, nausea and vomiting have been reported with intravenous administration of the agent (64). Emergence of resistant strains of herpes simplex virus and varicella-zoster virus has been reported with acyclovir (15).

Foscarnet

Foscarnet (Foscavir), a pyrophosphate analog, is the trisodium salt of phosphonoformic acid. Foscarnet differs from the nucleoside analogues, such as ganciclovir and acyclovir, in that it does not require phosphorylation to become active (78). DNA polymerase is inhibited by foscarnet, which precludes further viral DNA chain elongation (78–80). The drug binds to DNA polymerase, inhibiting the severing of pyrophosphate from deoxynucleoside triphosphates. The foscarnet-DNA polymerase complex appears to hinder either the enzyme release from, or translocation along, the template primer. Foscarnet-induced selective inhibition of DNA polymerase is reversible, and viral replication resumes when the drug is cleared from the infected cells (78, 81). Foscarnet also inhibits the reverse transcriptase of HIV in a noncompetitive reversible fashion (82). Foscarnet's inhibition of DNA polymerase and reverse transcriptase occurs at concentrations that do not affect host cellular division and enzymes (78, 81, 83).

Foscarnet has in vitro activity against cytomegalovirus, herpes simplex type 1 and type 2, varicella-zoster virus, and Epstein-Barr virus in decreasing order of concentrations required to inhibit DNA polymerase by 50% in cell culture systems. Foscarnet also inhibits hepatitis B DNA polymerase, but at concentrations higher than those required to inhibit herpes simplex virus DNA polymerase (78). The in vitro concentration of foscarnet needed to inhibit 50% of HIV reverse transcriptase activity is similar to that needed to inhibit 50% of cytomegalovirus DNA polymerase (78, 81). In human cell lines, when foscarnet is combined with zidovudine, additive inhibition of cytomegalovirus is observed (84).

Pharmacokinetic data on oral foscarnet are limited. Sjovall and colleagues (85) studied oral foscarnet absorption in six HIV-positive patients receiving 4000 mg of the agent every 6 hours, and found that only 17% of the drug was absorbed. It is theorized that oral absorption was poor in these HIV-positive patients because of nutrient malabsorption, saturation of intestinal sodium cotransport mechanisms, and the slow distribution of the drug into cells. Studies of foscarnet plasma levels during continuous intravenous infusion have reported great variation from patient to patient, but there is little variation within each individual (85–87). Plasma levels of foscarnet during 3-hour infusions of maintenance therapy for 5 days show a vast interpatient and intrapatient variability (86). Data on the distribution of foscarnet are limited, but the drug is distributed throughout the plasma compartment.

Animal data indicate that approximately 30% of a dose is retained, mainly in bone, with some in the kidney, heart, and lung (88). The drug is deposited in the bone matrix and displaces phosphate from the bone matrix, thus explaining the triphasic half-life of foscarnet. It has two short elimination periods, ranging from 0.5–1.4 hours to 3.3–6.8 hours, followed by a long final phase reflecting sequestration in the bones and ranging from 36–196 hours (78, 89). The initial short distribution phases of foscarnet require that it be given as a continuous infusion or as recurrent short infusions. Foscarnet is eliminated almost entirely through the kidneys via both glomerular filtration and tubular secretion (78, 88–90).

Toxicity of foscarnet includes renal insufficiency, hypocalcemia, and anemia. Renal insufficiency is reversible and is more common in patients receiving a continuous infusion of foscarnet as compared to bolus therapy (87, 89, 91). The renal complications are manifested by polyuria and polydipsia in patients receiving continuous infusions and an elevation of serum creatinine in patients receiving both continuous and bolus therapy. The polyuria and polydipsia appear to be due to foscarnet-induced nephrogenic diabetes insipidus (92). Elevation of serum creatinine has been reported to occur in as many as 40–60% of foscarnet-treated patients (78, 87, 91), but hemodialysis is rarely required (86, 91). The renal insufficiency is characterized by a normal urinary sediment, and no proteinuria. Histologically, acute tubular necrosis and interstitial nephritis have been identified, and crystals have been found in the glomerular capillaries, which have physicochemical properties of crystalline foscarnet (93, 94). Hydration before and during foscarnet therapy and dose-adjustment based on renal function will minimize renal insufficiency.

Serum calcium elevations have been reported in up to 66% of patients receiving foscarnet (87, 95), but hypercalcemia has also been reported in patients with untreated cytomegalovirus infections. In contrast, reversible symptomatic hypocalcemia (occasionally with tetany and seizures) has also been reported in patients receiving foscarnet (78, 96). Symptoms of hypocalcemia with normal total serum calcium levels and decreased ionized calcium levels have been reported, and probably reflect the ability of foscarnet to chelate calcium. Nauss-Karol and colleagues (97) reported that serum calcium levels remained normal in 10 AIDS patients treated with foscarnet despite elevations of parathyroid hormone levels. Foscarnet therapy increases serum phosphate levels (78, 87, 94), either because foscarnet replaces phosphate from bone or inhibits sodium and phosphate cotransport across proximal renal tubular membranes (98).

A decrease in hemoglobin concentration of >10 g/l has been reported (86, 87, 95) in 20–50% of foscarnet-treated patients, and blood transfusions are occasionally required. Thrombocytopenia has been an uncommon complication (78, 86). There have been several reports of penile ulcerations in AIDS patients receiving foscarnet therapy (78, 99, 100). These ulcers resolve after discontinuation of therapy and recur with retreatment. They may be due to accumulation of foscarnet in the subpreputial space producing a contact dermatitis (78, 99, 100).

USE OF ANTIVIRAL AGENTS

Herpes Simplex Virus Infection

Acyclovir is the treatment of choice for herpes simplex virus esophagitis, although there are limited published data on the effectiveness, dose, and duration of acyclovir therapy and the need for maintenance therapy in such patients. Foscarnet also shows activity against herpes simplex virus and can be used for patients who do not respond to acyclovir treatment. Foscarnet is especially useful in cases of acyclovir-resistant herpes simplex virus, as demonstrated by culture (15).

Much of the literature on treatment of herpes simplex virus esophagitis consists of a small series of HIV-negative immunosuppressed individuals (101–103), in whom acyclovir therapy appeared extremely effective for herpes simplex virus esophagitis and for whom acyclovir resulted in prompt symptomatic response. Isolated case reports have also shown foscarnet to be effective (104, 105).

Whether to use intravenous or oral acyclovir therapy is determined by the patient's symptoms. Patients with severe symptoms such as inability to swallow pills, fevers, and upper gastrointestinal bleeding are treated intravenously. The oral dosage of acyclovir is 200 mg five times a day for 10–14 days; intravenous dosage can also be given as 200 mg five times per day or as 5–10 mg/kg every 8 hours for 10–14 days. Foscarnet, at a dose of 60 mg/kg every 8 hours for 10–14 days, is used for treatment "failures." In patients who do not respond to acyclovir, it may be useful to repeat esophagoscopy to obtain herpes simplex virus-infected material to culture and test for sensitivities of the virus to the various available agents. Patients who respond to therapy are followed expectantly; full therapy is reinstituted for relapse and is followed by maintenance acyclovir therapy (400 mg twice a day). Foscarnet-treated patients with herpes simplex virus do well on maintenance acyclovir therapy, since only small numbers of the initial infecting virus are resistant to acyclovir as a rule, and these are killed by foscarnet.

Treatment of herpes simplex proctitis is similar to that for esophagitis, with oral acyclovir being the principal therapy and intravenous acyclovir used for severe cases. Foscarnet can be used for acyclovir failures.

Cytomegalovirus Infection

Ganciclovir is the treatment of choice for cytomegalovirus esophagitis and colitis. Foscarnet can be used for patients not responding to ganciclovir.

The usual ganciclovir induction dosage for acute cytomegalovirus esophagitis is 2.5 mg/kg every 8 hours or 5 mg/kg every 12 hours, given intravenously for 2–3 weeks. As with acyclovir therapy of herpes simplex virus esophagitis, there are limited data on the ideal duration of therapy, its effectiveness, and the role of maintenance therapy. When the data are combined from four studies (106–109), however, ganciclovir appears to be effective in 80% (range 50–86%) of patients with cytomegalovirus esophagitis. Foscarnet (60 mg/kg every 8 hours or 0.08 mg/kg/minute as a continuous infusion) can be used for ganciclovir "failures." In a recent paper, Nelson and colleagues (110) reported that foscarnet induced complete loss of symptoms and healing of ulcers in 15 of 18 episodes of cytomegalovirus esophagitis within 2 weeks. Three relapses occurred during follow-up, of which two were successfully retreated.

Our treatment protocol for patients with cytomegalovirus esophagitis is to treat the patient with ganciclovir for 2–3 weeks, after which repeat esophagoscopy is performed. If the esophagitis and ulcers have shown no response to ganciclovir, treatment is changed to foscarnet. If there is improvement, but not complete resolution of the infection, then ganciclovir is administered for another 2–3 weeks, after which the patient is reassessed again. If the cytomegalovirus esophagitis has resolved, one can discontinue ganciclovir, reinstitute zidovudine, and observe the patient for recurrent cytomegalovirus esophagitis. Alternatively, maintenance therapy with ganciclovir can be used in a dosage of 5 mg/kg daily. Zidovudine therapy can be given during ganciclovir maintenance, but lower than usual doses are required with careful monitoring for hematologic toxicity.

Preferred treatment for cytomegalovirus colitis is ganciclovir with foscarnet as a second drug for patients who do not respond. The doses used for induction therapy are the same as those for cytomegalovirus esophagitis. Dieterich et al. (109), using an open-label protocol, treated 46 HIV-positive patients with cytomegalovirus colitis using administration of 2 weeks of ganciclovir. Of 46 patients, 35 improved, 7 stabilized, and 4 did not respond. Jacobson et al. (107) reported that 8 of 11 cytomegalovirus colitis patients responded to ganciclovir therapy. In a double-blind trial lasting 2 weeks, the courses of 32 patients treated with ganciclovir (5 mg/kg every 12 hours) was compared with that of 30 placebo-treated patients (111). Ganciclovir-treated patients had less weight loss and a greater improvement in the colonic mucosa as determined by repeat colonoscopy at day 14. No ganciclovir-treated patient developed extracolonic cytomegalovirus, whereas, 4 placebo-treated patients developed cytomegalovirus retinitis and 1 developed cytomegalovirus pneumonia. There was no difference in diarrhea improvement between ganciclovir and placebo-treated patients.

In an open-label trial by Nelson and colleagues, 22 patients were treated with foscarnet at a dosage of 200 mg/kg of body weight given as a continuous infusion over a 24-hour period for 3 weeks (110). Complete and partial responses were defined by the absence of microscopic and macroscopic evidence of cytomegalovirus colitis; partial responders continued to have diarrhea. Of the 22 patients, 4 died during therapy, 11 had complete remission, 6 had partial remission, and 1 failed to have a microscopic or macroscopic resolution of the cytomegalovirus infection. All partial responders had a second pathogen to account for their continued diarrhea.

A major unanswered question is whether maintenance ganciclovir therapy is indicated after the acute gastrointestinal cytomegalovirus infection has been resolved. Randomized, controlled trials have shown that maintenance ganciclovir therapy delays the progression of cytomegalovirus retinitis (112). The initial data on recurrence of cytomegalovirus colitis reported by Deiterich and colleagues (109) showed that 47% (22/47) of patients had a recurrence of symptoms at a median of 9 weeks after induction therapy and that all patients responded to a second course of ganciclovir. In a second study, Dieterich and Rahmin (112) reported recurrence of cytomegalovirus colitis in 4 of 7 patients not treated with maintenance ganciclovir compared with 0 of 32 treated with maintenance ganciclovir therapy. Thus, the decision to treat a patient with maintenance therapy is a balance of risks and benefits. The benefits of ganciclovir maintenance therapy are a decrease in the risk of recurrent gastrointestinal and extracolonic cytomegalovirus. The risks of maintenance ganciclovir therapy include the need for a central catheter (with its attendant risk of infection) and the fact that coincident zidovudine (AZT) must be stopped or reduced in dose.

The limited data do suggest that recurrent gastrointestinal cytomegalovirus will respond to a second course of therapy; full-dose AZT therapy can be reinstituted if maintenance treatment is not utilized.

AGENTS USED TO TREAT PROTOZOAN INFECTIONS

The protozoa most commonly encountered in HIV positive patients include *cryptosporidia*, *Isospora belli*, *microsporidia* (*Enterocytozoon bienusei*), *Entamoeba histolytica*, *Giardia lambia*, and *Blastocystis hominis*, although the last three are not markers of immunocompromise.

Currently there is no proven effective therapy for *Cryptosporidia* (15). More than fifty different agents have been shown to be ineffective in treating this protozoan (113, 114). Improvement in immune function, with an increase in the CD_4 count, is probably the key to eradication of *Cryptosporidium* infection (115, 116). Reports of hyperimmune bovine colostrum (117), spiramycin (118), and diclazuril (118) being effective for treatment of cryptosporidiosis have not been proven in controlled trials. Paromomycin (120) and fluconazole (121) have recently been reported to be effective in small uncontrolled trials. Currently, therapy is supportive and includes nonspecific antidiarrheal agents and nutritional supplementation. Octreotide, a somatostatin analog, may be helpful in some patients (15).

Isospora belli is a common protozoan pathogen in tropical and subtropical climates that is a common cause of diarrhea in HIV-positive Haitian patients. Initial therapy with trimethoprim (160 mg) and sulfamethoxazole (800 mg) four times a day for 10–14 days is effective in eradicating the acute infection (122). Maintenance therapy, which is required to prevent relapse, consists of administration of trimethoprim (160 mg) and sulfamethoxazole (800 mg) daily (122). Patients who are intolerant of sulfonamides respond to pyrimethamine (75 mg daily) with folinic acid (123).

There are multiple species of *Microsporidia*, but the one identified by electron microscopy on duodenal biopsies of HIV-positive patients with diarrhea is *Enterocytozoon bienēusi*. Currently, there is no specific antimicrosporidial agent. Fluconazole has been reported to be effective in 2 patients with corneal *Microsporidia* (124) and there has been one questionable response to pyrimethamine in a patient with small intestinal *Microsporidia* (125). In one report, 4 of 5 patients with intestinal microsporidiosis treated with albendazole had resolution of diarrhea sufficient to allow discontinuation of antidiarrheal agents, while the fifth patient was able to halve the dose of antidiarrheal agents (126). Eeftinck Schattenkerk and Van Gool (127) reported that metronidazole was effective in relieving diarrhea in 10 of 13 patients with intestinal microsporidiosis. A small number of the patients whose symptoms were successfully treated with either metronidazole or albendazole underwent repeat upper endoscopy, which showed that no patient had eradication of the microsporidia infection (126, 127). As with cryptosporidiosis, therapy is supportive.

Giardia lambia therapy consists of either quinacrine HCl (100 mg three times a day for 5–7 days) or metronidazole (250 mg three times a day for 7–10 days). Both regimens result in a greater than 90% cure rate, and in contrast to *I. belli*, chronic suppressive therapy is not required in HIV-positive patients.

Entameba histolytica is rarely invasive in homosexuals and therefore is essentially a nonpathogen in such individuals. In a patient with invasive disease, metronidazole (750 mg three times a day for 7 days) is adequate therapy. In the asymptomatic cyst passer, diloxinide (500 mg 3 times a day for 10 days) is the therapy of choice.

Blastocystis hominis is occasionally identified in the stool of HIV-positive patients and is usually considered a nonpathogen. If it is decided to treat a patient in whom *B. hominis* was identified in the stool, the drug of choice is Iodoquinol (650 mg three times a day for 20 days). An alternative regimen is metronidazole (750 mg three times a day for 10 days).

AGENTS USED TO TREAT BACTERIAL INFECTIONS

Mycobacterium avium complex is the only bacterial infection of the gastrointestinal tract that is HIV specific; *M. avium* infection effectively establishes the diagnosis of AIDS. In contrast to *Mycobacteria tuberculosis*, there is no antimicrobial regimen that can eradicate *M. avium*. Chiu and colleagues (128) reported that 4 weeks of intravenous amikacin (7.5 mg/kg) and 12 weeks of ethambutol (1000 mg daily), ciprofloxacin (750 mg twice daily), and rifampin (600 mg daily) can decrease the bacterial load and improve patient symptoms. Kemper and colleagues (129) reported that rifampin (600 mg daily), ethambutol (15 mg/kg of body weight), ciprofloxacin (750 mg twice daily), and clofazamine (100 mg daily) was also effective in decreasing the MAI bacterial load and resulted in a rapid reduction of symptoms. It is currently recommended that therapy for disseminated *M. avium* complex include either azithromycin or clarithromycin in combination with ethambutol and one or more of the following agents: clofazimine, rifampin, rifabutin, ciprofloxacin or amikacin. Importantly, INH and pyrazinamide have no role in the treatment of *M. avium* complex (130). A recent report suggests that rifabutin (mycobutin), a semisynthetic rifamycin, reduces the frequency of dissemination of *M. avium* complex when given prophylactically to AIDS patients with CD4 counts ≤200 per cubic millimeter (131).

Other bacterial infections such as *Clostridium difficile*, *Shigella flexneri*, *Salmonella species (Salmonella typhimurium and Salmonella enteritidis)*, and *Campylobacter jejuni* are not specific HIV pathogens but do have a higher incidence in AIDS patients. These bacterial infections may behave differently in the immunosuppressed HIV-infected individual, exhibit a more prolonged course and a higher incidence of recurrence and bacteremia, and show a frequent need for maintenance suppressive therapy.

Treatment for *C. difficile* diarrhea includes discontinuing the causative antibiotics when possible, and administering oral vancomycin (125–500 mg four times a day for 10–14 days) or oral metronidazole (250 mg four times a day for 10–14 days) (121). Metronidazole is significantly less expensive than vancomycin and patients who do not respond to metronidazole therapy usually do respond to vancomycin. Relapses can occur in up to 25% of patients and repeated courses of therapy may be required (132).

The treatment of choice for *Shigella* is ciprofloxacin (500 mg twice daily for 7 days) or norfloxacin (400 mg for 7 days) with trimethoprim sulfamethoxazole (one double strength tablet twice daily for 7–14 days) as an alternative. For acute, severe, shigellosis, intravenous ceftriaxone or trimethoprim sulfamethoxazole can be used.

Treatment options for acute *Salmonella* infection include intravenous ampicillin, trimethoprim-sulfamethoxazole, a third-generation cephalosporin, chloramphenicol, and the fluoroquinones. Treatment options for suppression include trimethaprim/sulfamethoxazole, ampicillin, and ciprofloxacin. Selection of antibiotic therapy should be guided by sensitivity of the organism in in vitro testing.

The treatment of choice for *Campylobacter jejuni* consists of ciprofloxacin (500 mg twice a day) with erythromycin (250–500 mg four times a day for seven days) as an alternative.

CONCLUSION

New agents are continually being developed and tested to treat the gastrointestinal disorders and opportunistic infections that occur in AIDS patients. It is hoped that specific agents will be developed to eradicate microsporidia, cryptosporidia, and *M. avium* complex, and that less toxic, more effective oral antiviral agents soon will be available to treat gastrointestinal tract viral infections.

REFERENCES

1. Santangelo WC, Krejs GJ. Southwestern Internal Medicine Conference: Gastrointestinal manifestations of the acquired immunodeficiency syndrome. Am J Med Sci 1976;292:328–334.
2. Cello JP. Gastrointestinal manifestations of HIV infection. Inf Dis Clin North Am 1988:2:235–245.
3. Rodgers VD, Kagnoff MF. Gastrointestinal manifestations of the acquired immunodeficiency syndrome. West J Med 1987;146:57–67.
4. Bennet J. "antifungal agents." In: Gilman A, Rall T, Nies A, Taylor P, eds., Goodman and Gillman's Pharmacological basis of therapeutics. ed. 8. New York: Pergamon Press, 1990;1165–1182.
5. Van Den Bossche H, Willemsens G, Cools W, Cornelissen F, Lauwers W, Van Cutsem J. In vitro and in vivo effects of the antimycotic drug ketoconazole on sterol synthesis. Antimicrob Agents Chemother 1980;17:922–928.
6. Janssen PAJ, Van den Bossche H. Mode of action of cytochrome P-450 monooxygenase inhibitors: focus on azole derivatives. Arch Pharm Chem Sci Ed 1987;15:23–40.
7. Grant S. Fluconazole: a review. Drugs 1990;39:1–33.
8. Walsh TJ, Hamilton SR, Belitsos N. Esophageal candidiasis: managing an increasingly prevalent infection. Postgrad Med 1988;83:193–205.
9. Brass C, Galgiani JN, Campbell SC, Stevens DA. Therapy of disseminated or pulmonary coccidioidomycosis with ketoconazole. Rev Infect Dis 1980;2:656–660.
10. Maksymiuk AW, Levine HB, Bodey GP. The pharmacology of ketoconazole, a new orally administered antifungal. In: Proceedings of the 20th Interscience Conference on Antimicrobial Agents and Chemotherapy, New Orleans, September 22–24, 1980.
11. Espinel-Ingroff A, Shadomy S, Porter D, Steltz M. Dismukes W, and CMSC Group. Ketoconazole: serum levels as determined by bioassay. In: Proceedings of the 21st Interscience Conference on Antimicrobial agents and Chemotherapy, Chicago. 4–6 November 1981.
12. Heel RC, Brogden RN, Carmine A, Morley P, Speight T, Avery G. Ketoconazole: a review of its therapeutic efficacy in superficial and systemic fungal infections. Drugs 1982;23:1–36.
13. Lake-Bakaar G, Tom W, Lake-Bakaar D, et al. Gastropathy and ketoconazole malabsorption in the acquired immunodeficiency syndrome (AIDS). Ann Intern Med 1988;109:471–473.
14. Blum RA, D'Andrea DT, Florentino BM, et al. Increased gastric pH and the bioavailability of fluconazole and ketoconazole. Ann Intern Med 1991;114:755–757.
15. Drugs for AIDS and associated infections. Med Lett 1993;35:79–86.
16. Daneshmend TK, Warnock DW, Turner A, Roberts CJ. Pharmacokinetics of ketoconazole in normal subjects. Journal of Antimicrobial Chemotherapy 1981;8:299–304.
17. Engelhard D, Stutman HR, Marks MI. Interaction of ketoconazole with rifampin and isoniazid. New Engl J Med 1984;311:1681–1683.
18. Macnair AL, Gascoigne E, Heap J, Schuermans V, Symoens J. Hepatitis and ketoconazole therapy. Br Med J 1981;283:1058.
19. Heiberg JK, Svejgaard E. Toxic hepatitis during ketoconazole treatment. Br Med J 1981;283:825–826.
20. Firebrace D. Hepatitis and ketoconazole therapy. Br Med J 1980;283:1058–1059.

21. De Felice R, Johnson DG, Galgiani JN. Gynecomastia with ketoconazole. Antimicrob Agents Chemother 1981;19:1073–1074.
22. Humphrey MJ, Jevons S, Tarbit MH. Pharmacokinetic evaluation of UK-49, 858, a metabolically stable triazole antifungal drug, in animals and humans. Antimicrob Agents Chemother 1985;28:648–653.
23. Brammer KW, Farrow PR, Faulkner JK. Pharmacokinetics and tissue penetration of fluconazole in humans. Rev Infect Dis 1990;12(suppl 3):S318–S326.
24. Fouids G, Wajszczuk C, Weidler DJ, Garg DC, Gibson P. Steady state parenteral kinetics of fluconazole in man. In: Proceedings of the First International Conference on Drug Research in Immunologic and Infectious Diseases. Antifungal drugs: synthesis—preclinical and clinical evaluation [Abstract P6]. Oct 8–18, 1987.
25. Mitchell AS, Holland JT. Fluconazole and phenytoin: a predictable interaction. Br Med J 1989;298:1315–1316.
26. Isalska BJ, Stanbridge TN. Fluconazole in treatment of candidal prosthetic valve endocarditis. Br Med J 1988;297:178–179.
27. Collignon P, Hurley B, Mitchell D. Interaction of fluconazole with cyclosporin. Lancet 1989;1:1262.
28. Kruger HU, Schuler U, Zimmerman R, Ehninger G. No severe drug interaction of fluconazole, a triazole antifungal agent, with cyclosporin. Bone Marrow Transplant 1988;3(suppl 1):271–273.
29. Holmes J, Clements D. Jaundice in a HIV-positive haemophiliac. Lancet 1989;1:1027–1029.
30. Grant M, Clissold P. Itraconazole. A review of its pharmacodynamic and pharmacokinetic properties, and therapeutic use in superficial and systemic mycoses. Drugs 1989;37:310–344.
31. Hardin TC, Graybill JR, Fetchick R, Woestenborghs RR, Michael G, Huhn JG. Pharmacokinetics of itraconazole following oral administration to normal volunteers. Antimicrob Agents Chemother 1988;32:1310–1313.
32. Heykants J, van Peer A, van de Velde V, et al. The clinical pharmacokinetics of itraconazole: an overview. Mycoses 1989;32(suppl 1):67–87.
33. Sugar AM, Stern JJ, Dupont B. Treatment of cryptococcal meningitis: reviews of infectious diseases 1990;12(suppl 3):S338–S348.
34. Heykants J, Michiels M, Meuldermans W, et al. The pharmacokinetics of itraconazole in animals and man: an overview. In: Fromtling RA, ed. Recent trends in the discovery, development and evaluation of antifungal agents. Barcelona: JR Prous 1987:223–249.
35. Hay RJ, Clayton YM, Moore MK, Midgely G. An evaluation of itraconazole in the management of onychomycosis. Br J Dermatol 1986;119:359–366.
36. Rex J. Itraconazole-digoxin interaction. Ann Intern Med 1992;116:525.
37. Trenk D, Brett W, Jahnchen E, Birnbaum D. Time course of cyclosporine/itraconazole interaction. Lancet 1987;2:1335–1336.
38. Novakova I, Donnelly P, DeWitte T, et al. Itraconazole and cyclosporin nephrotoxicity. Lancet 1987;2:920–921.
39. Saag MS, Dismukes WE. Azole antifungal agents: emphasis on new triazoles. Antimicrob Agents Chemother 1988;32:1–8.
40. Sharkey PK, Rinaldi MG, Dunn JF, Hardin TC, Fetchick RJ, Graybill JR. High-dose itraconazole in the treatment of severe mycoses. Antimicrobial Agents and Chemotherapy 1991;35:707–713.
41. Bennett JE. Antifungal Agents. In: Mandell GL, Douglas RG, Jr., Bennett JE., eds. Principles and practice of infectious diseases. ed. 3. New York: Churchill Livingstone, 1990:361–370.
42. Bindschadler DD, Bennett JE. A pharmacologic guide to the clinical use of amphotericin. B J Infect Dis 1969;120:427–436.
43. Craven PC, Ludden TM, Drutz DJ, Rogers W, Haegele KA, Skrdlant HB. Excretion pathways of amphotericin B J Infect Dis 1979;140:329–341.
44. Christiansen KJ, Bernard EM, Gold JM, Armstrong D. Distribution and activity of amphotericin B in humans. J Infect Dis 1985;152:1037–1043.
45. Collette N, van der Auwere P, Lopez AP, Haymans C, Meunier F. Tissue concentrations and bioactivity of amphotericin B in cancer patients treated with amphotericin B deoxycholate. Antimicrob Agents Chemother 1989;33:362–368.
46. Kennedy M, Deeg H, Siegal M, Crowley J, Storb R, Thomas E. Acute renal toxicity with combined use of amphotericin B and cyclosporine after bone marrow transplantation. Transplantation 1983;35:211–215.
47. Sawyer P, Brogden R, Pinder P, Speight T, Avery G. Clotrimazole: a review of its antifungal activity and therapeutic efficacy. Drugs 1975;9:424–427.
48. Laine L, Conteas C, DeBruin M, DeBruin M, Multicenter Study Group. A prospective, randomized, double blind trial of fluconazole vs ketoconazole for *Candida* esophagitis [Abstract]. Gastroenterology 1991;100:A591.
49. Smith DE, Midgley J, Allan M, Connolly GM, Gazzard BG. Itraconazole versus ketoconazole in treatment of oral and oesophageal candidiasis in patients infected with HIV. AIDS 1991;5:1367–1371.
50. Smee DF. Interaction of 9-(1,3-dihydroxy-2-propoxymethyl)guanine with cytosol and mitochondrial deoxyguanosine kinases: possible role in ant-cytomegalovirus activity. Molecular and Cellular Biochemistry 1985;69:75–81.
51. Smee DF, Boehme R, Chernow M, Binko BP, Matthews TR. Intracellular metabolism and enzymatic phosphorylation of 9-(1,3-dihydroxy-2-propoxymethyl)guanine and acyclovir in herpes simplex virus-infected and uninfected cells. Biochem Pharmacol 1985;34:1049–1056.

52. Faulds D, Heel RC. Ganciclovir: a review of its antiviral activity, pharmacokinetic properties and therapeutic efficacy in cytomegalovirus infections. Drugs 1990;39:597–638.

53. Cheng Y-C, Grill SP, Dutschman GE, et al. Effects of 9-(1,3-dihydroxy-2-propoxymethyl)guanine, a new antiherpesvirus compound, on synthesis of macromolecules in herpes simplex virus infected cells. Antimicrob Agents Chemother 1984;26:283–288.

54. Biron KK, Stanat SC, Sorrell JB, et al. Metabolic activation of the nucleoside analog 9-{[2-hydroxy-1-(hydroxymethyl)ethoxy]methyl}guanine in human diploid fibroblasts infected with human cytomegalovirus. Proc Natl Acad Sci USA 1985;82:2473–2477.

55. Laskin OL, Cederberg DM, Mills J, et al. Ganciclovir for the treatment and suppression of serious infections caused by cytomegalovirus. Am J Med 1987;83:201–207.

56. Weller S, Liao SHT, Cederberg DM, de Miranda P, Blum MR. The pharmacokinetics of ganciclovir in patients with cytomegalovirus (CMV) infections. J Pharmaceut Sci 1987;76:S120.

57. Fletcher C, Sawchuk R, Chinnock B, de Miranda P, Balfour HH Jr. Human pharmacokinetics of the antiviral drug DHPG. Clin Pharmacol and Ther 1986;1:281–286.

58. Lake KD, Fletcher CV, Love KR, et al. Ganciclovir pharmacokinetics during renal impairment. Antimicrob Agents Chemother 1988;32:1899–1900.

59. Ho WG, Winston DJ, Champlin RE. Tolerance and efficacy of ganciclovir in the treatment of cytomegalovirus infections in immunosuppressed patients. Transplant Proc 1989;21:3103–3106.

60. Buhles WC, Mastre Jr BJ, Tinker AJ. Ganciclovir treatment of life-or sight-threatening cytomegalovirus infection: experience in 314 immunocompromised patients. Rev Infect Dis 1988;10(suppl 3):S495–S506.

61. Jacobson MA, de Miranda P, Gordon SM, et al. Prolonged pancytopenia due to combined ganciclovir and zidovudine therapy. J Infect Dis 1988;158:489–490.

62. O'Brien JJ, Campoli-Richards DM. Acyclovir: an updated review of its antiviral activity, pharmacokinetic properties and therapeutic efficacy. Drugs 1989;37:233–309.

63. Furman PA, St. Clair MH, Spector T. Acyclovir triphosphate is a suicide inactivator of the herpes simplex virus DNA polymerase. Journal of Biological Chemistry 1984;259:9575–9579.

64. Richards DM, Carmine AA, Brogden RN, Heel RC, et al. Acyclovir: a review of its pharmacodynamic properties and therapeutic efficacy. Drugs 1983;26:378–438.

65. Elion GB. Acyclovir. In Becker Y, ed. Antiviral drugs and interferon: the molecular basis of their activity. Boston: Martinus Nijhoff Publishing, 194:71–88.

66. de Miranda P, Blum MR. Pharmacokinetics of acyclovir after intravenous and oral administration. J Antimicrob Agents Chemother 1983;12(suppl B):29–37.

67. Brigden D, Whiteman P. The clinical pharmacology of acyclovir and its prodrugs. Scand J Infect Dis 1985;47(suppl):33–39.

68. Whitley RJ, Blum MR, Barton N, de Miranda P. Pharmacokinetics of acyclovir in humans following intravenous administration. Acyclovir Symposium. Am J Med 1982;73:165–170.

69. Wade JC, Hintz M, McGuffin RW, et al. Treatment of cytomegalovirus pneumonia with high-dose acyclovir. Acyclovir Symposium. Am J Med 1982;73:249–255.

70. de Miranda P, Good SS, Krasny HC, et al. Metabolic fate of radioactive acyclovir in humans. Acyclovir Symposium. Am J Med 1982;73:215–220.

71. Laskin OL, Longstreth JA, Whelton A, et al. Acyclovir kinetics in end-stage renal disease. Clin Pharmacol Therap 1982;31:594–601.

72. Seth SK, Visconti JA, Hebert LA, Krasny HC. Acyclovir pharmacokinetics in a patient on continuous ambulatory peritoneal dialysis. Clin Pharm 1985;4:320–322.

73. Mertz GJ, Jones CC, Mills J, et al. Long term acyclovir suppression of frequently recurring genital herpes simplex virus infection. A multicenter double-blind trial. JAMA 1988;260:201–206.

74. Robinson GE, Weber J, Griffiths C, et al. Cutaneous adverse reactions to acyclovir: case reports. Genitourin Med 1985;61:62–63.

75. Grattan CEH, Boyle J. Reaction to oral acyclovir. Br Med J 1984;289:1424.

76. Krigel RL. Reversible neurotoxicity to oral acyclovir in a patient with chronic lymphocytic leukemia. J Infect Dis 1986;189:154–157.

77. Wade JC, Meyers JD. Neurological symptoms associated with parenteral acyclovir treatment after bone marrow transplantation. Ann Intern Med 1983;98:921–925.

78. Chrisp P, Clissold C. Foscarnet. A review of its antiviral activity, pharmacokinetics properties and therapeutic use in immunocompromised patients with cytomegalovirus retinitis. Drugs 1991;41:104–129.

79. Eriksson B, Oberg B, Wahren B. Pyrophosphate analogues as inhibitors of DNA polymerases of cytomegalovirus, herpes simplex virus and cellular origin. Biochim Biophys Acta 1982;696:115–123.

80. Eriksson B, Larson A, Helgstrand E, Johansson NG, Oberg B. Pyrophosphate analogues as inhibitors of herpes simplex virus type I DNA polymerase. Biochim Biophys Acta 1980;607:53–64.

81. Oberg, B. Antiviral effects of phosphonoformate. Pharmacology and Therapeutics 1989;40:213–285.

82. Sandstrom EG, Kaplan JC, Byington RE, Hirsch MS. Inhibition of human T-cell lymphotropic virus type III in vitro by phosphonoformate. Lancet 1985;1:1480–1482.

83. Stenberg K, Skog S, Tribukait B. Concentration-dependent effects of foscarnet on the cell cycle. Antimicrob Agents Chemother 1985;28:802–806.

84. Eriksson BFH, Schinazi RF. Combinations of 3'-azido-3'-deoxythymidine (zidovudine) and phosphonoformate (foscarnet) against human immunodeficiency virus type I and cytomegalovirus replication in vitro. Antimicrob Agents Chemother 1989;33:663–668.

85. Sjovall J, Karlsoon A, Ogenstad S, Sandstrom E, Saarimaki M. Pharmacokinetics of foscarnet and distribution to cerebrospinal fluid after intravenous infusion in patients with human immunodeficiency virus infection. Antimicrob Agents Chemother 1988;44:65–73.

86. Fanning MM, Read SE, Benson M, et al. Foscarnet therapy of cytomegalovirus retinitis in AIDS. J Acq Immu Def Syndr 1990;3:472–479.

87. Gaub J, Pederson C, Poulsen AG, et al. The effect of foscarnet (phosphonoformate) on human immunodeficiency virus isolation, T-cell subsets and lymphocyte function in AIDS patients. AIDS 1987; 1:27–337.

88. Helgstrand E, Eriksson B, Johansson NG, et al. Trisodium phosphonoformate, a new antiviral compound. Science 1978;201:819–821.

89. Sjovall J, Bergdahl S, Movin G, Ogenstad S, Saarimaki M. Pharmacokinetics of foscarnet and distribution to cerebrospinal fluid after intravenous infusion in patients with human immunodeficiency virus infection. Antimicrob Agents Chemother 1989;33:1023–1031.

90. Aweeka F, Gambertoglio J, Mills J, Jacobson MA. Pharmacokinetics of intermittently administered intravenous foscarnet in the treatment of acquired immunodeficiency syndrome patients with serious cytomegalovirus retinitis. Antimicrob Agents Chemother 1989;33:742–745.

91. Cacoub P, Deray G, Baumelou A, et al. Acute renal failure induced by foscarnet: 4 cases. Clin Nephrol 1988;29:315–318.

92. Farese RV, Schambelan M, Hollander H, Stringari S, Jacobson MA. Nephrogenic diabetes insipidus associated with foscarnet treatment of cytomegalovirus retinitis. Ann Intern Med 1990;112:955–956.

93. Nyberg G, Blohme I, Persson H, Svalander C. Foscarnet-induced tubulointerstitial nephritis in renal transplant patients. Transplant 1990;22:241–246.

94. Beaufils H, Deray G, Katlama C, et al. Foscarnet and crystals in glomerular capillary lumens [Correspondence]. Lancet 1990;336:755.

95. Jacobson MA, O'Donnell JJ, Mills J. Foscarnet treatment of cytomegalovirus retinitis in patients with the acquired immunodeficiency syndrome. Antimicrob Agents Chemother 1989;33:736–741.

96. Youle MS, Clarbour J, Gazzard B, Chanas A. Severe hypocalcaemia in AIDS patients treated with foscarnet and pentamidine [Correspondence]. Lancet 1989;1:1455–1456.

97. Nauss-Karol C, Redding K, Sagaties H, Gray W, Ussery F. Effects of foscarnet on calcium homeostasis in man [Abstract Th.B.439]. Sixth International Conference on AIDS, San Francisco, June 20–24, 1990.

98. Webster S, Szczepanska-Konkel M, Yusufi ANK, Dousa TP. Inhibition of renal phosphate (Pi) reabsorption in vivo by phosphonoformic acid (PFA) [Abstract 2254]. Fed Proceed 1986;45:541.

99. Hoyle G, Nelson M, Barton S, et al. Penile Ulceration with foscarnet. Lancet 1990;335:547–548.

100. Connolly GM, Gazzard BG, Hawkins DA. Fixed drug eruption due to foscarnet. Genitourin Med 1990;66:97–98.

101. Agha FP, Horchang HL, Nostrant TT. Herpetic esophagitis: a diagnostic challenge in immunocompromised patients. Am J Gastroenterol 1986; 81(4):246–255.

102. Kadakia SC, Oliver GA, Peura DA. Acyclovir in endoscopically presumed viral esophagitis. Gastrointest Endosco 1987;33:33–35.

103. Connolly GM, Hawkins D, Harcourt-Webster JN, Parsons PA, Gazzard B. Oesophageal symptoms, their causes, treatment, and prognosis in patients with the acquired immunodeficiency syndrome. Gut 1989;30:1033–1039.

104. Youle M, Hawkins D, Collins P, et al. Acyclovir resistant herpes in AIDS treated with foscarnet. Lancet 1988;2:341–342.

105. Erlich KS, Jacobson M, Koehler J, et al. Foscarnet therapy for severe acyclovir resistant herpes simplex type 2 in patients with AIDS. Ann Intern Med 1989;110:710–713.

106. Wilcox CM, Diehl CL, Cello JP, Margasetten W, Jacobson M. Cytomegalovirus esophagitis in patients with AIDS: a clinical, endoscopic, and pathologic correlation. Ann Intern Med 1990;113:589–593.

107. Jacobson M, O'Donnell J, Porteous D, Brodie H, Fiegal D, Mills J. Retinal and gastrointestinal disease due to cytomegalovirus in patients with AIDS: prevalence, natural history and response to ganciclovir therapy. Q J Med 1988;65:463–486.

108. Chachoua A, Dieterich D, Kranski D, et al. 9-(1,3-dihydroxy-2-propoxymethyl) guanine for cytomegalovirus gastrointestinal disease in the acquired immunodeficiency syndrome. Ann Intern Med 1987;107:133–137.

109. Dieterich DT, Chachoua A, Lafleut F, Worrel C. Ganciclovir treatment of gastrointestinal infections caused by cytomegalovirus in patients with AIDs. Rev Infect Dis 1988;10(suppl 3):S532–537.

110. Nelson MR, Connolly GM, Hawkins DA, Gazzard B. Foscarnet in the treatment of cytomegalovirus infection of the esophagus and colon in patients with

the acquired immune deficiency syndrome. Am J Gastroenterol 1991;86:876–881.

111. Jacobson MA, O'Donnell JJ, Brodie HR, Wofsy C, Mills J. Randomized prospective trial of ganciclovir maintenance therapy for cytomegalovirus retinitis. J Med Virol 1988;25:339–349.

112. Dieterich DT, Rahmin M. Cytomegalovirus colitis in AIDS: presentation in 44 patients and a review of the literature. J AIDS 1991;4(suppl 1):S29–S35.

113. Tzipori S. Cryptosporidiosis in animals and humans. Microbiol Rev 1983; March:84–96.

114. Fayer R, Ungar BLP. Cryptosporidium spp. and cryptosporidiosis. Microbiol Rev 1986; Dec:458–483.

115. Greenburg R, Mir R, Bank S, Siegal F. Resolution of intestinal cryptosporidiosis after treatment with AZT. Gastroenterology 1989;97:1327–1330.

116. Simon D, Weiss L, Tanowitz H, Wittner M. Resolution of cryptosporidium infection in an AIDS patient after improvement of nutritional and immune status with octreotide. Am J Gastroenterol 1991; 86:615–619.

117. Ungar BLP, Ward DJ, Fayer R, et al. Cessation of cryptosporidium-associated diarrhea in an acquired immunodeficiency syndrome patient after treatment with hyperimmune bovine colostrum. Gastroenterology 1990;98:486–490.

118. Menichetti F, Moretti MV, Marroni M, et al. Diclazuril for cryptosporidiosis in AIDS. Am J Med 1991;90:271–272.

119. Moskovitz BL, Stanton TL, Kusmierek JJE. Spiramycin therapy for cryptosporidial diarrhoea in immunocompromised patients. J Antimicrob Chemother 1988;22(suppl B):189–191.

120. Gathe J, Piot D, Bernal A, et al. The effectiveness of paromomycin in the treatment of gastrointestinal cryptosporidiosis [abstract MB 2270]. Seventh International Conference on AIDS, Florence, Italy, 1991.

121. Leoncini F, Carbonai S, D'Elia D, et al. Successful treatment with fluconazole of cryptosporidium enteritis in AIDS [abstract MB2199]. Seventh International Conference on AIDS, Florence, Italy, 1991.

122. Pape JW, Verdier R, Johnson WD. Treatment and prophylaxis of isospora belli infection in patients with the acquired immunodeficiency syndrome. New Engl J Med 1989;1044–1047.

123. Weiss LM, Perlman DC, Sherman J, Tanowitz H, Wittner M. Isospora belli infection: treatment with pyrimethamine. Ann Intern Med 1988;109:474–475.

124. Bryan RT, Cali AN, Owen RL, Spencer H. Microsporidia: opportunistic pathogens in patients with AIDs. Progress in Clinical Parasitol 1991;2:1–2.

125. Rijpstra AC, Canning EU, Van Ketel RJ, Schattenkerk J, Laarman J. Use of light microscopy to diagnose small-intestinal microsporidiosis in patients with AIDS. J Infect Dis 1988;157:827–831.

126. Blanshard C, Peacock C, Ellis D, Gazzard B. Treatment of intestinal microsporidiosis with albendazole [Abstract WB2265]. Seventh International AIDS Conference, Florence, Italy, 1991.

127. Eftinck Schattenkerk JK, Van Gool T, et al. Clinical significance of small-intestinal microsporidiosis in HIV-1-infected individuals. Lancet 1991;337:895–898.

128. Chiu J, Nussbaum J, Bozzette S. Treatment of disseminated mycobacterium avium complex infection in AIDS with amikacin, ethambutol, rifampin, and ciprofloxacin. Ann Intern Med 1990;113:358–361.

129. Kemper C, Yze-Chiang M, Nussbaum J, et al. Treatment of *Mycobacteria avium* complex bacteremia in AIDS with a four drug oral regimen. Ann Intern Med 1992;116:466–472.

130. Masur H, and the Public Health Service Task Force. Recommendations on prophylaxis and therapy for disseminated *Mycobacterium avium* complex disease in patients infected with the human immunodeficiency virus. N Engl J Med 1993;329;898–904.

131. Nightingale SD, Cameron DW, Gordin FM, et al. Two controlled trials of rifabutin prophylaxis against *Mycobacterium avium* complex infection in AIDS. N Engl J Med 1993;329:828–833.

132. Bartlett J. *Clostridium difficile*: Clinical observations. Rev Infect Dis 1990;12:S243–251.

PANCREATOBILIARY DISORDERS

17

Drug Treatment of Acute and Chronic Pancreatitis

SCOTT TENNER, ROBERT S. LEVINE and WILLIAM M. STEINBERG

ACUTE PANCREATITIS

Acute pancreatitis is usually a mild, self-limiting illness that responds to simple supportive therapy in the form of intravenous fluids and analgesics. While supportive therapy remains the basis of management, the morbidity and mortality from severe pancreatitis remains a significant problem. No specific pharmacologic agents have been shown to affect the course of severe pancreatitis. Many of the controlled studies in this area, however, have been limited because too few patients have been investigated and many patients have had only mild disease (1). This chapter will review the pharmacologic therapies that have been employed in the treatment of acute pancreatitis, specifically focusing on controlled clinical trials in humans with emphasis on the most recent studies in the literature.

Inhibitors of Pancreatic Secretion

A commonly used initial treatment for acute pancreatitis involves agents that inhibit pancreatic secretion. The rationale for this approach is to place the pancreas "at rest." Drugs that indirectly or directly reduce pancreatic secretion have been tested. H_2-blockers that inhibit acid secretion are indirect inhibitors of acid secretion. Anticholinergics are both direct and indirect inhibitors because they also directly inhibit pancreatic secretion. Direct inhibitors of pancreatic secretion that have also been used include somatostatin, glucagon, and calcitonin.

Four studies have tested the value of H_2-blockers in the treatment of mild acute pancreatitis (2–5). None showed any benefit of these agents in ameliorating the pain of the illness or the length of hospitalization, however.

The rationale behind the use of anticholinergics in the treatment of acute pancreatitis relies on the ability of vagal stimulation to suppress pancreatic secretion. Although small uncontrolled studies have shown favorable outcomes with the use of atropine, one controlled study demonstrated no difference in morbidity or mortality (6). However, no conclusions can be made given the small sample size. The limitation of side effects such as tachycardia and prolongation of ileus discourages their use in randomized controlled trials.

GLUCAGON

Glucagon has a suppressive effect on pancreatic function in vitro and can relax the sphincter of Oddi (7). Several animal studies suggested that glucagon might have a role in treating acute pancreatitis (8, 9). One early uncontrolled study of humans (7) reported an apparent benefit with the use of glucagon in acute pancreatitis. However, four subsequent controlled studies have reported no statistically significant effect of glucagon on mortality or complication rate (10–13).

SOMATOSTATIN

Somatostatin was first isolated by Brazeau et al. in 1973 (14). Its first name, growth hormone release-inhibiting peptide, was derived from its originally described action. Somatostatin has a ubiquitous extracranial role as an

Table 17.1
Controlled Trials in the Medical Treatment of Acute Pancreatitis[a]

Author	Reference	Treatment	Mortality (%) of control/treatment	P value
Broe et al.	2	H$_2$-blocker	1/0	NS
Loiudice et al.	3	H$_2$-blocker	0/0	NS
Meshkinpour et al.	4	H$_2$-blocker	0/0	NS
Cameron et al.	6	Atropine	0/0	NS
Medical Research Council	10	Glucagon Aprotinin	11/12	NS
Waterworth et al.	11	Glucagon	11/0	NS
Durr et al.	12	Glucagon	6/0	NS
Kronberg et al.	13	Glucagon	42/30	NS
Trapnell et al.	36	Aprotinin	25/7	.05
Trapnell et al.	37	Aprotinin	8/15	NS
Inrie et al.	38	Aprotinin	9/9	NS
Larvin et al.	39	Aprotinin	17/27	NS
Buchler et al.	42	Foy	18/15	NS
Usadel et al.	22	Somatostatin	17/11	NS
Choi et al.	23	Somatostatin	1/2	NS
Goebell et al.	26	Calcitonin	0/0	NS
Paul et al.	25	Calcitonin	0/0	NS
Standfield and Kakkar	32	Prostaglandin	0/0	NS
Ebbehoj et al.	29	Indomethacin	0/0	NS
Finch et al.	45	Ampicillin	0/1	NS
Craig et al.	46	Ampicillin	0/0	NS
Howes et al.	47	Ampicillin	0/0	NS
Leese et al.	49	Fresh-frozen plasma	8/9	NS
Sax et al.	53	Total parenteral nutrition	0/0	NS

[a]NS, no significant difference.

inhibiting peptide. Infusions of this substance have been shown to suppress the release of a variety of pancreatic and gastrointestinal peptides including glucagon, gastrin, vasoactive intestinal peptide, pancreatic polypeptide, motilin, cholecystokinin, and secretin (15, 15a, 16). The basis for the use of somatostatin's (and its analog octreotide) in the treatment of pancreatitis lies in its ability to suppress pancreatic secretion (17).

Somatostatin has been used to treat animal models of acute pancreatitis. However, only one study has been shown to result in improved survival in animals with experimentally induced pancreatitis (18). Somatostatin has also been used in the setting of endoscopic retrograde cholangiopan-creatography (ERCP). One report has shown that this agent reduces the hyperamylasemia associated with ERCP (19). However, this study was too small to detect any change in the incidence of clinical pancreatitis.

Two small uncontrolled trials of somatostatin in human acute pancreatitis demonstrated improvements in pain and in amylase and lipase levels (20, 21). However, two other double-blind controlled trials reported no benefit. The first of these, by Usadel et al. (22), showed no statistically significant improvement in mortality, although there was a trend toward a favorable outcome in the treated patients. In a more recent controlled trial, described by Choi et al. (23), 35 patients with acute pancreatitis were randomized to treatment with somatostatin (250 μg bolus followed by constant infusion of 100 μg/hour) for a total of 48 hours (Table 17.1). Thirty-six other patients served as control subjects. Six of the controls and nine of the treatment patients had severe pancreatitis. There was no statistically significant difference in mortality and/or complications between the treatment and control groups. Moreover, the study was limited since neither group was blinded.

CALCITONIN

Calcitonin can both decrease pancreatic enzyme secretion and lower serum calcium in an attempt to prevent saponification (24). Calcitonin has been the subject of two clinical double-blind trials in the evaluation of acute pancreatitis (25, 26). In neither trial was there any apparent effect on survival and no statistically significant difference in complication rates was seen. At the present time, the use of calcitonin in the setting of acute pancreatitis cannot be recommended. However, it has been suggested that perhaps calcitonin could be used as an adjunct to other therapies (24).

Prostaglandin Inhibitors and Prostaglandins

Treating animals with experimentally induced pancreatitis with prostaglandin inhibitors has had mixed outcomes. Both increased (27) and decreased (28) survival rates have been observed. One controlled clinical trial in humans with acute pancreatitis treated with indomethacin has been described (29). Although there was no difference in mortality between treated and untreated patients in the study (all of whom had mild disease), there were significantly fewer days of pain in patients treated with indomethacin suppositories (50 mg twice daily). There is no way of discerning whether these results were due to the analgesic effects of indomethacin or specific pancreatic effects related to prostaglandin inhibition, however.

On the opposite side of the equation, there has been interest in the cytoprotective benefits of prostaglandins in the treatment of acute pancreatitis (30–32). Stanfield and Kakkar, after first showing improved survival of acute pancreatitis in mice with prostaglandins, treated 47 patients with acute pancreatitis who were randomized to receive either saline or 0.1 mg/kg of a continuous prostaglandin E_2 infusion over a 3-day period. Although there was no reported difference in the clinical outcome, patients treated with prostaglandins demonstrated laboratory evidence of a more rapid improvement.

Protease Inhibitors

The more severe forms of acute pancreatitis are characterized by necrosis of the pancreas. This is believed to be the result of intrapancreatic activation of digestive enzymes, including trypsinogen. This pathogenic mechanism has led to studies in which proteolytic enzyme inhibitors are administered in an attempt to reduce the mortality associated with the extreme forms of acute pancreatitis (33).

Originally introduced more than 40 years ago, aprotinin (Trasylol) has been used in several clinical studies to treat acute pancreatitis. This antiprotease is produced from bovine parotid gland and acts on a diverse number of proteases, including trypsin, chymotrypsin, and thrombin. Previous work with animals demonstrated that aprotinin was effective in the treatment of experimental pancreatitis in the mouse and rat (34, 35).

Intravenous aprotinin has been used in five controlled clinical trials to treat acute pancreatitis in humans (10, 33, 36–38). All but one (36) have failed to show that administration of this inhibitor alters the course of acute pancreatitis (10, 33, 37, 38). In the one positive study described by Trapnell et al. (36), 60,000 U/kg of aprotinin was given over 4 days to patients presenting with severe disease. A statistically significant improvement in survival was reported. Whereas only 75% of untreated patients survived the attack of acute pancreatitis, 93% of the treated groups survived. A recent controlled, randomized study, however, failed to show any benefit of peritoneally administered aprotinin in the amelioration of severe pancreatitis (39).

Gabexate mesilate (also known as Foy) has certain theoretical advantages over aprotinin. It inhibits more pancreatic enzymes, including trypsin, kallikrein, plasmin, thrombin, and phospholipase A2 (40). Foy also has a lower molecular weight, allowing better tissue penetration, and it relaxes the sphinctor of Oddi (40).

Foy has been shown to reduce the enzyme elevation in pancreatic tissue injury of experimental pancreatitis (41). In uncontrolled clinical trials in humans, Singer and Goebell (40) have noted alleviation of pain, nausea, vomiting, and abdominal distension in patients treated with Foy. However, a recent randomized, controlled clinical trial conducted in Germany showed no efficacy for Foy in alleviating the morbidity and mortality of severe pancreatitis (42).

Antibiotics

Necrotizing pancreatitis can become secondarily infected and pancreatic abscesses can develop as a late complication of acute pancreatitis. Both of these conditions are associated with significant morbidity and mortality (43, 44). Unfortunately, the use of antibiotics to prevent these feared complications has not been properly evaluated. Three early controlled trials using ampicillin in mild forms of alcoholic pancreatitis showed this medication to have no effect on the course of the illness (45–47). A recent randomized controlled study suggests that imipenem can reduce the pancreatic sepsis that can complicate severe pancreatitis (48). At the present time, the use of antibiotics in all patients presenting with acute pancreatitis cannot be justified. However, the use of these agents in patients with severe, necrotizing acute pancreatitis is a matter of clinical judgment. If antibiotics are chosen, they should be directed against the common bacteria that are pathogenic to this site of infection, including *Escherichia coli, Klebsiella, Enterobacter, Proteus, Pseudomonas, Bacteroides,* and *Clostridium species.*

Fresh Frozen Plasma

α-2-Macroglobulin, an important serum protein, plays a central role in the elimination of proteases that may be liberated from the pancreas into the systemic circulation during acute pancreatitis (12). Fresh-frozen plasma (FFP) has been shown to reduce the fall in serum α-2-macroglobin levels in this illness and has been proposed as a specific therapy for acute pancreatitis. A controlled animal study suggested that FFP replenished the circulating antiprotease system and an uncontrolled clinical study suggested that the mortality of acute pancreatitis was reduced (49).

However, Leese et al. (50) performed a randomized study of 202 patients with acute pancreatitis in which FFP afforded no discernible benefit on the outcome of pancreatitis despite less reduction in the serum α-2-macroglobin in the patients receiving FFP.

Total Parenteral Nutrition

Patients are routinely kept NPO (nothing by mouth) when presenting with acute pancreatitis. The desire to minimize nausea and vomiting while decreasing the stimuli for pancreatic secretion led investigators to study the use of early total parenteral nutrition (TPN) in patients with severe acute pancreatitis (51). This randomized study demonstrated no significant benefit regarding morbidity or mortality. TPN, however, remains an important nutritional therapy for patients who are expected to receive no oral nutrition for >7 days.

Summary

Despite numerous controlled clinical trials, few pharmacologic agents have shown significant value in decreasing the morbidity and/or mortality from acute pancreatitis at the present time. Recent early data, however, suggest that the use of broad-spectrum antibiotics may reduce the rate of pancreatic sepsis. Large, multicenter, clinical trials involving patients with severe disease are needed to evaluate potential therapies for this illness.

TREATMENT OF CHRONIC PANCREATITIS

Pharmacologic treatment of chronic pancreatitis involves the management of its two main clinical consequences: steatorrhea and chronic abdominal pain. The following section will review the various drugs employed in the treatment of these primary aspects of chronic pancreatic insufficiency, again focusing on controlled trials in humans.

Steatorrhea

Treating the patient with steatorrhea secondary to pancreatic insufficiency may seem simple. It would seem logical that if a patient is able to ingest exogenous pancreatic enzymes in sufficient quantity, then steatorrhea should be abolished. Unfortunately, it is not that simple. In practice, although it may be possible to eliminate malabsorption of protein, steatorrhea is usually only partially corrected (52–55). The major obstacle to the correction of steatorrhea is the hostile acidic environment of the stomach (51, 55, 56). Pancreatic enzymes require an alkaline pH for optimal activity. When ingested in pancreatic enzyme preparations, lipase is inactivated by gastric acid and pepsin (56). If intragastric or intraduodenal pH falls below 4.0, lipase is irreversibly denatured (52, 54, 58). In the patient with chronic pancreatic insufficiency, the pH in the duodenum may decrease to <4.0 (52–54, 60) because of the inability of the diseased pancreas to secrete a sufficient amount of bicarbonate.

In addition, the abnormal acidic intraluminal environment in patients with chronic pancreatic insufficiency causes precipitation of bile acids, which further aggravates fat malabsorption. Patients with cystic fibrosis are especially prone to have problems correcting their steatorrhea with enzymes. In particular, cystic fibrosis patients tend to be gastric acid hypersecretors and have increased fecal losses of bile acids.

A second obstacle to the correction of steatorrhea is the requirement that an adequate amount of pancreatic enzyme be ingested. To abolish steatorrhea, 5–10% of the maximal enzyme output of the pancreas must be delivered to the duodenum (55, 61). Thus if no inactivation occurs in the stomach, approximately 30,000 IU of lipase must be taken with every meal. This could mean ingesting up to 27 tablets per meal of a conventional pancreatic enzyme preparation. Administration of lesser amounts of enzyme will decrease but not abolish steatorrhea.

A third reason for incomplete correction of steatorrhea is the timing of administration of enzyme replacement. There has been controversy for years over the optimal dosing schedule for administration of enzyme replacement.

Early studies found hourly doses superior to ingestion with meals (62) but later studies showed that prandial dosing was as effective as hourly administration in decreasing steatorrhea and perhaps more effective in abolishing azotorrhea (52, 63).

CLINICAL STUDIES

Several pharmacologic approaches have been tried in order to minimize steatorrhea. These include: first, the addition of antacids or H_2-blockers to enzyme replacement therapy in order to diminish gastric acidity and subsequently preserve enzyme activity; second, the use of enteric coated tablets that would release enzymes only in an alkaline environment with the hope that enzymes would only be released in the small intestine; third, the development of microspheres containing small enteric coated granules, which would pass readily from the stomach into the alkaline medium of the duodenum where they would be activated; fourth, the development of acid stable lipases (ie, lingual lipase and fungal lipase), which are stable over a broad pH range.

CONVENTIONAL ENZYMES PLUS ACID INHIBITORY AGENTS (Table 17.1)

Therapy designed to protect enzymes from inactivation and thus to enhance efficacy must maintain a gastric and duodenal pH >4.0 for at least 60 minutes postprandially (54, 64).

Acid inhibitory agents such as bicarbonate, antacids, or H_2-blockers, when added to conventional pancreatic enzyme preparations, do not enhance the treatment of steatorrhea in patients with chronic alcoholic pancreatitis as well as they do in patients with cystic fibrosis.

Alcoholic Chronic Pancreatitis

Of four studies performed with this population, two showed no benefit of acid inhibitory agents in ameliorating steatorrhea. One study (65), however, showed that sodium bicarbonate and aluminum hydroxide antacids improved steatorrhea and another study (55) showed that cimetidine improved this problem.

Graham (65) compared the addition of sodium bicarbonate, aluminum hydroxide, magnesium hydroxide, calcium carbonate, or cimetidine as supplements to pancreatic enzyme therapy. Interestingly, he found that only sodium bicarbonate and aluminum hydroxide significantly reduced the amount of steatorrhea when compared with enzyme therapy alone. Magnesium- and calcium-containing antacids, when used in conjunction with enzymes, actually worsened steatorrhea. This is in keeping with previous findings that calcium or magnesium ion may increase fecal fat excretion by the formation of calcium/magnesium soaps or the intraluminal precipitation of glycine conjugates of bile salts (66, 67).

Regan et al. (55), failed to show any improvement in steatorrhea with the addition of bicarbonate or antacid to conventional enzyme therapy (Table 17.2). This was due to the fact that bicarbonate failed to maintain the gastric and duodenal pH >4.0. However, these same investigators found that cimetidine 300 mg taken 30 minutes before each meal, significantly reduced steatorrhea because of its ability to maintain the postprandial pH values in the stomach and duodenum at >4.

Although most early studies employing an H_2-blocker as an adjunct to the treatment of steatorrhea involved cimetidine, a more recent trial compared conventional enzyme replacement with ranitidine (68). The patients were all adults with chronic pancreatitis secondary to alcohol abuse. Although overall the authors found that ranitidine plus enzymes did not reduce steatorrhea more than enzymes alone (Tables 17.2 and 17.3), a subset of patients who were hypersecretors of acid did benefit from the addition of ranitidine.

There have also been two papers published on the use of omeprazole as an adjunct to pancreatic enzyme replacement therapy. The first (69) was an anecdotal report of two patients who responded dramatically to the addition of omeprazole. Both patients had been taking large doses of pancreatic enzyme replacement (10 g of pancreatic granulate with 225,000 IU of lipase) and H_2-blocker therapy with continued steatorrhea. One of these patients had the Zollinger-Ellison syndrome. It was of note that acid suppression was not fully achieved with cimetidine in the patient with Zollinger-Ellison syndrome. However, omeprazole 40 mg/day with enzymes dramatically reduced steatorrhea from approximately 100–30 g/day of fecal fat. The second omeprazole paper will be discussed below under "Cystic fibrosis."

Cystic Fibrosis

Of the six studies of patients with cystic fibrosis, five showed that acid inhibitory agents, when added to enzyme therapy, improved steatorrhea as compared with enzyme therapy alone (Table 17.3). One of these showed that bicarbonate improved steatorrhea, one showed Mg-Al antacid helped, and four showed that cimetidine ameliorated steatorrhea. As mentioned earlier, the difference between cystic fibrosis patients and alcoholic pancreatitis patients in response to acid inhibitory agents is thought to be due to the differences in the gastric acid secretory status of these patients. Patients with alcohol-induced chronic pancreatitis tend to have decreased acid production (70–72), whereas gastric acid secretion in patients with cystic fibrosis may be normal or greater than normal (70, 73, 74).

Other reasons for differences in the response of patients to these various agents include the quantity and timing of acid inhibitory agents such as sodium bicarbonate and the amount of enzyme given with each meal. Smaller doses of bicarbonate (2.5 g) may not be as efficacious as higher doses (3.6 g). Likewise, enzyme preparations containing ≥30,000 IU of lipase are likely to be more efficacious than smaller amounts (65).

Other factors that may be responsible for cimetidine's failure to completely abolish steatorrhea in patients with cystic fibrosis are the presence of bile acid deficiency (as discussed above) and small intestinal mucosal disease. Small intestinal mucosal injury associated with dissacharidase deficiency, as well as impaired amino acid and fatty acid transport have been reported in patients with cystic fibrosis (75–77).

Table 17.2
Conventional Enzyme Therapy in Adults with Chronic Pancreatitis[a]

Author	Therapy	No. of patients	Lipase/meal (IU)	Fecal fat/24° post-treatment (g)
Regan et al. (54)	Viokase	6	31,000	
	Viokase + HCO_3			NS
	Viokase + Maalox		31,000	NS
	Viokase + cimetidine		31,000	$P < .05$[b]
Staub et al. (152)	Eurobiol	23	52,120	20.33 ± 3.15
	Eurobiol + cimetidine (400 mg 30 min after meals)		52,120	18.93 ± 3.4
Graham (64)	Ilozyme	8	10,800	29.0 ± 4
	Ilozyme + $NaHCO_3$ (1.3 g)	8	10,800	16.6 ± 3[c]
	Ilozyme + $AlOH_3$	8	10,800	18.4 ± 5[c]
	Ilozyme + $MgOH_3$	8	10,800	36.3 ± 11
	Ilozyme + $CaCO_3$	8	10,800	39.0 ± 11
	Ilozyme + cimetidine (300 mg)	8	10,800	32.1 ± 9
Marotta (67)	Viokase	12	17,000	
	Viokase + ranitidine	12	17,000	NS[d]

[a]NS, no significant difference.
[b]Statistically significant difference compared to Viokase alone.
[c]Statistically significant difference compared to Ilozyme alone, $P = .029$.
[d]Statistically significant difference with the addition of ranitidine only in those patients with high or normal acid outputs, $P < .001$, but overall there was no significant difference.

Table 17.3
Conventional Enzyme Therapy in Cystic Fibrosis[a]

Author	Therapy	No. of patients	Lipase/meal (IU)	Fecal fat/24° post-treatment (g)
Durie (52)	Cotazyme	21	12,100	31.3 ± 15.5
	Cotazyme + cimetidine (300 mg)	21	12,100	20.3 ± 12.6[b]
	Cotazyme + $NaHCO_3$ (3.6 g)	21	12,100	19.3 ± 12.7[c]
	Cotazyme + $NaHCO_3$ + cimetidine (300 mg)	21	12,000	18.0 ± 10.7[c]
De Bieville (153)	Viokase	13	Not given	19.1
	Viokase + cimetidine (150–200 mg)	13	Not given	14.7
Hubbard (154)	Cotazyme or Viokase	8	Not given	16
	Cotazyme or Viokase + cimetidine	8	Not given	9[d]
Cox (72)	Cotazyme or Viokase	10	5,370 (Cotazyme)	25.3
	Cotazyme or Viokase + cimetidine (150–200 mg)	10	4,090 (Viokase)	17.3[e]
Boyle (155)	Viokase	7	9,816	39 ± 7
	Viokase + cimetidine (300 mg)	7	9,816	30 ± 6[f]
Nassif (88)	Cotazyme	11	12,084	34 ± 3
	Cotazyme + Maalox	11	12,084	24 ± 2[a]

[a]NS, no significant difference.
[b]Statistically significant difference compared to Cotazyme alone, $P < .01$.
[c]Statistically significant difference compared to Cotazyme alone, $P < .001$.
[d]Statistically significant difference compared to Cotazyme or Viokase alone, $P < .01$.
[e]Statistically significant difference compared to Cotazyme or Viokase alone, $P < .05$.
[f]Statistically significant difference compared to Viokase alone, $P < .05$.

Table 17.4
Enteric-Coated Enzyme Treatment in Adult Pancreatic Insufficiency[a]

Author	Therapy	No. of patients	Lipase/meal (IU)	Fecal fat/24° post-treatment (g)
Graham (77)	Ilozyme	6	10,800	
	Ilozyme	6	21,600	NS
	Ilozyme	6	43,200	NS
	Pancrease (ECM)	6	6,015	NS
Dutta (81)	Pancreatin	6	6,840	19 ± 1
	Cotazyme	6	35,000	15 ± 5
	Pancrease (ECM)	6	19,730	13 ± 5
	Pancrease (ECM)	6	39,500	11 ± 4[b]
Dutta (82)	Pancreatin	7	6,840	19 ± 4
	Pancrease (ECM)	7	19,730	13 ± 5
	Cotazyme-S (ECM)	7	22,848	9 ± 2
Schneider (83)	Pancreon	17	120,000	30.4
	Creon (ECM)	17	33,000	38.6
Marotta (67)	Viokase	12	17,000	
	Viokase + ranitidine (150 mg)	12	17,000	NS[c]
	Pancrease (ECM)	12	3,600	NS
	Creon (ECM)	12	4,800	NS
Jorgensen (84)	Pankreatin	23	180,000	15
	Pancrease (ECM)	23	12,400	21.5
	Pankreon (ECM)	23	16,000	17.5

[a]NS, no significant difference.
[b]Statistically significant difference compared to Pancreatin alone, $P < .01$.
[c]Statistically significant difference with the addition of ranitidine. Only in those patients with high or normal acid outputs, $P < .001$ but overall there was no significant difference.

ENTERIC COATED PREPARATIONS

Enteric coating is based upon the premise of delivering enzymes through the hostile environment of the stomach without inactivation. Once in the small intestine, the enteric coating is designed to dissolve at a pH >5.5.

The first enteric coated preparations were in tablet form. In an early study, Graham (78) concluded that despite their theoretical advantage, enteric coating might reduce clinical effectiveness because of limited bioavailability. One of the problems encountered was that some patients with pancreatic insufficiency have an acidic duodenum and upper jejunum (79) that may denature the pancreatic enzymes. A second problem encountered was the size of the tablets. Large tablets would not pass as quickly as smaller food particles into the small intestine, and thus would not be available to aid in digestion (78).

Microencapsulated enteric-coated preparations were developed to improve the delivery of enzymes into the duodenum. They are designed to pass into the duodenum and to become active at pH >5.0. They are not fully effective in situations where there are significant swings from an alkaline to an acidic environment. An example of this is the individual who is a normosecretor of acid and in whom intragastric pH rises rapidly to 6.0 during the meal and then falls to <4.0 shortly after the meal. In this situation, the enteric coating will dissolve at the near-alkaline pH, and the enzymes will liberate and then be inactivated when the pH lowers to the acidic range. Patients who are either hyposecretors or hypersecretors of acid will benefit more than those who are normosecretors from enteric-coated microspheres because the former have lesser shifts of intragastric pH during and after the meal (80).

Meyer et al. (81) determined that the optimal size of enzyme microspheres should be approximately 1 mm in diameter to effectively

Table 17.5
Enteric-Coated Enzymes in Cystic Fibrosis

Author	Therapy	No. of patients	Lipase/meal (IU)	Fecal fat/24° post-treatment (g)
Nassif (88)	Cotazyme	11	12,084	Exact numbers not given
	Cotazyme + Maalox	11	12,084	c
	Pancrease (ECM)	11	6,015	c
Gow (85)	Cotazyme	10	40,280	86.5 ± 12 mmol/24 hr
	Pancrease (ECM)	10	16,040	26.9 ± 4 mmol/24 hr[c]
	Pancrease + cimetidine (20 mg/kg/day)	10	16,040	30.1 ± 4 mmol/24 hr[c]
	Pancrease + antacid	10	16,040	22.0 ± 3 mmol/24 hr[c]
Mischler (156)	Placebo	10		67.9 ± 41
	Cotazyme	10	4,028	29.9 ± 22.2[d]
	Pancrease (ECM)	10	4,010	17.3 ± 9.3[e]
Mitchell (157)	Viokase	12	29,400	14.5 ± 7.5
	Viokase	12	58,800	17.3 ± 9.1
	Pancrease (ECM)	12	21,333	11.5 ± 6.9
	Pancrease (ECM)	12	42,666	8.7 ± 4.1[f]
Stead (89)	Pancrex V Forte	23	b	27.1
	Creon (ECM)	23	b	15.2[g]
Dutta (86)	Cotazyme	8	35,216	19.2 ± 5.7
	Pancrease (ECM)	8	39,464	5.9 ± 2.0[e]
Heijerman (90)	Pancrease (ECM)	9	10,000	22.3
	Pancrease + omeprazole (20 mg/day)	9	10,000	16.4
	Pancrease (ECM)	9	20,000	19.6
	Pancrease + omeprazole (20 mg/day)	9	20,000	10.7[h]

[a]NS, no significant difference.
[b]Exact amounts not given but doses were equivalent.
[c]Statistically significant difference compared to conventional enzyme alone, $P < .001$.
[d]Statistically significant difference compared to placebo, $P < .005$.
[e]Statistically significant difference compared to conventional enzyme alone, $P < .05$.
[f]Statistically significant difference compared to conventional enzyme alone (V16 or V32), $P < .02$.
[g]Statistically significant difference compared to standard enteric coated tablet (Pancrex V), $P < .01$.
[h]Statistically significant difference compared to Pancrease 10,000 IU/meal and 20,000 IU/meal, $P < .01$ as well as 10,000 IU/meal + omeparazole 20 mg/day, $P < .05$.

and consistently empty from the stomach independently of the composition of the meal. Microspheres >2 mm may not empty well at the pylorus. Some of the commercially available microsphere preparations have smaller particle size than others, which might supply these products with theoretical advantages.

Alcoholic Chronic Pancreatitis

Of the six studies (Table 17.4) that have compared enteric-coated microspheres to conventional pancreatic enzymes, only one (82) showed an advantage to the former preparation in treating steatorrhea (55, 69, 82–85). Studies in this population have not shown en-

teric-coated microsphere preparations to be more efficacious than conventional enzyme preparations presumably due to the fact that these patients tend to be gastric acid hyposecretors. However, they are equally efficacious in controlling steatorrhea with far fewer numbers of pills or capsules.

Cystic Fibrosis

Patients with cystic fibrosis, unlike those with alcoholic chronic pancreatitis, are more likely to respond to enteric-coated microspheres with a significant reduction in steatorrhea when compared to conventional enzymes because of their greater intragastric acid secretion (86–89). All six studies in this area showed that enteric-coated microspheres were superior to conventional enzymes (Table 17.5).

In several of the above studies, it has also been noted that patients prefer enteric-coated microsphere capsules to conventional enzymes (57, 82, 83, 86, 87, 90). Reasons for this include: (a) reduced capsule requirement (87–90) (b) better control of diarrhea (87, 90) and flatulence (87), and (c) improved palatability (82, 83).

The addition of acid inhibitory agents to enteric-coated preparations has not been extensively studied. A recent controlled investigation added omeprazole 20 mg/day to high-dose (83) pancrease (20,000 IU of lipase per meal) and found a significant reduction in steatorrhea as compared with treatment with enzymes alone.

Acid Stable Lipases

The investigation of acid stable lipases as a therapy in pancreatic insufficiency is based upon the hypothesis that if an enzyme preparation could be stable over a broad pH range (ie, 3.0–7.0), fat digestion might be optimized (58). Acid-stable lipase activity believed to be from the lingual von Ebner glands and the gastric mucosa (91) has been documented in the gastrointestinal tract for many years. Fungi such as *Rizopus arrhizus* and *Aspergillus niger* have been found to be sources of acid-stable lipases.

Schneider et al. (84) compared the efficacy of a conventional, an enteric-coated microsphere preparation, and an acid-stable fungal preparation, Nortase, in reducing steatorrhea in patients with alcoholic pancreatic insufficiency. The acid-stable fungal enzyme preparation was equal to, but not superior to, the conventional or enteric-coated microsphere preparations.

In a more recent report, Zentler-Munro et al. (93) compared an acid-resistant fungal lipase prepared from *A. niger*, an enteric-coated microsphere preparation, Creon, and a placebo. They found Creon to be superior to the acid-resistant fungal lipase and the placebo. Table 17.6 lists the commonly used pancreatic enzymes as well as their enzyme contents and price.

Summary

In general, adults with pancreatic insufficiency secondary to alcoholic pancreatic insufficiency will benefit most from large amounts of conventional pancreatic enzyme replacement (30,000 IU of lipase/meal). This will in most cases significantly decrease but not completely abolish steatorrhea. The addition of an agent to suppress or neutralize acid is usually not needed in these patients as they tend to be hyposecretors of acid. Those patients who do not respond to conventional enzyme therapy alone and continue to have steatorrhea may benefit from the addition of an H_2-blocker, sodium bicarbonate, or aluminum-only-containing antacid. Enteric coated pancreatic enzyme microspheres treat steatorrhea just as well as conventional preparations with fewer numbers of pills needed per day. This may enhance patient compliance and, thus, increase efficacy.

In children with cystic fibrosis, because of their higher gastric acidity, enteric-coated microspheres appear to be more efficacious than conventional enzyme therapy and should be the therapy of choice. If therapy is not successful, the addition of an H_2-blocker or omeprazole may improve the benefit of the regimen.

PAIN

In chronic pancreatitis, pain is a common and disabling symptom. It occurs either chronically or intermittently. Frequently, narcotic medications are needed for pain relief (94). The cause of pain is thought to be multifactorial. Some of the possible causes include: (a) increased pancreatic-ductal or parenchymal tissue pressure as a result of outflow obstruction; (b) inflammation of both pancreatic and/or peripancreatic neurons; (c) autodigestion with tissue necrosis; (d) pseudocyst formation; (e) ischemia and intraparenchymal acidosis. Increased intraductal pressure secondary to continued pancreatic secretion in the face of ductal obstruction caused by strictures and/or

Table 17.6
Pancreatic Enzyme Comparisons[a]

Enzyme	Lipase[b]	Amylase[b]	Protease[b]	Cost index ($)[c]
Conventional				
Cotazyme	8,000	30,000	30,000	0.16
Ilozyme	11,000	30,000	30,000	0.26
Viokase	8,000	30,000	30,000	0.17
Enteric coated				
Cotazyme-S	5,000	20,000	20,000	0.22
Enteric-coated microspheres				
Creon	8,000	30,000	30,000	0.24
Creon 25	25,000	74,700	62,500	1.24
Entolase	4,000	20,000	20,000	NA
Entolase HP	8,000	40,000	50,000	0.46
Kuzyme HP	8,000	30,000	30,000	0.26
Pancrease	4,000	20,000	25,000	0.27
Pancrease MT4	4,000	12,000	12,000	0.21
Pancrease MT10	10,000	30,000	30,000	0.53
Pancrease MT16	16,000	48,000	48,000	0.85
Pancrease MT25	25,000	75,000	75,000	1.49
Zymase	12,000	24,000	24,000	0.45
Acid-stable fungal lipases				
Nortase	7,500	10,000	700	NA

[a]NA, not available.
[b]Units per pill or capsule.
[c]Cost per pill or capsule.

intraductal stones (95) is thought to be one of the most common etiologies. This theory has been supported by several surgical as well as endoscopic studies (96–103).

Analgesia

Despite the importance of analgesics in the relief of pain in chronic pancreatitis, surprisingly, there are no controlled trials assessing the comparative efficacies of any particular preparations.

Empirically, the physician should begin with peripherally acting agents, that is, spasmolytics or analgesics such as nonsteroidals. Tranquilizers, in low doses, such as amitriptyline at bedtime, may be useful adjuncts.

Most often, however, the patient requires opiate derivatives for pain relief. Although morphine causes constriction of the sphincter of Oddi and should not be used in the treatment of acute pancreatitis, long-acting morphine derivatives are quite effective for managing chronic pain, but addiction remains an important concern.

Enzyme Replacement

A pharmacologic approach to the treatment of pain with enzymes was first suggested in 1977 (104) when the protease-specific feedback regulation of pancreatic secretion was suggested in man. The authors suggested that there might be an association between pancreatic enzyme replacement and the reduction of pain by a protease-induced negative feedback control on pancreatic secretion. This feedback control had before and since been described in rats, chickens, pigs, and calves (105–109), but seems to be absent in dogs (110). There have been several studies in man that confirm a feedback control of exocrine pancreatic secretion (104, 111–121). A low concentration of enzymes in the duodenum, as would be expected in patients with chronic pancreatitis, leads to a release of cholecystokinin (CCK) by enterocytes in this region. This in turn causes increased pancreatic secretion into the duodenum, which negatively inhibits CCK secretion (122). It is thought that the serine proteases—trypsin, chymotrypsin, and elastase (123)—are responsible for this response, lipase and amylase having no effect. If enzymes containing large amounts of the serine proteases are given exogenously, this would theoretically lead to suppression of CCK release and inhibition of pancreatic secretion, which would put the "pancreas to rest" and reduce pain. Evidence for and against this theory exists. Folsch et al. (124) found that diversion of bile and pancreatic juice from the intestines and perfusion of the duodenum with a trypsin inhibitor, aprotinin, resulted in a significant increase of both plasma CCK and pancreatic enzyme levels. However, studies by Dlugosz et al. (125) and Hotz et al. (126) could not demonstrate increases in pancreatic secretion when aprotinin was infused into the duodenum. It must be pointed out, however, that aprotinin is an inhibitor only of trypsin, and that active chymotrypsin and/or elastase in the duodenal lumen will also suppress CCK (126).

There have been two double-blind placebo-controlled trials (120, 128) demonstrating effective relief of pain in patients taking pancreatic enzyme supplementation. Isakkson and Ihse (128) treated 19 patients with chronic pancreatitis with a conventional enzyme preparation, (7.5 ml of pankreon granules) or placebo in a double-blind crossover study. They found that 15 of 19 patients had pain relief during the week of pankreon treatment as compared with the week of placebo treatment ($P < .05$). There was an average reduction of 70% of the pain in the 10 "good" responders, whereas overall there was a 30% reduction in pain intensity. Furthermore, there was a statistically significant decrease in the number of painful attacks in patients being treated with enzyme therapy as compared with placebo.

Slaff et al. (120) studied 20 patients with chronic pancreatitis (alcohol-induced or idiopathic) in a double-blind placebo-controlled crossover study for 60 days. They used a conventional enzyme preparation pancrelipase (Ilozyme) (six tablets four times daily) and found an overall reduction in pain in 9 of 12 patients with mild to moderate pancreatic disease, most of whom had idiopathic pancreatitis, compared with only 2 of 8 with severe disease (steatorrhea), most of whom had alcoholic pancreatitis.

In contrast to the above studies, Halgreen et al. (128) did not find a statistically significant reduction in pain relief when 20 patients were treated with an enteric microsphere preparation, pancrelipase (Pancrease). A recent study by Campbell and associates in 52 patients with alcoholic and idiopathic chronic pancreatitis also failed to demonstrate any reduction of plasma CCK levels or any benefit in pain relief when another enteric-coated microsphere preparation, Creon, was given in large doses (130). It is theorized that enteric-coated preparations do not work well for pain because they release their enzymes too distally in the small bowel to interrupt the CCK-mediated proximal bowel negative feedback loop of pancreatic secretion.

Summary

Patients with mild to moderate chronic pancreatitis, especially of the idiopathic type, may experience relief of pain with conventional pancreatic enzyme supplementation. If high doses of a conventional enzyme are not effective, adding an acid-inhibiting agent such as sodium bicarbonate, an H_2-blocker, or omeprazole may be helpful. Patients with more severe alcoholic pancreatitis with steatorrhea tend not to respond to enzyme therapy. Enteric-coated microsphere preparations may also be tried but do not appear to be as helpful as conventional enzymes in pain relief.

Dissolution of Pancreatic Stones

Pancreatic stone dissolution has been reported both in animals and humans. Noda et al. (131) reported that the antiepileptic agent trimethadione, when given orally to dogs at a dose of 1.0–1.5 g daily, caused the disappearance of pancreatic calculi in 13 of 15 animals. The authors stated that scanning electron microscopy, elemental analysis, and powder X-ray diffractometry of pancreatic calculi in this model revealed that the calculi closely resembled human pancreatic calculi and concluded that oral trimethadione treatment may have potential for dissolving human pancreatic calculi. In a later study of 14 humans, Noda (133) reported that trimethadione reduced the number of pancreatic stones in five and unequivocally decreased the size of the stone in a sixth patient. The authors stated that five of the eight patients with pain (six had painless stones) had disappearance of the pain, with an average follow-up observation of 55 months. There have been no follow-up studies to these intriguing observations.

PANCREATIC ASCITES AND PSEUDOCYSTS

In 1951, Davis and Kelsey (133) wrote the classical paper describing pancreatic ascites. Their young patient with chronic pancreatitis continued to reaccumulate significant ascites despite repeated paracenteses and drainage of fluid at laparotomy. Pancreatic ascites is believed to result from the spontaneous decompression of a pseudocyst or interruption of the pancreatic ductal system with direct communication into the peritoneal cavity (134–139).

Traditionally, therapy has first been directed at conservative measures. These include: (a) avoidance of oral intake; (b) sealing of the leak by repeated paracentesis, allowing adjacent organs to seal the leak; (c) improving nutritional status by intravenous hyperalimentation; and (d) suppressing pancreatic secretions with drugs such as atropine and acetazolamide. Cameron (136) reported that 8 of 17 patients (41%) sealed their leaks with this regimen. However, 4 of the 17 patients (24%) died during the trial from gastrointestinal bleeding, sepsis, and sudden unexplained causes.

The conservative approach has met with a <50% success rate (134, 140) and a significant mortality. In addition, conservative management is not recommended for longer than 2–3 weeks. If the ascites has not resolved by this time, it is unlikely to do so (139), and surgical therapy (i.e., internal drainage or distal pancreatectomy) is advised after endoscopic retrograde pancreatography to demonstrate the site of the leak.

Somatostatin has been described by several authors as useful in the management of exter-nal gastrointestinal fistulas. It has been reported to increase the healing rate and to shorten the time of fistula closure (141–144). It also has been reported to decrease exocrine pancreatic secretion (145–147) and to be beneficial in the healing of external pancreatic fistulae (148). Recently, there have been three case reports of continuous infusion of somatostatin for the treatment of pancreatic ascites (149, 150). In all three cases, the patients had failed medical management of at least 4 weeks duration. Each was treated with either somatostatin or a somatostatin analog (Sandostatin), 250 μg/hour for 9 to 14 days. Ascites resolved spontaneously in all three patients after the first few days of somatostatin therapy. At 6, 9, and 18 months, the patients all remained in good health without any recurrence of ascites. This early experience should encourage future studies with somatostatin.

There has been only one report (151) describing the use of octreotide (Sandostatin) for treatment of pancreatic pseudocysts. Seven patients were given this drug, 100 μg subcutaneously three times per day, for 2 weeks. In four patients, the pseudocyst decreased in size by a mean of 42%, and pain disappeared completely. The pseudocysts completely disappeared in two patients. However, in one of these patients retreatment was necessary for the reaccumulation of fluid. Obviously, the role of octreotide in the treatment of this complication of pancreatitis needs further evaluation.

REFERENCES

1. Steinberg WM, Schlesselman SE. Treatment of acute pancreatitis. Gastroenterology 1987;93:1420–1427.
2. Broe PJ, Zinner MJ, Cameron JL. A clinical trial of cimetidine in acute pancreatitis. Surg Gynecol Obstet 1982;154:13–16.
3. Loiudice TA, Lang J, Mehta H, et al. Treatment of acute pancreatitis: the roles of cimetidine and nasogastric suction. Am J Gastroenterol 1984;79:553–558.
4. Meshkinpour H, Molinari M, Gardner L, et al. Cimetidine in the treatment of acute alcoholic pancreatitis. Gastroenterology 1979;77:687–690.
5. Hadas N, Wapnick S, Grosberg SJ, Sugaar S. Cimetidine-induced mortality in experimental pancreatitis. Gastroenterology 1979;76:1148.

6. Cameron JL, Mehigan D, Zuidema GD. Evaluation of atropine in acute pancreatitis. Surg Gynecol Obstet 1979;148:206–208.

7. Knight MJ, Condon JR, and Smith R. Possible role of glucagon in the treatment of pancreatitis. Br Med J 1972;1:1097–1099.

8. Condon RE, Woods JH, Poulin TL, Wagner WG, Pissiotis CA. Experimental pancreatitis treated with glucagon or lactated Ringers. Arch Surg 1974; 109:154–158.

9. Lankisch PG, Wincklerk, Bokermann M, Schmidt H, Creutzfeldt W. The influence of glucagon on acute experimental pancreatitis in the rat. Scand J Gastroenterol 1974;9:725–729.

10. Medical Research Council Working Party: Death from acute pancreatitis. Multicenter trial of glucagon and aprotinin. Lancet 1977;2:632–634.

11. Waterforth MW, Barbezat GO, Bank S. Glucagon treatment of acute pancreatitis. Lancet 1974;1:123.

12. Durr HK, Maroske D, Zedler O, Bode J. Glucagon therapy in acute pancreatitis. Gut 1978;19:175–179.

13. Kronberg O, Bulow S, Jorgensen PM, Svendsen LB. A randomized controlled trial of glucagon in the treatment of first attack of severe acute pancreatitis without associated biliary disease. Am J Gastroenterol 1980;73:423–425.

14. Brazeau P, Vale W, Burgus R, et al. Hypothalamic peptide that inhibits immunoreactive pituitary growth hormone. Science 1973;179:77–79.

15. Bloom SR, Mortimer CH, Thorner MO, et al. Inhibition of gastrin and gastric acid secretion. Lancet 1974;2:1106–1109.

15a. Pederson R, Dryburg J, Brown J. The effect of somatostatin on human gastric polypeptide secretion, Can J Physiol Pharmacol 1977;53:1200–1205.

16. Osei K, O'Dorisio T. Effects of somatostatin and gastroenteropancreatic hormone in a malignant insulinoma patient. Clin Res 1985;33:312A.

17. Fahrenkrug J, Schaffalitzky OB, Holst JJ, et al. Vasoactive intestinal polypeptide in vagally mediated pancreatic secretion of fluid and bicarbonate. Am J Physiol 1979;237:535–540.

18. Baxter JN, Jenkins SA, Day DW, et al. Effects of somatostatin and a long-acting somatostatin analgue on the prevention and treatment of experimentally induced acute pancreatitis in the rat. Br J Surg 1985;72:382–385.

19. Bordas J, Toledo V, Mondelo F, et al. Prevention of pancreatic reactions by volus somatostatin administration in patients undergoing ERCP. Horm Res 1988;29:106–108.

20. Raptis S, Schlegel W, Lehmann E, et al. Effects of somatostatin on the exocrine pancreas and the release of duodenal hormones. Metabolism 1978; 27:1321–1328.

21. Limburg B, Komerfell B. Treatment of acute pancreatitis with somatostatin. N Eng J Med 1980; 303:284–289.

22. Usadel KH, Uberla KK, Leuschner U. Treatment of acute pancreatitis with somatostatin: results of a multicenter double-blind trial. Dig Dis Sci 1985; 30:992.

23. Choi TK, Mok G, et al. Somatostatin in the treatment of acute pancreatitis: a prospective randomized controlled trial. Gut 1989;30:223–227.

24. Durr HK. Acute pancreatitis. In: Howat HF, Sarles H, eds. Exocrine pancrease. Philadelphia: Saunders; 1979:352–401.

25. Paul F. Ohnhaus E, Hesch RD. Einfluss von salmcalcitonin auf der verlauf der akuten pancreatitis. Dsch Med Wochenschr 1979;104:615–622.

26. Goebel H, Ammann R, Herfarthe C. A double blind trial of synthetic salmon calcitonin in the treatment of acute pancreatitis. Scand J Gastroenterol 1979; 14:881–889.

27. Olazabal A, Nascimento L. J Lab Clin Med 1980; 96:570–574.

28. Coelle EF, Adham N, Elashoff J, Lewin K, Taylor IL. Gastroenterology 1983;85:1307–1312.

29. Ebbehoj N, Friss J, Svendsen LB, Bulow S, Madsen P. Indomethacin treatment of acute pancreatitis. Scand J Gastroenterology 1985;20:789–793.

30. Miller TA, Jacobson ED. Gastrointestinal cytoprotection by prostaglandins. Gut 1979;20:75–87.

31. Robert A. Cytoprotection by prostaglandins. Gastroenterology 1979;77:761–767.

32. Stanfield NJ, Kakkar VV. Prostaglandins and acute pancreatitis experimental and clinical studies. Br J Surg 1983;70:573–576.

33. Manabe T, Steer ML. Protease inhibitors and experimental acute hemorrhagic pancreatitis. Ann Surg 1979;190:13–19.

34. Lombardi B, Rao NK. Acute hemorrhagic pancreatic necrois in mice. Am J Pathol 1975;81:87–93.

35. McCutcheon AD, Race D. Experimental pancreatitis: use of a new antiproteolytic substance, tyrasylol. Ann Surg 1963;158:223–228.

36. Trapnell JE, Rigby CC, Talbot CH, et al. A controlled trial of Trasylol in the treatment of acute pancreatitis. Br J Surg 1974;61:177–182.

37. Trapnell JE, Talbot CH, Chir M, et al. Traysylol therapy in primary acute pancratitis. Am J Dig Dis 1967;12:409–412.

38. Inrie CW, Benjamin IS, Ferguson JC, et al. A single centre double-blind trial of Trasylol therapy in primary acute pancreatitis. Br J Surg 1978;65:337–342.

39. Larvin M, Wilson C, Heath D, Alexander D, McMahon MJ, and Imrie CW. A prospective, multicenter, randomized trial of intraperitoneal antiprotease therapy for acute pancreatitis. Gastroenterology 1992;112:274A.

40. Singer MV, Goebell H. Antiproteases: effective treatment with gabexate mesilate. In Beger H, Buchler M, eds. Acute pancreatitis. Berlin: Springer-Verlag, 1987:272–277.

41. Wisner JR, Renner IG, Grendell JH, Niederau C, Ferrell L. Gabexate mesilate Foy protects against

ceruletide induced acute pancreatitis in the rat. Pancreas 1987;2:181–186.

42. Buchler M, Malferheiner P, Uhl W, Stockmann F. The German Multicenter double-blind randomized study of gabexate-mesilate in acute pancreatitis. Gastroenterology 1993;104:1165–1170.

43. Stanten R, Frey CF. Comprehensive management of acute necrotizing pancreatitis and pancreatic abscess. Arch Surg 1990;125:1269–1275.

44. Berger HG, Bittner R, Block S. Bacterial contamination of pancreatitis necrosis. Gastroenterology 1986;91:433–438.

45. Finch WT, Sawyer JL, Scheuker S. A prospective study to determine the efficacy of antibiotics in acute pancreatitis. Ann Surg 1976;183:667–671.

46. Craig RM, Dordal E, Myles L. The use of ampicillin in acute pancreatitis. Ann Intern Med 1975; 83:831–840.

47. Howes R, Zuidema GD, Cameron JL. Evaluation of prophylactic antibiotics in acute pancreatitis. J Surg Res 1975;18:197–204.

48. Pederzoli P, Bassi C, Vesentini S, et al. A randomized multicenter clinical trial of antibiotic prophylaxis of septic complications in acute necrotizing pancreatitis with imipenem. Surg Gynecol Obstet 1993;176:480–483.

49. Cuschieri A, Wood RAB, Cumming JRG, Meehan SE, Mackie CR. The treatment of acute pancreatitis with fresh frozen plasma. Br J Surg 1983;70:710–712.

50. Lesse T, Holliday M, Heath D, Hall AW, Bell PR. Multicenter clinical trial of low volume fresh frozen plasma therapy in acute pancreatitis. Br J Surg 1987;74:907–911.

51. Sax HC, Warner BW, Talamini MA, et al. Early total parenteral nutrition in acute pancreatitis: lack of beneficial effects. Am J Surg 1987;153:117–124.

52. DiMagno EP, Malagelada JR, Go VLW, Moertel CG. Fate of orally ingested enzymes in pancreatic insufficiency. N Engl J Med 1977;296:1318–1322.

53. Durie P, Bell L, Corey ML, Forstner GG. Effect of cimetidine and sodium bicarbonate on pancreatic replacement therapy in cystic fibrosis. Gut 1980; 21:778–786.

54. Graham DY. Enzyme replacement therapy of exocrine pancreatic insufficiency in man. N Engl J Med 1977;296:1314–1317.

55. Regan PT, Malagelada Jr, DiMagno EP, Glanzmann SL, Go VLW. Comparative effects of antacids, cimetidine and enteric coating on the therapeutic response to oral enzymes in severe pancreatic insufficiency. N Engl J Med 1977;297:854–858.

56. Go VLW, Poley JR, Hofmann AF, Summerskill DM. Disturbances in fat digestion induced by acidic jejunal pH due to gastric hypersecretion in man. Gastroenterology 1970;58:638–646.

57. Heizer WD, Cleavland CR, Iber FL. Gastric inactivation of pancreatic supplements. Bull Johns Hopkins Hosp 1965;116:261–270.

58. Roberts IN. Enzyme therapy for malabsorption in exocrine pancreatic insufficiency. Pancreas 1989; 4:496–503.

59. Dutta SK, Russell RM, Iber FL. Impaired acid neutralization in the duodenum in pancreatic insufficiency. Dig Dis Sci 1979;24:775–780.

60. Dutta SK, Russell RM, Iber FL. Influence of exocrine pancreatic insufficiency on the intraluminal pH of the proximal small intestine. Dig Dis Sci 1979;24:529–534.

61. DiMagno EP, Go VLW, Summerskill WHJ. Relations between pancreatic enzyme outputs and malabsorption in severe pancreatic insufficiency. N Engl J Med 1973;288:813–815.

62. Jordon PH Jr, Grossman MI. Effect of dosage schedule on the efficacy of substitution therapy in pancreatic insufficiency. Gastroenterology 1959; 36:447–451.

63. Kalser MH, Leite CA, Warren WD, et al. Fat assimilation after massive distal pancreatectomy. N Engl J Med 1968;279:570–576.

64. DiMagno EP. Medical treatment of pancreatic insufficiency. Mayo Clin Proc 1979;54:435–442.

65. Graham DY. Pancreatic enzyme replacement. Dig Dis Sci 1982;27:485–490.

66. Drenick EJ. The influence of ingestion of calcium and other soap-forming substances of fecal fat. Gastroenterology 1961;41:242–244.

67. Hoffman AF, Small DM. Detergent properties of bile salts: correlation with physiological function. Annu Rev Med 1967;18:333.

68. Marotta F, O'Keefe SJD, Marks IN, et al. Pancreatic enzyme replacement therapy: importance of gastric acid secretion, H$_2$-antagonists, and enteric coating. Dig Dis Sci 1989;34:456–461.

69. Lamers CB, Jansen JB. Omeprazole as adjunct to enzyme replacement treatment in severe pancreatic insufficiency. Br Med J 1986;293:994.

70. Banks S, Marks IN, Groll A. Gastric acid secretion in pancreatic disease. Gastroenterology 1966; 51:649–655.

71. Kravetz RE, Spieo HM. Gastric secretion in chronic pancreatitis. Ann Intern Med 1965;63:776–782.

72. Chey WY, Kusakcioglu I, Dinoso V, Lorber SH. Gastric secretion in patients with chronic pancreatitis and in chronic alcoholics. Arch Intern Med 1968;122:399–403.

73. Cox KL, Isenberg JN, Osher AB, Dooley RR. The effect of cimetidine on maldigestion in cystic fibrosis. J Pediatr 1979;94:488–492.

74. Wormsley KG, Mahoney MP. Acid and bicarbonate secretion in health and disease. Lancet 1967;1:657–658.

75. Antonowicz I, Lebenthal E, Scwachman H. Disaccharidase activities in small intestinal mucosa in patients with cystic fibrosis. J Pediatr 1978;92:214.

76. Morin CL, Roy CC, Lasalle R, et al. Small bowel mucosal dysfunction in patients with cystic fibrosis. J Pediatr 1976;88:213.

77. Reemtsma K, di Sant'Agnese PA, Malm JR, et al. Cystic fibrosis of the pancreas: intestinal absorption of fat and fatty acids labeled with I^{131}. Pediatrics 1958;22:525.

78. Graham DY. An enteric-coated pancreatic enzyme that works. Dig Dis Sci 1979;24:906–909.

79. Benn A, Cooke WT. Intraluminal pH of duodenum and jejunum in fasting subjects with normal and abnormal gastric or pancreatic function. Scand J Gastroenterol 1971;6:313–317.

80. DiMagno EP. Controversies in the treatment of exocrine pancreatic insufficiency [Editorial]. Dig Dis Sci 1982;27:481–484.

81. Meyer JH, Elashoff J, Porter-Fink V, Dressman J, Amidon G. What should be the size of pancreatic microspheres [Abstract]? Gastroenterology 1987; 92:1533.

82. Dutta LK, Rubin J, Harvey J. Comparative evaluation of the therapeutic efficacy of a pH-sensitive enteric coated pancreatic enzyme preparation with conventional pancreatic enzyme therapy in the treatment of exocrine pancreatic insufficiency. Gastroenterology 1983;84:476–482.

83. Dutta SK, Tilley DK. The pH-sensitive enteric-coated pancreatic enzyme preparations: an evaluation of therapeutic efficacy in adult patients with pancreatic insufficiency. J Clin Gastroenterol 1983;5:51–54.

84. Schneider MU, Knoll-Ruzicka ML, Domschke S, et al. Pancreatic enzyme replacement therapy: comparative effects of conventional and enteric-coated microspheric Pancreatin and acid-stable fungal enzyme preparations on steatorrhoea in chronic pancreatitis. Hepato-gastroenterol 1985;32:97–102.

85. Jorgensen BB, Pedersen NT, Worning H. Monitoring the effect of substitution therapy in patients with exocrine pancreatic insufficiency. Scand J Gastroenterol 1991;26:321–326.

86. Gow R, Bradbear R, Francis P, Shepherd R. Comparative study of varying regimens to improve steatorrhea and creatorrhea in cystic fibrosis: effectiveness of an enteric-coated preparation with and without antacids and cimetidine. Lancet 1981; 2:1071–1074.

87. Dutta SK, Hubbard VS, Appler M. Critical examination of therapeutic efficacy of a pH-sensitive enteric-coated pancreatic enzyme preparation in treatment of exocrine pancreatic insufficiency secondary to cystic fibrosis. Dig Dis Sci 1988;33:1237–1244.

88. Beverley, DW, Kelleher J, Macdonald A, et al. Comparison of four pancreatic extracts in cystic fibrosis. Arch Dis Child 1987;62:564–568.

89. Nassif EG, Younoszai MK, Weinberger MM, Nassif CM. Comparative effects of antacids, enteric coating, and bile salts on the efficacy of oral pancreatic enzyme therapy in cystic fibrosis. J Pediatr 1981;98:320–323.

90. Stead RJ, Skypala I, Hodson ME, Batten JC. Enteric coated microspheres of pancreatin in the treatment of cystic fibrosis: comparison with a standard enteric coated preparation. Thorax 1987;42:533–537.

91. Heiferman HG, Lamers CB, Bakker W. Omeprazole enhances the efficacy of pancreatin (Pancrease) in cystic fibrosis. Ann Intern Med 1991;114:200–201.

92. Abrams CK, Hamosh M, Dutta SK, et al. Role of nonpancreatic lipolytic activity in exocrine pancreatic insufficiency. Gastroenterology 1987;92: 125–129.

93. Zentler-Munro PL, Assoufi BA, Balasubramanian K, et al. Therapeutic potential and clinical efficacy on acid-resistant fungal lipase in the treatment of pancreatic steatorrhoea due to cystic fibrosis. Pancreas 1992;7:311–319.

94. The Copenhagen Pancreatitis Study Group. An interim report from a prospective epidemiological multicenter study. Scand J Gastroenterol 1981; 16:305–312.

95. Chronic pancreatitis. In: Go VLW, Gardner J, Brooks F, DiMagno E, eds. The exocrine pancreas: biology, pathobiology, and disease. New York: Raven Press, 1986.

96. Bradley EL. Pancreatic duct pressure in chronic pancreatitis. Am J Surg 1982;144:313–316.

97. Sato T, Miyashita E, Yamauchi H, Matsuno S. The role of surgical treatment for chronic pancreatitis. Ann Surg 1986;203:266–271.

98. Madsen P, Winkler K. The intraductal pancreatic pressure in chronic obstructive pancreatitis. Scand J Gastroenterol 1982;17:553–554.

99. Banks PA. Pancreatitis. New York: Plenum, 1979.

100. Sarles H, Sahel J, Staub JL, et al. Chronic pancreatitis. In: Howat HT, Sarles H, eds. The exocrine pancreas. Philadelphia: Saunders, 1979:402–439.

101. Ammann RW, Largiader F, Akovbiantz A. Pain relief by surgery in chronic pancreatitis? Scand J Gastroenterol 1979;14:209–215.

102. Prinz RA, Greenlee HB. Pancreatic duct drainage in 100 patients with chronic pancreatitis. Ann Surg 1981;194:313–320.

103. Wolfson P. Surgical management of inflammatory disorders of the pancreas. Surg Gynecol Obstet 1980;151:689–698.

104. Ihse I, Lilja P, Lundquist I. Feedback regulation of pancreatic enzyme secretion by intestinal trypsin in man. Digestion 1977;15:303–308.

105. Greene GM, Lyman RI. Feed-back regulation of pancreatic enzyme secretion as a mechanism for trypsin inhibition-induced hypersecretion in rats. Proc Soc Exp Biol Med 1972;140:6–12.

106. Holmberg JT, Isaksson G, Ihse I. Long-term results of pancreaticojejunostomy in chronic pancreatitis. Surg Gynecol Obstet 1985;160:339–346.

107. Alumot E, Nitsan Z. The influence of soybean antitrypsin on the intestinal proteolysis of the chick. J Nutr 1961;73:71–77.

108. Ihse I, Lilja P. Effects of intestinal amylase and trypsin on pancreatic secretion in the pig. Scand J Gastroenterol 1979;14:1009–1013.

109. Davicco MJ, Lefaivre J, Thivend P, Bartlet JP. Feedback regulation of pancreatic secretion in the young milk-fed calf. Ann Anim Biochem Biophys 1979;19:1147–1152.

110. Sale JK, Goldberg DM, Fawcett AN, Wormsley KG. Chronic and acute studies indicating absence of exocrine pancreatic feedback inhibition in dogs. Digestion 1977;15:540–555.

111. Adler G, Mullenhoff A, Bozkuft T, et al. Comparison of the effect of single and repeated administration of a protease inhibitor (camostate) on pancreatic secretion in man. Scand J Gastroenterol 1988;23:158–162.

112. Adler G, Mullenhoff A, Koop I, et al. Stimulation of pancreatic secretion in man by a protease inhibitor (camostate). Eur J Clin Invest 1988;18:98–114.

113. Adler G, Reinshagen M, Koop J, et al. Differential effects of atropine and a cholecystokinin receptor antagonist on pancreatic secretion. Gastroenterology 1989;96:1158–1164.

114. Boyd EJ, Cumming JG, Cushieri A, Wormsley KG. Aspects of feed-back control of pancreatic secretion in man. Ital J Gastroenterol 1956;17:18–22.

115. Calan J, Bojarski JC, Spriner CJ. Raw soya-bean flour increases cholecystokinin release in man. Br J Nutr 1987;58:175–179.

116. Hanssen L, Osnes M, Myren J. Pancreatic secretion obtained by endoscopic cannulation of the main pancreatic duct and secretin release after duodenal acidification in man. Scand J Gastroenterol 1986; 13:325–330.

117. Liener JE, Goodale RL, Deshmukh A, et al. Effect of a trypsin inhibitor from soya-beans (Bowman-Birk) on the secretory activity of the human pancreas. Gastroenterology 1988;94:419–427.

118. Owyang C, Louie D, Tatum D. Feed-back regulation of pancreatic enzyme secretion. J Clin Invest 1986;77:2042–2047.

119. Owyang C, May D, Louie D. Trypsin suppression of pancreatic enzyme secretion. Gastroenterology 1986;91:637–643.

120. Slaff J, Jacobson D, Tillman CR, Curlington C, Toskes P. Protease-specific suppression of pancreatic exocrine secretion. Gastroenterology 1984; 87:44–52.

121. Yasui A, Nimura Y, Hayakawa N, et al. Feed-back regulation of basal pancreatic secretion in humans. Pancreas 1988;6:681–687.

122. Owyang C, Leksell K, May D, et al. Intraduodenal trypsin inhibits cholecystokinin release and pancreatic enzyme secretion in man. Gastroenterology 1983;84:1268.

123. Ihse I, Lilja P, Lundquist I. Intestinal concentrations of pancreatic enzymes following pancreatic replacement therapy. Scand J Gastroenterol 1980; 15:137–144.

124. Folsch HR, Wilms H, Schatmayer, et al. The negative feedback mechanism of pancreatic enzyme secretion is accompanied by elevated CCK plasma concentration. Dig Dis Sci 1984;29:A11.

125. Dlugosz J, Folsch UR, Creutzfeldt W. Inhibition of intraduodenal trypsin does not stimulate exocrine pancreatic secretion in man. Digestion 1983; 26:197–204.

126. Hotz J, Ho SB, Go VLW, et al. Short-term inhibition of duodenal tryptic activity does not affect human pancreatic, biliary or gastric function. J Lab Clin Med 1983;101:488–495.

127. Pitchumoni CS, Toskes PP. Controversies, dilemmas and dialogues: Is there an effective nonsurgical treatment for pain in chronic pancreatitis? Am J Gastroenterol 1991;86:26–29.

128. Isaksson G, Ihse I. Pain reduction by an oral pancreatic enzyme preparation in chronic pancreatitis. Dig Dis Sci 1983;28:97–102.

129. Halgreen H, Thorsgaard-Pedersen N, Worning H. Symptomatic effect of pancreatic enzyme therapy in patients with chronic pancreatitis. Scand J Gastroenterol 1986;21:104–108.

130. Campbell D, Jadunandan I, Curlington C, et al. Alcoholic and idiopathic patients with painful chronic pancreatitis do not experience suppression of CCK levels or pain relief following treatment with enteric-coated pancreatin. Gastroenterology 1992; 102:A259.

131. Noda A, Shibata T, Ogawa Y, et al. Dissolution of pancreatic stones by oral trimethadione in a dog experimental model. Gastroenterology 1987;93:1002–1008.

132. Noda A. Dissolution of pancreatic stones. Tropical Gastroenterol 1990;11:76–86.

133. Davis ML, Kelsey WM. Chronic pancreatitis in childhood. Am J Dis Child 1951;81:687–692.

134. Barkin JS. Ascites as a complication of chronic pancreatic disease. Postgrad Med 1978;64:195–200.

135. Cameron JL. Chronic pancreatic ascites and pancreatic pleural effusions. Gastroenterology 1978; 74:134–140.

136. Cameron JL, Kieffer RS, Anderson WJ, Zuidema GD. Internal pancreatic fistula: pancreatic ascites and pleural effusions. Ann Surg 1976;184:587–593.

137. Jones AM, Jacobs LA, Bowman DL, Weaver DW. Outcome after peritoneous-jugular shunting of pancreatic ascites. Am Surg 1984;50:386–389.

138. Sileo AV, Chawia SK, Lopresti PA. Pancreatic ascites: diagnostic importance of ascitic lipase. Dig Dis Sci 1975;20:1110–1114.

139. Weaver DW, Watt AJ, Sugawa C, Bowman DL. A continuing appraisal of pancreatic ascites. Surg Gynecol Obstet 1982;154:845–848.

140. Kozarek RA, Ball TJ, Patterson DJ, et al. Endoscopic transpapillary therapy for disrupted pancreatic duct and pseudocyst. Gastrointest Endosc 1990;36:203A.

141. Scott NA, Finnegan S, Irving MH. Octreotide and gastrointestinal fistulae. Digestion 1990;45:591–602.

142. Pederzoli P, Bassi C, Falconi M, et al. Conservative treatment of external pancreatic fistulas with parenteral nutrition alone or in combination with continuous intravenous infusion of somatostatin, glucagon or calcitonin. Surg Gynecol Obstet 1986; 163:428–432.

143. Geerdsen JP, Pedersen WM, Kjaergard HK. Small bowel fistula treated with somatostatin. Surgery 1986;100:811–814.

144. Saari A, Schroder T, Kivilaakso E, et al. Treatment of pancreatic fistula with somatostatin and total parenteral nutrition. Scand J Gastroenterol 1989; 24:859–862.

145. Boden G, Sivitz MC, Owen OE. Somatostatin suppresses secretin and pancreatic exocrine secretion. Science 1975;190:163–164.

146. Hanssen LE, Hanssen KF, Myren J. Inhibition of secretin release and pancreatic bicarbonate secretion by somatostatin infusion in man. Scand J Gastroenterol 1977;12:391–394.

147. Folsch UR, Lankisch PG, Creutzfeldt W. Effect of somatostatin on basal and stimulated pancreatic secretion in rat. Digestion 1978;17:194–203.

148. Costanzo JD, Cano N, Martin J. Somatostatin in persistent gastrointestinal fistula treated by total parenteral nutrition Lancet 1932;2:338–339.

149. Oktedalen O, Nygaard K, Osnes M. Somatostatin in the treatment of pancreatic ascites. Gastroenterology 1990;99:1520–1521.

150. Gislason H, Gronbech JE, Soreide O. Pancreatic ascites: treatment by continuous somatostatin infusion. Am J Gastroenterol 1991;86:519–521.

151. Gullo L, Barbara L. Treatment of pancreatic pseudocysts with octreotide. Lancet 1991;338:540–541.

152. Staub JL, Sarles H, Soule JC, et al. No effects of cimetidine on the therapeutic response to oral enzymes in severe pancreatic insufficiency. NEJM 1981;304:1364–1365.

153. de Bieville F, Neijens HJ, Fernandes J, et al. Cimetidine as an adjuct to oral enzymes in the treatment of malabsorption due to cystic fibrosis. Acta Paediatr Scand 1981;70:33–37.

154. Hubbard VS, Dunn GD, Lester LA. Effectiveness of cimetidine as an adjunct to supplemental pancreatic enzymes in patients with cystic fibrosis. Am J Clin Nutrition 1980;33:2281–2286.

155. Boyle BJ, Long WB, Balistreri WF, et al. Effect of cimetidine and pancreatic enzymes on serum and fecal bile acids and fat absorption in cystic fibrosis. Gastroenterology 1980;78:950–953.

156. Mischler EH, Parrell S, Farrell PM, et al. Comparison of effectiveness of pancreatic enzyme preparations in cystic fibrosis. Am J Dis Child 1982; 136:1060–1063.

157. Mitchell EA, Quested C, Marks RE, et al. Comparative trial of viokase, pancreatin and Pancrease pancrelipase (enteric coated beads) in the treatment of malabsorption in cystic fibrosis. Aust Paedtr J 1982;18:114–117.

HEPATIC DISORDERS

18

Interferon Therapy of Chronic Viral Hepatitis

ADRIAN M. DI BISCEGLIE

UNDERSTANDING CHRONIC VIRAL HEPATITIS

At least three distinct forms of chronic viral hepatitis exist, each caused by a different viral agent. These include chronic hepatitis B, chronic δ-hepatitis, and chronic hepatitis C. These forms of hepatitis can be distinguished from each other and from other forms of chronic liver disease by a series of serologic tests for detecting viral antigens, nucleic acid, and antibodies in serum (Table 18.1). α-Interferon has emerged as the most promising therapy of chronic hepatitis B and C to date. This chapter will review the clinical aspects of chronic viral hepatitis, followed by a discussion of interferon for use in this setting.

Chronic Hepatitis B

The hepatitis B virus (HBV) is found in serum as the 42 nm Dane particle. This comprises a nucleocapsid (hepatitis B core antigen, HBcAg) coated with hepatitis B surface antigen (HBsAg). The viral nucleocapsid contains the double-stranded viral DNA and a viral DNA polymerase (1). The presence of HBV infection is determined by finding HBsAg in serum. Patients with high levels of viral replication may also have hepatitis B e antigen (HBeAg) and HBV DNA detectable in serum. Antibody to HBcAg (anti-HBc) appears very early in the course of HBV infection and probably persists indefinitely. Antibody to HBsAg (anti-HBs) usually appears after recovery from HBV infection. Antibody to HBeAg (anti-HBe) is only found in patients who are negative for HBeAg in serum (2).

The HBV is a major cause of chronic liver disease worldwide. In some endemic areas, most of the population is infected at some time and as many as 15% may be carriers of the virus. In these areas, infection with HBV often occurs in infancy, either "vertically" from mother to infant or "horizontally" between children. In contrast, in the United States and other developed countries, HBV infection is less common and occurs predominantly in certain high-risk groups such as homosexual men, intravenous drug abusers, health care workers, and immigrants from endemic areas (3).

Progression in liver disease in individuals chronically infected with HBV appears to be related to the persistence of high levels of HBV replication (as indicated by the presence of HBeAg or HBV DNA) (4). In contrast, patients with only HBsAg in their serum and no evidence of HBV replication usually have normal serum aminotransferase activities and no evidence of progressive liver disease (5). Thus, therapy for chronic hepatitis B has been aimed at eliminating HBV replication. Indeed, the response to therapy has been defined by the loss of HBeAg and HBV DNA from serum. This is usually associated with normalization of serum aminotransferases and, eventually, improvement in liver histopathology.

ANTI-VIRAL THERAPY OF CHRONIC HEPATITIS B

Several antiviral agents have been tested for activity against HBV (Table 18.2). These include adenine arabinoside (ARA-A) and its

331

Table 18.1
Viruses Responsible for Chronic Hepatitis

	Hepatitis B	δ-Hepatitis	Hepatitis C
Virus	HBV	HDV	HCV
Nucleic acid	DNA (3.2 kb)	RNA (1.7 kb)	RNA (9.0 kb)
	Surface (HBsAg)		
	Core (HBcAg)		
Antigens	e (HBeAg)	HDAg	Unknown
	Anti-HBc		Anti-C100
	Anti-HBs		Anti-core (c22)
Antibodies	Anti-HBe	Anti-HDV	Anti-C33c

monophosphate derivative (ARA-AMP), α-interferon, γ-interferon, acyclovir, ribavirin, and dideoxyinosine (DDI). Some of these agents appeared to inhibit levels of HBV replication, but so far, only ARA-AMP and α-interferon were found to be able to eliminate it. The use of ARA-AMP was associated with unacceptable toxicity, however, and it is no longer used (6).

Small quantities of purified *α-interferon* were tested in patients with chronic hepatitis B in the mid-1970s. Interferon was found to suppress HBV DNA polymerase activity in serum (7). It was only when larger quantities of recombinant α-interferon became available early in the 1980s that large-scale clinical trials could be conducted. In an early pilot study, 43% of a group of patients treated with very high doses of α-interferon responded by clearing HBeAg and HBV DNA polymerase from their serum (8).

A series of controlled trials followed, using varying types of α-interferon at a range of doses for different periods of time (9–16) (Table 18.3). Indeed, the response rates in these studies varied markedly too, ranging between 0 and approximately 40%. In a trial conducted at the National Institutes of Health (NIH), 45 patients were randomized to receive either α-interferon (at a dosage of 5 million units daily or 10 million units on alternate days) or to be untreated control subjects (14). All patients had HBsAg in their serum for at least 1 year with stable serum levels of HBV DNA prior to therapy. During the 4-month treatment period, 10 of 31 (32%) treated patients but only

1 of 14 control subjects (7%) became negative for HBV DNA. All 10 patients who lost HBV DNA subsequently had a marked improvement in serum aminotransferase activities and lost HBeAg from their serum.

A comparison of responders and nonresponders indicated that female sex and high initial levels of serum aspartate aminotransferase (AST) correlated best with response (Fig. 18.1). These findings have been confirmed in several other studies. In addition, other predictive factors have been suggested, as follows: factors that may correlate with a lack of response include male homosexuality and human immunodeficiency virus infection. Furthermore, Asian patients do not appear to respond well to interferon. Some positive predictive factors include having a history of acute hepatitis, a short duration of hepatitis, and low levels of HBV DNA in the serum prior to therapy (17). However, none of these factors appears to be reliable in predicting the outcome of therapy in individual patients. Preliminary analysis of a second controlled trial done at NIH indicates that 44% of treated patients cleared HBeAg compared to 5% of untreated control subjects. In this study too, serum AST levels correlated very well with response. Thus, the response rate was 55% in those with serum AST >100 U/L and only 33% in those with lower AST values (16).

Patients who initially respond to therapy usually appear to have a long-term response. At follow-up examination, few, if any, appear to relapse with the reappearance of HBeAg and HBV DNA. In a long-term follow-up

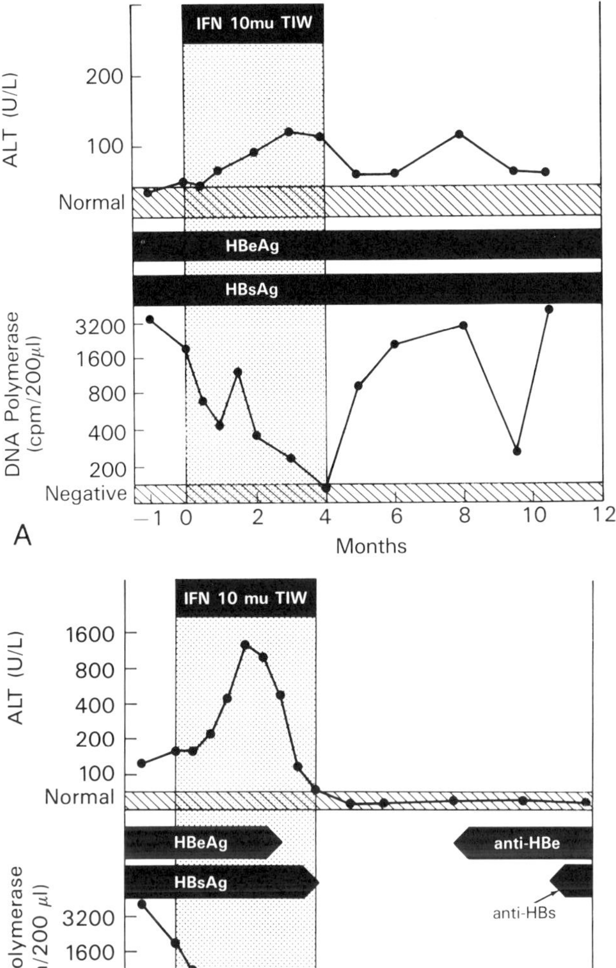

Figure 18.1. Changes in serum biochemical and virologic markers associated with therapy for chronic hepatitis B virus (HBV). (*A*) A representative nonresponder. HBV DNA polymerase levels decrease during therapy and transiently become normal. However, when interferon is stopped, viral markers return to pretreatment levels. Hepatitis B e and surface antigen (HBeAg, HBsAg) remain positive throughout therapy. (*B*) A representative responder. HBV DNA polymerase activity becomes undetectable in serum after 2 months of therapy. Shortly thereafter, HBeAg and then HBsAg become undetectable, to be replaced by antibody to HBeAg (anti-HBe) and antibody to HBsAg (anti-HBs) eventually.

Table 18.2
Drugs Used in Therapy of Chronic Hepatitis B[a]

Proven benefit	Possible benefit	Little or no benefit
α-Interferon	Ribavirin	Corticosteroids
		ARA-A, ARA-AMP
	3′Thiacytidine	Acyclovir
	Thymosin	Phyllanthus amarus
		γ-Interferon
		Levamisole

[a]Abbreviations: ARA-A, adenosine arabinoside (monophosphate).

Table 18.3
Results of Two Recent Controlled Trials in the United States of α-Interferon for Chronic Hepatitis B[a]

				Loss of HBeAg (%)		Loss of HBsAg (%)	
Reference	No. of patients	Dose	Duration	Treated patients	Control subjects	Treated patients	Control subjects
Di Bisceglie et al. (16)	47	10 tiw	16	44	5	16	0
Petrillo et al. (15)	169	5 dly	16	37	7	12	0

[a]tiw, three times weekly; dly, daily; HBeAg, hepatitis B e antigen; HBsAg, hepatitis B surface antigen.

Table 18.4
Features of "Typical" Patients with Chronic Hepatitis B Who Are Suitable for α-Interferon Therapy[a]

Raised aminotransferases (for >6 months)
HBeAg and HBV DNA in serum
Anti-HDV negative
Anti-HIV negative
Compensated liver disease[b]
No other serious medical illnesses

[a]Anti-HDV, antibody to the hepatitis δ-virus; Anti-HIV, antibody to the human immunodeficiency virus.
[b]Absence of ascites, history of variceal bleeding, encephalopathy, jaundice.

study conducted at NIH, the outcome of patients who had cleared HBeAg in response to interferon therapy was observed and compared with that of patients who had cleared HBeAg spontaneously (18). Among 64 patients treated with α-interferon, 23 (36%) responded with loss of HBeAg and improvement in serum aminotransferase levels. During follow-up, 3 of 23 patients relapsed, all within 1 year of therapy. The remaining 20 patients remained in remission, although 3 had minimal elevations of serum aminotransferases. Thirteen patients (65%) became negative for HBsAg during follow-up between 0.2 and 6 years after losing HBeAg.

Attempts have been made to improve the results of interferon therapy, most often by combining it with other antiviral or immunomodulatory agents such as ARA-AMP, acyclovir, or prednisone. However, these combinations have not usually realized their initial promise. In a multicenter U.S. study in which treatment with α-interferon alone (5 million units daily) was compared with treatment with interferon preceded by a 1-month course of prednisone, the response rate in the two groups was identical. Clearance of HBeAg and HBV DNA occurred in 36% of patients given prednisone plus interferon and 37% of those given interferon alone (19).

TREATMENT OF DECOMPENSATED CIRRHOSIS DUE TO CHRONIC HEPATITIS B

Most of the patients included in the studies cited above were in good general health with well-compensated liver disease (Table 18.4). Patients with decompensated cirrhosis (those with jaundice, ascites, encephalopathy, or bleeding esophageal varices) have been excluded from most studies. However, these are often the patients in greatest need of effective therapy. A few such patients have been treated outside of the usual protocols at the NIH (20). Eighteen patients were treated with α-interferon at doses of 2–5 million units daily. In 6 treated patients, there was a sustained loss of HBV DNA and HBeAg and a decrease of serum aminotransferases into the normal or near-normal range. In follow-up observation of these 6 patients all symptoms of cirrhosis were resolved and all are alive and fully active. In contrast, the 12 patients who did not respond to therapy have had evidence of progressive liver disease: 6 have died and 4 underwent hepatic transplantation. Side effects of interferon were common in this group and included bacterial infections and exacerbations of disease.

HBV-ASSOCIATED GLOMERULONEPHRITIS

Another form of HBV infection that may respond to interferon therapy is HBV-associated membranous glomerulonephritis (21). The cause of renal injury in such cases is uncertain but is probably related to the deposition of viral antigen-antibody complexes in the kidney. This complication often affects children and may resolve spontaneously. We have treated 7 adults with HBV-related glomerulonephritis and nephrotic syndrome. All had chronic HBV infection with HBsAg, HBeAg, and HBV DNA in serum, together with elevated serum aminotransferase activities. All had persistent proteinuria of >2 g/day, an active urine sediment, and histologic changes consistent with either membranous or membranoproliferative glomerulonephritis. They were treated with α-interferon (5 million units daily) for 16 weeks. In those patients who cleared HBeAg and HBV DNA (5 of 7), marked improvement was noted in the nephrotic syndrome with a return to normal of serum albumin, cholesterol, and aminotransferase levels.

TREATMENT OF E ANTIGEN-NEGATIVE ("MUTANT") HBV

A form of hepatitis B associated with active liver disease, raised serum aminotransferases, and detectable HBV DNA but without HBeAg in serum recently has been described (22). This syndrome has been found to be most common in Mediterranean countries, although cases have also been noted in the Far East. This syndrome has been attributed to infection with a variant of HBV. This variant appears to be due a mutation of the virus in the precore region of the viral genome. This mutation, often of a single nucleotide, disrupts the secretion of HBeAg from serum. This variant appears to cause more severe liver disease than the wild-type HBV. In addition, this form of hepatitis was initially reported to respond poorly to interferon therapy. Brunetto and coworkers noted that α-interferon treatment resulted in only a temporary suppression of HBV DNA and ALT levels, with a relatively low long-term response rate (23). However, in a more recent study conducted in Italy, researchers found that 53% of patients treated with α-interferon (5 million

units/m² for 6 months), cleared HBV DNA with normalization of serum ALT activities compared with only 17% of untreated control subjects (24).

In summary, α-interferon in a dose of 10 million units three times weekly or 5 million units daily for 16 weeks is effective in clearing HBV viremia in approximately 35–40% of patients with chronic hepatitis B. The presence of high serum aminotransferase activities is useful in predicting a response. The response rate in Asian patients and those with HIV infection has not been very good. Although patients with decompensated cirrhosis due to HBV infection may have dramatic improvement, therapy in this group may also be associated with severe complications and should only be administered with extreme caution. Patients with HBV-related glomerulonephritis may also benefit from α-interferon therapy if they clear HBV replication. Finally, selected patients with chronic liver disease who are serologically positive for HBV DNA but negative for HBeAg may also have a long-term response to interferon.

Chronic Delta (δ)-Hepatitis

The hepatitis-δ virus (HDV) is a defective negative-stranded, RNA virus that causes hepatitis in the presence of HBV. Thus, virtually all patients with δ-hepatitis have HBsAg in their serum. Its genome is approximately 1,700 nucleotides in length and encodes a viral protein, the hepatitis-δ antigen (HDAg) (25). HDV may be acquired at the same time as HBV (coinfection) or it may be acquired by individuals already chronically infected with HBV (superinfection). Following superinfection, chronic δ-hepatitis develops in most patients.

HDV infection is relatively uncommon in most parts of the world, affecting less than 10% of patients with HBV infection. Areas endemic for HDV infection appear to be Mediterranean countries such as Italy (particularly in the south), Greece, and parts of the Middle East (26). In addition, outbreaks of HDV infection have been noted in regions of the Amazon basin in South America. In the developed Western World (including the United States), HDV infection occurs most commonly in various high-risk groups including intravenous drug addicts and multiply transfused individuals.

HDV infection may be diagnosed by the presence of viral RNA or protein in serum or liver or by the presence of antibodies to HDAg in serum (27). The "gold standard" of diagnosis of HDV infection is hepatic HDAg, which may be detected by various methods of immunostaining. HDAg may be detected in serum by Western blot analysis or enzyme-linked immunoassay (ELISA). Western blot appears to be the more sensitive of the two tests, but is technically difficult to do and is only tested for in research laboratories (28). Using ELISA, HDAg is often present in the serum of patients with acute HDV infection but is usually undetectable in the serum of chronically infected patients. Antibody to HDAg (anti-HD) is readily detected by immunoassays in serum of infected individuals. Very high titers are found in chronically infected patients, whereas lower levels are noted in patients with acute δ-hepatitis (29). Interestingly, the appearance of anti-HD in serum following acute δ-coinfection may be short-lived and only very low levels may be present for short periods. IgM anti-HD may also be detected in acute δ-hepatitis and may also be present in the serum of some patients with chronic HDV infection. Indeed, the presence of IgM anti-HD may be a useful marker of HDV replication. The presence of IgM HBcAb (core antibody) can be used to distinguish acute coinfection from superinfection with the δ agent in a chronic HBsAg carrier.

The mechanism by which HDV results in hepatocellular injury is uncertain, although it has been suggested that HDV is directly cytopathic because very high levels of HDV replication are noted within hepatocytes. However, the role of the immune system in δ-hepatitis has not been well explored. The significance of HDV infection is that it very often seems to aggravate the injury caused by HBV infection. Thus, in acute δ-hepatitis, fulminant liver failure is more often likely to result from δ-coinfection or superinfection than from HBV infection alone (30). Similarly, chronic HDV infection appears to accelerate the injury caused by HBV and results in cirrhosis and liver failure more often and more rapidly than HBV alone (31, 32).

TREATMENT OF δ-HEPATITIS

No effective form of therapy is available for HDV infection. The effect of *corticosteroids* in the treatment of chronic δ-hepatitis has been examined in a retrospective analysis and found to be of little benefit (31). *α-Interferon* has been tested in patients with chronic delta hepatitis. Initial reports suggested that some patients appeared to benefit from α-interferon therapy with decreases in serum aminotransferase activities and the disappearance of HDV RNA and HDAg from serum. This was associated with an improvement in liver disease in approximately 50% of patients, with a decrease in serum aminotransferase activities, sometimes into the normal range. However, when interferon was stopped, HDV infection appeared to relapse; HDV RNA and HDAg reappeared in serum associated with a rise in serum aminotransferase activities again (33–35). Rosina and colleagues in Italy conducted a controlled trial of α-interferon therapy in chronic δ-hepatitis (36). In a preliminary analysis of that study, they found that 15 of 26 treated patients (58%) showed a significant decrease in serum alanine aminotransferase levels. But only 4 of 26 (15%) transiently cleared HDV RNA from serum during therapy (Table 18.5).

More recently, Farci and colleagues conducted a controlled trial of α-interferon in chronic δ-hepatitis using higher doses of interferon than those used by Rosina et al. (37). A total of 42 patients with chronic δ-hepatitis were enrolled in this study: 14 received α-interferon 9 million units three times weekly, 14 received 3 million units three times weekly, and 14 were untreated control subjects. After 12 months, serum ALT values were normal in 71% of those treated with 9 million units, 28% of those treated with 3 million units, and

Table 18.5
Controlled Trials of α-Interferon for Chronic Delta (δ)-Hepatitis[a]

Reference	No. of patients	IFN type	Dose	Duration (mo)	Normal ALT (%)	Loss of HDV RNA (%)
Rosina et al. (35)	24	2b	5 mu tiw Control	3	33	NA
				3	0	NA
Rosina et al. (36)	65	2b	5 mu, then 3 mu	4		NA
				8	0	NA
			9 mu tiw			
			3 mu tiw			
Farci et al. (37)	42	2a	Control	12	71	71
				12	29	36
				12	8	8

[a]NA, data not available; IFN, type of interferon α used; tiw, three times weekly; ALT, alanine aminotransferase; HDV, hepatitis δ-virus; mu, million units.

8% of the control subjects. Preliminary analysis suggests that a significant proportion of patients treated with the higher dose of interferon appear to have persistently normal serum aminotransferase levels, although HDV RNA is still present in serum.

Thus, very few patients with chronic δ-hepatitis appear to derive long-term benefit from a short course of interferon therapy. Only those who clear HBsAg from serum are not at risk of relapse when interferon is stopped. It has been suggested that patients with chronic δ-hepatitis may need long-term or permanent treatment with interferon to suppress HDV replication and significantly ameliorate liver disease. Unfortunately, many patients with chronic δ-hepatitis have severe liver disease with complications of cirrhosis, and they may not tolerate interferon very well, particularly at the high doses that appear to be needed.

Interestingly, patients with chronic δ-hepatitis may be good candidates for liver transplantation because the HBV and HDV infection recurs in the transplanted liver relatively infrequently (38). In those patients in whom recurrence of HDV has been noted, it has been found that HDAg is the first marker to reappear in the liver, often within only a few weeks of transplantation. This does not appear to be associated with significant liver injury. It is only when the HBV recurs that liver injury begins.

Chronic Hepatitis C

The hepatitis C virus is a recently discovered, positive-stranded RNA virus that appears to be responsible for most cases of blood-borne non-A, non-B hepatitis (39). Its genome is approximately 9,000 nucleotides in length and has a single open reading frame that appears to code for several proteins, including both structural and nonstructural viral peptides (40).

HCV infection is most often acquired through parenteral contact with blood and blood products by means of transfusions, intravenous drug use, and needlestick injuries among health care workers (41). In addition, a significant proportion of cases of HCV infection are found in individuals who deny contact with blood or blood products through one of the mechanisms listed above. This is referred to as "sporadic" hepatitis C (42).

Acute HCV infection is usually silent and asymptomatic, although it may occasionally cause jaundice (43). It is marked by a very high propensity to become chronic (in up to 70% of cases). The chronic disease state is also very often asymptomatic, although some patients have nonspecific complaints such as fatigue, arthralgias, and nausea. Long-term prospective studies have shown that up to 20% of cases of chronic hepatitis C may result in cirrhosis. Eventually, this may result in progressive liver disease and liver failure in up to 10% of patients observed for at least 10 years (44).

TREATMENT OF HEPATITIS C

Until recently, no effective form of therapy was available for hepatitis C. Corticosteroids did not appear to be of benefit and an early trial of high doses of acyclovir did not show any effect (45). *α-Interferon* was tested against hepatitis C in the mid-1980s, as it had been shown to be of benefit in some cases of hepatitis B and other viral infections (46, 47). These pilot studies were done before the discovery of the HCV when the condition was still being referred to as non-A, non-B hepatitis. The serum aminotransferase values were the only markers available to evaluate the disease and its response to therapy. In a pilot study of 10 patients treated with α-interferon, Hoofnagle and colleagues noted that 8 patients responded with a decrease in serum aminotransferase values to normal or near-normal levels while 2 patients had no change (46). After only 4 months of treatment, the hepatitis appeared to relapse when interferon was stopped, but after therapy was prolonged for up to 12 months, some long-term responses were noted (Fig. 18.2).

Because of promising results from several similar pilot studies, a series of randomized, controlled trials was launched to confirm the efficacy of α-interferon in the treatment of chronic hepatitis C. In two studies from the United States it was reported that approximately 50% of patients with chronic non-A, non-B hepatitis responded to a 6-month course of interferon with normalization of serum aminotransferase activities (48, 49). In a study conducted at NIH, 41 patients were treated in a randomized, double-blind placebo-controlled trial of α-interferon (2 million units three times weekly) vs. placebo (48). During treatment, serum alanine aminotransferase activities became normal in 48% of interferon-treated patients but in only 5% of controls. Serum aminotransferase activities decreased rapidly during α-interferon treatment; maximal changes were achieved after 1 to 2 months. Other biochemical liver tests, such as serum bilirubin, albumin, total protein, and prothrombin usually yielded normal results before therapy and did not change ap-

preciably with interferon treatment. In a multicenter trial, Davis and colleagues evaluated the efficacy of two different dosages of interferon, 1 million units and 3 million units respectively, three times weekly (49). They found that serum aminotransferases became normal in 46% of patients receiving 3 million units, in 28% receiving 1 million units, and in 8% of untreated control subjects. The long-term response rate after interferon was stopped was somewhat disappointing, and only 10–25% of patients had persistently normal aminotransferase levels after post-treatment with interferon. Table 18.6 summarizes results from several controlled trials of α-interferon for chronic hepatitis C (48–51).

α-Interferon therapy of chronic non-A, non-B hepatitis was also associated with improvement in the degree of hepatic injury seen histologically. After 6 months of therapy, liver samples were noted to have significantly less acinar injury, piecemeal necrosis, and portal inflammation.

When the studies described above were initiated, the HCV had not yet been discovered and patients with chronic non-A, non-B hepatitis were treated only if they had no evidence of other forms of liver disease and if they had a history of parenteral exposure to blood or blood products. Retrospective testing of stored serum samples from these trials has shown that 80–90% of patients had anti-HCV detectable in serum.

The development of methods to detect HCV infection has permitted an evaluation of changes in viral markers with therapy. The titers of anti-HCV decrease during therapy, although it is unusual for anti-HCV to disappear entirely. Assessment of anti-HCV titers has not therefore been useful for monitoring therapy of hepatitis C. Measurement of HCV RNA in serum appears to be a better way of monitoring therapy (52). Normalization of serum aminotransferases is often associated with the disappearance of HCV RNA from serum. In patients who do not respond, no change is noted in serum HCV RNA levels. HCV RNA reappears in the serum of patients

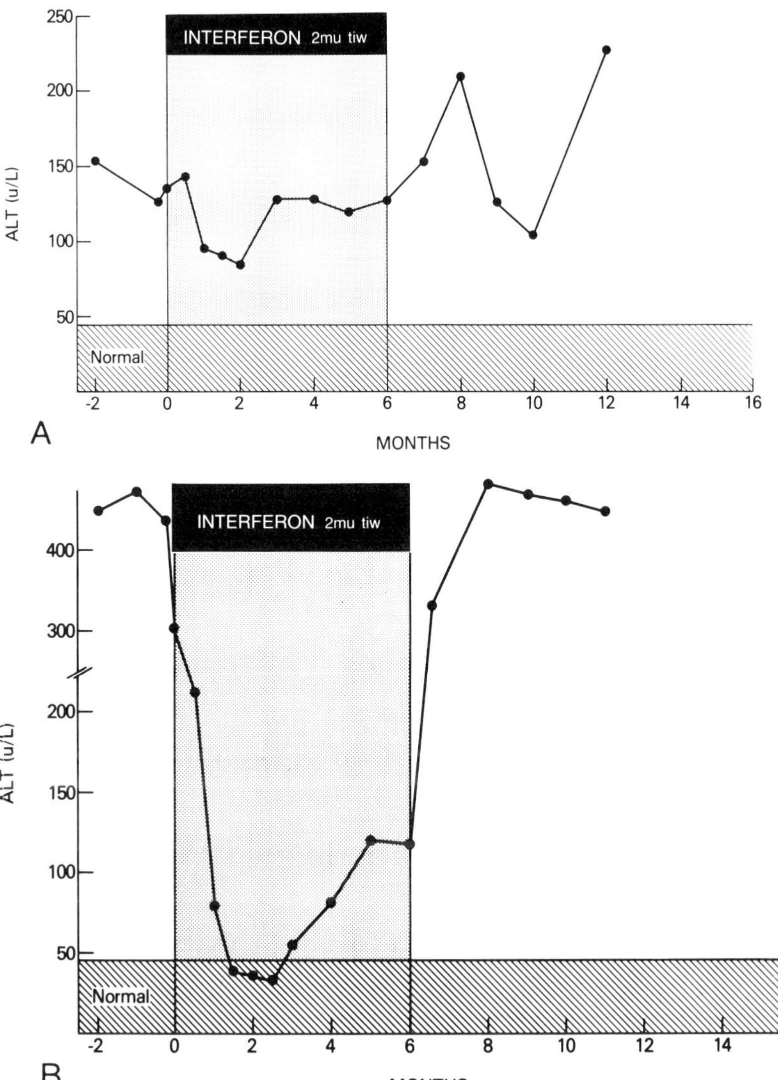

Figure 18.2. Types of responses seen with α-interferon therapy for chronic hepatitis C. (*A*) A nonresponder. Serum alanine aminotransferase (ALT) values remain unchanged throughout a 6-month course of therapy. (*B*) A partial responder. In this patient, serum ALT values transiently become normal but then drift upward during therapy. (*C*) A response with relapse. Serum ALT values promptly become normal during therapy and remain so until interferon is stopped, when they promptly return to baseline levels. (*D*) A long-term (sustained)-response. Normal serum ALT levels persist for at least 6 months after interferon is stopped. *C* and *D* have been reproduced from reference [60] with permission.

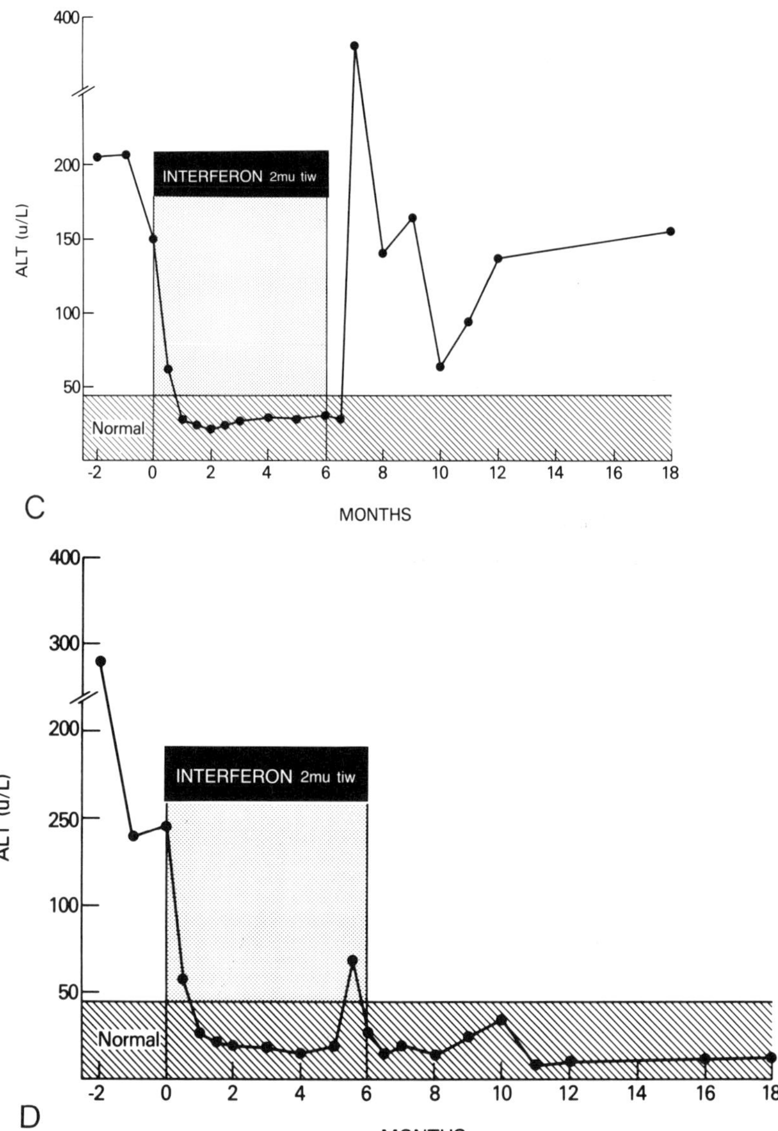

Figure 18.2 Continued. Types of responses seen with α-interferon therapy for chronic hepatitis C. (*A*) A nonresponder. Serum alanine aminotransferase (ALT) values remain unchanged throughout a 6-month course of therapy. (*B*) A partial responder. In this patient, serum ALT values transiently become normal but then drift upward during therapy. (*C*) A response with relapse. Serum ALT values promptly become normal during therapy and remain so until interferon is stopped, when they promptly return to baseline levels. (*D*) A long-term (sustained)-response. Normal serum ALT levels persist for at least 6 months after interferon is stopped. *C* and *D* have been reproduced from reference [60] with permission.

Table 18.6
Controlled Trials of Interferon Alfa-2b for Chronic Hepatitis C[a]

Reference	No. of patients	Dose (mu)	Response Rate (%) Treated patients	Control subjects
Di Bisceglie et al. (48)	41	2	48	0
Davis et al. (49)	166	3	46	8
		1	28	
Marcellin et al. (50)	60	3	39	0
		1	45	
Saracco et al. (51)	80	3	69	4
		1	66	

[a]Abbreviations: mu, million units.

Table 18.7
Indications for α-Interferon Therapy for Chronic Hepatitis C[a]

- Elevated serum aminotransferases (for >6 months)
- Evidence of hepatitis C virus (HCV) infection (anti-HCV, parenteral exposure to blood, exclusion of other forms of liver disease)
- Clinically significant liver disease (as assessed by symptoms, marked elevations of serum aminotransferases, severe hepatitis histologically, or evidence of progressive liver disease on repeat liver biopsy)

[a]All three features should be present prior to initiating therapy.

who initially respond to therapy and then relapse.

Long-term follow-up observation patients with chronic hepatitis C treated with α-interferon shows that among those in whom serum aminotransferase levels remain normal after interferon is stopped, the majority appear to have sustained improvement in their condition with persistently normal aminotransferases up to 6 years after treatment. HCV RNA has remained undetectable in the serum of these patients (53).

PATIENT SELECTION CRITERIA

The selection of patients with chronic type C hepatitis for α-interferon therapy remains somewhat controversial (Table 18.7). It has been suggested that patients with severe or progressive hepatitis should be considered for treatment and that patients with very mild hepatitis that does not appear to be progressing could simply be observed (54). Interferon therapy has not been evaluated in patients with decompensated cirrhosis due to hepatitis C. Their disease may be too severe to benefit

from therapy and they may be more likely to experience complications from interferon such as thrombocytopenia and bacterial infections. Similarly, the role of interferon in treating immunosuppressed patients with hepatitis C has not been evaluated. Patients with human immunodeficiency virus (HIV) infection, those on renal dialysis, and patients after organ transplantation often have evidence of HCV infection and may be candidates for antiviral therapy.

In most patients with chronic hepatitis C who do not respond to interferon, the activity of the hepatitis remains unchanged. However, there are isolated reports of patients having an exacerbation of disease activity associated with interferon therapy. It was initially suspected that these were patients with autoimmune hepatitis who had been incorrectly diagnosed as having hepatitis C. However, a recent report illustrates an exacerbation of hepatitis in a patient with well-documented hepatitis C viral infection (55).

Because α-interferon is not universally effective in patients with hepatitis C and may be

Table 18.8
Schedule for Monitoring Patients with Chronic Viral Hepatitis Treated with α-Interferon[a]

Pretreatment	During therapy	Post-treatment
Hepatitis C		
Anti-HCV	Blood count, aminotransferases (weekly × 2, then monthly)	Blood count, aminotransferases
Blood count		
Aminotransferases		
TSH, fT$_4$	TSH, fT$_4$ week 12	TSH, fT$_4$ week 24
Hepatitis B		
HBsAg, HBeAg,	Blood count, aminotransferases (weekly × 2, then monthly)	
HBV DNA		HBsAg, HBeAg, HBV DNA at 6 mos
Blood count		
Aminotransferases		
TSH, fT$_4$	TSH, fT$_4$ week 12	TSH, fT$_4$ week 24

[a]This schedule represents the minimum amount of monitoring suggested. Additional tests might be required and more frequent monitoring might be appropriate in individual patients.
Abbreviations: Anti-HCV, antibody to hepatitis C virus; TSH, thyroid-stimulating hormone; fT$_4$, free thyroxine.

associated with significant side effects, alternative therapies are being sought. *Ribavirin* (an orally administered nucleoside analog) appears to have promise. In a pilot study of ribavirin conducted at NIH, 13 patients were treated with escalating doses for 24 weeks. Serum aminotransferase levels decreased in all patients and became normal in 4 (31%). Levels of HCV RNA in serum decreased significantly, although HCV RNA did not become undetectable in any patient (56). Phase III trials of ribavirin are currently underway.

α-INTERFERON

The interferons are a group of naturally occurring protein cytokines with important immunomodulatory, antiproliferative, and antiviral actions. There are three groups of interferons, including α-(leukocyte) interferon, β-(fibroblast) interferon and γ-(immune) interferon (57). Most studies in viral hepatitis have used α-interferons. γ-Interferon does not appear to be particularly effective against viral hepatitis and is associated with severe side effects. β-Interferon must be given intravenously, although some newer preparations are being tested that are stable enough to be given by subcutaneous injection.

Several forms of α-interferon are available. They include alfa-2a (Roferon, Hoffman La-Roche), alfa-2b (Intron-A, Schering Corpo-

ration) and lymphoblastoid interferon (Wellferon, Wellcome). In the United States to date, only interferon alfa-2b (Intron-A) is approved for use in chronic viral hepatitis (types B and C) by the FDA although the other types have been tested extensively both in the United States and abroad and appear to have similar beneficial effects.

α-Interferon is usually given by subcutaneous injection daily for hepatitis B or three times weekly for hepatitis B or C. Patients can readily be taught to give themselves the interferon injections but they do need to be monitored frequently to check for changes in serum aminotransferase levels and blood count (Table 18.8). In addition, serum levels of thyroid-stimulating hormone and free thyroxine should be checked prior to and at the end of therapy or if signs or symptoms of thyroid dysfunction occur.

Approximately 2–3% of patients treated with α-interferon for chronic viral hepatitis will develop autoimmune thyroid disease. This takes the form of Grave disease or Hashimoto thyroiditis and results in hyper- or hypothyroidism (58). The major side effects of α-interferon are listed in Table 18.9 (59). Early side effects include fever, headache, and an influenza-like syndrome. These usually occur with the first few doses of interferon but soon fade. The development of late side ef-

Table 18.9
Common Side Effects of α-Interferon

Fever
Headache
Muscle aching
Fatigue[a]
Depression[a]
Emotional lability[a]
Organic brain syndrome[a]
Bone marrow depression[a]
Hair loss
Bacterial infections
Autoimmune thyroid disease

[a]Frequent reasons for decreasing the dose or discontinuing interferon therapy.

fects is somewhat unpredictable because not all patients experience them, the time of onset is variable, and they occur in some individuals with more severity than in others. In general, most patients are able to continue their normal work and life activities while taking interferon. Occasional patients find the side effects difficult to tolerate and either require a reduction in dose or early discontinuation of therapy. The side effects of α-interferon tend to clear quite rapidly after decreasing the dose or stopping therapy. Hair loss or "thinning" occurs in less than 10% of patients and may continue for some weeks after treatment but is almost always reversible. The development of thyroid dysfunction may persist and require continuing therapy after stopping interferon.

CONCLUSIONS

Three distinct forms of chronic viral hepatitis can be distinguished on the basis of specific serologic testing. All three forms can lead to progressive liver disease and thus require therapy. α-Interferon is the most promising form of therapy for all three types, although its effects are somewhat limited and not all patients will derive benefit from therapy. Successful treatment is associated with clearance of viral antigens and nucleic acid from serum with normalization of serum aminotransferase activities. Improvement in liver histopathology often follows. Long-term follow-up studies suggest that these improvements may be sustained indefinitely in a substantial proportion of patients and may beneficially alter the long-term outcome of these conditions.

Although significant progress certainly has been achieved to date, the optimal treatment of chronic viral hepatitis rests with newer therapies and future developments that will undoubtedly be made in this rapidly advancing field.

REFERENCES

1. Tiollais P, Pourcel C, Dejean A. The hepatitis B virus. Nature 1985;317:489–495.
2. Hoofnagle JH, Di Bisceglie AM. Serologic diagnosis of acute and chronic viral hepatitis. Sem Liver Dis 1991;11:73–83.
3. Hoofnagle JH, Alter HJ. Chronic viral hepatitis. In: Vyas GN, Dienstag JL, Hoofnagle JH, eds. Viral hepatitis and liver disease. Orlando, FL: Grune and Stratton, 1984:97–113.
4. Liaw YF, Tai D-I, Chu C-M, Chen T-J. The development of cirrhosis in patients with chronic type B hepatitis: a prospective study. Hepatology 1988;8:493–496.
5. Hoofnagle JH, Shafritz DA, Popper H. Chronic type B hepatitis and the "healthy" hepatitis B surface antigen carrier state. Hepatology 1987;7:758–763.
6. Garcia G, Smith CI, Weissberg JI, et al. Adenine arabinoside monophosphate (vidarabine phosphate) in combination with human leukocyte interferon in the treatment of chronic hepatitis B. Ann Intern Med 1987;107:278–285.
7. Greenberg HB, Pollard RB, Lutwick LI, Gregory PB, Robinson WS, Merigan TC. Effect of human leucocyte interferon on hepatitis B virus infection in patients with chronic active hepatitis. N Engl J Med 1976;295:517–522.
8. Dusheiko G, Di Bisceglie A, Bowyer S, et al. Recombinant leucocyte interferon treatment of chronic hepatitis B. Hepatology 1985;5:556–560.
9. Lai C-L, Lin H-J, Yeah E-K, Lok AS-F, Wu P-C, Yeung C-Y. Placebo-controlled trial of recombinant α2-interferon in Chinese HBsAg-carrier children. Lancet 1987;2:877–880.
10. McDonald JA, Caruso L, Karayiannis P, et al. Diminished responsiveness of male homosexual chronic hepatitis B virus carriers with HTLV-III antibody to recombinant α-interferon. Hepatology 1987;7:719–723.
11. Anderson MG, Harrison TJ, Alexander G, Zuckerman AJ, Murray-Lyon IM. Randomised controlled trial of lymphoblastoid interferon for chronic active hepatitis B. Gut 1987;28:619–622.
12. Alexander GJ, Brahm J, Fagan EA, et al. Loss of HBsAg with interferon therapy in chronic hepatitis B virus infection. Lancet 1987;2:66–68.
13. Lok ASF, Wu P-C, Lai C-L, Leung EKY. Long-term follow-up in a randomised controlled trial of

recombinant α2-interferon in Chinese patients with chronic hepatitis B infection. Lancet 1988;2:298–302.

14. Hoofnagle JH, Peters M, Mullen KD, et al. Randomized, controlled trial of recombinant human α-interferon in patients with chronic hepatitis B. Gastroenterology 1988;95:1318–1325.

15. Perrillo RP, Schiff ER, Davis GL, et al. A randomized, controlled trial of interferon alfa-2b alone and after prednisone withdrawal for the treatment of chronic hepatitis B. N Engl J Med 1990;323:295–301.

16. Di Bisceglie AM, Fong T-L, Fried MW, et al. A randomized, controlled trial of recombinant alpha interferon for chronic hepatitis B. Am J Gastroenterol (in press).

17. Brook MG, Karayiannis P, Thomas HC. Which patients with chronic hepatitis B virus infection will respond to α-interferon therapy? A statistical analysis of predictive factors. Hepatology 1989;10:761–763.

18. Korenman J, Baker B, Waggoner JG, Everhart JE, Di Bisceglie AM, Hoofnagle JH. Long-term remission in chronic hepatitis B following alpha interferon therapy. Ann Intern Med 1991;114:629–634.

19. Perrillo RP, Regenstein FG, Peters MG, et al. Prednisone withdrawal followed by recombinant alpha interferon in the treatment of chronic type B hepatitis. Ann Intern Med 1988;109:95–100.

20. Hoofnagle JH, Di Bisceglie AM, Waggoner JG, Park Y. Alpha interferon for patients with clinically apparent cirrhosis due to chronic hepatitis B. Gastroenterology 1993;104:1116–1121.

21. Lisker-Melman M, Webb D, Di Bisceglie AM, et al. Treatment of glomerulonephritis due to chronic hepatitis B virus infection with recombinant human alpha interferon. Ann Intern Med 1989;111:479–483.

22. Carman WF, Hadziyannis S, McGarvey MJ, et al. Mutation preventing formation of hepatitis B e antigen in patients with chronic hepatitis B infection. Lancet 1989;2:588–590.

23. Brunetto MR, Oliveri F, Rocca G, et al. Natural course and response to interferon of chronic hepatitis B accompanied by antibody to hepatitis B e antigen. Hepatology 1989;10:198–202.

24. Fattovich G, Farci P, Rugge M, et al. A randomized controlled trial of lymphoblastoid interferon-α in patients with chronic hepatitis B. Hepatology 1991;15:584–589.

25. Hoofnagle JH. Type D (delta) hepatitis. JAMA 1989;261:1321–1325.

26. Rizzetto M, Ponzetto A, Forzani I. Epidemiology of hepatitis delta virus: Overview. In: Gerin JL, Purcell RH, Rizzetto M, eds. The hepatitis delta virus. New York: Wiley-Liss, 1991:1–20.

27. Di Bisceglie AM, Negro F. Diagnosis of hepatitis delta virus infection [Editorial]. Hepatology 1989;10:1014–1016.

28. Buti M, Esteban R, Jardi R, et al. Chronic delta hepatitis: detection of hepatitis delta virus antigen in serum by immunoblot and correlation with other markers of delta viral replication. Hepatology 1989;10:907–910.

29. Aragona M, Caredda F, Lavarini C, et al. Serological response to the hepatitis delta virus in hepatitis D. Lancet 1987;1:478–480.

30. Govindarajan S, Chin KP, Redeker AG, et al. Fulminant B viral hepatitis: role of delta agent. Gastroenterology 1984;86:1416–1420.

31. Rizzetto M, Verme G, Recchia S, et al. Chronic HBsAg hepatitis with intrahepatic expression of delta antigen: an active and progressive disease unresponsive to immunosuppressive therapy. Ann Intern Med 1983;98:437–441.

32. Arico S, Rizzetto M, Zanetti A, et al. Clinical significance of antibody to the hepatitis delta virus in symptomless HBsAg carriers. Lancet 1985;2:356–358.

33. Di Bisceglie AM, Martin P, Lisker-Melman M, et al. Therapy of chronic delta hepatitis with interferon alfa-2b. J Hepatol 1990;11:S151–S154.

34. Farci P, Karayiannis P, Brook MG, et al. Treatment of chronic hepatitis delta virus (HDV) infection with human lymphoblastoid alpha interferon. Q J Med 1989;73:1045–1054.

35. Rosina F, Saracco G, Lattore V, et al. Alpha-2 recombinant interferon in the treatment of chronic hepatitis delta virus (HDV) hepatitis. In: Rizzetto M, Gerin JL, Purcell RH, eds. The hepatitis delta virus and its infection. New York: Alan R. Liss; 1987:299–303.

36. Rosina F, Pintus C, Rizzetto M, et al. Long-term interferon treatment of chronic hepatitis D: a multicentre Italian study. J Hepatol 1990;11:S149–S150.

37. Farci P, Mandas A, Lai ME, et al. A randomized controlled trial of high and low doses of interferon (IFN) α-2a (Roferon A) in chronic HDV hepatitis: An interim report. In: Hollinger FB, Lemon SM, Margolis HS, eds. Viral hepatitis and liver disease. Baltimore: Williams & Wilkins, 1991:672–673.

38. Grendele M, Gridelli B, Colledan M, et al. Good news about HBV-HDV reinfection in liver transplant patients. In: Hollinger FB, Lemon SM, Margolis HS, eds. Viral hepatitis and liver disease. Baltimore: Williams & Wilkins, 1991:495–497.

39. Choo Q-L, Kuo G, Weiner AJ, Overby LR, Bradley DW, Houghton M. Isolation of a cDNA clone derived from a blood-borne non-A, non-B viral hepatitis genome. Science 1989;244:359–362.

40. Houghton M, Weiner A, Han J, Kuo G, Choo Q-L. Molecular biology of the hepatitis C viruses: implications for diagnosis, vaccine development and control of viral disease. Hepatology 1991;14:381–388.

41. Esteban JI, Esteban R, Viladomiu L, et al. Hepatitis C virus antibodies among risk groups in Spain. Lancet 1989;2:294–297.

42. Alter MJ, Coleman PJ, Alexander WJ, et al. Importance of heterosexual activity in the transmission of

hepatitis B and non-A, non-B hepatitis. JAMA 1989;262:1201–1205.

43. Feinman SV, Berris B, Bojarski S. Posttransfusion hepatitis in Toronto, Canada. Gastroenterology 1988;95:464–469.

44. Di Bisceglie AM, Goodman ZD, Ishak KG, Hoofnagle JH, Melpolder JJ, Alter HJ. Long-term clinical and histopathological follow up of chronic posttransfusion hepatitis. Hepatology 1991;14:969–974.

45. Pappas SC, Young N, Straus SE, Jones EA. Treatment of chronic non-A, non-B hepatitis with acyclovir: pilot study. J Med Virol 1985;15:1–9.

46. Hoofnagle JH, Mullen KD, Jones DB, et al. Treatment of chronic non-A, non-B hepatitis with recombinant human alpha interferon: a preliminary report. N Engl J Med 1986;315:1575–1578.

47. Thomson BJ, Doran M, Lever AML, Webster ADB. Alpha-interferon therapy for non-A, non-B hepatitis transmitted by gammaglobulin replacement therapy. Lancet 1987;1:539–541.

48. Di Bisceglie AM, Martin P, Kassianides C, et al. Recombinant interferon alfa therapy for chronic hepatitis C: a randomized double-blind placebo-controlled trial. N Engl J Med 1989;321:1506–1510.

49. Davis GL, Balart LA, Schiff ER, et al. Treatment of chronic hepatitis C with recombinant interferon alfa: a multicenter randomized, controlled trial. N Engl J Med 1989;321:1494–1500.

50. Marcellin P, Boyer N, Giostra E, et al. Recombinant human α-interferon in patients with chronic non-A, non-B hepatitis: a multicenter randomized controlled trial from France. 1991;13:393–397.

51. Saracco G, Rosina F, Torrani Cerenzia MR, et al. A randomized controlled trial of interferon alfa-2b as therapy for chronic non-A, non-B hepatitis. J Hepatol 1990;11:S43–S49.

52. Shindo M, Di Bisceglie AM, Cheung L, et al. Decrease in hepatitis C viral RNA during alpha-interferon therapy for chronic hepatitis C. Ann Intern Med 1990;115:700–704.

53. Shindo M, Di Bisceglie AM, Hoofnagle JH. Long-term follow up of patients with chronic hepatitis C treated with alpha-interferon. Hepatology 1992;15:1013–1016.

54. Di Bisceglie AM, Hoofnagle JH. Therapy of chronic hepatitis C with α-interferon: the answer? or more questions? Hepatology 1991;13:601–603.

55. Shindo M, Di Bisceglie AM, Hoofnagle JH. Acute exacerbation of liver disease during alpha interferon therapy for chronic hepatitis C. Gastroenterology 1992;102:1406–1408.

56. Di Bisceglie AM, Shindo M, Fong TL, et al. A pilot study of ribavirin therapy for chronic hepatitis C. Hepatology 1992;16:649–654.

57. Peters M. Mechanisms of action of interferons. Semin Liver Dis 1989;9:235–239.

58. Lisker-Melman M, Di Bisceglie AM, Usala SJ, Weintraub B, Murray L, Hoofnagle JH. Autoimmune thyroid disease associated with recombi-fj nant human alpha-interferon therapy in patients with chronic viral hepatitis. Gastroenterology 1992;102:2155–2160.

59. Renault P, Hoofnagle JH. Side effects of alpha interferon. Semin Liver Dis 1989;9:273–278.

60. Di Bisceglie AM, Martin P, Kassianides C, et al. A randomized, double-blind, placebo-controlled trial of recombinant human α-interferon therapy for chronic non-A, non-B (type C) hepatitis. J Hepatol 1990;11:S36–S42.

19

Treatment of Alcoholic Liver Disease

ANNA MAE DIEHL and THOMAS G. TIETJEN

Alcoholic liver disease remains the major cause of clinically significant chronic liver disease in the United States (1). Despite several decades of work, effective therapies for most alcoholic patients with liver disease have not been developed. Success has been thwarted by several obstacles, including gaps in our understanding of the disease pathogenesis and, most notably, the failure of many patients to abstain from alcohol once liver injury has occurred. This chapter will briefly review current concepts concerning the pathogenesis of liver disease in alcoholic individuals and then present recommendations for treatment of patients at various stages of alcohol-induced liver disease.

PATHOGENESIS

Historical Perspective. The hepatotoxicity of alcohol had been suspected for centuries. Physicians such as Laennec, alerted the medical community to the potential hazards of alcohol by carefully documenting the high prevalence of cirrhosis among alcoholic individuals. Later, large epidemiologic surveys confirmed this association between liver disease and alcoholism. For example, in the United States, deaths from cirrhosis were found to decline during the Prohibition era. Conversely, deaths from cirrhosis have been noted to correlate with per capita consumption of alcohol in many countries (2).

Basic Science Advances. For the past three decades, mounting biochemical and pharmacotoxicologic evidence has clearly incriminated alcohol as a potent hepatotoxin (3). Alcohol can injure liver cells via several mechanisms. As a lipid-soluble molecule, it partitions in the lipid bilayer of cell membranes. This causes acute disorder in the membrane structure and, over time, results in adaptive reorganization of the membrane, which compromises physiologic, membrane-initiated signaling by multiple mediators, including various hormones, growth factors, and cytokines. Once in the cell, alcohol is efficiently oxidized by several enzyme systems (Table 19.1) to form potentially toxic intermediates. The latter are currently believed to play a major role in alcohol-induced liver injury. In nonalcoholic subjects most ethanol oxidation is accomplished by the cytosolic alcohol dehydrogenase-aldehyde dehydrogenase system (Fig. 19.1). However, chronic consumption of alcohol also induces certain microsomal cytochrome P-450 isozymes; hence, this pathway provides a supplemental route for ethanol disposal in alcoholic individuals. Both the cytosolic and microsomal ethanol-oxidizing enzymes generate acetaldehyde. Acetaldehyde is an extremely reactive intermediate that forms adducts with critical cellular constituents. Adduct formation has

Table 19.1
Ethanol-Metabolizing Enzymes

Alcohol dehydrogenase/acetaldehyde dehydrogenase
Microsomal enzyme-oxidizing system (MEOS)
Catalase
Fatty acid ethyl ester synthase

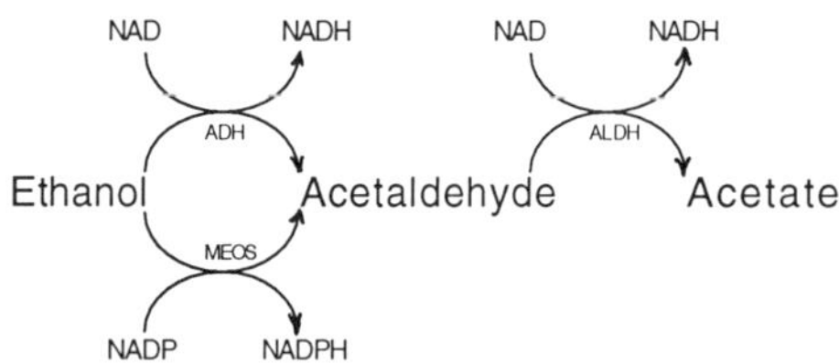

Figure 19.1. Principal oxidative pathways for ethanol. (ADH = alcohol dehydrogenase; ALDH = aldehyde dehydrogenase; MEOS = microsomal ethanol-oxidizing system).

been incriminated for many of the pathobiologic actions of alcohol, including Mallory body formation.

Alcohol/aldehyde dehydrogenase catalyzed oxidation of ethanol to acetaldehyde and eventually to acetate also generates excessive reducing equivalents. This, in turn, upsets the normal cellular oxidation-reduction (redox) balance and interferes with the intermediary metabolism of many nutrients. Oxidation of ethanol by microsomal enzyme oxidizing systems (MEOSs) is dependent on oxygen and hence creates a demand for oxygen that may compromise the viability of physiologically hypoxic, zone three hepatocytes that rim terminal hepatic venules. Since the MEOS also metabolizes other xenobiotics and drugs, ethanol induction of MEOS activity increases the probability of generating hepatotoxic intermediates from other substrates. The latter phenomenon explains the heightened sensitivity of alcoholic individuals to acetaminophen hepatotoxicity. Alcohol can also be metabolized by other cellular enzymes. Some of these (e.g., catalase) do not appear to be very important for ethanol disposal in humans, while the importance of others has been recognized only recently. For example, in tissues that lack active alcohol/aldehyde dehydrogenase and microsomal enzyme oxidizing systems, including the heart, fatty acid ethyl ester synthase metabolizes ethanol to the toxic intermediates which produce end-organ disease.

Host Characteristics

Although numerous cytotoxic actions of alcohol and its metabolites have been charac-

terized in experimental systems, toxicity appears to occur in only a minority of humans and animals that chronically consume the drug. Only about one-fifth of men will develop cirrhosis after drinking the equivalent of two six packs of beer daily for more than a decade (4, 5). Similarly, it has been difficult to establish animals models of alcohol-induced liver injury. Alcoholic hepatitis and cirrhosis occur infrequently, if at all, in most species of small mammals tested to date (6). Indeed, cirrhosis does not uniformly occur even in baboons that have been fed ethanol chronically (7).

In order to reconcile these apparent discrepancies between the in vitro and in vivo toxicity of alcohol, a working hypothesis has been developed. According to this theory, alcohol is a potential hepatotoxin. The evolution of liver disease in a given alcoholic individual depends on the balance between the hepatotoxic actions of alcohol and its metabolites and the presence or absence of several variables in the host. Several host characteristics have been identified that appear to modulate the propensity to alcohol-induced liver injury. These include: genetic polymorphisms of particular alcohol metabolizing enzymes, gender, coexposure to other drugs or infectious agents, immunologic factors, and nutritional status.

Genetic Polymorphisms. Several distinct isozymes of alcohol dehydrogenase (ADH) and aldehyde dehydrogenase (ALDH) have been characterized. These enzymes differ in the efficiency with which they can oxidize ethanol. The prevalence of certain ADH/ALDH isozymes appears to be variable among different ethnic groups. For example, the coinheritance of an isozyme of ADH that rapidly oxidizes ethanol to acetaldehyde and an isozyme of ALDH that only sluggishly converts acetaldehyde to acetate is common in Asians. When individuals with this pattern of alcohol metabolizing enzymes consume alcohol, acetaldehyde accumulates and produces a sense of dysphoria and flushing analogous to a disulfiram reaction. Habitual alcohol use, and consequently alcoholic liver disease, rarely occur in such individuals (3, 4). Identification of genetic polymorphisms for other alcohol metabolizing enzymes and correlation of the respective genotypes with the relative risk of alcoholism and alcoholic liver disease represents an area of active research.

Gender. Women appear to be more sensitive than men to alcohol-induced liver injury. The heightened sensitivity to alcohol cannot be attributed entirely to gender-related differences in tissue composition or volume of drug disposition. Recent identification of a gender-sensitive, gastric form of alcohol dehydrogenase may help explain female susceptibility to alcohol toxicity. Gastric ADH activity appears to be lower in women than in men. Hence, women detoxify less ethanol intragastrically, and a relatively greater fraction of each drink is absorbed "intact" into the portal circulation to be metabolized by the liver (8). This discovery could explain the seeming vulnerability of women to low doses of alcohol. However, it is important to note that the physiologic relevance of gastric ADH in either gender is, at present, hotly contested (8a).

Coexposure to Other Drugs and Infectious Agents. As noted above, chronic consumption of ethanol induces the activity of several microsomal enzymes and hence potentiates the metabolism of drugs and xenobiotics that normally serve as substrates for these enzymes. The potential importance of coexistent injury from other drugs to the pathogenesis of liver disease in alcoholic patients should not be underestimated. This is well-illustrated by both animal models and humans. When rats are treated with subtoxic doses of carbon tetrachloride (a compound that is metabolized to reactive intermediates by ethanol-inducible isozymes of cytochrome P-450), no liver disease ensues. Similarly, when rats are fed ethanol-containing diets chronically, no liver disease is apparent. However, when ethanol-fed rats are cotreated with typically subtoxic doses of carbon tetrachloride, cirrhosis ensues within 10 weeks (9).

Acetaminophen is a widely used and generally safe analgesic that is metabolized by ethanol-inducible P-450 enzymes. In-

deed, the main isoenzyme induced by ethanol (P4502EI) has been shown to be the one mainly involved in the metabolism of acetaminophen (9a). As a result, the threshold for acetaminophen-induced hepatocyte necrosis is significantly lowered by chronic alcohol use, and, in alcoholic individuals, lethal hepatotoxicity has been reported to follow the ingestion of doses that are typically well within the therapeutic range (10). These observations prompt serious concern about the possibility of occult, drug-induced liver injury in any individual who habitually consumes alcohol.

Infection with various hepatotrophic viruses is also more prevalent in alcoholic than in nonalcoholic individuals (11). While the basis for this predisposition remains obscure, it is clear that serologic markers of hepatitis B and C infection are common in alcoholic individuals. Not only is the prognosis of acute viral hepatitis worse in alcoholic patients, but the prevalence of viral markers also increases with the severity of the underlying chronic liver disease (12). These findings have prompted some workers to speculate that viral infections are intimately involved in the pathogenesis of alcohol-associated liver disease. Others have disputed this conjecture, noting that the full spectrum of alcoholic liver disease often occurs in the absence of documented viral infection. Nonetheless, it is likely that viral infection contributes to the liver-related morbidity and mortality in selected patients. Viral infections may also increase the risk of hepatocellular carcinoma in alcoholic patients with cirrhosis (13). In this regard, chronic infection with hepatitis C may prove to be a more widespread risk factor than is remote infection with hepatitis B.

Immunologic Factors. Immune dysfunction is a well-documented sequela of chronic alcohol consumption. Although impaired immunity is often cited as the basis for prevalent bacterial and viral infections in alcoholic individuals (14), recent attention has focused on two examples of alcohol-associated immune "hyper"-function. The first situation involves autoimmunity to liver cell antigens triggered by acetaldehyde-protein adducts. This process

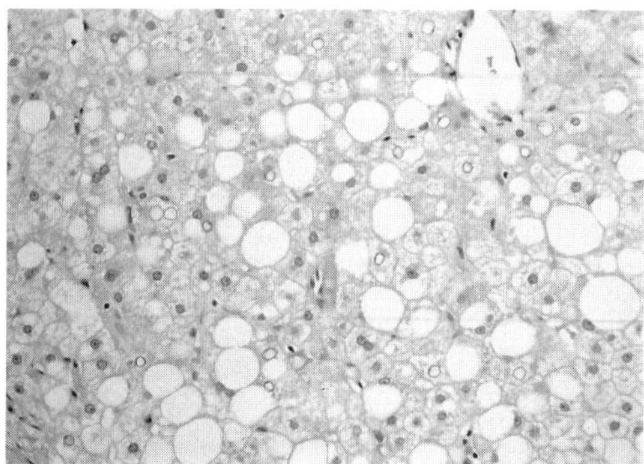

Figure 19.2. Photomicrograph of alcoholic fatty liver.

has been implicated as a basis for ongoing liver injury in some alcoholic individuals who have discontinued alcohol use (15). The second involves overproduction of certain proinflammatory cytokines by macrophages and monocytes. These cytokines have been incriminated as both hepatotoxic agents and effectors of the multiorgan failure response in patients with alcoholic hepatitis. Indeed, tumor necrosis factor α- and TNF-inducible cytokines have been shown to correlate with mortality in patients hospitalized with acute alcoholic hepatitis (16).

Nutritional Status. Classically, malnutrition has been recognized as an important variable in the progression of liver disease in alcoholic individuals. Chronic consumption impairs the intake, digestion, absorption, and storage of many macro- and micronutrients (17). At one point, alcohol-induced malnutrition was considered more important than alcohol itself in the pathogenesis of alcohol-related liver injury. However, attention was redirected in the early 1970s when Mak and coworkers demonstrated that baboons fed ethanol developed hepatic fibrosis despite ingesting a seemingly nutritious diet (7). The subsequent era of basic research also underscored the hepatotoxic potential of ethanol, and for a while the importance of malnutrition faded into the background. Ironically, some of these same workers have produced recent data that rekindles the old controversy. Coadministration of polyunsaturated lecithin has been shown to

prevent hepatic fibrogenesis in the alcohol-fed baboon model described above (18). The effect of choline supplements and cysteine prodrugs that potentiate the synthesis of reduced glutathione on alcohol-induced liver injury is currently being actively investigated. These efforts indicate that variability in host nutritional status influences the hepatotoxic potential of ethanol.

HISTOPATHOLOGY

No discussion about the pathogenesis of alcoholic liver disease would be complete without a brief review of alcohol-associated histopathology. This is important because histology provides unique insights into variable pathobiologic mechanisms that evolve over the course of the disease but are not reliably distinguished by clinical or noninvasive laboratory tests alone.

Three major histopathologic lesions have been associated with alcohol abuse—alcoholic fatty liver (steatosis), alcoholic hepatitis (steatonecrosis), and alcoholic cirrhosis (19). Alcoholic fatty liver (Fig. 19.2) is a reproducible consequence of ethanol oxidation. It results from the redox imbalance that follows ethanol oxidation and is seen in all humans and animals after consumption of large amounts of ethanol. Excessive reducing equivalents generated by the oxidation of ethanol favor lipid synthesis or accumulation relative to lipid degradation and result in the accumulation of large droplets of fat in hepatocytes. As the normal redox state is restored, this lipid is mobilized and the fatty liver resolves. Since this lesion is completely reversible, many do not consider it a true form of alcoholic liver injury. Nonetheless, it is indicative of the disordered intracellular metabolism that results from ethanol intoxication and has been associated with an acutely fatal outcome in occasional individuals.

The histopathology of alcoholic hepatitis is characterized by steatosis plus hepatocellular injury with associated acute inflammation plus or minus fibrosis (Fig. 19.3). As with alcoholic fatty liver, zone 3 of the hepatic acinus is most severely afflicated. Some injured hepatocytes

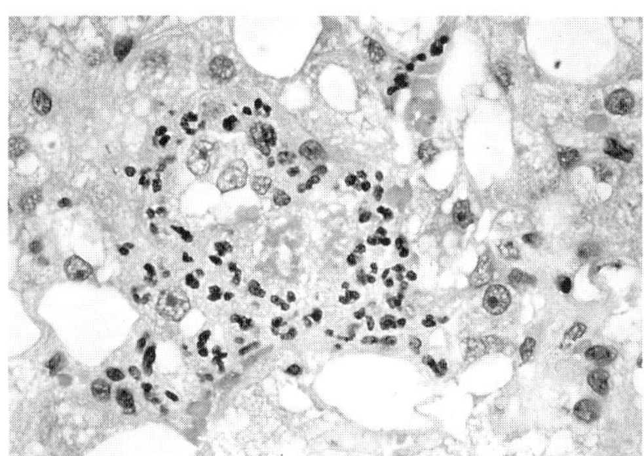

Figure 19.3. Photomicrograph of alcoholic hepatitis.

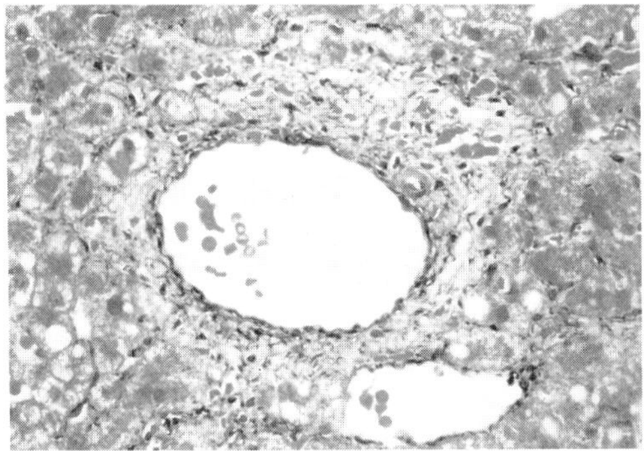

Figure 19.4. Photomicrograph of alcoholic fibrosis/cirrhosis.

contain eosinophilic fibrillar material, a condensation of cytoskeletal intermediary filaments that results when tublin-acetaldehyde adducts form (20). Such Mallory bodies, while typical of alcoholic hepatitis, are neither sensitive nor specific markers of that lesion. However, they do provide a graphic illustration of the ability of the alcohol to destroy normal mechanisms for intracellular trafficking, cell-to-cell, and cell-to-matrix communication. Intense lobular infiltration with polymorphonuclear leukocytes separates alcoholic hepatitis from most other forms of hepatitis (in which the inflammatory infiltrate is predominately periportal and mononuclear). The recent recognition that certain cytokines act as neutrophil chemotactic factors (21), coupled with data that correlate mortal-

ity in acute alcoholic hepatitis with circulating levels of proinflammatory cytokines, offers important insights into the pathogenesis of this lesion. At present, however, it is unclear whether alcoholic hepatitis is an inevitable consequence of heavy alcohol use or the prerequisite lesion for eventual alcoholic cirrhosis. Nonetheless, because of these suspicions and the fact that this lesion is sometimes associated with a characteristic clinical syndrome (i.e., fever, leukocytosis, tender hepatomegaly, and jaundice), it has been the target of multiple clinical treatment trials.

Cirrhosis, considered the final stage of alcohol-induced hepatic pathology, results after recurrent bouts of alcoholic hepatitis. Hepatocellular injury and perhaps direct actions of acetaldehyde on collagen-forming nonparenchymal cells induce a fibrogenic response. Collagen is deposited in a characteristic perivenular and pericellular distribution resulting in a chicken wire pattern of scarring (Fig. 19.4). Because chronic alcohol consumption impairs the hepatic regenerative response to injury (22), the regenerative nodules in alcoholic cirrhosis are typically small (micronodules).

Although it seems conceptually simplest to consider the evolution of alcoholic liver disease as a linear progression that begins with alcoholic fatty liver and moves through alcoholic hepatitis before culminating in alcoholic cirrhosis, this model is probably incorrect. Often varying "stages" of alcoholic liver disease coexist in a single patient. Conversely, many individuals never "progress" beyond the early stages of the disease despite continued alcohol abuse. Furthermore, features of alcoholic liver injury may mingle with those of nonalcoholic etiologies in individuals with superimposed viral or drug-induced hepatitis or biliary tract obstruction.

DIAGNOSIS

The clinical features of patients with alcoholic liver disease cover a broad spectrum, ranging from completely asymptomatic to the florid features of advanced parenchymal cell failure and portal hypertension. Fever, jaundice, and

Table 19.2
Composite Clinical and Laboratory Index Scoring[a]

Sign/symptom	Score
Hepatomegaly	1
Splenomegaly	1
Ascites	
1+	1
2+	2
3+	3
Encephalopathy	
Grade I	1
Grade II	2
Grade III	3
Clinical bleeding	1
Spider nevi	1
Palmar erythema	1
Collateral circulation	1
Peripheral edema	1
Anorexia	1
Weakness	1
SGOT >20 U	1
SGPT	
>100 U	1
>200 U	2
Alkaline phosphatase >80 U	1
Serum albumin <2.59%	1
Prothrombin time[b]	
<3	1
3–5	2
>5	3
Bilirubin (mg %)	
1.2–2	1
2.1–5	2
>5	3

[a]Adapted from Orrego et al. (24).
[b]Seconds above control.

tender hepatomegaly, typical of the classical syndrome of alcoholic hepatitis (23), occur in only a minority of individuals. Indeed, the dearth of pathognomonic symptoms and signs in alcoholic liver disease mandates the elimination of other potential etiologies of liver injury before a diagnosis of alcoholic liver disease can be established. There is no predictable level of alcohol consumption above which alcoholic liver disease can be presumed inevitable. Although studies suggest that the risk of alcohol-induced hepatic disease increases progressively when habitual intake exceeds 80 g/day of ethanol in men and 20 g/day in women, significant liver disease occurs in only a minority of individuals who drink 2 to 3 times these amounts (4, 5). None-

theless, alcohol should be considered a potential contributor to liver disease in all individuals, regardless of how little they consume. In addition to the history of habitual alcohol use, the pattern of aminotransferase abnormalities also provides a useful clue to alcohol-induced disease. Typically, the AST is elevated two to three times greater than the ALT and neither enzyme activity exceeds 300–400 IU/l. Leukocytosis should also suggest an alcohol-induced etiology of liver disease, once infection and biliary tract disease have been excluded. While liver biopsy can be used to confirm the clinical suspicion of alcoholic liver disease, it is seldom necessary, especially if noninvasive tests (e.g., liver ultrasound, hepatitis serology, iron studies) are ordered to complement a careful history and physical examination.

It is important to realize that liver enzyme patterns and histology are most helpful in the *diagnosis* of alcoholic liver disease. Unfortunately, neither the degree of abnormality of the serum aminotransferases nor the histopathology accurately predicts the gravity of the clinical illness. Rather, the immediate outcome for patients hospitalized with alcoholic liver disease is better estimated by combinations of tests that delineate both the severity of acute alcohol-induced metabolic disarray and the severity of fixed disease in vital organs such as the liver. Two groups of investigators have independently developed formulas for use in estimating the short-term prognosis of patients with alcoholic liver disease. Orrego and coworkers have defined a group of clinical and laboratory parameters which correlate with mortality in hospitalized patients with alcoholic liver disease (24) (Table 19.2; Fig. 19.5). These factors have been assigned a numerical value based on their importance as predictors of outcome. Summing the value of each variable generates a composite clinical laboratory index (CCLI). Patients with a low CCLI are likely to survive, while those with a high CCLI are at increased risk of dying during hospitalization. Hence, calculation of the CCLI is useful because it permits a linear estimate of acute mortality in patients with alcoholic liver disease. However, the disadvan-

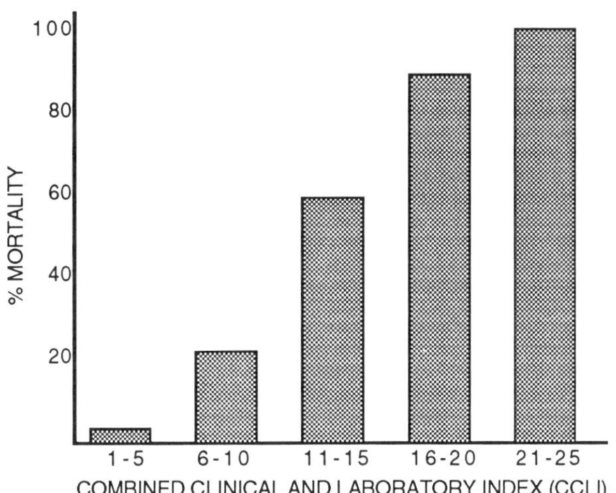

Figure 19.5. Combined clinical and laboratory index (CCLI) and mortality from alcoholic hepatitis. Adapted from Oreggo et al. (24).

tage of this approach is the large number of variables that must be scored and the complexity of the calculation itself. Maddrey and coworkers have simplified assessment of outcome in alcoholic liver disease by developing a discriminant function (DF). According to their formula, patients in whom 4.6 × prothrombin time + bilirubin level (mg/dl) exceeds 93 have a greater than 50% chance of dying during hospitalization (25). The utility of the DF has been prospectively validated (26) and offers the advantage of few variables and simple computation. Hence, it is the formula that is most often used in clinical practice. Nonetheless, it is important to recognize the relative imprecision of the DF. At best, it provides a crude estimate of mortality: if about half the patients with a DF >93 will die, the other half with a similar DF will live. Recent evidence that serum concentrations of tumor necrosis factor α and certain tumor necrosis factor (TNF)-inducible cytokines (interleukin-6 and interleukin-8) correlate with mortality in patients hospitalized with alcoholic liver disease (27) suggests that these parameters may also provide useful prognostic information. At present, however, these tests are not available for routine clinical use. Furthermore, the predictive value of serum cytokine concentrations has not been compared with that of the two form-

ulas currently employed to gauge the prognosis of patients with alcoholic liver disease.

The outcome for patients who survive hospitalization for alcoholic liver disease is also variable and, again, seems to be dictated by the severity of residual end-organ damage and whether the patient continues to drink. Two studies indicate that at least some (10%) patients hospitalized with alcoholic hepatitis can regain normal hepatic histology and function. Such "cures" require complete discontinuation of alcohol use. However, abstinence does not always guarantee resolution of liver disease. Almost half the patients hospitalized with precirrhotic alcoholic hepatitis will go on to develop cirrhosis. The risk of progression to cirrhosis increases with increasing histopathologic severity of the index bout of alcoholic hepatitis. Female gender conveys an independent risk of disease progression. Cirrhosis is likely to develop in women hospitalized with alcoholic hepatitis even if they had relatively mild disease initially and even if they become abstinent (28, 29).

Alcohol consumption continues to influence prognosis even after cirrhosis has developed. The 5-year survival of patients with clinically compensated cirrhosis approaches 90% if they abstain from alcohol, but decreases to 60% if they continue to drink. Abstinent patients with decompensated cirrhosis can expect a 60% 5-year survival rate, whereas similar patients who continue to drink have, at best, a 30% chance of living 5 years (28).

TREATMENT

Optimal treatment for most patients with alcoholic liver disease revolves around discontinuation of alcohol use and the resumption of a nutritious diet. Such therapy seldom requires hospitalization, although vigorous efforts should be made to enroll the patient in a detoxification program.

Selected subsets of patients with alcoholic liver disease definitely benefit from hospitalization. Such patients include those with features suggesting a high risk of acute mortality. Admission provides an opportunity to treat withdrawal symptoms and coexistent infections, to manage intercurrent gastrointestinal bleeding, and to correct fluid, electrolyte, and nutritional deficiencies.

The decision to intervene with pharmacologic therapy aimed at the underlying alcoholic liver disease should be based on the anticipated risks of morbidity and mortality as will be discussed (Table 19.3). Several meta-analyses and two prospectively, randomized and controlled clinical trials also indicate that, once infections and gastrointestinal bleeding have been controlled, severely ill, recently drinking patients with alcoholic liver disease benefit from treatment with corticosteroids (26, 30, 31). Although multiple trials (32–35) have failed to demonstrate that hyperalimentation improves the mortality of such patients, it is now evident that restricted intake of nutrients is associated with a poor prognosis (36). Hence, patients should be encouraged to eat and be given supplemental enteral (or, if necessary, parenteral) nutrition if they cannot. There is no evidence that providing adequate amounts of nitrogen triggers uncontrollable encephalopathy in these patients. Similarly, expensive, branched, chain-enriched mixtures of amino acids offer no proven advantage over standard mixtures of amino acids or even over a regular hospital diet. Because patients who drank alcohol until shortly before hospital-

ization are often depleted of potassium, magnesium, and phosphate, these elements should be replenished promptly. If glucose-containing fluids are administered as a vehicle for these elements, it is also critically important to provide supplemental thiamine in order to avoid triggering Wernicke's encephalopathy.

Norfloxacin should be given to cirrhotic patients who suffer portal hypertensive bleeding, since recent evidence indicates that this reduces inpatient morbidity and mortality in this subset of individuals (37). Similarly, patients with a previous episode of spontaneous bacterial peritonitis or low concentrations of ascitic fluid protein (<1 g/dl) should also receive norfloxacin prophylaxis (38). It is intriguing to speculate that such selective gut decontamination may also reduce the detrimental cytokine response in patients with alcoholic hepatitis, but the latter has not yet been evaluated. Severely ill patients should remain hospitalized until they demonstrate definite signs of clinical improvement and are able to ingest an adequate diet. It is unnecessary to defer discharge until histopathologic recovery occurs, since clinical improvement typically precedes resolution of hepatic necroinflammation by several weeks (19). Ideally, such patients can be transferred to an inpatient alcoholic rehabilitation unit to ensure a period of supervised abstinence while recovery continues.

Multiple other treatments have been tested in acutely ill patients with alcoholic liver disease, including treatments targeted to improve the regenerative response (anabolic steroids [39–42], insulin and glucagon infusions [43–46]), to scavenge free radicals (propylthiouracil [24,47,48], cyanidanol [49–51]), and to prevent fibrosis (D-penicillamine [52], colchicine [53–55]). None has reproducibly improved short-term survival. However, it is impossible to conclude that these approaches are totally devoid of merit, since most of the trials included relatively small numbers of heterogeneous patients and few actually determined whether the treatment beneficially influenced the targeted process.

Table 19.3
Potential Medical Therapy for Alcoholic Liver Disease[a]

Agent & reference	Dose/duration	Indication	Reported benefits	Commentary
Corticosteroids (30) Methylprednisone	32 mg/d × 1 mo 1 g/d iv × 3 d	Severe AH	Reduced short-term (30 d) mortality in some trials	May be useful in patients who are extremely ill but do not have active infections or acute GI bleeding
Prednisone	40 mg/d × 1 mo	Severe AH	Clinical improvement, but no effect on progression of fibrosis	
Anabolic steroids (41, 42) Testosterone	200 mg tid p.o.	Cirrhosis	Decrease in gynecomastia; increase in hemoglobin; reduction in serum hemoglobin; no effect on LFTs or survival	Not recommended for routine use
Oxandrolone	80 mg/d × 30 d	Severe AH	No effect on short term (30 d) survival but improved long-term (1 yr) survival	
Antifibrotic agents (54, 55) Colchicine	1 mg/d 5 d/wk ⩽14 yr	Cirrhosis	5-year survival prolonged vs. placebo (75 vs. 34%); decrease in fibrosis in 18%; general clinical improvement seen only after 30 mo of treatment	Can be used in selected abstinent patients; side effects uncommon
Antimetabolites (24, 56) Propylthiouracil	75 mg q 6 hr 150 mg bid × 2 yr (q 3 months in 4)	Severe AH Cirrhosis	No short-term benefit in inactive cirrhosis; improved survival in patients with low T_3 levels treated long-term; treatment hypothyroidism group	Not recommended at present; risk of bone marrow and liver toxicity; possible hypothyroidism
Antibiotics (37, 38) Norfloxacin	400 mg bid p.o. × 7 d	Prevents SBP after GI bleed	Reduced infection rate from 37%–10%	Recommended in patients at risk for SBP
	400 mg daily p.o.	Prophylaxis of SBP	Reduced infection rate from 42%–3% in hospitalized patients	
	400 mg daily p.o.	Prevent SBP recurrence	Reduced recurrence from 35%–12% over 1–19 mo	
Nutritional support (32–36) Amino acids	Parenteral or oral	Severe AH	Improved nutritional and biochemical parameters; no increase in encephalopathy seen with protein supplements	Amino acid formulations are expensive; encourage consumption of nutritionally balanced meals taken at regular intervals
Thiamine	100 mg iv daily	Severe AH	Prevents Wernicke's encephalopathy	
Vitamin K	10 mg/daily	Severe AH	Corrects hypoprothrombinemia	

[a]Abbreviations: severe AH = alcoholic hepatitis with encephalopathy, jaundice, hypoprothrombinemia; SBP = spontaneous bacterial peritonitis; GI = gastrointestinal ; iv, intravenous; tid, three times daily; p.o., orally; q = every.

Even fewer long-term treatment trials of patients with alcoholic liver disease have been conducted (55, 56). Those that have been accomplished are plagued by difficulties in assessing abstinence and compliance with therapy. Drop-out rates have also been relatively steep. These factors severely confound interpretation of the results. However, to date, two prospectively randomized, controlled trials have reported that treatment improves 5–10 year survival in patients with alcoholic liver disease. A survival advantage was noted in Mexican patients with alcoholic cirrhosis who received daily colchicine therapy (55). A Canadian group has also reported long-term survival benefits in a group of patients with varying degrees of alcoholic liver disease who were treated with propylthiouracil (56). Treatment-related toxicity was reportedly infrequent in both studies. However, given the relatively small number of patients who completed each trial, it is quite possible that the power of the studies was inadequate to detect potentially serious adverse reactions. Since the cost and potential toxicity of colchicine are less than those of propylthiouracil, the former seems a better choice when "maintenance" therapy of patients with alcoholic cirrhosis is considered.

Orthotopic liver transplantation improves the survival of patients with decompensated alcoholic cirrhosis when compared with historical, medically treated control subjects (57–60). No magic interval of abstinence has proven to be necessary before transplantation. However, given the extraordinary value and scarcity of donor organs, most transplant centers require that patients demonstrate commitment to lifelong sobriety before transplantation is offered as a therapeutic option. This screening process appears to have been generally successful since recidivism has been reported to occur in <10% of transplanted alcoholic patients. Emerging evidence suggests that alcoholic liver disease may follow an accelerated course in the few patients who resume alcohol use post-transplantation (59 and D. VanThiel and J. Gavaler, University of Oklahoma, personal communication). If confirmed, this would underscore the importance of careful pretransplantation screening to select individuals who are unlikely to resume alcohol use postoperatively.

Even if liver transplantation can effectively salvage many patients with advanced alcoholic liver disease, the morbidity, mortality, and expense of this therapy demand continued efforts to prevent alcoholic liver disease. Public education to increase awareness about potentially harmful, habitual alcohol use is a simple strategy that should not be overlooked. Alcoholic liver disease occurs in many individuals who consider themselves social drinkers and who could control their alcohol consumption if motivated to do so. Effective treatments of alcoholism remain much more elusive and, until available, ensure that alcoholic liver disease will remain a major public health problem, even if it occurs in a minority of heavy drinkers. In the next decade, attention will be directed to developing treatments that eradicate coexistent viral infections (e.g., interferon and other antiviral agents), improve cellular tolerance to oxidative stress (e.g., antioxidants and prodrugs of reduced glutathione), block excessive cytokine responses (e.g., pentoxiphylline, soluble cytokine receptors, anticytokine antibodies), and optimize the hepatic regenerative response to liver injury (e.g., supplemental polyamines and growth factors). These advances should offer novel strategies to control, if not eliminate, this ancient disease.

REFERENCES

1. U.S. Department of Health and Human Services/Public Health Services. Surveillance and assessment of alcohol-related mortality-United States, 1980. MMWR 1985;34:161–163.
2. Grant BF, Dufour MC, Hartford TC. Epidemiology of alcoholic liver disease. Semin Liver Dis 1988;8:12–25.
3. Lieber CS. Hepatic, metabolic and toxic effects of ethanol: 1991 update. Alcoholism 1991;15:573–592.
4. Pequignot G, Tuyns AJ, Berta JL. Ascitic cirrhosis in relation to alcohol consumption. Int J Epidemiol 1978;7:113–120.
5. Lelbach WK. Epidemiology of alcoholic liver disease. Progr Liver Dis 1976;5:494–515.
6. Diehl AM. Alcoholic liver disease. Med Clin North Am 1989;73:815–830.

7. Mak KM, Leo MA, Lieber CS. Alcoholic liver injury in baboons: transformation of lipocytes to transitional cells. Gastroenterology 1984;87:188–200.

8. Frezza M, di Padova C, Pozzato G, Terpin M, Baraona E, Lieber CS. High blood alcohol levels in women: The role of decreased gastric alcohol dehydrogenase activity and first pass metabolism. N Engl J Med 1990;322:95–99.

8a. Smith T, DeMaster EG, Furne JK, Springfield J, Levitt MD. First-pass gastric mucosal metabolism of ethanol is negligible in the rat. J Clin Invest 1992;89:1801–1806.

9. Hall P, Plummer JL, Ilsley AH, Cousins MJ. Hepatic fibrosis and cirrhosis after chronic administration of alcohol and "low-dose" carbon tetrachloride vapor in the rat. Hepatology 1991;13:815–819.

9a. Watkins PB. Role of cytochromes P450 in drug metabolism and hepatotoxicity. Semin Liver Dis 1990;10:235–250.

10. Seeff LB, Cuccherini BA, Zimmerman HJ, Adler E, Benjamin SB. Acetaminophen hepatotoxicity in alcoholics: a therapeutic misadventure. Ann Intern Med 1986;104:399–404.

11. Brechot C, Degos P, Lugassy C, et al. Hepatitis B virus DNA in patients with chronic liver disease and negative tests for hepatitis B surface antigen. N Engl J Med 1985;312:270–276.

12. Mendenhall CL, Seef L, Diehl AM, et al. Antibodies to hepatitis B virus and hepatitis C virus in alcoholic hepatitis and cirrhosis: their prevalence and clinical relevance. Hepatology 1991;14:581–589.

13. Inoe K, Kojima T, Koyata H, et al. Hepatitis B virus antigen and antibodies in alcoholics: Etiological role of HBV in liver disease of alcoholic patients. Liver 1985;5:247–252.

14. Zetterman RK, Sorrell MF. Immunologic aspects of alcoholic liver disease. Gastroenterology 1981;81:616–624.

15. Galambos J. Natural history of alcoholic hepatitis III: Histologic changes. Gastroenterology 1972;63:1026–1035.

16. Shedolfsky SI, McClain CJ. Hepatic dysfunction due to cytokines. In: Kimball ES, ed. Cytokines and inflammation. Boca Raton, FL: CRC Press; 1991;235–273.

17. Mezey E. Alcoholic liver disease. Progr Liver Dis 1982;7:555–572.

18. Li J, Kim CI, Leo MA, Mak KM, Rojkind M, Lieber CS. Polyunsaturated lecithin prevents acetaldehyde-mediated hepatic collagen accumulation by stimulating collagenase activity in cultured lipocytes. Hepatology 1992;15:373–381.

19. Boitnott JK, Maddrey WC. Alcoholic liver disease, 1: Interrelationships among histologic features and the histologic effects of prednisolone therapy. Hepatology 1981;1:599–612.

20. Tsukamoto H, Matsuoka M, French SW. Experimental models of hepatic fibrosis: a review. Semin Liver Dis 1990;10:56–65.

21. Hill D, Marsano L, Cohen D, Allen J, Shedolfsky S, McClain CJ. Increased plasma interleukin-6 activity in alcoholic hepatitis. J Lab Clin Med 1992;119:547.

22. Diehl AM, Yang SQ, Cote P, Wand GS. Chronic ethanol consumption disturbs G-protein expression and inhibits cyclic AMP-dependent signaling in regenerating rat liver. Hepatology 1992;15:1212–1219.

23. Levi AJ, Chalmer TM. Recognition of alcoholic liver disease in a district general hospital. Gut 1978;19:521–525.

24. Orrego H, Kalant H, Israel Y, et al. Effect of short-term therapy with propylthiouracil in patients with alcoholic liver disease. Gastroenterology 1979;76:105–115.

25. Maddrey WC, Boitnott JK, Bedine MS, et al. Corticosteroid therapy of alcoholic hepatitis. Gastroenterology 1978;75:193–199.

26. Carithers RL, Herlong HF, Diehl AM, et al. Methylprednisolone therapy in patients with severe alcoholic hepatitis: a randomized multicenter trial. Ann Intern Med 1989;110:685–690.

27. McClain C, Hill D, Schmidt J, Diehl AM. Cytokines and alcoholic liver diseases. Semin Liver Dis 1993;13:170–182.

28. Galambos J. Natural history of alcoholic hepatitis III: Histologic changes Gastroenterology 1972;63:1026–1035.

29. Pares A, Caballeria J, Bruguera M, et al. Histological course of alcoholic hepatitis: Influence of abstinence, sex, and extent of hepatic damage. J Hepatol 1986;2:33–42.

30. Imperiale TF, McCullough AJ. Do corticosteroids reduce mortality from alcoholic hepatitis? A meta-analysis of the randomized trials. Ann Intern Med 1990;113:299–307.

31. Ramond M-J, Poynard T, Rueff B, et al. A randomized trial of prednisolone in patients with severe alcoholic hepatitis. N Engl J Med 1992;326:507–512.

32. Diehl AM, Boitnott JK, Herlong HF, et al. Effect of parenteral amino acid supplementation in alcoholic hepatitis. Hepatology 1985;5:57–63.

33. Naveau S, Pelletier G, Poynard T, et al. A randomized clinical trial of supplementary parenteral nutrition in jaundiced alcoholic cirrhotic patients. Hepatology 1986;6:270.

34. Calvey H, Davis M, Williams R. Controlled trial of nutritional supplementation, with and without branched chain amino acid enrichment, in treatment of acute alcoholic hepatitis. J Hepatol 1985;1:141–151.

35. Mezey E, Caballeria J, Mitchell MC, et al. Effect of parenteral amino acid supplementation on short-term and long-term outcomes in severe alcoholic hepatitis: a randomized controlled trial. Hepatology 1991;14:1090–1096.

36. Mendenhall CL, Tosch T, Weesner RE, et al. VA cooperative study on alcoholic hepatitis, II: prognostic significance of protein-calorie malnutrition. Am J Clin Nutr 1986;43:213–218.

37. Soriano G, Guarner C, Tomas A, et al. Norfloxacin prevents bacterial infection in cirrhotics with gastrointestinal hemorrhage. Gastroenterology 1992;103:1267–1272.

38. Soriano G, Guarner C, Teixido M, et al. Selective intestinal decontamination presents spontaneous bacterial peritonitis. Gastroenterology 1991;100: 477–481.

39. Wells R. Prednisolone and testosterone propionate in cirrhosis of the liver: a controlled trial. Lancet 1960;2:1416–1417.

40. Fenster LF. The nonefficacy of short-term anabolic steroid therapy in alcoholic liver disease. Ann Intern Med 1966;65:738–744.

41. Mendenhall CL, Anderson S, Garcia-Pont P. Short-term and long-term survival in patients with alcoholic hepatitis treated with oxandrolone and prednisone. N Engl J Med 1984;311:1464–1470.

42. The Copenhagen Study Group for Liver Diseases. Testosterone treatment of men with alcoholic cirrhosis: a double-blind study. Hepatology 1986;6:807–813.

43. Baker AL, Jaspan JB, Haines NW, et al. A randomized clinical trial of insulin and glucagon infusion for treatment of alcoholic hepatitis: progress report in 50 patients [Abstract]. Gastroenterology 1982;8:1154.

44. Feher J, Cornides A, Romany A, et al. A prospective multi-center study of insulin and glucagon infusion therapy in acute alcoholic hepatitis. J Hepatol 1987;5:224–231.

45. Radvan G, Kanel G, Redeker A. Insulin and glucagon infusion in acute alcoholic hepatitis [Abstract]. Gastroenterology 1982;8:1954.

46. Trinchet J-C, Balkau B, Poupon RE, et al. Treatment of severe alcoholic hepatitis by infusion of insulin and glucagon: a multicenter sequential trial. Hepatology 1992;15:76–81.

47. Israel Y, Walfish PG, Orrego H, et al. Thyroid hormones in alcoholic liver disease: effect of treatment with 6-n-propylthiouracil. Gastroenterology 1979;76:116–122.

48. Halle P, Pare P, Kapstein E, et al. Double-blind, controlled trial of propylthiouracil therapy in severe acute alcoholic hepatitis. Gastroenterology 1982;82:925–931.

49. Colman JC, Morgan MY, Scheuer PJ, Sherlock S. Treatment of alcohol-related liver disease with (+)-cyanidanol-3: a randomized double-blind trial. Gut 1980;21:965–969.

50. Marshall AW, Graul RS, Morgan MY, et al. Treatment of alcohol-related liver disease with thioctic acid: a six-month randomized double-blind trial. Gut 1982;23:1088–1092.

51. Morgan MY. Hepatoprotective agents in alcoholic liver disease. Acta Med Scand 1985;703:225–233.

52. Resnick R, Boitnott J, Iber F, et al. Preliminary observations of D-penicillamine therapy in acute alcoholic liver disease. Digestion 1974;11:257–265.

53. Galambos JT, Riepe SP. Use of colchicine and steroids in the treatment of alcoholic liver disease. Rec Dev Alcohol 1984;2:181–194.

54. Kershenobich D, Uribe M, Suarez O, et al. Treatment of cirrhosis with colchicine: a double-blind randomized trial. Gastroenterology 1984;77:532–536.

55. Kershenobich D, Vargas F, Garcia-Tsao G, et al. Colchicine in the treatment of cirrhosis of the liver. N Engl J Med 1988;318:1709–1713.

56. Oreggo H, Blake JE, Blendis LM, Compton KV, Israel Y. Long-term treatment of alcoholic liver disease with propylthiouracil. New Engl J Med 1987;317:1421–1427.

57. Starzl TE, Van Theil D, Tzakis AG, et al. Orthotopic liver transplantation for alcoholic cirrhosis. JAMA 1988;260:2542.

58. Bird GIA, O'Grady JG, Harvey FAH, et al. Liver transplantation in patients with alcoholic cirrhosis: Selection criteria and rates of survival and relapse. Br Med J 1990;301:15–17.

59. Kumar S, Stauber RE, Gavaler JS, et al. Orthotopic liver transplantation for alcoholic liver disease. Hepatology 1990;11:159–164.

60. Lucey MR, Merion RM, Henley KS, et al. Selection for and outcome of liver transplantation in alcoholic liver disease. Gastroenterology 1992;102: 1736–1741.

20

Treatment of Metabolic Liver Disease

BRUCE R. BACON and SPENCER C. Y. LI

The three inherited metabolic liver diseases that can result in chronic liver disease in the adult are hereditary hemochromatosis, Wilson's disease, and α_1-antitrypsin deficiency. In all three disorders, liver damage culminating in cirrhosis is one of the major manifestations of the disease in which other organ systems are also affected. Treatment for hereditary hemochromatosis and Wilson's disease is fairly straightforward; however, good therapeutic agents do not exist for the treatment of α_1-antitrypsin deficiency. Various forms of secondary iron overload are also difficult to treat. Other metabolic disorders that will be considered in this chapter include the hepatic porphyrias, α_1-antitrypsin deficiency, and the hepatic complications of total parenteral nutrition.

IRON OVERLOAD

Classification of Iron Overload

Classification of iron overload is based on the cause and the distribution of the increased iron deposition (Table 20.1). Since humans have no excretory pathway for iron, iron overload occurs either as a result of an increase in intestinal iron absorption or from the parenteral administration of iron either as medicinal iron chelates or as iron in hemoglobin from transfused red blood cells. *Hereditary hemochromatosis (HHC)* refers to the disorder in which there is homozygous inheritance of both alleles of the HHC gene. This results in increased iron absorption from the gut with subsequent deposition in parenchymal cells in

the liver, heart, pancreas, and other organs (1, 2). *Secondary iron overload* encompasses a variety of clinical disorders in which there is an underlying condition that results in an increase in intestinal iron absorption. The best examples of secondary iron overload are the various disorders of ineffective erythropoiesis, such as β-thalassemia, sideroblastic anemia, and aplastic anemia. In these disorders, anemia is the underlying condition that results in an increase in iron absorption (3). Secondary iron overload is also seen in patients with a variety of liver diseases, including alcoholic cirrhosis (4), viral hepatitis with and without cirrhosis (5), following portocaval shunts (6), and in porphyria cutanea tarda (7). How the underlying liver disease results in increased iron deposition in these conditions is unknown.

Parenteral iron overload refers to the situation in which individuals receive excessive amounts of iron in the form of injectable iron chelates (e.g., iron dextran) or from chronic red blood cell (RBC) transfusion in the absence of blood loss. Most patients with ineffective erythropoiesis have a combination of both secondary and parenteral iron overload, since RBC transfusion is often necessary. In parenteral iron overload, iron is initially deposited in reticuloendothelial cells, but with enough iron loading, redistribution to parenchymal cells occurs (8). Finally, *African iron overload* has been described in sub-Saharan Africa. Recent studies suggest that this is an inherited form of iron overload that is genetically distinct from HHC (i.e., not

Table 20.1
Causes of Iron Overload

Hereditary hemochromatosis (HHC)
(primary, genetic, idiopathic)

Secondary iron overload
  Ineffective erythropoiesis
    β-Thalassemia
    Sideroblastic anemia
    Aplastic anemia
    Pure red cell aplasia
  Liver disease
    Alcoholic cirrhosis
    Viral hepatitis, cirrhosis
    Following portocaval shunt
    Porphyria cutanea tarda
  Associated with excessive medicinal iron therapy

Parenteral iron overload
  Red blood cell transfusion
  Excessive iron chelate (e.g., iron-dextran) therapy
  Associated with hemodialysis
  African iron overload
  Neonatal hemochromatosis

histocompatibility leukocyte antigen (HLA)-linked) and can be exaggerated by the ingestion of home-brewed beer, which is rich in iron (9, 10).

Hereditary Hemochromatosis

PATHOGENESIS

The gene responsible for HHC has not been precisely localized but is known to be on the short arm of chromosome 6 in close proximity to the HLA-A locus (1, 2). Pedigree analysis and population screening studies in North America, Australia, and Europe have shown that the gene frequency is approximately 5%, with homozygotes being described in 0.2–0.7% and heterozygotes in 8–14% of the population (11). Although the disorder is not sex-linked, the disease is more pronounced and presents at an earlier age in males than in females. Excessive iron accumulation in females is usually delayed by as much as 10 years when compared with that in males, due in part to physiologic losses of iron from menstruation and pregnancy. The main organs that are affected in HHC include the liver, heart, pancreas, joints, and pituitary. In homozygotes, coincident alcohol ingestion seems to accel-erate the progression of the liver disease; thus, cirrhosis can be found at lower hepatic iron concentrations in those who drink excessive amounts of alcohol than in those who do not. Approximately 25% of heterozygotes for HHC will have minor increases in hepatic iron content with alterations in blood tests of iron status, but progressive tissue damage does not occur (12).

CLINICAL FEATURES AND DIAGNOSIS

Detailed analysis of the clinical manifestations of HHC is beyond the scope of this chapter, and the reader is referred to several recent reviews (1, 2). Typical presenting symptoms are often nonspecific and include weight loss, fatigue, weakness, apathy, and lack of libido. Other clinical findings and symptoms seen in HHC include arthritis, impotence, diabetes, amenorrhea, cirrhosis, and heart failure. These findings can mimic symptoms and findings seen in other common disorders, and, as a result, diagnosis and treatment are frequently delayed. With the advent of increased awareness of the disease and the introduction of multiphasic screening that includes serum iron levels, the diseases are now being detected in many patients prior to the development of symptoms. Once the diagnosis is suggested either by screening studies or assessment of symptoms, blood studies for iron metabolism, including serum iron, transferrin, and ferritin levels, will suggest those who should go on to have liver biopsy with quantitative iron determination.

TREATMENT

Once the diagnosis is confirmed by liver biopsy, the treatment of HHC is relatively straightforward. The vast majority of patients with HHC can be successfully treated with regular, intensive phlebotomy therapy (1, 2). The principal goal of therapy is to remove excess tissue iron prior to the development of complications. If this occurs (i.e., before fibrosis or cirrhosis develops), patients can expect normal survival (13). At the time of diagnosis, most symptomatic patients with HHC will have 15–30 g of excess storage iron (normal iron stores are ≈1 g). Typically, asymptomatic or younger individuals will be less loaded with iron (5–10 g). Since each unit of blood contains about 250 mg of iron, these patients will require extended phlebotomy regimens. During phlebotomy therapy, the goals are to remove excess iron quickly without compromising the patient's well-being. Most patients can tolerate weekly phlebotomy of 450–500 ml of whole blood. Younger patients may be able to tolerate removal of 2 units (1,000 ml) of blood per week, whereas some older patients can only tolerate phlebotomy of 250 ml every other week. Phlebotomy is continued until patients develop mild anemia. Although not absolutely necessary, transferrin saturation and ferritin levels can be determined every 6–8 weeks; these will predict the eventual return to normal iron stores. The ferritin level gradually decreases proportional to the decrease in tissue iron stores, whereas the transferrin saturation will remain elevated until normal iron stores are achieved.

Once iron stores have reached low normal, as evidenced by a ferritin level of <50 ng/ml and a transferrin saturation of less than 50%, maintenance phlebotomies will be required in most patients every 3–4 months. Post-treatment liver biopsy is not necessary unless questions about the persistence of fibrosis exist. The rate of reaccumulation of iron varies among individuals, and some patients may not require repeat phlebotomy for quite some time. The goal of maintenance therapy should be to keep the serum ferritin level <50 ng/ml. Dietary manipulations are not necessary, since the amounts of iron that can be reduced are insignificant when compared with what can be removed by phlebotomy.

The nonspecific symptoms of malaise, fatigue, and right upper quadrant abdominal pain usually improve with phlebotomy therapy (1, 2). Additionally, heart disease, diabetes mellitus, skin pigmentation, and abnormal liver enzymes with hepatomegaly virtually always reverse with careful phlebotomy therapy. In contrast, symptoms due to arthritis, established cirrhosis, and hypogonadism do not improve. In noncirrhotic patients who are suc-

cessfully treated, the risk of hepatocellular cancer (HCC), which is increased two hundred-fold in patients with untreated HHC, is reduced to normal (13). However, treated cirrhotic patients are still at risk for HCC and should be screened at 6-month intervals with hepatic ultrasound and α-fetoprotein levels.

Chelating Agents

In treating patients with HHC, chelating agents such as deferoxamine (DFO) are usually not necessary. Rarely, however, individuals who present with significant cardiac dysfunction due to HHC constitute a medical emergency, and should receive intravenous deferoxamine in addition to phlebotomy therapy at the initiation of their treatment regimen (1, 14). As mentioned above, phlebotomy removes approximately 250 mg of iron per unit of blood removed, whereas chelation therapy with continuous subcutaneous infusion of DFO results in urinary excretion of approximately 50–100 mg of iron per 24 hours (14, 15). Thus, while the amount of iron removed weekly is roughly comparable between the two modalities, phlebotomy is much simpler, cheaper, and quicker than continuous parenteral deferoxamine therapy.

Occasionally, patients with hemochromatosis will have anemia that precludes aggressive phlebotomy therapy. In this setting, cautious phlebotomy is recommended. Even with caution, phlebotomy may not be tolerated by an occasional patient. If so, then chelation therapy should be considered.

Secondary Iron Overload, Parenteral Iron Overload

In contrast to patients with HHC, patients with chronic anemia and secondary and/or parenteral iron overload due to ineffective erythropoiesis and chronic RBC transfusions cannot be treated by phlebotomy; and thus, iron chelation therapy with deferoxamine is used. These patients are not difficult to diagnose, since their underlying hematologic condition is known and their total body iron burden is easily determined by counting their

Table 20.2
Characteristics of Deferoxamine (Desferal) (105, 106)

Binding properties	1 g of deferoxamine can bind 85 mg of iron
	Greatest affinity (K = 10^{31}) for ferric iron to form ferrioxamine, a water-soluble chelate
Molecular weight	656
Solubility	Water soluble
Other atoms it binds	Zinc, aluminum
Origin	*Streptomyces pilosus*
Uptake in GI tract	Poor, <15% absorption; binds intraluminal iron
Usual mode of delivery	Subcutaneous, but may also be given intravenous or intramuscular
Uptake by hepatocytes	Yes
Biliary excretion	One-third of serum ferrioxamine—Fe complex
Urinary excretion	Two-thirds of serum ferrioxamine—Fe complex (orange-red urine)
Metabolism	Mostly by plasma enzymes

Table 20.3
Toxicity of Deferoxamine (105, 106)

Subcutaneous administration—local histamine-like reactions and induration
Intravenous administration (rapid)—hypotension, tachycardia, urticaria
Visual—decreased acuity, peripheral field loss, decreased dark adaptation, retinal vessel thinning, abnormal visual evoked response. More common with high doses (107)
Auditory—high frequency, sensorineural hearing loss. More common with high doses (107)
Growth retardation (if given before age 3 yr) (108)
Mucormycosis (rare) (109)
Enhanced virulence of *Yersinia enterocolitica*

transfusions. As with HHC, hepatic and cardiac disease can develop in these individuals due to iron overload (16, 17), so therapy is imperative. From the experience with thalassemic children, it has been learned that concomitant use of DFO from the beginning of the transfusion regimen improves survival rates (17). Thus, all patients who are subjected to a chronic transfusion program (e.g., those with sickle cell anemia, sideroblastic anemia, thalassemia, pure red cell aplasia, etc.) who have an otherwise good prognosis should be considered for concomitant DFO therapy. Unfortunately, iron chelation therapy is often only considered in these patients after multiple transfusions of packed RBCs have been given, and patients are already grossly iron-loaded, with tissue damage due to excess iron.

The reluctance to begin a chronic chelation program is related to the fact that DFO must be given parenterally, because there are no effective oral iron chelators available for use. Nonetheless, chelation therapy with DFO should be provided for these patients.

DFO can be given either as an intramuscular injection or by intravenous or subcutaneous infusion (Table 20.2). Continuous subcutaneous infusion of 2–4 g/12 hours using an infusion pump is the method most commonly employed. This results in urinary excretion of approximately 50–100 mg of iron per 24 hours. Complications of DFO therapy include pain at the injection site, and, rarely, long-term visual and auditory impairment (Table 20.3). Ascorbic acid in doses of 100–200 mg/day can be administered to enhance iron excretion with DFO. This should only be given after the DFO has been begun because of reports of enhanced cardiac toxicity when ascorbic acid is given without DFO.

Oral iron chelators which could be readily absorbed and excreted in the urine, loaded with iron, have been contemplated and are in developmental stages at the present time. However, no effective oral iron chelators are currently being used, perhaps because the development of safe and effective oral iron chelators has not been a high priority for the pharmaceutical industry. Currently, the hydroxypridinone group of chelators has been the most tested, and one of these agents, 1,2-dimethyl-3-hydroxypyrid-4-one (L1), has been subjected to a few limited, uncontrolled clinical trials (18). Severe toxicity has led to discontinuation of some trials until further testing is completed.

Wilson's Disease

PATHOGENESIS

Like hemochromatosis, Wilson's disease is a potentially treatable liver disease. The incidence of Wilson's disease is estimated at about 1 in 30,000 individuals (19). Family studies have established that Wilson's disease is inherited as an autosomal recessive disorder, and linkage studies have shown that the gene for Wilson's disease is located on chromosome 13 near the esterase *d* locus (20). It has been speculated that the gene for the disease is a mutant of a single regulator gene that results in impairment of both ceruloplasmin synthesis and biliary copper excretion.

CLINICAL MANIFESTATIONS AND DIAGNOSIS

The clinical manifestations of Wilson's disease are usually not seen prior to the age of 6 years, and the typical hepatic and neurologic manifestations usually present in adolescence or early adult life. By 15 years of age, almost half of the patients with Wilson's disease will have symptoms referable to the disease. Of these symptomatic patients, approximately 40% present initially with hepatic manifestations, 35% with neurologic manifestations, and 10% with psychiatric manifestations. In approximately 25% of patients, presenting signs and symptoms originate from two or more organ systems (21). It is important to emphasize that patients presenting with neurologic disease all have evidence of pre-existing chronic liver disease. The hepatic manifestations of Wilson's disease are classified into four main clinicopathologic groups: (1) acute hepatitis with features of steatosis; (2) fulminant hepatitis with rapid progression; (3) chronic active hepatitis; and, (4) cirrhosis. Further information on clinical presentation and diagnosis of Wilson's disease can be found in several recent review articles (21–23).

Once Wilson's disease is diagnosed by characteristic ceruloplasmin levels, 24-hour urinary copper determinations, hepatic histology, and quantitative hepatic copper determinations, then therapy with copper chelating drugs should be initiated. Because Wilson's disease is one of the few serious metabolic disorders for which a specific and effective treatment is available, all patients, whether they are asymptomatic or whether they have established disease, should be given the benefit of decoppering therapy.

TREATMENT

D-Penicillamine. The chelating agent, D-penicillamine, is the drug of choice in Wilson's disease and was first used by Walshe in 1956 (24). It replaced the use of dimercaprol which had good chelating capability but had many toxic side effects. The D-isomer of penicillamine is more effective than the L-isomer, and is used clinically. In the reduced state, D-penicillamine is highly water-soluble and is rapidly excreted by the kidneys (Table 20.4). However, D-penicillamine is also degraded by the liver, and metabolites are seen in both urine and stool. Bioavailability is excellent with a 50–70% rate of absorption from the gastrointestinal tract, and peak concentrations are reached at approximately 1–3 hours after ingestion. Food, antacids, and medicinal iron can reduce absorption, so it is best taken between meals. The mechanisms of action of D-penicillamine have been widely studied, and in addition to its copper chelating effects, D-penicillamine induces synthesis of hepatic metallothionein (25–27), a cellular copper-binding protein. Chelation of nonceruloplasmin-bound copper in the serum results in an efficient cupriuresis. Finally, some studies have shown that D-penicillamine has efficacy as an antiinflammatory agent based on its effects on lymphocyte function (28).

Dosage of D-penicillamine in patients with Wilson's disease varies with the age and size of the patients as well as with the severity of the disease. In uncomplicated adults, the recommended initial dosage is 1–2 g/day in four divided doses (29). Some patients with neu-

Table 20.4
Characteristics of D-Penicillamine (Cuprimine) (110)

Binding properties	1 g of D-penicillamine can bind 200 mg of copper
Molecular weight	149
Solubility	Water soluble, slightly soluble in alcohol
Other atoms it binds	Iron, mercury, lead, gold, arsenic, pyridoxine, zinc
Origin	Inactive metabolic byproduct of penicillin isolated from urine; now manufactured synthetically
Uptake in GI tract	Good, 40–70% absorbed; decreased by antacids, foods, iron. Peak serum concentration 1.5–4 hr after oral ingestion
Usual mode of delivery	Oral
Uptake by hepatocytes	Yes, but poor binding of hepatocellular copper
Biliary excretion	Yes
Urinary excretion	Yes, major route of excretion
Metabolism	Hepatic biotransformation; renal excretion, unchanged

rologic disease may experience a deterioration during the first several weeks of high-dose D-penicillamine therapy. This is thought to be due to a transient rise in serum and brain copper levels during the initial treatment period (30). To circumvent this unfortunate situation, some authorities recommend an initial starting dose of 250 mg/day, which is gradually increased by 250 mg/day every 3–4 days until there is sufficient negative copper balance as evidenced by 24-hour urinary copper excretion in excess of 2 mg (30, 31). Since D-penicillamine is a pyridoxine antimetabolite, supplemental vitamin B_6 is usually recommended during periods of stress such as growth, pregnancy, and concomitant illness (32). The dose of vitamin B_6 is 50 mg weekly or 10 mg daily (23). D-Penicillamine therapy is not useful in acute Wilsonian crises, such as fulminant hepatic failure or hemolysis. In these settings, orthotopic liver transplantation is the only successful form of therapy (33).

Once initial therapy is begun, maintenance therapy is designed to keep the dose as low as possible to maintain effective cupriuresis. This can be accomplished by following 24-hour urinary copper excretion, expecting 500–1,000 μg/24 hours (23). This can usually be accomplished with a dose of 375–500 mg twice a day and should be continued for life. Patient compliance with this medical regimen needs to be life-long and is particularly critical, since abrupt reduction of therapy has led to catastrophic and sometimes irreparable or-

gan damage or death (34). Strict dietary restrictions are probably unnecessary, but avoidance of foods with high copper content such as liver, chocolate, nuts, shellfish, mushrooms, broccoli, and enriched cereals is prudent (35). In general, the average Western diet contains approximately 1 mg of copper per day. The daily obligatory copper loss is approximately 0.6–0.8 mg/day; thus, negative copper balance with D-penicillamine is fairly easily achieved. Prognosis is excellent when maintenance therapy is well-tolerated, provided patients are compliant and closely monitored.

Although efficacy with D-penicillamine is high, approximately 60% of patients have some adverse effects (Table 20.5) and approximately 10% will have intolerance to the drug. Hematologic, nephrologic, rheumatologic, or dermatologic complications are those most likely to lead to cessation of therapy with D-penicillamine. When complications of D-penicillamine therapy develop, there are several approaches that can be contemplated. One is to discontinue D-penicillamine altogether and change to another form of decoppering therapy such as trientine, zinc, therapy, or tetrathiomolybdate. For more severe side effects such as leukopenia, aplastic anemia, and severe nephropathy, this is the preferred approach. Alternatively, patients can be temporarily withdrawn from D-penicillamine to allow the side effects to ameliorate, followed by gradual reinstitution at very low doses (10

Table 20.5
Toxicity of D-Penicillamine

Organ system	Clinical feature	Reference
Hematologic	Leukopenia, aplastic anemia, agranulocytosis, pancytopenia, thrombocytopenia[a]	29, 111
	IgA deficiency	112
	Acute lymphoblastic leukemia[a]	113
Renal	Proteinuria[a]	114–116
	Goodpasture's syndrome[a]	117
Dermatologic	Maculopapular rash, urticaria	29, 118–120
	Pemphigoid lesions[a]	120
	Elastosis perforans serpiginosa[a]	121
	White papules at venipuncture[a]	118
	Dermatopathy $\pm$ lymphangiectasia[a]	122
Hepatic	Liver enzyme elevation (mild)	123
	Toxic hepatitis[a]	123
	Cholestatic jaundice[a]	124
Gastrointestinal	Nausea, vomiting, diarrhea	29
	Ileal stenosis	125
Rheumatologic	Arthropathy[a] (delayed hypersensitivity reaction)	126
Neurologic	Myasthenia gravis[a]	127
	Optic neuritis[a]	127

[a]Withdrawal of D-penicillamine beneficial.

mg/day). Subsequently, doses are increased in accordance to the patient's tolerance. Finally, some patients can have their drug therapy withdrawn and then reinstituted at low doses with the concomitant administration of prednisone (23, 36).

D-Penicillamine is an effective drug for initial and maintenance therapy, but it has a high toxicity profile. It is useful in symptomatic, as well as presymptomatic cases. With adequate patient compliance, prognosis is usually excellent, because the drug is successful in reducing tissue copper levels and preventing disease progression.

Trientine. An alternative copper chelating agent to D-penicillamine is trientine, which has recently been approved by the FDA and has been used in patients with Wilson's disease who are intolerant of D-penicillamine (36). Trientine can effectively chelate copper bound to albumin, but is unable to enter hepatocytes to bind intracellular copper (37). Initial cupriuresis by trientine is comparable to that exhibited for D-penicillamine; however, the level of cupriuresis progressively declines as trientine therapy continues (36). Despite this observation, patients treated with

trientine remain in remission, suggesting that other mechanisms (as yet unknown) may contribute to favorable copper balance during trientine therapy. Initial therapy is with 250 mg four times a day, which should be given either 1 hour before or 2 hours after meals (38). Experience with trientine as an initial form of therapy for Wilson's disease, is limited and it has more commonly been used as an alternative therapy for patients which are intolerant of D-penicillamine. To date, no documented neurologic or hepatologic decompensation has been seen with trientine, as is known to occur with initial therapy with D-penicillamine. However, this may relate to the fact that trientine has not been used very often as initial therapy. Once effective cupriuresis is induced, maintenance therapy with trientine can be achieved with approximately 500 mg–1 g given daily. Goals are to keep 24-hour urinary copper excretion at about 200–700 μg (23). Adverse effects of trientine are relatively minor and are shown in Table 20.6.

In summary, trientine has been used as a substitute therapy for patients intolerant of D-penicillamine. Its efficacy as initial therapy is

Table 20.6
Toxicity of Trientine

Organ system	Clinical feature	Reference
Hematologic (iron chelation)	Iron deficiency	128
	Sideroblastic anemia (copper deficiency)	38
Gastrointestinal (hypersensitivity)	Dyspepsia	129
Dermatologic (hypersensitivity)	Skin rash	129
Musculoskeletal (hypersensitivity)	Acute rhabdomyolysis	129

as yet unproven. More studies to determine its potential for side effects and usefulness as induction therapy are necessary.

Zinc. The other major form of treatment for Wilson's disease has been the use of zinc acetate. Zinc supplementation for treatment of Wilson's disease was first described in the early 1960s by Schouwink (39) and has been extensively studied by Brewer and colleagues (40, 41). Its principal mechanism of action appears to be an induction of intestinal metallothionein (42, 43), which leads to increased binding of copper in the intestine, making it unavailable for absorption. Zinc has also been shown to induce hepatic metallothionein (44), which can then bind hepatocellular copper and reduce the toxic consequences of increased cytosolic copper. Dosing studies have been performed, and it appears that the best negative copper balance is achieved with a dose of 50 mg of zinc as the acetate form given three times a day between meals. Simultaneous administration of D-penicillamine with zinc does not result in increased efficacy of therapy, because zinc interferes with the intestinal absorption of D-penicillamine (45).

Maintenance therapy with zinc acetate is well-tolerated and is effective in keeping patients in negative copper balance. It should be considered for those patients who are intolerant of D-penicillamine or trientine. Some authorities recommend zinc acetate as the maintenance therapy of choice after initial decoppering therapy has been achieved with either D-penicillamine or trientine.

Whether or not zinc acetate should be used as initial therapy for Wilson's disease is still controversial. Initial studies have shown that it can be an effective form of therapy; however, patient numbers are small and D-penicillamine has a long track record in this situation. Current recommendations are to use traditional copper chelating drugs as initial therapy and to reserve use of zinc for those who are either intolerant of D-penicillamine or trientine or as maintenance therapy after initial decoppering therapy has been achieved. As with D-penicillamine, prognosis is excellent if patients are compliant. Monitoring of clinical efficacy of zinc therapy relies on 24-hour urinary copper excretion studies. Most patients who receive zinc maintenance therapy have 24-hour urinary copper excretion in excess of 150 μg (46). Adverse effects from zinc therapy are trivial and are listed in Table 20.7.

Tetrathiomolybdate. One of the biggest problems in treatment of patients with Wilson's disease is arriving at successful initial therapy that does not lead to increased neurologic deterioration. Zinc compounds have delayed onset of action and are of questionable efficacy in induction therapy in patients with severe disease. D-Penicillamine can often induce neurologic deterioration, and in some patients, this may be irreversible. Trientine has not been used in large numbers of individuals as induction therapy. These problems have led to the consideration of tetrathiomolybdate for use as initial therapy. Tetrathio-

Table 20.7
Toxicity of Zinc

Organ system	Clinical feature	Reference
Hematologic (high dose)	Suppression of chemotaxis, phagocytosis by polymorphonuclear leukocytes	130
	Decreased lymphocyte response to phytohemagglutinin	130
Metabolic (high dose)	Elevation of low-density lipoprotein level	130
	Reduction of high-density lipoprotein level	130
	Increase in atherogenic indices	130
Musculoskeletal resorption (rats)	Hypocalcemia, increased bone	131
Gastrointestinal	Decreased appetite, diarrhea, jaundice, dehydration (calves)	132

molybdate is a copper chelating agent that has been extensively tested in animal models (47–49) and is thought to have at least three mechanisms of action in the treatment with copper overload. First, it binds with copper in the gastrointestinal tract, thus prevent ing absorption (47–49), and secondly, it binds with nonceruloplasmin-bound copper in the plasma (50), making this form of copper unavailable for cellular uptake. Finally, it is known to interact with hepatic metallothionein resulting in a reduction in hepatic copper content and enhanced biliary excretion of copper (50).

It has been suggested that tetrathiomolybdate be given with meals to block copper absorption and between meals to bind the nonceruloplasmin copper found in serum (51). The daily dose is 2–3 mg/day; this is distributed as one-third given with meals and two-thirds given between meals. Inhibition of copper absorption is immediate, but to completely reduce serum nonceruloplasmin levels of copper, 2–3 weeks of therapy are necessary. To date, no toxicity or adverse effects have been reported, and in small studies, stabilization of neurologic status has been achieved with favorable outcomes.

Tetrathiomolybdate may be a promising new copper chelating agent for the initial treatment of Wilson's disease, but larger studies are needed to compare it with other copper chelating agents. Its use as a maintenance therapy is as yet unproven.

PREGNANCY AND WILSON'S DISEASE

Because Wilson's disease has its primary manifestations in adolescence and young adulthood and because drug therapy is life-long, a special consideration is the effect of Wilson's disease therapy on pregnancy. Untreated Wilson's disease can result in infertility, spontaneous abortion, and premature delivery (52, 53). However, patients who have Wilson's disease successfully treated prior to the development of end-stage hepatic and/or neurologic complications have normal fertility, and the possibility of full-term pregnancy is quite high (52, 54, 55). In normal pregnancies, serum ceruloplasmin and serum copper levels can increase two- to fourfold, and even in adequately treated patients with Wilson's disease who are relatively copper-deficient, pregnancy can cause a 50% increase in serum nonceruloplasmin copper and in urinary copper excretion (56). These elevated levels usually return to prepregnancy levels by 6 months after delivery. It is reassuring that D-penicillamine, the most commonly used drug in patients with Wilson's disease, appears to be relatively safe in pregnancy (53, 57); however, teratogenic effects of D-penicillamine have been described. Birth defects related to connective tissue abnormalities such as cutis laxa and increased joint mobility may be due to D-penicillamine's known interference of collagen cross-linking (58). No strong recommendations for trientine can be made, since so few patients have used trientine while pregnant.

There are no known teratogenic effects of zinc therapy, and tetrathiomolybdate has not been studied.

In summary, the teratogenic effects of therapies for Wilson's disease appear quite limited, and cessation of therapy can precipitate acute decompensation, placing both mother and fetus at risk for increased morbidity or perhaps mortality. For these reasons, copper chelating therapy should be continued through pregnancy. Pyridoxine (vitamin B_6) should be given as supplemental therapy if D-penicillamine is used during pregnancy, and serum zinc levels should be checked periodically during chelation therapy to avoid clinical deficiency. Finally, there have been reports of spontaneous regression of Wilson's disease during pregnancy (59, 60), perhaps due to increased serum ceruloplasmin levels as an acute phase response and/or the effect of fetal development on removing maternal copper. This is controversial, since the fetal requirements for copper are negligible compared with the total maternal storage amounts of copper.

The Porphyrias

The porphyrias are a group of metabolic disorders characterized by various inherited or acquired enzyme deficiencies that result in abnormalities in heme biosynthesis. Specific enzyme deficiencies have been identified for each of the several types of porphyria (Table 20.8). Synthesis of heme is required by all cells, but the bone marrow and the liver are the only organs that are quantitatively important in the overproduction of porphyrins and porphyrin precursors in these various conditions. The major clinical manifestations of the porphyrias are dermatologic, neurologic, and hepatic disorders (61). The dermatologic conditions result from the photosensitizing effects of accumulated porphyrins which are deposited in the skin or found in the dermal circulation. The neurologic disturbances occur in those types of porphyria that are complicated by acute attacks of abdominal pain, believed to be caused by an autonomic neuropathy that affects the gastrointestinal tract.

Porphyria cutanea tarda (PCT) is the most common type of porphyria. Abdominal pain is not seen, but hepatic dysfunction with structural damage can occur. The biochemical defect in either the more common, acquired form or the rare, inherited form of PCT is a deficiency in the activity of the enzyme, uroporphobilinogen decarboxylase, which results in an increase in tissue and urinary uroporphyrins and hepatocarboxyl porphyrins. Patients with PCT have a variety of cutaneous manifestations including blisters, vesicles, and sores that develop at sites of mild trauma and in sun-exposed areas like the hands, forehead, ears, and neck. In addition to the accumulation of porphyrin in the liver, PCT is associated with excessive hepatic iron deposition in about 75% of patients. The cause of the iron overload is unknown, but the role of the increased iron in the pathogenesis of symptomatic PCT is well-established (62). Diminution of iron stores by phlebotomy therapy ameliorates the biochemical and symptomatic manifestations of the disease, and replenishment of iron stores after successful therapy causes biochemical relapse.

The mainstays of therapy for PCT are to remove excess iron by phlebotomy and to avoid any drugs such as alcohol or estrogens that have been implicated in the clinical expression of the disease. Excess iron stores in PCT are not as great as those seen in hereditary hemochromatosis, and weekly phlebotomy will usually result in iron deficiency after 4–6 months (4–6 g of excess iron). Chloroquine has also been advocated in reduced dosages (125 mg two to three times per week) for those patients who do not respond to phlebotomy therapy. Chloroquine appears to work by enhancing the removal of porphyrins from tissues with subsequent urinary excretion.

The other form of porphyria that is amenable to pharmacologic therapy is *acute intermittent porphyria* (AIP) caused by a defect in porphobilinogen deaminase. Patients with AIP do not have structural liver disease but can present with recurrent episodes of acute abdominal pain that can be quite distressing.

Table 20.8
Classification and Diagnosis of the Porphyrias[a]

Disease	Enzyme defect	Structural hepatic involvement	Acute abdominal pain	Diagnostic findings						
				Urinary				Fecal		
				ALA	PBG	Uro	Copro	Uro	Copro	Proto
ALA dehydrase deficiency	ALA dehydrase	−	+	↑↑	↑	↑	↑↑	nl	nl	nl
Acute intermittent porphyria	Porphobilinogen deaminase	−	+	↑	↑	nl-↑	nl-↑	nl-↑	nl-↑	nl-↑
Congenital erythropoietic porphyria	Uroporphyrinogen III synthase	+	−	nl	nl	↑↑	↑	↑↑	↑↑	nl
Porphyria cutanea tarda	Uroporphyrinogen decarboxylase	+	−	nl	nl	↑↑	↑	↑	↑	nl
Hepatoerythropoietic porphyria	Uroporphyrinogen decarboxylase (severe)	+	−	nl	nl	↑↑	↑	↑	↑	↑
Hereditary coproporphyria	Coproporphyrinogen oxidase	−	+	nl-↑↑	nl-↑↑	nl-↑	↑↑	nl	↑	↑
Variegate porphyria	Protoporphyrinogen oxidase	−	+	nl-↑↑	nl-↑↑	nl-↑	↑↑	nl	↑	↑↑
Protoporphyria	Ferrochelatase	+	−	nl	nl	nl-↑	nl-↑	nl	nl-↑	↑↑
Normal values:				<3[b]	<2.5[b]	10–60[c]	50–250[c]	0–5[d]	Tr-50[d]	Tr-120[d]

[a]From Reference (81) with permission from the authors. Abbreviations: ALA-aminolevulinic acid; nl, normal; Tr, trace; PBG, porphobilinogen; Uro, uroporphyrin; Copro, coproporphyrin; Proto, protoporphyrin.
[b]mg/g of creatinine.
[c]μg/g of creatinine.
[d]μg/g of dry weight stool.

The usual therapeutic approach in these individuals has been to try to prevent attacks by avoiding offending drugs such as estrogen, phenobarbital, and alcohol. Some patients respond to carbohydrate loading (at least 300 g/day). If patients continue to have attacks of abdominal pain despite avoidance of drugs and carbohydrate loading, some investigators have proposed the use of intravenous hematin (63, 64). Infusions of hematin have resulted in prompt decreases in the hepatic overproduction of aminolevulinic acid (ALA) and porphobilinogen (PBG). Symptoms of abdominal pain usually improve as well. (See [64] for a more detailed discussion of hematin use in acute porphyria).

α_1-Antitrypsin Deficiency

α_1-Antitrypsin (α_1-AT) is a glycoprotein synthesized primarily by the liver which functions in the plasma and extracellular fluids as a protease inhibitor (65). In addition to trypsin, α_1-AT also inhibits chymotrypsin, renin, urokinase, elastase, collagenase, and the proteases found in polymorphonuclear neutrophils. The clinical relevance of α_1-AT deficiency was first recognized in the early 1960s when an association between low levels of α_1-AT and early onset pulmonary emphysema was described (66). In 1969, Sharp et al. described an association between neonatal hepatitis and childhood cirrhosis and a deficiency of α_1-AT (67). Since then, it has been recognized that α_1-AT deficiency is more common than initially suspected, is easily diagnosed, and can present in adult life as cryptogenic cirrhosis without an antecedent history of liver disease in infancy.

There are at least 32 different alleles for the α_1-AT gene, resulting in numerous types of phenotypic expression due to the different combinations of alleles. The most common allele is PiMM, with a frequency in Americans of approximately 95% (68). Normal serum concentrations of α_1-AT are seen in individuals with homozygous PiMM phenotype. The most severe deficiency of α_1-AT is associated with the PiZZ homozygous state in which the circulating α_1-AT concentration is only about 15% of normal. This phenotype is present in approximately 0.03% of the population (69). The vast majority of patients with clinical liver disease due to α_1-AT deficiency have this phenotype, although there are many individuals with PiZZ phenotype who have no disease. α_1-AT of the Z phenotype exhibits a selective defect in transport of α_1-AT from the endoplasmic reticulum to the Golgi apparatus, resulting in accumulation of α_1-AT in the endoplasmic reticulum. This defect in secretion is attributed to a single amino acid substitution with replacement of glutamic acid by lysine at the 342 position. It appears that liver injury is a direct consequence of the intracellular accumulation of the mutant α_1-AT molecules (70).

Previously, therapy for α_1-AT deficiency had been directed toward increasing synthesis of α_1-AT by the use of either estrogen, progesterone, contraceptives (71), danazol (72), tamoxifen (73), or phenobarbital (65). Some authorities have been concerned that liver damage may be potentiated by an increased synthesis and accumulation of α_1-AT without there being a concomitant increase in secretion caused by the basic defect in the protein (65). More importantly, no clinical improvement has been identified in individuals who received any of these forms of therapy. Gene transfer therapy has been considered for treatment of α_1-AT deficiency (74, 75). The objective here is to introduce sufficient M genes to the liver of an α_1-AT-deficient individual and to convert them to either an MM homozygous or MZ heterozygous state. Use of this form of therapy in a practical fashion is not yet available. Presently, orthotopic liver transplantation is the treatment of choice, since it provides an effective treatment for the complications of chronic liver disease and results in a cure for α_1-AT deficiency (76, 77). Following transplantation, long-term survival for children and adults is relatively good with 5-year survival greater than 60% (76). After liver transplantation, the recipient converts to the phenotype of the donor (78). This conversion appears to be permanent, as reversion to the original phenotype has not been reported. Additionally, transplant recipients normalize their serum α_1-AT levels (76, 77, 79) and no longer develop pulmonary or other complications of α_1-AT deficiency (70).

Total Parenteral Nutrition-Induced Liver Disease

Total parenteral nutrition (TPN) is a commonly employed means of providing nutrition in a wide variety of clinical settings. With its increasing use, complications of TPN have become more precisely characterized, and their effective management is important. Abnormalities in liver function constitute a major complication of TPN. Usually, TPN-related hepatotoxicity only consists of fatty liver similar to nonalcoholic steatosis related to obesity, but more advanced lesions such as steatonecrosis, portal fibrosis, and cirrhosis have been described (80–83). In addition, a unique cholestatic syndrome may complicate the use of TPN.

Fatty liver most commonly presents within 3 weeks from institution of TPN (81). Individuals are asymptomatic and serum aminotransferase elevations are the most frequent clinical manifestation. The pathogenetic mechanisms are probably multifactorial, but are associated with an imbalance between deposition and mobilization of neutral fat into and from the liver (82). Other clinical factors may contribute to the imbalance including the infusion of excessive glucose-containing solutions leading to secondary hyperinsulinism (80). Additionally, essential fatty acid deficiency can occur that will interfere with fat mobilization from the liver and impede transport of long-chain fatty acids into hepatic mitochondria (84). Finally, excessive caloric intake in conjunction with low nitrogen intake can result in fatty liver (85). Treatment that has been suggested for fatty liver due to TPN is to decrease the concentration of glucose that is being infused and to substitute the caloric requirement with either lipids or amino acids (82). In addition, a reduction of excessive caloric infusion can be instituted, and attempts to achieve a more balanced calorie to

nitrogen intake ratio of approximately 150 kcal to 1 g of nitrogen should be tried (82). Infusion of 10% lipid emulsions is an effective means for treating essential fatty acid deficiency and, as mentioned above, lipid emulsion can be substituted for glucose for one-third to one-half of total calories (84). Finally, cyclic TPN therapy is also advocated with administration of TPN nightly over a 10–12 hour infusion (86). The majority of patients who develop aminotransferase elevations within 3 weeks of TPN therapy return to normal with continuation of TPN therapy, and there are no known reports of progressive liver damage once plasma alanine aminotransferase (ALT) levels return to normal.

The other hepatic abnormality that occurs in patients receiving chronic TPN is the development of cholestasis (82, 83). This is the predominant hepatic lesion in patients who receive TPN for more than 3 weeks. It is characterized by an increase in alkaline phosphatase and an elevation in bilirubin with modest increases in aminotransferases. In the majority of patients, serum bilirubin is in the 2–5 mg/dl range (87). When liver biopsies are performed, lymphocytic infiltrates and periportal canalicular bile plugs with mild triaditis are seen. Occasionally, an increase in portal fibrosis has been identified (80). The pathogenetic factors are poorly understood, but many theories have been proposed. These include the development of bacterial overgrowth due to diminished intestinal motility during the fasting state, resulting in portal endotoxemia and/or the conversion of chenodeoxycholic acid to the more pathogenic lithocholic acid (80, 88). When lithocholic acid constitutes as much as 7–15% of the total bile acid pool, it has been shown to induce hepatic histologic changes in experimental animals similar to those seen in patients with TPN cholestasis (88). Alternatively, some have suggested that the increase in lipid infusion is the cause of cholestasis due to TPN (87), whereas others have questioned deficiencies of taurine (89), which interferes with bile salt formation, conjugation, and subsequent excretion. Deficiency of choline (90), methionine (91), molybdenum (83), or antioxidants (92) have all been implicated.

Treatment modalities include the exclusion of correctable extrahepatic obstruction such as gallstones using either ultrasonography or endoscopic cholangiography. Empiric trials of metronidazole given at doses of 500 mg intravenously each 6–8 hours have been used to treat (93) and prevent intestinal anaerobic infection (94–96). Alterations in lipid infusions and/or cyclic parenteral nutrition have been suggested as effective therapies (86). Finally, searches for possible deficiencies of certain amino acids or trace elements in the infusate and subsequent correction should be considered. There is no proven efficacy of empiric supplementation with antioxidants. If at all possible, consideration should be given to discontinuation of TPN and resumption of oral feedings (80). Virtually all cases of TPN cholestasis improve or normalize with initiation of enteral nutrition. Rare complications of TPN cholestasis such as fibrosis and cirrhosis (97, 98) have been described. Thus, this is a disorder that should be taken seriously.

Whenever patients receiving long-term TPN are evaluated for cholestasis, one should keep in mind that extrahepatic obstruction needs to be effectively considered and excluded. The cases of these patients are usually complex. Frequently, the patients have multiple medical and/or surgical problems and are susceptible to the development of cholelithiasis (99), gallbladder sludge (100), or acalculous cholecystitis (101). In fact, by 6 weeks of TPN therapy, virtually all patients will have gallbladder sludge identified by ultrasonography (100). If cholestasis is found to be due to gallstones, treatment is by the usual methods, either by cholecystectomy or with endoscopic sphincterotomy (83). Perhaps more important than treating the complications is prevention of the development of complications. Recommendations include ingestion of small amounts of lipid and/or protein to periodically stimulate gallbladder contraction (83, 102). Some investigators have suggested the use of intravenous cholecystokinin on a daily basis; however, this is costly (103). In-

fusion of a large volume of crystalline amino acids may stimulate endogenous cholecystokinin secretion, which in turn would promote gallbladder contraction and emptying (83). Finally, agents that increase bile flow such as ursodeoxycholic acid have not had a significant impact on reducing the incidence of sludge formation due to the already abnormal cholesterol secretion and increased total bile acid pools that are found in these patients (100). Fortunately, acalculous cholecystitis is an infrequent complication (<5%) in patients receiving chronic TPN. However, mortality is high because of other comorbid medical conditions and delayed diagnosis (104).

OVERALL SUMMARY

There are several major categories of inherited and metabolic liver disorders that are amenable to specific therapies. The principal form of therapy for hereditary hemochromatosis remains aggressive phlebotomy. Some individuals require concomitant use of deferoxamine. Alternatively, in secondary and/or transfusional iron overload, therapy with parenteral iron chelators such as deferoxamine is all that is available. Hopefully, safe and effective oral iron chelators will become available in the future. Treatment of Wilson's disease with copper chelating drugs such as D-penicillamine and trientine is fairly well-established, and maintenance therapy with zinc acetate supplementation appears to be highly efficacious. Treatment of the porphyrias is limited and revolves around prevention of induction of heme synthesis by avoidance of certain drugs. Hematin has a limited role in acute intermittent porphyria. Unfortunately, there is no good pharmacologic therapy for α_1-antitrypsin deficiency despite a vastly increased knowledge of the pathophysiologic mechanisms of this protein abnormality. Orthotopic liver transplantation remains the treatment of choice. Finally, total parenteral nutrition results in specific hepatic lesions that are amenable to alterations in the infusate and treatment with metronidazole for the cholestatic form of this disease. As our knowledge of pharmacology and pathophysiology improves, we will expect to see new therapies available for the treatment of these diseases.

REFERENCES

1. Tavill AS, Bacon BR. Hemochromatosis: iron metabolism and the iron overload syndromes. In: Zakim D, Boyer TD, eds. Hepatology: a textbook of liver disease. Philadelphia: Saunders, 1990:1273–1299.
2. Nichols GM, Bacon BR. Hereditary hemochromatosis: pathogenesis and clinical features of a common disease. Am J Gastroenterol 1989;84:851–862.
3. McLaren GD, Nathanson MH, Jacobs A, Trevett D, Thomson W. Regulation of intestinal iron absorption and mucosal iron kinetics in hereditary hemochromatosis. J Lab Clin Med 1991;117:390–401.
4. Chapman RW, Morgan MY, Laulicht M, Hoffbrand AV, Sherlock S. Hepatic iron stores and markers of iron overload in alcoholics and patients with hemochromatosis. Dig Dis Sci 1982;27:909–916.
5. Di Bisceglie AM, Axiotis CA, Hoofnagle JH, Bacon BR. Measurements of iron status in patients with chronic hepatitis. Gastroenterology 1992;102:2108–2113.
6. Conn HO. Portacaval anastomosis and hepatic hemosiderin deposition: a prospective, controlled investigation. Gastroenterology 1972;62:61–72.
7. Bonkovsky HL. Porphyrin and heme metabolism and the porphyrias. In: Zakim D, Boyer TD, eds. Hepatology. a textbook of liver disease. Philadelphia: Saunders 1990:378–423.
8. Sibille J-C, Kondo H, Aisen P. Interactions between isolated hepatocytes and Kupffer cells in iron metabolism: a possible role for ferritin as an iron carrier protein. Hepatology 1988;8:296–301.
9. Gordeuk V, Mukiibi J, Hasstedt SJ, et al. Iron overload in Africa: interaction between a gene and dietary iron content. N Engl J Med 1992;326:95–100.
10. Bacon BR. Causes of iron overload. N Engl J Med 1992;326:126–127.
11. Edwards CQ, Griffen LM, Kaplan J, Kushner JP. Twenty-four hour variation of transferrin saturation in treated and untreated hemochromatosis homozygotes. J Intern Med 1989;226:373–379.
12. Bassett ML, Halliday JL, Powell LW. HLA typing in idiopathic hemochromatosis: distinction between homozygotes and heterozygotes with biochemical expression. Hepatology 1981;1:120–126.
13. Niederau C, Fischer R, Sonnenberg A, Stremmel W, Trampisch HJ, Strohmeyer G. Survival and causes of death in cirrhotic and in noncirrhotic patients with primary hemochromatosis. N Engl J Med 1985;313:1256–1262.
14. Cohen A, Witzleben C, Schwartz E. Treatment of iron overload. Semin Liver Dis 1984;4:228–238.
15. Propper RD, Cooper B, Rufo RR, et al. Continuous subcutaneous administration of deferoxamine in patients with iron overload. N Engl J Med 1977;297:418–423.
16. Cohen A, Martin M, Schwartz E. Depletion of excessive liver iron stores with desferrioxamine. Br J Haematol 1984;58:369–373.
17. Wolfe L, Olivieri N, Sallan D, et al. Prevention of cardiac disease by subcutaneous deferoxamine in patients with thalassemia major. N Engl J Med 1985;312:1600–1603.
18. Porter JB, Hider RC, Huehns ER. Update on the hydroxypyridinone oral iron-chelating agents. Semin Hematol 1990;27:95–100.
19. Scheinberg IH, Sternlieb I. Wilson's disease. In: Smith LH, ed. Major problems in internal medicine series. Philadelphia: Saunders, 1984.
20. Frydman M, Bonné-Tamir B, Farrer LA, et al. Assignment of the gene for Wilson disease to chromosome 13: linkage to the esterase D locus. Proc Natl Acad Sci USA 1985;82:1819–1821.
21. Sternlieb I. Perspectives on Wilson's disease. Hepatology 1990;12:1234–1239.
22. Stremmel W, Meyerrow KW, Niederau C, Hefter H, Kreuzpaintner G, Strohmeyer G. Wilson's disease: clinical presentation, treatment, and survival. Ann Intern Med 1991;115:720–726.
23. Brewer GJ, Yuzbasiyan-Durkan V. Wilson's disease: an update, with emphasis on new approaches to treatment. Dig Dis Sci 1989;7:178–193.
24. Walshe JM. Penicillamine: a new oral therapy for Wilson's disease. Am J Med 1956;21:487–495.
25. Scheinberg IH, Sternlieb I. Penicillamine may detoxify copper in Wilson's disease. Lancet 1987;2:95.
26. Goering PL, Tanden SK, Kassasen CD. Induction of hepatic metallothionein in mouse liver following administration of chelating agents. Toxicol Appl Pharmacol 1985;30:467–472.
27. Heilmaier HE, Jiang JL, Greim H, Schramel P, Summer KH. D-Penicillamine induces rat hepatic metallothionein. Toxicology 1986;42:23–31.
28. Stern RB, Wilkinson SP, Howorth PJN, Williams R. Controlled trial of synthetic D-penicillamine in maintenance therapy for active chronic hepatitis. Gut 1977;18:19–22.
29. Klaassen CD. Heavy metals and heavy metal antagonists. In: Gilman AG, Rall TW, Nies AS, Taylor P, eds. Goodman and Gillman's The pharmacological basis of therapeutics. New York: Pergamon Press, 1990:1610–1611.
30. Brewer GJ, Terry CA, Aisen AM. Worsening of neurological syndrome in patients with Wilson's disease with initial penicillamine therapy. Arch Neurol 1987;44:490–494.
31. Glass J, Reich SG, DeLong M. Wilson's disease-development of neurological disease after beginning penicillamine therapy. Arch Neurol 1990;47:595–596.
32. Walshe JM. Brief observations on the management of Wilson's disease. Proc R Soc Med 1977;70:1–3.

33. Sternlieb I. Wilson disease: Indications for liver transplant. Hepatology 1984;4:155–175.

34. Walshe JM, Dixon AK. Dangers of non-compliance in Wilson's disease. Lancet 1986;1:845–847.

35. Hook L, Brandt IA. Copper content of some low-copper foods. J Am Diet Assoc 1966;49:202–203.

36. Brewer GJ, Yuzbasiyan-Gurkan V, Young AB. Treatment of Wilson's disease. Semin Neurol 1987;7:209–220.

37. Bothwick TR, Benson GD, Schugar HJ. Copper chelating agents: a comparison of cupriuretic responses to various tetramines and D-penicillamine. J Lab Clin Med 1980;95:575–580.

38. Scheinberg IH, Jaffe ME, Sternlieb I. Trientine in Wilson's disease. N Engl J Med 1987;317:209–213.

39. Schouwink G. De hepato-cerebrale degeneratie. Met een onderzoek de zink stofwisseling. Academish Proefschrift Amsterdam van den Wiel, Arnheim, Ph.D. diss., 1961 doctoral thesis.

40. Brewer GJ, Hill GM, Prasad AS, Cossack ZT, Rabbani P. Oral zinc therapy for Wilson's disease. Ann Intern Med 1983;99:314–320.

41. Brewer GJ, Yuzbasiyan-Gurkan V, Lee DY. Use of zinc-copper metabolic interactions in the treatment of Wilson's disease. J Am Coll Nutr 1990;9:487–491.

42. Menard MP, McCormick CC, Cousins RJ. Regulation of intestinal metallothionein biosynthesis in rats by dietary zinc. J Nutr 1981;111:1353–1361.

43. Fischer WF, Giroux A, L'Abbe MR. Effects of zinc on mucosal copper binding and on kinetic of copper absorption. J Nutr 1983;113:462–469.

44. Lee D-Y, Brewer GJ, Wang Y-X. Treatment of Wilson's disease with zinc, VII: Protection of liver from copper toxicity by zinc-induced metallothionein in a rat model. J Lab Clin Med 1989;114:639–645.

45. Hill GM, Brewer GJ, Prasad AS, Hydrick CR, Hartmann DE. Treatment of Wilson's disease with zinc, I: oral zinc therapy regimen. Hepatology 1987;7:522–528.

46. Brewer GJ, Hill GM, Prasad A, Dick R. The treatment of Wilson's disease with zinc, IV: efficacy monitoring using urine and plasma copper (42499). Proc Soc Exp Biol Med 1987;184:446–455.

47. Mills CF, El-Gallad TT, Bremner I. Effects of molybdate, sulfide, and tetrathiomolybdate on copper metabolism in rats. J Inorgan Biochem 1981;14:189–207.

48. Bremner I, Mills CF, Young BW. Copper metabolism in rats given di- or trithiomolybdates. J Inorg Biochem 1982;16:109–119.

49. Mills CF, El-Gallad TT, Bremner I, Weham G. Copper and molybdenum absorption by rats given ammonium tetrathiomolybdate. J Inorg Biochem 1981;14:163–175.

50. McQuaid A, Mason J. A comparison of the effects of penicillamine, trientine, and trithiomolybdate on [35S]-labelled metallothionein in vitro; implications for Wilson's disease therapy. J Inorg Biochem 1990;41:87–92.

51. Brewer GJ, Dick RD, Yuzbasiyan-Gurkan V, Tankanow R, Young AB, Kluin KJ. Initial therapy of patients with Wilson's disease with tetrathiomolybdate. Arch Neurol 1991;48:42–47.

52. Walshe JM. Pregnancy in Wilson's disease. Quart J Med 1977;181:73–83.

53. Scheinberg IH, Sternlieb I. Pregnancy in penicillamine-treated patients with Wilson's disease. N Engl J Med 1975;293:1300–1302.

54. Walshe JM. The management of pregnancy in Wilson's disease treated with trientine. Q J Med 1986;58:81–87.

55. Marĕcek J, Graf M. Pregnancy in penicillamine-treated patients with Wilson's disease. N Engl J Med 1976;295:841–842.

56. Burrows JS, Pekala B. Serum copper and ceruloplasmin in pregnancy. Am J Obstet Gynecol 1971;109:907–909.

57. Dupont P, Irion O, Beguin F. Pregnancy in a patient with treated Wilson's disease: a case report. Am J Obstet Gynecol 1990;163:1527–1528.

58. Nimmi ME, Bavetta LA. Collagen defect induced by penicillamine. Science 1965;150:905–909.

59. Albukerk JN. The pregnant woman with Wilson's disease. N Engl J Med 1976;294:670–671.

60. March L, Fraser FC. Chelating agents and teratogenesis. Lancet 1973;2:846.

61. Bloomer JR, Bonkovsky HL. The porphyrias. Disease-A-Month 1989;35:13–54.

62. Lundvall O, Weinfeld A, Lundin P. Iron storage in porphyria cutanea tarda. Acta Med Scand 1970;188:37–53.

63. Lamon JM, Frykholm BC, Hess RA, Tschudy DP. Hematin therapy for acute porphyria. Medicine 1979;58:252–269.

64. Dhar GJ, Bossenmaier I, Petryka ZJ, Cardinal R, Watson CJ. Effects of hematin in hepatic porphyria: further studies. Ann Intern Med 1975;83:20–30.

65. Hussain M, Mielli-Vergani G, Mowat AP. Alpha-1-antitrypsin deficiency and liver disease: clinical presentation, diagnosis, and treatment. J Inherited Metab Dis 1991;14:497–511.

66. Laurell CB, Eriksson S. The electrophoretic alpha-1-globulin pattern of serum in alpha-1-antitrypsin deficiency. Scand J Clin Lab Invest 1963;15:132–140.

67. Sharp HL, Bridges RA, Krivit W, Freier EF. Cirrhosis associated with alpha-1-antitrypsin deficiency: A previous unrecognized inherited disorder. J Lab Clin Med 1969;73:934–939.

68. Pierce JA, Eradro B, Dew TA. Antitrypsin phenotypes in St. Louis. JAMA 1975;231:609–612.

69. Sverger T. Liver disease in alpha-1-antitrypsin detected by screening of 200,000 infants. N Engl J Med 1976;294:1315.

70. Birrer P, McElvancy NG, Chang-Strohman LM, Crystal RG. Alpha-1-antitrypsin deficiency and

liver disease. J Inherited Metab Dis 1991;14:512–525.

71. Laurell CB, Kullander S, Thorell J. Effect of administration of a combined estrogen-progestin contraceptive on the level of individual plasma proteins. Scand J Clin Lab Invest 1967;21:337–343.

72. Gadek JE, Fulmer JD, Gelfand JA, Frank MM, Petty TL, Crystal RG. Danazol-induced augmentation of serum alpha-1-antitrypsin levels in individuals with marked deficiency of this antiprotease. J Clin Invest 1980;66:82–87.

73. Wewers MD, Brantly ML, Casolaro MA, Crystal RG. Evaluation of tamoxifen as a therapy to augment alpha-1-antitrypsin concentrations in Z homozygous alpha-1-antitrypsin-deficient subjects. Am Rev Resp Dis 1987;135:401–402.

74. Crystal RG. Alpha-1-antitrypsin deficiency, emphysema, and liver disease. J Clin Invest 1990;85:1343–1352.

75. Perlmutter DH. The cellular basis for liver injury in alpha-1-antitrypsin deficiency. Hepatology 1991;13:172–185.

76. Esquivel CO, Marino IR, Fioravanti V, Van Thiel DH. Liver transplantation for metabolic disease of the liver. Gastroenterol Clin N Am 1988;17:167–177.

77. Putnam CW, Porter KA, Peters RL, Aschcavai M, Redeker AG, Starzl TE. Liver replacement for alpha-1-antitrypsin deficiency. Surgery 1977;81:258–261.

78. van Furth R, Kramps JA, van der Putten AB, Krom RA, Gips CH. Change in alpha-1-antitrypsin phenotype after orthotopic liver transplant. Clin Exp Immunol 1986;66:669–672.

79. Esquivel CO, Mash JW, Van Thiel DH. Liver transplantation for chronic cholestatic liver disease in adults and children. Gastroenterol Clin N Am 1988;17:145–155.

80. Baker AL, Rosenberg IH. Hepatic complications of total parenteral nutrition. Am J Med 1987;82:489–497.

81. Gholson CF, Bacon BR. Diseases of the liver and the biliary tract. In: Gitnick G, LaBrecque DR, Moody FR, eds. Metabolic and systemic diseases. St. Louis: Mosby-Year Book, 1992:489–523.

82. Bower RH. Hepatic complications of parenteral nutrition. Semin Liver Dis 1983;3:216–224.

83. Klein S, Nealon WH. Hepatobiliary abnormalities associated with total parenteral nutrition. Semin Liver Dis 1988;8:237–246.

84. Meguid MM, Schimmel E, Johnson WC, et al. Reduced metabolic complications in total parenteral nutrition: pilot study using fat to replace one-third of glucose calories. JPEN 1982;6:304–307.

85. Lowry SR, Brennan MF. Abnormal liver function during parenteral nutrition: relation to infusion excess. J Surg Res 1979;26:300–307.

86. Matuchansky C, Morichau-Beauchant M, Druart F, Tapin J. Cyclic (nocturnal) total parenteral nutrition in hospitalized adult patients with severe digestive diseases: report of a prospective study. Gastroenterology 1981;81:433–437.

87. Allardyce DB, Slavian AJ, Quenville NF. Cholestatic jaundice during total parenteral nutrition. Can J Surg 1978;21:332–339.

88. Mallory A, Kern F, Smith S, Savage D. Patterns of bile acids and microflora in human small intestine. Gastroenterology 1973;64:26–42.

89. Brown RS. Cholestasis in association with short-term parenteral alimentation. Crit Care Med 1976;4:313–316.

90. Kukis A, Mookerja S. Choline. Nutr Rev 1978;36:201–207.

91. Belli DC, Fournier LA, Lepage G, et al. Total parenteral nutrition-associated cholestasis in rats: comparison of different amino acid mixtures. JPEN 1987;11:67–73.

92. Berger HM, Ouden ALD, Calame JJ. Pathogenesis of liver damage during parenteral nutrition: is lipofuscin a clue? Arch Dis Childhood 1985;60:774–776.

93. Elleby H, Solhaug JH. Metronidazole, cholestasis, and total parenteral nutrition. Lancet 1983;1:1161.

94. Capron JP, Gineston JL, Herve MA, Baillon A. Metronidazole in prevention of cholestasis associated with total parenteral nutrition. Lancet 1983;1:446–447.

95. Lambert JR, Thomas SM. Metronidazole prevention of serum liver enzyme abnormalities during total parenteral nutrition. JPEN 1985;9:501–503.

96. Freund HR, Muggia-Sullam J, La France R, Enrione EB, Popp MB, Bjornson MS. A possible beneficial effect of metronidazole in reducing TPN-associated liver function derangements. J Surg Res 1985;38:356–363.

97. Stanko RT, Nathan G, Mendelow H, Adibi SA. Development of hepatic cholestasis and fibrosis in patients with massive loss of intestine supported by prolonged parenteral nutrition. Gastroenterology 1987;92:197–202.

98. Bowyer BA, Fleming CR, Ludwig J, Petz J, McGill DB. Does long-term home parenteral nutrition in adult patients cause chronic liver disease? JPEN 1985;9:11–17.

99. Holzbach RT. Gallbladder stasis: consequence of long-term parenteral hyperalimentation and risk factor for cholelithiasis. Gastroenterology 1983;84:1055–1058.

100. Messing B, Bories C, Kunstinger F, Bernier IJ. Does total parenteral nutrition induce gallbladder sludge formation and lithiasis? Gastroenterology 1983;84:1012–1019.

101. Peterson SR, Sheldon GF. Acute acalculous cholecystitis: a complication of hyperalimentation. Am J Surg 1979;138:814–817.

102. Lucas A, Bloom SR, Aynsky-Green A. Gut hormones and minimal enteral feeding. Acta Paediatr Scand 1986;75:719–723.

103. Sitzmann JV, Pitt HA, Steinborn PA, Pasha ZR, Sanders RC. Cholecystokinin prevents parenteral nutrition-induced biliary sludge in humans. Surg Gynec Obstet 1990;170:25–31.

104. Orlando R, Gleason E, Drezter AD. Acute acalculous cholecystitis in critically ill patients. Am J Surg 1983;145:472–475.

105. Cohen A. Current status of iron chelation therapy with deferoxamine. Semin Hematol 1990;27:86–90.

106. Drugs used in the management of poisoning. In: Ambre JJ, Bennett DR, Cranston JW, et al. Drug Evaluations Annual of 1992. Chicago: American Medical Association, 1992:57–61.

107. Olivieri NF, Buncic JR, Chew E, et al. Visual and auditory neurotoxicity in patients receiving subcutaneous deferoxamine infusion. N Engl J Med 1986;314:869–873.

108. De Virgillis S, Congia M, Frau F, et al. Deferoxamine-induced growth retardation in patients with thalassemia major. J Pediatr 1988;113:661–669.

109. Daly AL, Velazquez LA, Bradley SF, Kauffman CA. Mucormycosis: Association with deferoxamine therapy. Am J Med 1989;87:468–471.

110. Joyce DA. D-Penicillamine pharmacokinetics and pharmacodynamics in man. Pharmacol Ther 1989;42:405–427.

111. Hill HFH. Penicillamine in rheumatoid arthritis: Adverse effect. Scand J Rheum 1979;28:94–99.

112. Proesmans W, Jaeken J, Eeckels R. D-Penicillamine-induced IGA deficiency in Wilson's disease. Lancet 1976;2:804–805.

113. Gilman PA, Holtzman NA. All in a patient receiving D-Penicillamine for Wilson's disease. JAMA 1982; 248:467–468.

114. Adams DA, Goldman R, Maxwell MH, Latta H. Nephrotic syndrome associated with penicillamine therapy of Wilson's disease. Am J Med 1964;36: 330–336.

115. Sternlieb I. Penicillamine and nephrotic syndrome: results in patients with hepatolenticular degeneration. JAMA 1966;198:1311–1312.

116. Henningsen B, Maintz J, Basedow M, et al. Nephrotishes syndrome durch penicillamin. Dtsch Med Wochenschr 1973;98:1768–1772.

117. Sternlieb I, Bennett B, Scheinberg IH. D-Penicillamine-induced Goodpasture's syndrome. Ann Intern Med 1975;82:673–676.

118. Greer KE, Askew FC, Richardson D. Skin lesions induced by penicillamine. Arch Dermatol 1976; 112:1267–1269.

119. Gollan JL. Copper metabolism, Wilson's disease, and hepatic copper toxicosis. In: Zakim B, Boyer TD, eds. Hepatology: A textbook of liver disease. Philadelphia: Saunders, 1990:1249–1272.

120. Levy RS, Fisher M, Alter JN. Penicillamine: Review and cutaneous manifestation. J Am Acad Dermatol 1983;8:548–558.

121. Pass F, Goldfischer S. Elastosis perforans serpiginosa during penicillamine therapy for Wilson's disease. Arch Dermatol 1973;108:713–715.

122. Goldstein JB, McNutt NS, Hambrick GW, Hsu A. Penicillamine dermatopathy with lymphangiectasia. Arch Dermatol 1989;125:92–97.

123. Wolheim FA, Lindstrom CG. Liver abnormalities in penicillamine-treated rheumatoid arthritis. Scand J Rheumatol 1979;28:100–107.

124. Barzilai D, Dickstein G, Enat R, Bassan H, Gellei B. Cholestatic jaundice caused by D-penicillamine. Ann Rheumatol Dis 1978;37:98–100.

125. Wassef M, Galian A, Pepin B, et al. Unusual digestive lesions in a patient with Wilson's disease treated with long-term penicillamine. N Engl J Med 1985;313:49.

126. Walshe JM, Golding DN. Penicillamine-induced arthropathy in Wilson's disease. Proc Roy Soc Med 1977;70(suppl 3):4–6.

127. Buchnall RC, Dawkins RL. Myasthenia associated with D-penicillamine therapy in rheumatoid arthritis. Scand J Rheumatol 1979;28:91–93.

128. Walshe JM. Treatment of Wilson's disease with trientine (triethylene tetramine) dihydrochloride. Lancet 1982;1:643–647.

129. Epstein O, Sherlock S. Triethylene tetramine dihydrochloride toxicity in primary biliary cirrhosis. Gastroenterology 1980;78:1442–1445.

130. Chandra RK. Excessive intake of zinc impairs immune responses. JAMA 1984;252:1443–1446.

131. Yagamuchi M, Takahasi K, Okada S. Zinc-induced hypoclademia and bone resorption in rats. Toxicol Appl Pharmacol 1983;46:224–228.

132. Wentlick GH, Spierenburg TJ, de Graaf GJ, van Exsel AC. A case of chronic zinc poisoning in calves fed with zinc-contaminated roughage. Vet Q 1985;7:153–157.

21

Management of Hepatic Encephalopathy

E. ANTHONY JONES and KEVIN D. MULLEN

Hepatic encephalopathy (HE), or portal-systemic encephalopathy (PSE), is a complex neuropsychiatric syndrome that occurs as a result of acute or chronic hepatocellular failure, and is associated with increased delivery of gut-derived constituents of portal venous plasma to peripheral blood plasma (1, 2) (Fig. 21.1). Fulminant hepatic failure (FHF) is defined as the syndrome of acute liver failure complicated by HE. Acute HE in a cirrhotic patient is usually associated with a clearly definable precipitating factor and typically resolves when the precipitating factor is removed (3). The term chronic PSE is often applied to a patient with cirrhosis in whom HE is persistent or episodic with or without complete resolution of the encephalopathy between episodes. HE is considered to be a reversible metabolic encephalopathy (2). This classification tends to exclude structural changes in neurons or neuronal degeneration as constituting a component of the syndrome (4).

The spectrum of psychiatric and neurologic abnormalities that occur in HE is broad (2, 4–9). The earliest subclinical phase of HE may only be detected by psychometric (10–12) or electrophysiologic testing. Visual event-related (P-300) potentials, which depend on cognitive function, are likely to be superior to an electroencephalogram (EEG) or conventional visual-evoked potentials in detecting the earliest stages of HE (13). The earliest clinical signs of HE are psychiatric and behavioral changes that may be more apparent to the patient's family members and close friends than to the physician (14). These changes are primarily due to subtle impairment of intellectual function that reflects predominantly bilateral forebrain dysfunction. An inverted sleep pattern may occur. As HE progresses, intellectual abilities further deteriorate, motor function becomes impaired, asterixis is frequently present, and consciousness decreases. With further progression, coma ensues. Evolution of overt HE is associated with progressive slowing of the frequency of the EEG, an increase followed by a decrease in its amplitude, and frequent triphasic waves in late stages (15).

It is clear that a normally functioning liver is necessary to maintain normal brain function. HE is considered to be due primarily to a failure of the liver to adequately remove certain substances from plasma, particularly gut-derived nitrogenous substances (1, 2), which have the ability, directly or indirectly, to depress the function of the central nervous system (CNS). The overall manifestations of HE appear to be due primarily to a net increase in neuronal inhibition. The pathogenesis of HE is considered to be multifactorial (16). Several hypotheses of the pathogenesis of HE have been proposed, none of which is necessarily mutually exclusive (16). The validity of none of them has been definitively proved experimentally, but evidence for an involvement of the γ-aminobutyric acid (GABA$_A$) benzodiazepine (BZ) receptor complex has steadily accumulated during the past decade (17, 18). In the treatment of this syndrome, the goal is to normalize mental function. The following

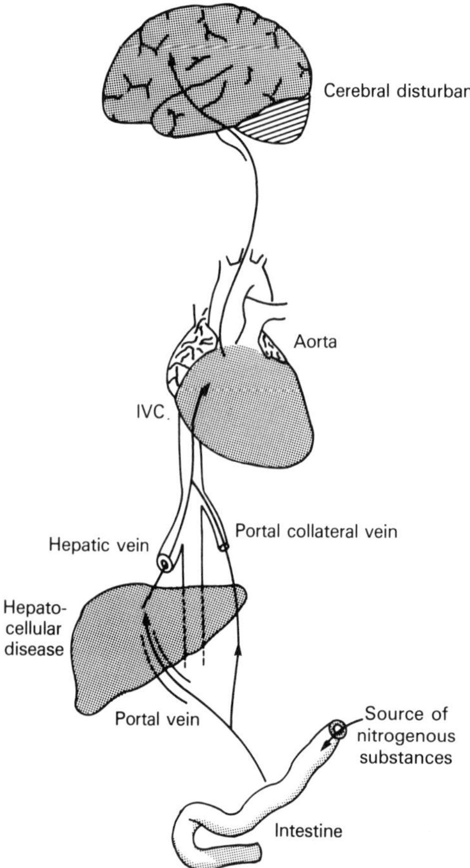

Figure 21.1. The concept of portal-systemic encephalopathy. In liver disease increased amounts of gut-derived nitrogenous substances in portal venous plasma gain access to peripheral blood plasma as a consequence of impaired hepatic extraction and/or passage through intrahepatic or extrahepatic collateral venous channels. If such substances are neuroactive and if they can cross the blood-brain barrier they may modulate brain function. A variety of substances may have these properties. Reproduced with minor modification from Sherlock et al. (1).

general principles are relevant in developing an approach to the management of a patient with HE: (*a*) removal or correction of any precipitating factor; (*b*) reduction of absorption of nitrogenous substances from the gastrointestinal tract; (*c*) reduction of increased portal-systemic shunting of blood; and (*d*) reversal of contributing neuropathophysiologic events with drugs that act directly on the brain. Approaches (*a*) and (*b*) are routine, (*c*) is practical only in rare instances, and (*d*) is experimental (Table 21.1).

ROUTINE MANAGEMENT

Acute Hepatic Encephalopathy

REMOVAL OR CORRECTION OF PRECIPITATING FACTORS

A large number of factors tend to precipitate or exacerbate HE (3) (Table 21.2). In general, these factors are better recognized in patients with chronic rather than acute liver disease. With the exception of sedative-hypnotic drugs acting on the $GABA_A$/benzodiazepine receptor complex (eg, benzodiazepines, barbiturates) (16), the relationship between common precipitating factors and pathogenesis is poorly understood. The hypersensitivity of patients with liver disease to benzodiazepines is due, not only to impaired drug metabolism, but also to increased cerebral sensitivity (19–21).

Treatment of HE should begin with a search for and appropriate management of precipitating factors. Any infection should be treated, with special attention to pneumonia and spontaneous bacterial peritonitis. Aminoglycoside antibiotics should be avoided whenever possible because of the high incidence of nephrotoxicity in cirrhotic patients (22). Electrolyte, acid-base, and hemodynamic disturbances should be corrected. Gastrointestinal hemorrhage should be sought and vigorously controlled. Blood in the gastrointestinal tract should be removed by aspiration and enemas. Diuretic therapy, a common cause of electrolyte disturbance, should be discontinued. Diuretic-induced hypokalemia and metabolic alkalosis are often associated with precipitation or exacerbation of HE (23). Hypokalemia can be corrected by the cautious administration of potassium chloride intravenously (e.g., 20–40 mEq KCl/l fluid administered) with rechecking of potassium levels. Intravenous fluid replacement is particularly important if there is diarrhea or vomiting, the causes of which should be sought and corrected. Dextrose is given to provide

Table 21.1
Treatment of Hepatic Encephalopathy

Correction or removal of precipitating factors	Mandatory
Institution of maneuvers to minimize absorption of nitrogenous substances	
Protein restriction	
Evacuation of the bowel	Routine
Lactulose (or a related sugar) or antibiotics	
Reduction of portal-systemic shunting	Rarely practical
Direct reversal of neuropathophysiology	Experimental
Flumazenil	

Table 21.2
Factors That May Precipitate Hepatic Encephalopathy

Oral protein load	
Upper gastrointestinal bleed	Acting through gut factors
Constipation	
Diarrhea and vomiting	Dehydration; electrolyte
Diuretic therapy	and acid/base imbalance
Paracentesis	(eg, hypokalemic alkalosis)
Hypoxia	
Hypoglycemia	Adverse effect on both
Anemia	liver and brain function
Hypotension	
Sedative/hypnotic drugs	
Azotemia	
Infection	

calories. Blood glucose should be checked, frequently in cases of FHF, and hypoglycemia corrected by additional intravenous dextrose. Massive quantities of dextrose may be necessary to correct hypoglycemia complicating FHF (24). Transfusion of blood may be indicated for anemia or hemorrhage into the gastrointestinal tract. Hypoxia is an indication for oxygen by face mask; specific causes of hypoxia (e.g., pneumonia) should be sought and corrected. Meticulous attention is paid to maintaining fluid and electrolyte balance and an adequate urine flow. Administration of any sedative-hypnotic drug, such as an opiate (25) or a benzodiazepine (19) should be discontinued. Consideration should be given to administering an appropriate antidote, for example, naloxone (0.4 ng intravenously) or flumazenil (<7 mg intravenously over a 30-minute period; see below).

MINIMIZING ABSORPTION OF NITROGENOUS SUBSTANCES

Diet

In acute HE, dietary intake of protein is completely withheld. Protein intake should be increased promptly but gradually with improvement and return of protein tolerance (e.g., in increments of 20 g/day) to minimize the duration of negative nitrogen balance (26).

Evacuation of the Bowel

The bowel is evacuated by administering cathartics (e.g., magnesium sulfate) by mouth and/or by rectum. The aim of this maneuver is to remove from the intestine neuroactive nitrogenous compounds that may precipitate or exacerbate HE. In patients predisposed to develop renal failure, magnesium sulfate

Table 21.3
Potential Beneficial Actions of Lactulose for Hepatic Encephalopathy

Cathartic effect. Shortened intestinal transit time limits potential for production and absorption of neuroactive substances from gut bacterial-substrate interactions
Acidification effect. Reduces production of ammonia by colonic flora and promotes ammonia incorporation into bacterial proteins
Alternation of spectrum of colonic bacterial flora
Promotion of colonic production of short-chain fatty acids from a variety of substrates
Inhibition of bacterial catabolism
Reduced intestinal production of ammonia due to inhibition of glutamine transport into enterocytes
Possible enhanced zinc absorption

should be given with caution because of the risk of hypermagnesemia developing (27).

Lactulose and Related Sugars

Lactulose has become a standard therapy for acute HE. Its use was originally based on the ammonia hypothesis (see below), and it is traditionally supplied in the form of a syrup contaminated with lactose and other sugars. There is no disaccharidase on the microvillus membrane of enterocytes in the small intestine that hydrolyzes lactulose (28); hence lactulose undergoes minimal absorption (29). Metabolism of lactulose in the colon leads to the production of lactic and other organic acids which can lead to an osmotic diarrhea (30), and to a fall in the pH of colonic contents (31) which stimulates peristalsis (32). The effects of lactulose on colonic metabolism have been extensively studied (33–36). However, the relationship between lactulose-induced changes in colonic metabolism and HE remain uncertain (37) (Table 21.3) and the therapeutic value of lactulose may depend largely on its cathartic properties (38).

In a controlled study, lactulose has been shown to be as effective as a combination of neomycin and sorbitol in the management of acute HE in cirrhotic patients (39). It is usually given orally (e.g., 30 ml tid) but may also be given rectally (40). Lactulose is used in the treatment of FHF based on experience with its use for patients with chronic liver disease. Intolerance of lactulose is a problem in some patients. Diarrhea and abdominal bloating are indications for dose reduction (41). Lactulose therapy can induce hypernatremia (serum so-

dium >145 mEq/l) which is associated with increased mortality. The hypernatremia is considered to be due to increased fecal water loss (osmotic diarrhea). If large doses of lactulose are given, a liberal amount of water should be administered and serum electrolytes checked regularly (30, 42).

Lactitol is a nonabsorbed disaccharide analog of lactulose for which there is also no disaccharidase on the microvillus membrane of enterocytes (43). Its metabolism in the colon is similar to that of lactulose (44). It is produced in the form of a fine crystalline powder that is less sweet and hence tastes better than lactulose (43, 45). Lactitol has been shown to be as effective as lactulose in the management of acute HE in cirrhotic patients (41, 46). In addition, lactitol (acidifying) enemas have been shown to be more effective than tap water (nonacidifying) enemas in ameliorating acute HE (47). The cathartic effect of lactitol appears to be more predictable and rapid than that of lactulose (43).

It is possible that other nonabsorbed sugars, such as sorbitol or mannitol, may be as effective as lactulose in the management of acute HE (38). Metabolism of sorbitol and lactulose in the colon are similar (48), and sorbitol has the same laxative threshold as lactitol (44).

Antibiotics

The rationale for administering oral broad-spectrum antibodies in HE is to reduce the production of nitrogenous substances by enteric bacteria in the colon (26). Oral neomycin (4–6 g daily) which is effective against aerobes appears to mediate a therapeutic effect in acute HE in cirrhotic patients and its use in this clinical situation and in FHF is rationalized by its apparent greater effectiveness than purgation alone in chronic HE (49). Another potential mechanism of action would be related to neomycin-induced villous atrophy and malabsorption (50). Other broad-spectrum antibiotics, such as paromomycin and kanamycin, are alternatives to neomycin (51, 52). Some neomycin is absorbed when it is given orally or rectally (51–54). Neomycin levels tend to be higher in the presence of impaired renal function (52) and ototoxicity may occur (53, 55). Other side effects of neomycin include diarrhea (49) and staphylococcal enterocolitis (56). Neomycin abolishes acidification of colonic contents by lactulose and lactitol and consequently may reduce the laxative effect of these sugars (43, 44). Metronidazole, a chemotherapeutic agent, which, in contrast to neomycin, is effective against anaerobes such as bacteroides, may be used in the management of acute HE based on its apparent effectiveness in chronic HE (57).

Chronic Portal-Systemic Encephalopathy (PSE)

The diagnosis of chronic PSE is an indication to advise the patient not to undertake certain activities such as driving a car (58).

REMOVAL OR CORRECTION OF PRECIPITATING FACTORS

Factors that precipitate chronic PSE and acute HE are similar. Hypokalemia may be chronic and necessitate long-term potassium supplementation.

MINIMIZING ABSORPTION OF NITROGENOUS SUBSTANCES

Diet

In a patient with chronic hepatocellular disease, a nutritious diet, including a high intake of good quality protein, if tolerated, should be encouraged to help maintain a positive nitrogen balance and a good nutritional status. However, in the presence of poor hepatocellular function, an oral protein load may pre-

cipitate HE (2, 26). Protein intolerance usually responds to a reduction of dietary protein intake. Protein tolerance may be increased by lactulose, lactitol, or antibiotic therapy. Long-term protein intake of <40 g/day is likely to induce a negative nitrogen balance and consequently should be avoided.

It has been suggested that vegetable protein may be better tolerated than animal protein (59–62) and that milk and milk products are better tolerated than meat and eggs (63) in chronic PSE. Use of vegetable protein diets in patients with chronic PSE and diabetes mellitus is associated with improved glucose tolerance (64). Apparent beneficial effects of vegetable protein diets on chronic PSE may be attributable to the laxative effect of their high fiber content (60). These diets do not have an established place in the management of chronic PSE.

There is some limited evidence that a deficiency of zinc may exacerbate HE (65). An apparent beneficial effect of oral zinc supplements on chronic HE in one controlled study (66) was not confirmed in another (67).

Avoidance of Constipation

In chronic PSE, complete evacuation of the bowel is not indicated, but it is important to avoid constipation by the prudent use of laxatives or lactulose or lactitol (see below).

Lactulose and Related Sugars

There is a wide consensus that lactulose mediates a beneficial effect on chronic PSE (68–73). Lactulose appears to be as effective as a combination of neomycin and sorbitol (74) or a combination of neomycin and magnesium sulphate (75) in the management of patients with chronic PSE. Furthermore, lactulose and lactitol have similar effects on chronic PSE (76). In patients with chronic PSE who have lactase deficiency, lactose may be used instead of lactulose (77), and lactose has been shown to be as effective as lactitol in these patients (78). Side effects of lactulose or lactitol in chronic PSE include abdominal discomfort and diarrhea (70). The usual dose of lactulose for chronic PSE is about 30 ml three times daily; the dosage of lactulose or lactitol is adjusted to achieve about two semiformed motions daily. For a further discussion of lactulose and lactitol see above under Lactulose and Related Sugars.

Antibiotics

Neomycin administration for chronic PSE has been associated with clinical and electrophysiologic improvements in the encephalopathy (49). The usual dose of neomycin is 2–4 g daily. Because of its side effects, notably ototoxicity (53, 55) and the tendency for high levels to develop if renal function is impaired (52), neomycin tends to be given only when lactulose or lactitol are poorly tolerated. The combination of neomycin and lactulose or lactitol may be contraindicated (43, 44). Patients treated with neomycin chronically should have frequent assessment of serum blood urea nitrogen (BUN), creatinine, urinalysis, and audiometry. Metronidazole has been shown to be as effective as neomycin (57), but attempts at altering the colonic bacterial flora by the dietary administration of lactobacillus acidophilus were shown to be less effective than neomycin (79) in the management of chronic PSE.

REVERSAL OF INCREASED PORTAL-SYSTEMIC SHUNTING

For the occasional patient with intractable chronic PSE associated with a large surgically induced or spontaneous portal-systemic shunt, it may be possible to reverse portal venous blood flow from hepatofugal to hepatopedal by the invasive radiologic technique of balloon occlusion of the main shunt coupled with coronary vein embolization. Restoration of portal perfusion in this way can improve hepatocellular function appreciably and achieve a dramatic and sustained amelioration of PSE (80). Rarely, it may be possible to improve portal perfusion by surgical suppression of a shunt (81, 82).

DRUGS ACTING DIRECTLY ON THE BRAIN

Attempts to reverse pathophysiologic events in neurons that contribute to HE by administration of drugs that act directly on the brain are currently experimental. Two classes of drugs of this type have received attention as potential therapeutic modalities for HE—dopaminergic drugs and benzodiazepine antagonists. These two classes of drugs are considered below in relation to the hypotheses of pathogenesis that provide a rationale for their use.

THERAPIES DEPENDENT ON SPECIFIC HYPOTHESES OF PATHOGENESIS

Ammonia Hypothesis

Ammonia is an established neurotoxin that is widely believed to play a role in the pathogenesis of HE. The gastrointestinal tract is one of the major sites of ammonia production. It is formed by enteric bacterial and intestinal enzymes that degrade amines, amino acids, and urea. Normally ammonia is converted into either urea or glutamine in the liver. With liver failure, hepatocellular dysfunction and intra- and extrahepatic portal-systemic shunting of blood are associated with increased levels of ammonia in peripheral blood plasma (16).

Several factors can be cited in support of the ammonia hypothesis: (*a*) Ammonia accumulates in liver failure and its uptake by the brain is increased (83). (*b*) Ammonia can induce encephalopathy. (*c*) Encephalopathy occurs in children with hyperammonemia due to congenital deficiencies of enzymes in the Krebs-Henseleit urea cycle. (*d*) Therapies that lead to a reduction in intestinal absorption of ammonia tend to induce ameliorations of HE in patients with cirrhosis (15).

Issues of concern with the ammonia hypothesis include the following: (*a*) Plasma levels of ammonia correlate poorly with the stage of HE. (*b*) Experimental hyperammonemia does not reproduce the behavioral or electrophysiologic manifestations of HE and is characterized by a preconvulsive state followed by seizures and postictal coma (84, 85). (*c*) Seizures are common in the congenital hyperammonemia syndromes, but are unusual in HE because of acute or chronic liver failure (16).

There are several mechanisms by which ammonia may interfere with CNS function. The effects of ammonia on the tricarboxylic acid cycle may decrease cerebral energy metabolism. However, a change in energy status may be a result rather than a cause of ammonia-induced encephalopathy (86). Metabolism of ammonia in the brain promotes glutamine formation from glutamate, and it has been suggested that decreased availability of glutamate may lead to decreased glutamatergic excitatory neurotransmission (87), and hence a relative increase in neural inhibition. The direct electrophysiologic effects of ammonia include the induction of neuronal excitation (dysinhibition) by impairing Cl^- extrusion from neurons and thereby blocking the formation of inhibitory postsynaptic potentials (88). Thus, increased brain levels of ammonia have documented neurochemical and electrophysiologic effects. However, the contribution of ammonia-induced modulation of neuronal function in liver failure to the clinical syndrome of HE remains poorly defined.

There are two main pathways of metabolic ammonia detoxification: the synthesis of urea through the Krebs-Henseleit cycle in the liver, and the synthesis of glutamine from ammonia through α-ketogutamate and glutamate in liver, muscle, brain, and other tissues (89). Therapies with the goal of accelerating these pathways have been popular since the 1950's, and include:

Arginine, Ornithine, and Glutamate. These amino acids have been used to promote ammonia detoxification. The combination of ornithine with α-ketoglutamate was reported anecdotally to be effective in ameliorating HE (90). However, L-arginine was ineffective in ameliorating HE in a controlled study (91).

Sodium Benzoate. Benzoate combines with ammonia to form hippuric acid, which is excreted in urine. In studies with controlled designs, administration of sodium benzoate has been shown to lower blood ammonia, be as effective as lactulose in ameliorating acute HE (92), and be associated with improvement in chronic HE (93).

Urease Inhibitors. Urease inhibitors have been used with the aim of inhibiting intestinal ammonia production. In one controlled study, administration of the competitive urease inhibitor, niotinohydroxomate, was reported to be associated with amelioration of HE (90).

However, none of these treatments specific for the ammonia hypothesis has an established place in the treatment of HE.

False Neurotransmitter Hypothesis

With liver failure, the ratio of serum concentrations of branched-chain amino acids (BCAA) to those of aromatic amino acids (AAA) decreases. BCAAs and AAAs compete for a common transport carrier at the blood brain barrier (BBB). The decreased BCAA:AAA ratio, together with an increased efflux of glutamine from the brain as a result of increased cerebral ammonia metabolism, are thought to be responsible for an accumulation of AAAs in the brain. Of the AAAs, phenylalanine and tyrosine at high concentrations may inhibit tyrosine hydroxylase, the key enzyme for the synthesis of dopamine and noradrenaline. Thus the production of normal catecholaminergic neurotransmitters would be decreased. False neurotransmitters, such as octopamine and β-phenylethanolamine would then be synthesized through an alternative pathway and would compete with normal catecholaminergic neurotransmitters for their receptor sites. The ultimate result of these changes would be decreased catecholaminergic neurotransmission. Another AAA, tryptophan, would increase the synthesis of serotonin, and consequently may also contribute to the manifestations of HE (16, 94).

BASES FOR THE HYPOTHESIS

False neurotransmitters accumulate in liver failure. The plasma BCAA:AAA ratio tends to be decreased in patients with cirrhosis. In animal models of HE, efflux of glutamine from the brain occurs (94).

ISSUES OF CONCERN WITH THE HYPOTHESIS

The intraventricular administration of octopamine to rats induced profound depletion of noradrenaline from the brain, but no obvious change in consciousness (95). The plasma BCAA:AAA ratio in patients with cirrhosis correlates poorly with HE (96). Although subject to reservations inherent in all brain autopsy studies, patients with cirrhosis dying in HE were found to have increased noradrenaline and dopamine concentrations and decreased octopamine concentrations in the brain (97). Nevertheless, therapies designed at improving the BCAA:AAA ratio have been advocated as discussed below:

BRANCHED CHAIN AMINO ACIDS

Administration of BCAA has been shown to correct the decreased BCAA:AAA ratio in HE. This should prevent increased transfer of AAAs into the brain and hence reverse events leading to increased production of false neurotransmitters. However, controlled trials of the administration of BCAAs or amino acid preparations enriched in BCAA either orally or intravenously have not shown that this form of therapy consistently induces an amelioration of acute HE or chronic PSE in patients with chronic liver disease (98, 99). However, BCAA may be useful in improving the nutritional status of cirrhotic patients and may permit a higher dietary intake of amino acid nitrogen to be achieved without precipitating overt HE (100). α-Keto analogs of BCAA have also been ineffective in producing robust ameliorations of HE in cirrhotic patients (98).

DOPAMINERGIC DRUGS

Dopaminergic drugs such as L-dopa and bromocriptine would tend to normalize decreased dopaminergic neurotransmission postulated in this hypothesis. However, controlled clinical trials have not shown that L-dopa is effective in reversing acute HE in cirrhotic patients (101) or that bromocriptine is consistently superior to standard therapy for chronic PSE (102–104).

γ-Aminobutyric Acid (GABA)-ergic Neurotransmission Hypothesis

GABA is the principal inhibitory neurotransmitter in the brain (105). Increased neuro-

transmission mediated by GABA is associated with impaired motor function and decreased consciousness (106). Because these behavioral phenomena are prominent features of HE, it has been suggested that increased GABA-ergic tone may contribute to this syndrome (107).

The $GABA_A$/benzodiazepine (BZ) receptor/chloride ionophore complex is an oligomeric glycoprotein complex that has been pharmacologically and biochemically subdivided into three components: $GABA_A$-receptors, central BZ-receptors and chloride ionophores. These units are allosterically linked to form a "supramolecular" complex (Fig. 21.2). Binding of GABA to the $GABA_A$-receptor increases neuronal membrane permeability to Cl^- by opening the Cl^- ionophore. When the Cl^- resting potential of the neuron is more negative than the neuronal resting membrane potential, Cl^- enters the neuron, causing membrane hyperpolarization. This phenomenon prevents neuronal membrane depolarization in response to stimuli and hence causes neuronal inhibition. These receptor and membrane events are the basis of GABA-ergic inhibitory neurotransmission. The BZ-receptor modulates the efficacy of GABA in opening the Cl^- ionophore. BZ-receptor agonists (e.g., diazepam) increase the frequency of GABA-gated Cl^- channel openings. It is believed that the anxiolytic, sedative, muscle relaxing, and anticonvulsant properties of BZ-receptor agonists are mediated through this mechanism. Potential mechanisms of increased GABA-ergic tone in HE include increased availability of GABA at $GABA_A$-receptors, and/or the presence of agonist ligands (e.g., BZs) that potentiate the action of GABA (16).

BASES FOR THE GABA HYPOTHESIS IN ANIMAL MODELS OF FHF

The visual-evoked response (VER) changes associated with HE are similar to those associated with encephalopathies induced by drugs that increase GABA-ergic tone, including BZ-agonists, but differ from those in encephalopathies due to drugs or toxins that are

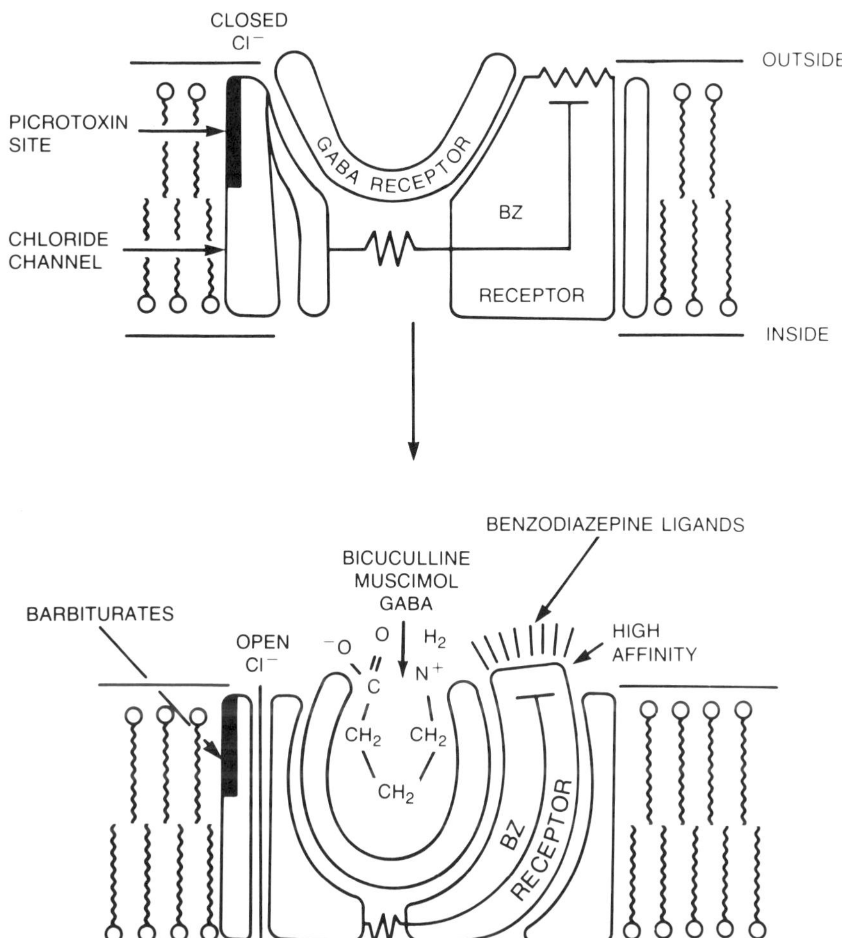

Figure 21.2. Diagramatic representation of γ-aminobutyric acid (GABA$_A$) benzodiazepine (BZ) receptor chloride ionophore complex in postsynaptic neural membranes in the central nervous system (CNS). Receptors are depicted for GABA and GABA$_A$-receptor ligands (eg, muscimol, bicuculline), picrotoxin and barbiturates, and central BZ-receptor ligands (eg, diazepam, flumazenil). A: *Top*, The receptor complex in a nonactivated state with the chloride channel closed. *Bottom*, The receptor complex in the activated state with the chloride channel open. Activation is induced by GABA or a GABA agonist (eg, muscimol) binding to GABA$_A$-receptors. Activation is associated with conformational changes and opening of the chloride channel. These phenomena promote chloride conductance across the cell membrane and hyperpolarize the neuron. This mechanism is the basis of GABA-ergic inhibitory neurotransmission. The "gating" of the chloride channel by GABA can be allosterically modulated by BZ-receptors that exist in the form of different subtypes. BZ-receptor ligands have different BZ-receptor subtype specificities. (Reproduced from Biological Psychiatry 1981;16:213–229). Basile et al. show a more current model of the GABA$_A$-receptor complex that incorporates the configuration of subunits (16).

not considered to mediate their behavioral effects primarily via the GABA$_A$/BZ-receptor complex (106). HE is associated with increased resistance to the induction of seizures by drugs that decrease GABA-ergic tone (106). Isolated CNS neurons from rabbits with HE are three to five times more sensitive to depression by agonists of the GABA$_A$/BZ-receptor complex than control neurons (21). The administration of BZ receptor antagonists significantly increases the spontaneous activity of neurons from rabbits with HE at doses that had no effect or depressed the activity of control neurons (21). Administration of antagonists of the GABA$_A$/BZ-receptor complex, including BZ-antagonists, induce ameliorations of the behavioral and VER changes of HE (106, 108, 109).

Together, these findings provide strong evidence of a functional increase in GABA-ergic tone in animal models of HE due to FHF. They also suggest that this phenomenon is mediated allosterically through the BZ-receptor (110). Strong support for this hypothesis has been provided by finding increased levels of BZ-agonists, including diazepam, in the brains of animal models of HE (111–113) and humans with HE due to FHF (114). Increased levels of BZ-receptor binding activity and immunoreactive BZs have also been found in cerebrospinal fluid (CSF), sera, and urine in patients with decompensated cirrhosis who had not ingested prescription BZs. The levels of BZs in these patients correlated with the degree of HE (115). Thus, a rationale exists for the administration of a BZ-receptor antagonist, such as flumazenil, in HE.

ISSUES OF CONCERN WITH THIS HYPOTHESIS

Direct evidence for increased availability of GABA at GABA$_A$-receptors is lacking, although increased plasma-to-brain transfer of GABA has been documented in one model of FHF (116). Some patients dying of FHF do not have increased brain BZ levels (114). Brain levels of BZs appear to be insufficient to account for all of the manifestations of HE

(16), although the distribution of BZs in the brain is heterogenous (117). Nevertheless, as mentioned below, treatment with a benzodiazepine receptor antagonist may be quite effective in ameliorating HE, and merits in-depth consideration.

FLUMAZENIL

Pharmacology

Structurally, flumazenil is a 1,4-imidazobenzodiazepine (Fig. 21.3). Functionally, it is BZ-receptor antagonist with high specificity and affinity for central BZ-receptors. It does not interact directly with GABA$_A$-receptors, barbiturate binding sites, or peripheral BZ-receptors. It competitively antagonizes the actions of BZs and other compounds that directly bind to central BZ-receptors. All effects of BZ-receptor agonists such as diazepam can be blocked by flumazenil. The potency of flumazenil as an antagonist is approximately the same as that of diazepam as an agonist. The effects of a BZ-agonist can be reversed by the intravenous administration of 0.25–0.5 mg of flumazenil (16, 118).

Flumazenil is lipid soluble and rapidly traverses the blood-brain barrier. It is taken up by gray matter structures in the brain, its initial distribution reflecting blood flow. Thus it promptly reaches BZ-receptors in the brain. Flumazenil is effective at lower doses after intravenous than after oral administration. This difference in efficacy reflects the low bioavailability of the orally administered drug (about 16%), which is attributable to the high first-pass hepatic extraction of enterically absorbed flumazenil. After oral administration flumazenil is rapidly and almost completely absorbed, with peak plasma concentrations occurring after 20–90 min (16, 118).

Binding of flumazenil to plasma proteins is about 40%. The drug is rapidly distributed with a high apparent volume of distribution, consistent with substantial tissue uptake. It is rapidly metabolized into inactive polar metabolites that are completely eliminated within 48–72 hrs. When labeled flumazenil is given intravenously or orally 90–95% of the label

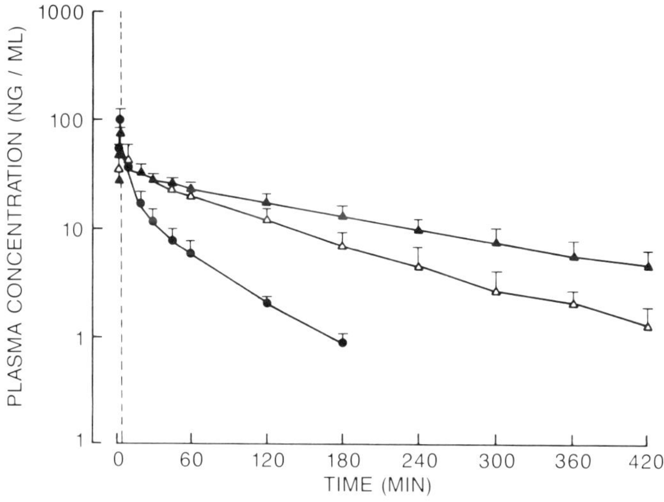

Figure 21.3. The chemical structures of midazolam and flumazenil (Ro 15–1788). Midazolam is a 1,4-substituted benzodiazepine (BZ) that acts as an antagonist at central BZ-receptors. Flumazenil is an imidazobenzodiazepine that acts as an antagonist (and at high doses/concentrations, a weak partial agonist) at central BZ-receptors.

Figure 21.4. Concentration-time curves of flumazenil. Flumazenil (2 mg) was infused intravenously over a 5-minute period: *dotted line*, end of infusion; *closed circles*, normal volunteers; *open triangles*, cirrhotic patients with moderate liver dysfunction; *closed triangles*, cirrhotic patients with severe liver dysfunction. Data are given as means ± SD. The plasma half-life of flumazenil is markedly prolonged in patients with advanced cirrhosis. Reproduced from Pomier-Layrarques et al. (119).

appears in urine and 5–10% in feces. Plasma clearance is rapid, the plasma half-life being about 46 minutes in normal subjects (119) (Fig. 21.4). Rapid metabolism is the main factor determining the duration of the antagonistic effect which lasts 2–3 hours in normal subjects. Clearance of the drug is attributed largely to hepatic extraction and metabolism, although it is an ester and metabolism by serum esterases may be important (16, 118).

In studies of the fate of ^{11}C-labeled flumazenil in normal subjects, the label rapidly

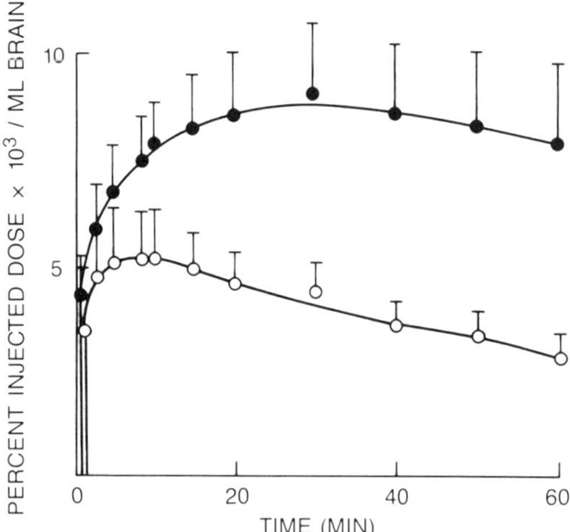

Figure 21.5. Kinetics of ¹¹C-flumazenil in human temporal cortex determined by position emission tomography following an intravenous bolus injection of a tracer dose of ¹¹C-flumazenil. *Closed circles*, patients with cirrhosis and history of hepatic encephalopathy (HE) within the previous month (N = 4); *open circles*, control subjects (N = 8). Data are given as means ± SD. The prolonged brain retention of flumazenil in cirrhotic patients may be attributable to its slower metabolism by the diseased liver. Reproduced with minor modifications from Samson et al. (120).

reaches and binds to BZ-receptors in the brain. It can be rapidly removed from these receptors by administering an unlabeled BZ-receptor ligand, as determined by position emission tomography (16, 118). Cerebral retention of the label of ¹¹C-flumazenil is prolonged in patients with advanced cirrhosis (120) (Fig. 21.5). This finding probably reflects impaired metabolism of flumazenil in chronic liver disease with consequent increase in the plasma half-life of the drug (119) (Fig. 21.4).

When flumazenil is given intravenously, the minimum effective dose is 0.1 mg, and a clinical effect attributable to its BZ-receptor antagonist action can usually be detected within 1 minute. An infusion of 0.1 mg/hour can induce a consistent BZ-receptor antagonist effect (16, 118).

Flumazenil has a high therapeutic index. Extensive use of flumazenil in animal studies and appreciable experience with the adminis-

tration of this drug to human subjects suggests that it is very safe. Doses of as much as 600 mg orally and 100 mg intravenously have been tolerated well by normal subjects. Transient mild anxiety has been observed following the administration of flumazenil to normal subjects and a patient with chronic PSE (see below). This effect is probably attributable to displacement of agonist ligands from BZ-receptors, because flumazenil does not appear to have any intrinsic neuronal activating properties. Indeed, at high doses it has partial agonist (i.e., weak diazepam-like) actions and no convulsive potential (16, 118).

Clinical Application

In 1985, Bansky and colleagues described amelioration of HE in a 58-year-old woman with cirrhosis. Before treatment she had stage IV HE (ie, hepatic coma) and continuous 1–2 Hz triphasic wave EEG activity. Forty seconds after the intravenous administration of 0.3 mg flumazenil, the encephalopathy had improved clinically to stage II and the EEG showed more rapid 4–5 Hz continuous background θ-activity (121) (Fig. 21.6). Similar findings in a patient with HE due to FHF were simultaneously reported (122). Anecdotal uncontrolled reports of the administration of flumazenil to more than 80 patients with HE have appeared (16, 123). The overall response rate has been about 60%. The responses were not only clinical but also electrophysiologic as assessed by EEG findings and evoked responses. In none of these reports was previous ingestion of synthetic BZ-agonist drugs implicated in the flumazenil-induced remissions of encephalopathy in patients with liver disease. Sometimes when flumazenil is given intravenously to patients with hepatic coma the patient becomes conscious and starts talking with dramatic rapidity. Such responses occur from 28 seconds–30 minutes after the injection of flumazenil and last for 0.6–4 hours (16). No other therapeutic modality for HE is associated with such rapid responses. Responses of HE to intravenous flumazenil are comparable to responses of hypoglycemic coma to intravenous dextrose.

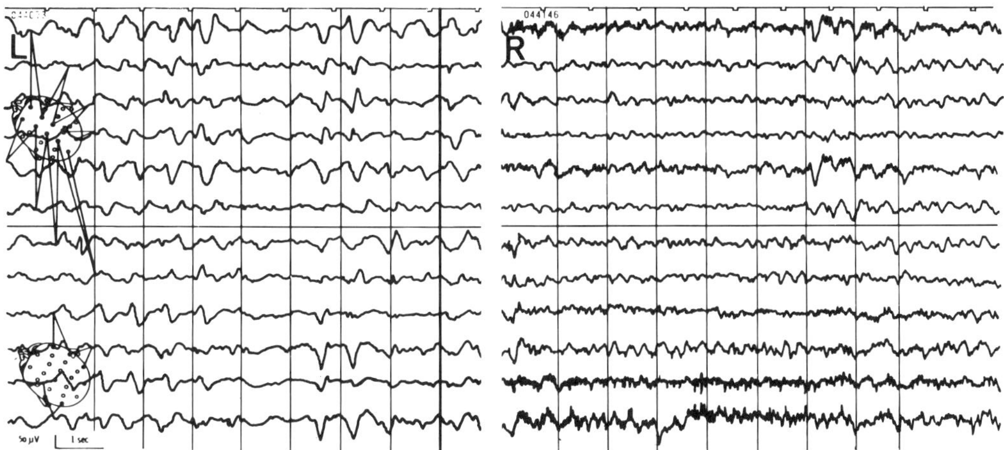

Figure 21.6. Amelioration of hepatic encephalopathy (HE) in a 58-year-old woman with cirrhosis following the administration of the benzodiazepine receptor antagonist flumazenil. *Left*, before treatment, when the patient was in stage IV HE (coma), the encephalogram (EEG) showed continuous 1- to 2-Hz triphasic wave activity; right, 40 seconds after the intravenous administration of 0.3 mg of flumazenil, the patient's degree of HE had improved to stage II, and the EEG showed more rapid 4- to 5-Hz θ background activity. Reproduced with modifications from Bansky et al. (121, 125).

Table 21.4
Flumazenil-Induced Improvements of Human Hepatic Encephalopathy (HE)[a]

Reference	Grade of HE				Response/ No. of patients
	I	II	III	IV	
Meier and Gyr (128)		2/3	1/1		3/4
Grimm et al. (124)	0/1	1/1	7/7	4/11	12/20
Bansky et al. (125)		1/1	3/3	6/10	10/14
Pidoux et al. (129)	1/1	1/1	1/2	3/4	6/8
van der Rijt et al. (130)	2/2		2/2	1/5	5/9
Case reports (118, 131)				2/3	2/3
Total	3/4 (75)	5/6 (83)	14/15 (93)	16/33 (48)	38/58 (66)

[a]Numbers in parentheses are percentages.

Current experience suggests that the incidence of responses of HE to flumazenil is similar in patients with cirrhosis or FHF (16). In two of the largest studies (124, 125), 19 of 31 (61%) patients with HE responded to flumazenil with an average improvement of 1.4 ± 0.1 HE stage units or 2.8 ± 0.38 units on the Glasgow coma scale (mean ± SEM) (Table 21.4).

There are several potential reasons why the intravenous administration of flumazenil may not always lead to an improvement in the degree of HE. Even though increased levels of BZs may be present in the brain, a response may not occur if the dose is inadequate, if additional CNS complications of FHF are present (such as raised intracranial pressure, hypoxic brain damage, or hypoglycemia), or if many factors are contributing to the encephalopathy in the agonal stages of liver failure. With regard to dose, there are numerous instances of substantial ameliorations of HE following administration of 0.2–1.0 mg of flumazenil and recent evidence suggests that 7 mg is sufficient to occupy the majority of central BZ-receptors (126). Another reason for a

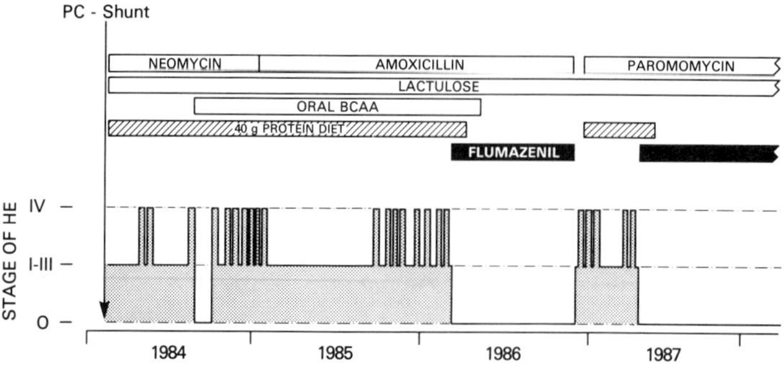

Figure 21.7. Remissions of chronic intractable portal systemic encephalopathy (PSE) in a 42-year-old woman associated with the oral administration of flumazenil. Degrees of encephalopathy are depicted as 0 (clinically normal mental function), stages I–III, and stage IV (coma). A two-thirds hepatectomy and end-to-side portacaval shunt were followed by the development of chronic incapacitating encephalopathy with episodes of coma. Treatment with oral broad-spectrum antibiotics, lactulose, and dietary protein restriction did not appreciably ameliorate the encephalopathy. Addition of oral branched-chain amino acids (BCAA) therapy was associated with a transient improvement in the encephalopathy. In contrast, flumazenil administration (25 mg orally twice a day) was associated with a complete and sustained remission of the encephalopathy, which induced a normalization of tolerance to dietary protein. Discontinuing flumazenil therapy precipitated a recurrence of the encephalopathy; reinstituting it was followed by a further complete and sustained remission. Reproduced with modifications from Ferenci et al. (127).

lack of response of HE to flumazenil is the presence of normal brain levels of BZ-receptor ligands (114). Indeed, in the absence of complicating factors responsiveness of HE to flumazenil may depend primarily on brain levels of BZ-ligands (16).

Flumazenil has also been administered to a patient who apparently had chronic intractable PSE in the absence of established chronic liver disease (127). The patient was a 42-year-old woman who underwent a two-thirds hepatectomy and end-to-side portacaval shunt for an inflammatory mass in the liver. Postoperatively, chronic incapacitating encephalopathy soon developed and she had 18 episodes of coma during the ensuing 2 years. The encephalopathy was refractory to standard treatment with a reduced dietary protein intake, oral broad-spectrum antibiotics, lactulose, and oral branched-chain amino acids. When flumazenil 25 mg orally twice daily was started 2 years after the surgery she rapidly became and remained free from evidence of encephalopathy in spite of unrestricted dietary protein intake (as much as 150 g/day). After 9 months of flumazenil, use of the drug was discontinued when she developed a fever of unknown

origin. The fever resolved spontaneously but she again became chronically encephalopathic and had several further episodes of coma over a 4-month period in spite of a comprehensive regimen of conventional therapy. Reinstitution of flumazenil was again associated with a complete and sustained remission of encephalopathy and normal dietary protein tolerance (Fig. 21.7). Flumazenil therapy in this patient was associated with reversal of abnormalities of event-related auditory-evoked potentials. In this study, flumazenil induced a consistent side effect; 25–40 minutes after the ingestion of 25 mg of flumazenil, she regularly experienced a feeling of anxiety that subsided after 30–60 minutes (127). This side effect can be explained by the anxiogenic effect of a decrease in GABA-ergic tone occurring as a consequence of disinhibition of neurons because of flumazenil-induced displacement of endogenous BZ-agonist ligands.

There appear to be several potential uses for intravenously administered flumazenil in the management of patients with acute HE. First, it may be used to reverse the effects of any exogenously administered BZ. Second, the response to flumazenil may indicate whether the encephalopathy is potentially reversible and hence may have prognostic and therapeutic implications. The drug may be given, perhaps by intravenous infusion, to optimize brain function in the presence of liver failure. Finally, orally administered flumazenil may decrease dietary protein intolerance in patients with chronic PSE.

CONCLUDING PERSPECTIVES

The pathogenesis of HE is considered to be multifactorial. Of the many factors that suggested as contributors to HE, those that have been recognized as clinically important are certain identifiable precipitating factors and certain (poorly defined) gut-derived nitrogenous substances that bypass the diseased liver and accumulate in plasma. Conventional management aimed at restoring normal mental function in a patient with HE requires the application of two cardinal traditional principles. First, it is essential to determine which precipitating or exacerbating factors are contributing to the HE and to take appropriate clinical measures to remove or correct such factors. Second, the absorption of nitrogenous substances from the gastrointestinal tract is minimized by reducing dietary protein intake, purgation, and the administration of nonabsorbed disaccharides or a poorly absorbed broad-spectrum antibiotic. The relative merits of different disaccharides (e.g., lactulose, lactitol) are being assessed. Neomycin remains the most popular antibiotic for use in the treatment of HE. Much remains to be learned concerning the relevance of the multiple actions of disaccharides such as lactulose and lactitol, and of antibiotics in relation to correcting manifestations of HE.

Reduction of portal-systemic shunting of blood is a desirable objective in the management of HE. This approach is only practical in a rare patient with chronic intractable PSE. Improvement of hepatocellular function is another desirable objective. This approach is being most actively pursued in the context of FHF by experimental attempts to decrease hepatocellular necrosis (e.g., with postaglandins) and stimulate hepatic regeneration (e.g., with

hepatotrophic factors). Treatments for manifestations of encephalopathy attributable to raised intracranial pressure in FHF such as mannitol and thiopental are logically classified separately from treatments for uncomplicated HE.

Application of pharmacologic principles in the management of HE seems likely to be more important as new experimental treatments are applied than with the administration of traditional therapeutic modalities. The most promising experimental treatment for HE at the time of writing is the BZ-antagonist flumazenil. The rationale for the use of this drug in the treatment of HE is evidence that endogenous BZ-agonists contribute to the manifestations of HE by allosterically potentiating the action of GABA. Currently, flumazenil is the only BZ-antagonist available for clinical use. Proof of its efficacy in the management of HE must await the results of appropriately designed controlled clinical trials. However, flumazenil may not be the ideal BZ-receptor ligand for use in patients with HE. Other BZ-receptor ligands with antagonist properties are available for evaluation in animal models and new drugs of this type continue to be synthesized. Such drugs can be selected for their safety and the efficacy with which they reverse the manifestations of HE. In addition to an absence of serious side effects, which would include a lack of significant intrinsic activity, important properties of an ideal BZ-receptor ligand for use in the management of HE would be much slower metabolism than flumazenil and high affinity and specificity for central BZ-receptors. Another important determinant of the efficacy of such a drug may be its BZ-receptor subtype specificity. If important roles for neurotransmitter systems other than the $GABA_A$-receptor complex become defined, it is possible that centrally acting drugs other than BZ-antagonists may be shown to have a useful role in the management of HE.

REFERENCES

1. Sherlock S, Summerskill WHJ, White LP, Phear EA. Portal-systemic encephalopathy: neurological

complications of liver disease. Lancet 1954;2:453–457.

2. Summerskill WHJ, Davidson EA, Sherlock S, Steiner RE. The neuropsychiatric syndrome associated with hepatic cirrhosis and an extensive portal collateral circulation. Q J Med 1956;25:245–266.

3. Sherlock S. Hepatic encephalopathy. In: Disease of the Liver and Biliary System. 8th ed. Blackwell Scientific, Oxford, 1989;95–115.

4. Read AE, Sherlock S, Laidlaw J, Walker JG. The neuropsychiatric syndromes associated with chronic liver disease and an extensive portal-systemic collateral circulation. Q J Med 1967;36:135–150.

5. Adams RD, Foley JM. The neurological disorder associated with liver disease. Res Publ Assn Res Nerv Ment Dis 1953;32:198.

6. Davidson EA, Summerskill WHJ. Psychiatric aspects of liver disease. Postgrad Med J 1956;32:487.

7. Havens LL, Child III CG. Recurrent psychosis associated with liver disease and elevated blood ammonia. N Engl J Med 1955;252:756–759.

8. Tarter RE, Hegedus AM, van Thiel DH, Schade RR. Portal-systemic encephalopathy: neuropsychiatric manifestations. Int J Psych Med 1985;15:265–274.

9. Mullen KD. Hepatic encephalopathy. In: Rector WG Jr, ed. Complications of chronic liver disease. St. Louis: Mosby-Year Book, 1992:127–160.

10. Conn HO. Trailmaking and number-connection tests in the assessment of mental state in portal systemic encephalopathy. Am J Dig Dis 1977;22:541–550.

11. Tarter RE, Hegedus AM, van Thiel DH, Schade RR, Gavaler JS, Starzl TE. Nonalcoholic cirrhosis associated with neuropsychological dysfunction in the absence of overt evidence of hepatic encephalopathy. Gastroenterology 1984;86:1421–1427.

12. Gitlin N, Lewis DC, Hinkley L. The diagnosis and prevalence of subclinical hepatic encephalopathy in apparently healthy, ambulant non-shunted patients with cirrhosis. J Hepatol 1986;3:75–82.

13. Kügler CFA, Petter J, Wensing G, Taghavy A, Hahn EG, Fleig WE. Visual event-related P300 potentials in early portal-systemic encephalopathy. Gastroenterology 1992;103:302–310.

14. Gazzard BG, Price H, Dawson AM. Detection of hepatic encephalopathy. Postgrad Med J 1986;62:163–166.

15. Parsons-Smith BG, Summerskill WHJ, Dawson AM, Sherlock S. The electroencephalograph in liver disease. Lancet 1957;2:867–871.

16. Basile AS, Jones EA, Skolnick P. The pathogenesis of hepatic encephalopathy: Evidence for the involvement of benzodiazepine receptor ligands. Pharmacol Rev 1991;43:27–71.

17. Jones EA, Skolnick P. Benzodiazepine receptor ligands and the syndrome of hepatic encephalopathy. In: Popper H, Schaffner F, eds. Progress in liver diseases. Philadelphia: Saunders, 1990;9:345–370.

18. Jones EA. Benzodiazepine receptor ligands and hepatic encephalopathy: further unfolding of the GABA story. Hepatology 1991;14:1286–1290.

19. Bakti G, Fisch HV, Karlaganis G, Minder C, Bircher J. Mechanism of the excessive sedative response of cirrhosis to benzodiazepines: model experiments with triazolam. Hepatology 1987;7:629–638.

20. Basile AS, Gammal SH, Mullen KD, Jones EA, Skolnick P. Differential responsiveness of cerebellar Purkinje neurons to GABA and benzodiazepine receptor ligands in an animal model of hepatic encephalopathy. J Neurosci 1988;8:2414–2421.

21. Püspök A, Herneth A, Steindl P, Ferenci P. Hepatic encephalopathy in rats with thioacetamide induced liver failure is not mediated by endogenous benzodiazepines. Gastroenterology 1993;105:851–857.

22. Moore RD, Smith CR, Lietman PS. Increased risk of renal dysfunction due to the interaction of liver disease and aminoglycosides. Am J Med 1986;80:1093–1097.

23. Read AE, Laidlaw J, Haslam RM, et al. Neuropsychiatric complications following chlorothiazide therapy in patients with hepatic cirrhosis: possible relation to hypokalemia. Clin Sci 1959;18:409–423.

24. Samson RI, Trey C, Timme AM, Saunders SJ. Fulminating hepatitis with recurrent hypoglycemia and hemorrhage. Gastroenterology 1967;53:291–300.

25. Laidlaw J, Read AE, Sherlock S. Morphine tolerance in hepatic cirrhosis. Gastroenterology 1961;40:389–396.

26. Summerskill WHJ, Wolfe SJ, Davidson CS. The management of hepatic coma in relation to protein withdrawal and certain specific measures. Am J Med 1957;23:59–76.

27. Collinson PO, Burroughs AK. Severe hypermagnesaemia due to magnesium sulphate enemas in hepatic coma. Br Med J 1986;293:1013–1014.

28. Dahlquist A, Gryboski JD. Inability of the human small intestinal lactase to hydrolyse lactulose. Biochem Biophys Acta 1965;110:635–636.

29. Carrulli M, Salvioli GF, Manenti F. Absorption of lactulose in man. Digestion 6:139–145.

30. Nanji AA, Lauener RM. Lactulose-induced hypernatremia. Drug Intell Clin Pharm 1984;18:70–71.

31. Brown RL, Gibson JA, Sladen GE, Hicks B, Dawson AM. Effects of lactulose and other laxatives on ileal and colonic pH as measured by a radiotelemetry device. Gut 1974;15:999–1004.

32. Bennett A, Eley KG. Intestinal pH and propulsion: an explanation of diarrhea in lactase deficiency and laxation by lactulose. J Pharm Pharmacol 1976;28:192–195.

33. Vince A, Zeegan R, Drinkwater JE, O'Grady F, Dawson AM. The effect of lactulose on the fecal flora of patients with hepatic encephalopathy. J Med Microbiol 1974;7:163–168.

34. Florent CH, Flourie B, Leblond A, Rautureau M, Bernier J-J. Influence of chronic lactulose in man. J Clin Invest 1985;75:608–613.

35. Mortensen PB, Rasmussen HS, Holtug K. Lactulose detoxifies in vitro short-chain fatty acid production in colonic contents induced by blood: implications for hepatic coma. Gastroenterology 1988;94:750–754.

36. Weber FL Jr, Banwell JG, Fresard KM. Nitrogen in fecal bacterial, fiber and soluble fractions of cirrhotic patients: effects of lactulose and lactulose plus neomycin. J Lab Clin Med 1988;110:259–263.

37. Schafer DF. In hepatic coma, the problem comes from the colon, but will the answers come from there? J Lab Clin Med 1987;110:253–254.

38. Heubel KA. Lactulose works, but why? Gastroenterology 1973;65:349–351.

39. Atterbury CE, Maddrey WC, Conn HO. Neomycin-sorbitol and lactulose in the treatment of acute portal-systemic encephalopathy: a controlled, double-blind clinical trial. Am J Dig Dis 1978;23:398–406.

40. Kersh ES, Rifkind H. Lactulose enemas. Ann Intern Med 1973;78:81–84.

41. Morgan MY, Hawley KM. Lactitol versus lactulose in the treatment of acute hepatic encephalopathy in cirrhotic patients: a double-blind, randomized trial. Hepatology 1987;7:1278–1284.

42. Nelson DC, McGrew WRG, Hoyumpa AM. Hypernatremia and lactulose therapy. JAMA 1983;249:1295–1298.

43. Patil DH, Grimble GK, Silk DBA. Lactitol, a new hydrogenated lactose derivative; intestinal absorption and laxative threshold in normal human subjects. Br J Nutr 1987;57:195–199.

44. Patil DH, Westaby D, Mahida YR. Comparative modes of action of lactitol and lactulose in the treatment of hepatic encephalopathy. Gut 1987;28:255–259.

45. Lanthier PL, Morgan MY. Lactitol in the treatment of chronic hepatic encephalopathy: an open comparison with lactulose. Gut 1985;26:415–420.

46. Heredia D, Caballeria J, Arroyo V, Ravelli G, Rodes J. Lactitol versus lactulose in the treatment of acute portal systemic encephalopathy. J Hepatol 1987;4:293–298.

47. Uribe M, Campollo O, Vargas F, et al. Acidifying enemas (lactitol and lactulose) versus nonacidifying enemas (tap water) to treat acute portal-systemic encephalopathy: a double-blind, randomized clinical trial. Heptology 1987;7:639–643.

48. Beaven J, Bjorneklett A, Jenssen E, Blomhoff JP, Skrede S. Pulmonary hydrogen and methane and plasma ammonia after the administration of lactulose or sorbitol. Scand J Gastroenterol 1983;18:343–347.

49. Dawson AM, McLaren J, Sherlock S. Neomycin in the treatment of hepatic coma. Lancet 1957;2:1263–1268.

50. Falloon WW, Paesk K, Woolfolk D, Nankin H, Wallace K, Haro EN. Effect of neomycin and kanomycin upon intestinal absorption. Ann NY Acad Sci 1966;132:879–887.

51. Fast BB, Wolfe SJ, Stormont JM, Davidson CS. Antibiotic therapy in the management of hepatic coma. Arch Intern Med 1958;101:467–475.

52. Kunin CM, Chalmers TC, Leevy CM, Sebastyen SC, Lieber CS, Finland M. Absorption of orally-administered neomycin and kanamycin with special reference to patients with severe hepatic and renal disease. N Engl J Med 1960;262:380–385.

53. Last PM, Sherlock S. Systemic absorption of orally administered neomycin in liver disease. N Engl J Med 1960;262:385–389.

54. Breen KJ, Bryant RE, Levinson JD, Shenker S. Neomycin absorption in man. Studies of oral and enema administration and effect of intestinal ulceration. Ann Intern Med 1972;76:211–218.

55. Berk DP, Chalmers T. Deafness complicating antibiotic therapy of hepatic encephalopathy. Ann Intern Med 1970;73:393–396.

56. Tisdale WA, Fenster LF, Klatskin G. Acute staphylococcal enterocolitis complicating oral neomycin therapy in cirrhosis. N Engl J Med 1960;263:1014–1016.

57. Morgan MH, Read AE, Speller DCE. Treatment of hepatic encephalopathy with metronidazole. Gut 1982;23:1–7.

58. Schomerus H, Hamster W, Blunck H, Reinhard U, Mayer K, Dolle W. Latent portal systemic encephalopathy, I: nature of cerebral functional defects and their effect on fitness to drive. Dig Dis Sci 1981;26:622–630.

59. Greenburger NJ, Carley J, Schenker S, Bettinger I, Stamnes C, Beyer P. Effect of vegetable and animal protein diets in chronic hepatic encephalopathy. Am J Dig Dis 1977;22:845–855.

60. Uribe M, Marquez MA, Garcia Ramos G, et al. Treatment of chronic portal-systemic encephalopathy with vegetable and animal protein diets: a controlled crossover study. Dig Dis Sci 1982;27:1109–1116.

61. Bruijn KM, Blendis LM, Zilm DH, Carlen PL, Anderson GH. Effect of dietary protein manipulations in subclinical portal systemic encephalopathy. Gut 1983;24:53–60.

62. Keshavarzian A, Meek J, Sutton VM, Emery VM, Hughes EA, Hodgson HJF. Dietary supplementation from vegetable sources in the management of chronic portal systemic encephalopathy. Am J Gastroenterol 1984;79:945–949.

63. Fenton JCB, Knight EJ, Humpherson PL. Milk and cheese diet in portal systemic encephalopathy. Lancet 1966;1:164–166.

64. Uribe M, Dibildox M, Malpica S, et al. Beneficial effect of vegetable protein diet supplemented with psyllium plantago in patients with hepatic encephalopathy and diabetes mellitus. Gastroenterology 1985;88:901–907.

65. Rijt van der CCD, Schalm SW, Shat H, Foeken K, de Jonge G. Overt hepatic encephalopathy precipitated by zinc deficiency. Gastroenterology 1991;100:1114–1118.

66. Reding P, Duchateu J, Bataille C. Oral zinc supplementation improves hepatic encephalopathy: results of a randomized controlled trial. Lancet 1984; 2:493–495.

67. Riggio O, Ariosto F, Merli M, et al. Short term oral zinc supplementation does not improve chronic hepatic encephalopathy. Dig Dis Sci 1991;36:1204–1208.

68. Bircher J, Miller J, Guggenheim P, Haemmerli UP. Treatment of chronic portal-systemic encephalopathy with lactulose. Lancet 1966;1:890–893.

69. Elkington SH, Floch MH, Conn CO. Lactulose in the treatment of chronic portal-systemic encephalopathy: a double-blind clinical trial. N Engl J Med 1969;281:408–412.

70. Zeegan R, Drinkwater JE, Fenton JCB, Vince A, Dawson AM. Some observations on the effects of treatment with lactulose on patients with chronic hepatic encephalopathy. Quart J Med 1970;39:245–263.

71. Simmons F, Goldstein H, Boyle JD. A controlled clinical trial of lactulose in hepatic encephalopathy. Gastroenterology 1970;59:827–832.

72. Bircher J, Haemmerli UP, Scollo-Lavizzari G, Hoffmann K. Treatment of chronic portal-systemic encephalopathy with lactulose. Am J Med 1971; 51:148–159.

73. Kardel T, Olsen PZ, Stigsby B, Tonnesen K. Hepatic encephalopathy evaluated by automatic period analysis of the electroencephalogram during lactulose treatment. Acta Med Scand 1972;192:493–498.

74. Conn HO, Leevy CM, Vlahcevic ZR, et al. Comparison of lactulose and neomycin in the treatment of chronic portal-systemic encephalopathy. Gastroenterology 1977;72:573–583.

75. Orlandi F, Freddara U, Candelaresi MT, et al. Comparison between neomycin and lactulose in 173 patients with hepatic encephalopathy: a randomized clinical study. Dig Dis Sci 1981;26:498–506.

76. Morgan MY, Hawley KE, Stambuk D. Lactitol versus lactulose in the treatment of chronic hepatic encephalopathy: a double-blind, randomized crossover study. J Hepatol 1987;4:236–244.

77. Uribe M, Marquez MA, Garcia Ramos G, et al. Treatment of chronic portal-systemic encephalopathy with lactose in lactase-deficient patients. Dig Dis Sci 1980;25:924–929.

78. Uribe M, Toledo H, Perez E, et al. Lactitol, a second-generation disaccharide for the treatment of chronic portal-systemic encephalopathy: a double-blind, crossover randomized clinical trial. Dig. Dis Sci 1987;32:1345–1353.

79. Read AE, McCarthy CF, Heaton KW, Laidlaw J. Lactobacillus acidophilus (Enpac) in treatment of hepatic encephalopathy. Br Med J 1966;1:1267–1269.

80. Potts III JR, Henderson JM, Millikan WJ Jr, Sones P, Warren WD. Restoration of portal venous perfusion and reversal of encephalopathy by balloon occlusion of portal systemic shunt. Gastroenterology 1984;87:208–212.

81. Bismuth H, Houssin D, Grange D. Suppression of the shunt and esophageal transaction: a new technique for the treatment of disabling post shunt encephalopathy. Am J Surg 1983;146:392–396.

82. Chandler JG, Fechner RE. Hepatopedal flow restoration in patients intolerant of total portal diversion. Ann Surg 1983;197:574–583.

83. Lockwood AH, MacDonald JM, Reiman RE, et al. The dynamics of ammonia metabolism in man: effects of liver disease and hyperammonemia. J Clin Invest 1979;63:449–460.

84. Pappas SC, Ferenci P, Schafer DF, Jones EA. Visual-evoked potentials in a rabbit model of hepatic encephalopathy, II: comparison of hyperammonemic encephalopathy, postictal coma, and coma induced by synergistic neurotoxins. Gastroenterology 1984;86:546–551.

85. Jones DB, Mullen KD, Roessle M, Maynard T, Jones EA. Hepatic encephalopathy: application of visual evoked responses to test hypotheses of its pathogenesis in rats. J Hepatol 1987;4:118–126.

86. Hawkins RA, Mans AM. Brain energy metabolism in hepatic encephalopathy. In: Butterworth RF, Pomier-Layrarques G, eds. Hepatic encephalopathy: pathophysiology and treatment. Clifton, NJ: Humana Press, 1989:159–170.

87. Butterworth RF, Lavoie J, Peterson C, Cotman CW, Szerb JC. Excitatory amino acids and hepatic encephalopathy. In: Butterworth RF, Pomier-Layrarques G, eds. Hepatic encephalopathy: pathophysiology and treatment. Clifton, NJ: Humana Press, 1989:417–433.

88. Raabe W. Neurophysiology of ammonia intoxication. In: Butterworth RF, Pomier-Layrarques G, eds. Hepatic encephalopathy: pathophysiology and treatment. Clifton, NJ: Humana Press, 1989:49–77.

89. Cooper AJL, Plum F. Biochemistry and physiology of brain ammonia. Physiol Rev 1987;67:440–519.

90. Conn HO, Lierbethal MM. The hepatic coma syndromes and lactulose. Baltimore: Williams & Wilkins, 1978.

91. Reynolds TB, Redeker AG, Davis P. A controlled study of the effects of l-arginine on hepatic encephalopathy. Am J Med 1958;25:359–367.

92. Mendenhall CL, Rouster S, Marshall L, Weesner R. A new therapy for portal systemic encephalopathy. Am J Gastroenterol 1986;81:540–543.

93. Sushma S, Dasarathy S, Tandon RK, Jain S, Gupta S, Bhist MS. Sodium benzoate in the treatment of acute hepatic encephalopathy: a double-blind randomized trial. Hepatology 1992;16:138–144.

94. James JH, Ziparo V, Jeppson B, Fischer JE. Hyperammonemia, plasma amino acid imbalance and blood-brain amino acid transport: a unified theory of portal-systemic encephalopathy. Lancet 1979; 2:772–775.

95. Zieve L, Olsen RL. Can hepatic coma be caused by a reduction of brain noradrenalin and dopamine? Gut 1977;18:688–691.

96. Morgan MY, Milsom JP, Sherlock S. Plasma ratio of valine, leucine and isoleucine to phenylalanine and tyrosine in liver disease. Gut 1978;19:1068–1073.

97. Cuilleret G, Pomier-Layrarques G, Pons F, Cadilhac J, Michel H. Changes in brain catecholamine levels in human cirrhotic hepatic encephalopathy. Gut 1981;21:565–569.

98. Eriksson LS, Conn HO. Branched-chain amino acids in the management of hepatic encephalopathy: an analysis of variants. Hepatology 1989;10:228–246.

99. Alexander WF, Spindel E, Harty RF, Cerda JJ. The usefulness of branched chain amino acids in patients with acute and chronic hepatic encephalopathy. Am J Gastroenterol 1989;84:91–96.

100. Horst D, Grace ND, Conn HO, et al. Comparison of dietary protein with an oral, branched chain-enriched amino acid supplement in chronic portal-systemic encephalopathy: a double-blind controlled trial. Hepatology 1984;4:279–287.

101. Michel H, Solere M, Granier P, Cauvet JP, Bali JP, Bellet-Herman H. Treatment of cirrhotic hepatic encephalopathy with l-dopa: a controlled trial. Gastroenterology 1980;79:207–211.

102. Uribe M, Farca A, Marquez MA, Garcia-Ramos G, Guevara L. Treatment of chronic portal-systemic encephalopathy with bromocriptine: a double-blind controlled trial. Gastroenterology 1979;76:1347–1351.

103. Morgan MY, Jakobovits AW, James IM, Sherlock S. Successful use of bromocriptine in the treatment of chronic hepatic encephalopathy. Gastroenterology 1980;78:663–670.

104. Uribe M, Garcia-Romos G, Ramos M, et al. Standard and higher doses of bromocriptine for severe chronic portal-systemic encephalopathy. Am J Gastroenterology 1983;78:517–522.

105. Roberts E. The establishment of GABA as a neurotransmitter. In: Squires RF, ed. GABA and benzodiazepine receptors, volume 1. Boca Raton, FL: CRC Press, 1988:1–21.

106. Bassett ML, Mullen KD, Skolnick P, Jones EA. Amelioration of hepatic encephalopathy by pharmacologic antagonism of the GABA$_A$-benzodiazepine receptor complex in a rabbit model of fulminant hepatic failure. Gastroenterology 1987; 93:1069–1077.

107. Jones EA. Hepatic encephalopathy and GABAergic neurotransmission. In: Conn HO, Bircher J, eds. Hepatic encephalopathy: management with lactulose and related carbohydrates. East Lansing, MI: Medi-Ed Press, 1988:61–80.

108. Jones EA, Bassett ML, Mullen KD. Hepatic encephalopathy. In: Arias IM, Frenkel M, Wilson JHP (eds). The liver annual, vol. 5. Amsterdam, Elsevier, 1986:274–313.

109. Gammal SH, Basile AS, Geller D, Skolnick P, Jones EA. Reversal of the behavioral and electrophysiological abnormalities of an animal model of hepatic encephalopathy by benzodiazepine receptor ligands. Hepatology 1990;11:371–378.

110. Mullen KD, Mendelson WB, Martin JV, Roessle M, Maynard TF, Jones EA. Could an endogenous benzodiazepine ligand contribute to hepatic encephalopathy? Lancet 1988;1:457–459.

111. Basile AS, Pannell L, Jaonni T, et al. Brain concentrations of benzodiazepines are elevated in an animal model of hepatic encephalopathy. Proc Natl Acad Sci USA 1990;87:5263–5267.

112. Basile AS. The contribution of endogenous benzodiazepine receptor ligands to the pathogenesis of hepatic encephalopathy. Synapse 1991;7: 141–150.

113. Olasmaa M, Rothstein JD, Guidotti A, et al. Endogenous benzodiazepine receptor ligands in human and animal hepatic encephalopathy. J Neurochem 1990;55:2015–2023.

114. Basile AS, Hughes RD, Harrison PM, et al. Elevated brain concentrations of 1,4-benzodiazepines in fulminant hepatic failure. N Engl J Med 1991;325:473–478.

115. Mullen KD, Szauter KM, Kaminsky-Russ K. "Endogenous" benzodiazepine activity in body fluids of patients with hepatic encephalopathy. Lancet 1990;336:81–83.

116. Bassett ML, Mullen KD, Scholz B, Fenstermacher JD, Jones EA. Increased brain uptake of γ-aminobutyric acid in a rabbit model of hepatic encephalopathy. Gastroenterology 1990;98:747–757.

117. Basile AS, Ostrowsky NL, Gammal SH, Jones EA, Skolnick P. The GABA$_A$ receptor complex in hepatic encephalopathy: autoradiographic evidence for the presence of an endogenous benzodiazepine receptor ligand. Neuropsychopharmacol 1990; 3:61–71.

118. Jones EA, Basile AS, Mullen KD, Gammal SH. Flumazenil: potential implications for hepatic encephalopathy. Pharmacol Ther 1990;40:331–343.

119. Pomier-Layrarques G, Giguere J-F, Lavoie J, Willems B, Butterworth RF. Pharmakokinetics of benzodiazepine antagonist Ro 15–1788 in cirrhotic patients with moderate or severe liver dysfunction. Hepatology 1989;10:969–972.

120. Samson Y, Bernau J, Puppata S, Chavoix C, Baron JC, Maziere MA. Cerebral uptake of benzodiazepines measured by positron emission tomography in hepatic encephalopathy. N Engl J Med 1987; 316:414.

121. Bansky G, Meier PJ, Ziegler WH, Walser H, Schmid M, Huber M. Reversal of hepatic coma by benzodiazepine antagonist (Ro 15–1788). Lancet 1985;1:1324–1325.
122. Scollo-Lavizzari G, Steinmann E. Reversal of hepatic coma by benzodiazepine antagonist (Ro 15–1788). Lancet 1985;1:1324.
123. Jones EA, Ferenci P. Hepatic encephalopathy and GABAergic neurotransmission In: Medi-Ed Press, Hepatic encephalopathy: management with non-absorbed carbohydrates and other innovative therapies. Bloomington, IL: Conn HO, Bircher J, eds. (in press).
124. Grimm G, Ferenci P, Katzenschlager R, Madl C, et al. Improvement of hepatic encephalopathy treated with flumazenil. Lancet 1988;2:1392–1394.
125. Bansky G, Meier PJ, Riederer E, Walser H, Ziegler WH, Schmid M. Effects of the benzodiazepine receptor antagonist flumazenil in hepatic encephalopathy in humans. Gastroenterology 1989;97:744–750.
126. Savic I, Widen L, Stone-Elander S. Feasibility of reversing benzodiazepine tolerance with flumazenil. Lancet 1991;337:133–137.
127. Ferenci P, Grimm G, Meryn S, Gangl A. Successful long-term treatment of portal-systemic encephalopathy by the benzodiazepine antagonist flumazenil. Gastroenterology 1989;96:240–243.
128. Meier R, Gyr K. Treatment of hepatic encephalopathy with the benzodiazepine antagonist flumazenil: a pilot study. Eur J Anaesthesiol 1988;2(suppl):139–146.
129. Pidoux B, Zylberberg PH, Valla D, et al. Ètude électroencéphalographique de l'effet d'un antagoniste des benzodiazépines dans l'encéphalopathie hépatique. Neurophysiol Clinique 1989;19:469–476.
130. van der Rijt CCD, Schalm SW, Meulstee J, et al. Flumazenil therapy for hepatic encephalopathy: a double-blind cross-over study. Hepatology 1989;10:590.
131. Burke DA, Mitchell KW, Al Mardini H, et al. Reversal of hepatic coma with flumazenil with improvement in visual evoked potentials. Lancet 1988;1:505–506.

22

Pruritus of Cholestasis: Empiric Therapeutic Approaches and Rationale for Use of Opioid Antagonists

NORA V. BERGASA and E. ANTHONY JONES

Pruritus is a distressing complication in many patients with cholestatic liver diseases (1). This form of pruritus is not readily relieved by scratching, it may be intermittent or persistent, and it can be generalized or localized to particular parts of the body. In some patients, this symptom is mild and does not interfere with normal activities. In others, it is more severe and may lead to sleep deprivation. All current conventional therapies are empiric and none of them reliably ameliorates the pruritus. Consequently, the pruritus of cholestasis is often a major problem to manage. When unrelieved it can be an indication for liver transplantation (2).

The pathogenesis of the pruritus of cholestasis remains unknown. A major factor that retards progress in studying this symptom is its inherent subjectivity. The perception of itch may be influenced by a variety of factors, such as mood and distractions, and descriptions of the itching sensation vary widely. It is difficult to assess whether an apparent amelioration of pruritus is attributable to a therapeutic response to a treatment, to a spontaneous decrease in the intensity of the pruritus, or to a placebo effect. Furthermore, there are major deficiencies in methods that have been applied to assess the pruritus of cholestasis in clinical studies.

THE CONCEPT OF PRURITUS OF PERIPHERAL ORIGIN

The Bile Acid Hypothesis

The dominant hypothesis for the pathogenesis of the pruritus of cholestasis during the past 25 years has implicated bile acids (3).

It has been suggested that the pruritus of cholestasis may arise peripherally as a result of the interaction between nerve endings in the skin and one or more substances retained in plasma in cholestasis, including in particular bile acids (4). Although the itch sensation is perceived in the brain, it is conventionally considered to arise as a consequence of stimulation of nonmyelinated C nerve endings and is transmitted via the lateral spinothalamic tract to the thalamus and the sensory cortex, as is the sensation of pain (5). The types of stimuli that can induce pruritus are diverse and include many inflammatory disorders of the skin, in which the source of the pruritus appears to be peripheral (6, 7). Bile acids have been considered to be likely candidate substances in the pathogenesis of the pruritus of cholestasis following the demonstration of a correlation between their recovery from the skin surface and the apparent intensity of pruritus in cholestatic patients (8, 9). Furthermore, the administration of bile acids under highly artificial conditions has been reported

Table 22.1
Treatments for the Pruritus of Cholestasis[a]

Treatment	Potential mechanisms of action	Controlled trials	Quantification of Scratching activity	References
Cholestyramine	Decreased enterohepatic	Y	N	19–21
Colestipol	circulation; choleresis	N	N	
Antihistamines	Histamine antagonism; sedation	Y	N	4–30
Phenobarbital	Hepatic enzyme induction; choleresis, sedation	Y	N	17, 31, 37
Rifampicin	Hepatic enzyme induction	Y	N	33–37
Flumecinol		Y	N	32
S-Adenosylmethionine	Anticholestasis	Y	N	39
Charcoal hemoperfusion	Removal of "substances" from plasma	N	N	40
Plasmapheresis		N	N	41
Partial external diversion	Removal of "substances" secreted in bile	N	N	42
Phototherapy	?	N	N	43, 44
Lignocaine	?	N	N	45
Androgens	?	N	N	46
Hydroxyethylrutosides	?	N	N	47
Carbamazepine	?	N	N	48
Ursodeoxycholic acid	?	Y	N	49
Naloxone	Opiate antagonism	Y	Y	86, 87, 91
Nalmefene		Y	Y	70

[a]?, unknown; Y, yes; N, no.

to induce pruritus in humans (10, 11). However, skin surface bile acid levels may not be relevant, because the site at which nerve endings are excited in pruritus of peripheral origin is at or below the dermoepithelial junction, which is separated from the surface by the slowly maturing dermis and the impermeable stratum corneum (6). Furthermore, bile acid levels in skin tissue obtained at surgery and bile acid levels measured in skin interstitial fluid do not appear to correlate with the pruritus of cholestasis, suggesting that this symptom is not primarily related to bile acids in skin (12–16). Apparent relief of pruritus may occur without a decrease in serum bile acid levels (17). These levels remain high as chronic cholestatic liver disease progresses, although the pruritus may subside spontaneously (18). It has been suggested that this development may portend the onset of hepatocellular failure (4). In addition, serum bile acid levels may be elevated in patients with chronic cholestasis who do not complain of itching (18). Whereas there appears to be a general consensus that the oral administration of bile acid sequestering resins, such as cholestyramine or colestipol, effectively ameliorates pruritus in a large proportion of cholestatic patients (19–22), the results of clinical trials of these resins and several experimental therapies for the pruritus of cholestasis (Table 22.1) have failed to definitely implicate bile acids or any other specific class of substance in the pathogenesis of the pruritus. Potentially pruritogenic substances removed by cholestyramine or colestipol may not necessarily be bile acids, since these agents have been reported to induce apparent ameliorations of pruritus in patients with uremia (23) and polycythemia rubra vera (24), conditions that are not associated with bile acid retention.

Empiric Therapies

BILE ACID SEQUESTERING RESINS

Since 1960, the most widely administered treatment for this syndrome has been the basic anion exchange resin cholestyramine (19–22). More recently, colestipol, another resin with similar properties, has also been used. These agents, which are given by mouth, are hydrophilic but insoluble in water. They are unaffected by digestive enzymes, remain unchanged in the gastrointestinal tract, and are not absorbed (25). They bind bile acids and other compounds in the intestine, with the result that the fecal excretion of bound substances is increased (26). Cholestyramine has also been reported to mediate a choleretic effect and thus may promote the biliary clearance of a variety of compounds (27). The net result of administering one of these resins is to decrease the plasma concentrations of a variety of substances by decreasing their enterohepatic circulation and/or facilitating their biliary clearance. It is generally recommended that these resins be taken before and after breakfast to take advantage of the gallbladder filling with bile during the overnight fast. This would result in maximal binding of constituents of the enterohepatic circulation in the intestine, which may include putative pruritogens. These resins may also be given after lunch and dinner. To avoid malabsorption of orally administered drugs due to adsorption to resin, drugs should not be given at times close to those of resin administration. It is suggested that the total dose should not exceed 16 g/day. The main side effects are bloating, constipation, and an exacerbation of the malabsorption syndrome secondary to cholestasis. Whether substances that contribute to the pruritus of cholestasis also undergo resin-induced changes in their metabolism is unknown.

There appears to be a general consensus that the administration of one of these resins effectively ameliorates pruritus in a large proportion of cholestatic patients. In many patients, troublesome pruritus seems to be rendered tolerable by long-term therapy with one of these resins. However, in many cholestatic patients itching is not relieved by resin treatment.

ANTIHISTAMINES

Antihistamines are often administered to pruritic patients with cholestasis. Histamine is a potent pruritogen (5). It induces the classical wheel and flare reaction in skin and mediates pruritus in many inflammatory skin disorders. However, whereas excoriations may occur in patients with the pruritus of cholestasis (28) and serum histamine levels have been reported to be elevated in them (29), no skin changes consistent with histamine-mediated effects are found, and antihistamines do not consistently induce amelioration of the itching (30).

HEPATIC ENZYME INDUCERS

Hepatic enzyme inducers that have been used in the treatment of patients with the pruritus of cholestasis include phenobarbital, flumecinol, and rifampicin. In some patients, phenobarbital appears to partially ameliorate pruritus (17, 31), but this effect seems not to be sustained for longer than a few weeks or months. Flumecinol has also been reported to induce amelioration of the pruritus of cholestasis in a controlled study (32). Rifampicin has also been tried with variable results (33–37). In three of four controlled studies, an apparent beneficial effect of rifampicin on pruritus was reported. In one of the controlled studies, this drug appeared to be more effective than phenobarbital in inducing ameliorations of pruritus (37). The mechanism of this reported effect is unknown. It seems unlikely that it would be due to an effect on bile acids since this drug has been shown to increase serum concentrations of bile acids (38) (Fig. 22.1).

SEDATIVES

Antihistamines and phenobarbital could have a nonspecific beneficial effect due to their sedative rather than their other properties.

CHOLERETICS

Both cholestyramine (27) and phenobarbital (31) have been reported to have choleretic properties and may induce a relevant effect as a consequence of promoting bile flow.

ANTICHOLESTATIC AGENTS

S-Adenosylmethionine has been reported to reverse the effects of cholestatic agents and to ameliorate the pruritus of cholestasis (39).

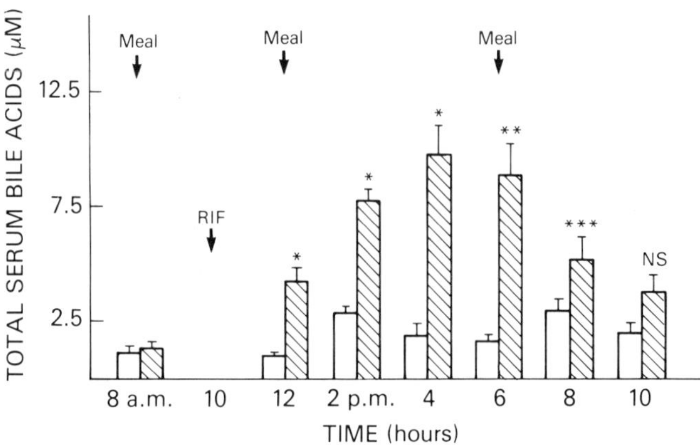

Figure 22.1. Fasting and postprandial total serum bile acid levels in normal subjects the day before (*open bars*) and the day of rifampicin administration in a single 900-mg dose (*hatched bars*). *$P < .0005$; **$P < .005$; ***$P < .05$. Reproduced with permission from Galeazzi et al. (38).

REMOVAL OF SUBSTANCES FROM THE BODY

Some experimental therapies are designed to remove substances from the body that are considered to contribute to the pruritus either directly or indirectly. Such therapies, which include charcoal hemoperfusion (40), plasmapheresis (41), and partial external diversion of bile (42) have been reported to induce apparent transient ameliorations of pruritus in some patients in uncontrolled studies. The nature of any relevant substance removed by these therapeutic approaches has not been defined.

UNCLASSIFIED TREATMENT MODALITIES

Some experimental therapies that have been tried appear to lack any readily expressible rationale. These include phototherapy (43, 44), lignocaine (45), androgens (4, 46), hydroxyethylrutosides (47), and carbamazepine (48). These therapeutic modalities have also been reported to induce transient ameliorations of pruritus in some patients in uncontrolled trials. Furthermore, in a controlled trial, administration of ursodeoxycholic acid (Actigall) has been associated with amelioration of pruritus in some patients (49). The mechanism of such ameliorations is unknown.

It should be emphasized that nonspecific treatment modalities that lower the plasma concentrations of a variety of substances (such as cholestyramine, colestipol, charcoal hemoperfusion, plasmapheresis, partial external diversion of bile, and drugs that induce hepatic enzymes) have the potential of ameliorating the pruritus of cholestasis by lowering the circulating levels of an undefined pruritogen or a factor responsible for inducing the primary mechanism of the pruritus.

THE CONCEPT OF PRURITUS OF CENTRAL ORIGIN

Whereas it has been traditional to consider that the pruritus of cholestasis is of peripheral origin, our current lack of understanding of the pathogenesis of this disorder is so profound that it is necessary to consider other mechanisms that induce pruritus. One possibility is that a significant component of the pruritus of cholestasis may be of neurogenic central origin. This possibility has received little attention. It is well recognized that certain psychiatric (5) and neurologic (7) disorders are associated with pruritus. In cholestatic liver disease, it is conceivable that pruritus could be mediated centrally by the opioid system.

The Opioid System

Although opiate agonist drugs such as morphine have been used in medical practice for

Table 22.2
Simplified Classification of Opioids

Opioid receptor ligand	Chemical classification	Origin	Pharmacologic classification	Relevant opioid receptors	Some Important physiological effects
Morphine	Alkaloid	Exogenous	Opioid agonist	μ	Supraspinal and spinal analgesia
β-Endorphin	Peptide	Endogenous	Opioid agonist	μ	Sedation; tolerance; decreased gastrointestinal motility, respiratory depression
Metenkephalin	Pentapeptide	Endogenous	Opioid agonist	μ and δ	
Leuenkephalin	Pentapeptide	Endogenous	Opioid agonist	δ	Spinal and stress analgesia, respiratory depression
Dynorphin	Peptide	Endogenous	Opioid agonist	κ	Dysphoria, sedation, appetite stimulation
Naloxone	Alkaloid	Exogenous	Opioid antagonist	$\mu > \delta > \kappa$	Reversal of effects of opioid agonists, opiate withdrawal syndrome in opiate addiction
Nalmefene	Alkaloid	Exogenous	Opioid antagonist	μ, δ, κ	

Morphine **Naloxone** **Nalmefene**

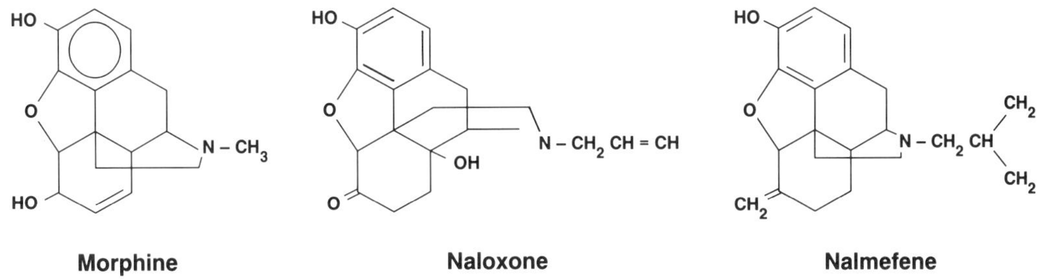

Figure 22.2. Chemical structures of morphine, naloxone, and nalmefene. Morphine is an alkaloid and a potent agonist at opioid receptors. Naloxone and nalmefene are antagonists at opioid receptors. In contrast to naloxone, nalmefene is bioavailable when given by mouth (72). Nalmefene is also a more potent antagonist and has a longer half-life than naloxone (69).

decades, it was the discovery of opioid receptors in the central nervous system that stimulated a search for endogenous ligands of opioid receptors. In 1973, Pert and Snyder (50) demonstrated opioid receptor binding, its confinement to the nervous system, and a close correlation between the pharmacologic potency of opiates and their affinity for opioid receptors. The existence of opioid receptors was independently confirmed by the demonstration of stable, stereospecific binding of an active narcotic analgesic (^{3}H-etorphine) (51). Three classes of endogenous opioid ligands are currently recognized: enkephalins, endorphins, and dynorphins. These ligands are classified as opioid peptides, with some pharmacologic activity similar to morphine.

However, their chemical structure is distinct from that of morphine-like opiates, which are alkaloids (52) (Table 22.2; Fig. 22.2). The functional status of the opioid system is related to the concentrations of specific ligands at opioid receptors, their receptor affinities, and the number of opioid receptors (53).

Centrally Mediated Pruritus Induced by Opiates

Several observations implicate opiate agonist ligands in the mediation of pruritus. The administration of morphine (0.2–0.5 mg/kg) intracisternally to cats (54) or the administration of morphine (0.03 µg) (DA Thomas, personal communication) or the μ-opioid analog DAMGO (3.1–25 ng) into the medullary dor-

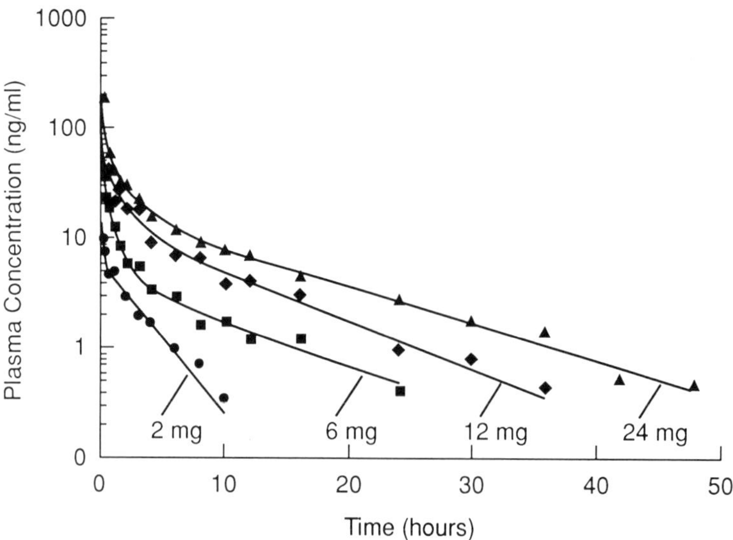

Figure 22.3. Plasma concentration-time data for nalmefene in normal subjects after the intravenous injection of different doses. Reproduced with permission from Dixon et al. (69).

sal horn of monkeys (55) all induce dramatic scratching activity. The scratching induced in monkeys is reversed by intramuscular administration of the opiate antagonist naloxone (55). Pruritus is a recognized side effect of morphine in man (56–58). Furthermore, other opiate receptor agonists have also been reported to induce pruritus, for example, diamorphine, meperidine, methadone, fentanyl, hydromorphone, pethidine, and butorphanol (59–66). The intraspinal administration of an opiate agonist has been reported to induce itching in the distribution of the facial nerve (62). In addition, blocking of opiate agonist-induced itching by naloxone has been reported in humans (58, 60, 67). It appears that "central modulators of pruritus, such as systemic morphine, cause itch . . . by acting on central opiate receptors" (7).

Central Opiatergic Tone Is Increased in Cholestasis

If the opioid system in the brain is implicated in the pathogenesis of the pruritus of cholestasis, one would expect certain relevant abnormalities of the opioid system to be present in patients with liver disease. This postulate

has been partially confirmed. An alteration of central opioid homeostasis in liver disease was first suggested by the observation that patients with cirrhosis and impaired hepatocellular function exhibit increased sensitivity to morphine (68). More recently, a specific disturbance of central opioid function in cholestasis has been suggested by the effects of nalmefene in patients with chronic cholestatic liver disease. Nalmefene is a specific opiate antagonist devoid of intrinsic activity (69) (Fig. 22.2). It is more potent and has a more prolonged pharmacologic action than naloxone (Fig. 22.3). When nalmefene was administered orally (5 mg twice daily to 20–40 mg three times daily) to 11 patients with cirrhosis, 9 of whom had predominantly cholestatic disease, all experienced a reaction that began within 1 hour of the first dose (70). The reaction invariably consisted of anorexia, nausea, colicky abdominal pain, constipation, pallor, cool skin, an increase in blood pressure, and a decrease in pulse rate. Some patients also experienced changes in mood and symptoms that could be classified as unpleasant cerebral effects. The cerebral effects included visual and auditory hallucinations. Descriptions of side effects experienced by two patients were as follows: "Heavy trembling limbs. Dream-like state. No energy. No concentration. Heavy eyelids. Wanted to sleep but couldn't. Didn't want to be bothered by anyone. Couldn't think. No appetite"; and "Cold sweat. Dizzy. Very dry mouth. My mind felt white inside. Slept really badly. Just catnapped. Too pepped up." These reactions were always temporary, often becoming minimal after 2 or 3 days despite continued administration of nalmefene (70). Furthermore, side effects of nalmefene in cholestatic patients observed in another study included transient difficulty in visual focusing precipitated by a dose increase weeks after starting the drug and chronic goose bumps of the skin (71, and NV Bergasa unpublished observations). In addition, two patients clearly described a transient dysphoric reaction to nalmefene, which was characterized by an unrealistic relationship to their own self (NV Bergasa, unpublished observations). Such side effects were not observed when nalmefene was given to patients with various other nonhepatic diseases. Furthermore, when a large dose of nalmefene (300 mg) was given to normal subjects, only minor side effects occurred (70, 72).

It should be emphasized that the side effects that occurred in the patients with chronic liver disease were produced at one-sixtieth of the dose that produces occasional minor cerebral effects (eg, light-headedness) in healthy subjects (70). The reaction that followed the administration of nalmefene to the cirrhotic patients is strikingly similar to the withdrawal reaction of opiate addiction precipitated by naloxone (73–75). Small doses of naloxone produce intense withdrawal symptoms in opiate addicts (76), but this drug induces no subjective effects in normal subjects, even at high doses (77). These observations strongly suggest that the patients with cholestasis were chronically exposed to increased levels of opioid agonists in the absence of exogenously administered drugs of this class.

There is no animal model of the pruritus of cholestasis. However, data obtained in an animal model of cholestasis strongly support the inference that cholestasis is associated with increased opioid agonist-mediated activity (78). A major function of the opioid system is the mediation of analgesia, which can be induced by exogenous opiate agonist ligands, such as morphine (53). Using the tail flick test to assay endogenous opioid activity, rats with acute cholestasis 5 days after bile duct resection have been shown to exhibit a greater degree of antinociception than sham-resected control rats. This state of antinociception in cholestasis was stereoselectively reversed by naloxone (ie, it was reversed by (−) naloxone, but not by its inactive enantiomer (+) − naloxone) (78). Increased antinociception was also demonstrated in a rat model of acute hepatocellular necrosis, but in contrast to the cholestatic model, the antinociception associated with hepatocellular necrosis was not reversed by (−) − naloxone. These observations indicate that the antinociception associated with cholestasis, but not that associated with acute hepatocellular necrosis, is due to increased opioidergic tone mediated by opioid receptors.

The mechanism for increased opioidergic tone in cholestasis is unknown. However, a major possible mechanism is the accumulation of endogenous opioids. Increased serum levels of methionine and leucine enkephalin have been reported in humans with chronic cholestatic liver disease (70, 79–81). Furthermore, in the bile duct resected rat model of cholestasis, serum methionine enkephalin levels are 17-fold higher than in normal rats. However, methionine enkephalin accounts for only 5% of the increased total serum opioid activity that occurs in this model (82) (Fig. 22.4). The nature of specific endogenous opioids that contribute to increased opioidergic tone in cholestasis has yet to be determined.

As chronic administration of an opiate agonist to rats has been shown to induce a decrease in opioid receptors in the rat (83), an accumulation of opioid ligands in cholestasis may also be associated with a decrease in opioid receptors. This hypothesis has been tested in the bile duct resected rat model using

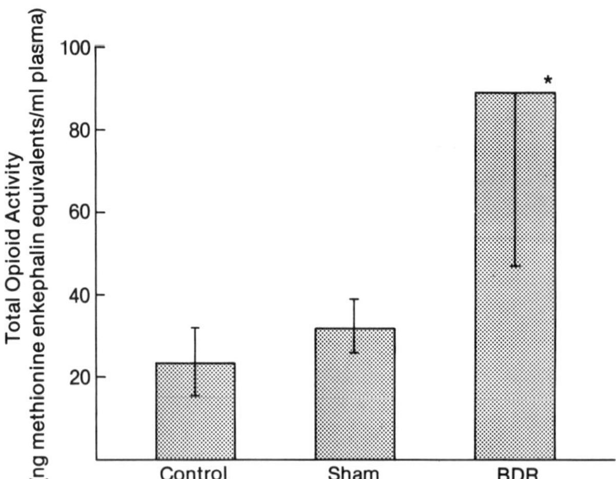

Figure 22.4. Total plasma opioid activity in cholestasis. Opioid activity was determined by measuring the inhibition by plasma extracts of the binding of the opioid receptor ligand ^{3}H-DAMGO to rat brain-lysed synaptosomal preparations. Plasma was obtained from unoperated (*control*) rats and rats 5 days after sham (*sham*) bile duct resection or bile duct resection (*BDR*). Data are expressed as means ± SEM. Opioid activity is greater in rats with cholestasis due to BDR than in control or sham-resected groups ($P < .05$). Reproduced with permission from Gastroenterology (82).

a standard ligand-receptor binding assay. The densities of (μ and δ) opioid receptors in the brain was found to be significantly less in this model than in sham-resected control rats (84, 85) (Fig. 22.5). These observations are consistent with a response of the central opioid system to increased exposure of opioid receptors to endogenous opioids.

Initial Trials of Opiate Antagonists for the Pruritus of Cholestasis

If the hypothesis that increased action of opioid agonist ligands contributes to the pruritus of cholestasis is correct, it should be possible to induce amelioration of the pruritus by administering an opiate antagonist. Preliminary reports suggest that this hypothesis is correct. Naloxone (0.8 mg) was reported to relieve severe itching from 5 minutes to 1.5–2.5 hours after its subcutaneous administration to a patient with primary biliary cirrhosis, whereas injection of saline had no effect (86). In a double-blind, placebo-controlled trial involving 20 patients with pruritus caused by chronic cholestatic liver disease, the effects of intravenous injections of naloxone (2 mg) and saline were compared. Two methods to assess pruritus were applied: visual analog scores and

measurements of limb movements at night. Nine patients appeared to have a placebo response without any apparent response to naloxone. In most of the other 11 patients, in whom no placebo response was apparent, administration of naloxone appeared to be associated with an amelioration of pruritus (87). In this study, the duration of any effect attributable to an intravenous injection of naloxone would be expected to be of short duration. In a third study, nalmefene was administered orally to 9 patients with primary biliary cirrhosis (70). A placebo-controlled, randomized, double-blind crossover design could not be completed because of the florid opiate withdrawal-like reaction that developed after the first dose of the drug. Nevertheless, as judged subjectively in that study, which employed visual analog scores, administration of the drug appeared to be associated with a rapid amelioration of pruritus that was sustained throughout a 6-month period of drug administration (70) (Fig. 22.6). It seems likely that this apparent beneficial effect of nalmefene on the pruritus of cholestasis is due to its central action on the opioid system, since it does not appear to have any direct antipruritic effect in pruritic skin disorders (70, 88).

THE PROBLEM OF ACCURATELY ASSESSING PRURITUS IN CHOLESTATIC PATIENTS

Most studies of the pruritus of cholestasis have relied on subjective assessments of the itch sensation. These have involved the use of descriptive terms (e.g., mild, moderate, severe) (31), questionnaires (40), and visual analog

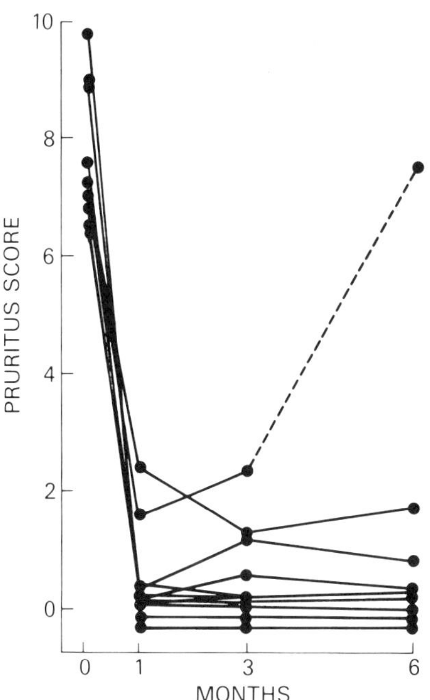

Figure 22.6. Effect of orally administered nalmefene on a visual analog score of pruritus in nine patients with primary biliary cirrhosis. Reproduced with permission from Br Med J (70).

scores (33, 35, 39). Application of a visual analog score in this context is an attempt to quantify pruritus. The patient is asked to record the severity of pruritus by making a mark on a 10-cm horizontal line (0 cm representing "no itching" and 10 cm representing "worst itching ever"). This approach has the appeal that numerical values are generated. However, a visual analog score requires the patient not only to integrate the perception of itch over a time interval, but also to translate this perception, which is inherently subjective, into a visuospatial score that is subject to individual differences in its conceptualization (89). There is a tendency for patients not to treat the visual-analog scale as a continuum, with the result that clustering of marks at the extremes or center of the scale may occur (89). Visual analog scores may not be a reliable index of the severity of pruritus, particularly in short-term studies (90, 91). As itching is defined as the need to scratch, it is a perception

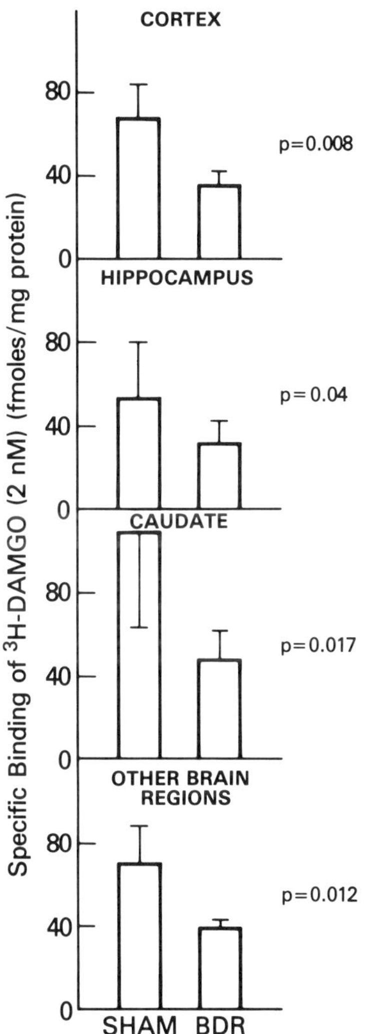

Figure 22.5. Specific binding of the mu opioid receptor ligand 3H-DAMGO to membranes prepared from different brain regions of rats with cholestasis due to bile duct resection and sham-resected control rats. The data are consistent with a global down-regulation of mu opioid receptors in the brain in cholestasis. Reproduced with permission from J Hepatol (84).

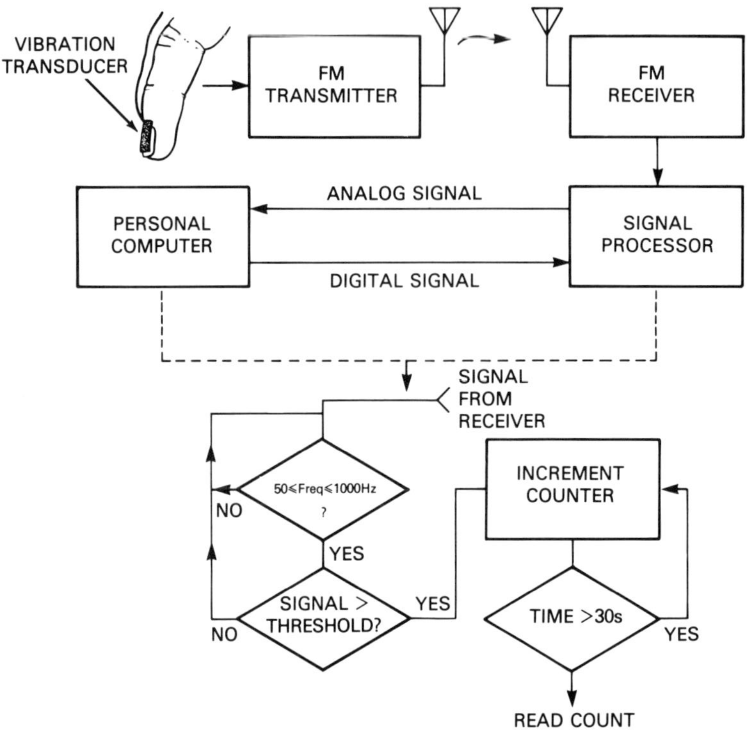

Figure 22.7. Block diagram of scratching activity monitoring system with flow chart of signal processor. Only the vibration transducer and FM transmitter are attached to the patient. Reproduced with permission from Gastroenterology (91).

that cannot be quantified directly. However, the behavioral manifestations of the pruritus of cholestasis is scratching activity that, in contrast to itching, can be quantified. Thus, the problem of assessing the subjective perception of itch can be obviated by objectively quantifying scratching activity (3).

In 1975, Felix and Shuster described the application of a device to measure limb movements in a study of pruritus in patients with itchy skin disorders (92) and, subsequently, Summerfield and Welch applied a sophisticated apparatus to measure limb movements in a study of pruritus in patients with cholestatic liver disease (93). The development of these pioneer methods reflected the need to apply objective quantitative methods in clinical studies of pruritus. Unfortunately, measurements of limb movements record activities other than scratching activity. Ideally,

scratching activity should be quantified independently of limb movements. Recently, a scratching activity-monitoring system has been designed to achieve this objective (94). The system consists of a vibration (scratch) transducer, an FM transmitter and receiver, a custom-made signal processor, and a personal computer (Fig. 22.7). The vibration transducer, which is taped to the middle finger of the patient's dominant hand, consists of a square piece of piezoelectric film, 28-μm thick, and metalized on both sides with silver ink. It is connected by a wire to a transmitter box which is attached to the arm by a Velcro cuff (Fig. 22.8). The transducer has the property of converting physical strain into electrical voltage. Physical strain is derived from the bending of the transducer induced by vibrations of the fingernail as it transverses the skin in the act of scratching. The electrical signal

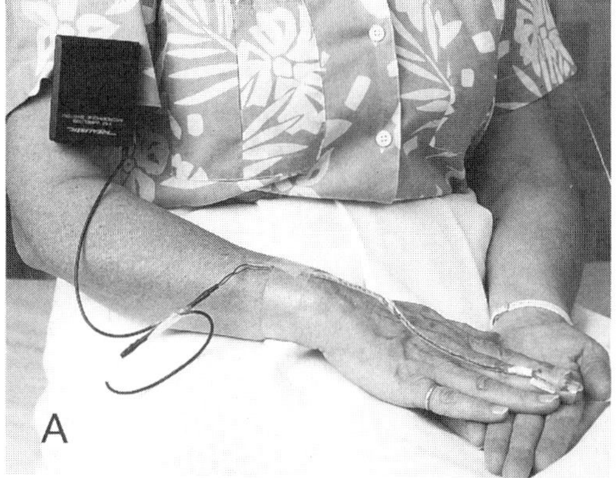

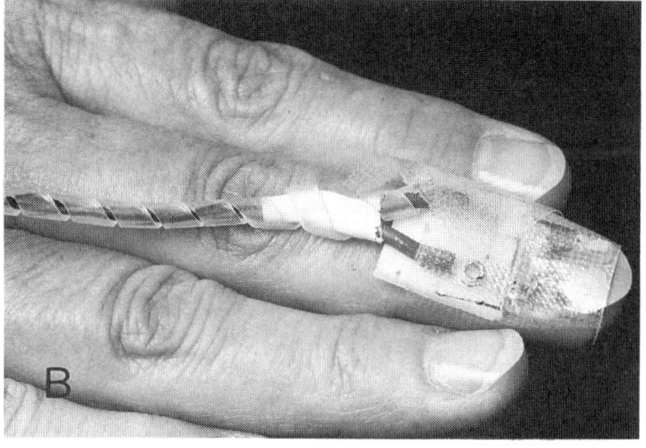

Figure 22.8. Patient wearing vibration transducer and transmitter box. Reproduced with permission from Am J Gastroenterol (1991;86:1404–1412).

is transmitted by the transmitter across the room, where it is received, processed, and logged by the personal computer as a scratching activity index in counts per 30-second intervals. Fourier analysis of demodulated signals indicated that frequencies associated with vibrations of the fingernail derived from scratching activity are between 50 and 1000 Hz. Only signals above a set threshold and within this frequency band are used to generate a numerical index of the degree of scratching activity. Thus, low frequencies associated with body movements are not recorded (Fig. 22.9). This device is well tolerated by patients and enables the behavioral manifestation of the pruritus of cholestasis to be detected and quantified continuously throughout the day and night, irrespective of whether the patient complains of itching or perceives the itch sensation. The validity of

applying the device to measure scratching activity has been verified by demonstrating a close concordance between the index generated by the device (counts per unit time) and independent direct observations and video tapes of scratching activity. In particular, it was consistently observed that counts were not recorded by the device during gross movements of the hand that were not associated with the interaction between fingernails and the skin, and that counts were recorded during the act of scratching by the hand to which the transducer was taped. The device in its present form enables more meaningful quantitative studies of the pruritus of cholestasis to be conducted than has hitherto been possible (91, 94).

EFFECTS OF OPIATE ANTAGONISTS ON SCRATCHING ACTIVITY IN CHOLESTATIC PATIENTS

To test more conclusively the hypothesis that opioid agonists contribute to the pruritus of cholestasis, the effect of intravenous infusions of naloxone on scratching activity was studied in eight female patients with primary biliary cirrhosis in whom chronic pruritus had not been relieved by conventional medications (91). Naloxone is the drug of choice in most situations in which an opiate antagonist effect is required (Fig. 22.2). It is a competitive antagonist at μ-, δ-, and κ-receptors. Because of its low oral bioavailability, it is necessary to administer naloxone parenterally (58). Each patient received one or two 24-hour infusions of naloxone and one or two 24-hour infusions of a placebo solution. The infusions were administered consecutively in a non-predetermined order. The patients, but not the attending staff members, were unaware of their content. Scratching activity was recorded continuously throughout the infusions, using the newly developed scratching activity monitoring system (94) (Fig. 22.10). Only data obtained between identical times of the day and night during both naloxone and control infusions were analyzed to obviate any possible effects of diurnal rhythms of scratching activity on the results. The infusion rate of na-

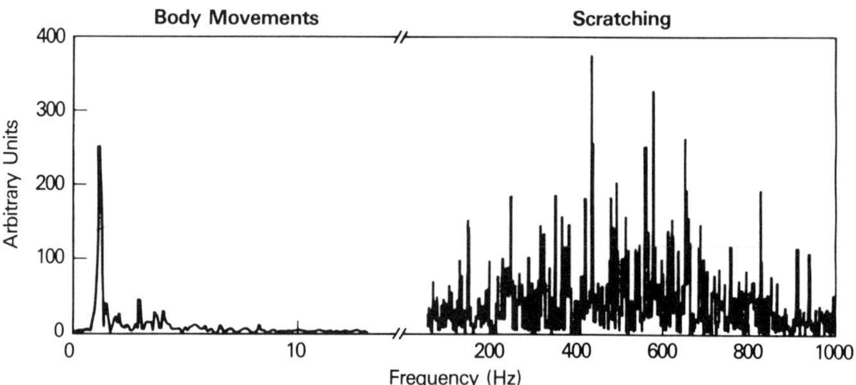

Figure 22.9. Results of Fourier analysis of demodulated signals generated by the scratching activity monitoring system (see Fig. 22.7) indicating that frequencies associated with gross body movements are <50 Hz and those associated with the scratching fingernail are between 50 and 1000 Hz. Reproduced with permission from Bergasa et al. (91).

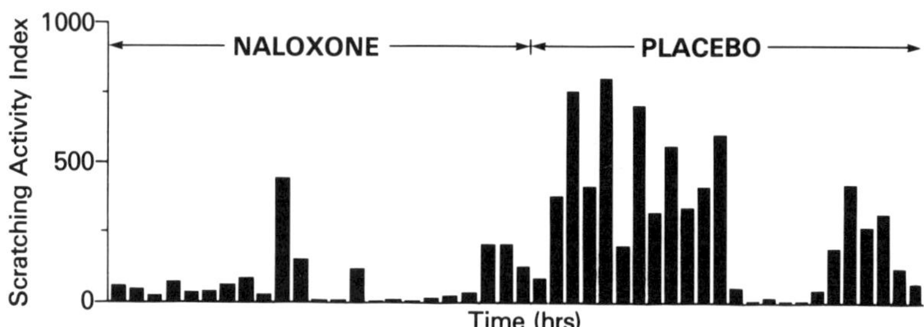

Figure 22.10. Representative data on scratching activity index in a patient with primary biliary cirrhosis during intravenous infusions of a placebo solution and naloxone (0.2 μ/kg/minute). Reproduced with permission from Bergasa et al. (91).

loxone, determined after conducting a pilot dose finding study, was 0.2 μg/kg/minute. This infusion rate is four times that necessary to reverse morphine anesthesia (95). No pattern of side effects suggestive of an opiate withdrawal syndrome occurred. Interestingly, mean values for a visual analog score of pruritus during naloxone and placebo infusions did not correlate with the scratching activity index, indicating that the visual analog score is an unreliable indicator of scratching activity in short-term studies. Naloxone infusions were consistently associated with a decrease in values for the scratching activity index. The magnitude of the decrease varied between 26% and 96%, the mean decrease being 50%

$(P < .001)$ (91) (Fig. 22.11). The results of this study provide further support for the hypothesis that a major component of the pruritus of cholestasis is attributable to the action of opioid agonists at opioid receptors in the central nervous system. The findings in this study have been confirmed in a double-blind, randomized, controlled trial, (96).

Naloxone infusions may be beneficial for the emergency treatment of intractable pruritus due to cholestasis. For the long-term treatment of the pruritus of chronic cholestasis, however, it would be desirable to administer an opiate antagonist that is effective when given orally (72). Nalmefene is much more bioavailable when given orally, is a more po-

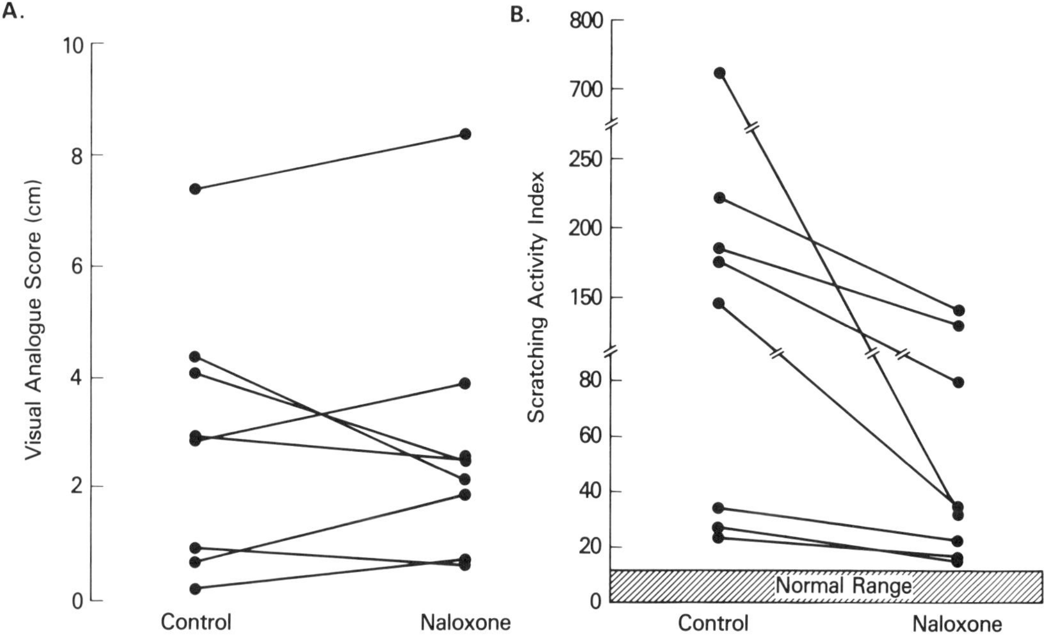

Figure 22.11. The effects of the intravenous infusion of naloxone on scratching activity index and on a visual analog score (VAS) of pruritus in eight patients with primary biliary cirrhosis. Naloxone infusions were associated with a decrease in scratching activity in all eight patients ($P < .001$) and a decrease in VAS in four of the patients (pNS). Data in each patient have been reported by Bergasa et al. (91).

tent opiate antagonist, and has a longer half-life than naloxone (69, 72). Preliminary data from an open-label trial of oral nalmefene for the pruritus of chronic cholestasis were encouraging (71) (Fig. 22.12) and the association of oral nalmefene therapy with the relief of this form of pruritus has been confirmed in a double-blind randomized placebo-controlled trial (97).

CONCLUDING PERSPECTIVES

Progress in understanding the pathogenesis of the pruritus of cholestasis has been hampered by a lack of objective quantitative methods for assessing this syndrome. All attempts to assess the perception of itch are inherently subjective and, hence, unreliable. In contrast, scratching activity, which can be defined as the behavioral manifestation of the pruritus of cholestasis, can be objectively quantified, independent of gross body movements, using a scratching activity-monitoring system (94).

The hypothesis that retained bile acids play a major role in the pruritus of cholestasis has not been experimentally verified.

Most current conventional and experimental therapies are empiric and lack a sound rationale. However, of potential interest are preliminary observations, using subjective methods for assessing pruritus, that suggest that opiate antagonists may induce ameliorations of pruritus in patients with cholestatic liver disease (70, 86, 87). Consequently, they suggest that opioid receptors may be involved in the mediation of this form of pruritus and that the opioid system is altered in liver disease. Several additional observations provide support for this notion: (a) Exogenous opiate agonist ligands induce pruritus that can be reversed by naloxone (58, 60, 67); (b) patients with cirrhosis exhibit hypersensitivity to morphine (68); (c) an opiate antagonist has been reported to induce an opiate withdrawal-like reaction in patients with cirrhosis and/or chronic cholestasis (70); (d) acute cholestasis,

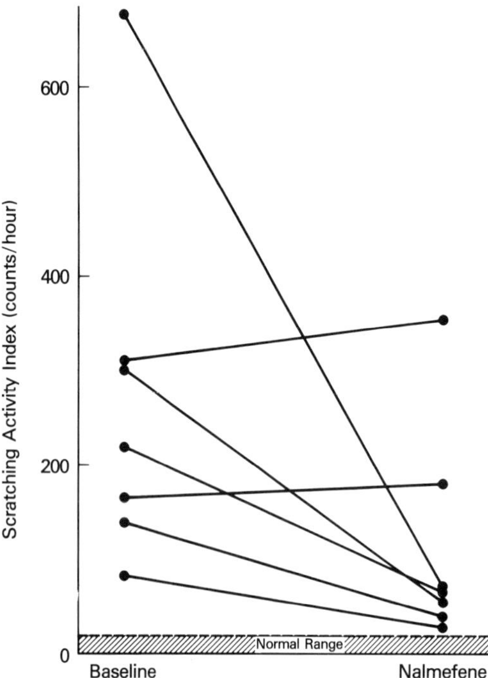

Figure 22.12. The effects of orally administered nalmefene on the scratching activity index (SAI) in seven patients with pruritus due to chronic cholestatic liver diseases. Maintenance doses of nalmefene were 16–200 daily. The second SAI was obtained 1–4 months after starting therapy. Nalmefene therapy was associated with a decrease in SAI in five of seven patients and with a decrease in the mean SAI for the whole group ($P <$ .025). These data have been reported in abstract form (71).

but not acute hepatocellular necrosis, in rats is associated with antinociception that can be stereoselectively reversed by naloxone (78); and (e) central μ- and δ-opioid receptors are down-regulated in rats with acute cholestasis (84, 85). One major potential mechanism of increased activity of the opioid system in cholestasis would be increased availability of endogenous opioid agonists at opioid receptors in the brain. Total opioid activity and metenkephalin levels are increased in plasma in an animal model of cholestasis (82) and plasma enkephalin levels are also increased in patients with chronic cholestasis (70, 79–81). Thus, in cholestasis, abnormalities of the opioid system are being defined both within and outside the

central nervous system. As cholestasis originates in the liver, the primary disturbance of the opioid system is presumably outside the central nervous system. It is not clear whether the peripheral changes in opioids are responsible for signaling the changes in opioid function in the brain. If such signaling were to involve plasma-to-brain transfer of opioids, this process would have to occur irrespective of any nonspecific change in the status of the blood-brain barrier in cholestasis (98).

Further support for the hypothesis that increased opioid agonist action contributes to the pruritus of cholestasis comes from a single-blind controlled study of naloxone infusions in pruritic patients with primary biliary cirrhosis in which scratching activity was objectively quantified. Naloxone infusions were consistently associated with a reduction in scratching activity (91). This finding, which was recently confirmed in a double-blind controlled trial, implies that the pruritus of cholestasis can be ameliorated by blocking central opioid receptors to reduce opioid-induced effects. This finding also provides a rationale for the long-term treatment of patients with pruritus due to chronic cholestatic disorders with an opiate antagonist, such as nalmefene (71), which is effective when given orally. The results of an open label study (71) and of a double-blind randomized placebo-controlled trial (97) suggest that therapy with oral nalmefene is associated with the relief of the pruritus of cholestasis.

REFERENCES

1. Sherlock S. Cholestasis. In: Diseases of the liver and biliary system. ed. 8. Oxford: Blackwell, 1989;248–272.
2. Maddrey W, van Thiel DH. Liver transplantation: an overview. Hepatology 1988;8:948–959.
3. Jones EA, Bergasa NV. The pruritus of cholestasis: from bile acids to opiate agonists. Hepatology 1990;11:884–887.
4. Lloyd-Thomas HGL, Sherlock S. Testosterone therapy for the pruritus of obstructive jaundice. Br Med J 1952;2:1289–1291.
5. Domonkos AN, Arnold HL, Odom RB. Pruritus and neurocutaneous dermatosis. In: Andrews' diseases of the skin. Philadelphia: Saunders, 1982;56–74.

6. Shelley WB, Arthur RP. The neurohistory and neurophysiology of the itch sensation in man. Arch Dermatol 1957; 76:296–323.

7. Parker F. Skin diseases. In: Wyngaarden JB, Smith LH, eds. Cecil textbook of medicine, 18th ed. Philadelphia: Saunders, 1988;2300–2353.

8. Schoenfield LJ, Sjovall S, Perman E. Bile acids on the skin of patients with pruritic hepatobiliary disease. Nature 1967;213:93–94.

9. Stiehl A. Bile acids and bile acid sulfates in the skin of patients with cholestasis and pruritus. Z Gastroenterol 1974;12:121–124.

10. Varadi DP. Pruritus induced by crude bile and purified bile acids: experimental production of pruritus in human skin. Arch Dermatol 1974;109:678–681.

11. Kirby J, Heaton KW, Burton JL. Pruritic effect of bile salts. Br Med J 1974;4:693–695.

12. Ghent CN, Bloomer JR, Klatskin G. Elevations in skin tissue levels of bile acids in human cholestasis: relation to serum levels and to pruritus. Gastroenterology 1977;73:1125–1130.

13. Freedman MR, Holzbach RT, Ferguson DR. Pruritus in cholestasis: no direct causation role for bile acid retention. Am J Med 1981;70:1011–1016.

14. Ghent CN, Bloomer JR, Itch in liver disease: facts and speculation. Yale J Biol Med 1979;52:77–82.

15. Bartholomew TC, Summerfield JA, Billing BH, et al. Bile acid profiles of human serum and skin interstitial fluid and their relationship to pruritus studied by gas chromatography-mass spectrometry. Clin Sci 1982;63:65–73.

16. Ghent CN. Pruritus of cholestasis is related to effects of bile salts on the liver, not the skin. Am J Gastroenterol 1987;82:117–118.

17. Ghent CN, Bloomer JR, Hsia YE. Safety and efficacy of long term treatment of familial intrahepatic cholestasis with phenobarbital. J Pediatr 1978;93:127–132.

18. Murphy GM, Ross A, Billing BH. Serum bile acids in primary biliary cirrhosis. Gut 1972;13:201–206.

19. Carey JB Jr. Lowering of serum bile acid concentrations and relief of pruritus in jaundiced patients fed a bile acid sequestering resin. J Lab Clin Med 1960;56:797–798.

20. Carey JB, Williams G. Relief of the pruritus of jaundice with a bile sequestering resin. JAMA 1961; 176:432–435.

21. van Itallie TB, Hashim SA, Cramton RS, et al. Treatment of pruritus and hypercholesterolemia of primary biliary cirrhosis with cholestyramine. N Engl J Med 1961;265:469–474.

22. Datta DV, Sherlock S. Cholestyramine for long term relief of the pruritus complicating intrahepatic cholestasis. Gastroenterology 1966;50:323–332.

23. Silverberg DS, Iaina A, Reisin E, et al. Cholestyramine in uraemic pruritus. Br Med J 1977;1:752–753.

24. Chanarin I, Szur I. Relief of intractable pruritus in polycythaemia rubra vera with cholestyramine. Br J Haematol 1970; 29:669–670.

25. Brown MS, Goldstein JL. Drugs used in the treatment of hyperlipoproteinemias. In: Gilman AG, Goodman LS, Rall TW, et al., eds. The pharmacological basis of therapeutics. 7th ed. New York: 1985:827–845.

26. Thompson WG, Grant W. Cholestyramine. Can Med Assoc J 1971;104:305–309.

27. Garbutt JT, Kenney TJ. Effect of cholestyramine on bile acid metabolism in normal man. J Clin Invest 1972;51:2781–2789.

28. Reynolds TB. The "butterfly" sign in patients with chronic jaundice and pruritus. Ann Intern Med 1973;78:545–546.

29. Gittlen SD, Schulman ES, Maddrey WC. Raised histamine concentrations in chronic cholestatic liver disease. Gut 1990;31:96–99.

30. Duncan JS, Kennedy HJ, Trigger DR. Treatment of pruritus due to chronic obstructive liver disease. Br Med J 1984;289:22.

31. Bloomer JR, Boyer JL. Phenobarbital effects in cholestatic liver disease. Ann Intern Med 1975;82:310–317.

32. Turner JB, Rawlins MD, Nagy JT, et al. Flumecinol improves pruritus in cholestatic liver disease: a double-blind placebo controlled trial [Abstract]. J Hepatol 1990;11(suppl 2):S63.

33. Ghent CN, Caruthers SG. Treatment of pruritus in primary biliary cirrhosis with rifampin: results of a double-blind cross-over randomized trial. Gastroenterology 1988;94:488–493.

34. Hoensch HP, Balzerk K. Dylewizc P, et al. Effect of rifampicin on hepatic drug metabolism and serum bile acids in patients with primary biliary cirrhosis. Eur J Clin Pharmacol 1985;28:475–477.

35. Woolf GM, Reynolds TB. Failure of rifampicin to relieve pruritus in chronic liver disease. J Clin Gastroenterol 1990;12:174–177.

36. Cynamon HA, Andres JM, Iafrate PR. Rifampin relieves pruritus in children with cholestatic liver disease. Gastroenterology 1990;98:1013–1016.

37. Bachsl LM, Montserrat E, Piera C, et al. Comparison of rifampicin with phenobarbitone for treatment of pruritus in biliary cirrhosis. Lancet 1989;1:574–576.

38. Galeazzi R, Lorenzini I, Orlandi F. Rifampicin-induced elevation of serum bile acids in man. Dig Dis Sci 1980;25:108–112.

39. Frezza M, Surrenti C, Manziello G, et al. Oral S-adenosylmethionine in the symptomatic treatment of intrahepatic cholestasis. Gastroenterology 1990; 99:211–215.

40. Lauterburg BT, Pineda AA, Burgstadler EA, et al. Treatment of pruritus of cholestasis by plasma perfusion through USP-charcoal-coated glass beads. Lancet 1980;2:53–55.

41. Cohen LB, Ambinder EP, Wolke AM, et al. Role of plasmapheresis in primary biliary cirrhosis. Gut 1985;26:291–294.

42. Whitington PF, Whitington GL. Partial external diversion of bile for the treatment of intractable pruri-

tus associated with intrahepatic cholestasis. Gastroenterology 1988;95:130–136.

43. Hanid MA, Levi AJ. Phototherapy for pruritus in primary biliary cirrhosis [Letter]. Lancet 1980;2:530.

44. Maggiore G, Grifeo S, De Giacomo C, et al. Phototherapy for pruritus in chronic cholestasis of childhood. Eur J Pediatr 1982;139:90–91.

45. Watson WC, Intravenous lignocaine for relief of intractable itch [Letter]. Lancet 1973;1:211.

46. Walt RP, Daneshmend TK, Fellows IW, et al. Effect of stanozolol on itching in primary biliary cirrhosis. Br Med J 1988;296:607.

47. Hishon S, Rose JD, Hunter JO. The relief of pruritus in primary biliary cirrhosis by hydroxyethylrutorides. Br J Dermatol 1981;105:457–459.

48. Donovan GK, Kidwell M. Benign recurrent intrahepatic cholestasis: relief of pruritus with carbamazepine [Abstract]. Gastroenterology 1988;94:A536.

49. Poupon RE, Balkav B, Eschwege E, et al. A multicenter, controlled trial of ursodiol for the treatment of primary biliary cirrhosis. N Engl J Med 1991;324:1548–1553.

50. Pert C, Snyder S. Opiate receptor: demonstration in nervous tissue. Science 1973;179:1011–1014.

51. Simon EJ, Hiller JM, Edelman J. Stereospecific binding of the potent narcotic analgesic [³H] etorphine to rat-brain homogenate. Proc Natl Acad Sci USA 1973;70:1947–1949.

52. Evans CJ, Hammond DL, Frederickson RCA. The opioid peptides. In: Pasternak GW, ed. The opiate receptor. Clifton, NJ: Humana Press, 1988:23–71.

53. Blanchard SG, Chang KT. Regulation of opioid receptors. In: Pasternak GW, ed. The opiate receptor. Clifton, NJ: Humana Press, 1988:425–439.

54. Koenigstein H. Experimental study of itch stimuli in animals. Arch Dermatol Syph 1948;57:828–849.

55. Thomas DA, Williams GM, Iwata K et al. Effects of central administration of opioids on facial scratching in monkeys. Brain Res 1992;585:315–317.

56. Reiz S, Westberg M. Side effects of epidural administration of opioids. Anesthesiology 1980;2:203–204.

57. Cousins MJ, Mather LE. Intrathecal and epidural administration of opioids. Anesthesiology 1984; 62:276–310.

58. Jaffe JH, Martin WR. Opioid analgesics and antagonists. In: Gilman AG, Goodman LS, Rall TW, et al., eds. The pharmacologic basis of therapeutics, 7th ed. New York: Macmillan, 1985:491–531.

59. Ballantyne JC, Loach AB, Carr DB. Itching after epidural and spinal opiates. Pain 1988;33:149–160.

60. Bromage PR. The price of intraspinal narcotic analgesia: basic constraints. Anesth Analg 1988;60:461–463.

61. Bernstein JE, Grinzi RA. Burtorphanol-induced pruritus antagonized by naloxone. J Am Acad Dermatol 1981;5:227–228.

62. Scott PV, Fischer HBJ. Spinal opiate analgesia and facial pruritus: a neural theory. Postgrad Med J 1982;58:531–535.

63. Justins DM, Reynolds F. Intraspinal opiates and itching: a new reflex? Br Med J 1982;284:1401.

64. Welchew EA, Thornton JA. Continuous thoracic epidural fentanyl: a comparison of epidural fentanyl with intramuscular papaveretum for postoperative pain. Anaesthesia 1983;37:309–315.

65. Brownridge PR. Epidural and intrathecal opiates for postoperative pain relief. Anaesthesia 1983;38:74–75.

66. Shipton EA, Hugo JM, Muller FO. Epidural fentanyl in the management of postoperative pain. S Afr Med J 1986;13:325–328.

67. Bromage PR, Camporesi EM, Durant PA, et al. Nonrespiratory side effects of epidural morphine. Anesth Analg 1982;61:490–495.

68. Laidlaw J, Read AE, Sherlock S. Morphine tolerance in hepatic cirrhosis. Gastroenterology 1961;40:389–396.

69. Dixon R, Howes J, Gentile J, et al. Nalmefene: intravenous safety and kinetics. Clin Pharmacol Ther 1986;39:49–53.

70. Thornton JR, Losowsky MS. Opioid peptides and primary biliary cirrhosis. Br Med J 1988;297:1501–1504.

71. Bergasa NV, Alling DW, Talbot TL, et al. Relief from the intractable pruritus of chronic cholestasis associated with oral nalmefene therapy [Abstract]. Hepatology 1991;4:154A.

72. Gal TJ, DiFarzio CA, Dixon R. Prolonged blockade of opioid effect with oral nalmefene. Clin Pharmacol Ther 1986;40:537–542.

73. Gold MS, Redmond DE, Kleber HD. Clonidine blocks acute opiate-withdrawal symptoms. Lancet 1978;2:599–602.

74. Washton AM, Resnick RB. Clonidine for opiate detoxification: outpatient clinical trials. Am J Psychiatry 1980;137:1121–1122.

75. Charrey DS, Heninger GR, Kleber HD. The combined use of clonidine and naltrexone as a rapid, safe and effective treatment of abrupt withdrawal from methadone. Am J Psychiatry 1986;143: 831–837.

76. Resnick RB, Kestenbaum RS, Washton A, et al. Naloxone-precipitated withdrawal: a method for rapid induction onto naltrexone. Clin Pharmacol Ther 1977;21:409–413.

77. Grossman A, Stubb WA, Gaillard RC, et al. Studies of the opiate control of prolactin, GH and TSH. Clin Endocrinol 1981;14:381–382.

78. Bergasa NV, Vergalla J, Jones EA. Acute cholestasis in the rat is associated with antinociception: reversal by naxolone. J Hepatol 1993 (in press).

79. Thornton JR, Dean H, Losowsky MS. Is ascites caused by impaired hepatic inactivation of bloodborne endogenous opioid peptides? Gut 1988; 29:1167–1172.

80. Thornton JR, Losowsky MS. Plasma methionine enkephalin concentration and prognosis in primary biliary cirrhosis. Br Med J 1988;297:1241–1242.

81. Thornton JR, Dean HG, Losowsky MS. Do increased catecholamines and plasma methionine enkephalin in cirrhosis promote bleeding oesophageal varices? Q J Med 1988;68:541–551.

82. Swain MG, Rothman RB, Xu H, et al. Endogenous opioids accumulate in plasma in a rat model of acute cholestatis. Gastroenterology 1992;103:630–635.

83. Tao P-L, Law P-Y, Loh HH. Decrease in delta and mu opioid receptor binding capacity in rat brain after chronic etorphine treatment. J Pharmacol Exp Ther 1987;240:809–816.

84. Bergasa NV, Rothman RB, Vergalla J, et al. Central mu-opioid receptors are down-regulated in a rat model of cholestasis. J Hepatology 1992;15:220–224.

85. Bergasa NV, Rothman RB, Vergalla J, et al. Down-regulation of delta opioid receptors in bile duct resected rats: further evidence for alteration in the opioid system in cholestasis [Abstract]. Gastroenterology 1992;102:A946.

86. Bernstein JE, Swift R. Relief of intractable pruritus with naloxone. Arch Dermatol 1979;115:1366–1367.

87. Summerfield JA. Naloxone modulates the perception of itch in man. Br J Clin Pharmacol 1980;10:180–182.

88. Burch JR, Harrison PV. Opiates, sleep and itch. Clin Exp Dermatol 1988;13:418–419.

89. McCormack HM, de L'Horne DJ, Sheather S. Clinical applications of visual analogue scales: a critical review. Psycholog Med 1988;18:1007–1019.

90. Bergasa NV, Alling D, Talbot T, et al. Assessment of the pruritus of cholestasis: an appraisal of the visual analogue scale [Abstract]. Hepatology 1990;12:887.

91. Bergasa NV, Talbot TL, Alling DW, et al. A controlled trial of naloxone infusions for the pruritus of chronic cholestasis. Gastroenterology 1992;102:544–549.

92. Felix R, Shuster S. A new method for the measurement of itch and the response to treatment. Br J Dermatol 1975;93:303–312.

93. Summerfield JA, Welch ME. The measurement of itch with sensitive limb movement meters. Br J Dermatol 1980;102:275–281.

94. Talbot TL, Schmitt JM, Bergasa NV, et al. Application of piezofilm technology for the quantitative assessment of pruritus. Biomed Instrumentation Tech 1991;25:400–403.

95. Johnstone RE, Jobes DR, Kennell EM, et al. Reversal of morphine anesthesia with naloxone. Anesthesiology 1974;41:361–367.

96. Bergasa NV, Alling DW, Talbot TL, et al. Naloxone ameliorates the pruritus of cholestasis: results of a double-blind randomized placebo-controlled trial [Abstract]. Hepatology 1992;16:152A.

97. Bergasa NV, Alling DW, Talbot TL, et al. Nalmefene therapy is associated with the relief of the pruritus of cholestasis: results of a double-blind randomized placebo-controlled trial [Abstract]. Hepatology 1993 (in press).

98. Wahler JB, Swain MG, Carson R, et al. Blood brain barrier permeability is markedly decreased in a classical rat model of cholestasis. Hepatology 1993;17:1103–1108.

23

Medical Management of Ascites

RICHARD V. BENYA and LEONARD B. SEEFF

Ascites is a common and often dramatic physical response to a heterogeneous group of disorders that affects millions of people worldwide. Indeed, the extent of the problem may not be fully recognized. Many patients with ascites have insufficient abdominal distension to cause gross disfigurement, and only 10–20% of patients with ascites are handicapped by intractable disease (1). By far the predominant cause of ascites is chronic liver disease following long-term alcohol (ethanol) abuse; however, the differential diagnosis for ascites is extensive and includes malignancy, infection, cardiac and pancreatic dysfunction, as well as a host of miscellaneous disorders (Table 23.1). The prognosis for many patients with ascites is poor, and in the case of ascites due to alcohol abuse, no treatment modality has been demonstrated to prolong survival. Consequently, many clinicians view this condition with pessimism. The ever-expanding pharmacopeia, however, continues to generate new treatment options. In this chapter, we review the pathophysiology of, the diagnostic approach to, and the various medical therapies available for the patient with ascites. For comparison purposes, selected nonpharmacologic approaches to ascites also are reviewed.

PATHOPHYSIOLOGY

The pathophysiology of the disease process is often disregarded in considering the care of individuals with ascites. Yet the survival of the patient with ascites due to liver dysfunction depends on the severity of the underlying liver disease (2), or on the origin of the ascites when not due to liver disease. A patient with massive ascites secondary to congestive heart failure has a poor prognosis, with a life expectancy measured in months; whereas one with ascites due to an infectious process such as tuberculosis can have a normal life expectancy if the underlying disease is diagnosed and treated. It is evident, therefore, that the pathophysiology of ascites varies depending on its origin and that treatment will need to be tailored accordingly. For the purposes of the present discussion, we classify ascites as due to alcoholic cirrhosis, peritoneal disease, obstructive disorders of the vascular and lymphatic systems, and miscellaneous entities. Not every etiologic process listed in Table 23.1 will be discussed in detail, except to clarify principles pertinent to understanding the pathogenetic mechanisms underlying ascites formation.

Alcoholic Cirrhosis

In the United States, alcohol-induced cirrhosis is the most common cause of ascites, and ascites is the most frequent physical manifestation of alcoholic cirrhosis. Fifty percent of alcoholic cirrhotics who die have ascites (3). Individuals with alcohol-related ascites have a 1-year survival rate of 50%, and a 5-year survival rate of 20% (4). Their demise is due to variceal hemorrhage (25%), hepatorenal syndrome-induced renal failure (10%), and the adverse effects of their medical therapy (10%) (3). These grim figures demand that the clinician have a thorough knowledge of the mechanisms responsible for ascites, as well as of the multiple agents available for its control.

Table 23.1
Differential Diagnosis of Ascites

Alcoholic cirrhosis

Peritoneal disease
   Malignant
      Peritoneal carcinomatosis
      Solid tumors with or without peritoneal
         involvement
         Ovary
         Endometrium
         Breast
         Colon
         Stomach
         Pancreas
   Non-malignant
      Sarcoid
      Mesothelioma
      Crohn's disease
      Systemic lupus erythematosus
      Infection
         Tuberculosis
         Fungal
         Parasitic

Mechanical obstruction of blood and/or lymph
   Cirrhosis
      Alcohol
      Viral hepatitis B, C
      Hemochromatosis
      α_1-Antitrypsin deficiency
      Wilson's disease
   Congestive heart failure
   Hepatic vein obstruction (Budd-Chiari syndrome)
      Polycythemia vera
      Hepatocellular carcinoma
      Renal cell carcinoma
      Idiopathic
   Veno-occlusive disease of the liver
   Infection
      Schistosomiasis

Miscellaneous
   Pancreatic ascites
   Hypothyroidism
   Chylous ascites

The precise basis for the production of ascites is not yet fully understood. One aspect of the physiologic state that is generally accepted and noncontroversial concerns the circulatory derangements observed in cirrhotic patients with ascites. These patients have a decreased total vascular resistance, decreased mean arterial blood pressure, and an increased cardiac index with normal to increased plasma volume (5–7). Although patients with ascites have increased activation of their plasma pressor systems (8–10), including increased splanchnic sympathetic output (11), they also exhibit splanchnic vasodilation. This vasodilation is a direct consequence of portal hypertension (12, 13), but also may be due to an as yet undefined neurohumoral factor(s). Cirrhosis does not seem to be an absolute prerequisite for portal hypertension, however, since patients with alcoholic hepatitis but without histologic evidence of cirrhosis also have been described with ascites (14). Presumably, this is due to the venous outflow obstruction that results from the central hyaline necrosis encircling the terminal hepatic venules (14). Unfortunately, the hormonal abnormalities observed are not consistently seen in all patients, perpetuating our ongoing inability to precisely describe the pathogenesis of ascites.

The multiple hormonal derangements that do exist directly influence renal function. Among these, the renin-angiotensin-aldosterone (RAA) system has received the most attention. Early investigators believed that ascites developed as a consequence of a generalized activation of the RAA system, leading to a state of "hyperaldosteronism." It is now clear that this phenomenon is due primarily to faulty renal function. Arterial renins are elevated in decompensated cirrhosis because of their increased synthesis by cells within the juxtaglomerular (JG) complex, and not because of decreased degradation by the liver (15). It is this increase in renin that results in an overall increase in circulating aldosterone. A correlation exists between plasma aldosterone concentrations and blood volume, and between aldosterone concentrations and the ability of the kidney to excrete an Na^+ load (16, 17). Furthermore, inhibition of aldosterone by medical (spironolactone) or surgical (adrenalectomy) means reliably reverses the Na^+-avid state of the kidney, provided that irreversible renal failure has not yet occurred (18).

That alterations in plasma aldosterone concentration may not be the central hormonal derangement is suggested by the fact that only 35–50% of patients with ascites have increases in plasma aldosterone levels (19). Indeed, early evidence of altered renal function exists at a time when there is an overall suppression of the RAA system (20, 21). Also conflicting with this theory is aldosterone's variable interaction with the kallikrein-kininogen-kinin system. In normal individuals, the elevation in aldosterone levels acts to increase serum kinin concentrations; this in turn acts to increase the glomerular filtration rate and blocks distal tubular Na^+ uptake. In cirrhotics, however, a decrease in kinin excretion has been observed that is independent of plasma renin activity, aldosterone, or Na^+ excretion (22).

Other hormonal abnormalities include elevated norepinephrine (but not epinephrine) levels (23), elevated plasma arginine-vasopressin levels (24), and normal to increased concentrations of plasma atrial natiuretic peptide (ANP) (25–27). Receptors for ANP have been shown to be significantly down-regulated in the glomerular cells of patients with ascites, resulting in the diminished ability of ANP to maintain sodium and water homeostasis (28).

Together these identified hormonal aberrations, along with as yet undiscovered hormonal imbalances, result in increased proximal tubular Na^+ resorption (29) and reduced filtrate delivery to the distal tubule (30). Thus, the primary defect in patients with cirrhotic ascites is the excessive retention of Na^+ by the kidney. What actually induces this Na^+-avid state, however, is still not known. Despite nearly a century of research, it remains unclear whether it is ascites that is the primary event, leading to a decrease in plasma volume that secondarily promotes kidney Na^+ retention, or whether the Na^+-avid state is the primary defect that secondarily results in ascites. A panoply of conflicting physiologic data can be mustered to support either viewpoint. This has led to the proposal of two separate mechanisms by which ascites is formed, these being the underfill and the overflow theories.

UNDERFILL THEORY

In this original model for ascites formation, portal hypertension leads to splanchnic vasodilation, with subsequent exudation of plasma into the peritoneal cavity. Ascites formation reduces intravascular volume, which secondarily induces the kidney to become Na^+-avid. The temporarily reconstituted intravascular space exacerbates the portal hypertension, leading to further ascites formation. Although plasma volume has not been found to be decreased in patients with ascites (29), proponents of the underfill theory argue that it is a decrease in "effective" blood volume that is of importance.

According to this view, stretch receptors located within the atria and volume sensors located within the JG complex (26) are activated by the decrease in effective plasma volume. Activation of these stretch and volume receptors results in increased sympathetic tone, increased release of arginine-vasopressin, and of ANP (25, 30). These peptides, along with increased sympathetic activity, permit blood volume maldistribution within the various components of the vascular system. Arteriolar vasodilation and increased capacitance of the venous circulation together offset any increases in overall plasma volume, resulting in a decreased effective plasma volume.

Studies that artificially increase plasma volume partially support the underfill hypothesis. Head-out immersion of the body into water causes a redistribution of blood away from dependent extremities, thereby increasing central plasma volume and activating atrial stretch receptors. This maneuver increases renal perfusion and temporarily improves urine output in most patients, although a certain percentage of patients will fail to respond to this method of increasing renal perfusion. However, concomitant administration of epinephrine, an adrenergic agonist, increases vascular tone and decreases arteriolar vascular capacity, normalizing urine Na^+ excretion in otherwise unresponsive patients (31). This suggests that plasma volume reconstitution alone is not sufficient to correct the renal defect in all patients with ascites. Although ANP levels are increased in patients with decompensated cirrhosis compared with normal volunteers, the levels are less than those seen in patients with cardiac or renal failure (32). With placement of a portal-venous shunt, central blood volume is restored to normal, and serum ANP levels increase dramatically (33, 34). Thus, if ascites were a problem primarily of renal Na^+ handling (overflow theory), increasing central blood volume instead would be expected to worsen ascites, leaving ANP levels unchanged. That ANP levels are elevated at all is explained by the underfill theory proponents as being due to multiple events including diuretic therapy, hypersensitive atrial stretch receptors, decreased ANP metabolism, and decreased atrial pressure gradients induced by the ascites (35).

Finally, statistical analysis seems to lend additional support to the underfill theory. This is based on the evidence that patients with cirrhotic ascites can be stratified into two groups: those who excrete more and those who excrete less than 15 mmol Na^+ per day. Although poor Na^+ excreters have higher plasma levels of renin, aldosterone, and of arginine-vasopressin, multiple regression analysis associates the development of ascites only with low blood pressure and with high plasma aldosterone levels (36). These results indirectly support the view that Na^+ retention in decompensated cirrhosis is due to a contraction of effective blood volume.

OVERFLOW THEORY

The underfill theory is tenable for patients who show activation of their RAA system, but it cannot satisfactorily explain the pathophysiology of patients with normal aldosterone levels. Important work by Levy suggests that Na^+ retention by the kidney precedes ascites formation (37). The mechanism by which the kidney is signaled to retain Na^+ is not clear, but may relate to the increase in hepatic venous pressure triggering an as yet unidentified splanchnic baroreceptor. In animal studies, this hepatorenal reflex causes increased Na^+ and water retention by the kidney (38, 39). Human studies by Lieberman et al. (29, 40, 41) also suggest that volume contraction alone does not totally account for the kidney's aberrant handling of Na^+. In these investigations,

diuresis in the face of saline infusion, but not albumin infusion, fails to worsen renal function.

Human studies suffer from the fact that they are conducted among patients who already have ascites, thus precluding patients in the early phase of ascites development from study. One method of overcoming this temporal limitation would be to stratify patients with cirrhosis and without ascites into groups of patients who have had or have never had ascites in the past. Using this approach, Warner et al. (26) studied serum ANP levels in patients administered diets with varying amounts of Na^+. The investigators found that renal resistance to ANP is evident in the group with a history of ascites, and that this resistance is associated with increased Na^+ retention as diets of increasing Na^+ content are administered. This group concludes that in such patients, high Na^+ diets increase intra-sinusoidal pressure and directly cause the kidney to retain Na^+, and that Na^+ homeostasis ordinarily is maintained by gradual elevations in ANP levels.

PERIPHERAL VASODILATION HYPOTHESIS

These varied and sometimes conflicting observations suggest that ascites in patients with alcohol-induced cirrhosis may not be attributable to only one pathogenetic mechanism. Clinical observation alone suggests that two patient groups exist, namely those who can tolerate diuretic therapy without renal impairment and those who cannot tolerate such therapy (42). Yet attempts to present a unified hypothesis persist. Perhaps the most logical of these is the peripheral vasodilation hypothesis proposed by Schrier et al. (43). In this model, the initiating event is arteriolar vasodilation, which results in moderate hypotension. This vasodilation activates the RAA system as well as inducing the release of other pressor peptides, with renal sodium retention occurring later, but before clinically apparent ascites develops. With time, a proportion of patients (ie, those without evidence of hyperaldosteronism) should "correct" their vasodilated state by retaining sufficient Na^+ and water. Recent work by Albillos et al. (44) confirms this chronology. Rats undergoing portal vein ligation first expand their intra-arterial space, and 24 hours later increase their total body Na^+. Although the putative vasodilatory agent in cirrhosis is unknown, preliminary animal investigations support a possible role for nitrous oxide (45).

MISCELLANEOUS MECHANISMS

A variety of other mechanisms have been identified that could contribute to ascites formation in patients with cirrhosis. Foremost of these mechanisms are arginine-vasopressin hypersecretion, endotoxemia, and diminished renal eicosanoid production. The kidney in patients with cirrhosis and ascites, in addition to being Na^+-avid, is unable to excrete free water. This defect, which clinically results in hyponatremia, originally was believed to be secondary to a low filtered Na^+; consequently, near-total Na^+ resorption occurs in the proximal convoluted tubule (46). The potent vasoconstrictor arginine-vasopressin, however, also has been shown to be elevated in patients with cirrhotic ascites, there being an inverse relationship between the concentration of this hormone and the ability of the kidney to excrete free water (47). Two arginine-vasopressin receptor subtypes have been identified in the kidney: V_1 receptors that are present in the vascular smooth muscle and which mediate vasoconstriction, and V_2 receptors located on epithelial cells of the collecting duct that mediate the antidiuretic effects of this peptide (48). Receptor-specific antagonists have recently been isolated and used in animal models of cirrhotic ascites. Using a V_2-specific antagonist in the rat, Claria et al. demonstrate that this agent normalizes water excretion without changing water metabolism in the overwhelming majority of animals (30). Accordingly, they conclude that the concentration of arginine-vasopressin is the most important factor responsible for the inability of the cirrhotic patient to appropriately excrete free water.

Chronic endotoxemia may also play a role in the ascites of cirrhosis because of its tendency to alter renal eicosanoid concentrations. Eicosanoids normally synthesized by the kidney include vasodilators (PgE_2, PgI_2) and vasoconstrictors (leukotrienes, thromboxane A_2 [TxA_2]). The vasodilatory eicosanoids, especially PgE_2, play a critical role in maintaining renal perfusion, and renal production of all of these compounds is increased in patients with ascites (49). In circumstances where there is an alteration in the relative concentration of these compounds, as occurs with administration of prostaglandin synthetase inhibitors (ie, nonsteroidal anti-inflammatory drugs [NSAIDs]), renal function may become seriously impaired. The role of endotoxemia and of TxA_2 in mediating renal arteriolar vasoconstriction is less clear. Theoretically, elevated portal pressures promote increased bacterial translocation across the gut, and portosystemic shunting extant in the cirrhotic prevents adequate removal of lipopolysaccharide endotoxin moieties by Kupffer cells (50). These lipopolysaccharides activate eicosanoid production, predominantly TxA_2. However, recent data also suggest that while TxA_2 levels are increased in patients with ascites, the levels are not significantly higher than those observed in patients with a similar degree of hepatic dysfunction and preserved renal function (51). Whether serum TxA_2 can serve as a marker for future or impending renal insufficiency, however, is currently unknown.

HEPATORENAL SYNDROME

Although the pathogenesis of ascites in alcoholic liver disease has not been precisely elucidated, it is clear that the kidney plays a central role in creating and in maintaining this extravascular fluid accumulation. Furthermore, the same factors that act on the kidney to retain Na^+ and water also result in progressive renal failure. This continuum in impaired renal function, when made clinically obvious by a reduced urine output, is labeled the hepatorenal syndrome (HRS). The major clinical features of this syndrome include its occurrence in the hospitalized patient without obvious precipitating factors and marked oliguria with a nearly total absence of urinary

Na$^+$ (52). Of note is the fact that the clinical features and urinary abnormalities of HRS are difficult to distinguish from those of prerenal azotemia.

The blood flow to the kidney in cirrhosis is maintained by a delicate balance between vasoconstrictor agents attempting to restore intravascular volume and vasodilatory agents attempting to preserve renal perfusion. The vasodilatory factors, largely prostaglandins (Pgs), are produced within the kidney and act to antagonize the vascular effects of angiotensin II, norepinephrine, ANP, etc. These vasoconstricting peptides themselves also act to enhance renal Pg synthesis. In patients with cirrhosis and ascites but without HRS, this fragile equilibrium is maintained (53). Evidence supporting a central role for renal Pgs in maintaining renal blood flow in the face of the vasoconstrictor onslaught include the following two observations: (a) Patients with HRS have increased plasma levels of vasoconstrictor peptides and decreased urinary Pg levels (50). (b) Administration of Pg synthetase inhibitors such as NSAIDs can result in the HRS (54).

It is probable that other factors also play a role in the pathogenesis of HRS. In persons with alcoholic cirrhosis, cardiomyopathy may contribute to poor cardiac output and thus result in impaired renal blood flow (55). Furthermore, patients abusing ethanol are known to suffer multiple nutritional deficiencies, some of which can impair both cardiac and renal function. One such nutrient is thiamine, deficiency of which results in the well-known cardiomyopathy of dry beriberi. Thiamine deficiency has recently been associated with the development of HRS by some (56) but not all investigators (57).

Thus, factors that play a role in the pathogenesis of ascites also can result in a decreased glomerular filtration rate (GFR); relatively small perturbations in GFR in a patient with ascites may be all that is necessary to precipitate clinically evident renal failure (Fig. 23.1). By further reducing intravascular volume, diuretic therapies designed to reduce ascites can result in GFRs incompatible with mainte-nance of renal function. Unfortunately, definitive therapies do not exist for the management of HRS, and prevention therefore remains the prime objective for the physician. Injudicious use of diuretics, NSAIDs, aminoglycosides, and other drugs that interfere with renal function may account for most cases of HRS, so that most of these agents should only be used with caution and others should not be used at all.

Peritoneal Disease

Diseases of the peritoneum that may be associated with ascites formation include malignant processes, granulomatous disorders, infections, and the vasculitides. Each category includes a variety of diseases, yet similar general principles appear to govern ascites formation within each broad grouping. Although noncirrhotic ascites has been studied in less detail than cirrhotic ascites, relatively precise pathogenetic mechanisms nonetheless have been established to account for these abnormal extravascular fluid collections.

MALIGNANCY

Malignant tumors that arise within the abdomen as well as those that metastasize to the peritoneum are capable of causing ascites. These include, in decreasing order of frequency, ovarian, endometrial, breast, colonic, gastric, and pancreatic carcinoma (58). These tumors account for more than 80% of the ascites observed with malignancy, although almost any tumor involving the abdomen can be associated with ascites. Solitary tumors and widespread peritoneal carcinomatosis can induce ascites by similar mechanisms.

Mechanical obstruction of the lymphatic glands is commonly cited as a basis for the development of ascites of malignant origin. In both animal and human studies, it has been observed that there is decreased uptake of ^{51}Chromium-labeled erythrocytes (59) and of ^{99}Technetium-labeled sulfur colloid (60) through diaphragmatic lymph channels. This decreased uptake is observed prior to the actual development of ascites. Other mecha-

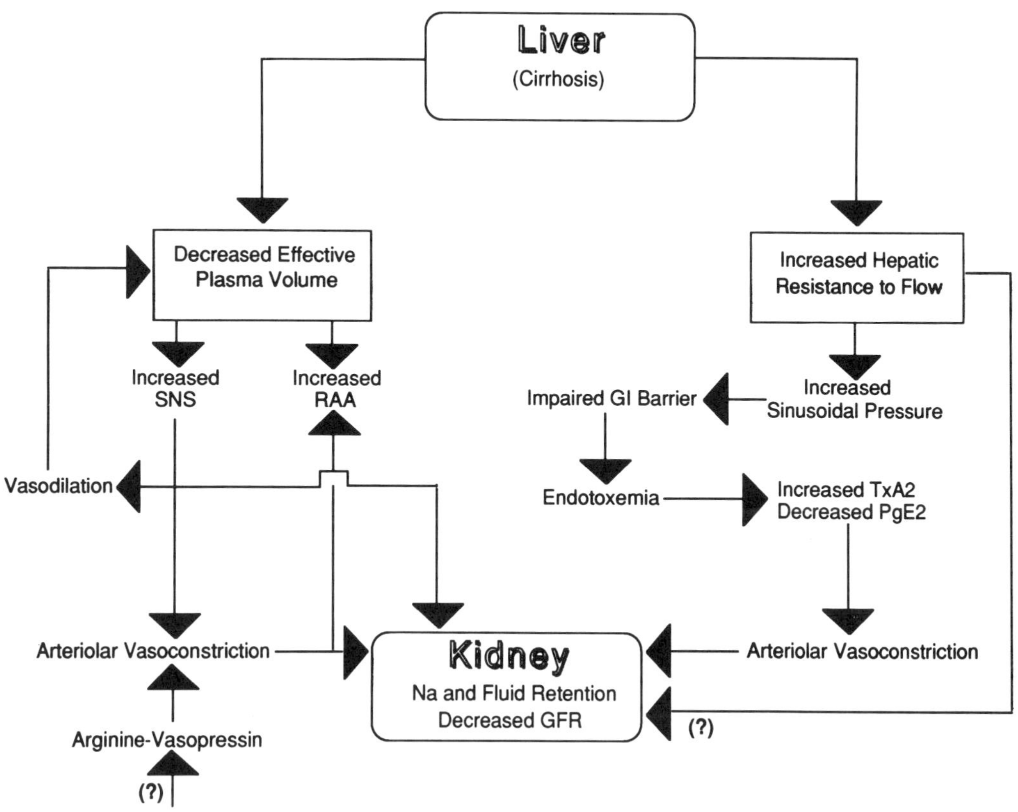

Figure 23.1. Summary of various processes resulting in ascites secondary to alcoholic cirrhosis. Processes of uncertain action or significance are indicated by a question mark. *SNS*, sympathetic nervous system; *RAA*, renin-angiotensin-aldosterone system.

nisms of malignant ascites formation independent of altered lymph flow also exist, however. For example, there is evidence that in patients with peritoneal carcinomatosis, protein-rich fluid leaks from the peritoneum in quantities equivalent to that found in patients with cirrhosis (61). Indeed, a well-known phenomenon observed in patients with malignant ascites is increased endothelial permeability with increased fluid production from tumor-free areas of the peritoneal surface (62, 63). Moreover, a variety of kinins and proteases have been identified in malignant ascites that can act directly to increase the permeability of peritoneal endothelial cells. These include plasminogen, α-2 antiplasmin, antithrombin III, factor V, and α-1 protease inhibitor (64). These peptides, either singly or in concert

with other agents, permit the exudation of plasma into the peritoneum.

One group of proteins, the bradykinins, seem to play a particularly critical role in inducing a leaky vascular endothelium. Bradykinin is formed from kininogen by activated factor XII (Hageman factor) and by kallikrein. Interestingly, this species of bradykinin contains hydoxylproline, suggesting that it was synthesized from a source rich in proline, such as collagen (65). This information can be used to generate a theoretical construct for malignant ascites formation (Fig. 23.2). Kallikrein extravasates into the peritoneum, perhaps facilitated in some way by malignant cells, whereupon it is acted upon by kininogen present in the peritoneum. This reaction is usually inhibited by aprotinin, α_2- macroglobulin, and

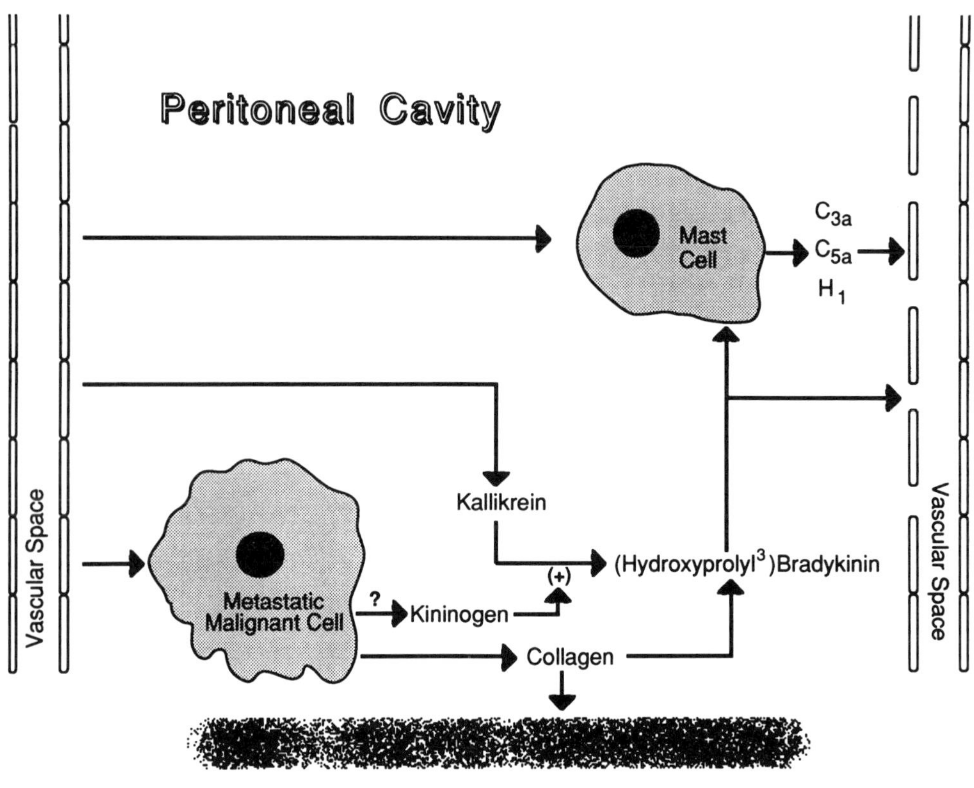

Figure 23.2. A proposed format for malignant ascites formation involving the kallikrein-kinin-kininogen system. Metastatic tumor cells attach to the extracellular matrix, which contains collagen. The basic amino acid structure for collagen is X-proline-glycine; local remodeling of the matrix by malignant tissues makes proline available for incorporation into kinins (ie, [hydroxyprolyl^3]bradykinin). Only kininogen would require initial extravasation into the peritoneum, where it could be acted upon by kallikrein in the absence of protease inhibitors normally present in the serum. Bradykinin so created would act directly to increase vascular endothelial permeability, as well as to stimulate histamine (H) and complement (C_{3a}, C_{5a}) release from mast cells.

α-antitrypsin, large molecular weight structures that are not readily found in the peritoneal cavity. In the peritoneum, no such inhibition of the kallikrein-kinin-kininogen cascade would be expected. Generation of bradykinin would appear to take place in close proximity to the extracellular matrix, itself synthesized in situ by malignant cells (66), given the proline component of this kinin. This suggests that the kininogen present in the peritoneum may originate from the malignant cell. Bradykinin could then act directly upon the vascular endothelium, increasing permeability, or it could act upon mast cells.

Mast cells in response to bradykinin stimulation release complement and histamine, each of which can further promote ascites formation (67). Neovascularization induced by the tumor probably does not play a major role in ascites formation, since the aforementioned permeability factors have been demonstrated to act on neovascular as well as endogenous endothelium (68). Accordingly, pharmacologic agents that suppress neovascularization (ie, protamine sulfate) are not likely to play an important role in the evolving therapy of malignant ascites.

Finally, a recent report suggests that certain chemotherapeutic agents themselves can induce ascites formation, independently of the underlying malignancy. Kemeny et al. (69) document that the combination of 5-fluorouracil and *N*-phosphonacetyl-L-aspartate (PALA) used in the treatment of colon cancer can result in a syndrome consisting of ascites, hyperbilirubinemia, and hypoalbuminemia. This drug combination produces an ascites with a high serum-ascites albumin gradient that responds to diuretics and discontinuation of the offending medications. Thus, it is important to realize that the occurrence of ascites in the patient with malignancy need not reflect tumor progression, but may be a consequence of therapy.

NONMALIGNANT DISEASE OF THE PERITONEUM

Although a number of diseases resulting in granuloma formation have been associated with ascites, including tuberculosis (TB), sarcoidosis, mesothelioma, and Crohn's disease, the precise pathogenetic mechanism remains unclear. Detailed studies of the components of the ascitic fluid similar to those performed in the study of malignant ascites have not been performed. At present, the most tenable theory to explain ascites formation in granulomatous disease of the peritoneum is that the lesions themselves directly exude plasma-rich fluid. The same mechanism may account for the rare instances of ascites found in patients with vasculitic disorders such as systemic lupus erythematosis.

A variety of parasitic and fungal organisms can cause ascites by invading into and directly irritating the peritoneum. Fungal organisms predominantly include *Candida, Histoplasma,* and *Cryptococcus*; parasites include *Entamoeba histolytica, Ascaris,* and *Strongyloides* (70). Infection with these organisms is uncommon and suggests gastrointestinal tract perforation. Even more uncommonly, it may result as a complication of peritoneal dialysis (70).

Disorders That Mechanically Obstruct Blood and/or Lymph Flow

Ascites in patients with cirrhosis, regardless of etiology, derives in part from increased resistance to blood flow through the fibrotic liver. Obstruction to blood flow is clearly a major determinant of ascites formation, as mechanical devices such as the portal-venous shunt are effective in eliminating ascites in many instances simply by bypassing the high-resistance liver. In the same way that blood pressure is regulated by the arterioles, which represent the largest component of the systemic vasculature, portal pressure is controlled by the hepatic sinusoids, which represent the largest component of the intrahepatic vasculature. In conjunction with the overall increase in splanchnic blood flow, there is greatly increased hydrostatic pressure across the sinusoidal epithelium. This results in a loss of sinusoidal permselectivity (71), meaning that molecules of almost any size and charge can traverse the sinusoidal barrier. Consequently, fluid accumulates within the space of Disse, and this results in increased drainage by the hepatic lymphatics. When the sinusoidal pressure rises above that of lymphatic pressure, direct exudation of lymph begins to occur from surface lymphatics (72). This phenomenon is consistent with the observation at surgery that patients with cirrhosis exude fluid directly from the liver surface.

Mechanical causes for impedence of blood flow include, in addition to cirrhosis, right-sided congestive heart failure (73), constrictive pericarditis (74), hepatic vein obstruction (Budd-Chiari syndrome), and obstruction of the inferior vena cava. Cardiac ascites has been estimated to be responsible for approximately 6% of all cases of ascites in the United States, thus representing the third leading cause of ascites after cirrhosis and malignancy (75). It is probable that the frequency of cardiac ascites is actually higher, given the high prevalence of both cardiac disease and of alcohol abuse in the United States. Indeed, autopsy studies reveal that upwards of 40% of patients with heart disease have ascites (76).

Diseases causing hepatic vein obstruction, referred to as the Budd-Chiari syndrome, represent an important cause of hepatomegaly and refractory ascites. A variety of disease processes can result in the Budd-Chiari syndrome, including malignancy (hepatocellular carcinoma, renal cell carcinoma), myeloproliferative disorders (polycythemia vera) and other hypercoagulable states and drugs (e.g., oral contraceptives). Anatomic abnormalities such as idiopathic membranous obstruction and congenital venous leaflets, as well as macronodular cirrhosis, have also been associated with hepatic vein thrombosis (77). Finally, small vessel hepatic veno-occlusive disease can be caused by ingestion of pyrrolizidine alkaloids, agents unique to "bush" and comfrey teas made with plants of the family *Crotilaria* (78). Veno-occlusive disease is rare in the United States, but must be kept in mind for patients who are herbalists or hail from developing countries.

Parasitic infections such as that due to *Schistosoma* also result in ascites by mechanically obstructing portal flow to the liver. Schistosomal infection can cause ascites by peritoneal irritation, but more commonly does so by directly obstructing portal flow at the presinusoidal level. The associated inflammatory reaction to infection induces granuloma formation and hence presinusoidal obstruction (79). The inflammatory nature of this lesion lends itself to therapy with corticosteroids.

Other Diseases

HYPOALBUMINEMIA

Many patients with ascites also have depressed serum albumin concentrations. Because albumin is the predominant serum protein and is the prime determinant of serum oncotic pressure in normal individuals, hypoalbuminemia is often held responsible in the pathogenesis of ascites. Although the notion is intellectually appealing, the role of hypoalbuminemia by itself, in ascites formation, is not clear and is certainly not proven.

Serum albumin concentration is determined by its rate of synthesis, its volume of distribution, and its rate of catabolism. Each of these factors needs to be considered in the cirrhotic patient. First, the cirrhotic patient will have impaired synthetic capability, although with the ability of the liver to generate 120–200 mg/kg of body weight of albumin per day, tremendous synthetic reserve exists (80). Second, the majority of albumin is extravascular (60%) in the normal individual (81). As serum levels decline, a shift of protein to the intravascular space occurs. With this hepatic synthetic capacity and whole body albumin reserve, precipitous drops in serum albumin concentration due to cirrhosis alone should not occur, enabling other factors to play increasingly important roles in maintaining oncotic pressure. The relative role of albumin in determining serum oncotic pressure would therefore be expected to become progressively smaller. Indeed, chronic hypoalbuminemia as observed in other disease states does not necessarily result in ascites formation: patients born analbuminemic do not manifest ascites (82), nor do all patients with nephrotic syndrome, renal failure on hemodialysis, or patients with severe protein-calorie malnutrition. Thus, low serum albumin by itself is not likely to result in ascites, although hypoalbuminemia may facilitate ascites formation by acting as a co-factor with other previously discussed pathogenetic mechanisms.

PANCREATIC ASCITES

Only recently has pancreatic ascites been recognized as a specific entity. The most complete reviews of this condition (83–86) suggest that 66–91% of cases of pancreatic ascites are observed in patients who abuse alcohol. Such patients often have pseudocysts, which have been found radiographically or at surgery to be leaking. Pancreatic ascites also has been described as a consequence of nonpenetrating abdominal trauma, both with and without evidence of a leaking pancreatic duct. Traumatic origin is usually observed in children, but this cause has been reported in adults, albeit rarely (86). Other even rarer etiologies associated with pancreatic ascites include pancreatic duct stones, choledochal cysts, and ampullary stenosis (87). The diagnosis of pancreatic ascites requires the presence of massive amounts of peritoneal fluid (86), in order to distinguish this entity from the smaller amounts of ascites that may accompany acute pancreatitis.

Evidence suggests that mechanisms other than simple drainage are responsible for pancreatic ascites formation. Early experiments with dogs in which a direct pancreatic duct leak into the peritoneum was created failed to generate ascites (88). Additionally, ascitic amylase and lipase concentrations, although high, rarely reach the levels seen in pancreatic juice and may occasionally be only marginally elevated (87). Evidence now suggests a supporting role for phospholipase A_2 (PLA_2) in the pathogenesis of pancreatic ascites, independently of etiology. PLA_2 is a pancreatic enzyme that is exuded into the peritoneum in large quantities in experimental models of acute pancreatitis (89). This enzyme, furthermore, has been shown to markedly increase peritoneal permeability in a rat model (89). Administration of PLA_2 in animals force-fed alcohol results in peritoneal fluid accumulations, whereas this does not occur in control (ie, healthy) rat populations. This suggests that alcohol is an essential cofactor for PLA_2 activity (90). This finding further supports the contention that mechanical processes alone are not responsible for pancreatic ascites formation. While pancreatic ascites is currently considered a surgical disease, the disorder might be appropriately treated with PLA_2 inhibitors when they become available for use in humans.

CHYLOUS ASCITES

The major cause of chylous ascites is rupture of the thoracic duct, either due to an operative complication or to chest trauma. Iatrogenic rupture of the thoracic duct is uncommon and is usually associated with abdominal aortic procedures or with surgery of the posterior mediastinum (91, 92). Chylous ascites also can be associated with neoplasms obstructing the thoracic duct (93), as well as with tuberculosis (93), chronic pancreatitis (94), severe right-sided heart failure (95), and yellow nail syndrome (96). Chylous ascites, furthermore, has been associated with cirrhosis (97, 98), and this is probably due to the increased portal pressures being directly transmitted to the abdominal lymphatics.

HYPOTHYROIDISM

Ascites is a well-known yet infrequently observed complication of myxedema. The pathogenetic mechanisms responsible for the ascites are completely unknown, and accurate diagnosis is often difficult (99). Once diagnosed, however, thyroid replacement therapy results in an immediate and total resorption of the ascites.

DIAGNOSTIC EVALUATION

PHYSICAL EXAMINATION

Initial suspicion of the presence of ascites comes from the history and physical examination. Shifting dullness, a "U"-shaped pattern of dullness extending from the hypogastrium to the lateral quadrants, and bulging flanks, when present, make the diagnosis obvious. Cattau et al. (100) evaluated 21 patients referred specifically because the diagnosis of ascites was in doubt. These investigators found flank dullness to percussion to be the most sensitive but least specific physical finding, whereas the presence of a fluid wave was the most specific but least sensitive finding. The high specificity of the fluid wave was confirmed by Cummings et al. (101), but this group found that the most sensitive component of the physical examination was the presence of shifting dullness. Unfortunately, neither of these studies determined the positive predictive value of each maneuver. In the only prospective study available, Simel et al. (102) evaluated the ability of house officers to correctly diagnose ascites in 1515 patients at a major medical center. It was gratifying to find that the overall clinical evaluation accurately discriminated between the presence and absence of ascites in most instances. Their evidence even suggests that listening to the patient can be of value: the patient's subjective impression as to whether abdominal size was increasing or not was as helpful in making the diagnosis as was the presence of a fluid wave or shifting dullness (102).

Ultrasonography clearly has improved our diagnostic ability for detecting ascites, with all the studies reviewed above having used ultrasound as their "gold" standard. Although certain maneuvers during the physical examination have been described that supposedly can detect as little as 120 ml of peritoneal fluid (103), this achievement likely exceeds the abilities of most clinicians. Ultrasound, however, has been demonstrated to reliably detect 100 ml or less of ascitic fluid (104). The cost of ultrasonography, however, can exceed $250 for a "quick look" when attempting to localize fluid for paracentesis and $350 for a complete hepatobiliary examination. A British study demonstrated that auscultation performed in conjunction with a hand-held Doppler ultrasound machine detects ascites with a diagnostic accuracy similar to that of regular ultrasound evaluation (105). In this method the clinician places the transducer just above the level of the pubis, while rapidly depressing and releasing the abdominal wall. Detection of the air-fluid interface, when present, is readily discernable as the level of abdominal percussion is lowered caudad.

ASCITIC FLUID ANALYSIS

All patients with ascites of recent onset require diagnostic paracentesis, regardless of the patient's overall medical condition. When performed with ultrasound localization, paracentesis is a very safe procedure, and risks to the patient are minimal even when there is an underlying coagulopathy (106). In addition to newly diagnosed ascites, paracentesis is required of all cirrhotic patients readmitted to the hospital, and of any patient with ascites whose clinical condition deteriorates.

Initial laboratory evaluation of ascites should include cytology, glucose, cell count, and albumin concentration; simultaneous serum albumin concentration also should be determined. Because cytologic diagnostic accuracy is increased when large quantities of fluid can be processed for cells, a minimum of 1000 ml of fluid should be removed, if possible, at the time of the initial diagnostic paracentesis. The usefulness of ascites total protein concentrations is minimal, even though many authors continue to classify ascites as an exudate or transudate. These latter terms are outdated and should not be used. Currently, ascites should be characterized on the basis of the serum-ascites albumin gradient (SAAG) (107–109). This diagnostic approach is based on the fact that portal pressure is directly proportional to the oncotic pressure gradient between the splanchnic vasculature and the ascites (110), albumin being the prime determinant of these oncotic pressures. Ascitic fluid with a high SAAG has been shown to accurately identify the patient population with portal hypertension, and is thus useful in differentiating ascites secondary to cirrhosis from that due to malignancy. It should be appreciated that the former exudate/transudate classification fails to discriminate patients on the basis of portal hypertension. Patients with cirrhosis may have either low or high absolute total protein concentrations in their ascites, but in either instance will have an appropriately elevated SAAG (107). The separation of ascites into exudates and transudates is arbitrary and is totally without physiological basis (110).

Pare et al. (108) were the first to perform a systematic study of the SAAG. They found this parameter to clearly differentiate between patients with cirrhotic and malignant ascites due to peritoneal carcinomatosis. Subsequent studies have been able to associate high SAAGs with hepatic malignancy (110), right ventricular failure (112), Budd-Chiari syndrome (110), and fulminant hepatic failure (110). In addition to peritoneal carcinomatosis, low SAAGs have been observed with peritoneal tuberculosis (113), hollow organ leakage, and in patients with hypoalbuminemia secondary to a variety of disorders (114) (Table 23.2).

The SAAG is not, however, without its limitations. The gradient should not be used in isolation from the remainder of the clinician's evaluation or specific diagnoses will not be forthcoming and "mixed" cases may be mis-

Table 23.2
Serum-Ascites Albumin Gradient[a]

High SAAG	Low SAAG	Mixed/misleading
Cirrhosis	Tuberculosis	Portal vein thrombosis
HCC	Hypoalbuminemia	Diuretic therapy
Heart failure	Visceral leak	High serum globulins
Budd-Chiari syndrome	Peritoneal carcinomatosis	Cirrhosis plus tuberculosis
Fulminant hepatic failure		Non-steady state

[a]High SAAG defined as >1.1 g/dl, and low SAAG defined as <1.0 g/dl. Mixed or misleading conditions can result in inappropriate SAAG, such as may exist in patients receiving diuretics or in a clinical non-steady state. HCC, hepatocellular carcinoma.

leading. Rector (110) has counseled that misleadingly high SAAGs may be obtained with heart failure, portal venous thrombosis, and cirrhosis complicated by peritoneal tuberculosis. A study from Pittsburgh also casts doubt on the absolute correlation of portal pressure with the SAAG. Thirty-five patients requiring orthotopic liver transplantation, both with and without alcoholic liver disease, underwent SAAG determination at the time hepatic venous wedge pressures were measured (115). Although a good correlation between SAAG and portal pressure was observed in patients with alcohol-induced cirrhosis, no correlation was seen in patients without alcoholic liver disease. As pointed out by the authors, the SAAG reliably reflects the oncotic pressure gradient only when the serum globulin level is between 3.2 and 4.5 mg/dl, with high globulin levels acting to narrow the SAAG. Furthermore, the SAAG can be misleading during diuretic therapy or when the patient is in a non-steady state condition (115). Regardless of these caveats concerning SAAG use, its measurement clearly remains the most helpful parameter for assessing the origin of ascites. Albillos et al. (116), in a prospective study of 285 patients conducted over a 2-year period, found the SAAG to be 99% accurate in differentiating ascites in patients with cirrhosis from those with peritoneal carcinomatosis. With this level of precision, SAAG measurements that do not fit with the remainder of the evaluation cannot be ignored, but rather mandate further investigation into the pathogenesis of the ascites.

Other elements in the ascitic fluid have been identified in association with malignant ascites. Prieto et al. (117) found the presence of ascitic cholesterol and fibronectin superior to the SAAG in differentiating malignant from cirrhotic ascites. Fibronectin is a protein that exists in both soluble and insoluble forms, plays a role in mediating cell-cell and cell-basement membrane attachment, and has been found to be elevated in some malignant conditions. Additional support for a role for fibronectin in diagnosing malignant ascites comes from Salerno et al. (118), who studied 133 consecutive patients with ascites. Patients with peritoneal carcinomatosis were found to have higher concentrations of fibronectin as well as of carcinoembryonic antigen (CEA) in their ascitic fluid than did patients with other causes for their ascites. Although these parameters were not helpful in identifying patients with cirrhosis and hepatocellular carcinoma, the latter did manifest elevations in ascitic α-fetoprotein levels in 28 of 32 cases (118). Finally, ascitic sialic acid has been examined as a marker of malignant ascites. Colli et al. (119) compared ascitic sialic acid concentrations with ascitic fibronectin and cholesterol levels and found that the diagnostic accuracies of both sialic acid and fibronectin were high for the identification of ascites generated by peritoneal carcinomatosis. Unfortunately, these measurements were unhelpful for establishing the diagnosis of hepatocellular carcinoma.

Currently, the real value of these markers in elucidating the origin of ascites remains unclear. Hence, they should be considered experimental and should not be routinely determined at the present time. Rather, determination of ascitic fluid cholesterol, fibronectin, CEA, α-fetoprotein, and sialic acid should be limited to diagnostically challenging patients enrolled in experimental protocols. When necessary, such determinations should be performed by a laboratory with appropriate experience.

Peritoneal tuberculosis resulting in ascites remains a difficult diagnosis, with proof often requiring laparoscopic documentation of peritoneal granulomas ("studding") and positive culture from granulomous material. Even arriving at the decision to perform laparoscopy can be difficult since much of the information derived from history, physical examination, and initial laboratory assessment is nonspecific. Ascitic fluid analysis has generally been unhelpful for the diagnosis of tuberculosis, and ascitic fluid cultures are almost always negative for *Mycobacteria* (120). Low SAAGs are consistent with, but unfortunately not diagnostic for, peritoneal tuberculosis. Recently, it has been reported that ascitic adenosine deaminase can be of value in making this diagnosis. Dwivedi et al. (121) compared patients in India with ascites due to tuberculosis to those with ascites due to cirrhosis and malignancy and found that adenosine deaminase levels were 6- to 8-fold higher in ascitic fluid of tuberculous origin. Indeed, they found that adenosine deaminase levels greater than 33 U/L established a sensitivity of 100%, a specificity of 97%, and a positive predictive value of 95% for the diagnosis of tuberculosis ascites. Whether this high positive predictive value holds true for countries with lesser frequencies of tuberculosis is unknown and awaits further investigation. Determining ascitic fluid adenosine deaminase concentration, however, may ultimately prove to be a useful prelude to laparoscopic evaluation.

SERUM ANALYSIS

As part of the initial diagnostic evaluation of patients with ascites, blood should be obtained for the determination of serum electrolytes and creatinine. Depending on the prevailing circumstances, specific diagnostic markers for

viral hepatitis, ceruloplasmin, ferritin, and α₁-antitrypsin also can be determined. In the patient with known pre-existing cirrhosis, new onset of ascites or clinical deterioration can be a feature of hepatocellular carcinoma, so that serum α-fetoprotein determinations are justifiable in these patients. Whether or not early diagnosis of hepatocellular carcinoma affects patient prognosis, however, remains to be determined.

In addition, serum biochemical markers recently have been described for assessing patient prognosis. A study by Llach et al. (122) evaluated 139 patients hospitalized with ascites due to alcohol abuse to determine which parameters were most useful for predicting survival. Interestingly, this group found that hemodynamic parameters appeared superior to tests reflecting hepatic function. Specifically, decreased mean arterial pressure and increased plasma norepinephrine concentrations, along with decreased urine Na$^+$ excretion and glomerular filtration rates (GFR), independently and accurately predicted patient prognosis. Recurrence of ascites in this population can be predicted by serum levels of CA-125, a tumor-associated antigen originally thought to be helpful in differentiating malignant from cirrhotic ascites (123). Elevations in serum CA-125 were found to predict the recurrence of ascites in patients with cirrhosis, even among those without evidence of underlying malignancy (124). Thus, serum CA-125 may prove useful in determining which patients with cirrhosis are ascites-prone, and thereby permit the clinician to tailor more aggressive therapeutic regimes.

URINE ANALYSIS

Urinary electrolytes and creatinine should be obtained as a guide to the patient's pharmacologic management. Urine Na$^+$ and K$^+$ are especially helpful in assessing renal function and responsiveness to spironolactone. The urine Na$^+$:K$^+$ ratio was originally proposed as a means of assessing the effect of aldosterone on the kidney, and of establishing whether the patient remained sensitive to treatment with the aldosterone inhibitor spironolactone

(125). Patients with a ratio >1 were found to respond well to spironolactone 100 mg/day, whereas patients with a ratio that was <1 responded poorly to doses as high as 1000 mg/day (125). Consequently, little would appear to be gained by increasing the daily spironolactone dose in patients whose urinary $Na^+:K^+$ ratio is <1. Urine Na^+ alone reflects the degree to which various counter-regulatory forces are attempting to maintain intravascular volume. Its measurement has also been advocated by some as a guide to diuretic therapy. Urinary Na^+ levels of <20 mEq/L imply that severe renal refractoriness to spironolactone alone exists (126), and suggests the need for small amounts of additional loop diuretics (82, 127).

Another measure of renal Na^+ handling is the fractional excretion of sodium (FE_{Na}). This parameter is calculated as the (urine Na^+/plasma Na^+)/(urine creatinine/plasma creatinine) $\times$ 100; values <1 usually are associated with intravascular volume depletion. In patients with cirrhotic ascites, this parameter would be expected to reflect the avidity of the kidney for Na^+. Knauf et al. (128) found the FE_{Na} useful in predicting the potential failure of diuretic therapy, as patients with a FE_{Na} <0.2% were ultimately found to be unresponsive to any combination of diuretics. Urinary electrolytes, therefore, provide the clinician with important information regarding the patient's medical management and should be obtained as part of the initial evaluation.

INVASIVE PROCEDURES

Laparoscopy has experienced a recent renaissance in popularity. Laparoscopy is a procedure with low morbidity that has high diagnostic yields and can be of significant importance when evaluating the diagnostically difficult patient (129–131). This procedure permits visualization of the viscera and peritoneum and facilitates the obtaining of biopsies. In women, visualization of the ovaries is particularly important to rule out malignancy, although this aspect of the procedure is often neglected by nongynecologists performing laparoscopy.

Finally, Swann-Ganz catheterization can be used to cannulate the hepatic vein, and may be useful in measuring wedged and free hepatic pressures. Insel et al. (132) studied 11 patients with anasarca of unknown etiology using Swann-Ganz catheterization in precisely this manner. They found that, while all patients had evidence of pulmonary hypertension, 6 patients also had evidence of portal hypertension. Only 3 of these patients had previous clinical evidence of liver disease. Swann-Ganz catheterization of patients with ascites of unknown origin could conceivably become standard procedure, given the prevalence of both cardiac and pulmonary disease. The procedure would then include determination of hepatic vein pressures in addition to the standard ventricular and pulmonary pressures.

MEDICAL MANAGEMENT

The most common cause of ascites is alcoholic cirrhosis, followed by malignancy and heart disease. Accordingly, the bulk of this section will focus on the treatment of cirrhosis-induced ascites, although other therapies including that for malignant ascites will be reviewed. Certain nonpharmacologic treatment modalities recently have gained in popularity including paracentesis and peritoneovenous shunting, so that these options, too, will be explored.

Treatment of Cirrhotic Ascites

GENERAL

Cirrhotic ascites should be managed in a stepwise fashion. This approach commences with dietary modifications, bedrest, and proceeds to increasingly aggressive diuretic interventions. Dietary modifications can work (133), but often fail if the clinician does not recognize the degree to which sodium restriction must be implemented, or because the relatively well patient with preserved appetite rejects the draconian restrictions necessary to achieve Na^+ balance. The average American diet contains significantly >4 g Na^+/day (>9 g of salt), the standard hospital no-added salt diet provides 3–4 g Na$^+$/day, and a low salt diet contains 2 g of Na$^+$/day. (The nomenclature is so confusing that it is a wonder the correct diet is ever consumed by the patient. For the record, 1 tsp salt = 5 g salts; 1 g Na$^+$ = 2.2 g salt = 100 mEq Na$^+$; and 1 mEq Na$^+$ = 1 mmole Na$^+$, the latter being the unit of choice when using the Système International [SI]. Because most clinicians and dietitians discuss diets in terms of g of Na$^+$, we have chosen to use this particular unit of measure.) The patient with resistant ascites might lose <500 mg Na$^+$/day, meaning that any quantity provided in excess of this amount will be retained (134). In this instance, the oft-prescribed 2-g Na$^+$ diet is destined to fail the patient, even one receiving concomitant diuretic therapy. Instead, the administration of a 250–500 mg Na$^+$ diet will be necessary to restore sodium balance to a neutral state. The healthy individual, however, will reject such an unpalatable diet; whereas hospitalized patients with hepatic dysfunction commonly suffer loss of taste or may be so ill that they are unable to maintain a normal intake, regardless of the Na$^+$ content of the diet. Paradoxically, low-sodium diets can adversely effect the cirrhotic patient once the ascites has resolved. Simon et al. (135) compared patients on regular diets to those on diets containing 1 g of Na$^+$/day. The Na$^+$-restricted patients with cirrhosis and no ascites showed significant increases in plasma norepinephrine levels as compared to similar patients eating a regular diet. These elevated norepinephrine levels resulted in significant decreases in mean arterial pressure with clinically evident hypotension.

Recent investigations suggest that nutritional support is of considerable benefit to hospitalized patients with alcoholic liver disease. Early studies comparing patients with alcoholic hepatitis having low Na$^+$ diets to those who were administered high calorie and protein supplements did not demonstrate any difference in 30-day mortality between the two groups (136). Placement of a nasogastric feeding tube, however, ensures that adequate nutrients are delivered to these notoriously

anorectic patients. Cabre et al. (137) were able to decrease in-hospital 30-day mortality by 74% in patients with alcoholic hepatitis by using nasogastric tubes to deliver at least 2000 calories per patient per day. Unfortunately, these tube-fed patients failed to show any resolution of ascites, a not surprising fact since the formula used contained excessive amounts of Na$^+$ (1 g Na$^+$/day). Kearns et al. (138) monitored physical and biochemical parameters in patients with alcoholic hepatitis who were receiving tube feeding. This diet also contained excessive Na$^+$ (2 g of Na$^+$/day) so that their ascites similarly did not decrease; however, significant improvement in hepatic reserve was seen only in the group of patients receiving enteral nutritional support. Because aggressive nutritional support appears to benefit the patient with alcoholic liver disease, future studies should attempt to restrict Na$^+$ intake to 250–500 mg/day in order to determine whether the ascites also can be ameliorated with total enteral nutrition.

Bedrest is often prescribed for ascites mobilization because it increases GFR and decreases the proximal tubular reabsorption of Na$^+$ (139). The effect of posture in optimizing ascites mobilization was systematically evaluated by Karnad et al. (140), who found that the best position consisted of a 10° leg elevation and a 10° head-down tilt. This position improves urine output and creatinine clearance, and increases total urinary Na$^+$ compared with the sitting and supine positions. Unfortunately, the supine position, particularly when supplemented with tilting, cannot be maintained indefinitely. These positional maneuvers, however, should be kept in mind for the patient resistant to standard pharmacologic therapies. Otherwise, bedrest only predisposes the patient to decubiti, and should not be routinely employed in the management of ascites.

DIURETIC THERAPY

Early subscription to the underfill theory of ascites production resulted in preferential use of aldosterone antagonists, especially *spironolactone*. Activation of aldosterone receptors by its agonist increases distal renal tubular reabsorption of Na^+ and Cl (141). Increased K^+ excretion also occurs, because aldosterone increases K^+ uptake by cells lining the distal nephron from the peritubular fluid; an electrochemical gradient then facilitates the diffusion of K^+ into the collecting duct (141). Spironolactone increases Na^+ excretion by up to 2% of the filtered Na^+ load (142), a lesser amount than is observed with loop diuretics such as *furosemide*. However, 50% of patients receiving furosemide fail to mobilize their ascites (142), whereas spironolactone is effective in most cirrhotics without pre-existing renal failure (143).

Loop and thiazide diuretics act in the proximal nephron, whereas aldosterone exerts its effect more distally. A possible explanation for the failure of proximally acting agents could be that any Na^+ escaping their action is subsequently taken up in the distal nephron because of increased aldosterone concentrations (144). This increased Na^+ reabsorption in the distal nephron would alter Na^+ gradients within the loop of Henle, and would thereby decrease the effectiveness of the proximally acting diuretics. This theory is substantiated by the finding that, in contrast to responders, most patients who are not helped by loop diuretics have higher plasma aldosterone (142). Conversely, nonresponders to spironolactone have lower pretreatment urinary Na^+ concentrations (126) and manifest markedly enhanced rates of proximal tubular Na^+ reabsorption (126, 128). Although nonresponders have higher plasma aldosterone levels than do responders (128, 142), the failure of spironolactone in these patients suggests that there are other factors independent of the RAA system activation that are involved in the observed severe Na^+ retention. This refractoriness to spironolactone therapy also indicates that additional diuretic agents are necessary for many patients with ascites.

Loop diuretics, particularly furosemide, can adversely affect renal function in patients with ascites. Daskalopoulos et al. (145) demonstrate that renal clearance of para-aminohippurate, a marker of renal blood flow, is decreased immediately after furosemide administration to cirrhotic patients with ascites, but not when it is given to cirrhotic patients without ascites. This effect on blood flow may be mediated by thromboxane A_2, a potent vasoconstrictor that reduces renal blood flow, and which is directly increased by furosemide (146). Consequently, loop diuretics must be administered with caution to patients with ascites.

Combination diuretic therapy has been studied in only a few trials. Perez-Ayoso et al. (143) studied patients with preserved renal function and found that responsiveness to spironolactone alone was similar to that with combination therapy with furosemide. Sarin et al. (147) also studied nonazotemic patients who were treated with spironolactone, the loop diuretic *bumetanide*, or a combination of these two agents. Diuretic response was as rapid in patients receiving bumetanide alone as it was in patients receiving combination therapy, although fewer electrolyte abnormalities occurred in the combination therapy group. In contradistinction, Fogel et al. (148) evaluated combination therapy in patients with varying degrees of renal insufficiency. Furosemide, spironolactone, or combination therapy initially were equally effective, but over time, an increasing number of patients failed to respond to spironolactone monotherapy. These latter patients required increasing doses of furosemide to ensure adequate diuresis. In this study, patients with prestudy evidence of renal insufficiency required as much as 400 mg/day of spironolactone and 1600 mg/day of furosemide, and severe electrolyte disturbances were common (148). These studies suggest that patients with preserved renal function can be treated with spironolactone monotherapy, whereas patients with pre-existing renal insufficiency will require combination therapy with a loop diuretic. Unfortunately, the latter group will likely require increasing doses of both agents in order to maintain their diuresis, and diuretic therapy will eventually fail this group. Given the potency of loop diuretics, their initial dosage should be low. The starting dose of furosemide, for example, should not exceed 10–20 mg/day. Management thereafter should be guided by urine Na^+ concentrations, with the dose of furosemide needing to be increased if spot values are <20 mEq/l. Once furosemide dosage rises significantly above 100 mg/day, however, severe renal drug resistance is evident (126), and eventual failure of diuretic management is certain.

The success of diuretic therapy in decreasing ascites is limited by the fact that the peritoneal lining absorbs <1000 ml/day, and can approach as little as 100 ml/day (144). Should urine output exceed peritoneal reabsorption, therefore, the result would be azotemia. Unfortunately, this complication affects approximately 25% of cirrhotics who receive diuretics (149). Diuretic-induced azotemia generally is reversible, but in 20% of instances, the cirrhotic patient will either develop the hepatorenal syndrome or will suffer adversely from diuretic therapy (3). Electrolyte imbalances similarly occur with great frequency, although their effect on the patient depends on the implicated electrolyte. For example, chronic hyponatremia frequently complicates the management of the patient with cirrhotic ascites, but usually does not alter the patient's clinical situation. Indeed, some authorities counsel against sodium restriction unless the serum Na^+ level drops to <120 mEq/l or encephalopathy ensues (82). Alterations in serum K^+ concentration can be more serious, with hyper- or hypokalemia commonly complicating spironolactone and furosemide therapy, respectively. Fortunately these shifts in serum K^+ can be minimized by using combination diuretic therapy.

Metabolic acidosis commonly occurs with diuretic therapy because these agents alter transcellular electrochemical gradients, which in time impairs [H^+] secretion into the tubular space (150). Injudicious diuretic therapy may also induce hepatic encephalopathy. The mechanism is not clear, although it has been believed to be related to increased serum ammonia concentrations. The kidneys are a rich source of NH_3, and elevated levels have been detected within the renal veins of cirrhotic patients receiving diuretics (151). The increase in renal NH_3 production may be drug-specific and avoidable by selecting specific pharmaceutical agents. As measured by urine output, creatinine, and serum renin activities, the new loop diuretic *torasemide*, has been shown to influence renal function with potency equal to that of furosemide (152). However, increases in serum NH_3 are significantly less after torasemide than after furosemide administration (152). Spironolactone therapy also may lead to complications, a consequence of its generalized antiandrogenic activity. Spironolactone usage has been associated with gynecomastia, impotence, and decreased libido (141). A new aldosterone inhibitor, *canrenoate*, has been compared with spironolactone as therapy for cirrhotic ascites. This newer agent is as effective in promoting diuresis and naturesis as spironolactone, but has significantly less antiandrogenic activity (153).

Overall, only 7% of patients will fail diuretic therapy (154), so that this is the sole therapeutic approach necessary for most patients with cirrhosis and ascites. Diuretic therapy can result in significant electrolyte imbalance and intravascular depletion, necessitating frequent clinic visits and appropriate serum biochemical determinations. Since therapy of the ascites is largely for cosmetic and comfort purposes—diuretic therapy will not prolong life expectancy—overly aggressive treatment needs to be avoided. If carefully managed, medical treatment should not by itself be reason for reducing the lifespan of the cirrhotic patient.

NONDIURETIC MEDICAL THERAPY

Although diuretics remain the mainstay of pharmacological therapy for cirrhotic ascites, a variety of other agents are being investigated (Table 23.3). *Atrial natriuretic peptide* is one such agent. As previously discussed, this peptide has been observed to be insufficiently elevated in cirrhotic patients as compared with patients with heart or kidney failure, but its concentration rises dramatically with placement of a portal-venous shunt (32–34). Studies using normal human volunteers have dem-

Table 23.3
Therapies for Alcohol-Related Ascites[a]

| | Pharmaceutical | | |
	Oral	Parenteral	Nonpharmaceutical
Accepted	Spironolactone Canrenoate Furosemide Bumetanide	Furosemide	PVS Paracentesis
Investigational	Torasemide Misoprostol Ibopramine Captopril Clonidine	Fenoldopam Ornipressin Naloxone Somatostatin Clonidine	TIPS
Without benefit	ANP TxA_2 antagonists Saralasin	Dopamine	

[a]Pharmaceuticals listed under investigational are of potential benefit for reabsorbing ascites, but differ widely in their possible therapeutic benefit. ANP, atrial naturetic peptide, PVS, peritoneovenous shunt, TIPS, transjugular intrahepatic portosystemic shunt, TxA_2 = thromboxane A_2.

onstrated that the infusion of recombinant human ANP (hANP) induces diuresis, naturesis, and vasodilation while simultaneously inhibiting aldosterone secretion (155). In cirrhotic patients, however, hANP had no such effect when delivered by single injection (156), and promotes naturesis in only 45% of patients when administered by continuous infusion (157, 158). Some investigators speculate that this absence of response to continuous hANP is secondary to ANP-induced hypotension, and reflects these patients' depleted intravascular volume. However, it is unlikely that volume status alone accounts for the failure of hANP to promote diuresis. Gines et al. (158) corrected the low mean arterial pressure in nonresponders by concomitantly administering norepinephrine; this maneuver failed to reverse the lack of renal response to ANP. Many cirrhotic patients also express decreased numbers of glomeruli ANP receptors (28), possibly because prolonged exposure to high ANP levels results in receptor down-regulation. Finally, animal studies suggest that even if the problem of altered ANP receptor density could be overcome, long-term administration of this peptide will still likely fail. Withrington et al. (159) demonstrate that in dogs, ANP has equal potency to isoproteranol in increasing hepatic arterial flow. This alteration in hepatic hemodynamics favors trans-sinusoidal fluid exchange, and results in an expanded extravascular space (159). Chronically administered ANP thus would be expected to encourage ascites formation.

Alterations in prostanoid concentrations within the kidney, including decreased levels of the vasodilator PgE_1 and increased levels of the vasoconstrictor thromboxane A_2 (TxA_2), have led to strategies using agonists and antagonists of these compounds. *Misoprostol*, a synthetic PgE_1 analog currently used in the treatment and prevention of NSAID-induced gastric ulceration, has been used in a limited fashion for the treatment of the hepatorenal syndrome. Fevery et al. (160) studied four consecutive patients in whom the hepatorenal syndrome developed while they were hospitalized for problems other than those related to their alcoholic cirrhosis. All patients produced <400 ml/day of urine, had a urinary Na^+ of <10 mEq/l, and did not respond to volume expansion using saline and albumin infusion. Administration of 400 µg of misoprostol four times a day (orally) increased the mean urine output from 328 ml/day to 1529 ml/day. Diuresis was pronounced, and was observed within 24 hours of drug administration. Naturesis was less dramatic, possibly reflecting the profound serum hyponatremia extant prior to therapy. Misoprostol also has been evaluated in cirrhotic patients with preserved renal function and who had been given the NSAID indomethacin (161). Misoprostol attenuated the fall in urinary Na^+ when given together with indomethacin, suggesting a possible role for this prostaglandin analog in patients with cirrhosis and ascites who absolutely require NSAID therapy.

The use of *TxA₂ antagonists* has been less successful. Zipser et al. (162) administered dazoxiben to patients with the hepatorenal syndrome. Although they observed significantly decreased production of TxA_2, there was no increase in diuresis or naturesis. Gentilli et al. (163) used another TxA_2 inhibitor, OKY-046, in nonazotemic cirrhotic patients. Again this resulted in decreased TxA_2 production—and GFR increased by approximately 20%—but without any observable effect on Na^+ or water balance. These findings support the contention that Na^+ retention in cirrhotic patients is not due to alterations in filtered load (10). Other TxA_2 antagonists are not likely, therefore, to be of clinical benefit to the patient.

Dopamine receptors have long been known to be present in the renal arteries, and to be involved in renal Na^+ processing (164). Indeed, a variety of clinical disorders associated with Na^+ retention have been associated with aberrant renal dopamine regulation, including essential hypertension (165) and chronic renal failure (166). Early attempts at pharmacologic management of patients with the hepatorenal syndrome included dopamine administration (167, 168). Aside from being ineffective in these studies, the value of dopamine is severely limited by the fact that until recently it has been available only as an intravenous preparation requiring continuous infusion. *Ibopramine* is an oral dopamine nonspecific agonist that has been subjected to comparative study with intravenous dopamine in cirrhotic patients both with and without renal insufficiency (169). In patients able to excrete more than 20 mmol/day of Na^+, ibopramine clearly

increases GFR, decreases serum aldosterone levels, and improves diuresis and naturesis (169). This effect is not observed in patients with evidence of severe Na^+ retention. Two dopamine receptor types have been isolated, namely, postsynaptic DA_1 receptors that mediate renal vasodilation, and presynaptic DA_2 receptors that inhibit sympathetic discharges and norepinephrine release. *Fenoldopam*, an experimental DA_1 selective agonist currently available in intravenous form, has been studied in patients with severe Na^+ retention (170). This agent, unfortunately, like dopamine and ibopramine before it, is not successful in patients who have severe Na^+ retention. Perhaps a role will exist for an oral fenoldopam cogener in patients without evidence of severe Na^+ retention.

Because patients with cirrhosis and related renal failure have both a decrease in systemic vascular resistance and an increase in renal vascular resistance, vasoconstrictor therapy has only a limited role (171). However, the use of vasopressor substances that are selective for the splanchnic vascular bed, such as 8-ornithin vasopressin (*ornipressin*) can induce a significant improvement in naturesis and diuresis. Lenz et al. (172) studied 11 patients with decompensated cirrhosis and deteriorating renal function. Patients who were given ornipressin had a dramatic improvement in naturesis (increased 259%) and in fractional excretion of sodium (FE_{Na} increased 130%). Ornipressin increased systemic vascular resistance while simultaneously increasing renal blood flow. Although the complete pharmacology of ornipressin is not known, it appears that this agent does not interact with the vasopressin V_1 or V_2 receptors located within the kidney (48).

Management of the patient with severe renal Na^+ retention remains an ongoing challenge. Several pharmaceutical agents, available for the treatment of unrelated disorders, are currently being evaluated for the treatment of patients with HRS. *Naloxone*, a nonspecific opioid partial antagonist, has been successfully used to increase diuresis and naturesis. Leehey et al. (173) evaluated the effect of intravenous continuous naloxone administration in alcoholic cirrhotics and in healthy volunteers. Naloxone increased diuresis by 50% and naturesis by 100% in cirrhotic patients as compared with control subjects, without adversely affecting mean arterial pressure or heart rate. These investigators postulate that naloxone exerts its effect by increasing GFR as well as by decreasing distal tubular Na^+ reabsorption (173). A new long-acting analog of *somatostatin*, SMS 201-995, has been evaluated in patients with decompensated cirrhosis and oliguria (174). Although this agent also requires intravenous administration, significant increases in creatinine clearance and in urine output have been observed, persisting for as long as 24 hours after drug delivery. Unfortunately, SMS 201-995 did not increase naturesis. Whether other commercially available somatostatin analog, such as octreotide, will also benefit the patient with HRS, remains to be determined.

The well-recognized process of activation of the RAA system in cirrhotic ascites has made this a natural target for pharmacologic manipulation. Original reports using standard doses of angiotensin-converting enzyme inhibitors such as *captopril* resulted in severe systemic hypotension and decreased urine output (175, 176). Brunkhorst et al. (177) used low-dose captopril (6.25 mg every 6 hours) in 14 cirrhotic patients who had become refractory to other diuretic therapy. Although mean arterial pressure still decreased with low-dose captopril, no patient suffered clinically significant hypotension. Therapy increased naturesis, diuresis, and weight loss in all patients; discontinuation of drug caused urinary Na^+ levels to decrease to pretreatment levels within 3 days (177). Unfortunately, this study was limited to patients with high plasma aldosterone concentrations, so it is not clear whether low-dose captopril therapy is of similar benefit for patients with normal or minimally elevated renin concentrations. Use of the angiotensin II antagonist saralasin, however, did not result in clinical improvement (178). This potent agent results in decreased renal function, which may be

secondary to marked hypotension induced by this drug.

Sympathetic nervous system activation is well-appreciated in alcoholic cirrhosis (11), but the clinical consequences of this activation are unclear. Esler et al. (179) administered intravenous *clonidine*, a centrally acting α_1 agonist, to patients with biopsy-proven cirrhosis and to normal volunteers. These investigators demonstrated that the hepatomesenteric circulation was more sensitive to clonidine than was the systemic circulation. Cirrhotic patients treated with clonidine manifested decreased renal vascular resistance but increased their GFR; decreased portal pressures were also observed. Albillos et al. (180) provided cirrhotic patients with oral clonidine, but were unable to demonstrate a consistent decrease in portal pressures. Unfortunately, neither study addressed ascites reabsorption per se. However, if future investigators are able to consistently increase GFR and decrease portal pressure using oral clonidine, this agent could become a mainstay in the pharmacologic therapy of cirrhotic ascites.

In the final analysis, the best long-term therapy for alcohol-related ascites is abstinence. In a unique study, Capone et al. (181) observed patients with decompensated cirrhosis and ascites who survived for >2 months after their initial hospitalization. Of these patients, 11 resumed drinking and 5 died of hepatic causes within 10 months; all 11 patients had recurrence of their ascites. In contradistinction, 7 patients completely avoided alcohol; all were alive 33 months later, and all had total resolution of their ascites. The beneficial effect of alcohol avoidance is confirmed in a 20-year prospective study of cirrhotic patients. Saunders et al. (182) show that no method of therapy other than abstinence effects long-term patient survival, with 5-year survival rates being twice as high in patients refraining from alcohol as in patients continuing to drink.

NONMEDICAL THERAPY

Peritoneovenous Shunts (PVS). Although the PVS was originally limited to patients with intractable ascites, an ever-expanding list of conditions have been treated with this device, including recurrent ascites, ascites with intractable hydrothorax, and pancreatic, malignant, and chylous ascites (183). Six prospective randomized trials have been performed on patients with alcoholic cirrhosis comparing PVS to medical therapy (184–190). All but one (189) used the LeVeen shunt, and all but one (184) failed to demonstrate any difference in survival between patients receiving PVS and patients receiving standard diuretic therapy. Wapnick et al. (184) claimed that patients undergoing PVS placement lived 3 weeks longer than medically treated patients. Although the difference between the two groups was statistically significant, the extent of the gain in longevity was actually trivial. In all the studies, there was a rapid resolution of ascites, and an overall decrease in subsequent hospitalizations required for ascites management. An analysis of all published studies on PVS demonstrates that these devices are associated with an 18% perioperative mortality, and result in significantly improved diuresis in only 59%. Overall, shunt failure complicates 19% of all placements, and in single series is reported to occur in as many as 50–75% of recipients (183, 189, 191).

Because of these conflicting data, a large Veterans Administration (VA) cooperative trial was initiated to compare PVS with medical therapy. A total of 299 men with alcoholic ascites and severe or recurrent ascites were assigned randomly to either PVS or diuretic therapy (190). The patients were stratified into three groups: group 1 had normal or mildly abnormal liver dysfunction; group 2 had more severe liver dysfunction or a history of previous complications; and group 3 had severe prerenal azotemia without evidence of kidney disease. In comparison to medically treated patients, PVS prolonged the time to recurrence of ascites by 12 months in group 1 and by 9 months in group 2. Similarly, initial hospitalization was significantly longer in medically treated patients (6.1 weeks) than in surgically treated patients (2.4 weeks). Group 3 was too small to permit significant conclu-

sions. Overall, however, there was no difference in patient survival in either treatment group. Survival depended solely on the degree of liver dysfunction prior to study enrollment, with a median survival of 1093 days for patients in group 1, 222 days for patients in group 2, and 37 days for patients in group 3.

Transjugular Intrahepatic Portosystemic Shunts (TIPS). Invasive radiologists are now able to produce the same mechanical bypass around the high resistance liver by percutaneously placing expandable metallic stents directly through the liver. To date, the bulk of TIPS have been inserted to decrease portal pressure and as primary therapy for esophageal varices (193, 194). Although this device has not been specifically evaluated for the therapy of ascites, ascites reabsorption has nonetheless been an unexpected benefit of TIPS placement. However, this therapy remains in the initial stage of evaluation, and it is premature to comment as to the future usefulness of TIPS placement for patients with ascites.

Paracentesis. Over the past few years, large volume paracentesis has become an accepted therapy for cirrhotic ascites. Gines et al. (195) have shown that large volume paracentesis, arbitrarily defined as the removal of 5 liters of ascites, is well-tolerated and is faster in ameliorating ascites than standard diuretic therapy. In patients with evidence of peripheral edema, these taps are safe, whereas in patients without edema, plasma expanders need to be concurrently administered to prevent intravascular depletion (196). Indeed, by providing intravenous albumin, Tito et al. (197) have successfully and safely performed total paracentesis, removing an average of 10 l of ascites. Intravenous albumin, however, is expensive, and as a blood product, it is obtained from paid donors. The Barcelona group, therefore, compared Dextran-70 with albumin in patients undergoing total paracentesis (198). Although neither plasma expander was associated with adverse changes in renal function, the use of Dextran-70 resulted in increased plasma renin and aldosterone concentrations (198). Whether these changes, reflecting depleted intravascular volume, are of clinical significance has yet to be determined. If not, Dextran-70 may well replace albumin as the plasma expander of first choice.

The surprising results of the VA cooperative trial that compared PVS to diuretic therapy (190) prompted the Barcelona group to compare the PVS with large-volume paracentesis (199). In this prospective, randomized study, 89 patients with refractory ascites underwent repeated large volume paracentesis or PVS placement (199). Patients undergoing paracentesis had total elimination of their ascites, and were hospitalized for a shorter period of time than were PVS patients (11 ± 5 days versus 19 ± 9 days). Although the paracentesis group required significantly more subsequent hospitalizations, total hospital time did not differ between the two groups. Not surprisingly, survival time poststudy entry was similar for both treatment groups.

Treatment of Malignant Ascites

MEDICAL THERAPY

Ovarian cancer is the major cause of malignant ascites, although any malignant process metastatic to the peritoneum can result in increased peritoneal fluid formation. Malignant ascites can be massive, and result in significant dyspnea, anorexia, and indigestion. Diuretic therapy can be of value for some patients with malignant ascites. Greenway et al. (200) treated patients with ascites due to a variety of tumors, who were no longer responsive to systemic chemotherapy, with *spironolactone* and bedrest. Fully one-half of such patients responded to spironolactone therapy, and relief was maintained for an average of 4 months. In general, diuretics are used as adjunctive therapy, since patient responsiveness is difficult to predict, and since monotherapy is not as effective as intraperitoneal chemotherapy for palliating malignant ascites (Table 23.4).

Intraperitoneal chemotherapy, using agents specific for the tumor or using sclerosing agents, has become a common approach to palliating malignant ascites. Because of the toxicity of these drugs and the high frequency of ascites loculation, it is essential that free communication of fluid throughout the peri-

Table 23.4
Potential Therapies for Malignant Ascites[a]

Oral	Spironolactone
Intraperitoneal	Calcium-calmodulin inhibitors
	Nicardipine
	Chemotherapeutic agents
	Cis-platinum
	Cytosine arabinoside
	5-FU
	Adriamycin
	Cytokines
	Interleukine-2
	Interferon
	Tumor necrosis factor-α
	Immunomodulation
	C. parvum
	OK-432
	Monoclonal antibodies
	DAL-D29
	Photodynamic therapy
	Sclerosing agents
	Bleomycin
Mechanical	Paracentesis
	Tenckhoff catheter
	PVS (except for ovarian cancer)
	Denver shunt

[a]PVS, peritoneovenous shunt; 5-FU, 5-fluorouracil.

toneum be documented prior to instituting therapy. This can be done by introducing a small amount of ^{99}Tc into the peritoneum via the drainage catheter, followed by imaging to demonstrate uniform distribution (201). The best chemotherapeutic results seem to be obtained by draining the peritoneum of malignant fluid, instilling the drug(s) of choice into a large volume of fluid (i.e., 2 l), and draining the peritoneal cavity after 15–30 minutes (202). This approach permits retreatment, as well as avoids complications associated with high systemic concentrations of drug (202).

Not all chemotherapeutic agents undergo significant peritoneal absorption, so that limited time exposure to a drug is not always necessary. Kirmani et al. (203) evaluated prolonged intraperitoneal infusion of *cytosine arabinoside* (Ara-C) in a phase I study. Fourteen patients with a variety of tumors refractory to standard therapy were given continuous intraperitoneal Ara-C for as long as 3 weeks; 40 mg/M² was the highest dose tolerated by all patients without side effects. Higher doses resulted in a chemical peritonitis, as well as in sufficient systemic absorption to cause myelosupression (203). Other drugs including *cisplatin, 5-fluorouracil* and *adriamycin* also have been used to palliate malignant ascites (204, 205), but no controlled studies have been performed evaluating these agents. *Bleomycin*, however, has been more rigorously investigated and appears to have great promise for the therapy of malignant ascites. Bleomycin is a sclerosing agent that is frequently used to palliate patients with pleural effusions resistant to other agents. In patients with a variety of intra-abdominal tumors refractory to standard chemotherapy, bleomycin achieved a 50% prolonged response rate and was associated with few side effects (206). This may become the intraperitoneal chemotherapeutic agent of choice as a palliative for patients with malignant ascites.

Resistance to traditional chemotherapeutic agents commonly limits the usefulness of these agents. Calmodulin is a calcium-binding regulatory protein that has been shown to be increased during periods of cell growth. Consequently, great interest exists in being able to inhibit calmodulin activity in malignant cells. In an animal model, intraperitoneal administration of the calcium channel blocker *nicardipine* potentiates the effect of adriamycin in Ehrlich ascites tumor cells (207). Direct inhibitors of calmodulin, including *calmidazolium, naphthalenesulfonamide* (W-7), and *trifluoperazine* similarly inhibit protein synthesis in Ehrlich ascites tumor cells (208). It is unclear, however, whether these agents act by inhibiting all aspects of calmodulin's growth regulatory effects or whether these agents specifically inhibit the *p*-glycoprotein multidrug resistance gene product. These agents may subsequently play an adjunctive role in intraperitoneal chemotherapy.

Increasing the efficacy of standard chemotherapeutic agents also can be attempted by using *monoclonal antibodies*. Antibodies targeted against various tumor cell-specific antigens can be generated, and then linked to a lipid vesicle that acts as a vehicle for the appropriate drug. This approach has been employed in preliminary animal studies using DAL-K29, a monoclonal antibody specific to renal carcinoma cells, which is linked to vesicles containing methotrexate (209, 210). This approach permits higher local concentrations of methotrexate directed at the malignant cell itself, and can actually result in tumor resolution; renal cell carcinoma has previously been considered refractory to standard intraperitoneal chemotherapy.

Malignant cells within the peritoneal cavity synthesize a variety of autologous growth factors and cytokines (211). Those growth factors present within the ascitic fluid support the growth of existing cells, but also increase the resistance of malignant cells to chemotherapy. *Intraperitoneal immunostimulation* has been used to alter abdominal cavity cytokine concentrations in order to enhance malignant cell drug sensitivities. *Corynebacterium parvum* was the first of the agents to be used in ascites-directed immunostimulation therapy. Although the mechanism for its action remains unclear, tumor regression has been observed with its usage (212). Unfortunately numerous side effects are associated with intraperitoneal *Corynebacterium* therapy, including abdominal pain, nausea, vomiting, and fever. A purified streptococcal preparation, OK-432, has been used in the treatment of peritoneal malignancies. This agent has been shown to activate complement, to increase polymorphonuclear leukocyte migration into the peritoneal cavity (213), and to increase endogenous synthesis of interleukins and of tumor necrosis factor (TNF)-α (214, 215). Pure preparations of these latter cytokines, generated using recombinant DNA technology, also have been given directly to the patient with malignant ascites. *Interleukin-2* has been administered together with lymphokine-activated killer (LAK) cells to patients with ovarian carcinoma (216). Although the frequency of side effects of this therapy were high (including nausea, vomiting, anorexia, and anemia), a decrease in ascites was achieved (216). Similarly, *TNF-α* was used in patients with a variety of malignancies and intractable ascites (217). In contrast to interleukin-based therapy, no dose-limiting toxicities were observed. Furthermore, 55% of this diverse group of patients had complete, and 21% had partial resolution of their malignant ascites (217). Clearly, cytokines are not all the same, and future cytokine-directed therapy will require a determination of the optimal agent for each ascites-producing tumor.

Many tumor types appear to respond to *interferons* (218). In one study of 24 patients with advanced ovarian cancer otherwise resistant to therapy, 9 patients were able to withstand the fever, fatigue, and leukopenia of intraperitoneal α-interferon (219). Of these 9 patients, 4 had ascites, and marked reduction in ascites volume was recorded in 3 patients. Bezwoda et al. (220) specifically evaluated the usefulness of α-interferon in patients with less bulky tumor mass. These investigators found that the greatest reduction in ascites occurs in patients given α-interferon with the smallest tumor burden. Growth suppression of tumor cells explanted onto agar plates correlates well with the magnitude of subsequent reductions in ascites volume, suggesting that this test may be useful in deciding whether or not to use this particular form of intraperitoneal therapy. Interferon therapy, however, will not replace intraperitoneal chemotherapy, but will likely be used concomitantly with other chemotherapeutic agents. Bezwoda et al. (221) further demonstrate that the clinical response to interferon therapy is due to tumor cell growth inhibition and is not due to a direct cytotoxic effect. Indeed, significantly improved responses are observed in patients treated with interferon and cisplatin as compared with those treated with interferon alone (221).

Finally, intraoperative *photodynamic therapy* can palliate malignant ascites, and may well supplant other intraperitoneal chemotherapy-based techniques. Using phototherapy, patients receive dihematoporphyrin ethers intravenously 48–72 hours prior to laparotomy (222). After tumor debulking, 630-nm red light from an argon dye laser is delivered to the entire peritoneal lining. In preliminary studies, 75% of patients so treated remained disease- and ascites-free for as many as 18 months after therapy (222). Routine use of intraoperative photodynamic therapy may reduce the subsequent incidence of malignant ascites.

NONMEDICAL THERAPY

Paracentesis. Although paracentesis can occasionally result in permanent resolution of the problem of malignant ascites (201), repeated paracentesis is often necessary. Adhesions due to previous abdominal surgery or due to the tumor itself can make paracentesis-related bowel perforation a significant risk of the procedure (201). Permanent peritoneal access can be achieved by placing a Tenckhoff catheter that permits frequent drainage (223). Unfortunately, fluid loculation is common in malignant ascites, and repeated Tenckhoff catheter placements may be necessary (201). Often, the use of Tenckhoff catheters is reserved for delivery of intraperitoneal chemotherapy.

Peritoneovenous Shunts. Short-term improvement in palliating malignant ascites can be achieved by PVS placement, while long-term palliation is significantly more difficult to attain because of shunt malfunction. In the largest series designed to evaluate PVS for malignant ascites, there was a mean shunt survival time of approximately 2 months (224), with an observed 20% of patients surviving to 6 months (225). Shunt type appears to predict future patency. Oosterlee (226) compared LeVeen shunts to Denver shunts in 20 patients with malignant ascites. Thirty percent of the LeVeen shunts failed whereas there was no malfunction with Denver shunts (226), suggesting that Denver shunts should be used for palliating malignant ascites. Ovarian cancer is the most frequent cause of malignant ascites, and PVS may be contraindicated in this group of patients. Several reports identify fatal pulmonary artery tumor embolization in patients with ovarian cancer shortly after shunt placement (227, 228).

Other Disorders

Although the role of steroids is more restricted than previously, steroid therapy still plays a role in specific disease states. *Chronic lupus peritonitis* can be difficult to treat with diuretic therapy alone, but appears to respond to high-dose pulse steroid administration (229). Evidence suggests that an excellent response can be observed when methylprednisone (1 g/M² weekly, times four doses) is administered to lupus patients with otherwise intractable ascites (230). Parasitic infections of the liver, such as can be due to *schistosomiasis*, result in ascites formation as a consequence of the secondary inflammatory response mounted against the organism. A large study by el-Zayadi et al. (231) compared short-term prednisone therapy to diuretic therapy in patients with schistosomal liver disease and resistant ascites. This randomized prospective trial demonstrates that patients receiving steroids and diuretics (n = 18) dramatically increase their diuresis and naturesis as compared to patients treated with diuretics alone (n = 19).

Chylous ascites is usually refractory to conservative therapy. This disorder can complicate abdominal surgery with significant subsequent patient morbidity and even mortality if not aggressively treated. Recent studies suggest that PVS is the best approach for patients with chylous ascites, and that excellent long-term survival can be expected (92, 93, 232).

The treatment of *pancreatic ascites* is traditionally considered to be surgical, but recent insights into the pathogenesis of this disorder encourage a pharmacologically based approach. Recent reports of the use of the somatostatin analog, octreotide, are encouraging, although anecdotal in nature (233, 234). Its supposed mechanism of action is to decrease exocrine gland secretions. Since phospholipase A_2 appears to play a major role in pancreatic ascites (90), we await further studies using PLA_2-inhibitors as primary therapy for this surprisingly common disorder.

CONCLUSIONS

Cirrhosis secondary to alcohol abuse is the most common cause of ascites in the United States. Therapy will not alter patient prognosis, and is pursued largely for reasons of cosmetic concern and comfort. Diuretic therapy is usually successful and, along with Na^+ restriction, is the first line of approach in ascites therapy. Severe or intractable ascites also can be successfully treated using large-volume paracentesis or by placing a peritoneovenous shunt; the data do not suggest that one therapy is superior to the other. Finally, many newer pharmacologic agents are being evaluated that may be of benefit in managing cirrhotic ascites.

Malignancy is the second most common cause of ascites. A variety of agents and devices have been evaluated, but none alter patient prognosis. Intraperitoneal chemotherapy appears successful for patient palliation, and the patient may benefit from the additional infusion of various immunomodulatory agents. Paracentesis, PVS, and permanent peritoneal drainage catheters are less effective than in cirrhotic ascites, largely because of fluid loculation and the propensity for catheter occlusion.

Finally, other clinical conditions resulting in ascites can respond to specific pharmacologic therapies. This underscores the importance of accurately diagnosing the cause of the ascites. Future pharmacologic advances will depend on a thorough understanding of the underlying pathophysiology specific to each condition resulting in ascites.

REFERENCES

1. Conn HO. A rational approach to the hepatorenal syndrome. Gastroenterology 1973;65:321–340.
2. Stanley MM, Ochi S, Lee KK, et al. The Veterans Administration co-operative study on treatment of alcoholic cirrhosis with ascites: peritovenous shunting as compared with medical treatment in patients with alcoholic cirrhosis and massive ascites. N Engl J Med 1989;321:1632–1638.
3. Trey C, Trey G. Complications of cirrhosis: ascites and hepatic encephalopathy. Curr Opin Gastroenterol 1990;6:365–369.
4. LaVilla G, Arroyo V. Pathophysiology and treatment of ascites in cirrhosis. Trop Gastroenterol 1990;11:56–75.

5. Benoit J, Granger DN. Splanchnic hemodynamics in chronic portal hypertension. Semin Liver Dis 1986;6:287–298.

6. Kontos HA, Shapiro W, Mauck HP, et al. General and regional circulatory alterations in cirrhosis of the liver. Am J Med 1964;37:526–535.

7. Bosch J, Arroyo V, Rodes J. Hepatic and systemic hemodynamics and the renin-angiotensin-aldosterone system in cirrhosis. In: Epstein M, ed. The kidney in liver disease. New York: Elsevier Biomedical, 1983:353–376.

8. Henriksen JH, Ring-Larsen H, Christensen NJ. Circulating noradrenaline and central hemodynamics in patients with cirrhosis. Scand J Gastroenterol 1985;20:1185–1190.

9. Epstein M, Levinson R, Sancho J, et al. Characterization of the renin-aldosterone system in decompensated cirrhosis. Circ Res 1977;41:818–829.

10. Epstein M. The renin-angiotensin system in liver disease. In: Epstein M, ed. The kidney in liver disease. New York: Elsevier Biomedical, 1983:353–376.

11. Floras JS, Legault L, Morali GA, et al. Increased sympathetic outflow in cirrhosis and ascites: direct evidence from intraneural recordings. Ann Intern Med 1991;114:373–380.

12. Caramelo C, Schrier RW. A critical update on the pathogenesis of ascites and renal failure in cirrhosis. In: Rodes J, ed. Pathophysiology of ascites and functional liver failure. Barcelona: Salvat Editores, 1987:47–58.

13. Vorobioff J, Bredfelt JE, Groszmann RJ. Increased blood flow through the portal system in cirrhotic rats. Gastroenterology 1984;87:1120–1126.

14. Reynolds TB, Hidemura R, Michel H, Peters R. Portal hypertension without cirrhosis in alcoholic liver disease. Ann Intern Med 1969;70:497–506.

15. Rector WG, Hossack KF. Splanchnic and hepatic renin metabolism in alcoholic cirrhosis: lack of evidence of a splanchnic source of production or of significantly impaired hepatic clearance. J Hepatol 1988;7:93–97.

16. Bernadini M, Trevisani F, Santini C, et al. Aldosterone related blood volume expansion in cirrhosis before and during the early phase of ascites formation. Gut 1983;24:761–766.

17. Bichet D, Szatalowkz V, Chaimaavitz C, et al. Role of vasopressin in abnormal water excretion in cirrhotic patients. Ann Intern Med 1982;96:413–417.

18. Marson FGW. Total adrenalectomy in hepatic cirrhosis with ascites. Lancet 1954;2:847–848.

19. Wilkinson SP, Jowett TP, Slater JDH, et al. Renal sodium retention in cirrhosis: relation to aldosterone and nephron site. Clin Sci 1979;56:169–177.

20. Wilkinson SP, Smith IK, Williams R. Changes in plasma renin activity in cirrhosis: a reappraisal based on studies in 67 patients with "low renin" cirrhosis. Hypertension 1979;1:521–524.

21. Arroyo V, Bosch J, Mauri M, et al. Renin, aldosterone and renal haemodynamics in cirrhosis with ascites. Eur J Clin Invest 1979;9:69–73.

22. Solomon R, Azar P, Trebbin W, et al. The kallikrein-kininogen-kinin system in patients with liver disease and ascites. Nephron 1988;50:39–44.

23. Hasegawa M, Yamada S, Hirayama C. Fasting plasma caffeine levels in cirrhotic patients: relation to plasma levels of catacholamines and renin activity. Hepatology 1989;10:973–977.

24. Linas SL, Anderson RJ, Guggenhein SJ, et al. Role of vasopressin in impaired water excretion in conscious rats with experimental cirrhosis. Kidney Int 1981;20:173–180.

25. Elias AN, Vaziri ND, Domurat ES, et al. Atrial natriuretic peptide, arginine vasopressin, aldosterone and plasma renin activity in carbon tetrachloride-induced cirrhosis in rats. J Pharmacol Exp Ther 1990;252:438–441.

26. Warner LC, Campbell PJ, Morali GA, et al. The response of atrial natriuretic factor and sodium excretion to dietary sodium challenges in patients with chronic liver disease. Hepatology 1990;12:460–466.

27. La Villa G, Asbert M, Jimenez W, et al. Natriuretic hormone activity in the urine of cirrhotic patients. Hepatology 1990;12:467–475.

28. Gerbes AL, Kollenda MC, Vollmar AM, et al. Altered density of glomerular binding sites for atrial natriuretic factor in bile duct-ligated rates with ascites. Hepatology 1991;13:562–566.

29. Leiberman FL, Denison EK, Reynolds TB. The relationship of plasma volume, portal hypertension, ascites and renal sodium retention in cirrhosis. The overflow theory of ascites formation. Ann NY Acad Sci 1970;170:202–212.

30. Claria J, Jimenez W, Arroyo V, et al. Blockade of the hydroosmotic effect of vasopressin normalizes water excretion in cirrhotic rats. Gastroenterology 1989;97:1294–1299.

31. Shapiro MD, Nicholls KM, Groves BM, et al. Interrelationship between cardiac output and vascular resistance as determinants of effective arterial blood volume in cirrhotic patients. Kidney Int 1985;28:206–211.

32. Nozuki M, Mouri T, Itoi K, et al. Plasma concentrations of atrial natriuretic peptide in various diseases. Tokohu J Exp Med 1986;148:439–447.

33. Campbell P, Skorecki K, Logan A, et al. Acute effect of peritoneovenous shunting on plasma atrial natriuretic peptide in cirrhotic patients with massive refractory ascites. Am J Med 1988;84:112–119.

34. Klepetko W, Muller CH, Harter E, et al. Plasma atrial natriuretic factor in cirrhotic patients with ascites. Gastroenterology 1988;95:764–770.

35. Witte CL, Witte MH. The portocardiorenal axis and refractory ascites: the underfilled cup runneth over. Hepatology 1989;10:114–119.

36. Gentile S, Angelico M, Chiappini MG, et al. Clinical and hormonal conditions associated with so-

dium retention in cirrhotic patients with ascites: evaluation by univariate and multivariate analyses. Dig Dis Sci 1987;32:569–576.

37. Levy M. Sodium retention and ascites formation in dogs with experimental portal cirrhosis. Am J Physiol 1977;233:F572–F585.

38. Levy M, Allotery JBK. Temporal relationship between urinary salt retention and altered systemic hemodynamics in dogs with experimental cirrhosis. J Lab Clin Med 1978;92:560–569.

39. Unikowski B, Wexler MJ, Levy M. Dogs with experimental cirrhosis of the liver but without intrahepatic hypertension do not retain sodium or form ascites. J Clin Invest 1983;72:1594–1604.

40. Lieberman FL, Ito S, Reynolds TB. Effective plasma volume in cirrhosis with ascites: evidence that a decreased volume does not account for renal sodium retention, a spontaneous reduction in glomerular filtration rate (GFR), and a fall in GFR during drug-induced diuresis. J Clin Invest 1969;48:975–981.

41. Lieberman FL, Reynolds TB. Plasma volume in cirrhosis of the liver: its relation to portal hypertension, ascites, and renal failure. J Clin Invest 1967;46:1297–1308.

42. Lebrec D, Kotelanski B, Cohn JN. Splanchnic hemodynamic factors in cirrhosis with refractory ascites. J Lab Clin Med 1979;93:301–309.

43. Schrier RW, Arroyo V, Bernardi M, et al. Peripheral arterial vasodilation hypothesis: a proposal for the initiation of renal sodium and water retention in cirrhosis. Hepatology 1988;8:1151–1157.

44. Albillos A, Colombato LA, Groszmann RJ. Vasodilation and sodium retention in prehepatic portal hypertension. Gastroenterology 1992;102:931–935.

45. Wilkinson SP, Moore KP, Arroyo V. Pathogenesis of ascites and hepatorenal syndrome. Gut 1991;37(suppl):S12–S17.

46. Epstein M. Derangements of renal water handling in liver disease. Gastroenterology 1985;89:1415–1425.

47. Bichet D, Van Putten VJ, Schrier RW. Potential role of increased sympathetic activity in impaired sodium and water excretion in cirrhosis. N Engl J Med 1982;307:1552–1557.

48. Kinter LB, Huffman WF, Stassen FL. Antagonists of the antidiuretic activity of vasopressin. Am J Physiol 1988;254:F165–F177.

49. Rimola A, Gines P, Arroyo V, et al. Urinary excretion of 6-keto-prostaglandin F_{1alpha}, thromboxane B_2 and prostaglandin E_2 in cirrhosis with ascites: relationship to functional renal failure (hepatorenal syndrome). J Hepatol 1986;3:111–117.

50. Rolando N, Harvey F, Brahm J, et al. Prospective study of bacterial infection in acute liver failure: an analysis of 50 patients. Hepatology 1990;11:49–53.

51. Moore KP, Ward P, Taylor GW, et al. Urinary excretion of systemic and renal metabolites of prostacyclin and thromboxane in decompensated liver disease and hepatorenal syndrome. Gastroenterology 1991;100:1069–1077.

52. Epstein M. The hepatorenal syndrome. Hosp Pract 1989;24:65–76.

53. Arroyo V, Gines P. Prostaglandins and the treatment of hepatorenal syndrome in cirrhosis. J Hepatol 1990;11:142–144.

54. Boyer TD, Zia P, Reynolds TB. Effects of indomethacin and prostaglandin Al in renal function and plasma renin activity in alcoholic liver disease. Gastroenterology 1979;77:215–222.

55. Limas CJ, Guiha NH, Lekagul O, et al. Impaired left ventricular function in alcoholic cirrhosis with ascites: ineffectiveness of ouabain. Circulation 1974;49:754–760.

56. Anderson SH. Thiamine deficiency as a cause of hepatorenal syndrome. Lancet 1984;2:644.

57. Vaamonde CA. Thiamine deficiency and hepatorenal syndrome. Nephron 1988;49:261–263.

58. Mauch PM, Ultmann JE. Treatment of malignant ascites. In: De Vita VT, Hollman S, Rosenberg SA, eds. Cancer: principles and practice of oncology. New York: Lippincott, 1988:2150–2153.

59. Feldman GB, Knapp RO, Order SE, et al. The role of lymphatic obstruction in the formation of ascites in a murine ovarian carcinoma model. Cancer Res 1972;32:1663–1666.

60. Feldman GB, Knapp RC. Lymphatic drainage of the peritoneal cavity and its significance in ovarian cancer. Am J Obstet Gynecol 1974;119:991–994.

61. Pockros PJ, Woods. Malignant ascites from peritoneal carcinomatosis is immobile in comparison to cirrhotic ascites. Hepatology 1988;8:1450.

62. Garrison RN, Galloway R, Heuser LS. Mechanisms of malignant ascites production. J Surg Res 1987;42:126–132.

63. Hirabayshi KI, Graham J. Genesis of ascites in ovarian carcinoma. Am J Obstet Gynecol 1970;109:492–497.

64. Scholmerich J, Zimmermann U, Kottgen E, et al. Proteases and antiproteases related to the coagulation system in plasma and ascites: an approach to differentiate between malignant and cirrhotic ascites. Klin Wochenschr 1987;65:634–638.

65. Maeda H, Matsumura Y, Kato H. Purification and identification of [hydroxyprolyl³] bradykinin in ascitic fluid from a patient with gastric cancer. J Biol Chem 1988;263:16051–16054.

66. Watt FM. Cell culture models of differentiation. Fed Am Sci Exp Biol J 1991;5:287–294.

67. White MJ, Miller FN, Heuser LS, et al. Human malignant ascites and histamine-induced protein leakage from the normal microcirculation. Microvasc Res 1988;35:63–72.

68. Heuser LS, Miller FN, Gilley-Pietsch C. Protein leak from normal vasculature due to human malignant ascites. Am J Surg 1988;155:765–769.

69. Kemeny N, Seiter K, Martin D, et al. A new syndrome: ascites, hyperbilirubinemia, and hypoalbu-

minemia after biochemical modulation of fluorouracil with N-phosphonacetyl-l-aspartate (PALA). Ann Intern Med 1991;115:946–951.

70. Bender MD. Diseases of the peritoneum, mesentary, and diaphragm. In: Sleisenger MH, Fordtran JS, eds. Gastrointestinal disease. 4th ed. Philadelphia: Saunders, 1989:1932–1967.

71. Granger DM, Miller T, Allen R, Parker RE, Parker JC, Taylor AE. Permselectivity of cat liver blood-lymph barrier to endogenous macromolecules. Gastroenterology 1979;77:103–109.

72. Levy M. Pathophysiology of ascites formation. In: Epstein M, ed. The kidney in liver disease, ed 3. Baltimore: Williams & Wilkins, 1988:209–243.

73. Runyon BA. Cardiac ascites: a characterization. J Clin Gastroenterol 1988;10:410–412.

74. Fowler NO. Constrictive pericarditis. In: Fowler NO, ed. The pericardium in health and disease. New York: Futura, 1985:304–305.

75. Berner C, Fred HL, Riggs S, Davis JS. Diagnostic probabilities in patients with conspicuous ascites. Arch Intern Med 1964;113:687–690.

76. Lefkowitch JH, Mendez L. Morphologic features of hepatic injury in cardiac disease and shock. J Hepatol 1986;2:313–327.

77. Mitchell MC, Boitmott JK, Kaufman S, et al. Budd-Chiari syndrome: aetiology, diagnosis and management. Medicine 1982;61:199–218.

78. McDermott WV, Ridker PM. The Budd-Chiari syndrome and hepatic veno-occlusive disease: recognition and treatment. Arch Surg 1990;125:525–527.

79. Hidayst MA, Wanid HA. A study of the vascular changes in bilharzic hepatic fibrosis and their significance. Surg Gynecol Obstet 1971;132:997–1004.

80. Kirsch R, Frith L, Black E, Hoffenberg R. Regulation of albumin synthesis and catabolism by alterations of dietary protein. Nature 1968;217:578–579.

81. Rothschild MA, Oratz M, Schreiber SS. Albumin synthesis. N Engl J Med 1972;286:748–757.

82. Runyon BA. Cirrhotic ascites: pathogenesis and treatment. AGA Postgraduate Course 14 May 1989:166–172.

83. Donowitz M, Kerstein MD, Spiro HM. Pancreatic ascites. Medicine 1974;53:183–195.

84. Sankaran S, Walt AJ. The natural and unnatural history of pancreatic pseudocysts. Br J Surg 1975;62:37–44.

85. Sankaran S, Walt AJ. Pancreatic ascites: recognition and management. Arch Surg 1976;111:430–434.

86. Uchiyama T, Yamamoto E, Mizuta E, et al. Pancreatic ascites: a collected review of 37 cases in Japan. Hepato-Gastroenterol 1989;36:244–249.

87. MacLaren IF. Pancreatic ascites. In: Howard JM, Jordan GL, Reber HA, eds. Surgical diseases of the pancreas. Philadelphia: Lea & Febiger, 1987:591–602.

88. Dragstedt LR, Haymond HE, Ellis JC. Pathogenesis of acute pancreatitis. Arch Surg 1934;28:233–242.

89. Zirngibl H, Mann S, Schild A, et al. Phospholipase A activities in ascites, serum, lymph, and urine in acute pancreatitis following pancreas stimulation with secretin-ceruletid. Klin Wochenschr 1989;67:141–143.

90. Svensson C, Sjodhl R, Lilja I, et al. The role of ascites and phospholipase A_2 on peritioneal permeability changes in acute experimental pancreatitis. Int J Pancreatol 1990;6:71–79.

91. Williams RA, Vetto J, Quinones-Baldrich W, Bongard FS, Wilson SE. Chylous ascites following abdominal aortic surgery. Ann Vasc Surg 1991;5:247–252.

92. Heyl A, Veen HF. Iatrogenic chylous ascites: operative or conservative approach. Netherlands J Surg 1989;41:5–7.

93. Press OW, Press NO, Kaufman SD. Evaluation and management of chylous ascites. Ann Intern Med 1982;96:358–364.

94. Goldfarb JP. Chylous effusions secondary to pancreatitis: case report and a review of the literature. Am J Gastroenterol 1984;79:13–135.

95. Hurley MK, Emilani VJ, Comer GM, et al. Dilated cardiomyopathy associated with chylous ascites. Am J Gastroenterol 1989;84:1567–1569.

96. Tan WC. Dietary treatment of chylous ascites in yellow nail syndrome. Gut 1989;30:1622–1623.

97. Dumont AE, Mulholland JH. Alterations in thoracic duct lymph flow in hepatic cirrhosis: significance in portal hypertension. Ann Surg 1962;156:668–677.

98. Malagelada JR, Iber FL, Linscheer WG. Origin of fat in chylous ascites of patients with liver cirrhosis. Gastroenterology 1974;67:878–886.

99. Kinney EL, Wright RJ, Caldwell JW. Value of clinical features for distinguishing myxedema ascites from other forms of ascites. Comput Biol Med 1989;19:55–59.

100. Cattau EL, Benjamin SB, Knuff TE, et al. The accuracy of the physical examination in the diagnosis of suspected ascites. JAMA 1972;247:1164–1166.

101. Cummings S, Papadakis M, Melnick J, et al. The predictive value of physical examinations for ascites. West J Med 1985;142:633–636.

102. Simel DL, Halvorsen RA, Feussner JR. Quantitating bedside diagnosis: clinical evaluation of ascites. J Gen Int Med 1988;3:423–428.

103. Jason JD, Weissbein AS. The puddle sign: an aid in the diagnosis of minimal ascites. N Engl J Med 1959;260:652–654.

104. Rosenberg BB, Goodman GA, Clearfield HR. Evaluation of ascites by ultrasound. Radiology 1970;96:15–22.

105. McLean ACL. Diagnosis of ascites by auscultatory percussion and hand-held ultrasound unit. Lancet 1987;2:1526–1527.

106. Runyon BA. Paracentesis of ascitic fluid, a safe procedure. Arch Intern Med 1986;146:2259–2261.
107. Sampliner RE, Iber FL. High protein ascites in patients with uncomplicated hepatic cirrhosis. Am J Med Sci 1974;267:275–279.
108. Pare P, Talbot J, Hoefs TC. Serum-ascites albumin concentration gradient: a physiologic approach to the differential diagnosis of ascites. Gastroenterology 1983;85:240–244.
109. Hoefs TC. Serum protein concentration and protal pressure determine the ascitic fluid protein concentration in patients with chronic liver disease. J Lab Clin Med 1983;102:260–273.
110. Rector WG. An improved diagnostic approach to ascites. Arch Intern Med 1987;147:215.
111. Runyon BA, Hoefs JC, Morgan TR. Ascitic fluid analysis in malignancy-related ascites. Hepatology 1988;8:1104–1109.
112. Mauer K, Manzione N. Usefulness of serum-ascites albumin difference in separating transudative from exudative ascites: another look. Dig Dis Sci 1988;33:1208–1213.
113. Marshall JB, Vogele KA. Serum-ascites albumin difference in tuberculous peritonitis. Am J Gastroenterol 1988;83:1259–1261.
114. Hoefs JC. Diagnostic paracentesis: a potent clinical tool. Gastroenterology 1990;98:230–236.
115. Kajani MA, Yoo YK, Alexander JA, et al. Serum-ascites albumin gradients in nonalcoholic liver disease. Dig Dis Sci 1990;35:33–37.
116. Albillos A, Cuervas-Mons C, Millan I, et al. Ascitic fluid polymorphonuclear cell count and serum to ascites albumin gradient in the diagnosis of bacterial peritonitis. Gastroenterology 1990;98:134–140.
117. Prieto M, Gomea-Lechon MJ, Melchor H, et al. Diagnosis of malignant ascites: comparison of ascitic fibronectin, cholesterol, and serum-ascites albumin difference. Dig Dis Sci 1988;33:833–838.
118. Salerno F, Restelli B, Incerti P, et al. Utility of ascitic fluid analysis in patients with malignancy related ascites. Scand J Gastroenterol 1990;25:251–256.
119. Colli A, Buccino G, Cocciolo M, Parravini R, et al. Diagnostic accuracy of sialic acid in the diagnosis of malignant ascites. Cancer 1989;63:912–916.
120. Manobar A, Simjee AE, Haffejee AA, Pettengell KE. Symptoms and investigative findings in 145 patients with tuberculous peritonitis diagnosed by peritoneoscopy and biopsy over a five-year period. Gut 1990;31:1130–1132.
121. Dwivedi M, Misra SP, Misra V, Kumar G. Value of adenosine deaminase estimation in the diagnosis of tuberculous ascites. Am J Gastroenterol 1990;85:1123–1125.
122. Llach J, Gines P, Arroyo C, et al. Prognostic value of arterial pressure, endogenous vasoactive systems, and renal function in cirrhotic patients admitted to the hospital for the treatment of ascites. Gastroenterology 1988;94:482–487.
123. Bergmann JF, Bidart JM, George M, et al. Elevation of CA 125 in patients with benign and malignant ascites. Cancer 1987;59:213–217.
124. Aguilar-Reina J, Rey-Romero C, Ortega-Vinas M, et al. Cancer antigen 125 levels in serum can predict the recurrence of ascites in patients with cirrhosis of the liver. Hepato-Gastroenterol 1990;37(suppl 2):163–165.
125. Eggert RC. Spironolactone diuresis in patients with cirrhosis and ascites. Br Med J 1970;4:401–403.
126. Gatta A, Angeli P, Caregaro L, Menon F, Sacerdoti D, Merkel C. A pathophysiological interpretation of unresponsiveness to spironolactone in a stepped-care approach to the diuretic treatment of ascites in nonazotemic cirrhotic patients. Hepatology 1991;14:231–236.
127. Bourgeois N, Devares S, Adler M, Cremer M. Use of diuretics in the treatment of ascites in patients with cirrhosis. Acta Gastroenterol Belg 1990;53:256–260.
128. Knauf H, Wenk T, Scholmerich J, et al. Prediction of diuretic mobilization of cirrhotic ascites by pretreatment fractional sodium excretion. Klin Wochenschr 1990;68:545–551.
129. Mauk PM, Schwartz JT, Lowe JE, et al. Diagnosis and course of nephrogenic ascites. Arch Intern Med 1988;148:1577–1579.
130. Sackier JM, Berci G, Paz-Partlow M. Elective diagnostic laparoscopy. Am J Surg 1991;161:326–331.
131. Hoefs JC and Jonas GM. Diagnostic paracentesis. Adv Intern Med 1992;37:391–409.
132. Insel JM, Mookherjee S, Smulyan H, Warner RA. Use of hepatic vein catheterization in the evaluation of patients with anasarca. Am J Med Sci 1990;299:245–249.
133. Pecikyan R, Kanzank G, Berger EY. Electrolyte excretion during the spontaneous recovery from the ascitic phase of cirrhosis of the liver. Am J Med 1967;42:359–367.
134. Shear L. Ascites in cirrhosis: a medical or surgical problem? Hepatology 1990;11:323–325.
135. Simon MA, Diez J, Prieto J. Abnormal sympathetic and renal response to sodium restriction in compensated cirrhosis. Gastroenterology 1991;101:1354–1360.
136. Mendenhall C, Bongrovanni G, Goldberg S, et al. VA cooperative study on alcoholic hepatitis III: changes in protein-calorie malnutrition associated with 30 days of hospitalization with and without enteral nutrition therapy. JPEN 1985;9:590–596.
137. Cabre E, Gonzales-Huix F, Abad-Lacruz A, et al. Effect of total enteral nutrition on the short-term outcome of severely malnourished cirrhotics: a randomized, controlled trial. Gastroenterology 1990;98:725–720.
138. Kearns PJ, Young H, Garcia G, et al. Accelerated improvement of alcoholic liver disease with enteral nutrition. Gastroenterology 1991;102:200–205.

139. Bernardi M, Santini C, Trevisani F, et al. Renal function impairment induced by change in posture in patients with cirrhosis and ascites. Gut 1985;26:629–635.

140. Karnad DR, Tembulkar P, Abraham P, Desai N. Head-down tilt as a physiological diuretic in normal controls and in patients with fluid-retaining states. Lancet 1987;2:525–527.

141. Gilman AG, Goodman LS, Gilman A. The pharmacologic basis of therapeutics. ed. 6. New York: Macmillan, 1980:907–908.

142. Suki WN, Stinebaugh BJ, Frommer JP, Eknoyan G. Physiology of diuretic action. In: Seldin DW, Giebisch G, eds. The kidney: physiology and pathophysiology. New York: Raven Press, 1985.

143. Perez-Ayuso RM, Arroyo V, Planas R, et al. Randomized comparative study of efficacy of furosemide versus spironolactone in nonazotemic cirrhosis with ascites. Gastroenterology 1984;84:961–968.

144. Arroyo V, Gines P, Planas R, Panes J, Rodes J. Management of patients with cirrhosis and ascites. Semin Liv Dis 1986;6:353–369.

145. Daskalopoulos G, Laffi G, Morgan T, et al. Immediate effects of furosemide on renal hemodynamics in chronic liver disease with ascites. Gastroenterology 1987;92:1859–1862.

146. Pinzani M, Laffi G, Meacci E, La Villa G, Cominelli F, Gentilini P. Intrarenal thromboxane A2 generation reduces the furosemide-induced sodium and water diuresis in cirrhotics with ascites. Gastroenterology 1988;95:1081–1087.

147. Sarin SK, Sachdev G, Mishra SP, et al. Bumetanide, spironolactone and a combination of the two, in the treatment of ascites due to liver disease: a prospective, controlled, randomized trial. Digestion 1988;41:101–107.

148. Fogel MR, Sawhney VK, Neal EA, et al. Diuresis in the ascitic patient: a randomized controlled trial of three regimens. J Clin Gastroenterol 1981; 3(suppl 1):73–80.

149. Rodes J, Bosch J, Arroyo V. Clinical types and drug therapy of renal impairment in cirrhosis. Postgrad Med J 1975;55:492–497.

150. Hulter HN, Bonner EL, Glynn RD, Sebastian A. Renal and systemic acid-base effects of chronic spironolactone administration. Am J Physiol 1981; 240:F381–F387.

151. Baertl JM, Sancetta SM, Gabuzda GJ. Relation of acute potassium depletion to renal ammonium metabolism in patients with cirrhosis. J Clin Invest 1963;42:696–707.

152. Laffi G, Marra F, Buzzelli G, et al. Comparison of the effects of torasemide and furosemide in nonazotemic cirrhotic patients with ascites: a randomized, double-blind study. Hepatology 1991; 13:1101–1105.

153. Andriulli A, Attigoni A, Gindro T, et al. Canrenone and androgen receptor-active materials in plasma of cirrhotic patients during long-term K-canrenoate of

154. spironolactone therapy. Digestion 1989;44:155–162.

154. Nemchausky B, Stanley M, Juler G, et al. Ascites responds to short-term medical treatment in 59% of alcoholic cirrhotics, is intractable in 7%; remainder are critically ill. VA cooperative study: surgical peritoneovenous shunt versus medical treatment of ascites [Abstract]. Gastroenterology 1983;84:1387.

155. Cody RJ, Atlas SA, Laragh JH, et al. Atrial natriuretic factor in normal subjects and heart failure patients: plasma levels and renal, hormonal, and hemodynamic responses to peptide infusion. J Clin Invest 1986;78:1362–1374.

156. Laffi G, Marra F, Pinzani M, et al. Effects of repeated atrial natriuretic peptide bolus injections in cirrhotic patients with refractory ascites. Liver 1989;9:315–321.

157. Laffi G, Pinzani M, Meacci E, et al. Renal hemodynamic and natriuretic effects of human atrial natriuretic factor infusions in cirrhosis with ascites. Gastroenterology 1989;96:167–177.

158. Gines P, Tito L, Arroyo V, et al. Renal insensitivity to atrial naturetic peptide in patients with cirrhosis and ascites. Gastroenterology 1992;102:280–286.

159. Withrington PG, Dhume VG, Croxton R, Gerbes AL. The actions of human atrial natriuretic factor on hepatic arterial and portal vascular beds of the anaesthetized dog. Br J Pharmacol 1990;94:810–814.

160. Fevery J, Van Cutsem E, Nevens F, Van Steenbergen W, 1Verberckmoes R, De Groote J. Reversal of hepatorenal syndrome in four patients by peroral misoprostol (prostaglandin E$_1$ analogue) and albumin administration. J Hepatol 1990;11:153–158.

161. Antillon M, Cominelli F, Lo S, et al. Effects of oral prostaglandins on indomethacin-induced renal failure in patients with cirrhosis and ascites. J Rheumatol 1990;17(suppl 20):46–49.

162. Zipser RD, Krongerg IJ, Rector W, Reynolds T, Dakalopoulos G. Therapeutic trial of thromboxane synthesis inhibition in the hepatorenal syndrome. Gastroenterology 1984;87:1228–1232.

163. Gentilli P, Laffi G, Meacci E, et al. Effects of OKY 046, a thromboxane-synthase inhibitor, on renal function in nonazotemic cirrhotic patients with ascites. Gastroenterology 1988;94:1470–1477.

164. Oates NS, Ball SG, Perkins CM, Lee MR. Plasma and urine dopamine in man given sodium chloride in the diet. Clin Sci 1979;56:261–264.

165. Harvey JN, Casson IF, Clayden AD, et al. A paradoxical fall in urine dopamine output when patients with essential hypertension are given added dietary dalt. Clin Sci 1984;67:83–88.

166. Casson IF, Lee MR, Brown-John AM, et al. Failure of renal dopamine response to salt loading in chronic renal disease. Br Med J 1983;286:503–506.

167. Bernardo DE, Baldus WP, Maher FT. Effects of dopamine on renal function in patients with cirrhosis. Gastroenterology 1970;58:524–531.

168. Bennet WM, Deefe E, Melnick C, et al. Response to dopamine hydrochloride in the hepatorenal syndrome. Arch Intern Med 1975;135:964–971.

169. Salerno F, Incerti P, Badalamenti S, et al. Renal and humoral effects of ibopamine, a dopamine agonist, in patients with liver cirrhosis. Arch Intern Med 1990;150:65–69.

170. Hadengue A, Moreau R, Bacq Y, Gaudin C, Braillon A, LeBrec D. Selective dopamine DA_1 stimulation with fenoldopam in cirrhotic patients with ascites: a systemic, splanchnic and renal hemodynamic study. Hepatology 1991;13:111–116.

171. Epstein M. Treatment of refractory ascites. N Engl J Med 1989;321:1675–1677.

172. Lenz K, Hortnagl H, Druml W, et al. Ornipressin in the treatment of functional renal failure in decompensated liver cirrhosis. Gastroenterology 1991;101:1060–1067.

173. Leehey DJ, Gollapudi P, Deakin A, Reid RW. Naloxone increases water and electrolyte excretion after water loading in patients with cirrhosis and ascites. J Lab Clin Med 1991;118:484–491.

174. Mountokalakis T, Kallivretakis N, Mayopoulou-Symvoulidou D, Karvountzis G, Tolis G. Enhancement of renal function by long-acting somatostatin analogue in patients with decompensated cirrhosis. Nephrol Dial Transpl 1988;3:604–607.

175. Pariente EA, Bataille L, Bercoffe, Lebrec D. Acute effects of captopril on systemic and renal hemodynamics and on renal function in cirrhotic patients with ascites. Gastroenterology 1985;88:1255–1259.

176. Schlienger JL, Imbs JG, Chabrier G, Doffeil M, Imler M. Traitement de l'acite cirrhotique. Absence d'effet favorable du captopril. Nouv Presse Med 1982;11:1570–1573.

177. Brunkhorst R, Wrenger E, Kuhn K, Schmidt FW, Foch K. Effect of captopril therapy on sodium and water excretion in patients with liver cirrhosis and ascites. Klin Wochenschr 1989;67:774–783.

178. Schroeder ET, Anderson GH, Goldman SH, Streeten DHP. Effect of angiotensin II (AII) blockade with 1-Sar-8-Ala-AII (saralasin) in patients with cirrhosis and ascites. Kidney Int 1976;9:511–519.

179. Esler M, Dudley F, Jennings G, et al. Increased sympathetic nervous system activity and the effects of its inhibition with clonidine in alcoholic cirrhosis. Ann Intern Med 1992;116:446–455.

180. Albillos A, Banares R, Barrios C, et al. Oral administration of clonidine in patients with alcoholic cirrhosis: hemodynamic and liver function effects. Gastroenterology 1992;102:248–254.

181. Capone RR, Buhac I, Kohberger RC, et al. Resistant ascites in alcoholic liver cirrhosis: course and prognosis. Dig Dis 1978;23:267–271.

182. Saunders JB, Walters JRF, Davies P, et al. A 20-year prospective study of cirrhosis. Br Med J 1981;282:263–266.

183. Muskovitz M. The peritoneovenous shunt: expectations and reality. Am J Gastroenterol 1990;85:917–929.

184. Wapnick S, Grosber SJ, Evans MI. Randomized prospective matched pair study comparing peritoneovenous shunt and conventional therapy in massive ascites. Br J Surg 1979;66:667–670.

185. Linas SL, Schaefer JW, Moore EE, et al. Peritoneovenous shunt in the management of the hepatorenal syndrome. Kidney Int 1986;30:736–740.

186. Bories P, Compean G, Michel H, et al. The treatment of refractory ascites by the LeVeen shunt; a multi-centre controlled trial (57 patients). J Hepatol 1986;3:212–218.

187. Stanley MM. Peritoneovenous shunting vs medical treatment of alcoholic cirrhotic ascites [Abstract]. Hepatology 1985;5:980.

188. Stanley MM. Randomized clinical trials of treatment of ascites in alcoholic cirrhotics: medical treatment versus peritoneovenous shunting. ASAIO Trans 1989;35:174–176.

189. Ring-Larsen H, Siemssen O, Krintel JJ, et al. Denver shunt in the treatment of refractory ascites in cirrhosis: a randomized controlled trial [Abstract]. Gastroenterology 1989;96:A649.

190. Stanley MM, Ochi S, Lee KK, et al. Peritoneovenous shunting as compared with medical treatment in patients with alcoholic cirrhosis and massive ascites. Veterans Administration cooperative study on treatment of alcoholic cirrhosis with ascites. N Engl J Med 1989;321:1675–1677.

191. Bernhoft RA, Pellegrini CA, Way LW. Peritoneovenous shunt for refractory ascites: operative complications and long-term results. Arch Surg 1982;117:631–635.

192. Gleysteen JJ, Klamer TW. Peritoneovenous shunts: predictive factors of early treatment failure. Am J Gastroenterol 1984;79:654–658.

193. Richter GM, Noeldge G, Roessle M, et al. Transjugular intrahepatic portosystemic stent shunt (TIPSS). Radiology 1990;174:1027–1030.

194. Ring EJ, Lake JR, Roberts JP. Using transjugular intrahepatic portosystemic shunts to control variceal bleeding before liver transplantation. Ann Int Med 1992;116:304–309.

195. Gines P, Arroyo V, Quintero E, et al. Comparison between paracentesis and diuretics in the treatment of cirrhotics with tense ascites. Gastroenterology 1987;93:234–241.

196. Gines P, Tito LL, Arroyo V, et al. Randomized comparative study of therapeutic paracentesis with and without intravenous albumin in cirrhosis. Gastroenterology 1988;94:1493–1502.

197. Tito LL, Gines P, Arroyo V, et al. Total paracentesis associated with intravenous albumin in the management of patients with cirrhosis and ascites. Gastroenterology 1990;98:146–151.

198. Planas R, Gines P, Arroyo V, et al. Dextran-70 versus albumin as plasma expanders in cirrhotic patients with tense ascites treated with total paracentesis. Gastroenterology 1990;99:1736–1744.

199. Gines P, Arroyo V, Vargas V, et al. Paracentesis with intravenous infusion of albumin as compared with peritoneovenous shunting in cirrhosis with refractory ascites. N Engl J Med 1991;325:829–835.

200. Greenway B, Johnson PJ, Williams R. The control of malignant ascites with spironolactone. Br J Surg 1982;69:441–442.

201. Hird V, Thomas H, Stewart JSW, Epenetos AA. Malignant ascites: review of the literature, and an update on monoclonal antibody-targeted therapy. Eur J Obstetr Reprod Biol 1989;32:37–45.

202. Jones RB, Collins JM, Myers CE, et al. High volume intraperitoneal chemotherapy with methotrexate in patients with cancer. Cancer Res 1981;41:55–59.

203. Kirmani S, Zimm S, Cleary SM, Mowry J, Howell SB. Extremely prolonged continuous intraperitoneal infusion of cytosine arabinoside. Cancer Chemother Pharmacol 1990;25:454–458.

204. Markman M. Intraperitoneal chemotherapy as treatment of ovarian cancer: why, how and when? Obstet Gynecol Surg 1987;42:533–539.

205. Lind SE, Cashavelly B, Fuller AF. Resolution of malignant ascites after intraperitoneal chemotherapy in women with carcinoma of the ovary. Surg Gynecol Obstet 1988;166:519–522.

206. Ostrowski MJ. An assessment of the long-term results of controlling the reaccumulation of malignant effusions using intracavitary bleomycin. Cancer 1986;57:721–727.

207. Matsuoka H, Sugimachi K, Kuwano H, Yano K. Intratumoural injection of calcium channel blocker enhances cytotoxicity of adriamycin in Ehrlich ascites solid tumour. Eur J Surg Oncol 1989;15:224–231.

208. Kumar RV, Panniers R, Wolfman A, Henshaw EC. Inhibition of protein synthesis by antagonists of calmodulin in Ehrlich ascites tumor cells. Eur J Biochem 1991;195:313–319.

209. Singh M, Ghose T, Mesei M, Belitsky P. Inhibition of human renal cancer by monoclonal antibody targeted methotrexate-containing liposomes in an ascites tumor model. Cancer Lett 1991;56:97–102.

210. Singh M, Ghose T, Kralovec J, Blair AH, Belitsky P. Inhibition of human renal cancer by monoclonal-anti-body-linked methotrexate in an ascites tumor model. Cancer Immunol Immunother 1991;32:331–334.

211. Mills GB, May C, Hill M, Campbell S, Shaw P, Marks A. Ascitic fluid from human ovarian cancer patients contains growth factors necessary for intraperitoneal growth of human ovarian adenocarcinoma cells. J Clin Invest 1990;86:851–855.

212. Mantovani A, Sessa C, Peri G, et al. Intraperitoneal administration of *Corynebacterium parvum* in patients with ascitic ovarian tumors resistant to chemotherapy: effects on toxicity of tumors resistant to chemotherapy: effects on toxicity of tumor-associated macrophages and natural killer cells. Int J Cancer 1981;27:437–446.

213. Katano M and Torisu M. Inflammatory cell-mediated tumor-cell destruction. Surgery 1983;93:65–73.

214. Mori H, Itoh N, Yamada Y, Tamaya T. Induction of endogenous cytokines in ascites of patients with ovarian cancer by OK-432, a streptococcal preparation. Asia Oceania J Obstet Gynaecol 1989;15:281–289.

215. Mori H, Itoh N, Tamaya T. Mechanism of induction of endogenous tumor necrosis factor in ascites of ovarian cancer patients by OK-432, a streptococcal preparation. Immunopharmacol Immunotoxicol 1989;11:33–53.

216. Stewart JA, Belinson JL, Moore AL, et al. Phase I trial of intraperitoneal recombinant interleukin-2/lymphokine-activated killer cells in patients with ovarian cancer. Cancer Res 1990;50:6302–6310.

217. Rath U, Kaufmann M, Schmid H, et al. Effect of intraperitoneal recombinant human tumor necrosis factor alpha on malignant ascites. Eur J Cancer 1991;27:121–125.

218. Cherchi PL, Campliglio A, Rubattu A, Desole A, Andria G, Ambrosini A. Endocavitary beta-interferon in neoplastic effusions. Eur J Gynecol Oncol 1990;11:477–479.

219. Einhorn N, Ling P, Einhorn S, Strander H. A phase II study on escalating interferon doses in advanced ovarian carcinoma. Am J Clin Onc 1988;11:3–6.

220. Bezwoda WR, Seymour L, Dansey R. Intraperitoneal recombinant interferon-alpha 2b for recurrent malignant ascites due to ovarian cancer. Cancer 1989;64:1029–1033.

221. Bezwoda WR, Golombick T, Dansey R, Keeping J. Treatment of malignant ascites due to recurrent/refractory ovarian cancer: the use of interferon-alpha or interferon-alpha plus chemotherapy in vivo and in vitro. Eur J Cancer 1991;27:1423–1429.

222. Sindelar WF, DeLaney TF, Tochner Z, et al. Technique of photodynamic therapy for disseminated intraperitoneal malignant neoplasms. Phase I study. Arch Surg 1991;126:318–324.

223. Lomas DA, Wallis PJ, Stockley RA. Palliation of malignant ascites with a Tenckhoff catheter. Thorax 1989;44:828.

224. Akimaru K, Ueda Y, Shoji T. Peritoneovenous shunting for intractable cirrhosis and cancerous ascites using different types of shunting tubes. Jpn J Surg 1988;18:502–508.

225. Straus AK, Roseman DK, Shapiro TM. Peritoneovenous shunting in the management of malignant ascites. Arch Surg 1979;114:489–491.

226. Oosterlee J. Peritoneovenous shunting for ascites in cancer patients. Br J Surg 1980;67:663–666.

227. Maat B, Oosterlee J, Spaas JAJ, et al. Dissemination of tumor cells via LeVeen shunt [Letter]. Lancet 1979;1:988.

228. Berger A, Goldberg MI. Subcutaneous cancer growth complicating the peritoneovenous shunting of malignant ascites. Surgery 1983;93:374–376.

229. Ishiguro N, Tomino Y, Fujito K, Nakayama S, Koide H. A case of massive ascites due to lupus peritonitis with a dramatic response to steroid pulse therapy. Jpn J Med 1989;28:608–611.

230. Kaklamanis P, Vayopoulos G, Stamatelos G, Dadinas G, Tsokos GC. Chronic lupus peritonitis with ascites. Ann Rheum Dis 1991;50:176–177.

231. el-Zayadi A, Mohran Z, Haseeb N, Nagy N, Dabbous H. Short-term course of corticosteroids in the treatment of resistant ascites complicating schistosomal liver disease. Am J Gastroenterol 1991;86:53–56.

232. Ohri SK, Patec T, Desa LA, Spencer J. The management of postoperative chylous ascites: a case report and literature review. J Clin Gastroenterol 1990;12:693–697.

233. Gislason H, Gronbech JE, Soreide O. Pancreatic ascites: treatment by continuous somatostatin infusion. Am J Gastroenterol 1991;86:519–521.

234. Oktedalen O, Nygaard K, Osnes M. Somatostatin in the treatment of pancreatic ascites. Gastroenterology 1990;99:1520–1521.

MISCELLANEOUS TOPICS

24

The Use of Gastrointestinal Drugs in Renal Disease

WILLIAM M. BENNETT and MARY M. MEYER

The elimination of many therapeutic agents and their metabolites from the body requires adequate renal function. In addition, the kidney is more than a simple organ of waste excretion, because renal insufficiency impacts on other pharmacologic processes such as hepatic drug metabolism (1). Patients with gastrointestinal and/or hepatic disease with concomitant renal dysfunction represent a common and certainly challenging clinical subpopulation. The clinician managing these particular patients constantly walks a therapeutic tightrope in trying to achieve maximal drug efficacy while avoiding toxicity. In this chapter, basic pharmacologic principles will be examined as they apply under normal and uremic conditions. Dosage recommendations for common drugs used by the gastroenterologist including antiulcer, anticholinergic, antiemetic, antibiotic, immunosuppressive, and diuretic agents in patients with chronic renal failure will be presented in tabular form. The final section of the chapter will deal with special considerations in patients treated for renal disease that may trigger consultations with the gastroenterologist for help in management.

PHARMACOKINETICS AND DOSAGE ADJUSTMENTS IN THE PATIENT WITH RENAL INSUFFICIENCY

Drugs (and their metabolites) with elimination predominantly by renal excretion require dosage adjustments in the setting of renal insufficiency. However, dosage modification cannot simply be based on the extent of decreased renal drug excretion, because alter-

ations in other pharmacokinetic parameters, such as absorption, volume of distribution, protein binding, and metabolism also are affected in renal failure.

BIOAVAILABILITY

The amount and appearance kinetics of a drug in the central circulation compared with intravenous dosing of the drug define its bioavailability. Drugs given intravenously enter the central circulation directly and generally have a rapid onset of action. Drugs given by other routes must first traverse a series of membranes and may need to pass through important organs of elimination before entering the systemic circulation. Thus, only a fraction of the administered dose may reach the circulation and become available at the site of drug action.

Gastrointestinal absorption of drugs may decrease in patients with uremia. Gastrointestinal symptoms are common in uremia, but there is little specific information about bowel function in patients with renal failure. Salivary urea converted to ammonia by urease or by the use of alkalinizing histamine H_2-receptor antagonists may decrease the bioavailability of drugs that are best absorbed in an acidic environment (2). This effect is particularly relevant for patients receiving oral iron supplements that require conversion by gastric acid from ferrous to ferric forms for optimal absorption. The ingestion of milk, calcium supplements, or aluminum salts used as phosphate binders may also decrease drug absorption by chelation with the formation of

451

nonabsorbable complexes (3). In addition, uremic patients have decreased small bowel absorptive function (4). Uremia-induced vomiting, delayed gastric emptying, and sluggish gut motility secondary to diabetic neuropathic changes all may contribute to diminished absorption. Aluminum-containing phosphate binders can combine with various drugs to block absorption by forming insoluble compounds. Bowel wall edema, as encountered in cirrhotic patients, may also slow drug absorption.

First-pass hepatic metabolism may be altered in patients with uremia. Decreased biotransformation in the liver may lead to increased amounts of active drug in the systemic circulation with resulting enhanced bioavailability of some drugs. Conversely, impaired plasma protein binding allows more free drug to be available at the site of hepatic metabolism increasing the amount of drug removed during the first pass through the liver. The interactions of absorption and first-pass hepatic metabolism are complex. It is therefore not surprising that drug bioavailability varies more in patients with renal impairment than in patients without renal impairment.

DISTRIBUTION

After administration, a drug disperses through the body at a given rate. At equilibrium, the apparent volume of distribution is the ratio of the amount of drug in the body to its plasma concentration. This ratio does not correspond to a specific anatomic space but does provide an estimate for the initial dose of a drug needed to reach a given therapeutic plasma concentration. Highly protein-bound agents, or those that are water soluble, tend to be restricted to the extracellular fluid space and thus have small volumes of distribution. However, highly lipid-soluble drugs more easily penetrate body tissues and have large distribution volumes.

Renal insufficiency frequently alters drug distribution volume. Edema and ascites may increase the apparent volume of distribution of highly water-soluble or protein-bound drugs. Usual doses given to patients with edema can result in inadequate plasma levels. Conversely, dehydration or muscle wasting usually decreases the apparent volume of distribution of water-soluble drugs. In these cases, usual doses may result in unexpectedly high plasma concentrations.

The alteration of plasma protein binding in patients with renal insufficiency has an important effect on the volume of distribution of a drug, the quantity of free drug available for action, and the degree to which the agent can be excreted by the liver or kidneys. The binding of many acidic drugs is decreased in renal failure. However, binding of organic bases is less affected by uremia (5).

Reduced plasma protein binding in uremic patients has been attributed to a combination of decreased serum albumin concentration and reduction in drug affinity for albumin. Affinity may be influenced by either uremia-induced changes in the structural orientation of the albumin molecule or accumulation of endogenous inhibitors of protein binding that compete with drugs for their binding sites.

The therapeutic consequences of impaired plasma protein binding in uremia are important because the unbound fraction of several acidic drugs, such as salicylate and phenytoin, may be substantially increased. Serious toxicity can occur if the total plasma concentration is pushed into the "therapeutic range" by increasing the dose. For such drugs, both total and unbound plasma concentrations should be measured.

METABOLISM

Renal failure substantially affects drug biotransformation. Drugs metabolized by oxidation, conjugation, or both may be predisposed to decreased hepatic clearance in renal failure. Further, drug interactions may be important in adverse systemic effects of drugs metabolized by the liver. For example, verapamil and diltiazem inhibit cyclosporine metabolism resulting in high blood levels and decreased renal function for a given cyclosporine dose (6). The hepatic metabolism of metoclopramide is altered in patients with chronic renal failure and this must be considered in dosing for these patients (7). Intrinsic clearance by the liver of propranolol is reduced, resulting in higher bioavailability of a given oral dose in end stage renal disease patients (8). Other drugs or drug classes that have a high potential to have reduced nonrenal clearance in renal failure are lipophilic β-blockers, encainide, some calcium antagonists, captopril, nortriptyline, propoxyphene, desmethyldiazepam, zidovudine, and erythromycin (1). Drugs oxidized by the human cytochrome P-450 IID6 isozyme seem to be affected more by renal failure than other P-450 isozymes (6). Many active or toxic drug metabolites depend on renal function for elimination. The high incidence of adverse drug reactions seen in patients with renal failure may be explained in part by the accumulation of such pharmacologically active metabolites (9).

RENAL EXCRETION

Renal excretion of drugs depends on glomerular filtration as well as renal tubular secretion and reabsorption. Glomerular elimination of drugs also depends on the molecular size and protein-binding capacity of the agent. Although protein binding decreases the filtration of drugs, it may increase the amount that the renal tubule secretes. When glomerular filtration is impaired by renal disease, the clearance of drugs eliminated primarily by this mechanism is decreased, and the plasma half-life of the drug is prolonged.

Although tubular function is not routinely measured clinically, the secretion of drugs by active transport systems in the renal tubule will also be affected in patients with renal disease. As creatinine clearance decreases, drugs dependent on renal tubular secretion for elimination are excreted more slowly. Furthermore, because the proximal tubular secretion of some agents is carrier mediated and capacity limited, concurrent use of several drugs eliminated by renal tubular secretion may saturate these transport systems. For example, cimetidine competitively inhibits the tubular secretion of cations such as creatinine. Burgess et al. showed that creatinine clearance can be reduced without affecting glomerular filtra-

tion rate, the latter measured by the clearance of inulin (10). This needs to be kept in mind for patients on cimetidine so that true renal function is not underestimated based solely on a serum creatinine value. Ranitidine and other H_2 blockers do not alter measurement of renal function in this way (11).

DOSING FOR PATIENTS WITH RENAL DYSFUNCTION

A rational approach to drug dosing in patients with renal impairment begins with a thorough history and physical examination. Particularly important is the history of previous drug allergy or toxicity, the use of concurrently prescribed or nonprescription medications, and the ingestion of alcohol or other recreational drugs. Physical assessment should include an estimation of the extracellular fluid volume because the presence of edema, ascites, or dehydration alters drug dose. Body weight and height need to be measured. For obese patients, the ideal body weight should be calculated, and drug doses should be estimated accordingly. Evidence of impaired excretory organ function should be sought. Signs of chronic liver disease are a clue that the drug dose may need to be severely altered.

A specific diagnosis should be established before drug therapy is initiated. Patients with renal dysfunction receive many concurrent medications, often without specific indications; therefore medication lists should be reviewed frequently. Many adverse drug effects could be avoided if fewer agents were used and potential drug interactions recognized.

RENAL FUNCTION ASSESSMENT

When the necessity for drug therapy has been established, renal function should be measured. Because the rate of elimination of drugs excreted by the kidneys is proportional to the glomerular filtration rate, the serum creatinine or creatinine clearance can be used to estimate renal function. The equation of Cockroft and Gault (12) can be used to estimate the creatinine clearance, as shown below, if an actual measured creatinine clearance is not available.

Creatinine clearance

$$= \frac{(140 - \text{age}) \times (\text{ideal body weight in kg})}{72 \times \text{serum creatinine in mg/dl}}$$

This value should be multiplied by 0.85 for women.

Ideal body weight = 50.0 kg + 2.3 kg/inch over 5 feet tall (for men)

Ideal body weight = 45.5 kg + 2.3 kg/inch over 5 feet tall (for women)

Estimating the glomerular filtration rate from the serum creatinine level assumes that renal function is stable and that the serum creatinine measurement is constant. With changing renal function, the serum creatinine level will no longer reflect the true clearance rate; creatinine clearance should be measured with a timed urine collection using the midpoint value. If oliguria is present, the creatinine clearance should be estimated at less than 10 ml/minute for purposes of drug dosing adjustments.

The serum creatinine is a function of muscle mass as well as glomerular filtration rate. Serum creatinine measurements within the "normal" range are often erroneously used to establish the presence of "normal" renal function. Such an assumption can cause serious overdose and toxic drug accumulation in elderly or debilitated patients with diminished muscle mass.

INITIAL OR LOADING DOSE

If the physical examination suggests that the extracellular fluid volume is normal, the initial drug dose for a patient with renal failure is usually the same as that for a patient with normal renal function. However, if substantial edema or ascites is present, a larger initial dose may be necessary. Conversely, dehydrated or severely debilitated patients may require smaller initial doses. The purpose of the initial, or loading, dose is to rapidly produce a therapeutic plasma drug concentration. Subsequent doses may need to be decreased to maintain therapeutic levels below the toxic range.

When a loading dose is given, levels within the therapeutic range are rapidly achieved. If no loading dose is prescribed, three to four half-lives of the drug are needed before plasma levels reach a steady state. A loading dose should always be considered when the half-life of a drug is particularly long in a patient with renal failure or when rapid attainment of therapeutic plasma levels is critical.

MAINTENANCE DOSE

After the initial drug dose, subsequent doses may need modification in patients with diminished renal function. After measurement of renal function and determination of the drug dose for patients with normal renal function, a dose appropriate for patients with impaired renal function can be calculated.

A maintenance regimen in patients with renal failure may be determined by one of two methods. First, the dosing interval can be lengthened by the following formula:

Dosing interval

$$= \frac{\text{Normal } C_{Cr}}{\text{Patient's } C_{Cr}} \times \text{normal interval}$$

Alternatively, each individual dose can be reduced and given at standard intervals:

Reduced dose

$$= \frac{\text{Patient's } C_{Cr}}{\text{Normal } C_{Cr}} \times \text{normal dose}$$

The variable interval method can potentially lead to long periods of subtherapeutic drug levels. Conversely, reducing individual doses and keeping intervals between doses constant produces more constant drug levels but risks increased toxicity.

Guidelines for dosing drugs important to gastroenterologists in patients with impaired renal function are provided in tables following this chapter.

THERAPEUTIC DRUG MONITORING

Clinical application of pharmacokinetic principles to individualize dosage regimens defines therapeutic drug monitoring. Sensitive and specific assays for plasma drug concentrations and inexpensive computer technology are alternatives to drug dosing by trial and error. Appropriate pharmacokinetic application of drug level measurements can improve patient care at decreased cost (13).

Measurement of plasma drug concentrations may help in assessing a particular drug dosing regimen when the relationship between drug levels and efficacy or toxicity has been established. These measurements are particularly important for drugs with a narrow range between therapeutic and toxic levels and for drugs whose pharmacologic effects are not readily measured. Plasma level monitoring, however, has little value for drugs with a biologic effect that is easily measured or for which adverse reactions are not clinically serious. Most drugs that gastroenterologists use fall into this category.

ADVERSE DRUG REACTIONS

Despite increased awareness of uremia-induced changes in drug disposition, adverse drug responses remain common in patients with impaired renal function (14). Some toxicity can be eliminated by avoiding drugs known to cause adverse events as a result of direct toxicity of the drug or its metabolites, poor efficacy of the drug in patients with decreased renal function, or allowance for an increased metabolic load that diseased kidneys cannot excrete.

Knowing a drug's potential for direct renal toxicity is particularly important for patients with reduced renal function. Even a mild renal injury in a patient with diminished renal reserve can be catastrophic. Drugs may precipitate direct renal tubular toxicity, obstructive uropathy, glomerulonephritis, interstitial nephritis, or disturbances of sodium and water and acid-base balance. The accumulation of active or toxic metabolites may lead to unexpected drug reactions. Acute onset of any unexplained symptoms should alert the clinician to a possible adverse drug effect.

Patients with renal failure are heterogenous, and their responses to drug therapy are variable. Dosage nomograms, dosage tables, and computer-assisted dosing recommendations should not be used as a fixed approach, but only as an initial attempt to arrive at an effective dose regimen. In this chapter, recommendations are included for common drugs used by gastroenterologists in patients with renal dysfunction. Doses will vary with the specific needs of each patient. In addition, specific supplementary doses for patients undergoing hemodialysis, continuous ambulatory peritoneal dialysis, and continuous arteriovenous or venovenous hemofiltration are provided. Physicians using sound clinical judgment in caring for patients with renal disease evaluate each individual situation, choose a drug regimen based on all factors, and continually reevaluate response to therapy.

DOSAGE RECOMMENDATIONS FOR GASTROINTESTINAL DRUGS IN RENAL FAILURE

Drugs in this chapter are listed in Table 24.1 by generic name, in alphabetical order, under subdivisions based on similarity of pharmacologic action. For example, drugs in the H_2-blocker class and antiemetic class are grouped together.

Toxicity and Notes

Nephrotoxicity, systemic adverse effects, or information specifically related to patients with renal disease are listed directly under the generic drug name. Remarks common to all members of a class or group of drugs are listed under the name of the drug class and generally apply to each drug in the group.

Major Excretion Route

The second column in Table 24.1 lists the percentage of total drug excreted unchanged in the urine for patients with normal renal function. For some drugs, the second column gives the major route of elimination or metabolism.

Drugs extensively metabolized by the liver or extracted during initial circulation through the liver after gastrointestinal absorption have complex pharmacokinetics. For these drugs, the half-life given is for disappearance of ac-

Table 24.1
Dosage Guidelines in Renal Dysfunction for Drugs Used in Gastroenterology[a]

Drug, toxicity, notes	Amount excreted unchanged (%)	Half-life (normal/ESRD) (hr)	Plasma protein binding	Volume of distribution (l/kg)	Dose for normal renal function	Method[b]	>50[c]	10–50	<10	Supplement for dialysis
Anti-emetics and Motility Agents										
Cisapride (33) Can begin intra-peritoneally to CAPD patients	<5	7–10/7–10	98	2.4	5–10 qid po	D	100%	100%	100%	None
Granisetron (34)	8–15	6–10/6–10	?	2.2–3.3	40–160 ng/kd as 5–30 min i.v. infusion	D	100%	100%	100%	None
Metoclopramide (35)	10–25	2.5–4/14–15	40	2–3.5	10–15 mg qid p.o.	D	100%	75%	50%	None
Octreotide (36, 37)	30	1–1.5/?	?	0.4	50 ng bid sub-cutaneously	D	100%	100%	100%	None
Odansetron (38)	<5	3.5/5–9	70–75	2.1	0.15 mg/kg as 15-min infusion	D	100%	100%	100%	None
Antimicrobial Agents for Specific Conditions Used by Gastroenterologists (2)										
Aztreonam	75	1.7–2.9/6–8	55	0.1–2	1–2 q 8–12 hr	D	100%	50–75%	25%	0.5 g after dialysis
Chloramphenicol	5–15	1.6–3.3/3–7	60	0.6–1	12.5 mg/kg q 6 hr	D	100%	100%	100%	None
Ciprofloxacin Poorly absorbed with antacids, sucralfate and phosphate binders. IV dose 1/3 of oral dose	70	3–6/6–9	20–40	2.1	500–750 mg q 12 hr	D	100%	50%	33%	250 mg q 12 hr for Hemo and CAPD
Erythromycin Ototoxicity with high doses in ESRD Volume of distribution increases in ESRD	15	1.4/5–6	60–95	0.8	250–500 mg q 6–12 hr	D	100%	100%	50–75%	None
Imipenam Seizures in ESRD. Administered with Cilastatin to prevent nephrotoxicity of a metabolite	20–70	1/4	13–21	0.17–0.3	250 mg–1 g q 6 hr	D	100%	50%	25%	Dose after dialysis
Sulbactam	50–80	1/10–21	29	0.25–0.50	0.75–1.5 g q 6–8 hr	I	q 6–8 hr	q 12–24 hr	q 24–48 hr	Dose after dialysis CAPD 0.75–1.5 g q 24 hr
Sulfadiazine Alkalinization enhances drug excretion; hydration is important	57	9.9/14–16	54	0.29	2 g q 8 hr	I	q 6–8 hr	q 8 hr	q 12–24 hr	None
Sulfamethoxazole	70	10/20–50	50	0.28–0.38	1 g q 8 hr	I	q 12 hr	q 18 hr	q 24 hr	1 g after dialysis. CAPD 1 g q 24 hr
Sulfisoxazole Protein binding deceased in ESRD Use normal dosing for UTI in ESRD	70	3–7/6–12	85	0.14–0.28	1–2 g q 6 hr	I	q 6 hr	q 8–12 hr	q 12–24 hr	2 g after dialysis. CAPD 3 g/day

Tetracyclines Potentiate acidosis, increase BUN, phosphorus, anti-anabolic										
Doxycycline	33–45	15–24/18–25	80–93	0.75	100 mg q 24 hr	D	100%	100%	100%	None
Group drug of choice for decreased renal function. Not antianabolic										
Tetracyline	48–60	6–10/57–108	55–90	>0.7	250–500 mg bid	I	q 8–12 hr	q 12–24 hr	124 hr	None
Vancomycin	90	6–8/200–250	10	0.47–0.84	250–500 mg q 8 hr	I	q 24–72 hr	q 72–240 hr	q 240 hr	None
Little absorption when given orally										
Benzodiazepines (2) May cause excessive sedation and encephalopathy in ESRD										
Diazepam	<1	20–90/20–90	94–98	0.7–3.4	5–40 mg/day	D	100%	100%	100%	Hemo: None CAPD: Unknown CAVH: Unknown
Active metabolite; protein binding decreased and volume of distribution increased in ESRD										
Midazolam	<1	1.2–12.3/1.2–12.3	93–96	1–6.6	Individualized	D	100%	100%	50%	Not applicable
Protein binding decreased in ESRD										
H₂ Antagonists (2, 39)										
Cimetidine	50–70	1.5–2/5	20	0.8–1.3	400 mg bid or 400–800 mg qhs	D	75%	50%	25%	Hemo: 1/2 dose at end of dialysis CAPD: None CAVH: Unknown
Increases serum creatinine and decreases creatinine clearance by inhibition of tubular creatinine secretion, mental confusion in patients with renal or hepatic disease. Acute renal failure due to interstitial nephritis reported										
Famotidine	65–80	2.5–4/12–19	15–22	0.8–1.4	20–40 mg qhs	D	100%	75%	25–50%	Hemo: None CAPD: None CAVH: None
Nizatidine	54–65	1.3–1.6/5.3–8.5	28	1.1–1.3	150–300 mg qhs	I	75%	50%	25%	Hemo: Unknown CAPD: Unknown CAVH: Unknown
Pharmacologically active metabolite excreted by the kidney										
Ranitidine	80	1.5–3/6–9	15	1.1–1.9	150–300 mg qhs	D	75%	50%	25%	Hemo: 1/2 dose at end of dialysis CAPD: None CAVH: Unknown
Roxatidine acetate	70	4–8/12–24	10	1.7	150 mg bid or qhs	D	75%	50%	25%	Hemo: 1/2 dose CAPD: None CAVH: Unknown

Table 24.1 Continued
Dosage Guidelines in Renal Dysfunction for Drugs Used in Gastroenterology[a]

Drug, toxicity, notes	Amount excreted unchanged (%)	Half-life (normal/ESRD) (hr)	Plasma protein binding	Volume of distribution (l/kg)	Dose for normal renal function	Method[b]	Adjustment for renal failure GFR (ml/min) >50[c]	10–50	<10	Supplement for dialysis
Active metabolite roxatidine formed by esterases in small intestine, plasma and liver										
Immunosuppressive Drugs (2)										
Azathioprine	<2	0.16–1/Increased	20	0.55–0.8	1.5–2.5 mg/kg/day	D	100%	75%	50%	Hemo: Yes CAPD: Unknown
6-mercaptopurine is active metabolite										
Cyclophosphamide	10–15	4–7.5/10	14	0.6	1–5 mg/kg/day	D	100%	100%	75%	Hemo: 1/2 dose CAPD: Unknown
Hemorrhagic cystitis, bladder fibrosis and cancer										
Cyclosporine	<1	3–16/Unchanged	96–99	3.5–7.4	3–10 mg/kg/day	D	100%	100%	100%	Hemo: None CAPD: None
Nephrotoxic. Hypertension, seizures, tremor, inhibitors of hepatic metabolism increase blood concentration										
Corticosteroids										
May aggravate azotemia, sodium retention, glucose intolerance and hypertension										
Dexamethasone	8	3–4/Unknown	70	0.8–1	0.75–9 mg/day	D	100%	100%	100%	None
Hydrocortisone	<2	1.5–2/Unknown	Unknown	Unknown	20–500 mg/day	D	100%	100%	100%	None
Prednisone	34	2.5–3.5/Unknown	Saturable	2.2	5–60 mg/day	D	100%	100%	100%	None
Miscellaneous Drugs Commonly Used in Gastroenterology Practice (2)										
Cholestyramine	None	Not absorbed	None		4 g q 4–6 hr	D	100%	100%	100%	
Hyperchloremic acidosis										
Diuretics										
Bumetanide	33	1.2–1.5/15	96	0.2–0.5	1–2 mg q 8–12 hr	D	100%	100%	100%	
Furosemide	67	0.5–1.1/2–4	95	0.07–0.2	40–80 mg bid	D	100%	100%	100%	Hemo: None CAPD: None
Ototoxicity in combination with aminoglycosides. High doses effective in ESRD										

Drug					Dose					Supplement
Metolazone	70	4–20/Unknown	95	1.6	5–10 mg/day	D	100%	100%	100%	Hemo: None CAPD: None
High doses effective in renal failure										
Spironolactone	20–30	10–35/Unchanged	98	Unknown	25 mg tid-qid	I	q 6–12 hr	q 12–24 hr	Avoid	N/A
Active metabolites with long half-life Hyperkalemia common when GFR < 30 ml/min Hyperchloremic acidosis										
Thiazides	>95	6–8/12–20	40	3	25–50 mg bid	0	100%	100%	Avoid	N/A
Usually ineffective with GFR < 30 ml/min Hyperuricemia										
Propranolol (2)	<5	2–6/1–6	93	2.8	80–160 mg bid	D	100%	100%	100%	None
Ursodiol (40)	<5	?	?	?	4–5 ng/kg bid po	D	100%	100%	100%	None

Other Drugs Used for Peptic Disease

Antacids

Calcium, magnesium and aluminum salts all have absorption of constituent cations which have reduced elimination in renal failure producing hypercalcemia, hypermagnesemia and hyperalbuminuremia, respectively. Protracted use may cause nephrolithiasis, metabolic alkalosis and milk alkali syndrome. Calcium salts now drugs of choice as phosphate binders.

Drug					Dose					Supplement
Aluminum hydroxide					30–60 ml-2 as needed withmeals for phosphate binding	D	100%	100%	Avoid	
Calcium acetate					250–750 mg with meals for phosphate binding	D	100%	100%	100%	
Calcium carbonate					600-1 g with meals for phosphate binding	D	100%	100%	100%	
Enprostil (41)	50	3+/?	?	?	35 ng bid	D	100%	100%	100%	None
Magnesium hydroxide					30–60 mEq q 2 hr as needed	D	100%	100%	Avoid	

Table 24.1 Continued
Dosage Guidelines in Renal Dysfunction for Drugs Used in Gastroenterology[a]

Drug, toxicity, notes	Amount excreted unchanged (%)	Half-life (normal/ESRD) (hr)	Plasma protein binding	Volume of distribution (l/kg)	Dose for normal renal function	Method[b]	Adjustment for renal failure			Supplement for dialysis
							GFR (ml/min)			
							>50[c]	10–50	<10	
Misoprostol (42)	1–4	1.7/?	85	?	100–200 ng	D	100%	100% qid po	100%	None
Free acid metabolites have pharmacologic activity										
Omeprazole (43–44)	<5 aluminum	<1/<1	95	0.3	20–40 mg/day	D	100%	100%	100%	None required
Sucralfate (45–46) Contains aluminum which may be absorbed to produce dementia, renal osteodystrophy and anemia. Less than 5% of dose absorbed	~100%	?	?	?	1 g qid po	D	100%	Avoid	Avoid	Avoid

[a]ESRD, end stage renal disease; GFR, glomerular filtration rate; CAPD, chronic ambulatory peritoneal dialysis; Hemo, hemodialysis; CAVH, continuous anteriovenous or venovenous hemofiltration; q.i.d., four times daily; t.i.d., three times daily; b.i.d., twice daily; q, every; i.v., intravenous, p.o., oral; UTI, urinary tract infection; BUN, blood urea nitrogen; q.h.s., every night; N/A, not applicable; ?, unknown.
[b]Preferred method for dosage adjustment during renal failure indicated by D (dose reduction) or I (internal extension).
[c]GFR >50 implies a reduction from normal.

tive drugs after it has reach the general circulation. In patients with hepatic dysfunction, the· percentage of an administered dose metabolized by the "first pass" effect may be reduced. For these tables, it is assumed that liver function is normal and that other drugs that alter hepatic metabolism are not being given.

Pharmacokinetic Variables

Dosage adjustments for renal failure depend on knowledge of normal drug disposition. Pharmacokinetic variables in normal subjects are given in the tables. These variables include the major route of drug elimination by either excretion or metabolism, the plasma or biologic half-life for patients with normal renal function or end-stage renal disease, the extent of drug binding to plasma proteins, and the apparent volume of distribution. The volume of distribution and half-life given should be considered in estimating initial blood levels after loading, in finding the proper maintenance regimen, and in deciding the likelihood of drug removal by dialysis. It should be emphasized that complex pharmacokinetics and variability of drug disposition in patients with renal failure often cannot be adequately described by these simple parameters.

Dosage for Normal Renal Function

After the column listing pharmacokinetic variables, drug doses given to patients with normal renal function are listed. These recommendations are meant only as a guide and do not imply efficacy of a listed regimen.

Dosage Adjustment for Renal Failure

A loading dose should be considered when the half-life of a drug is particularly long in patients with impaired renal function. When the physical examination suggests that the extracellular fluid volume is normal, the loading dose of a drug given to a patient with renal insufficiency is the same as the initial dose given to a patient with normal renal function. Initial doses for most drugs requiring loading are already known. However, the loading dose may be calculated using the following formula:

Loading dose

$$= Vd \ (l/kg) \times Wt \ (kg) \times Cp \ (mg/l)$$

Vd = volume of distribution of the drug; Wt = patient's ideal body weight; Cp = desired plasma drug level.

If the patient has substantial edema or ascites, a somewhat larger loading dose may be required. Conversely, dehydrated or debilitated patients should receive smaller initial drug doses.

To adjust the maintenance dosage in patients with renal insufficiency, the intervals between individual doses can be lengthened (interval extension method), keeping the dose size normal. The calculated dose interval should be rounded off to create a convenient time schedule. This method is particularly useful for drugs with wide therapeutic ranges and long plasma half-lives in patients with renal impairment. Lengthening the interval will result in wide swings of the plasma drug concentrations from peak to trough levels. If the range between the therapeutic and toxic levels is too narrow, either toxic or subtherapeutic plasma concentrations may result.

Alternatively, the size of the individual doses can be reduced, keeping the interval between doses normal (dose reduction method). Decreasing the individual doses reduces the difference between peak and trough plasma concentrations. This effect is important to note for drugs with narrow therapeutic ranges and short plasma half-lives in patients with renal impairment. Decreasing dose size is recommended for drugs in which a relatively constant blood level is desired. The reduced dose should be rounded off to a convenient value.

In the tables, the preferred method for dosage adjustment is included for each drug. Dose reduction is indicated by "D," and interval extension by "I." After the recommended method for dosage adjustment, recommendations are given for levels of renal function as estimated by the glomerular filtration rate. For the dose-reduction method, the percentage of the usual dose to be given at the normal dose interval is shown. When the interval extension method is recommended, the number of hours between doses of normal size is given.

No controlled clinical trials have been done to compare the efficacy of the two methods for maintenance drug-dose alteration in patients with renal insufficiency. Prolonging the dose interval is often more convenient and less expensive. When the dose interval can safely be lengthened beyond 24 hours, extended parenteral therapy can be completed without prolonged hospitalization. In patients requiring chronic hemodialysis, many drugs need to be given only at the end of the dialysis treatment. Further, compliance with any drug regimen may be better when fewer doses can be taken at convenient times. In practice, a combination of interval prolongation and dose-size reduction is often effective and convenient. These recommendations are shown by the notation "D" and "I."

Dialysis Adjustment

The effect of standard clinical treatment on drug removal is shown for hemodialysis (Hemo), chronic ambulatory peritoneal dialysis (CAPD), and continuous arteriovenous or venovenous hemofiltration (CAVH). When known, specific recommendations for dose adjustment are given. Some drugs that have high dialysis clearance do notrequire supplemental doses after dialysis if the amount of drug removed is not significant. This would be the case if the volume of distribution is large. To insure efficacy when information about dialysis losses is not available and to simplify dosimetry, maintenance doses of most drugs should be given after dialysis.

Pharmacokinetic studies have led to the development of inclusive nomograms and tables of drug disposition and dosimetry for patients with renal impairment. The tables in this book contain dose recommendations based on the most current information available (2).

THE RENAL PATIENT— CONSIDERATIONS FOR THE GASTROENTEROLOGIST

Chronic renal failure is relatively common in the population with annual incidence figures of 50–75 patients per million population per year. There are approximately 100,000 patients receiving maintenance dialysis with another 10,000 renal transplants performed annually (15). Diabetes mellitus, chronic glomerulonephritis, hypertension, autosomal dominant polycystic kidney disease, and urinary obstruction/infection are common causes. All of these primary diagnoses may have gastrointestinal and/or hepatic signs and symptoms. It is beyond the scope of this chapter to cover these subjects in detail. In this section, the gastrointestinal manifestations of the renal patient that might involve evaluation or consultation by the gastroenterologist or hepatologist will be covered.

Considerations in Pre-End Stage Chronic Renal Failure

Gastrointestinal symptoms are frequent in patients with chronic renal disease particularly when glomerular filtration rate (GFR) is reduced to less than 25–30% of normal. These symptoms may alert the clinician to the need for renal replacement therapy with dialysis or transplantation. Early morning nausea, vomiting, hiccups, and alterations of taste are frequent. In diabetic patients with advancing nephropathy, it is difficult to distinguish these symptoms from autonomic neuropathy. Dyspeptic symptoms are also common and are often linked to medications such as iron supplements, or calcium and aluminum-containing phosphate binders. Primary gastrointestinal pathology such as peptic ulcer disease, gastritis, or diabetic gastroparesis is also common. Constipation due to dietary changes or phosphate binders is usually managed with an increase in dietary fiber and addition of docusate sodium. With refractory cases, particularly in the elderly who have a high prevalence of diverticular disease, sorbitol or mineral oil is useful.

Upper gastrointestinal bleeding is usually due to gastritis; however, other lesions are sufficiently frequent as to require an aggressive management approach including endoscopy. Persistent or major bleeding and/or persistent dyspeptic symptoms are indications for initiation of dialysis therapy. Telangiectasis and hypertrophic gastric folds have an increased frequency in chronic renal failure. The long term use of aluminum containing phosphate binders is discouraged because of aluminum-associated metabolic bone disease. Frequent use of magnesium containing antacids may produce hypermagnesemia that can cause neurologic and respiratory depression.

Lower gastrointestinal pathology such as telangiectasia, diverticulitis, colonic ulcers, and stercoral ulcers can be devastating if they are complicated by hemorrhage or perforation in the patient with chronic renal failure. Diabetics with autonomic neuropathy are particularly susceptible. Pancreatitis relating to renal failure per se has been described but is extremely rare. Stomatitis, oral ulcerations, and uriniferous breath are signs of advanced renal failure and in most cases would prompt referral for renal replacement therapy.

Dialysis Patients—Hemodialysis and Peritoneal Dialysis

Peritoneal dialysis has had renewed interest due to the emergence of new catheters and connectors in the past decade. A continuous form of therapy known as continuous CAPD now is a preferred way of instituting chronic dialysis with patient survival and quality of life comparable to the more traditional hemodialysis. The results of treatment with this and related peritoneal techniques allow high rates of subsequent transplantation and rehabilitation. The major complication remains peritonitis but intraperitoneal antibiotics administered by the patient or a nurse based on a preset algorithm is successful in >90% of cases without the requirement for catheter removal. Most episodes of peritonitis are due to indigenous skin flora such as *Staphylococcus epidermidis* and *Staphylococcus aureus*. A smaller percentage (about 20%) are due to bowel flora. Fungal, myobacterial, and chemical etiologies are possible and need to be considered in refractory cases (16). Clinically, abdominal pain and rebound tenderness are common. However, relatively asymptomatic patients may also have peritonitis. A cloudy dialysate effluent with a cell count of >100/mm^3 (75% polymorphonuclear cells) can also make the diagnosis. A specific etiologic diagnosis should be established as quickly as possible to insure optimal therapeutic results. Absorption of antibiotics from intraperitoneal dialysis solutions is rapid and it is generally not necessary to give parenteral antibiotics. Prophylactic antibiotics are not recommended because of the problem of selection of resistant organisms. If the patient accidentally contaminates his peritoneal dialysis system, the tubing should be changed and a short course of vancomycin or a cephalosporin prescribed. Full recommendations for treatment of CAPD peritonitis are published (17). A major chronic gastrointestinal complication of peritonitis is encapsulating and sclerosing peritonitis with recurrent abdominal pain, nausea, vomiting, and ultimately partial or complete bowel obstruction. Pleural effusions, intra-abdominal abscesses, and inguinal/abdominal hernias may also complicate long-term peritoneal dialysis.

Hemodialysis is the most popular form of treatment for chronic renal failure with older, more complex and challenging patients being accepted into treatment programs (18). Nausea and vomiting may occur in 5–10% of individual treatments. Diabetic gastroparesis and dialysis-induced hypotension are common etiologies. Short term use of promethazine, 25 mg intravenously or orally, cyproheptadine, 4 mg orally or metoclopramide, 5 mg orally may be helpful to improve symptoms. Other gastrointestinal complications are not specific for this form of end stage renal disease management. Guaiac positive stools should not simply be attributed to the intermittent anticoagulation necessary for dialysis treatments. A search for underlying sources of bleeding is required similar to other patients with gastrointestinal bleeding of unknown cause.

RENAL TRANSPLANTATION

Increasing success rates and new immunosuppressive drugs have resulted in long-term survival of most renal transplant patients. Consequently, internal medicine subspecialty consultants frequently are involved in the diagnosis and management of various chronic problems many of which involve the liver and gastrointestinal tract.

Colonic complications occur in 1–7% of transplant recipients (19). Ischemic colitis has a high mortality rate in this setting. The retroperitoneal placement of the renal allograft that interferes with colonic arterial collateral as well as the trauma of surgical dissection in this area may be predisposing factors (19). Most cases occur in the first four posttransplant months. Hypotension particularly induced by hemodialysis-associated fluid shifts may be precipitating factors (20). Chronic constipation and cation-exchange enemas (21) should be avoided if possible.

Infectious and nonspecific colitis can occur in the renal transplant setting. Specific treatment should be based on documented pathogens. *Clostridium difficile* should be sought and treated in all patients with persistent diarrhea. Cytomegalovirus (CMV) can produce severe diarrhea with crampy abdominal pain mimicking diverticulitis, ischemic bowel disease or intra-abdominal abscess. The diagnosis can only be confirmed by a rectal or colonic biopsy. Ulcerations, when present, may lead to fatal hemorrhage or perforation (22). CMV colitis may respond to reduced immunosuppression and ganciclovir.

Diverticulitis is the most common cause of bowel perforation in renal transplant recipients (23). Patients with polycystic kidney disease have a very high prevalence of the predisposing diverticulosis, although this is a common finding in other recipients as well. The diagnosis may be subtle in the presence of steroids and immunosuppressive drugs. A transplant patient with abdominal pain and/or sepsis needs urgent attention because delay in diagnosis undoubtedly contributes to high mortality observed. Once the diagnosis is made, immunosuppressive therapy should be reduced or stopped. After coverage with broad spectrum antibiotics and vigorous volume repletion, prompt resection of the affected colonic segment with a diverting colostomy is recommended. Colonic perforation may also occur spontaneously in renal allograft recipients without any known prior bowel pathology. Ischemia, fecal impaction, CMV-associated ulceration, other infection, and severe constipation are possible etiologic factors (24). The majority of cases occur within 3 months of transplantation associated with an episode of allograft rejection.

Inasmuch as patients with advanced renal failure are predisposed to gastrointestinal bleeding from angiodysplasia, significant colonic bleeding after transplantation from these sources may also occur. Other etiologies are also common and thus diagnosis usually requires angiography and/or colonoscopy. Patients may progress rapidly to a hemodynamically unstable state necessitating emergent bowel resection.

Upper gastrointestinal complications after renal transplantation are extremely common, particularly peptic ulcer disease and erosive gastritis. Renal dysfunction, corticosteroids, CMV, and acid hypersecretion are frequent. Rigorous efforts are usually made before transplant to exclude active peptic disease. Endoscopic documentation of healing of previously diagnosed pathology is demanded by most renal transplant centers before a patient's placement on a cadaver transplant waiting list. Prophylactic H_2-receptor blockers are used in the first 3 months posttransplant. Ranitidine is the preferred drug because cimetidine competes with creatinine for secretion and may confuse the diagnosis of allograft dysfunction. Ulcers that fail to heal posttransplant may be due to CMV and not the usual peptic ulcer diathesis (25). This is especially true if ulcerations occur during periods of heavy immunosuppression.

Oral and esophageal ulcerations may occur in transplant patients particularly at times of increased doses of immunosuppression. *Candida* and herpetic infections are frequently implicated. Upper gastrointestinal endoscopy

Table 24.2
Causes of Liver Dysfunction in Renal Transplant Recipients (24)

Viral hepatitis	Hepatitis B
	Hepatitis C
	Cytomegalovirus
	Epstein-Barr virus
	Adenovirus
	Herpes simplex
	Herpes zoster
Immunosuppressive drugs	Azathioprine
	Cyclosporine
Hepatic veno-occlusive disease	
Peliosis hepatis and nodular regenerative hyperplasia	

with appropriate biopsies and culture are indicated for patients with dysphagia, retrosternal pain, or occult blood loss. Prophylactic mycostatin or clotrimazole suspension/lozenges three or four times daily are used in the first 3 months posttransplant usually with a decrease in the incidence of oral-esophageal candidiasis. In patients with histories of herpes simplex, acyclovir 200 mg bid as prophylaxis is useful for 3–4 months after the allograft.

Chronic liver disease is an important cause of late mortality among recipients of long-surviving renal allografts. Causes of hepatic dysfunction in this setting are shown in Table 24.2. Many of these patients ultimately develop active hepatitis or cirrhosis. Donors and recipients should be screened pretransplant for hepatitis B and C. Any prospective recipient with a positive serology should have a liver biopsy to ascertain the hepatic risk of immunosuppression. In patients with liver dysfunction posttransplant, serial liver biopsies at 1- to 3-year intervals may reveal serious progressive pathology so that immunosuppression can be promptly reduced.

The incidence of hepatitis B posttransplant has been reduced by the use of fewer transfusions and vaccination of prospective recipients with recombinant hepatitis B vaccine. The prevalence of hepatitis B surface antigenemia in North American dialysis units is less

than 2.7%. From studies using proper serologic markers including hepatitis B virus (HBV) DNA polymerase, it is clear that transplant immunosuppression enhances viral replication or reactivation that in turn is associated with a high prevalence of chronic liver disease (26, 27). This clinical course is different from the general population of HB Ag$^+$ carriers who develop cirrhosis only 3–6% of the time. Hepatitis B virus appears to have a steroid sensitive enhancer sequence that favors viral replication in hepatocytes. In a Canadian study, 82% of HB Ag$^+$ patients progressed to chronic active hepatitis and/or cirrhosis with a 55% mortality rate (28). Mortality from hepatitis B is greater in transplant recipients than chronic hemodialysis patients. Initial liver biopsies and serum transaminases tend to underestimate the severity and activity of hepatitis B-associated liver disease (28). The effect of viral coinfection or delta agent infection on the excessive morbidity and mortality post transplant is unknown. Hepatitis B surface Ag$^+$ patients are probably best served by remaining on dialysis. If renal transplants are performed, patients should be followed with serial biopsies and serologies that can detect active viral replication (HBV DNA, DNA polymerase, HBe Ag). Immunosuppressive drugs should be withdrawn or reduced promptly if active viral replication is documented.

Hepatitis C is now the most common cause of hepatitis in patients and staff of hemodialysis units. Many cases of chronic liver disease in renal transplant recipients are undoubtedly due to this newly discovered virus or other non-A, non-B hepatitis viruses. Low level elevations of serum transaminases and mild symptoms of fatigue and weakness do not correlate well with the severity of underlying liver pathology. Furthermore, liver enzymes may be intermittently elevated with long periods of normality even in patients who ultimately develop active hepatitis or cirrhosis. Donors and recipients should be screened pre-transplant for hepatitis C. Any prospective recipient with a positive serology should have a liver biopsy to ascertain the hepatic risk of immunosuppression. In patients with liver dysfunction post transplant, serial liver biopsies at 1- to 3-year intervals may reveal serious progressive pathology so that immunosuppression can be promptly reduced.

CMV hepatitis usually occurs with other manifestations of systemic CMV infection. Mild elevations of alkaline phosphatase with normal bilirubin is usual. Rarely cholestasis dominates the clinical picture particularly in patients with AIDS in which sclerosing cholangitis complicates CMV infection. Ganciclovir is indicated for this tissue invasive form of CMV infection.

Herpes simplex hepatitis occurs in the setting of disseminated herpes simplex virus infection (29). Often, the mucocutaneous herpetic lesions are absent even with fulminant disease. The transaminases may be markedly elevated and the disease is usually rapidly fatal with hemorrhagic liver necrosis and disseminated intravascular coagulation. Early diagnosis by a characteristic liver biopsy or viral culture from liver tissue followed by intravenous acyclovir may avoid some fatalities.

Immunosuppressive drugs used in transplantation may cause hepatic dysfunction. Azathioprine may cause a spectrum of pathologic changes in the liver including acute reversible cholestatic hepatitis, acute focal hepatocellular necrosis, or chronic irreversible hepatic failure with portal hypertension, perisinusoidal fibrosis, and cirrhosis (30). Hepatic veno-occlusive disease has been linked to azathioprine. Biopsy findings are characteristic with fibrous obliteration of small hepatic venules and small sublobular veins. Patients are predominantly male and present within the first 2-years of transplantation with jaundice, vague abdominal pain, and portal hypertension (31). Viral hepatitis may predispose to this entity (31). Alkaline phosphatase is increased with little elevation of transaminase. Withdrawal of azathioprine may provide some clinical improvement but the clinical course is usually progressive, culminating in death from hepatic failure and/or portal hypertension (31).

Mild reversible elevations of bilirubin and transaminase are seen in 20–40% of transplant recipients treated with cyclosporine. A much smaller percentage of patients experience recurrent or persistent liver dysfunction. Liver biopsies show nonspecific changes (30, 32). Cyclosporine-treated recipients may be predisposed to cholelithiasis because of reduced bile flow and secretion rates.

Peliosis hepatis is a condition characterized by blood-filled cavities in the liver without endothelial lining randomly distributed in the liver parenchyma. It is most often seen in conjunction with nodular regeneration of the liver. In renal transplantation, these processes are thought to result from hepatotropic viruses (CMV) or azathioprine causing endothelial injury with compensatory regenerative changes. The pathogenesis and clinical course may be similar to hepatic veno-occlusive disease. Early liver biopsy for abnormalities of liver function and azathioprine withdrawal are key to any hope for reversibility.

Acute pancreatitis after renal transplantation occurs in 1–7% of cases and carries a high mortality, particularly if it occurs in the first 3 months post-transplant. Hypercalciuria frequently present postoperatively may promote pancreatic autodigestion by converting in active trypsinogen to active trypsin or by causing pancreatic ductal obstruction. In addition, parathyroid hormone (PTH) may be directly toxic to the pancreas. Azathioprine, cyclosporine, CMV, and possibly corticosteroids may be associated with pancreatitis. Withdrawal of offending agents, particularly azathioprine, often is necessary but the pathogenesis is often complex and difficult to assess.

REFERENCES

1. Touchette MA, Slaughter RL. The effect of renal failure on hepatic drug clearance. Drug Intell Clin Pharm 1991;25:1214–1224.
2. Bennett WM, Aronoff GR, Golper TA, Morrison GN, Singer I, Brater DC. Drug prescribing in renal failure. Philadelphia: American College of Physicians, 1991.
3. Hurwitz A. Antacid therapy and drug kinetics. Clin Pharmacokinet 1977;2:269–280.
4. Craig R, Murphy T, Gibson TP. Kinetic analysis of D-xylose absorption in normal subjects and in pa-

tients with chronic renal insufficiency. J Lab Clin Med 1983;101:496–506.

5. Reidenberg MM. The binding of drugs to plasma proteins and the interpretation of measurements of plasma concentration of drugs in patients with poor renal function. Am J Med 1977;62:466–470.

6. Brosen K. Recent development in hepatic drug oxidation: implications for clinical pharmacokinetics. Clin Pharmacokinet 1990;18:220–239.

7. Lehmann CR, Heironimus JD, Collins CB, et al. Metoclopramide kinetics in patients with impaired renal function and clearance by hemodialysis. Clin Pharmacol Ther 1985;37:284–289.

8. Bianchetti G, Graziani G, Brancaccio D, et al. Pharmacokinetics and effects of propranolol in terminal uremic patients and in patients undergoing regular dialysis treatment. Clin Pharmacokinet 1976;1:373–384.

9. Verbeeck RK, Branch RA, Wilkinson GR. Drug metabolites in renal failure: pharmacokinetic and clinical implications. Clin Pharmacokinet 1981;6:329–345.

10. Burgess E, Blair A, Kirchman K, Cutler RF. Inhibition of renal creatinine secretion by cimetidine in humans. Renal Physiol 1982;5:27–30.

11. Lin JH. Pharmacokinetic and pharmacodynamic properties of histamine H_2-receptor antagonists. Clin Pharmacokinet 1991;20:218–236.

12. Cockroft DW, Gault MH. Prediction of creatinine clearance from serum creatinine. Nephron 1976; 16:31–41.

13. Aronoff GR, Abel SR. Principles of administering drugs to patients with renal failure. In: Brenner BM, Stein JH, eds. Pharmacotherapy in renal disease and hypertension. New York: Churchill-Livingstone, 1986:1–19.

14. Jick H. Adverse drug effects in relation to renal function. Am J Med 1977;62:514–517.

15. United States Renal Data System Report. Bethesda, MD: The National Institutes of Health, The National Institutes of Diabetes, Digestive and Kidney Diseases, Division of Kidney, Urologic and Hematologic Diseases, 1990.

16. Khanna R, Oreopous D. Peritoneal dialysis. In: Levine D, ed. Care of the renal patient, Philadelphia: Saunders, 1991:187–219.

17. Keane WF, Everett ED, Fine RN, et al. CAPD related peritonitis management and antibiotic therapy recommendations. Peritoneal Dialy Bull 1987;7:55.

18. Ismail N, Hakim R. Hemodialysis. In: Levine D, ed. Care of the renal patient. Philadelphia: Saunders, 1991:220–246.

19. Flanigan RC, Reckard CR, Lucas BA. Colonic complications of renal transplantation. J Urol 1988;139: 503–506.

20. Jablonski U, Putzki H, Heymann H. Necrosis of the ascending colon in chronic hemodialysis patients. Dis Colon Rectum 1987;30:623–625.

21. Lillemoe KD, Romolo JL, Hamilton SR, Pennington LR, Burdick JF, Williams GM. Intestinal necrosis due to sodium polystyrene (Kay-exolate) in sorbitol enemas: clinical and experimental support for the hypothesis. Surgery 1987;101:267–272.

22. Sutherland D, Chan F, Foucar E, Simmons R, Howard R, Najarian J. The bleeding cecal ulcer in transplant patients. Surgery 1979;86:386–398.

23. Church JM, Fazio VW, Novack AC, Steenmuller DR. Perforation of the colon in renal hemograft recipients. Ann Surg 1986;203:69–76.

24. Komorowski R, Cohen E, Kauffman HM, Adams M. Gastrointestinal complications of renal transplant recipients. Am J Clin Pathol 1986;86:161–167.

25. Cohen E, Komorowski R, Kauffman HM, Adams M. Unexpectedly high incidence of cytomegalovirus infection in apparent peptic ulcers in renal transplant recipients. Surgery 1985;97:606–612.

26. DuSheiko G, Sung E, Bowyer S, et al. Natural history of hepatitis B virus infection in renal transplant recipients—a fifteen year follow-up. Hepatology 1983; 3:330–336.

27. Degos F, Lugassy G, Degott G, et al. Hepatitis B virus and hepatitis B-related viral infection in renal transplant recipients. Gastroenterology 1988;94: 151–156.

28. Parfrey PS, Forbes RDC, Hutchinson TA, et al. The impact of renal transplantation on the course of hepatitis B liver disease. Transplantation 1985;39:610–615.

29. Elliott WC, Houghton D, Bryant R, et al. Herpes simplex type I hepatitis in renal transplantation. Arch Intern Med 1980;140:1656–1660.

30. Haboubie NY, Hiam HAL, Whitwell HL, Ceckrill P. Role of endothelial cell injury in the spectrum of azathioprine-induced liver disease after renal transplant: light microscopy and ultra-structural observations. Am J Gastroenterol 1988;83:256–261.

31. Read A, Wiesner R, LaBrecque D, et al. Hepato veno-occlusive disease associated with renal transplantation and azothioprine therapy. Ann Intern Med 1986;104:651–655.

32. Mourad G, Bories P, Berthalemy C, Barneon G, Michel H, Mion C. Peliosis hepatis and nodular regeneration of the liver in renal transplants. Trans Proc 1987;19:3697–3698.

33. McCalium RW, Prakash C, Campoli-Richard DM, Goa KL. Cisapride: a preliminary review of its pharmacodynamic and pharmacokinetic properties, and therapeutic use as a prokinetic agent in gastrointestinal motility disorders. Drugs 1988;36:652–681.

34. Plosker GL, Goa KL. Granisetron: a review of its pharmacological properties and therapeutic use as an antiemetic. Drugs 1991;42:805–824.

35. Bateman DN. Clinical pharmacokinetics of metoclopramide. Clin Pharmacol 1983;8:523–529.

36. Battershill PE, Clissold SP. Octreotide: a review of its pharmacodynamic and pharmacokinetic properties, and therapeutic potential in conditions associated with excessive peptide secretion. Drugs 1989;38:658–702.

37. Rosenberg JM. Octreotide: a synthetic analog of somatostatin. Drug Intell Clin Pharm 1988;22:748–754.
38. Kohler DR, Goldspiel BR. Ondansetron: a serotonin receptor (5-HT$_3$) antagonist for antineoplastic chemotherapy-induced nausea and vomiting. DICP Ann Pharmacother 1991;25:367–380.
39. Murdoch D, McTavish D. Roxatidine acetate: a review of its pharmacodynamic and pharmacokinetic properties, and its therapeutic potential in peptic ulcer disease and related disorders. Drugs 1991;42:240–260.
40. Rosenbaum CL, Cluxton Jr RJ. Ursodiol: a cholesterol gallstone solubilizing agent. Drug Intell Clin Pharm 1988;22:941–946.
41. Goa KL, Monk JP. Enprostil: a preliminary review of its pharmacodynamic and pharmacokinetic properties, and therapeutic efficacy in the treatment of peptic ulcer disease. Drugs 1987;34:539–559.
42. Jones JB, Bailey Jr RT. Misoprostol: a prostaglandin E$_1$ analog with antisecretory and cytoprotective properties. DICP Ann Pharmacol 1989;23:276–282.
43. McTavish D, Buckley MM-T, Heel RC. Omeprazole: an updated review of its pharmacology and therapeutic use in acid-related disorders. Drugs 1991;42:138–170.
44. Maton PN. Omeprazole. N Engl J Med 324:965–975.
45. Richardson CT. Sucralfate. Ann Intern Med 1982;97:269–272.
46. McCarthy DM. Drug therapy. N Engl J Med 1991;325:1017–1025.

25

The Use of Gastrointestinal Drugs During Pregnancy and Lactation

GERALD G. BRIGGS and SUMNER J. YAFFE

One of the most difficult tasks facing a physician who is treating a pregnant woman is prescribing medications for that patient. In these situations there are always, at least, two patients; the woman and her fetus. The former has a disease process requiring the ministrations of the clinician, the second is a presumably healthy, developing living being who becomes a patient by default. In general, anything given to the mother will obtain measurable concentrations in her fetus. The task can be especially difficult in the first 14–56 days after conception because this portion of the embryonic period is the time of major organogenesis, and the period that chemicals, including drugs, can produce structural malformations. After the embryonic period, during the fetal period (i.e., late first, second, and third trimesters), defects of the central nervous system, genitourinary system, and skeleton (e.g., hypoplastic calvaria secondary to angiotensin converting enzyme inhibitors) are still possible. Moreover, the central nervous system is susceptible to drug-induced toxicity throughout the fetal period with modification of functional aspects possible for several years after birth. Other changes, such as intrauterine growth retardation, and fetotoxicity are possible right up to the time of birth. Thus, clinicians must carefully weigh the impact of their drug therapy on both the mother and her fetus throughout gestation and during the period she is nursing her infant.

In this chapter, the effects of medicinal agents used to treat maternal gastrointestinal disease on the second patient, the fetus and/or newborn, are evaluated. As is true with most biologic systems, drugs may exert an entire spectrum of fetal effects, ranging from no effect at all in the majority of cases, to reversible and irreversible toxicity, and to overt and covert structural malformations, many of which may not be detectable for years. Drug-induced fetal effects are dependent on the time of the exposure in relation to gestational age, the particular agent, the dose, the route of administration, the duration of exposure, and, often, the mother's genetic makeup. Animal studies may be predictive of the risk an individual drug represents, but the accuracy of the prediction depends greatly on the species used. For determination of human teratogenicity, the sensitivity and specificity of rodent studies is <60%, but those involving nonhuman primates are >90% (1). Unfortunately, studies using nonhuman primates are expensive, much more than rodent studies, and thus few drugs are evaluated in this way (1).

The sections below are organized by therapeutic class. An alphabetical listing of the drugs is shown in Table 25.1. The FDA risk factor and a common trade name for each drug are given with the drug name. Many of the drugs reviewed are available from multiple sources, but for simplicity, only one trade name (with an exception or two) has been listed. The use of a specific trade name does

Table 25.1
Listing of Drugs Evaluated by Class[a]

Drug (trade name)

Antacids
Aluminum carbonate (Basaljel)
Aluminum hydroxide (Amphojel)
Aluminum phosphate (Phosphaljel)
Calcium carbonate (Tums)
Dihydroxyaluminum sodium carbonate (Rolaids)
Hydroxymagnesium aluminate
Magnesium hydroxide
Magnesium oxide
Sodium bicarbonate

Anticholinergics
Atropine
Belladonna alkaloids
L-Hyoscyamine
Scopolamine
Quarternary anticholinergics
    Anisotropine (Valpin 50)
    Clidinium (Quarzan)
    Glycopyrrolate (Robinul)
    Hexocyclium (Tral)
    Isopropamide (Darbid)
    Mepenzolate (Cantil)
    Methantheline (Banthine)
    Methscopolamine (Pamine)
    Propantheline (Pro-Banthine)
    Tridihexethyl (Pathilon)

Antidiarrheals
Diphenoxylate/atropine (Lomotil)
Bismuth subsalicylate (Pepto-Bismol)
Kaolin/pectin (Kaopectate)
Lactobacillus (Lactinex)
Loperamide (Imodium)
Opium
Paregoric

Antiemetics
Piperazine antihistamines
    Buclizine (Bucladin-S)
    Cyclizine (Marezine)
    Hydroxyzine (Atarax; Vistaril)
    Meclizine (Antivert; Bonine)
Dimenhydrinate (Dramamine)
Diphenhydramine (Benadryl)
Droperidol (Inapsine)
Ondansetron
Prochlorperazine (Compazine)
Promethazine (Phenergan)
Trimethobenzamide (Tigan)

Antiflatulants
Simethicone (Mylicon)
Charcoal

Oral Anti-infective Agents
Metronidazole (Flagyl)
Vancomycin (Vancocin)

Antisecretory Agents
Histamine-2 receptor antagonists
    Cimetidine (Tagamet)
    Famotidine (Pepcid)

Table 25.1 Continued
Listing of Drugs Evaluated by Class[a]

Drug (trade name)

    Nizatidine (Axid)
    Ranitidine (Zantac)
Proton pump inhibitors
    Omeprazole (Prilosec)
Prostaglandin analogs
    Misoprostol (Cytotec)

Antispasmodics
Dicyclomine (Bentyl)
Oxyphencyclimine (Daricon)

Corticosteroids
Prednisolone
Prednisone

Digestive Enzymes
Pancreatin (Entozyme)
Pancrelipase (Entolase)
Papain (Panafil)
Pepsin (Entozyme)

Gallstone-Solubilizing Agents
Chenodiol (Chenix)
Monoctanoin (Moctanin)
Ursodiol (Actigall)

Gastric Acidifiers
Glutamic acid

Gastrointestinal Protectants
Sulcralfate (Carafate)

Gastrointestinal Stimulants
Metoclopramide (Reglan)
Dexpanthenol (Ilopan)
Dexpanthenol with choline bitartrate (Ilopan-Choline)

Agents Used for Inflammatory Bowel Disease
Azathioprine (Imuran)
Corticosteroids
Mercaptopurine (Purinethol)
Metronidazole
Sulfasalazine (Azulfidine)
Mesalamine (Rowasa)
Olsalazine (Dipentum)

Laxatives
Bulk laxatives
    Methylcellulose
    Polycarbophil (FiberCon)
    Psyllium (Metamucil)
Bile salts
    Dehydrocholic acid
Irritant/stimulants
    Bisacodyl (Dulcolax)
    Casanthranol
    Cascara sagrada
    Castor oil
    Danthron
    Phenophthalein (Ex-Lax; Feen-a-mint)
    Senna (Senokot)

Table 25.1 Continued
Listing of Drugs Evaluated by Class[a]

Drug (trade name)

Laxatives
  Lubricants
    Mineral oil
  Saline laxatives
    Magnesium citrate
    Magnesium hydroxide
    Magnesium sulfate
    Sodium phosphate
  Stool softeners
    Docusate (Surfak; Dialose; Colace)
  Glycerin
  Lactulose (Cephulac)

Sedatives
  Chlordiazepoxide (Librium)
  Phenobarbital

Miscellaneous Agents
  Cholestyramine (Questran)
  Penicillamine (Cuprimine)

[a]In some cases, agents are available under other trade names. The trade names used here are given as examples and no endorsement is implied.

not imply an endorsement of that product. The definition of the risk factors is shown in Table 25.2. Because they tend to oversimplify a complex topic, they should only be used in conjunction with the detailed discussion of the drug and should not be soley relied upon to make a decision whether or not a drug should be used during pregnancy.

Only drugs that are specific for the treatment of gastrointestinal disorders are included. Obviously, a large number of other medications may also be prescribed by gastroenterologists, and other sources should be consulted to determine the risk in pregnancy or lactation.

The primary reference sources used for the preparation of this chapter were as follows: (a) Briggs GG, Freeman RK, Yaffe SJ, eds. Drugs in Pregnancy and Lactation: A Reference Guide to Fetal and Neonatal Risk. ed. 3. Baltimore: Williams & Wilkins, 1990; (b) Shepard TH. Catalog of Teratogenic Agents. ed. 6. Baltimore: Johns Hopkins University Press, 1989; (c) Heinonen OP, Slone D, Shapiro S. Birth Defects and Drugs in Pregnancy. Littleton, CO: Publishing Sciences Group, 1977;

(d) the statement of the American Academy of Pediatrics on drug excretion in breast milk. Pediatrics 1989;84:924–936; and (e) information from the files of Anthony R. Scialli, M.D., Director, Reproductive Toxicology Center, Columbia Hospital for Women Medical Center, Washington, DC. A number of other sources were also consulted, but the bulk of our information originated from the five references listed above. Readers interested in expanding their professional libraries may wish to consult a 1991 reference that reviewed five current source books on developmental toxicology (2).

Data from the Collaborative Perinatal Project (CPP) (i.e., Birth Defects and Drugs in Pregnancy) are often cited in this chapter and, perhaps, some explanation of this study would be helpful. This large prospective, multicenter study, conducted between 1958 and 1965, involved over 50,000 mother-child pairs. The study was sponsored by the National Institute of Neurological and Communicative Disorders and Stroke and its primary purpose was to determine if factors occurring during pregnancy were related to the risk of cerebral palsy or other neurologic outcomes. This study made multiple comparisons between outcome and drug consumption and, although many statistical associations resulted, the authors emphasized throughout their work that causal relationships could not be inferred from the data without independent confirmation from other studies. We have also emphasized this throughout this chapter whenever we have cited their data.

ETIOLOGY AND INCIDENCE OF MALFORMATIONS

The etiology of congenital malformations is diverse and, in most cases, cannot be determined from our present state of knowledge. The mechanisms of teratogenesis are believed to be either errors in genetic programming or environmental agents or factors interacting with the developing embryo (3). This latter category includes such items as ionizing radiation, hyperthermia, drugs, chemicals, in-

Table 25.2
FDA Risk Factors

Category A: Controlled studies in women fail to demonstrate a risk to the fetus in the first trimester (and there is no evidence of a risk in later trimesters), and the possibility of fetal harm appears remote.

Category B: Either animal-reproduction studies have not demonstrated a fetal risk but there are no controlled studies in pregnant women or animal-reproduction studies have shown an adverse effect (other than a decrease in fertility) that was not confirmed in controlled studies in women in the first trimester (and there is no evidence of a risk in later trimesters).

Category C: Either studies in animals have revealed adverse effects on the fetus (teratogenic or embryocidal or other) and there are no controlled studies in woman or studies in women and animals are not available. Drugs should be given only if the potential benefit justifies the potential risk to the fetus.

Category D: There is positive evidence of human fetal risk, but the benefits from use in pregnant women may be acceptable despite the risk (e.g., if the drug is needed in a life-threatening situation or for a serious disease for which safer drugs cannot be used or are ineffective).

Category X: Studies in animals or human beings have demonstrated fetal abnormalities or there is evidence of fetal risk based on human experience or both, and the risk of the use of the drug in pregnant women clearly outweighs any possible benefit. The drug is contraindicated in women who are or may become pregnant.

Source: Federal Register 1980;44:37434-37467.

fections, disorders of maternal metabolic states, and mechanical factors (3). Approximately 60–65% of all defects do not have a known cause, but proposed etiologies within this category include polygenic, multifactoral (i.e., interactions between genetic makeup and nongenetic, usually unknown, environmental factors), spontaneous errors in development, and synergistic interactions of teratogens (3, 4). The causes that are known, and the approximate percentage each contributes to the population of infants with congenital malformations, are: (a) monogenic origin (i.e., autosomal genetic disease) (7.5–20%), (b) chromosomal abnormalities (i.e., cytogenic) (e.g., Down's syndrome) (5–6%), and (c) environmental agents and factors (8–9%) (3–5).

Although some believe that many of the malformations that fall within the unknown group are of polygenic origin (3), multifactoral etiologies involving drugs may be an important contributor. For example, one of the causes of the fetal hydantoin syndrome may be an inherited deficiency of the enzyme epoxide hydrolase that is required to eliminate the toxic oxidative metabolites (epoxides) of the anticonvulsant, phenytoin (6).

Among environmental factors, infectious agents, such as rubella, cytomegalovirus, toxoplasmosis, syphilis, herpesvirus hominis type II, varicella, Venezuelan equine encephalitis, and group B coxsackievirus account for about 1–3% of congenital malformations (3–5). The principle teratogenic maternal disease is diabetes mellitus, which accounts for more than 90% of the 1–4% of defects related to maternal disorders other than infections (3–5). Other teratogenic maternal disorders are phenylketonuria, virilizing tumors and other endocrinopathies, nutritional deficiences, starvation, hyperthermia, and drug and substance addiction (3–5). Fetal deformations (mechanical factors), such as abnormal cord constrictions, and disparity between uterine size and contents, are thought to contribute 1–2% to the total number of anomalies (3). Drugs and chemicals account for the remaining approximate 1–6% of known causes of congenital malformations, but less than two dozen such agents are proven human teratogens (3–5).

The exact incidence of congenital malformations is open to question, because it is dependent on such factors as the definition of the term (e.g., major versus minor congenital malformations), how detailed the examination is of the infant, and how long the exposed persons are followed after birth (4, 5). One review stated the reported incidence is in the range of 0.5–1.0%, but increases to 2–4% if hospital discharges are used (5). The incidence may rise to 10% if children are followed for several years (5). In general, however, a value many agree with is an incidence of major congenital malformations of 3% recognized at birth, and another 3% discovered in the months or years after birth (4). If minor malformations are also included, the incidence may be two to three times this number, and, as mentioned previously, adverse functional effects may occur not only in utero but at anytime thereafter.

GASTROINTESTINAL DRUGS

Antacids

Aluminum Carbonate (C) (Basaljel)
Aluminum Hydroxide (C) (Amphojel)
Aluminum Phosphate (C) (Phosphaljel)
Calcium Carbonate (C) (Tums)
Dihydroxyaluminum Sodium Carbonate (C) (Rolaids)
Hydroxymagnesium Aluminate (C)
Magnesium Hydroxide (C)
Magnesium Oxide (C)
Sodium Bicarbonate (C)

Antacids are used to neutralize gastric acid, thereby raising the pH of the stomach contents and, when above pH 4, inhibiting the proteolytic activity of pepsin. Little information in human or animal pregnancies is available for these preparations, and many large prospective studies do not include them in their data (7, 8). Antacids, however, are frequently consumed in pregnancy as noted in several reports (9–11).

A retrospective study evaluated the drug consumption patterns of 458 mothers who gave birth to infants with malformations compared to 911 mothers of normal infants (9). Significantly more mothers in the study group took antacids in comparison to controls for both major and minor abnormalities. Moreover, there was an association between the consumption of antacids in general during the first 56 days of pregnancy and both major and

minor congenital anomalies (9). There were no significant differences among the individual antacids and the association with defects. The antacids consumed, in order of frequency, were magnesium carbonate, aluminium hydroxide, sodium bicarbonate, magnesium trisilicate, propantheline bromide, kaolin, belladonna, and calcium carbonate (9). Two of these products, propantheline bromide and belladonna, are, of course, anticholinergics, and should not be classified as antacids, nor should the adsorbant aluminum silicate clay, kaolin, be included in this group.

A 1974 review warned that the use of certain antacids could produce toxicity in the mother and the fetus/newborn, based on the pharmacology of the products (12). Large, continuous use of the systemic antacid, sodium bicarbonate, may produce the "milk alkali syndrome" with resulting metabolic alkalosis, edema, and fluid overload leading to congestive heart failure. Magnesium trisilicate was classified as potentially damaging to fetal kidneys and possible of producing siliceous nephrolithiasis in the newborn (12). The ingestion of magnesium hydroxide was thought to potentially lead to magnesium toxicity and subsequent adverse effects on the fetal neurologic and neuromuscular systems, and impairment of the fetal cardiovascular system (12). There is no evidence, however, that any of these toxicities mentioned in this review have been observed, even after frequent ingestion of antacids during pregnancy.

Although toxicity with antacids is apparently rare, a case of baking powder (30% sodium bicarbonate with cornstarch, sodium aluminum sulfate, calcium acid phosphate, and calcium sulfate) pica resulting in maternal toxicity was described in 1992 (13). Maternal toxicity, consisting of hypertension, hypokalemia, and elevated liver function tests, occurred at least three times during gestation at 19.5, 33, and 40 weeks', with the last event occurring just before delivery. The symptoms, similar to those observed in preeclampsia, resolved during the first two hospitalizations. A normal, although alkalotic, 4235-g infant boy, with Apgar scores of 8 and 9 at 1 and 5 minutes, respectively, was delivered by cesarean section shortly after her third admission to the hospital.

High systemic concentrations of aluminum are toxic to animals and humans, but the use of aluminum antacids has not been reported to be harmful to the mother or the fetus. The effects of aluminum salts are discussed under Sucralfate (see under Gastrointestinal Protectant Agent). All of the antacids appear to be safe to consume during lactation.

ANTICHOLINERGICS

Atropine (C)

A study published in 1988 estimated the use of atropine during the first, second, and third trimesters to be 11.3, 6.7, and 6.3/1000 women, respectively (14). The CPP, a large multicenter study involving 50,282 mother-child pairs published in 1977, found 401 first-trimester exposures (7, pp. 346–353) and 1,198 exposures anytime during pregnancy to atropine among the study patients (7, p. 439). No association between atropine and congenital malformations was discovered.

Atropine rapidly crosses the placenta to the fetus (15–17) and may cause dose-related vagal inhibition with resulting fetal tachycardia (18). In one study, 0.5 mg atropine administered intravenously resulted in a decrease between 10 and 100% in fetal breathing in 13 of 15 fetuses, an increase of 300% in one fetus, and no effect in another (19). The decrease in fetal breathing occurred approximately 2 minutes after administration of the drug and lasted 5–10 minutes. No fetal hypoxia was observed nor was there an effect on fetal heart rate or beat-to-beat variation.

This anticholinergic has been used just before cesarean section in a dose of 0.01 mg/kg to reduce gastric secretions without effecting fetal heart rate or variability, uterine activity, or neonatal outcome (20, 21).

Atropine is probably excreted into breast milk, although this has never been fully documented (22). Neonates are particular sensitive to the effects of anticholinergics, but, interestingly, no adverse effects attributable to atropine have been reported and the American

Academy of Pediatrics classifies the drug as compatible with breast feeding (23).

Belladonna Alkaloids (C)

Belladonna is a mixture of the anticholinergic alkaloids from which atropine, hyoscyamine, scopolamine, and other minor alkaloids can be obtained. A total of 554 first trimester exposures (7, pp. 346–353) to this drug mixture was found by the CPP, as well as 1355 exposures anytime in pregnancy (7, p. 439). In contrast to the individual agents, possible associations with congenital malformations as a whole and with minor defects was found with first trimester belladonna exposure. Increased risks were observed for defects of the respiratory tract, hypospadias, and eye and ear. Interpretation of these data are difficult, however, because the authors of the study emphasized that even though some statistically significant associations occurred in their study, a cause and effect relationship could not be determined and independent confirmation of their results were required.

The appearance of the individual alkaloid components of belladonna in breast milk should be expected and anticholinergic effects may potentially occur in the nursing infant.

L-Hyoscyamine (C)

Little information is available for this agent in human pregnancy, but the anticholinergic effects on the fetus and newborn should be similar to atropine and scopolamine. Both placental transfer and excretion into breast milk probably occur to the same degree as other anticholinergics.

Scopolamine (C)

As with atropine, scopolamine readily crosses the placenta to the fetus and may produce characteristic fetal tachycardia (24–27). Newborn scopolamine toxicity consisting of fever, tachycardia, lethargy, and a "barrel chested" appearance without respiratory depression was reported in one case where the mother had received 1.8 mg scopolamine during labor (28). The CPP observed 309 first trimester (7, pp. 346–353) and 881 exposures anytime in pregnancy (7, p. 439) without evidence of association with adverse fetal outcome.

Although scopolamine excretion into breast milk has not been reported, the appearance of this anticholinergic in milk should be expected. Vagal blockade in the nursing infant is a theoretical possibility. The American Academy of Pediatrics classifies scopolamine as compatible with breast feeding (23).

Quaternary Anticholinergics

Anisotropine (C) (Valpin 50)
Clidinium (C) (Quarzan)
Glycopyrrolate (B) (Robinul)
Hexocyclium (C) (Tral)
Isopropamide (C) (Darbid)
Mepenzolate (C) (Cantil)
Methantheline (C) (Banthine)
Methscopolamine (C) (Pamine)
Propantheline (C) (Pro-Banthine)
Tridihexethyl (C) (Pathilon)

Quaternary anticholinergics, because they are ionized at physiologic pH, are poorly and erratically absorbed, and cross biologic membranes with difficulty. Little information is available on the use of these agents in human pregnancy, and much of this was obtained from the CPP (7, p. 346). From a total of 50,282 mother-child pairs studied, first trimester drug exposure included anisotropine methylbromide (N = 2), clidinium bromide (N = 4), glycopyrrolate (N = 4), isopropamide (N = 180), mepenzolate bromide (N = 1), methantheline bromide (N = 2), methscopolamine bromide (N = 2), propantheline bromide (N = 33), and tridihexethyl (N = 6). None of these agents was individually associated with a risk of malformations. Although this large study did find a statistically significant association between the total anticholinergic class of drugs, 2,323 exposures during the first trimester, and minor congenital anomalies, the authors cautioned that these data cannot be extrapolated to individual exposures because causal relationships were not established.

In pregnant sheep, the transfer of glycopyrrolate (0.025 mg/kg) across the placenta was significantly less than that of atropine (0.05 mg/kg) (29). Neither drug caused a change in maternal arterial pressure, fetal arterial pressure, fetal heart rate, or beat-to-beat variability. Similar effects were observed in pregnant dogs (30).

Four studies examined the effects of glycopyrrolate on the fetus when it was used before cesarean section to decrease maternal gastric secetions (20, 21, 31, 32). As predicted by its poor placental transfer, the drug had minimal effects on the fetal heart rate and variability, and no anticholinergic effects were observed in the newborn. In animal studies, a dose-related impairment of fertility and survival at weaning were noted, secondary to the potent anticholinergic effects, but the drug was not a teratogen (33, 34).

In animal studies, clidinium and mepenzolate did not impair fertility nor did they cause fetal harm (35, 36). Similarly, from limited data derived from marketing surveillance of both drugs, no adverse reports involving human pregnancies have been reported to the manufacturers (35, 36).

Because of the poor oral absorption of these compounds, little or no drug should appear in breast milk after their use. Intravenous use would produce higher maternal plasma concentrations, and possibly, higher milk concentrations, but the drug would still have to be absorbed from the infant's gastrointestinal tract to produce systemic effects. Thus, the probability of adverse effects in the nursing infant appears to be remote.

ANTIDIARRHEALS
Diphenoxylate/Atropine (C) (Lomotil)

No adverse fetal effects attributable to diphenoxylate, a derivative of meperidine, have been reported (atropine is discussed in *Anticholinergics*). In animal studies using up to 50 times the human dose, an adverse effect on fertility was noted but no teratogenicity (37). The CPP observed no malformed infants after seven first trimester exposures (7, p. 287). Studies of the combination have not been conducted, although there is no reason to expect fetal effects different from those observed with the individual drugs.

Specific information relating to the excretion of diphenoxylate and atropine into breast milk is lacking, but the manufacturer states that diphenoxylate is probably excreted into milk (37). Adverse effects, such as central nervous system depression, decreased gastrointestinal motility, and anticholinergic activity, may potentially occur in a nursing infant, but no reports of these problems have appeared.

Bismuth Subsalicylate (C)
(Pepto-Bismol)
Salicylates (C)

Bismuth subsalicylate is hydrolyzed in the gastrointestinal tract to bismuth salts and sodium salicylate (38, 39). Two tablets or 30 ml suspension of the compound yields 204 and 258 mg, respectively, of salicylate. Inorganic bismuth salts, in contrast to organic complexes of bismuth, are relatively water-insoluble and are poorly absorbed systemically, but significant absorption of salicylate does occur (38, 39). A limited study found minimal absorption of bismuth (exact serum concentrations not specified) from bismuth subsalicylate in 12 healthy subjects (40). However, a peak serum level of 0.050 μg/ml was measured after a dose of 216 mg of colloidal bismuth subcitrate in a single patient (40). Some bismuth absorption was documented across the normal gastric mucosa, but the primary absorption occurred from the duodenum (40). Other investigators, commenting on this study, believe the study design produced the observed results, and that bismuth absorption occurs only in the gastric antrum, not in the gastric body or duodenum (41).

Although absorption of bismuth salts formed by hydrolysis in the gastrointestinal tract is minimal, in a study of chronic administration of bismuth tartrate 5 mg/kg/day, one of four lambs born of treated ewes was stunted, hairless, and exophthalmic, and a second was aborted (42). Moreover, in one case report, the use of an extemporaneously compounded antidiarrheal mixture containing bismuth subsalicylate was associated with bis-

muth encephalopathy in a 60-year-old man who took an unknown amount of the preparation over a 1-month period (43). Encephalopathy was diagnosed by an electroencephalogram characteristics of bismuth toxicity and a blood bismuth level of 72 μg/l (upper limit of normal is 5 μg/l).

No reports of adverse fetal outcome after the use of commercially available bismuth subsalicylate have been located for humans. The CPP recorded 15 first-trimester exposures to bismuth salts (bismuth subgallate [N = 13], bismuth subcarbonate [N = 1], and milk of bismuth [N = 1]), but none to bismuth subsalicylate (7, pp. 384–387). These numbers are small, but no evidence was found to suggest any association with congenital abnormalities. For use anytime during pregnancy, 144 mother-child pairs were exposed to bismuth subgallate, and five of the in utero-exposed infants had inguinal hernia, a hospital standardized relative risk (SRR) of 2.6 (7, pp. 442, 497). A causal relationship, however, cannot be determined from these data.

In contrast to bismuth, salicylate is rapidly absorbed with more than 90% of the dose recovered in the urine. Data on the use of salicylates in human pregnancy, primarily acetylsalicylic acid (aspirin), is extensive. The main concerns from exposure to this drug during pregnancy include congenital defects, increased perinatal mortality from intracranial hemorrhage or premature closure of the ductus arteriosus in utero, intrauterine growth retardation, and salicylate intoxication.

A large prospective study found that 64% of 41,337 pregnant women used salicylates sometime during gestation (44). No evidence was discovered that this use was a cause of stillbirths, neonatal deaths, or reduced birth weight. The difference between the findings of this study and other studies that found positive evidence of fetotoxicity may have related to the chronic or intermittent use of higher doses.

Three large retrospective studies discovered that maternal salicylate use in the first trimester was more common in infants with congenital defects than in mothers of normal infants (9, 45, 46). Several biases have been identified in these studies that might have accounted for the results obtained (44). Moreover, data from the CPP indicated that 14,864 of the mother-child pairs used aspirin during the first trimester and 32,164 (64% of the total sample) used the drug anytime during pregnancy (47). No evidence was found for aspirin-induced teratogenicity, although the data could not exclude the possibility that very large doses were teratogenic. Negative findings for an association between salicylates and congenital anomalies were also reported in an earlier study (48).

Acetylsalicylic acid is known to affect blood clotting ability by suppressing collagen-induced platelet aggregation as a consequence of its antiprostaglandin activity. Due to this activity, an increased risk of intracranial hemorrhage in premature or low birth weight infants may be a potential complication of maternal aspirin use near delivery (49). However, other salicylates, including sodium salicylate, may not be a cause of this condition because the presence of the acetyl moiety is apparently required to suppress platelet function (50–52).

The use of salicylates (but not acetaminophen) in the second and third trimesters may cause premature closure of the ductus arteriosus, resulting in primary pulmonary hypertension of the newborn and, possibly, neonatal death in severe cases. When the fetal ductus arteriosus closes, blood is shunted from the right ventricle into the pulmonary vessels causing pulmonary arterial hypertrophy. After birth, persistent fetal circulation occurs due to the pulmonary hypertension forcing blood to be shunted through the foramen ovale, bypassing the lungs.

To summarize, the bismuth moiety apparently presents little or no risk to the fetus from normal therapeutic doses, but the data available for bismuth in pregnancy are poor and the actual fetal risk cannot be determined (53). However, the potential actions of salicylates on the fetus are complex and, although the risk for toxicity may be small, significant fetal adverse effects may result. Because of this, the use of bismuth subsalicylate during gestation

should be restricted to the first half of pregnancy, and then only in amounts that do not exceed the recommended dose.

The excretion of large amounts of exogenous bismuth into breast milk should not occur because of the poor absorption of bismuth into the systemic circulation. However, salicylates do appear in milk and are eliminated more slowly from milk than from plasma with milk:plasma ratios rising from 0.03–0.08 at 3 hours to 0.34 at 12 hours (54). Due to the potential for adverse effects in the nursing infant, the American Academy of Pediatrics recommends that salicylates should be used cautiously during breast feeding (23). A recent review also states that bismuth subsalicylate should be avoided during lactation because of systemic salicylate absorption (55).

Kaolin/Pectin (C) (Kaopectate)

Kaolin is a hydrated aluminum silicate clay used for its adsorbant properties in diarrhea and pectin is a polysaccharide obtained from plant tissues that is used as a solidifying agent. Neither agent is absorbed into the systemic circulation. Although no reports have related the use of the kaolin/pectin mixture in pregnancy with adverse fetal outcome, there have been reports of iron deficiency anemia and hypokalemia secondary to the eating of clays (i.e., geophagia) containing kaolin (56–58). The mechanism for this is thought to be either a reduction in the intake of foods containing absorbable iron or an interference with the absorption of iron. In humans, iron deficiency anemia may significantly enhance the chance for a low birth weight infant and preterm delivery (59).

Female rats fed a diet containing 20% kaolin became anemic and delivered pups with a significant decrease in birth weight (60). When an iron supplement was added to the kaolin fortified diet, no anemia or reduced birth weight was observed.

Other than producing anemia in the mother after prolonged, chronic use, the kaolin/pectin mixture should have no effect on lactation or the nursing infant.

Lactobacillus (C) (Lactinex)

Lactobacillus is a viable culture of the naturally occurring metabolic products produced by *Lactobacillus acidophilus* and *Lactobacillus bulgaricus*. No information is available on the use of this product in pregnancy or lactation, but the risks to the fetus and nursing infant are probably nil.

Loperamide (B) (Imodium)

The synthetic antidiarrheal agent, loperamide, acts directly in the bowel to slow intestinal motility and inhibit peristaltic activity. Not only is it poorly absorbed from the gastrointestinal tract, but it penetrates the central nervous system poorly (61). No information is available on the placental passage of this drug, but it is probably minimal due to the very low plasma concentrations (in the range of <2 ng/ml after a 2-mg dose) that occur after oral dosing. In animals, no evidence of impaired fertility or fetotoxic effects were observed with loperamide doses exceeding those used in humans (62).

Small amounts of loperamide are excreted in human breast milk. Six non-breast-feeding women, a mean 29 hours after delivery, were given loperamide oxide 4 mg 12 hours apart (63). Loperamide oxide is a pharmacologically inactive prodrug that is slowly converted in vivo to loperamide (63). Mean milk levels of loperamide and the milk:plasma ratios 12 hours after the first dose, and 6 and 36 hours after the second dose were 0.18 ng/ml (0.50), 0.27 ng/ml (0.37), and 0.19 ng/ml (0.35), respectively. Loperamide oxide was not detected in any of the milk samples. Although the amounts measured are very small, no data are available for loperamide excretion after administration of the active drug, or with either drug later in the postpartum period with more mature milk. The effects of the exposure on the nursing infant are also unknown, but are probably not clinically significant in full-term, normal weight infants.

Opium (B)

Opium is a mixture of alkaloids of which morphine is the most important agent responsible for the antidiarrheal properties. The CPP monitored 36 first trimester (7, pp. 287–295) and 181 anytime during pregnancy (7, pp. 434, 485) exposures to opium. Four of the newborns exposed in the first trimester had congenital anomalies and seven infants had an inguinal hernia after exposure anytime during gestation. No conclusions could be drawn from the first trimester data. After anytime use, a possible association between opium and inguinal hernia was suggested (SRR 2.9), but the numbers were too small to determine if a causal relationship existed. No reports associating the use of morphine in pregnancy with major congenital abnormalities have been located. However, in 448 exposures observed anytime during pregnancy, the CPP found a possible association (SRR 1.7) between morphine and inguinal hernia in 10 infants (7, p. 484).

As should be predicted, fetal addiction with neonatal withdrawal has been reported when the mother was treated with opium for prolonged periods in the latter part of pregnancy (64, 65). Only trace amounts of morphine enter breast milk and the American Academy of Pediatrics classifies morphine as compatible with breast feeding (23).

Paregoric (B)

Paregoric is a mixture of opium powder, anise oil, benzoic acid, camphor, glycerin, and ethanol. Its antidiarrheal effects, as with opium, are primarily due to morphine. In the CPP, 90 fetuses were exposed to paregoric during the first trimester (7, pp. 287–295) and 562 anytime during pregnancy (7, p. 434). No evidence was found to suggest a relationship to major or minor malformations or to individual defects. Prolonged use near term may lead to fetal addiction and resulting withdrawal symptoms in the newborn (66).

Morphine, the principle antidiarrheal agent of paregoric, is excreted in small amounts into milk. Alcohol, which freely passes into milk, may produce dose-related toxicity in a nursing infant but the small amounts contained in paregoric probably have no effect when normal doses of the antidiarrheal drug are consumed by the mother. No information is available on the other components of paregoric. The American Academy of Pediatrics classifies morphine as compatible with breast feeding (23).

ANTIEMETICS

Buclizine (C) (Bucladin-S)
Cyclizine (B) (Marezine)
Hydroxyzine (C) (Atarax; Vistaril)
Meclizine (B) (Antivert; Bonine)

These agents are piperazine antihistamines that are used as antiemetics. All are teratogenic in rats producing a syndrome consisting of cleft palate, micrognathia, microstomia, and glossopalatine fusion (67, pp. 388–389). The metabolite, norchlorcyclizine, may be the actual teratogenic agent (68, 69). The possible mechanism of the oral-facial malformations may be due to the edema produced by the drug and the resulting pressures induced by the fluid-enlarged tissues disrupting development (70). Ocular defects have also been observed after cyclizine exposure in rats, rabbits, and mice (67, pp. 388–389). Cleft palate was produced by hydroxyzine in mice (71). Hydroxyzine and cyclizine have caused abortions in nonhuman primate studies with monkeys (67, pp. 388–389; 72).

In the early 1960s, a large number of case reports and letters argued over the effects of meclizine on the human fetus (73–100). Several large prospective and retrospective studies, however, have provided evidence that this class of drugs is not teratogenic in humans (7, 9, 101–104).

The CPP observed a number of exposures to these agents both during and after the first trimester. Exposures to buclizine involved 44 during the first trimester (7, pp. 323–324) and 62 anytime during pregnancy (7, p. 437). Three infants with congenital malformations were noted after first trimester use, but the relationship between buclizine and the defects is unknown. Among 113 pregnancies exposed to miscellaneous antihistamines, cyclizine was used by 15 and a total of 5 infants from this group had congenital defects (7, pp. 323–324). Hydroxyzine exposure consisted of 50 during the first trimester (7, pp. 335–337) and 187 anytime during pregnancy (7, p. 438). Six of the exposed pregnancies delivered an infant with defects, but the significance of these findings cannot be determined from this study. The largest number of exposures recorded in this group of antihistamines was for meclizine with 1,014 exposed during the first trimester (7, p. 328) and 1,463 anytime during pregnancy (7, p. 437). No evidence was found in either case to suggest a relationship to large categories of major or minor malformations. Possible associations were discovered with individual defects, but the significance is unknown, and independent confirmation is required to determine the actual risk: respiratory defects (7 cases), eye and ear defects (7 cases), inguinal hernia (18 cases), hypoplasia cordis (3 cases), and hypoplastic left heart syndrome (3 cases).

The Food and Drug Administration's Over-the-Counter Laxative Panel, acting on the above data for cyclizine and meclizine, concluded that these two agents are not teratogenic (101). A study published in 1974 found no relationship between the cyclizine group of drugs and oral clefts (102). Another retrospective study, published 3 years earlier, actually found that fewer infants with anomalies were exposed to antihistamines/antiemetics in the first trimester as compared with control infants (9). Meclizine was the third most commonly used antiemetic and cyclizine was the fifth. Finally, two large prospective studies involving 613 (103) and 628 (105) first trimester exposures found no relationship between meclizine and congenital anomalies.

The use of hydroxyzine in labor (75 mg intramuscularly) has been associated with a clinically significant decrease in fetal heart rate variability (106). An isolated case of neonatal withdrawal lasting for approximately 5 days, presumably secondary to hydroxyzine, has been reported (107). The mother had taken 600 mg of the drug throughout gestation for severe eczema and asthma. The mother was also treated with phenobarbital during the last 3 weeks of pregnancy for mild preeclampsia.

The concentrations of hydoxyzine and phenobarbital in the cord blood were 1.8 μg/ml (usual therapeutic adult level 0.50 μg/ml) and 0.10 μg/ml, respectively (107).

Although no evidence has been found, after careful study, to support the original contention that these agents are teratogenic, use of antihistamines near the end of pregnancy may present a risk to the fetus/newborn. The use of antihistamines (specific agents were not identified) during the last 2 weeks of pregnancy has been associated with retrolental fibroplasia in otherwise normal premature infants weighing less than 1750 g and who survived for at least 24 hours after birth (108). Compared to 2940 controls, 324 (11%) of whom were affected, 19 of 86 (22%) study infants developed the disease. Adjustment for severity of disease did not change the estimated risk ratio.

None of this group of antihistamines has been studied during lactation, and it is not known if these agents cross into breast milk in sufficient quantities to produce adverse effects in a nursing infant.

Dimenhydrinate (B) (Dramamine)

Dimenhydrinate is the clorotheophylline salt of diphenhydramine. The antihistamine is not teratogenic at a dose of 75 mg/kg/day in rats (109). Human studies have also failed to implicate this agent with congenital malformations (7, 89, 105, 110).

Dimenhydrinate usage was compared in 266 infants with anomalies and two normal control groups of 266 each in a 1963 prospective study (89). No difference in the usage of the drug between the three groups was discovered. The CPP recorded 319 first trimester exposures (7, pp. 367–370) to dimenhydrinate and 697 anytime during pregnancy (7, p. 440). No evidence was found to suggest a relationship to large categories of major or minor abnormalities, but two possible associations were discovered for individual anomalies: cardiovascular defects (5 cases) and inguinal hernia (8 cases). Due to the design of this study, evaluation of the actual risk and statistical significance of these associations

cannot be determined. Use of the drug and various other antiemetics for the treatment of hyperemesis gravidarum in 64 women presenting with the condition before 13 weeks' gestation has been reported (110). Although the defects were not thought to be related to the drug therapy, three infants had integumentary abnormalities consisting of webbed toes with an extra finger (1 case), and skin tags (2 cases). A large cohort study conducted between 1964–1976 observed major malformations in only 11 infants who had been exposed to dimenhydrinate and three other antiemetics during the first 10 weeks' of gestation, compared to 12 infants from matched controls (105).

Intravenous dimenhydrinate during labor has been reported to produce oxytocic effects on the uterus (111). Moreover, use of any antihistamine in the final 2 weeks of gestation may be associated with retrolent fibroplasia in premature infants (see discussion under *Buclizine*).

No reports have been located that describe the effects, if any, on the nursing infant from dimenhydrinate obtained from breast milk. Similarly, it is not known if the drug is excreted into milk.

Diphenhydramine (C) (Benadryl)

As with its salt form above, diphenhydramine is not an animal teratogen in studies with rats and rabbits (112). During the CPP, a total of 595 women consumed the drug during the first trimester (7, pp. 323–337) and 2,948 exposures were recorded anytime during gestation (7, p. 437). No evidence was discovered to suggest a relationship to large categories of major or minor anomalies, but a number of possible associations were found for individual defects (7, pp. 323–337, 437, 475): genitourinary (other than hypospadias (5 cases), hypospadias (3 cases), eye and ear defects (3 cases), syndromes other than Down's syndrome (3 cases), inguinal hernia (13 cases), clubfoot (5 cases), any ventricular septal defect (open or closing) (5 cases), and malformations of the diaphragm (3 cases). Due to the design of the study, evaluation of the actual risk and statistical significance of these associations cannot be determined without confirming studies, which have not appeared.

A 1974 case control study of 599 children with cleft palate compared to 590 controls without clefts associated first trimester diphenhydramine usage with cleft palate, 20 cases versus 6 cases, a statistically significant difference (102). However, a 1971 study, in which diphenhydramine was the second most commonly used antihistamine, reported significantly fewer infants with malformations were exposed to antihistamines as compared to controls (9). A prospective study published in 1976 observed 46 women with nausea and vomiting in the first trimester who were treated with diphenhydramine (104). Four of the newborns had minor malformations and three had "insignificant major defects" (no description of the defects was given), but this did not differ statistically from controls (104). In a study of 6509 women, 270 consumed diphenhydramine during the first trimester and no association was found with congenital malformations (113).

Problems reported with diphenhydramine, other than congenital defects, include withdrawal in a newborn (mother consumed 150 mg/day during pregnancy) (114), and a possible interaction with temazepam resulting in fetal death (115). As with dimenhydrinate, intravenous use of diphenhydramine during labor has been shown to produce oxytocic effects (111). Finally, use of antihistamines in the last 2 weeks of gestation has been associated with retrolental fibroplasia in premature infants (see discussion under *Buclizine*).

Diphenhydramine is excreted into breast milk (116), but information as to the amounts appearing in milk has not been published. Newborn or premature infants are especially sensitive to antihistamines, and the avoidance of the drug during this period is probably best for the nursing infant.

Droperidol (C) (Inapsine)

Droperidol is a butyrophenone derivative that is structurally related to haloperidol. The drug is not teratogenic in animals, but a slight increase in newborn rat mortality was observed secondary to maternal central nervous system depression (117). No reports of adverse fetal outcome in humans have been located.

When used during labor as a sedative, droperidol crosses the placenta slowly (118). The agent has been used as a continuous intravenous infusion by the authors for the treatment of hyperemesis gravidarum (GG Briggs, unpublished data, 1993). No adverse effects in the fetus or newborn attributable to droperidol have been observed. An extrapyramidal syndrome, which has occurred in pregnant women treated with the drug (GG Briggs, unpublished data, 1993), has not been observed in the newborn exposed in utero to droperidol.

It is not known if droperidol is excreted into breast milk. The closely related drug, haloperidol, does appear in milk and excretion of droperidol should be expected. Sedation in the nursing infant is a potential adverse effect.

Ondansetron (C) (Zofran)

Ondansetron is a highly selective and potent $5-HT_3$-receptor antagonist that is used in the prevention of chemotherapy- and radiation therapy-induced emesis as well as for treatment of postoperative nausea and vomiting. It is not teratogenic in animals but there is only limited experience in human pregnancies. The drug was successfully used in a primigravida with life-threatening hyperemesis gravidarum unresponsive to other antiemetics (118a). Ondansetron in a dose of 8 mg was administered intravenously three times daily for 14 days during the 11th–13th weeks of gestation, until the patient could eat and drink normally. A full-term healthy infant was born without incident. At present, however, the manufacturer does not recommend its use in pregnancy, especially during the first trimester.

Prochlorperazine (C) (Compazine)

In one rat study, this piperazine phenothiazine produced significant postnatal weight decrease, increased fetal mortality, and minor behavioral changes, but no structural defects (119). In a second rat study, an increased incidence of cleft palate, a few anencephalic defects, and one double monster were observed (120).

Prochlorperazine readily crosses the placenta to the fetus (121). Several studies have found the drug to be safe during human gestation, including when it was used for the treatment of nausea and vomiting of pregnancy (9, 103, 104, 122–124). A prospective study published in 1976 observed 91 exposures to prochlorperazine in women with first trimester nausea and vomiting (104). Eight newborns had minor malformations and two had "insignificant major malformations" (descriptions of the defects were not given), but this did not differ statistically from controls (104). The CPP recorded 877 first trimester exposures and 2,023 anytime during gestation (123). Although two infants exposed in utero during the first trimester had defects (cleft palate, micrognathia, congenital heart defects, and skeletal defects in one; thanatophoric dwarfism or short limb syndrome in one), there was no evidence linking the use of prochlorperazine to these or other congenital anomalies, or adverse outcomes relating to perinatal mortality rate, birth weight, or intelligence quotient scores at 4 years old. The case of dwarfism was probably due to genetic factors. In another study, no increase in defects or pattern of malformations were observed in 74 infants exposed in utero to the antiemetic (124). In a 1971 retrospective study of 1369 pregnant women, significantly fewer mothers of infants with major anomalies took antiemetics during the first trimester in comparison to mothers of normal babies (9). Prochlorperazine was the third most commonly ingested antiemetic. An extrapyramidal syndrome, which may occur in the mother, has not been reported in the newborn after in utero exposure to prochlorperazine.

Four case reports have described limb defects in infants exposed in utero to prochlorperazine (125–128). A case of phocomelia of the upper limbs, reported in 1963, involved the use for 2–3 days of another phenothiazine

agent, trifluoperazine, at about 4 weeks of gestation (125). Prochlorperazine therapy was initiated at about 13 weeks' gestation and, thus, cannot be related to the defect. A second case report described an infant with hypoplasia of the left radius and ulnar bones with a vestigial wrist and hand after in utero exposure to prochlorperazine from 7–9 weeks of gestation (126). The third report involved two infants who were both exposed before 12 weeks of gestation to the antiemetic (127). A below-elbow amputation in one arm and a small atrophic hand attached to the stump was observed in one infant, whereas the second infant had a below-knee amputation with a rudimentary foot attached to the stump (127). The twin of the latter infant was normal. No evidence of amniotic bands was observed in either case. An infant girl had multiple defects composed of cleft palate, micrognathia, Wormian bones, congenital heart disease, dislocated hips, absent tibiae, bowed fibulae, preaxial polydactyly of the feet, and abnormal dermal patterns in a case involving exposure to congugated estrogens and prochlorperazine early in gestation (128). The authors of the report could not determine the cause of the malformations, except that a relationship to the drugs could not be excluded.

No reports relating to the passage of prochlorperazine into human breast milk have been located, but the drug has been found in the milk of lactating dogs (116). Inasmuch as other phenothiazines appear in human milk (e.g., chlorpromazine), excretion of prochlorperazine should be expected. Although sedation is a possible effect in the nursing infant, the amounts of phenothiazines that have been measured are so small that adverse effects are unlikely (129).

Promethazine (C) (Phenergan)

This phenothiazine antihistamine has been used as an antiemetic during pregnancy. The CPP observed 114 first trimester exposures (7, pp. 323–324) and 746 anytime during pregnancy (7, p. 437). No evidence associating this drug with large classes of major or minor defects or to individual anomalies was discovered. A 1964 report examined the effects of first trimester promethazine exposure in 165 cases and failed to find an association with congenital anomalies (130). In another study, mothers who consumed antiemetics during the first trimester, promethazine was the most common agent, actually had fewer infants with congenital defects when compared with control subjects (9).

A woman, who conceived after multiple courses of clomiphene for ovulation stimulation, was treated with promethazine during the first trimester for nausea and vomiting (131). She delivered a stillborn anencephalic female fetus who also had cervical spina bifida, pronounced kyphoscoliosis of the thoracic spine, and mild bilateral hydronephrosis (131). The association between the drugs and the defects cannot be determined. A prospective study of the treatment of nausea and vomiting in pregnancy was published in 1976 (104). A total of 617 women were treated with promethazine resulting in 538 normal newborns, 52 with "minor malformations," 16 with "insignificant major malformations," and 11 with "gross major malformations" (104). Descriptions of the defects observed in the promethazine-treated women were not given, except that antiemetics, primarily promethazine, were used by most of women delivering an infant with congenital dislocation of the hip. The investigators attributed the etiology to either endocrine disturbances, such as elevated maternal hormonal levels, or to genetic factors, but an association with promethazine could not be excluded (104).

At term, promethazine rapidly crosses the placenta and establishes equilibrium with the maternal circulation within 15 minutes (24). When used in labor, neonatal respiratory depression has been reported (132), but other large studies did not observe this adverse effect (133–135). A 1962 study, however, concluded that the use of the phenothiazines, promethazine or promazine, in labor could cause neonatal jaundice if the mother delivered a premature infant (136). The proposed mechanism for the adverse effect was fetal hypoxia

superimposed upon an immature liver (136). A study in four infants, ages 11–22 weeks, given promethazine syrup (1 mg/kg/day) found that the drug depresses the arousal and respiratory mechanisms during sleep, and could result in sudden death in apnea-prone infants (137).

Promethazine use during labor has also been shown to markedly impair platelet aggregation in the newborn, but less so in the mother (138, 139), and to produce a clinically significant reduction in fetal heart rate variability after an intravenous dose of 25 mg (140). The degree of platelet impairment in the newborn is comparable to that associated with a definite bleeding state, but the lack of additional studies of this effect prevents evaluation of its clinical significance. One author, however, concluded that promethazine should be avoided in labor because of the potential for respiratory depression and the effect on platelet aggregation (141).

No reports describing the passage of promethazine into human breast milk have been located, but the presence of this drug in milk should be expected. Sedation in the nursing infant is a potential adverse effect.

Trimethobenzamide (C) (Tigan)

Trimethobenzamide is not teratogenic in rats and rabbits, but an increase in embryonic resorptions and stillborns were observed (142). In two human studies, the use of trimethobenzamide to treat nausea and vomiting of pregnancy was not associated with adverse effects in the fetus or newborn (143, 144). In a third study, 193 women were treated with the antiemetic during the first trimester and the incidences of severe congenital defects at 1 month, 1 year, and 5 years were 2.6, 2.6, and 5.8%, respectively (103). The latter figure, in comparison to the 3.2% observed in controls, was statistically significant, but other factors, including the use of other antiemetics, may have contributed to the results. No reports describing the passage of trimethobenzamide into human breast milk have been located.

ANTIFLATULENTS

Simethicone (C) (Mylicon)

Although the manufacturer does not report animal studies, the silicone antiflatulent, simethicone, is apparently not absorbed from the gastrointestinal tract and presents minimal risk to the fetus from maternal use. Inasmuch as there is no systemic absorption of this agent, no excretion in breast milk can occur.

Charcoal (A)

This is a local-acting product with no known fetal risk in pregnancy or to the nursing infant during breast feeding.

ORAL ANTI-INFECTIVE AGENTS

Metronidazole (B) (Flagyl)

Metonidazole crosses the placenta to the fetus with a cord:maternal plasma ratio of approximately 1.0 (145–147). A 1960 study in pregnant rats using 100 mg/kg/day throughout gestation observed no changes in the number of viable offspring or malformations (148). Mutagenic activity was observed, however, in the *Salmonella typhimurium* test using urine from patients taking metronidazole (149). The value of this test is still open to question, according to some investigators who have found that about half of the chemicals found to be mutagenic in bacterial tests are animal teratogens (67, p. 426).

Because of the bacterial mutagenicity and carcinogenic effects in rodents, some authors have suggested that metronidazole should not be used in human pregnancy (150, 151). However, no association with human cancer and metronidazole has been proven (151, 152). Although human studies have not been reported, metronidazole has been shown to markedly potentiate the fetotoxicity and teratogenicity of alcohol in mice (153).

Two large reviews evaluated the published results of metronidazole exposure in over 3600 pregnancies (154, 155). No evidence was found in these studies for an increase in malformations, abortions, or stillbirths. In contrast, some studies have reported an increased incidence of congenital anomalies after exposure to metronidazole in the first trimester (7, 152, 156–158). The CPP observed four infants with defects after 31 first trimester exposures to the drug, a SRR of 2.02 (7, pp. 298, 299, 302). The significance of this finding is unknown. The use of metronidazole in 57 pregnancies, 23 during the first trimester, was described in 1979 (152). Three of the pregnancies were ended by spontaneous abortions, a normal incidence. In the remaining 20 cases, five infants had defects, some of which appeared to be related to genetic factors (152). Two mothers, treated with the anti-infective in the first trimester gave birth to infants with midline facial defects; holotelencephaly in one and unilateral cleft lip and palate in the other (156). One of the mothers had also received diiodohydroxyquinoline during the first trimester. In another case, an infant with a cleft of the hard and soft palate, optic atrophy, a hypoplastic, short philtrum, and a Sydney crease on the left-hand was exposed in utero to metronidazole between the 6th and 7th weeks of gestation (157). The relationship between the above anomalies and metronidazole is unknown.

In data collected between 1980 and 1983 from the Michigan Medicaid program involving 55,736 deliveries, 1,020 cases of first trimester metronidazole exposure for the treatment of vaginitis were not linked, and 63 cases were linked, with birth defects (158). The estimated relative risk of a birth defect, based on these data, was 0.92 (95% confidence limits 0.7–1.2). A total of 122 infants had oral clefts, none of whom were exposed to metronidazole. Of the 4,264 spontaneous abortions observed, 135 had been treated with metronidazole, an estimated relative risk of 1.67 (95% confidence limits 1.4–2.0). The investigators also cited data from the Food and Drug Administration involving 27 reports of adverse outcomes with metronidazole exposure during gestation including spontaneous abortions (three), brain defects (six), limb defects (five), genital defects (four), unspecified defects (three), and one each of craniostenosis, peripheral neuropathy, ventricular septal defects, retinoblastoma, obstructive uropathy, and a chromosomal defect (158).

Metronidazole is excreted into breast milk with milk:plasma ratios of approximately 1.0. A 2-g oral dose produces peak milk concentrations in the 50–60 μg/ml range (159). With normal breast feeding, after such a dose, an infant would ingest about 25 mg of metronidazole over the next 48 hours. Discontinuing feeding for 12 hours after a 2-g oral dose would reduce the infant's exposure to 9.8 mg, and to 3.5 mg if stopped for 24 hours (159). Divided oral doses of 600 or 1200 mg/day produces mean milk levels of 5.7 and 14.4 μg/ml, respectively (160). No adverse effects in nursing infants of mothers consuming metronidazole have been reported, except for a single case of diarrhea and secondary lactose intolerance in a breast-fed infant where the relationship between the effects and the drug could not be established (161). The American Academy of Pediatrics recommends discontinuing breast feeding for 12–24 hours if a single 2-g oral dose is given to the mother for the treatment of trichomonas (23). No recommendation is made, however, with other dosing regimens.

Vancomycin (C) (Vancocin)

Animal studies have not been conducted with vancomycin. After intravenous therapy in humans, vancomycin crosses the placenta (162). In two newborns, cord blood levels were 13.2 and 16.7 μg/ml, 2.5 and 6 hours, respectively, after a 1-g dose. Chronic intravenous dosing has the potential to produce ototoxicity and renal dysfunction in the fetus/newborn if toxic levels are maintained in the mother, but this has not been reported. The lack of reports may be more related to the relative infrequent use of this antibiotic in the pregnant patient and the prevention of toxic levels, rather than a statement of its potential toxicity.

In contrast to intravenous therapy, oral vancomycin treatment poses little risk to the fetus due to its very poor absorption from the gastrointestinal tract. Oral therapy is indicated only for staphylococcal enterocolitis and antibiotic-associated pseudomembranous colitis due to *Clostridium difficile*.

Vancomycin is excreted into breast milk after intravenous therapy with a milk:plasma ratio of nearly 1.0 (162). Appearance of the antibiotic in milk after oral therapy should not be expected due to the poor absorption.

ANTISECRETORY AGENTS

Cimetidine (B) (Tagamet)

This reversible histamine H_2-receptor antagonist has been used in all trimesters of pregnancy without causing adverse fetal effects attributable to the drug. In studies with multiple animal species, no evidence of impaired fertility or teratogenesis was observed with doses much greater than used in humans.

Cimetidine does have weak antiandrogenic effects in animals, as shown by a reduction in the size of testes, prostatic glands, and seminal vesicles (163, 164), and in humans, by reports of decreased libido and impotence (165). Conflicting reports on the antiandrogenic activity in animals exposed in utero to cimetidine have been published (166–170). Three references, all from the same research group, described the effects on male rats of exposure to cimetidine from in utero up to the time of weaning (166–168). The exposed rats had decreased weights of testicles, prostate glands, and seminal vesicles at 55 and 110 days of age as compared to nonexposed controls. Exposed animals also had reduced testosterone serum levels, lack of sexual motivation, and decreased sexual performance, but normal luteinizing hormone levels. The observed demasculinization effects were still present 35 days after discontinuation of the drug, indicating that exposure may have modified both central and end-organ androgen receptor activity or responsiveness (166–168). In contrast, researchers from the manufacturer treated rats similarly to the above reports and found no effect on any of the parameters described previously in male rats exposed to cimetidine in utero and during lactation (169). Another group found no effect of cimetidine exposure during gestation and lactation on masculine sexual development, except for an insensitivity of the pituitary gland to androgen regulation, and no effect at all on female pups (170). These authors concluded that cimetidine was not a teratogen.

Cimetidine crosses the placenta to the fetus (171–174). No placental metabolism of cimetidine occurs (171). At term, the peak fetal:maternal serum ratio, 0.84, occurred at 1.5–2.0 hours (172). An in vitro study using isolated perfused human placentas found a fetal:maternal ratio of 0.46 at 2 hours indicating that placental transfer of the drug was slow (175).

As of 1986, the manufacturer had received a number of reports on the use of cimetidine throughout gestation without causing fetal harm. Long-term follow-up of infants exposed in utero, however, have not been published. Although there was no evidence that cimetidine contributed to the outcomes, three infants with congenital defects had been reported: congenital heart disease, mental retardation detected later in life, and clubfoot (B. Dickson, personal communication, Smith Kline & French Laboratories, 1986). However, because of the lack of human data, an assessment of the teratogenic risk cannot be made (176).

The primary use of cimetidine in pregnancy is to prevent maternal gastric acid aspiration pneumonitis (Mendelson's syndrome) before delivery (174, 177–193). Transient liver impairment in a newborn was attributed to the antihistamine in a 1980 reference after in utero exposure to cimetidine at term (194). However, this adverse effect has not been confirmed by numerous other studies and case reports.

In a study using lactating mice, drug metabolizing enzymes in nursing pups were inhibited much more by cimetidine than those in the mother (195). Mouse dams were treated with cimetidine from the delivery date to 6 weeks, the time of weaning. Male pups were adversely affected from 4 weeks of age to 8 weeks, 2 weeks after cessation of exposure, although female pups were affected for a greater time, commencing at 2 weeks of age and continuing up to 8–10 weeks. The effects on enzyme activity were completely gone in both sexes at 10 weeks of age.

The pharmacokinetics of cimetidine transfer into the milk of rats and rabbits was studied in a 1992 reference (196). The study results indicated that cimetidine transport into rabbit milk was by simple diffusion, whereas the transfer into rat milk may involve active transport (196).

Cimetidine is concentrated in human breast milk after single and multiple dosing with milk concentrations up to seven-times that found in the mother's plasma (197). No adverse effects have been observed in nursing infants whose mothers were consuming the drug. Theoretically, several adverse effects may occur in the nursing infant, including an effect on gastric acidity, impaired drug metabolism (as indicated by the animal study described above), and central nervous system stimulation. Cimetidine was originally listed by the American Academy of Pediatrics as contraindicated during lactation (198). However, in the absence of adverse reports, the American Academy of Pediatrics has reclassified cimetidine as compatible with breast feeding (23, 199).

Famotidine (B) (Pepcid)

No reports on the use of the reversible histamine H_2-receptor antagonist, famotidine, in human pregnancy have appeared in the medical literature, but studies in rats and rabbits, using oral doses up to 2000 mg/kg/day and intravenous doses of 100–200 mg/kg/day, have found no evidence of impaired fertility, fetotoxic effects, or changes in postnatal behavior attributable to the drug (200, 201). The drug is known to cross the term human placenta based on in vitro studies (202).

Famotidine is more potent than cimetidine or ranitidine and, thus, smaller doses can be used with the advantage described in the section below for ranitidine. Due to the lack of human pregnancy experience with this agent, however, no recommendations can be made regarding its use during gestation.

Famotidine is concentrated in breast milk, but to a lesser degree than either cimetidine or ranitidine (203). After a single 40-mg dose administered to eight postpartum women who were not planning to breast feed, the mean milk:plasma ratios at 2, 6, and 24 hours were 0.41, 1.78, and 1.33, respectively. The mean peak milk concentration, 72 ng/ml, occurred at 6 hours compared with 2 hours for plasma (mean 75 ng/ml). Exposure of the nursing infant to famotidine via milk has not been reported and although a potential risk may exist for adverse effects, another drug in this class, cimetidine, is considered compatible with breast feeding by the American Academy of Pediatrics (see under *Cimetidine*).

Misoprostol (X) (Cytotec)

Misoprostol is a synthetic prostaglandin E_1 analog used to prevent gastric ulcers induced by nonsteroidal anti-inflammatory agents. The drug is contraindicated in pregnancy. Although not fetotoxic or teratogenic in rats and rabbits at doses much higher than those used in humans, misoprostol, in the pregnant patient, may induce uterine bleeding and contractions resulting in abortion (204).

Misoprostol has been combined with the antiprogestogen mifepristone (RU 486) to induce legal abortion (205–207), and, as a single agent, has been misused as an illegal abortifacient (208). This latter use was reportedly associated with an unusual congenital malformation in five infants consisting of an asymmetrical, well-circumscribed anomaly of the cranium and overlying scalp, exposing the dura mater and underlying cerebrum (209). Other investigators have not observed congenital abnormalities after first trimester attempts at abortion with misoprostol (210).

No studies evaluating the passage of misoprostol or its active metabolite, misoprostol acid, into milk have been found. The manufacturer considers the drug contraindicated during nursing because of the potential for severe, drug-induced diarrhea in the nursing infant (204).

Nizatidine (C) (Axid)

No reports on the use of this reversible histamine H_2-receptor antagonist in human pregnancy are known. The drug is three times more potent than cimetidine (211). In pregnant rats and rabbits given oral doses up to 506 mg/kg/day, no adverse effects were observed on fertility, and no teratogenic effects occurred with doses up to 1,500 mg/kg/day, although some abortions occurred in rabbits, but not rats, at the highest dose (212). In contrast, the manufacturer's product information describes congenital malformations observed in two fetuses of pregnant New Zealand white rabbits administered nizatidine intravenously in doses of 20 and 50 mg/kg, respectively (213). Defects in the fetus exposed to the lower dose consisted of cardiac enlargement, coarctation of the aortic arch, and cutaneous edema, and those after the higher dose were a ventricular anomaly, enlarged heart, distended abdomen, spina bifida, and hydrocephaly (213).

Based on studies in male humans (214) and animals (215, 216), nizatidine does not appear to have antiadrogenic effects such as those observed with cimetidine. Reversible impotence, however, has been described in men treated with nizatidine for therapeutic indications (217).

In an in vitro study, nizatidine crossed the human placenta at approximately the same rate and quantities observed for cimetidine, famotidine, and ranitidine (202). No clinical studies of placental transfer, however, have been published.

Although the above animal data relating to teratogenesis cannot be directly extrapolated to humans, it is probably safer to use either cimetidine or ranitidine in the pregnant woman, if a H_2-receptor antagonist is required, because neither of these agents is an animal teratogen and human experience with these drugs is much more extensive.

During lactation, very small amounts of nizatidine are excreted into breast milk (218). The total amount of excretion in milk collected over a 12-hour period after single and multiple doses of 150 mg was 0.064% of the mother's dose, an amount that probably presents minimal risks to a nursing infant.

Omeprazole (C) (Prilosec)

The antisecretory agent, omeprazole, suppresses gastric acid secretion by a direct inhibitory effect on the gastric parietal cell (219). In animals, doses up to approximately 375 times the normal human dose produced no evidence of teratogenicity, although dose-related fetotoxicity was observed (219). Omeprazole crosses both animal (220) and human placentas (221) to the fetus.

Twenty women were administered a single 80-mg oral dose the night before scheduled cesarean sections with a dosing to general anesthesia induction time interval mean of 853 minutes (range of 765–977 minutes) (221). At the time of surgery, maternal omeprazole levels ranged from 0–271 nmol/l. The drug concentration in 13 of the 20 infants (both arterial and venous umbilical samples were drawn in most cases) was either 0 or below the minimum detection limit (20 nmol/l). In the remaining seven infants, omeprazole cord blood concentrations ranged from 21–109 nmol/l. No adverse effects attributable to the drug were observed either at birth or at follow-up in 7 days.

No information is available on the excretion of omeprazole into breast milk. Suppression of gastric acid secretion is a potential effect in the nursing infant, but the clinical significance of this is undetermined.

Ranitidine (B) (Zantac)

The published experience in human pregnancy with raniditine is less than with cimetidine, but this reversible antihistamine H_2-antagonist also appears to be safe to use in the pregnant patient. Ranitidine crosses the placenta to the fetus with mean fetal:maternal ratios after 50 mg intravenously and 150 mg orally of 0.9 and 0.38, respectively (222–224).

Animal studies at doses much higher than those used in humans have revealed no evidence of impaired fertility or teratogenesis. In contrast to the controversy surrounding cimetidine, ranitidine apparently has no anti-

androgenic activity in humans (225) or in animals (226, 227). Another theoretical advantage is its greater potency in comparison to cimetidine. Because it is more potent, smaller doses can be used resulting in lower molar concentrations and less potential to induce reversible inhibition of oxidative enzymes in the mother and the fetus/newborn, such as cytochrome P-450 (228). Two other agents in this class, famotidine and nizatidine, are minimally bound to the cytochrome P-450 system (228).

As with cimetidine, the major obstetric use of ranitidine is to prevent Mendelson's syndrome in the mother at delivery. The use of ranitidine near term has had no effect on uterine contractions, fetal heart rate pattern, subsequent Apgar scores of the newborn, or neonatal gastric acidity at 24 hours of age (212–224, 229–234).

Ranitidine, similar to cimetidine, is concentrated in the mother's milk with levels up to nearly 24 times that of her plasma after single and multiple doses (235, 236). In a study involving multiple dosing, the peak concentration in the milk, 2610 ng/ml, and serum, 309 ng/ml, occurred at 5.5 hours (ratio 8.44) (236). Adverse effects in the nursing infant are possible, but have not been reported. One group recommended scheduling feedings between 1 and 2 hours after a dose to limit exposure to ranitidine (236).

ANTISPASMODICS

Dicyclomine (B) (Bentyl)

The tertiary ammonium agent, dicyclomine, is an anticholinergic, but lacks antimuscarinic activity and, thus, although it is a nonspecific smooth muscle relaxant, it has no effect on gastric acid secretion. The CPP observed over 1,000 exposures to the drug during the first trimester and found a significant association with minor malformations (SRR of 1.46); 21 malformed infants (expected 14.4) from 1,024 mothers (7, pp. 345–356, 439). An increased SRR (not statistically significant) was also found for polydactyly in black women; six cases (3.2 expected) from 277 women. As discussed previously, direct interpretation of these data are not possible in the absence of confirming studies. Almost 1,600 exposures to dicyclomine occurred anytime during pregnancy, and the SRR in this group was lower than unity (0.90).

A retrospective study published in 1971, involving more than 1,200 mothers, examined the relationship between drugs and congenital malformations (9). This investigation found that significantly fewer mothers of infants with major abnormalities, as compared to normal controls, took antiemetics during the first 56 days of pregnancy. Dicyclomine was the fourth most frequently ingested antiemetic.

Dicyclomine, at one time, was a component of Bendectin, an antinauseant used extensively in early pregnancy. In 1976, Bendectin was reformulated to remove dicyclomine because this agent did not contribute to the antiemetic effectiveness of the proprietary product. Several hundred cases of congenital defects have been attributed to the use of Bendectin (both old and new formulations) by various case reports and studies (231–248). Despite this, however, a large number of studies have found no or minimal evidence that the combination product was associated with malformations (103, 249–267). Moreover, the combination product is not teratogenic in animals (268).

No information has been published on the excretion of dicyclomine into breast milk. The manufacturer has received a case report of apnea in a 12-day-old breast-fed infant whose mother was receiving dicyclomine therapy (N.G. Dahl, personal communication, Marion Merrell Dow, 1992). After the adverse event, the mother was administered a single, 20-mg dose of dicyclomine and breast feeding was discontinued for 24 hours. Milk and plasma concentrations 2 hours after the dose were 131 and 59 ng/ml, respectively, corresponding to a milk:plasma ratio of 2.2. Although a causal relationship between the drug and the apnea was not established, similar adverse effects have been observed when dicyclomine was administered directly to infants (269). Consequently, dicyclomine should not be administered to nursing women.

Oxyphencyclimine (C) (Daricon)

No pregnancy or lactation data are available for this anticholinergic/antispasmodic agent that is used as adjunctive therapy in the treatment of peptic ulcer.

CORTICOSTEROIDS

Prednisolone (B)
Prednisone (B)

Prednisone is metabolized in the maternal liver to the biologically active corticosteroid, prednisolone. Conversely, placental β-dehydrogenase can oxidize prednisolone to inactive prednisone or less active cortisone (270). Moreover, after prednisone-to-prednisolone conversion in the maternal liver, prednisolone is bound to transcortin, which does not cross the placenta, thus further limiting the amount of active corticosteroid reaching the fetus (271). Both corticosteroids cross the placenta to the fetus, however, with prednisone concentrations higher than prednisolone, although the difference was not statistically significant in one study (272).

Six studies, involving rats, mice, and rabbits, were reviewed in a 1989 reference with the finding that corticosteroids were fetotoxic and teratogenic in these species, producing cleft palates, omphaloceles, umbilical hernias, decreased birth weight, and increased resorptions (67, pp. 520–521). In another study, cleft palate was not induced in rats with various doses of prednisolone, methylprednisolone, and cortisone, but dose-related methylprednisolone-induced cleft palate was observed in mice (273). A 1980 report found a decrease in birth weight of female mice exposed in utero to prednisone, but the difference in weight between the exposed pups and the controls had disappeared 21 days after birth (274). However, a permanent masculinization effect on behavior in later life was observed in the exposed female mice suggesting that prednisone had an androgenic effect on the fetus (274).

Prednisone, and its active metabolite, prednisolone, have been used in a large number of human pregnancies without evidence of an association with congenital malformations

(279–290). These agents are not considered human teratogens (291). An infant exposed to prednisone throughout pregnancy was born with congenital cataracts (292). The eye defect was consistent with reports of subcapsular cataracts observed in adults receiving corticosteroids. However, because this is an isolated case, the relationship between the cataracts and prednisone is doubtful. The CPP recorded 43 first trimester exposures to prednisone and 15 to prednisolone (7, pp. 389–391). No relationship to large categories of major or minor abnormalities, or to individual defects, was found.

Although no evidence has been found to suggest that prednisone and prednisolone are human teratogens, an adverse effect on birth weight cannot be entirely excluded (280, 293, 294). Other investigators, however, contend that intrauterine growth retardation is primarily attributable to the severity of the mother's disease, and not to the drug therapy (289, 295). The combination of prednisone and azathioprine has caused immunosuppression in the newborn (see under *Azathioprine* below). Single-dose therapy with prednisone has been used successfully to prevent neonatal respiratory distress syndrome when premature delivery occurs between 28 and 36 weeks of gestation (296). Other, more potent corticosteroids, such as betamethasone, or dexamethasone, are now commonly used for this purpose using a two-dose regimen administered over 24–48 hours.

High, prolonged doses of prednisolone (30 mg/day for at least 4 weeks) may damage spermatogenesis (297). Recovery may require 6 months after the drug is stopped.

Trace amounts of prednisone and prednisolone have been measured in breast milk (298–300). After a 10-mg oral dose of prednisone, milk concentrations of prednisone and prednisolone at 2 hours were 0.03 and 0.002 μg/ml, respectively (298). In a second study using radioactive-labeled prednisolone in seven patients, a mean of 0.14% of a 5-mg oral dose was recovered per liter of milk over 48–61 hours (299). This is equivalent to 0.007 μg/ml.

In six lactating women, prednisolone doses of 10–80 mg/day resulted in milk concentrations ranging from 5–25% of maternal serum levels (300). The milk:plasma ratio increased with increasing serum concentrations. For maternal doses of 20 mg once or twice daily, the authors concluded that the nursing infant would be exposed to minimal amounts of steroid. At higher doses, they recommended waiting at least 4 hours after a dose before nursing was performed. However, even at 80 mg/day, the nursing infant would ingest <0.1% of the dose, which corresponds to <10% of the infant's endogenous cortisol production (300).

Although nursing infants were not involved in the above studies, it is doubtful if these amounts are clinically significant. A 1984 case report observed no adverse effect in two infants nursing from mothers receiving methylprednisolone (301). One source recommends using prednisolone, rather than prednisone, when doses of more than 20 mg/day are used or prolonged therapy is anticipated, to avoid milk levels of both prednisolone and prednisone (55). This author also recommended waiting 3–4 hours after a dose before breast feeding. The American Academy of Pediatrics considers prednisone and prednisolone to be compatible with breast feeding (23).

DIGESTIVE ENZYMES

Pancreatin (C) (Entozyme)
Pancrelipase (C) (Entolase)
Papain (C) (Panafil)
Pepsin (C) (Entozyme)

Pancreatin and pepsin are natural digestive enzymes that are combined with bile salts to aid in the digestion of foods when a deficiency of these enzymes exist. Pancrelipase is a pancreatic enzyme concentrate containing lipase, protease, amylase, and other pancreatic enzymes that is used in deficiency states such as that encountered with cystic fibrosis and chronic pancreatitis. All are obtained from a bovine or porcine source. Papain is derived from the fruit of carica papaya and is applied topically to debride necrotic tissue. Little experience in pregnancy is available for any of these agents. The CPP observed 14 first trimester exposures to papain, 3 to pancreatin, and 1 to an unspecified proteolytic enzyme (7, p. 385). No infants exposed in utero to these products had congenital malformations. Diethyl phthalate, used in the enteric coating for the pancreatin/pepsin commercial product, has been reported to be teratogenic in rats when given in high intraperitoneal, but not oral, doses (271). However, the risk to the fetus or nursing infant from these nonabsorbable products is probably nil.

GALLSTONE-SOLUBILIZING AGENTS

Chenodiol (X) (Chenix)
Monoctanoin (C) (Moctanin)
Ursodiol (B) (Actigall)

Chenodiol (chenodeoxycholic acid) and ursodiol (ursodeoxycholic acid) are naturally occurring bile acids used orally to dissolve gallstones. Monoctanoin is a semisynthetic esterified glycerol that is administered by infusion of the common bile duct to produce dissolution of cholesterol gallstones.

Chenodiol is not teratogenic in animals. No congenital malformations were observed in rats and mice (302, 303), or in baboons (304), exposed in utero to the agent during organogenesis. Dose-related hepatotoxicity was observed in dams, but not newborn rats, in one study using three dosage levels (305), and no fetal hepatotoxicity was observed in a study in rats where the drug composed 0.25% of the maternal diet during pregnancy (306). However, hepatotoxicity was observed in newborn baboons (304), and rhesus monkeys (307) exposed to chenodiol during gestation. Extensive hemorrhagic necrosis of the adrenal glands and interstitial hemorrhage of the kidneys were also noted in the newborn rhesus monkeys (307). One study concluded that dihydroxy bile acids, such as chenodiol, are transferred, at least in rats, from the mother to the fetus (306). Based on the observed hepatotoxicity of this agent, the use of chenodiol is contraindicated during pregnancy.

No fetal adverse effects were observed when ursodiol was fed to pregnant rats (308). Embryotoxicity was observed in a rat study,

but this was less than with chenodiol, and no evidence of hepatotoxicity was observed at three dosage levels (305). In humans, inadvertent exposure during the first trimester to therapeutic doses in four women had no effect on their fetuses or newborns (309).

No data have been located for the use of monoctanoin in either animal or human pregnancies. Similarly, no data are available on the excretion of any of the above agents into breast milk.

GASTRIC ACIDIFIERS

Glutamic Acid (C)

This product provides a source of hydrochloric acid for disorders involving a deficiency of the acid in gastric contents. No effects on the fetus or nursing infant should be expected.

GASTROINTESTINAL PROTECTANTS

Sucralfate (B) (Carafate)

Sucralfate is an aluminum salt of a sulfated disaccharide that inhibits pepsin activity and protects against ulceration. It is a highly polar anion when solubilized in strong acid solutions that results in minimal absorption from the gastrointestinal tract. In animals, sucralfate has no effect on fertility and is not teratogenic with doses up to 38- and 50-times those used in humans, respectively (310). Sucralfate is a source of bioavailable aluminum (310, 311). Each 1-g tablet of sucralfate contains 207 mg of aluminum (311). The potential fetal toxicity from sucralfate relates to its aluminum content.

When administered parenterally to pregnant animals, aluminum accumulates in the fetus causing an increased perinatal mortality, and impaired learning and memory (313, 314). Teratogenic effects, however, were not observed (314). Prolonged exposure to the metal causes neurobehavioral and skeletal toxicity (315). A 1985 review of aluminum described these toxic effects on the brain and bone tissue as dialysis encephalopathy in patients with renal failure and an unique form of osteodystrophy in uremic patients (311). Aluminum received from intravenous fluids may also be related to osteopenia in premature infants (316). A 1991 report described the results of a study of 88 pregnancies in women exposed to high amounts of aluminium sulfate that had been accidently added to the city's water supply (317). Except for an increased rate of talipes (clubfoot) (four cases, one control; $P = .01$), there was no evidence that the exposure was harmful to the fetuses. Several theoretical explanations for the four cases of clubfoot were offered by the investigators, including the possibility that the observed incidence occurred by chance (317).

In patients with end stage chronic renal failure, the use of sucralfate to bind phosphate resulted in serum aluminum levels comparable to those obtained from the antacid, aluminum hydroxide (312). Administration of sucralfate to normal subjects did not increase plasma aluminum concentrations, but evidence of tissue aluminum loading was found in experiments with animals (311).

Analysis of 97 amniotic fluid samples, mostly from women undergoing amniocentesis for advanced maternal age, found a mean aluminum concentration of 93.4 µg/l (range 37–149 µg/l) (318). The authors of this study did not mention if the women were consuming aluminum-containing medications, and the measured levels are apparently the normal baseline for the patient population studied.

Although the toxicity of aluminum has been well documented, there is no evidence that normal doses of aluminum-containing medications, such as sucralfate, present a risk to the fetus of pregnant women with normal renal function. Oral absorption of aluminum is poor with only an average of 12% retained in one study of six normal subjects ingesting 1–3 g of aluminum per day (311). Moreover, no evidence has been found to suggest that aluminum is actively absorbed from the gastrointestinal tract (311). Because of these characteristics, no risk to the fetus is anticipated from recommended doses of sucralfate.

Lactating rabbits absorbed 0.7 and 1.9% of 4,000 and 20,000 µmol/kg oral doses, respectively (315). Limited distribution of aluminum into the milk occurred with less than 1% of the aluminum in the milk absorbed by the suckling offspring after the lower dose. A study published in 1989 measured the plasma aluminum content of healthy full-term infants from birth to 3 months of age (319). The infants were either entirely breast-fed (group 1) or formula-fed one of two soy-based infant formulas (groups 2 and 3). The soy-based formulas contained either 1.6 or 1.7 µg/ml of aluminum, compared to human milk that contains <0.005–0.45 µg/ml of the metal (319). Measurements of plasma aluminum at birth, 1 month, and 3 months of age were similar in the three groups, indicating that little of the aluminum in the formulas was absorbed. Inasmuch as very small amounts of aluminum are available from sucralfate, and oral absorption is poor, no risk to the nursing infant should be expected when the mother is ingesting normal doses.

GASTROINTESTINAL STIMULANTS
Metoclopramide (B) (Reglan)

At term, metoclopramide crosses the placenta to the fetus obtaining fetal concentrations that are approximately 60–80% of maternal levels (320–322). Studies have not been conducted at other gestational times, but passage to the fetus should be expected throughout pregnancy.

High doses, up to 250 times the human dose, in various species, and by various routes of administration, have not shown evidence of fertility impairment or adverse fetal effects. This lack of fetal toxicity has also been found in limited human experience, even when the drug was used in the mid-first trimester as an antiemetic (323–328). Several studies have documented the efficacy of metoclopramide in the prevention of Mendelson's syndrome during labor (320, 322, 329–335). Use of the drug in these cases had no effect on the course of labor, Apgar scores, or newborn neurobehavior. A single 10-mg dose during labor had no effect on maternal growth hormone levels (336).

Metoclopramide, at a dosage of 20–45 mg/day, has been used as a lactation stimulant in women with inadequate or decreased milk production due to its ability to stimulate the release of prolactin from the anterior pituitary (337–347). In one study of 11 patients, the drug did not effect serum levels of prolactin, thyroid-stimulating hormone, or free thyroxin in the nursing infants (345).

Metoclopramide is concentrated in breast milk due to ion trapping in the more acidic (as compared to plasma) milk with per volume concentrations about twice as much as found in plasma (337–339). In the case of a mother taking 30 mg/day, the estimated dose that a nursing infant would receive from the milk ranges up to 45 μg/kg/day, much less than the maximum dose recommended for infants (500 μg/kg/day) (323) or the 100 μg/kg/day dose that has been given to premature infants (348). However, mild intestinal discomfort was noted in two nursing infants where the mothers were consuming 30 and 45 mg/day, respectively (342, 343).

Although the lack of adverse reactions reported in the nursing infants of mothers consuming metoclopramide is reassuring, the American Academy of Pediatrics recommends caution with the use of the drug during breast feeding because of to the potent central nervous system effects that may occur (23).

Dexpanthenol (C) (Ilopan)

Dexpanthenol, also known as d-pantothenyl alcohol, is an analog of d-pantothenic acid, a B complex vitamin and a precursor of coenzyme A, the cofactor for enzyme-catalyzed reactions involving the transfer of acetyl groups. No animal studies have been reported for this agent. Moreover, the manufacturer has no information regarding the use of dexpanthenol in pregnancy or lactation (R.P. Fudge, personal communication, Adria Laboratories, 1992).

Dexpanthenol with Choline Bitartrate (C) (Ilopan-Choline)

Choline is a precursor of, and has the same pharmacologic actions as, acetylcholine. The only study relating to this substance in pregnancy was a 1957 report that found that a deficiency of choline was not teratogenic in mice (349). The manufacturer has no information regarding the use of this combination in human pregnancy or lactation (R.P. Fudge, personal communication, Adria Laboratories, 1992).

AGENTS USED FOR INFLAMMATORY BOWEL DISEASE

Azathioprine (D) (Imuran)

Azathioprine, an antineoplastic/immunosuppressant agent, is used for the treatment of inflammatory bowel disease either alone or combined with corticosteroids. Azathioprine rapidly crosses the placenta and it, and its active metabolite, 6-mercaptopurine, can be measured in fetal blood (350).

No congenital malformations were discovered in the offspring of pregnant mice and rats treated with azathioprine (293, 351), but an increase in resorptions and fetal growth retardation were observed in one of the studies (293). Pregnant rabbits treated with 5 mg/kg/day produced offspring with limb reduction deformities (351).

A large number of studies and reports have described the use of azathioprine in human pregnancy without causing fetal harm (270, 276, 354–370). Congenital malformations that have been reported in newborns exposed in utero to azathioprine, but not thought to be related to maternal drug therapy (369, 370), include: plagiocephaly with neurologic damage (360), bilateral pes equinovarus (360), congenital heart disease (mild mitral regurgitation) (360), cerebral palsy (frontal hemangioma) and cerebral hemorrhage (died at 2 days of age) in twins (360), hypospadias (360), pulmonary valvular stenosis (371), preaxial polydactyly (thumb polydactyly type) (372), and hypothyroidism and arial septal defect (azathioprine started in second trimester) (373). Two exposed newborns were infected with cytomegalovirus at birth (357, 360), and, although the relationship to azathioprine and the clinical significance are questionable,

Table 25.3
Concentrations of Drugs in Women at 16 Weeks' Gestation

	Amniotic Fluid	Maternal Plasma	Cord Plasma	Milk
Number of women	4	5	5	3
		(concentrations in μg/ml)		
Sulfasalazine	<0.05–1.5	3.2–43.3	3.2–25.7	<0.05–1.2
Sulapyridine	6.8–11.6	6.8–19.8	6.6–16.5	9.0–16.9
Acetyl SP	1.3–8.5	1.1–19.7	7.3–16.8	1.1–6.7
5-ASA	0.02–0.08	0.08–0.29	<0.02–0.10	0.02
Acetyl-5-ASA	0.07–0.77	0.31–1.27	0.29–1.80	1.13–3.44

three infants had chromosomal aberrations (360, 374).

Immunosuppression, characterized by lymphopenia, decreased survival of lymphocytes in culture, absence of immunoglobulin M, and reduced levels of immunoglobulin G, was observed in an infant exposed in utero to azathioprine and prednisone throughout gestation with recovery occurring at about 15 weeks (357). Another infant exposed to the combination was born with pancytopenia and severe combined immune deficiency, and died at 28 days of age from irreversible bone marrow and lymphoid hypoplasia (375). In contrast, five women, after kidney transplantation, were treated with azathioprine (100 mg/day in four, 125 mg/day in one) and prednisone throughout pregnancy and delivered infants with intact, functional, humeral immune systems (376). Reducing the dose of azathioprine at 32 week's gestation, based on the mother's leukocyte count, was found in one study to eliminate the occurrence of leukopenia and thrombocytopenia in their newborns (327). Intrauterine growth retardation has been suggested as an effect of maternal azathioprine therapy (293, 294), but other causes, including the combined use of corticosteroids, and the severity of the mother's disease, cannot be excluded (295).

Little information is available on the excretion of azathioprine or its metabolites into human milk. In three reports, a total of four infants were breast-fed although their mothers were taking the drug (25–100 mg/day) (301, 378, 379). The metabolite, 6-mercaptopurine (6-MP), but not azathioprine, was found in low levels in the milk: peaks 3.4 ng/ml (2 hours) and 4.5 ng/ml (8 hours) in one patient (378, 379), peak 18 ng/ml (2 hours) in one patient (378), and not determined in two patients (301). One reviewer stated that breast feeding could be undertaken during use of this drug if the infant was closely monitored (55).

Corticosteroids (B)

See under *Corticosteroids* above.

Mercaptopurine (Purinethol)

Mercaptopurine (6-MP) is an antineoplastic agent that is the active metabolite of azathioprine (see above). Animal studies of 6-MP and 13 purine analogs in the chick, mouse, rat, and rabbit were reviewed in a 1989 reference (67, pp. 396–397). 6-MP was teratogenic in the rat and chick, but in the rabbit, no morphologic changes were noted when it was administered during the ovulation and cleavage stages (67, pp. 396–397). A 1960 review described an earlier study in rabbits that also found no congenital malformations, but stunting occurred in up to 50% of the fetuses (380).

A large number of reports, describing the use of mercaptopurine in 89 human pregnancies, 36 during the first trimester, have been published (380–401). Excluding those cases ending in abortion or stillbirths, only one infant was reported to have congenital defects and, in this case, the anomalies were attributed to busulfan (390). Neonatal toxicity due to combination chemotherapy was observed in three other infants: pancytopenia (386), microangiopathic hemolytic anemia (389), and transient severe bone marrow hypoplasia (392).

No reports on the maternal use of mercaptopurine during breast feeding have appeared. However, small amounts of mercaptopurine were measured in the milk of four women who were being treated with 25–100 mg/day of azathioprine (see under *Azathioprine* above). Women who are breast feeding should probably not be treated with mercaptopurine because of the potential toxicity of this drug in the nursing infant.

Metronidazole (B)

See under *Oral Anti-infectives* above.

Sulfasalazine (B) (Azulfidine)
Mesalamine (B) (Rowasa)
Olsalazine (C) (Dipentum)

The oral compound, sulfasalazine (salicylazosulfapyridine), is used for the treatment of ulcerative colitis and Crohn's disease. It is partially metabolized in the large intestine to 5-aminosalicylic acid (mesalamine, 5-ASA) and sulfapyridine. Mesalamine is administered by either rectal suspension or suppository. Olsalazine is a sodium salt of a salicylate compound that is metabolized in the colon, after oral administration, to two molecules of 5-aminosalicylic acid. The history, pharmacology, and pharmacokinetics of mesalamine and olsalazine were extensively reviewed in a 1992 reference (402).

Although the parent compound and sulfapyridine are absorbed into the systemic circulation, only small amounts of mesalamine are absorbed from the cecum and colon, and most of this is rapidly excreted in the urine (403). Sulfasalazine and the metabolite, sulfapyridine, readily cross the placenta with fetal concentrations approximately the same as those in the mother (404–406). Mean cord blood concentrations in 11 infants were 4.6 and 18.2 μg/ml, respectively (407). These concentrations were not great enough to displace bilirubin from albumin (407). Moreover, mesalamine is bound to different sites on al-

bumin than bilirubin and, thus, has no bilirubin-displacing ability (408). A 1987 reference reported the results of a study in pregnant women being treated prophylactically with 3 g/day of sulfasalazine (409). Concentrations of sulfasalazine, sulfapyridine, acetyl sulfapyridine, 5-aminosalicylic acid, and acetyl-5-aminosalicylic acid in amniotic fluid at 16 weeks' gestation, maternal and cord plasma at term, and in breast milk after delivery were as shown in Table 25.3.

No fetal or nursing infant effect from the maternal drug therapy were mentioned. However, at doses used in humans, no cases of kernicterus or severe neonatal jaundice have been reported, even when sulfasalazine was given up to the time of delivery (407, 410, 411).

The use of sulfasalazine has been reported in a number of pregnancies without producing fetotoxicity or an increase in congenital defects (404–407, 410, 412–418). Five infants with severe congenital malformations, two of them stillborn and one dying after birth, have been described after in utero exposure to sulfasalazine, but a causal relationship between the drug, the disease, or a combination of these and other factors cannot be determined (419–421). The defects observed were bilateral cleft lip/palate, severe hydrocephalus, death; ventricular septal defect, coarctation of the aorta; Potter-type IIa polycystic kidney, rudimentary left uterine cornu, stillborn (first twin), Potter's facies, hypoplastic lungs, absent kidneys and ureters, talipes equinovarus, stillborn (second twin); ventricular septal defect, coarctation of the aorta, macrocephaly, gingival hypeplasia, small ears (latter two defects thought to be inherited). Neutropenia in a premature infant has also been attributed to maternal use of sulfasalazine during gestation (422).

Sulfasalazine may adversely affect spermatogenesis in males treated with the drug for inflammatory bowel disease (423–427). Stopping the drug, or changing therapy to mesalamine, allows recovery of spermatogenesis usually within 3 months (424–427).

Sulfapyridine is excreted into breast milk with concentrations approximately 40–60% of maternal serum levels (403, 406, 428). Except for a single case of bloody diarrhea, no adverse effects have been observed in nursing infants exposed to the drug via the milk. A mother, identified as a slow acetylator with a blood sulfapyridine concentration of 42.4 μg/ml (therapeutic range 20–50 μg/ml) was consuming 3 g/day of sulfasalazine while nursing her infant (429). Bloody diarrhea first occurred at 2 months of age in the exclusively breast fed infant, recurred 2 weeks later, and then persisted for the next 2 weeks. The condition stopped 2–3 days after the mother discontinued the drug. Based on this report, the American Academy of Pediatrics classifies sulfasalazine as a drug that should be given with caution during lactation because of the serious adverse effects that may occur (23).

Diarrhea in a nursing infant, apparently due to the rectal administration of mesalamine to the mother, has been reported (430). The mother had relapsing ulcerative proctitis and 6 weeks after childbirth, treatment was begun with 500 mg mesalamine suppositories twice daily. Her exclusively breast-fed infant developed watery diarrhea 12 hours after the mother's first dose. After 2 days of therapy, the mother stopped the suppositories and the infant's diarrhea stopped 10 hours later. Therapy was reinstituted on four occasions with diarrhea developing each time in the infant 8–12 hours after the first dose and stopping 8–12 hours after therapy was halted. Because of the severity of the mother's disease, breast feeding was discontinued and no further episodes of diarrhea were observed in the infant.

A 1990 report described the excretion of mesalamine and its metabolite, acetyl-5-ASA into breast milk (431). The woman was receiving 500 mg three times daily for ulcerative colits. A single plasma and milk sample was obtained 5.25 hours after a dose, milk and plasma levels of 5-ASA were 0.11 μg/ml and 0.41 μg/ml, respectively, a milk:plasma ratio of 0.27. Similar levels of the metabolite, acetyl-5-ASA, were 12.4 and 2.44 μg/ml, respectively, a ratio of 5.1.

LAXATIVES

Bulk Laxatives

Methylcellulose
Polycarbophil (FiberCon)
Psyllium (Metamucil)

The bulk-forming laxatives act by retaining water in the bowel and are poorly absorbed. They are considered safe for use in pregnancy (271) and during lactation (55).

Choleretics/Hydrocholeretics

BILE SALTS (C)
Dehydrocholic Acid (C)

These agents aid in the digestion of food, especially fat, and are indicated for the temporary relief of constipation, or as adjunctive therapy following surgery or diseases of the biliary tract. They have not been studied in pregnancy, although the CPP recorded 11 first trimester exposures to bile salts and six to dehydrocholic acid (7, p. 385). No evidence of an association with major or minor defects was found from this small sample. No data are available relating to the effect of these agents on the nursing infant, but the risk is probably negligible.

Irritant/Stimulant

Bisacodyl (Dulcolax)
Casanthranol
Cascara Sagrada
Castor Oil
Danthron
Phenolphthalein (Ex-Lax, Feen-A-mint)
Senna (Senokot)

Bisacodyl is a contact laxative that acts on the colonic mucosa to stimulate peristalsis (432). Small amounts may be absorbed from the small intestine after oral therapy, but absorption is negligible after the use of rectal suppositories (271). The drug is approved for use during pregnancy, labor, and the postpartum period. Stimulation of the pregnant uterus is not a problem (432).

The anthraquinone purgatives include cascara sagrada, casanthranol, danthron, and senna. In the CPP, 53 mother-child pairs were exposed to cascara, and 21 to casanthranol, during the first trimester (7, pp. 384–387).

Based on congenital defects in three infants, a hospital SRR of 1.90 was found for casanthranol. The authors of this study, however, concluded that there was no evidence that fetal exposure to drugs used for gastrointestinal disturbances during the first trimester increased the risk of malformations (7, p. 387). For exposure anytime during pregnancy, 188 and 109 were exposed to cascara and casanthranol, respectively (7, pp. 438, 442). An increased SRR, 2.03, was discovered for cascara based on seven infants with defects, but not for casanthranol. Three of the infants exposed to cascara in utero had benign tumors (7, p. 497). At least one of the anthraquinone laxatives, dihydroxyanthraquinone, crosses the placenta to the fetus and appears in the amniotic fluid and newborn's urine, when administered before the induction of labor (433). This information, combined with the CPP data cited above, led some to conclude that this class of laxatives should not be used during pregnancy (433).

The vegetable laxatives, sennaglucosides and sennosides A and B, have been studied in rats, rabbits, and sheep (434–437). The stereoisomers, sennosides A and B, are broken down in the large bowel to a glycone structure, monoanthrone, which is responsible for the laxative action (435). No effect on reproduction or the fetus was discovered in these studies. In pregnant sheep, senna produced a slight inhibition of contractions in both in vivo and in vitro experiments (436, 437). A 1992 review cited 10 studies involving 937 pregnant patients who were treated with senna preparations for 2 weeks to 9 months without any evidence of maternal or fetal harm (438). Two of the studies involved women with high risk pregnancies who were prone to premature labor and/or vaginal bleeding. No uterine stimulation, bleeding, or other effects were observed. The use of prophylactic senna during pregnancy has been recommended to prevent constipation and undue straining (439).

Danthron, a nonglucoside anthraquinone laxative, is readily absorbed from the bowel and crosses the placenta to the fetus and amniotic fluid (440). Combination with docusate salts may increase the absorption of danthron (441). Danthron can be detected in the newborn's urine when administered shortly before delivery, but no adverse effects, such as diarrhea, were observed.

Phenolphthalein was used by 236 mother-child pairs during the first trimester and 806 anytime during pregnancy in the CPP study (7, pp. 384–387, 442, 497). No evidence was found to associate the use of this drug with major or minor malformations.

Although not absorbed, castor oil is a very potent purgative and may initiate premature uterine contractions (271). The drug is used by some obstetricians to initiate uterine contractions in over-due pregnancies, but, except for this indication, should be avoided during gestation. It has not been studied, but castor oil is not expected to appear in breast milk and should be safe to use during lactation.

Because bisacodyl is not absorbed from the gastrointestinal tract, this agent should not appear in breast milk and is considered safe to give to the lactating woman (55). Neither are sennosides A and B absorbed systemically, although the metabolite, rhein, does appear in maternal serum in small amounts. A 1973 study failed to detect the laxative in breast milk (sensitivity limit 0.34 μg/ml) (442). A 1988 study, using a more sensitivity analysis, measured levels of the laxatively active metabolite, rhein, ranging from 0 to 0.027 μg/ml in 100 breast milk samples from 20 lactating women ingesting a senna preparation containing 15 mg/day of sennosides A and B (443). The majority of the samples (94%) contained less than 0.010 μg/ml of rhein. None of the nursing infants developed diarrhea or had an abnormal stool consistency (443). Use of senna during lactation has been reported in three studies, and although diarrhea occurred in some of the infants, this was probably due to other causes (442, 444, 445). In one of these studies, mothers, whose infants had developed diarrhea after maternal administration of a 100-mg dose (containing 8.6 mg of sennosides A and B), were given a 200-mg dose of senna (436). No diarrhea occurred after the higher dose. The American Academy of Pediatrics considers senna, cascara, and danthron to be compatible with breast feeding (23). Other reviewers have also concluded that the use of senna during lactation involves negligible risk to the breast-feeding infant (446, 447).

The use of danthron in lactating women has been associated with increased bowel activity in nursing infants (23, 445). This latter finding is interesting because in another study of 14 lactating women, danthron was detected in their urine but not in their milk or in their infant's urine (448). The authors of that study concluded that danthron, if it was excreted into milk at all, did so in such small quantities as to have no significant effect on the nursing infant. As mentioned above, the docusate salts will increase the absorption of danthron and greater amounts should pass into milk.

Conjugated phenolphthalein, but not unchanged phenolphthalein, was excreted into breast milk in concentrations up to 1.0 μg/ml after a single 200–800 mg dose in 22 lactating women (449). Bowel movements occurred in 16 of the women after the dose, but none of the nursing infants had diarrhea. In an analysis of this study, one group stated that conjugated phenolphthalein may undergo deconjugation in the infant's bowel and, thus by implication, produce diarrhea in the infant (447). No adverse reports, however, after use of this product during nursing have been located.

Lubricant

MINERAL OIL (C)

Mineral oil is an emollient laxative that is poorly absorbed from the bowel into the systemic circulation. Combination with docusate salts, however, may increase the absorption, and, thus the toxicity of mineral oil (441). Chronic use of mineral oil can decrease the absorption of fat-soluble vitamins, such as vitamins K, A, D, and E. No direct effect on the nursing infant is expected if an adequate maternal vitamin status is maintained.

Saline Laxatives

Magnesium Citrate
Magnesium Hydroxide
Magnesium Sulfate
Sodium Phosphate

All of the saline (osmotic) laxatives are poorly absorbed into the systemic circulation, but small, nontoxic amounts of the cations, magnesium and sodium, may be absorbed. These agents act in the small and large intestine to draw water into the bowel. Sodium retention in the mother is a potential complication (271). No studies on the use of these agents in either pregnancy or lactation have been located.

Stool Softeners (Surfactants)

Docusate Calcium (C) (Surfak)
Docusate Potassium (C) (Dialose)
Docusate Sodium (DSS) (C) (Colace)

These agents act throughout the intestine by softening the stool by a detergent-like action to allow a mixing of fat and water. They are poorly absorbed, if at all, into the systemic circulation. They should not be combined with danthron or mineral oil because the absorption of these latter agents will be increased (441).

The CPP recorded 30 cases of first trimester and 116 cases of anytime during gestation exposure to docusate sodium (7, pp. 384–387, 442). No increase in congenital malformations in either period was observed after the use of this laxative. In a later study, 319 first trimester exposures were observed and again, no increase in the incidence of congenital defects was noted (113).

No reports of adverse effects in nursing infants after the maternal use of stool softeners have been located. One review cites docusate as a preferred laxative during lactation if such an agent is required (55).

Miscellaneous Laxatives

GLYCERIN (C)

Glycerin suppositories act in the colon by a hyperosmotic action (similar to the saline cathartics) and local irritation, the latter effect due to the sodium stearate in the preparation. A liquid preparation that does not contain sodium stearate is also available for rectal use. No data are available for glycerin in either pregnancy or lactation, but since the product is nonabsorbable, the risk to the fetus and nursing infant is probably negligible.

LACTULOSE (B) (CEPHULAC)

Lactulose is a synthetic disaccharide that is biodegraded only by bacteria in the colon to the low molecular weight acids, lactic acid, formic acid, and acetic acid. Small amounts of lactulose, in the order of 3% of a dose, are absorbed after oral administration (450). No impairment of fertility or fetal harm have been observed in pregnant mice, rats, and rabbits using two to four times the usual human oral dose (450). No reports on the use of this product in human pregnancy or lactation have been located, but the risk to the fetus and the newborn appears to be negligible.

SEDATIVES

Chlordiazepoxide (D) (Librium)

Chlordiazepoxide is a member of the benzodiazepine class of sedatives. No congenital malformations were noted when pregnant rats were fed chlordiazepoxide 10–80 mg/kg/day (451). At 100 mg/kg/day, skeletal malformations were observed in some of the newborn rats.

Human experience with chlordiazepoxide is extensive. In a study evaluating 19,044 live births, the use of chlordiazepoxide was associated with a more than 4-fold increase in severe congenital anomalies (452). In 172 patients exposed to the drug during the first 42 days of gestation, defects were observed in four infants: mental deficiency; spastic diplegia and deafness; microcephaly and retardation; duodenal atresia and Meckel's diverticulum (452). Although not statistically significant, an increased fetal death rate was also found with maternal chlordiazepoxide ingestion (452). A survey of 390 infants with congenital heart disease matched with 1,254 normal infants found a higher rate of exposure

to several drugs, including chlordiazepoxide, in the offspring with defects (453). Other studies have not confirmed a relationship with increased defects or mortality (454–457).

The CPP observed 257 first trimester exposures to chlordiazepoxide (7, pp. 335–344, 439). No association with large classes of malformations or to individual defects was found. Similar results occurred for use anytime during pregnancy, when 740 exposures to chlordiazepoxide were observed (7, p. 438). SRR of 2.1, 2.7, and 1.6 were calculated for clubfoot (6 cases), pectus excavatum (seven cases), and inguinal hernia (16 cases), respectively, but there was no evidence that these non-uniform malformations were related to chlordiazepoxide therapy (7, p. 491).

Neonatal withdrawal consisting of severe tremulousness and irritability has been attributed to maternal use of chlordiazepoxide (458). The onset of withdrawal symptoms occurred on the 26th day of life.

Chlordiazepoxide readily crosses the placenta at term in an approximate 1:1 ratio (459–461). The drug has been used to reduce pain during labor, but the maternal benefit was not significant (462, 463). Marked depression was observed in three infants whose mothers received chlordiazepoxide within a few hours of delivery (460). The infants were unresponsive, hypotonic, hypothermic, and fed poorly. Hypotonicity persisted for up to a week. Although other studies have not seen newborn depression after use of chlordiazepoxide in labor (459, 460), the drug should not be used during this period. The adverse effects described above are termed the "floppy infant syndrome" and are a dose-related response to diazepam and other benzodiazepines (464–467).

No information has been published on the excretion of chlordiazepoxide in breast milk. The closely related benzodiazepine, diazepam, is excreted and accumulates in milk, and sedation has been observed in a nursing infant (468). The American Academy of Pediatrics classifies diazepam and other benzodiazepines (but does not mention chlordiazepoxide) as drugs whose effect on the nursing infant is unknown but may be of concern (23). Because of this, the use of chlordiazepoxide is not recommended during lactation.

Phenobarbital (D)

Phenobarbital has been used widely in clinical practice as a sedative, anticonvulsant, or hypnotic since 1912 (469). A 1989 reference reviewed several studies of the drug in mice, rats, and rabbits (67, pp. 494–495). Multiple defects were observed in these studies including cleft palate, and other anomalies involving the skeleton, heart, brain, and kidneys.

Phenobarbital administered to pregnant rats during the last several days of gestation produced delayed onset of puberty, disorders of the estrus cycle, and a 50% infertility rate in female offspring (470). These severe adverse effects have not been observed in humans, but preliminary results in one study indicate that long-term biologic and pharmacologic effects from in utero exposure to phenobarbital may also occur in humans (471). In a study conducted between 1968 and 1971 in Greece, 1522 mothers were treated with phenobarbital 100 mg/day, compared with 1,553 control subjects, from 34–36 weeks' gestation to delivery in an attempt to prevent neonatal hyperbilirubinemia (472). No adverse effects were observed in either the fetuses/newborns or the mothers. The first follow-up occurred between the ages of 5.1 and 6.8 years and involved a statistically selected sample of 415 children (233 exposed to phenobarbital and 182 controls) (471). Children exposed in utero to phenobarbital had a statistically significant greater height and scored higher on a Visuo-Motor Integration test compared with the control children. Approximately 10 years later, a second follow-up was conducted using the 415 children from the first evaluation (471). A total of 341 (phenobarbital group 198; controls 143) was available for this phase of the study. Although the data are still being analyzed, preliminary results indicate that males exposed to phenobarbital were significantly taller than control males and had a significantly lower mean testicular volume (471). The investigators could not determine, at this stage, if the latter finding had an effect on reproductive function.

Pregnant women with epilepsy, who are using phenobarbital either alone or in combination with other anticonvulsants, have a two to three times greater risk for delivering a child with congenital defects over the general population (470, 473–480). The reasons for this increased risk may include the disease state, genetic composition of the mother and the fetus, anticonvulsant medication, and/or an interaction between the drugs and the maternal/fetal genetic factors. A phenotype, as described for phenytoin in the fetal hydantoin syndrome (FHS), has not been identified for phenobarbital, but some of the minor malformations associated with the FHS have been observed in infants of mothers treated only with the barbiturate (481).

A retrospective study published in 1971 found that significantly more mothers of infants with major congenital anomalies consumed phenobarbital throughout pregnancy than did those mothers in a control group (9). During the first trimester, the number of exposed infants with major malformations (6.3%) was more than double that observed in controls (3.0%), but the difference was not statistically significant.

The CPP recorded 1,415 first trimester exposures to phenobarbital (7, pp. 336–344), and 8,037 exposures anytime during pregnancy (7, p. 438). No evidence was found to suggest a relationship to large categories of major or minor malformations. A statistically significant association was found with Down syndrome, but because this is a genetic defect (i.e., chromosomal abnormality), a cause and effect relationship is biologically implausible. Among individual malformations, SRR of >1.5 were found in the first trimester for microcephaly (SRR 2.2; 5 exposed of 77 cases), any ventricular septal defect (SRR 1.9; 9 exposed of 171 cases), and coarctation of aorta-preductal (SRR 5.6; 4 exposed of 26 cases) (7, pp. 475–476). For exposure anytime during pregnancy, SRR of >1.5 were found for microcephaly (SRR 1.7; 21 exposed of 77 cases), ductus arteriosus persistens (SRR 1.8; 12

exposed of 45 cases), hypoplasia of limb (SRR 1.7; 13 exposed of 51 cases), stenotic ureter (SRR 1.8; 7 exposed of 26 cases), hydronephrosis (SRR 4.3; 10 exposed of 23 cases), hydroureter (SRR 4.6; 9 exposed of 21 cases), coloboma (SRR 2.9; 5 exposed of 13 cases), hypoplasia/atrophy of adrenals (SRR 2.4; 8 exposed of 26 cases), and any malignant tumors (SRR 1.7; 6 exposed of 24 cases) (7, pp. 489–490). Although increased risks were observed for the above defects after in utero phenobarbital exposure, the authors of this study emphasized that the data cannot be used to infer a causal relationship, and that independent confirmation was required in each case (7, p. 468).

Phenobarbital withdrawal has been reported in newborns who were exposed to the drug during gestation (483). Infants were exposed to doses ranging from 64–300 mg/day, and the average onset of their symptoms was 6 days (range 3–14 days).

Early hemorrhagic disease of the newborn may be induced by chronic, long-term administration of phenobarbital (483–492). This potentially fatal complication, occurring during the first 24 hours after birth, may be due to phenobarbital induction of fetal liver microsomal enzymes that deplete the already low reserves of fetal vitamin K (492). Prophylactic vitamin K_1 (phytonadione) administered immediately after birth can prevent this disorder. Cronic use of phenobarbital may also induce folic acid deficiency in pregnant women and supplemental folic acid is recommended to prevent this deficiency (493–495).

In contrast to the above, short-term therapy with phenobarbital has been used to prevent intracranial hemorrhage in low birth weight, premature newborns (496–498). Other studies have not observed a beneficial effect on this potentially severe complication (499–501), and, thus, this therapy is not recommended until further studies have been completed.

Phenobarbital has been used in the latter half of gestation to treat cholestasis of pregnancy (502–504). No effect on the fetus or newborn was reported in these limited studies.

Based on the above data, phenobarbital use during pregnancy in nonepileptic women does not pose a major risk to the fetus, except for the possibilities of hemorrhage and addiction in the newborn. In epileptic women, the fetal risk of the drug also includes minor malformations, but the risk to the mother and fetus from seizure activity is greater and, thus, continued use of the drug during pregnancy, at the lowest therapeutic dose to control seizures, is recommended.

Phenobarbital is excreted in breast milk with milk:plasma ratios ranging from 0.4 to 0.6 (505–509). Because the infant eliminates phenobarbital slower than the mother, accumulation may occur to the point that levels in the infant exceed those in the mother (507). Sedation secondary to accumulation of the drug has been observed in nursing infants (505) and, as a consequence, nursing mothers should be instructed to watch for this adverse effect. One reference source recommends monitoring for changes in infant behavior, weight gain, and the measurement of phenobarbital levels in the nursing infant (55). The American Academy of Pediatrics classifies phenobarbital as a drug that has caused major adverse effect in some nursing infants, and it should be given to nursing women with caution (23).

MISCELLANEOUS AGENTS

Cholestyramine (C) (Questran)

Cholestyramine is a nonabsorable anion exchange resin indicated for the treatment of high serum cholesterol concentrations and for the relief of pruritis associated with partial biliary obstruction. The drug is not an animal teratogen (510–512), but may be a procarcinogen in rats (510, 511).

Limited experience in human pregnancies has noted no fetal adverse effects (503, 504, 513–515). Cholestyramine also binds fat-soluble vitamins, and long-term treatment could result in deficiencies of these agents in either the mother or the fetus. Because of this, the drug should be used cautiously during lactation. One source recommends the use of fat-soluble vitamin supplements and the periodic monitoring of prothrombin times in women treated with cholestyramine (271).

Penicillamine (D) (Cuprimine)

The chelating agent, penicillamine, is used for the treatment of Wilson's disease, cystinuria, and severe rheumatoid arthritis unresponsive to other therapies. In two rat studies reviewed in 1989, skeletal malformations were observed in rat fetuses whose mothers were administered the drug via the intraperitoneal route, and 40% of the offspring of rats gavaged with penicillamine had tracheobronchomegaly (67, pp. 487–488). A third study, however, found no defects after high oral dosing in rats (67, pp. 487–488). The manufacturer reports that cleft palates, skeletal defects, and resorptions occurred in the fetuses of rats fed six times the highest recommended human dose (516).

The human experience with penicillamine involves approximately 100 pregnancies, with defects observed in eight infants (517–530):

> Cutis laxa, hypotonia, hyperflexion of hips and shoulders, pyloric stenosis, vein fragility, varicosities, impaired wound healing, death (518)
> Cutis laxa, growth retardation, inguinal hernia, simian crease, perforated bowel, death (522)
> Cutis laxa (519)
> Cutis laxa, mild micrognathia, low-set ears, inguinal hernia (527)
> Cutis laxa, inguinal hernia (528)
> Marked flexion deformities of extremities, dislocated hips, hydrocephalus, intraventricular hemorrhage, death (529)
> Cerebral palsy, blindness, bilateral club feet, sudden infant death at 3 months (529)
> Hydrocephalus (529)

The relationship between the last three cases and penicillamine is controversial because they did not include connective tissue anomalies. The drug may be partially responsible, but other factors, such as maternal infections and surgery, may have a stronger association with the defects (529). A small ventricular septal defect was observed in another newborn but this was probably not related to penicillamine (527).

Penicillamine crosses the placenta to the fetus. A mother was treated for cystinuria throughout gestation with penicillamine hydrochloride 1050 mg/day (843 mg of penicillamine base) (517). The drug was found in the urine of her newborn infant. The baby's physical and mental development was normal at 3 months.

Although the evidence is incomplete, limiting the dose consumed by the mother inflicted with Wilson's disease during pregnancy may reduce the incidence of penicillamine-induced toxicity in the fetus and newborn. Two reports suggest a daily dose of 500 mg or less (521, 526), but the manufacturer recommends a daily dose of 1000 mg (510). If cesarean section is planned, the manufacturer suggests the dose be reduced to 250 mg/day 6 weeks before surgery and until wound healing is complete (516). Although authors of one review believe the drug should be avoided during pregnancy (531), others believe the consequences of untreated Wilson's disease is a greater risk to the mother and fetus than the drug therapy (271, 520, 523).

No information on the passage of penicillamine into milk is available, nor are reports describing breast feeding during maternal therapy with the drug. Authors of one review recommend avoiding penicillamine during lactation (531).

SUMMARY

Fortunately, drugs used for the treatment of gastrointestinal disorders, with only a few notable exceptions, do not present a risk to the fetus or newborn. When placed in the proper perspective, drug-induced fetotoxicity or teratogenesis is relatively uncommon in comparison to other known causes. Of course, avoidance of medications during gestation and lactation is the wisest course of action, but often this is not possible or desirable. If given the opportunity, however, the safest option is to delay prescribing medications, at least during the first trimester.

Among specific agents and classes of gastrointestinal medications, the benefits of drugs in the following categories to the mother probably outweigh the risks to the fetus and/or newborn:

antacids

anticholinergics

antidiarrheals (with the exception of bismuth subsalicylate and the prolonged use of opium or paregoric)

antiemetics (with the exception of promethazine immediately before delivery)

antiflatulents

oral anti-infective agents (metroniadazole and vancomycin)

antisecretory agents (avoid misoprostol)

antispasmodics

corticosteroids

digestive enzymes

gastric acidifiers

gastrointestinal protectants

gastrointestinal stimulants (use with caution during lactation)

agents used for inflammatory bowel disease

laxatives (avoid the use of castor oil and the combined use of stool softeners with other laxatives)

cholestyramine

Drugs that should be used with caution or avoided during pregnancy and nursing are:

gallstone solubilizing agents (chenodiol is contraindicated)

misoprostol (contraindicated)

sedatives (use with caution)

penicillamine (use with caution)

In sum, if the mother's condition requires medicinal therapy, the majority of gastrointestinal agents can be used without overdue concern for the safety of the fetus and/or newborn. The risks and benefits of drug treatment, of course, should be discussed thoroughly with the patient before commencing on any course of therapy, but the mother's condition should be the primary factor in the decision process.

REFERENCES

1. Little BB, Gilstrap LC III, Cunningham FG. Medication use during pregnancy, part 1: concepts of human teratology. In: Cunningham FG, MacDonald PC, Gant NF, eds. Williams Obstetrics, ed. 18. Norwalk, CT: Appleton & Lange, 1989 (suppl 10, Feb/March 1991).
2. Scialli AR. The proliferation of reference books in developmental toxicology. Reprod Toxicol 1991; 5:459–461.
3. Beckman DA, Brent RL. Mechanism of known environmental teratogens: drugs and chemicals. Clin Perinatol 1986;13:649–687.
4. Kalter H, Warkany J. Congenital malformations. Etiologic factors and their role in prevention, part I. N Engl J Med 1983;308:424–431.
5. Oakley GP Jr. Frequency of human congenital malformations. Clin Perinatol 1986;13:545–554.
6. Buehler BA, Delimont D, Van Waes M, et al. Prenatal prediction of risk of the fetal hydantoin syndrome. N Engl J Med 1990;322:1567–1572.
7. Heinonen OP, Slone D, Shapiro S. Birth Defects and Drugs in Pregnancy. Littleton, CO: Publishing Sciences Group, 1977.
8. Witter FR, King TM, Blake DA. The effects of chronic gastrointestinal medication on the fetus and neonate. Obstet Gynecol 1981;58:79S–84S.
9. Nelson MM, Forfar JO. Associations between drugs administered during pregnancy and congenital abnormalities of the fetus. Br Med J 1971;1:523–527.
10. Jacobs D. Maternal drug ingestion and congenital malformations. S Afr Med J 1975;49:2073–2080.
11. Bodendorfer TW, Briggs GG, Gunning JE. Obtaining drug exposure histories during pregnancy. Am J Obstet Gynecol 1979;135:490–494.
12. Schenkel B, Vorherr H. Non-prescription drugs during pregnancy: potential teratogenic and toxic effects upon embryo and fetus. J Reprod Med 1974;12:27–45.
13. Barton JR, Riely CA, Sibai BM. Baking powder pica mimicking preeclampsia. Am J Obstet Gynecol 1992;167:98–99.
14. Piper JM, Baum C, Kennedy DL, Price P. Maternal use of prescribed drugs associated recognized fetal adverse drug reactions. Am J Obstet Gynecol 1988;159:1173–1177.
15. Kivalo I, Saarikoski S. Placental transmission of atropine at full-term pregnancy. Br J Anaesth 1977;49:1017–1021.
16. Kanto J, Virtanen R, Iisalo E, Maenpaa K, Liukke P. Placental transfer and pharmacokinetics of atropine after a single maternal intravenous and intramuscular administration. Acta Anaesth Scand 1981;25:85–88.
17. Onnen I, Barrier G, d'Athis Ph, Surean C, Clive G. Placental transfer of atropine at the end of pregnancy. Eur J Clin Pharmacol 1979;15:443–446.
18. Hellman LM, Fillisti LP. Analysis of the atropine test for placental transfer in gravidas with toxemia and diabetes. Am J Obstet Gynecol 1965;91:797–805.
19. Roodenburg PJ, Wladimiroff JW, Van Weering HK. Effect of maternal intravenous administration of atropine (0.5 mg) on fetal breathing and heart pattern. Contr Gynecol Obstet 1979;6:92–97.
20. Roper RE, Salem MG. Effects of glycopyrrolate and atropine combined with antacid on gastric acidity. Br J Anaesth 1981;53:1277–1280.

21. Abboud T, Raya J, Sadri S, Crobler N, Stine L, Miller F. Fetal and maternal cardiovascular effects of atropine and glycopyrrolate. Anesth Analg 1983; 62:426–430.

22. Stewart JJ. Gastrointestinal drugs. In: Wilson JT, ed. Drugs in Breast Milk. Balgowlah, Australia: ADIS Press, 1981:65–71.

23. Committee on Drugs, American Academy of Pediatrics. Transfer of drugs and other chemicals into human milk. Pediatrics 1989;84:924–936.

24. Moya F, Thorndike V. The effects of drugs used in labor on the fetus and newborn. Clin Pharmacol Ther 1963;4:628–653.

25. Shenker L. Clinical experiences with fetal heart rate monitoring of one thousand patients in labor. Am J Obstet Gynecol 1973;115:1111–1116.

26. Boehm FH, Growdon JH Jr. The effect of scopolamine on fetal heart rate baseline variability. Am J Obstet Gynecol 1974;120:1099–1104.

27. Ayromlooi J, Tobias M, Berg P. The effects of scopolamine and ancillary analgesics upon the fetal heart rate recording. J Reprod Med 1980;25:323–326.

28. Evens RP, Leopold JC. Scopolamine toxicity in a newborn. Pediatrics 1980;66:329–330.

29. Murad SHN, Conklin KA, Tabsh KMA, Brinkman CR III, Erkkola R, Nuwayhid B. Atropine and glycopyrrolate: hemodynamic effects and placental transfer in the pregnant ewe. Anesth Analg 1981; 60:710–714.

30. Proakis AG, Harris GB. Comparative penetration of glycopyrrolate and atropine across the blood-brain and placental barriers in anesthetized dogs. Anesthesiology 1978;48:339–344.

31. Diaz DM, Diaz SF, Marx GF. Cardiovascular effects of glycopyrrolate and belladonna derivatives in obstetrics patients. Bull NY Acad Med 1980; 56:245–248.

32. Abboud TK, Read J, Miller F, Chen T, Valle R, Henriksen EH. Use of glycopyrrolate in the parturient: effect on the maternal and fetal heart and uterine activity. Obstet Gynecol 1981;57:224–227.

33. Product information. Robinul. A.H. Robins Co., 1992.

34. Kagiwada K, Ishizaki O, Saito G. Effects of glycopyrrolate on pre- and post-natal developments of the offsprings in pregnant mice and rats. Oyo Yakuri 1973;7:617–626. As cited by Shepard TH. Catalog of teratogenic agents. ed. 6. Baltimore: Johns Hopkins University Press, 1989:301.

35. Product information. Quarzan. Roche Products, 1992.

36. Product information. Cantil. Marion Merrell Dow, 1992.

37. Product information. Lomotil. GD Searle & Co, 1992.

38. Pickering LK, Feldman S, Ericsson CD, Cleary TG. Absorption of salicylate and bismuth from a bismuth subsalicylate-containing compound (Pepto-Bismol). J Pediatr 1981;99:654–656.

39. Feldman S, Chen S-L, Pickering LK, Cleary TG, Ericsson CD, Hulse M. Salicylate absorption from a bismuth subsalicylate preparation. Clin Pharmac Ther 1981;29:788–792.

40. Menge H, Brosius B, Lang A, Gregor M. Bismuth absorption from the stomach and small intestine. Gastroenterology 1992;102:2192.

41. Nwokolo CU, Pounder RE. Bismuth absorption from the stomach and small intestine [Reply]. Gastroenterology 1992;102:2192–2193.

42. James LF, Lazar VA, Binns W. Effects of sublethal doses of certain minerals on pregnant ewes and fetal development. Am J Vet Res 1966;27:132–135.

43. Hasking GJ, Duggan JM. Encephalopathy from bismuth subsalicylate. Med J Aust 1982;2:167.

44. Collins E. Maternal and fetal effects of acetaminophen and salicylates in pregnancy. Obstet Gynecol 1981;58(suppl):57S–62S.

45. Richards ID. Congenital malformations and environmental influences in pregnancy. Br J Prev Soc Med 1969;23:218–225.

46. Saxen I. Associations between oral clefts and drugs during pregnancy. Int J Epidemiol 1975;4:37–44.

47. Slone D, Heinonen OP, Kaufman DW, Siskind V, Monson RR, Shapiro S. Aspirin and congenital malformations. Lancet 1976;1:1373–1375.

48. Turner G, Collins E. Fetal effects of regular salicylate ingestion in pregnancy. Lancet 1975;2:338–339.

49. Rumack CM, Guggenheim MA, Rumack BH, Peterson RG, Johnson ML, Braithwaite WR. Neonatal intracranial hemorrhage and maternal use of aspirin. Obstet Gynecol 1981;58(suppl):52S–56S.

50. O'Brien JR. Effects of salicylates on human platelets. Lancet 1968;1:779–783.

51. Weiss HJ, Aledort ML, Shaul I. The effect of salicylates on the haemostatic properties of platelets in man. J Clin Invest 1968;47:2169–2180.

52. Bleyer WA. Maternal ingested salicylates as a cause of neonatal hemorrhage. J Pediatr 1974;85:736–737.

53. Friedman JM, Little BB, Brent RL, Cordero JF, Hanson JW, Shepard TH. Potential human teratogenicity of frequently prescribed drugs. Obstet Gynecol 1990;75:594–599.

54. Findlay JWA, DeAngelis RL, Kearney MF, Welch RM, Findley JM. Analgesic drugs in breast milk and plasma. Clin Pharmacol Ther 1981;29:625–633.

55. Anderson PO. Drug use during breast feeding. Clin Pharm 1991;10:594–624.

56. Mengel CE, Carter WA, Horton ES. Geophagia with iron deficiency and hypokalemia: cachexia africana. Arch Intern Med 1964;114:470–474.

57. Talington KM, Gant NF Jr, Scott DE, et al. Effect of ingestion of starch and some clays on iron absorption. Am J Obstet Gynecol 1970;108:262–267.

58. Roselle HA. Association of laundry starch and clay ingestion with anemia in New York City. Arch Intern Med 1970;125:57–61.

59. Scholl TO, Hediger ML, Fischer RL, Shearer JW. Anemia vs iron deficiency: increased risk of preterm delivery in a prospective study. Am J Clin Nutr 1992;55:985–988.

60. Patterson EC, Staszak DJ. Effects of geophagia (kaolin ingestion) on the maternal blood and embryonic development in the pregnant rat. J Nutr 1977;107:2020–2025.

61. Product information. Imodium. Janssen Pharmaceutica, 1992.

62. Marsboom R, Herin V, Verstraeten A, Vandesteene R, Fransen J. Loperamide (R 18 553): a novel type of antidiarrheal agent. Arzneim-Forsch Drug Res 1974;24:1645–1649. Cited by Shepard (67, p. 377).

63. Nikodem VC, Hofmeyr GJ. Secretion of the antidiarrhoel agent loperamide oxide in breast milk. Eur J Clin Pharmacol 1992;42:695–696.

64. Fisch GR, Henley WL. Symptoms of narcotic withdrawal in a newborn infant secondary to medical therapy of the mother. Pediatrics 1961;28:852–853.

65. Cotton MF et al. Neonatal apnoea due to propriety medicines—still a problem. S Afr Med J 1988;73:134.

66. Challier P, Larue M. Withdrawal syndrome in the newborn infant of a mother taking paregoric. Arch Fr Pediatr 1987;44:66.

67. Shepard TH. Catalog of Teratogenic Agents, ed. 6th. Baltimore: Johns Hopkins University Press, 1989.

68. Narrod SA, Wilk AL, King CTG. Metabolism of meclizine in the rat. J Pharmacol Exp Ther 1965; 147:380–384.

69. King CTG, Howell. Teratogenic effect of buclizine and hydroxyzine in the rat and chlorcyclizine in the mouse. Am J Obstet Gynecol 1966;95:109–111.

70. Posner HS, Darr A. Fetal edema from benzhydrylpiperazines as a possible cause of oral-facial malformations in rats. Toxicol Appl Pharmacol 1970; 17:67–75.

71. Walker BE, Patterson A. Induction of cleft palate in mice by tranquilizers and barbiturates. Teratology 1974;10:159–164.

72. Steffek AJ, King CTG, Wilk AL. Abortive effects and comparative metabolism of chlocyclizine in various mammalian species. Teratology 1968;1:399–406.

73. Watson GI. Meclozine ("Ancoloxin") and foetal abnormalities. Br Med J 1962;2:1446.

74. Smithells RW. "Ancoloxin" and foetal abnormalities. Br Med J 1962;2:1539.

75. Diggorg PLC, Tomkinson JS. Meclozine and foetal abnormalities. Lancet 1962;2:1222.

76. Carter MP, Wilson FW. "Ancoloxin" and foetal abnormalities. Br Med J 1962;2:1609.

77. Macleod M. "Ancoloxin" and foetal abnormalities. Br Med J 1962;2:1609.

78. Lask S. "Ancoloxin" and foetal abnormalities. Br Med J 1962;2:1609.

79. Leck IM. "Ancoloxin" and foetal abnormalities. Br Med J 1962;2:1610.

80. McBride WG. Drugs and foetal abnormalities. Br Med J 1962;2:1681.

81. Fagg CG. "Ancoloxin" and foetal abnormalities. Br Med J 1962;2:1681.

82. Barwell TE. "Ancoloxin" and foetal abnormalities. Br Med J 1962;2:1681–1682.

83. Woodall J. "Ancoloxin" and foetal abnormalities. Br Med J 1962;2:1682.

84. McBride WG. Drugs and congenital abnormalities. Lancet 1962;2:1332.

85. Lenz W. Drugs and congenital abnormalities. Lancet 1962;2:1332–1333.

86. David A, Goodspeed AH. "Ancoloxin" and foetal abnormalities. Br Med J 1963;1:121.

87. Gallagher C. "Ancoloxin" and foetal abnormalities. Br Med J 1963;1:121–122.

88. Watson GI. "Ancoloxin" and foetal abnormalities. Br Med J 1963;1:122.

89. Mellin GW, Katzenstein M. Meclozine and foetal abnormalities. Lancet 1963;1:222–223.

90. Salzmann KD. "Ancoloxin" and foetal abnormalities. Br Med J 1963;1:471.

91. Burry AF. Meclozine and foetal abnormalities. Br Med J 1963;1:1476.

92. Smithells RW, Chinn ER. Meclozine and foetal abnormalities. Br Med J 1963;1:1678.

93. O'Leary JL, O'Leary JA. Nonthalidomide ectromelia. Report of a case. Obstet Gynecol 1964; 23:17–20.

94. Smithells RW, Chinn ER. Meclozine and foetal malformations: a prospective study. Br Med J 1964;1:217–218.

95. Pettersson F. Meclozine and congenital malformations. Lancet 1964;1:675.

96. Yerushalmy J, Milkovich L. Evaluation of the teratogenic effect of meclizine in man. Am J Obstet Gynecol 1965;93:553–562.

97. Sadusk JF Jr, Palmisano PA. Teratogenic effect of meclizine, cyclizine, and chlorcyclizine. JAMA 1965;194:987–989.

98. Lenz W. Malformations caused by drugs in pregnancy. Am J Dis Child 1966;112:99–106.

99. Lenz W. How can the teratogenic action of a factor be established in man? South Med J 1971;64(Suppl 1):41–47.

100. Bokesoy I, Aksuyek C, Deniz E. Oromandibular limb hypogenesis/Hanhart's syndrome: possible drug influence on the malformation. Clin Genetics 1983;24:47–49.

101. Anonymous. Pink sheets. Meclizine, cyclizine not teratogenic. FDC Rep 1974:2.

102. Saxen I. Cleft palate and maternal diphenhydramine intake. Lancet 1974;1:407–408.

103. Milkovich L, Van den Berg BJ. An evaluation of the teratogenicity of certain antinauseant drugs. Am J Obstet Gynecol 1976;125:244–248.

104. Kullander S, Kallen B. A prospective study of drugs and pregnancy. Acta Obstet Gynecol Scand 1976; 55:105–111.

105. Michaelis J, Michaelis H, Gluck E, Koller S. Prospective study of suspected associations between certain drugs administered during early pregnancy and congenital malformations. Teratology 1983; 27:57–64.

106. Petrie RH, Yeh S-Y, Murata Y, et al. The effect of drugs on fetal heart rate variability. Am J Obstet Gynecol 1978;130:294–299.

107. Prenner BM. Neonatal withdrawal syndrome associated with hydroxyzine hydrochloride. Am J Dis Child 1977;131:529–530.

108. Zierler S, Purohit D. Prenatal antihistamine exposure and retrolental fibroplasia. Am J Epidemiol 1986;123:192–196.

109. McColl JD, Globus M, Robinson S. Effect of some therapeutic agents in the developing rat fetus. Toxicol Appl Pharmacol 1965;7:409–417.

110. Gross S, Librach C, Cecutti A. Maternal weight loss associated with hyperemesis gravidarum: a predictor of fetal outcome. Am J Obstet Gynecol 1989; 160:906–909.

111. Hara GS, Carter RP, Krantz KE. Dramamine in labor: potential boon or a possible bomb? J Kans Med Soc 1980;81:134–136.

112. Schardein JL, Hentz DL, Petrere JA, Kurtz SM. Teratogenesis studies with diphenhydramine HCl. Toxicol Appl Pharmacol 1971;18:971–976.

113. Aselton P, Jick H, Milunsky A, Hunter JR, Stergachis A. First-trimester drug use and congenital disorders. Obstet Gynecol 1985;65:451–455.

114. Parkin DE. Probable Benadryl withdrawal manifestations in a newborn infant. J Pediatr 1974;85:580.

115. Kargas GA, Kargas SA, Bruyere HJ Jr, Gilbert EF, Opitz JM. Perinatal mortality due to interaction of diphenhydramine and temazepam. N Engl J Med 1985;313:1417.

116. Knowles JA. Excretion of drugs in milk—a review. J Pediatr 1965;66:1068–1082.

117. Product information. Inapsine. Janssen Pharmaceutica Inc., 1992.

118. Zhdanov GG, Ponomarev GM. The concentration of droperidol in the venous blood of the parturients and in the blood of the umbilical cord of neonates. Anesteziol Reanimatol 1980;4:14–16.

118a. Guikontes E, Spantidbas A, Diakakis J. Ondansetron and hyperemesis gravidarum (Letter). Lancet 1992;340:1223.

119. Vorhees CV, Brunner RL, Butcher RE. Psychotropic drugs as behavioral teratogens. Science 1979;205:1220–1225. Cited by Shepard (67, p. 526).

120. Roux C. Action teratogene de la prochlorpemazine. Arch Fr Pediatr 1959;16:968–971. Cited by Shepard (67, p. 526).

121. Moya F, Thorndike V. Passage of drugs across the placenta. Am J Obstet Gynecol 1962;84:1778–1798.

122. Reider RO, Rosenthal D, Wender P, Blumenthal H. The offspring of schizophrenics. Fetal and neonatal deaths. Arch Gen Psychiatry 1975;32:200–211.

123. Slone D, Siskind V, Heinonen OP, Monson RR, Kaufman DW, Shapiro S. Antenatal exposure to the phenothiazines in relation to congenital malformations, perinatal mortality rate, birth weight, and intelligence quotient score. Am J Obstet Gynecol 1977;128:486–488.

124. Mellin GW. Report of prochlorperazine during pregnancy from the fetal life study bank [Abstract]. Teratology 1975;11:28A.

125. Hall G. A case of phocomelia of the upper limbs. Med J Aust 1963;1:449–450.

126. Freeman R. Limb deformities: possible association with drugs. Med J Aust 1972;1:606–607.

127. Rafla N. Limb deformities associated with prochlorperazine. Am J Obstet Gynecol 1987;156: 1557.

128. Ho C-K, Kaufman RL, McAlister WH. Congenital malformations. Cleft palate, congenital heart disease, absent tibiae, and polydactyly. Am J Dis Child 1975;129:714–716.

129. Ananth J. Side effects in the neonate from psychotropic agents excreted through breast-feeding. Am J Psychiatry 1978;135:801–805.

130. Wheatley D. Drugs and the embryo. Br Med J 1964;1:630.

131. Dyson JL, Kohler HG. Anencephaly and ovulation stimulation. Lancet 1973;1:1256–1257.

132. Crawford JS, as quoted by Moya F, Thorndike V. The effects of drugs used in labor on the fetus and newborn. Clin Pharmacol Ther 1963;4:628–653.

133. Powe CE, Kiem IM, Fromhagen C, Cavanagh D. Propiomazine hydrochloride in obstetrical analgesia. JAMA 1962;181:290–294.

134. Potts CR, Ullery JC. Maternal and fetal effects of obstetric analgesia. Am J Obstet Gynecol 1961; 81:1253–1259.

135. Carroll JJ, Moir RS. Use of promethazine (Phenergan) hydrochloride in obstetrics. JAMA 1958; 168:2218–2219.

136. Scokel III PW, Jones WN. Infant jaundice after phenothiazine drugs for labor: an enigma. Obstet Gynecol 1962;20:124–127.

137. Kahn A, Hasaerts, Blum D. Phenothiazine-induced sleep apneas in normal infants. Pediatrics 1985; 75:844–847.

138. Riffel HD, Nochimson DJ, Paul RH, Hon EH. Effects of meperidine and promethazine during labor. Obstet Gynecol 1973;42:738–745.

139. Corby DG, Shulman I. The effects of antenatal drug administration on aggregation of platelets of newborn infants. J Pediatr 1971;79:307–313.

140. Petrie RH, Yeh S-Y, Murata Y, et al. The effect of drugs on fetal heart rate variability. Am J Obstet Gynecol 1978;130:294–299.

141. Hall PF. Use of promethazine (Phenergan) in labour. Can Med Assoc J 1987;136:690–691.

142. Product information. Tigan. Beecham Laboratories, 1992.

143. Breslow S, Belafsky HA, Shangold JE, Hirsch LM, Stahl MB. Antiemetic effect of trimethobenzamide in pregnant patients. Clin Med 1961;8:2153–2155.

144. Winters HS. Antimetics in nausea and vomiting of pregnancy. Obstet Gynecol 1961;18:753–756.

145. Amon K, Amon I, Huller H. Maternal-fetal passage of metronidazole. In: Advances in Antimicrobial and Antineoplastic Chemotherapy. Proceedings of the VII International Congress of Chemotherapy, Prague, 1971:113–115.

146. Heisterberg L. Placental transfer of metronidazole in the first trimester of pregnancy. J Perinat Med 1984;12:43–45.

147. Karhunen M. Placental transfer of metronidazole and tinidazole in early human pregnancy after a single infusion. Br J Clin Pharmacol 1984;18:254–257.

148. Gauter P, Jolou L, Cosar C. Study on the action of metronidazole (No. 8823RP) on the genital system of the rat. Obstet Gynecol 1960;59:609–620.

149. Legator MS, Conner TH, Stoeckel M. Detection of mutagenic activity of metronidazole and niradazole in body fluids of humans and mice. Science 1975;188:1118–1119.

150. Anonymous. Is Flagyl dangerous? Med Lett Drugs Ther 1975;17:53–54.

151. Finegold SM. Metronidazole. Ann Intern Med 1980;93:585–587.

152. Beard CM, Noller KL, O'Fallon WM, Kurland LT, Dockerty MB. Lack of evidence for cancer due to use of metronidazole. N Engl J Med 1979;301:519–522.

153. Damjanov I. Metronidazole and alcohol in pregnancy. JAMA 1986;256:472.

154. Berget A, Weber T. Metronidazole and pregnancy. Ugeskr Laeger 1972;134:2085–2089. Cited by Shepard (67, p. 426).

155. Royer ME. Innocuite du metronidazole (Flagyl) prescrit pendant la grossesse. Med Malades Infect 1983;13:727–729. Cited by Shepard (67, p. 427).

156. Cantu JM, Garcia-Cruz D. Midline facial defect as a teratogenic effect of metronidazole. Birth Defects 1982;18:85–88.

157. Greenberg F. Possible metronidazole teratogenicity and clefting. Am J Med Genet 1985;22:825.

158. Rosa FW, Baum C, Shaw M. Pregnancy outcomes after first-trimester vaginitis drug therapy. Obstet Gynecol 1987;69:751–755.

159. Erickson SH, Oppenheim GL, Smith GH. Metronidazole in breast milk. Obstet Gynecol 1981;57:48–50.

160. Heisterberg L, Branebjerg PE. Blood and milk concentrations of metronidazole in mothers and infants. J Perinat Med 1983;11:114–120.

161. Clements CJ. Metronidazole and breast feeding. NZ Med J 1980;92:329.

162. Reyes MP, Ostrea EM Jr, Cabinian AE, Schmitt C, Rintelmann W. Vancomycin during pregnancy: does it cause hearing loss or nephrotoxicity in the infant? Am J Obstet Gynecol 1989;161:977–981.

163. Finkelstein W, Isselbacher KJ. Cimetidine. N Engl J Med 1978;299:992–996.

164. Pinelli F, Trivulzio S, Colombo R, et al. Antiprostatic effect of cimetidine in rats. Agents Actions 1987;22:197–201.

165. Sawyer D, Conner CS, Scalley R. Cimetidine: adverse reactions and acute toxicity. Am J Hosp Pharm 1981;38:188–197.

166. Anand S, Van Thiel DH. Prenatal and neonatal exposure to cimetidine results in gonadal and sexual dysfunction in adult males. Science 1982;218:493–494.

167. Parker S, Udani M, Gavaler JS, Van Thiel DH. Pre- and neonatal exposure to cimetidine but not ranitidine adversely affects adult sexual functioning of male rats. Neurobehav Toxicol Teratol 1984;6:313–318.

168. Parker S, Schade RR, Pohl CR, Cavaler JS, Van Thiel DH. Prenatal and neonatal exposure of male rat pups to cimetidine but not ranitidine adversely affects subsequent adult sexual functioning. Gastroenterology 1984;86:675–680.

169. Walker TF, Bott JH, Bond BC. Cimetidine does not demasculinize male rat offspring exposed in utero. Fund Appl Toxicol 1987;8:188–197.

170. Shapiro BH, Hirst SA, Babalola GO, Bitar MS. Prospective study on the sexual development of male and female rats perinatally exposed to maternally administered cimetidine. Toxicol Lett 1988;44:315–329.

171. Schenker S, Dicke J, Johnson RF, Mor LL, Henderson GI. Human placental transport of cimetidine. J Clin Invest 1987;80:1428–1434.

172. Howe JP, McGowan WAW, Moore J, McCaughey W, Dundee JW. The placental transfer of cimetidine. Anaesthesia 1981;36:371–375.

173. McGowan WAW. Safety of cimetidine in obstetric patients. J R Soc Med 1979;72:902–907.

174. Johnston JR, Moore J, McCaughey W, et al. Use of cimetidine as an oral antacid in obstetric anesthesia, Anesth Analg 1983;62:720–726.

175. Ching MS, Mihaly GW, Morgan DJ, Date NM, Hardy KJ, Smallwood RA. Low clearance of cimetidine across the human placenta. J Pharm Exp Ther 1987;241:1006–1009.

176. Friedman JM, Little BB, Brent RL, Cordero JF, Hanson JW, Shepard TH. Potential human teratogenicity of frequently prescribed drugs. Obstet Gynecol 1990;75:594–599.

177. Husemeyer RP, Davenport HT. Prophylaxis for Medelson's syndrome before elective caesarean sections: a comparison of cimetidine and magnesium trisilicate mixture regimens. Br J Obstet Gynaecol 1980;87:565–570.

178. Pickering BG, Palahniuk RJ, Cumming M. Cimetidine premedication in elective caesarean section. Can Anaesth Soc J 1980;27:33–35.

179. Howe JP, Dundee JW, Moore J, McCaughey W. Cimetidine: has it a place in obstetric anaesthesia? Anaesthesia 1980;35:421–422.

180. Dundee JW, Moore J, Johnston JR, McCaughey W. Cimetidine and obstetric anaesthesia. Lancet 1981;2:252.

181. Crawford JS. Cimetidine in elective caesarean section. Anaesthesia 1981;36:641–642.

182. McCaughey W, Howe JP, Moore J, Dundee JW. Cimetidine in elective caesarean section. Anaesthesia 1981;36:642.

183. McCaughey W, Howe JP, Moore J, Dundee JW. Cimetidine in elective caesarean section: effect on gastric acidity. Anaesthesia 1981;36:167–172.

184. Hodgkinson R, Glassenberg R, Joyce TH III, Coombs DW, Ostheimer CW, Gibbs CP. Safety and efficacy of cimetidine and antacid in reducing gastric acidity before elective cesarean section. Anesthesiology 1982;57:A408.

185. Ostheimer GW, Morrison JA, Lavoie C, Sopkoski C, Hoffman J, Datta S. The effect of cimetidine on mother, newborn and neonatal neurobehavior. Anesthesiology 1982;57:A405.

186. Johnston JR, McCaughey W, Moore J, Dundee JW. Cimetidine as an oral antacid before elective caesarean section. Anaesthesia 1982;37:26–32.

187. Johnston JR, McCaughey W, Moore J, Dundee JW. A field trial of cimetidine as the sole oral antacid in obstetric anaesthesia. Anaesthesia 1982;37:33–38.

188. Hodgkinson R, Glassenbery R, Joyce TH III, Coombs DW, Ostheimer GW, Gibbs CP. Comparison of cimetidine (Tagamet) with antacid for safety and effectiveness in reducing gastric acidity before elective cesarean section. Anesthesiology 1983;59:86–90.

189. Qvist N, Storm K. Cimetidine pre-anesthetic: a prophylactic method against Mendelson's syndrome in cesarean section. Acta Obstet Gynecol Scand 1983;62:157–159.

190. Okasha AS, Motaweh MM, Bali A. Cimetidine-antacid combination as premedication for elective caesarean section. Can Anaesth Soc J 1983;30:593–597.

191. Frank M, Evans M, Flynn P, Aun C. Comparison of the prophylactic use of magnesium trisilicate mixture B.P.C., sodium citrate mixture or cimetidine in obstetrics. Br J Anaesth 1984;56:355–362.

192. McAuley DM, Halliday HL, Johnston JR, Moore J, Dundee JW. Cimetidine in labour: absence of adverse effect on the high-risk fetus. Br J Obstet Gynaecol 1985;92:350–355.

193. Thorburn J, Moir DD. Antacid therapy for emergency caesarean section. Anaesthesia 1987;42:352–355.

194. Glade G, Saccar CL, Pereira GR. Cimetidine in pregnancy: apparent transient liver impairment in the newborn. Am J Dis Child 1980;134:87–88.

195. Kwanashie HO, Osuide G, Wambebe C, Ikediobi CO. Effects of maternally administered cimetidine during lactation on the development of drug metabolizing enzymes in mouse pups. Biochem Pharmacol 1989;38:204–206.

196. McNamara PJ, Burgio D, Yoo SD. Pharmacokinetics of cimetidine during lactation: species differences in cimetidine transport into rat and rabbit milk. J Pharmacol Exp Ther 1992;261:918–923.

197. Somogyi A, Gugler R. Cimetidine excretion into breast milk. Br J Clin Pharmacol 1979;7:627–629.

198. Bernshaw N. Cimetidine and breast-feeding. Pediatrics 1991;88:1294.

199. Berlin CM Jr. Cimetidine and breast-feeding [Reply]. Pediatrics 1991;88:1294.

200. Burek JD, Majka JA, Bokelman DL. Famotidine: summary of preclinical safety assessment. Digestion 1985;32(suppl 1):7–14.

201. Shibata M, Kawano K, Shiobara Y, et al. Reproductive studies on famotidine (YM 11170) in rats and rabbits. Oyo Yakuri 1983;26:489–97, 543–78, 831–40. Cited by Shepard (67, p. 273).

202. Dicke JM, Johnson RF, Henderson GI, Kuehl TJ, Schenker S. A comparative evaluation of the transport of H2-receptor antagonists by the human and baboon placenta. Am J Med Sci 1988;295:198–206.

203. Courtney TP, Shaw RW, Cedar E, Mann SG, Kelly JG. Excretion of famotidine in breast milk. Br J Clin Pharmacol 1988;26:639P.

204. Product information. Cytotec. G.D. Searle & Co., 1992.

205. Anonymous. Misoprostol and legal medical abortion. Lancet 1991;338:1241–1242.

206. Baird DT, Norman JE, Thong KJ, Glasier AF. Misoprostol, mifepristone, and abortion. Lancet 1992;339:313.

207. Norman JE, Thong KJ, Baird DT. Uterine contractility and induction of abortion in early pregnancy by misoprostol and mifepristone. Lancet 1991;338:133–136.

208. Schonhofer PS. Brazil: misuse of misoprostol as an abortifacient may induce malformations. Lancet 1991;337:1534–1535.

209. Fonseca W, Alencar AJC, Mota FSB, Coelho HLL. Misoprostol and congenital malformations. Lancet 1991;338:56.

210. Schuler L, Ashton PW, Sanseverino MT. Teratogenicity of misoprostol. Lancet 1992;339:437.

211. Callaghan JT, Bergstrom RF, Rubin A, et al. A pharmacokinetic profile of nizatidine in man. Scand J Gastroenterol 1987;22(suppl 136):9–17.

212. Morton DM. Pharmacology and toxicology of nizatidine. Scand J Gastroenterol 1987;22(suppl 136):1–8.

213. Product information. Axid. Lilly Research Laboratories, 1992.

214. Van Thiel DH, Gavaler JS, Heyl A, Susen B. An evaluation of the anti-androgen effects associated

with H_2 antagonist therapy. Scand J Gastroenterol 1987;22(suppl 136):24–28.

215. Neubauer BL, Goode RL, Best KL, et al. Endocrine effects of a new histamine H_2-receptor antagonist, nizatidine (LY139037), in the male rat. Toxicol Appl Pharmacol 1990;102:219–232.

216. Probst KS, Higdon GL, Fisher LF, McGrath JP, Adams ER, Emmerson JL. Preclinical toxicology studies with nizatidine, a new H_2-receptor antagonist: acute, subchronic, and chronic toxicity evaluations. Fundam Appl Toxicol 1989;13:778–792.

217. Kassianos GC. Impotence and nizatidine. Lancet 1989;1:963.

218. Obermeyer BD, Bergstrom RF, Callaghan JT, Knadler MP, Golichowski A, Rubin A. Secretion of nizatidine into human breast milk after single and multiple doses. Clin Pharmacol Ther 1990;47:724–730.

219. Product information. Prilosec. Merck Sharp & Dohme, 1992.

220. Ching MS, Morgan DJ, Mihaly GW, Hardy KF, Smallwood RA. Placental transfer of omeprazole in maternal and fetal sheep. Dev Pharmacol Ther 1986;9:323–331.

221. Moore J, Flynn RJ, Sampaio M, Wilson CM, Gillon KRW. Effect of single-dose omeprazole on intragastric acidity and volume during obstetric anaesthesia. Anaesthesia 1989;44:559–562.

222. McAuley DM, Moore J, Dundee JW, McCaughey W. Preliminary report on the use of ranitidine as an antacid in obstetrics. Ir J Med Sci 1982;151:91–92.

223. MaAuley DM, Moore J, McCaughey W, Donnelly BD, Dundee JW. Ranitidine as an antacid before elective caesarean section. Anaesthesia 1983;38:108–114.

224. McAuley DM, Moore J, Dundee JW, McCaughey W. Oral ranitidine in labour. Anaesthesia 1984;39:433–438.

225. Wang C, Wong KL, Lam KC, Lai CL. Ranitidine does not affect gonadal function in man. Br J Clin Pharmacol 1983;16:430–432.

226. Parker S, Udani M, Gavaler JS, Van Thiel DH. Pre- and neonatal exposure to cimetidine but not ranitidine adversely affects adult sexual functioning of male rats. Neurobehav Toxicol Teratol 1984;6:313–318.

227. Parker S, Schade RR, Pohl CR, Gavaler JS, Van Thiel DH. Prenatal and neonatal exposure of male rat pups to cimetidine but not ranitidine adversely affects subsequent adult sexual functioning. Gastroenterology 1984;86:675–680.

228. Garnett WR, Dukes GE Jr. Upper gastrointestinal disorders. In: Koda-Kimble MA, Young LY, eds. Applied therapeutics: the clinical use of drugs. ed. 5. Vancouver, WA: Applied Therapeutics, 1992: 19(1)–19(22).

229. Gillett GB, Watson JD, Langford RM. Ranitidine and single-dose antacid therapy as prophylaxis against acid aspiration syndrome in obstetric practice. Anaesthesia 1984;39:638–644.

230. Thompson EM, Loughran PG, McAuley DM, Wilson CM, Moore J. Combined treatment with ranitidine and saline antacids prior to obstetric anaesthesia. Anaesthesia 1984;39:1086–1090.

231. Gillett GB, Watson JD, Langford RM. Prophylaxis against acid aspiration syndrome in obstetric practice. Anesthesiology 1984;60:525.

232. Macnab MSP, Milne MK, Allison RH. Oral ranitidine in labour. Br J Anaesth 1985;57:1040–1041.

233. Mathews HML, Wilson CM, Thompson EM, Moore J. Combination treatment with ranitidine and sodium bicarbonate prior to obstetric anaesthesia. Anaesthesia 1986;41:1202–1206.

234. Ikenoue T, Iito J, Matsuda Y, Hokanishi H. Effects of ranitidine on maternal gastric juice and neonates when administered prior to caesarean section. Aliment Pharmacol Therap 1991;5:315–318.

235. Riley AJ, Crowley P, Harrison C. Transfer of ranitidine to biological fluids: milk and semen. In: Misiewicz JJ, Wormsley KG, eds. Proceedings of the 2nd International Symposium on Randitidine. Oxford, England: Medicine Publishing Foundation, 1981:78–81.

236. Kearns GL, McConnell RF Jr, Trang JM, Kluza RB. Appearance of ranitidine in breast milk following multiple dosing. Clin Pharm 1985;4:322–324.

237. Korcok M. The Bendectin debate. Can Med Assoc J 1980;123:922–928.

238. Soverchia G, Perri PF. Two cases of malformations of a limb in infants of mothers treated with an antiemetic in a very early phase of pregnancy. Pediatr Med Chir 1981;3:97–99.

239. Donaldson GL, Bury RG. Multiple congenital abnormalities in a newborn boy associated with maternal use of fluphenazine enanthate and other drugs during pregnancy. Acta Paediatr Scand 1982;71:335–338.

240. Grodofsky MP, Wilmott RW. Possible association of use of Bendectin during early pregnancy and congenital lung hypoplasia. N Engl J Med 1984;311:732.

241. Fisher JE, Nelson SJ, Allen JE, Holsman RS. Congenital cystic adenomatoid malformation of the lung: a unique variant. Am J Dis Child 1982;136:1071–1074.

242. Bracken MB, Berg A. Bendectin (Debendox) and congenital diaphragmatic hernia. Lancet 1983;1:586.

243. Ohga K, Yamanaka R, Kinumaki H, Awa S, Kobayashi N. Bendectin (Debendox) and congenital diaphragmatic hernia. Lancet 1983;1:930.

244. Eskenazi B, Bracken MB. Bendectin (Debendox) as a risk factor for pyloric stenosis. Am J Obstet Gynecol 1982;144:919–924.

245. Bendectin and pyloric stenosis. FDA Drug Bull 1983;13:14–15.

246. Mitchell AA, Schwingl PJ, Rosenberg L, Louik C, Shapiro S. Birth defects in relation to Bendectin use in pregnancy, II: pyrolic stenosis. Am J Obstet Gynecol 1983;147:737–742.

247. Aselton P, Jick H, Milunsky A, Hunter JR, Stergachis A. First-trimester drug use and congenital disorders. Obstet Gynecol 1985;65:451–455.

248. Zierler S, Rothman KJ. Congenital heart disease in relation to maternal use of Bendectin and other drugs in early pregnancy. N Engl J Med 1985; 313:347–352.

249. Holmes LB. Teratogen update: Bendectin. Teratology 1983;27:277–281.

250. Shapiro S, Heinonen OP, Siskind V, Kaufman DW, Monson RR, Slone D. Antenatal exposure to doxylamine succinate and dicyclomine hydrochloride (Bendectin) in relation to congenital malformations, perinatal mortality rate, birth weight, intelligence quotient score. Am J Obstet Gynecol 1977; 128:480–485.

251. Rothman KJ, Flyer DC, Goldblatt A, Kreidberg MB. Exogenous hormones and other drug exposures of children with congenital heart disease. Am J Epidemiol 1979;109:433–439.

252. Bunde CA, Bowles DM. A technique for controlled survey of case records. Curr Ther Res 1963;5:245–248.

253. Gibson GT, Collen DP, McMichael AJ, Hartshorne JM. Congenital anomalies in relation to the use of doxylamine/dicyclomine and other antenatal factors. An ongoing prospective study. Med J Aust 1981;1:410–414.

254. Correy JF, Newman NM. Debendox and limb reduction deformities. Med J Aust 1981;1:417–418.

255. Clarke M, Clayton DG. Safety of Debendox. Lancet 1981;2:659–660.

256. Harron DWG, Griffiths K, Shanks RG. Debendox and congenital malformations in Northern Ireland. Br Med J 1980;4:1379–1381.

257. Smithells RW, Sheppard S. Teratogenicity testing in humans: a method demonstrating safety of Bendectin. Teratology 1978;17:31–35.

258. Morelock S, Hingson R, Kayne H, et al. Bendectin and fetal development: a study at Boston City Hospital. Am J Obstet Gynecol 1982;142:209–213.

259. Cordero JF, Oakley GP, Greenberg F, James LM. Is Bendectin a teratogen? JAMA 1981;245:2307–2310.

260. Mitchell AA, Rosenberg L, Shapiro S, Slone D. Birth defects related to Bendectin use in pregnancy, I: oral clefts and cardiac defects. JAMA 1981; 245:2311–2314.

261. Fleming DM, Knox JDE, Crombie DL. Debendox in early pregnancy and fetal malformation. Br Med J 1981;283:99–101.

262. Greenberg G, Inman WHW, Weatherall JAC, Adelstein AM, Haskey JC. Maternal drug histories and congenital abnormalities. Br Med J 1977;2:853–856.

263. Aselton PJ, Jick H. Additional follow-up of congenital limb disorders in relation to Bendectin use. JAMA 1983;250:33–34.

264. McCredie J, Kricker A, Elliott J, Forrest J. The innocent bystander:doxylamine/dicyclomine/pyridoxine and congenital limb defects. Med J Aust 1984;140:525–527.

265. Hughes DT, Cavanagh N. Chromosomal studies on children with phocomelia, exposed to Debendox during early pregnancy. Lancet 1983;2:399.

266. David TJ. Debendox does not cause the Poland anomaly. Arch Dis Child 1982;57:479–480.

267. Brent RR. Editorial. The Bendectin saga: another American tragedy. Teratology 1983;27:283–286.

268. Gibson JP, Staples RE, Larson EJ, Kuhn WL, Holtkamp DE, Newberne JW. Teratology and reproduction studies with an antinauseant. Toxicol Appl Pharmacol 1968;13:439–447.

269. Product information. Bentyl. Marion Merrell Dow, 1992.

270. Fine LG, Barnett EV, Danovitch GM, et al. Systemic lupus erythematosus in pregnancy. Ann Intern Med 1981;94:667–677.

271. Lewis JH, Weingold AB, and the Committee on FDA-Related Matters, American College of Gastroenterology. The use of gastrointestinal drugs during pregnancy and lactation. Am J Gastroenterol 1985;80:912–923.

272. Beitins IZ, Bayard F, Ances IG, Kowarski A, Migeon CJ. The transplacental passage of prednisone and prednisolone in pregnancy near term. J Pediatr 1972;81:936–945.

273. Walker BE. Induction of cleft palate in rats with anti-inflammatory drugs. Teratology 1971;4:39–42.

274. Reinisch JM, Simon NG, Gandelman R. Prenatal exposure to prednisone permanently alters fighting behavior of female mice. Pharmacol Biochem Behav 1980;12:213–216.

275. Durie BGM, Giles HR. Successful treatment of acute leukemia during pregnancy: combination therapy in the third trimester. Arch Intern Med 1977;137:90–91.

276. Nolan GH, Sweet RL, Laros RK, Roure CA. Renal cadaver transplantation followed by successful pregnancies. Obstet Gynecol 1974;43:732–739.

277. Grossman JH III, Littner MR. Severe sarcoidosis in pregnancy. Obstet Gynecol 1977;50(suppl):81s–84s.

278. Cutting HO, Collier TM. Acute lymphocytic leukemia during pregnancy: report of a case. Obstet Gynecol 1964;24:941–945.

279. Hanson GC, Ghosh S. Systemic lupus erythematosus and pregnancy. Br Med J 1965;2:1227–1228.

280. Warrell DW, Taylor R. Outcome for the foetus of mothers receiving prednisolone during pregnancy. Lancet 1968;1:117–118.

281. Walsh SD, Clark FR. Pregnancy in patients on long-term corticosteroid therapy. Scott Med J 1967;12:302–306.

282. Zulman JI, Talal N, Hoffman GS, Epstein WV. Problems associated with the management of pregnancies in patients with systemic lupus erythematosus. J Rheumatol 1980;7:37–49.

283. Hartikainen-Sorri AL, Kaila J. Systemic lupus erythematosus and habitual abortion: case report. Br J Obstet Gynaecol 1980;87:729–731.

284. Minchinton RM, Dodd NJ, O'Brien H, Amess JAL, Waters AH. Autoimmune thrombocytopenia in pregnancy. Br J Haematol 1980;44:451–459.

285. Tozman ECS, Urowitz MB, Gladman DD. Systemic lupus erythematosus and pregnancy. J Rheumatol 1980;7:624–632.

286. Karpatkin M, Porges RF, Karpatkin S. Platelet counts in infants of women with autoimmune thrombocytopenia: effect of steroid administration to the mother. N Engl J Med 1981;305:936–939.

287. Pratt WR. Allergic diseases in pregnancy and breast feeding. Ann Allergy 1981;47:355–360.

288. Strother SV, Wagner AM. Prendisone in pregnant women with idiopathic thrombocytopenic purpura. N Engl J Med 1988;319:178.

289. Fitzsimons R, Greenberger PA, Patterson R. Outcome of pregnancy in women requiring corticosteroids for severe asthma. J Allergy Clin Immunol 1986;78:349–353.

290. Bongiovanni AM, McPadden AJ. Steroids during pregnancy and possible fetal consequences. Fertil Steril 1960;11:181–186.

291. Kalter H, Warkany J. Congenital malformations: second of two parts. N Engl J Med 1983;308:491–497.

292. Kraus AM. Congenital cataract and maternal steroid injection. J Pediatr Ophthalmol 1975;12:107–108.

293. Scott JR. Fetal growth retardation associated with maternal administration of immunosuppressive drugs. Am J Obstet Gynecol 1977;128:668–676.

294. Pirson Y, Van Lierde M, Ghysen J, Squifflet JP, Alexandre GPJ, Van Ypersele De Strihou C. Retardation of fetal growth in patients receiving immunosuppressive therapy. N Engl J Med 1985;313:328.

295. Hou S. Retardation of fetal growth in patients receiving immunosuppressive therapy [Reply]. N Engl J Med 1985;313:328.

296. Szabo I, Csaba I, Novak P, Drozgyik I. Single-dose glucocorticoid for prevention of respiratory-distress syndrome. Lancet 1977;2:243.

297. Mancini RE, Larieri JC, Muller F, Andrada JA, Saraceni DJ. Effect of predisolone upon normal and pathologic human spermatogenesis. Fertil Steril 1966;17:500–513.

298. Katz FH, Duncan BR. Entry of prednisone into human milk. N Engl J Med 1975;293:1154.

299. McKenzie SA, Selley JA, Agnew JE. Secretion of prednisone into breast milk. Arch Dis Child 1975;50:894–896.

300. Ost L, Wettrell G, Bjorkhem I, Rane A. Prednisolone excretion in human milk. J Pediatr 1985;106:1008–1011.

301. Grekas DM, Vasiliou SS, Lazarides AN. Immunosuppressive therapy and breast-feeding after renal transplantation. Nephron 1984;37:68.

302. Kitao T, Kamishita S, Yoshikawa H, Sakaguchi M. Teratogenicity studies of chenodeoxycholic acid in rats. Yakuri to Chiryo 1982;10:3887–3901, as cited by Shepard (67, p. 127).

303. Takahashi H, Miyashita T, Tozuka K. Effects of chenodeoxycholic acid, administered in the organogenetic period, on the pre- and post-natal development of rat's and mouse's offsprings. Oyo Yakuri (Pharmacometrics) 1978;15:1047–1055.

304. McSherry CK, Morrissey KP, Swarm RL, May PS, Niemann WH, Glenn F. Chenodeoxycholic acid induced liver injury in pregnant and neonatal baboons. Ann Surg 1976;184:490–499.

305. Celle G, Cavanna M, Bocchini R, Robbiano L. Chenodeoxycholic acid (CDCA) versus ursodeoxycholic acid (UDCA): a comparison of their effects in pregnant rats. Arch Int Pharmacodyn Ther 1980;246:149–158.

306. Sprinkle DJ, Hassan AS, Subbiah MTR. Effect of chenodeoxycholic acid feeding during gestation in the rat on bile acid metabolism and liver morphology. Proc Soc Exp Biol Med 1984;175:386–397.

307. Heywood R, Palmer AK, Foll CV, Lee MR. Pathological changes in fetal rhesus monkey induced by oral chenodeoxycholic acid. Lancet 1973;2:1021.

308. Toyoshima S, Fujita H, Sakurai T, Sato R, Kashima M. Reproduction studies of ursodeoxycholic acid in rats, II: teratogenicity study. Oyo Yakuri 1978;15:931–945. Cited by Shepard (675, p. 655).

309. Product information. Actigall. Summit Pharmaceuticals, 1992.

310. Product information. Carafate. Marion Merrell Dow, 1992.

311. Lione A. Aluminum toxicology and the aluminum-containing medications. Pharmacol Ther 1985;29:255–285.

312. Leung ACT, Henderson IS, Halls DJ, Dobbie JW. Aluminium hydroxide versus sucralfate as a phosphate binder in uraemia. Br Med J 1983;286:1379–1381.

313. Yokel RA. Toxicity of gestational aluminum exposure to the maternal rabbit and offspring. Toxicol Appl Pharmacol 1985;79:121–133.

314. McCormack KM, Ottosen LD, Sanger VL, Sprague S, Mayor GH, Hook JB. Effect of prenatal administration of aluminum and parathyroid hormone on fetal development in the rat (40493). Proc Soc Exp Biol Med 1979;161:74–77.

315. Yokel RA, McNamara PJ. Aluminum bioavailability and disposition in adult and immature rabbits. Toxicol Appl Pharmacol 1985;77:344–352.

316. Sedman AB, Klein GL, Merritt RJ, et al. Evidence of aluminum loading in infants receiving intravenous therapy. N Engl J Med 1985;312:1337–1343.

317. Golding J, Rowland A, Greenwood R, Lunt P. Aluminium sulphate in water in north Cornwall and

outcome of pregnancy. Br Med J 1991;302:1175–1177.

318. Hall GS, Carr MJ, Cummings E, Lee M. Aluminum, barium, silicon, and strontium in amniotic fluid by emission spectrometry. Clin Chem 1983;29:1318.

319. Litov RE, Sickles VS, Chan GM, Springer MA, Cordano A. Plasma aluminum measurements in term infants fed human milk or a soy-based infant formula. Pediatrics 1989;84:1105–1106.

320. Bylsma-Howell M, Riggs KW, McMorland GH, et al. Placental transport of metoclopramide: assessment of maternal and neonatal effects. Can Anaesth Soc J 1983;30:487–492.

321. Arvela P, Jouppila R, Kauppila A, Pakarinen A, Pelkonen O, Tuimala R. Placental transfer and hormonal effects of metoclopramide. Eur J Clin Pharmacol 1983;24:345–348.

322. Cohen SE, Jasson J, Talafre M-L, Chauvelot-Moachon L, Barrier G. Does metoclopramide decrease the volume of gastric contents in patients undergoing cesarean section? Anesthesiology 1984;61:604–607.

323. Lyonnet R, Lucchini G. Metoclopramide in obstetrics. J Med Chir Prat 1967;138:352–355.

324. Sidhu MS, Lean TH. The use of metoclopramide (Maxolon) in hyperemesis gravidarum. Proc Obstet Gynaecol Soc Singapore 1970;1:1–4.

325. Martynshin MYA, Arkhengel'skii AE. Experience in treating early toxicoses of pregnancy with metoclopramide. Akush Ginekol 1981;57:44–45.

326. Pinder RM, Brogden RN, Sawyer PR, Speight TM, Avery GS. Metoclopramide: a review of its pharmacological properties and clinical use. Drugs 1976;12:81–131.

327. Harrington RA, Hamilton CW, Brogden RN, Linkewich JA, Romankiewicz JA, Heel RC. Metoclopramide: an update review of its pharmacological properties and clinical use. Drugs 1983;25:451–494.

328. Milo R, Neuman M, Klein C, Caspi E, Arlazoroff A. Acute intermittent porphyria in pregnancy. Obstet Gynecol 1989;73:450–452.

329. McGarry JM. A double-blind comparison of the anti-emetic effect during labour of metoclopramide and perphenazine. Br J Anaesth 1971;43:613–615.

330. Howard FA, Sharp DS. Effect of metoclopramide on gastric emptying during labour. Br Med J 1973;1:446–448.

331. Brock-Utne JG, Dow TGB, Welman S, Dimopoulos GE, Moshal MG. The effect of metoclopramide on the lower oesophageal sphincter in late pregnancy. Anaesth Intensive Care 1978;6:26–29.

332. Hey VMF, Ostick DG. Metoclopramide and the gastro-oesophageal sphincter. Anaesthesia 1978;33:462–465.

333. Feeney JG. Heartburn in pregnancy. Br Med J 1982;284:1138–1139.

334. Murphy DF, Nally B, Gardiner J, Unwin A. Effect of metoclopramide on gastric emptying before elective and emergency caesarean section. Br J Anaesth 1984;56:1113–1116.

335. Vella L, Francis D, Houlton P, Reynolds F. Comparison of the antemetics metoclopramide and promethazine in labour. Br Med J 1985;290:1173–1175.

336. Robuschi G, Emanuele R, d'Amato L, et al. Failure of metoclopramide to release GH in pregnant women. Horm Metabol Res 1983;15:460–461.

337. Lewis PJ, Devenish C, Kahn C. Controlled trial of metoclopramide in the initiation of breast feeding. Br J Clin Pharmacol 1980;9:217–219.

338. Pelkonen O, Arvela P, Kauppila A, Koivisto M, Kivinen S, Ylikorkala O. Metoclopramide in breast milk and newborn [Abstract]. Acta Physiol Scand 1982 (suppl 502):62.

339. Kauppila A, Arvela P, Koivisto M, Kivinen S, Ylikorkala O, Pelkonen O. Metoclopramide and breast feeding: transfer into milk and the newborn. Eur J Clin Pharmacol 1983;25:819–823.

340. Sousa PLR. Metoclopramide and breast-feeding. Br Med J 1975;1:512.

341. Guzman V, Toscano G, Canales ES, Zarate A. Improvement of defective lactation by using oral metoclopramide. Acta Obstet Gynecol Scand 1979;58:53–55.

342. Kauppila A, Kivinen S, Ylikorkala O. Metoclopramide increases prolactin release and milk secretion in puerperium without simulating the secretion of thyrotropin and thyroid hormones. J Clin Endocrinol Metab 1981;52:436–439.

343. Kauppila A, Kivinen S, Ylikorkala O. A dose response relation between improved lactation and metoclopramide. Lancet 1981;1:1175–1177.

344. de Gezelle H, Ooghe W, Thiery M, Dhont M. Metoclopramide and breast milk. Eur J Obstet Gynecol Reprod Biol 1983;15:31–36.

345. Kauppila A, Anunti P, Kivinen S, Koivisto M, Ruokonen A. Metoclopramide and breast feeding: efficacy and anterior pituitary responses of the mother and the child. Eur J Obstet Gynecol Reprod Biol 1985;19:19–22.

346. Gupta AP, Gupta PK. Metoclopramide as a lactogogue. Clin Pediatr 1985;24:269–272.

347. Ehrenkranz RA, Ackerman BA. Metoclopramide effect on faltering milk production by mothers of premature infants. Pediatrics 1986;78:614–620.

348. Sankaran K, Yeboah E, Bingham WT, Ninan A. Use of metoclopramide in preterm infants. Dev Pharmacol Ther 1982;5:114–119.

349. Meader RD, Williams WL. Choline deficiency in the mouse. Am J Anat 1957;100:167–204. Cited by Shepard (67, p. 146).

350. Sarrikoski S, Seppala M. Immunosuppression during pregnancy: transmission of azathioprine and its metabolites from the mother to the fetus. Am J Obstet Gynecol 1973;115:1100–1106.

351. Tuchmann-Duplessis H, Mercier-Parot L. Foetopathes therapeutiques: production experimentale de

malformations des membres. Union Med Can 1968;97:283–288. Cited by Shepard (67, p. 63).

352. Gillibrand PN. Systemic lupus erythematosus in pregnancy treated with azathioprine. Proc R Soc Med 1966;59:834.

353. Board JA, Lee HM, Draper DA, Hume DM. Pregnancy following kidney homotransplantation from a non-twin: report of a case with concurrent administration of azathioprine and prednisone. Obstet Gynecol 1967;29:318–323.

354. Kaufmann JJ, Dignam W, Goodwin WE, Martin DC, Goldman R, Maxwell MH. Successful, normal childbirth after kidney homotransplantation. JAMA 1967;200:338–341.

355. Anonymous. Eleventh annual report of human renal transplant registry. JAMA 1973;216:1197.

356. Sharon E, Jones J, Diamond H, Kaplan D. Pregnancy and azathioprine in systemic lupus erythematosus. Am J Obstet Gynecol 1974;118:25–27.

357. Cote CJ, Meuwissen HJ, Pickering RJ. Effects on the neonate of prednisone and azathioprine administered to the mother during pregnancy. J Pediatr 1974;85:324–328.

358. Erkman J, Blythe JG. Azathioprine therapy complicated by pregnancy. Obstet Gynecol 1972;40:708–709.

359. Price HV, Salaman JR, Laurence KM, Langmaid H. Immunosuppressive drugs and the foetus. Transplantation 1976;21:294–298.

360. The Registration Committee of the European Dialysis and Transplant Association. Successful pregnancies in women treated by dialysis and kidney transplantation. Br J Obstet Gynaecol 1980;87:839–845.

361. Golby M. Fertility after renal transplantation. Transplantation 1970;10:201–207.

362. Rabau-Friedman E, Mashiach S, Cantor E, Jacob ET. Association of hypoparathyroidism and successful pregnancy in kidney transplant recipient. Obstet Gynecol 1982;59:126–128.

363. Myers RL, Schmid R, Newton JJ. Childbirth after liver transplantation. Transplantation 1980;29:432.

364. Williams PF, Johnstone M. Normal pregnancy in renal transplant recipient with history of eclampsia and intrauterine death. Br Med J 1982;285:1535.

365. Westney LS, Callender CO, Stevens J, Bhagwanani SG, George JPA, Mims OL. Successful pregnancy with sickle cell disease and renal transplantation. Obstet Gynecol 1984;63:752–755.

366. Ogburn PL Jr, Kitzmiller JL, Hare JW, et al. Pregnancy following renal transplantation in class T diabetes mellitus. JAMA 1986;255:911–915.

367. Marushak A, Weber T, Bock J, et al. Pregnancy following kidney transplantation. Acta Obstet Gynecol Scand 1986;65:557–559.

368. Key TC, Resnik R, Dittrich HC, Reisner LS. Successful pregnancy after cardiac transplantation. Am J Obstet Gynecol 1989;160:367–371.

369. Davison JM, Lindheimer MD. Pregnancy in renal transplant recipients. J Reprod Med 1982;27:613–621.

370. Kossoy LR, Herbert CM III, Wentz AC. Management of heart transplant recipients: guidelines for the obstetrician-gynecologist. Am J Obstet Gynecol 1988;159:490–499.

371. Nishimura H, Tanimura T. Clinical aspects of the teratogenicity of drugs. New York: American Elsevier, 1976:106–107.

372. Williamson RA, Karp LE. Azathioprine teratogenicity: review of the literature and case report. Obstet Gynecol 1981;58:247–250.

373. Burleson RL, Sunderji SG, Aubry RH, et al. Renal allotransplantation during pregnancy. Successful outcome for mother, child, and kidney. Transplantation 1983;36:334.

374. Leb DE, Weisskopf B, Kanovitz BS. Chromosome aberrations in the child of a kidney transplant recipient. Arch Intern Med 1971;128:441–444.

375. DeWitte DB, Buick MK, Cyran SE, Maisels MJ. Neonatal pancytopenia and severe combined immunodeficiency associated with antenatal administration of azathioprine and prednisone. J Pediatr 1984;105:625–628.

376. Cederqvist LL, Merkatz IR, Litwin SD. Fetal immunoglobulin synthesis following maternal immunosuppression. Am J Obstet Gynecol 1977;129:687–690.

377. Davison JM, Dellagrammatikas H, Parkin JM. Maternal azathioprine therapy and depressed haemopoiesis in the babies of renal allograft patients. Br J Obstet Gynaecol 1985;92:233–239.

378. Fagerholm MI, Coulam CB, Moyer TP. Breastfeeding after renal transplantation: 6-mercaptopurine content in human breast milk. Surg Forum 1980;31:447–449.

379. Coulam CB, Moyer TP, Jiang N-S, Zincke H. Breast-feeding after renal transplantation. Transplant Proc 1982;13:605–609.

380. Sokal JE, Lessmann EM. Effects of cancer chemotherapeutic agents on the human fetus. JAMA 1960;172:1765–1771.

381. Moloney WC. Management of leukemia in pregnancy. Ann NY Acad Sci 1964;114:857–867.

382. Nicholson HO. Cytotoxic drugs in pregnancy: review of reported cases. J Obstet Gynaecol Br Commonw 1968;75:307–312.

383. Gililland J, Weinstein L. The effects of cancer chemotherapeutic agents on the developing fetus. Obstet Gynecol Surv 1983;38:6–13.

384. Wegelius R. Successful pregnancy in acute leukaemia. Lancet 1975;2:1301.

385. Nicholson HO. Leukaemia and pregnancy: a report of five cases and discussion of management. J Obstet Gynaecol Br Commonw 1968;75:517–520.

386. Pizzuto J, Aviles A, Noriega L, Niz J, Morales M, Romero F. Treatment of acute leukemia during

pregnancy: presentation of nine cases. Cancer Treat Rep 1980;64:679–683.

387. Burnier AM. Discussion. In: Plows CW. Acute myelomonocytic leukemia in pregnancy: report of a case. Am J Obstet Gynecol 1982;143:41–43.

388. Dara P, Slater LM, Armentrout SA. Successful pregnancy during chemotherapy for acute leukemia. Cancer 1981;47:845–846.

389. McConnell JF, Bhoola R. A neonatal complication of maternal leukemia treated with 6-mercaptopurine. Postgrad Med J 1973;49:211–213.

390. Diamond J, Anderson MM, McCreadie SR. Transplacental transmission of busulfan (Myleran) in a mother with leukemia: production of fetal malformation and cytomegaly. Pediatrics 1960;25:85–90.

391. Khurshid M, Saleem M. Acute leukaemia in pregnancy. Lancet 1978;2:534–535.

392. Okun DB, Groncy PK, Sieger L, Tanaka KR. Acute leukemia in pregnancy: transient neonatal myelosuppression after combination chemotherapy in the mother. Med Pediatr Oncol 1979;7:315–319.

393. Doney KC, Kraemer KG, Shepard TH. Combination chemotherapy for acute myelocytic leukemia during pregnancy: three case reports. Cancer Treat Rep 1979;63:369–371.

394. Schleuning M, Clemm C. Chromosomal aberrations in a newborn whose mother received cytotoxic treatment during pregnancy. N Engl J Med 1987;317:1666–1667.

395. Turchi JJ, Villasis C. Anthracyclines in the treatment of malignancy in pregnancy. Cancer 1988; 61:435–440.

396. Feliu J, Juarez S, Ordonez A, Garcia-Paredes ML, Gonzales-Baron M, Montero JM. Acute leukemia and pregnancy. Cancer 1988;61:580–584.

397. Haerr RW, Pratt AT. Multiagent chemotherapy for sarcoma diagnosed during pregnancy. Cancer 1985;56:1028–1033.

398. Frenkel EP, Meyers MC. Acute leukemia and pregnancy. Ann Intern Med 1960;53:656–671.

399. Loyd HO. Acute leukemia complicated by pregnancy. JAMA 1961;178:1140–1143.

400. Lee RA, Johnson CE, Hanlon DG. Leukemia during pregnancy. Am J Obstet Gynecol 1962;84:455–458.

401. Coopland AT, Friesen WJ, Galbraith PA. Acute leukemia in pregnancy. Am J Obstet Gynecol 1969;105:1288–1289.

402. Segars LW, Gales BJ. Mesalamine and olsalazine: 5-aminosalicylic acid agents for the treatment of inflammatory bowel disease. Clin Pharm 1992; 11:514–528.

403. Berlin CM Jr, Yaffe SJ. Disposition of salicylazosulfapyridine (Azulfidine) and metabolites in human breast milk. Dev Pharmacol Ther 1980;1:31–39.

404. McEwan HP. Anorectal conditions in obstetric practice. Proc R Soc Med 1972;65:279–281.

405. Willoughby CP, Truelove SC. Ulcerative colitis and pregnancy. Gut 1980;21:469–474.

406. Azad Khan AK, Truelove SC. Placental and mammary transfer of sulphasalazine. Br Med J 1979; 2:1553.

407. Jarnerot G, Into-Malmberg MB, Esbjorner E. Placental transfer of sulphasalazine and sulphapyridine and some of its metabolites. Scand J Gastroenterol 1981;16:693–697.

408. Jarnerot G, Andersen S, Esbjorner E, Sandstrom B, Brodersen R. Albumin reserve for binding of bilirubin in maternal and cord serum under treatment with sulphasalazine. Scand J Gastroenterol 1981; 16:1049–1055.

409. Christensen LA, Rasmussen SN, Hansen SH, Bondesen S, Hvidberg EF. Salazosulfapyridine and metabolites in fetal and maternal body fluids with special reference to 5-aminosalicylic acid. Acta Obstet Gynecol Scand 1987;66:433–435.

410. Mogadam M. Sulfasalazine, IBD, and pregnancy [Reply]. Gastroenterology 1981;81:194.

411. Peppercorn MA. Sulfasalazine: pharmacology, clinical use, toxicity, and related new drug development. Ann Intern Med 1984;101:377–386.

412. Levy N, Roisman I, Teodor I. Ulcerative colitis in pregnancy in Israel. Dis Colon Rectum 1981; 24:351–354.

413. Mogadam M, Dobbins WO III, Korelitz BI, Ahmed SW. Pregnancy in inflammatory bowel disease: effect of sulfasalazine and corticosteroids on fetal outcome. Gastroenterology 1981;80:72–76.

414. Fielding JF. Pregnancy and inflammatory bowel disease. J Clin Gastroenterol 1983;5:107–108.

415. Sorokin JJ, Levine SM. Pregnancy and inflammatory bowel disease: a review of the literature. Obstet Gynecol 1983;62:247–252.

416. Baiocco PJ, Korelitz BI. The influence of inflammatory bowel disease and its treatment on pregnancy and fetal outcome. J Clin Gastroenterol 1984;6:211–216.

417. Fedorkow DM, Persaud D, Nimrod CA. Inflammatory bowel disease: a controlled study of late pregnancy outcome. Am J Obstet Gynecol 1989; 160:998–1001.

418. Mulder CJJ, Tytgat GNJ, Weterman IT, et al. Double-blind comparison of slow-release 5-aminosalicylate and sulfasalazine in remission maintenance in ulcerative colitis. Gastroenterol 1988; 95:1449–1453.

419. Craxi A, Pagliarello F. Possible embryotoxicity of sulfasalazine. Arch Intern Med 1980;140:1674.

420. Newman NM, Correy JF. Possible teratogenicity of sulphasalazine. Med J Aust 1983;1:528–529.

421. Hoo JJ, Hadro TA, Von Behren P. Possible teratogenicity of sulfasalazine. N Engl J Med 1988; 318:1128.

422. Levi S, Liberman M, Levi AJ, Bjarnason I. Reversible congenital neutropenia associated with maternal sulphasalazine therapy. Eur J Pediatr 1988; 48:174–175.

423. Freeman JG, Reece VAC, Venables CW. Sulphasalazine and spermatogenesis. Digestion 1982;23:68–71.

424. Toovey S, Hudson E, Hendry WF, Levi AJ. Sulphasalazine and male infertility: reversibility and possible mechanism. Gut 1981;22:445–451.

425. O'Morain C, Smethurst P, Dore CJ, Levi AJ. Reversible male infertility due to sulphasalazine: studies in man and rat. Gut 1984;25:1078–1084.

426. Chatzinoff M, Guarino JM, Corson SL, Batzer FR, Friedman LS. Sulfasalazine-induced abnormal sperm penetration assay reversed on changing to 5-aminosalicylic acid enemas. Dig Dis Sci 1988;33:108–110.

427. Delaere KP, Strijbos WE, Meuleman EJ. Sulphasalazine-induced reversible male infertility. Acta Urol Belg 1989;57:29–33.

428. Jarnerot G, Into-Malmberg MB. Sulphasalazine treatment during breast feeding. Scand J Gastroenterol 1979;14:869–871.

429. Branski D, Kerem E, Gross-Kieselstein E, Hurvitz H, Litt R, Abrahamov A. Bloody diarrhea—a possible complication of sulfasalazine transferred through human breast milk. J Pediatr Gastroenterol Nutr 1986;5:316–317.

430. Nelis GF. Diarrhoea due to 5-aminosalicylic acid in breast milk. Lancet 1989;1:383.

431. Jenss H, Weber P, Hartmann F. 5-Aminosalicylic acid and its metabolite in breast milk during lactation. Am J Gastroenterol 1990;85:331.

432. Product information. Dulcolax. Boehringer Ingelheim Pharmaceuticals, 1992.

433. Witter FR, King TM, Blake DA. The effects of chronic gastrointestinal medication on the fetus and neonate. Obstet Gynecol 1981;58:79S–84S.

434. Mizutani M, Izutsu M, Hoshimoto Y, Nagao T, Matsuda H. Effects of sennaglucosides on reproductive function and fetal development and differentiation in rats. Kiso to Rinsho 1980;14:380–396. Cited by Shepard (67, p. 574).

435. Mengs U. Reproductive toxicological investigations with sennosides. Arzneim Forsch 1986;36–42:1355–1358. Cited by Shepard TH. (67, p. 575).

436. Garcia-Villar R. Evaluation of the effects of sennosides on uterine motility in the pregnant ewe. Pharmacology 1988;36(suppl 1):203–211.

437. Odenthal KP, Ziegler D. In vitro effects of anthraquinones on rat intestine and uterus. Pharmacology 1988;36(suppl 1):57–65.

438. Leng-Peschlow E. Risk assessment for senna during pregnancy. Pharmacology 1992;44(suppl 1):20–22.

439. Burgess DE. Constipation in obstetrics. In: Jones FA, Godding EW, eds. Management of Constipation. Oxford, England: Blackwell Scientific Publications, 1972;176–188. Cited by Leng-Peschlow (438).

440. Blair AW, Burdon M, Powell J, Gerrard M, Smith R. Fetal exposure to 1:8 dihydroxyanthraquinone. Biol Neonate 1977;31:289–293.

441. Jinks MJ, Fuerst RH. Geriatric therapy. In: Koda-Kimble MA, Young LY, eds. Applied therapeutics: the clinical use of drugs. ed. 5. Vancouver, WA: Applied Therapeutics, 1992:79–112.

442. Werthmann MW Jr, Krees SV. Quantitative excretion of Senokot in human breast milk. Med Ann Dist Col 1973;42:4–5.

443. Faber P, Strenge-Hesse A. Relevance of rhein excretion into breast milk. Pharmacology 1988;36(suppl 1):212–220.

444. Baldwin WF. Clinical study of senna administration to nursing mothers: assessment of effects on infant bowel habits. Can Med Assoc J 1963;89:566–568.

445. Greenhalf JO, Leonard HSD. Laxatives in the treatment of constipation in pregnant and breast-feeding mothers. Practitioner 1973;210:259–263.

446. Leng-Peschlow E. Senna in the puerperium. Pharmacology 1992;44(suppl 1):23–25.

447. Bennett PN and the WHO Working Group, eds. Drugs and human lactation. New York: Elsevier, 1988:87.

448. Friebel H, Walkowiak L. Gehen anthrachinonhaltige Abführmittel in die Franenmilch über? Med Klin 1951;46:208–209. Cited by Leng-Peschlow (446).

449. Fantus B, Dyniewicz JM. Phenolphthalein administration to nursing women. Am J Dig Dis 1937;3:184–185. Cited by Bennett PN, et al. (447).

450. Product information. Cephulac. Marion Merrell Dow, 1992.

451. Product information. Librium. Roche Laboratories, 1992.

452. Milkovich L, van den Berg BJ. Effects of prenatal meprobamate and chlordiazepoxide hydrochloride on human embryonic and fetal development. N Engl J Med 1974;291:1268–1271.

453. Rothman KJ, Fyler DC, Golblatt A, Kreidberg MB. Exogenous hormones and other drug exposures of children with congenital heart disease. Am J Epidemiol 1979;109:433–439.

454. Crombie DL, Pinsent RJ, Fleming DM, Rumeau-Rouguette C, Goujard J, Huel G. Fetal effects of tranquilizers in pregnancy. N Engl J Med 1975;293:198–199.

455. Hartz SC, Heinonen OP, Shapiro S, Siskind V, Slone D. Antenatal exposure to meprobamate and chlordiazepoxide in relation to malformations, mental development, and childhood mortality. N Engl J Med 1975;292:726–728.

456. Bracken MB, Holford TR. Exposure to prescribed drugs in pregnancy and association with congenital malformations. Obstet Gynecol 1981;58:336–344.

457. Committee on Drugs, American Academy of Pediatrics. Psychotropic drugs in pregnancy and lactation. Pediatrics 1982;69:241–244.

458. Athinarayanan P, Pierog SH, Nigam SK, Glass L. Chlordiazepoxide withdrawal in the neonate. Am J Obstet Gynecol 1976;124:212–213.

459. Decancq HG Jr, Bosco JR, Townsend EH Jr. Chlordiazepoxide in labour: its effect on the newborn infant. J Pediatr 1965;67:836–840.

460. Mark PM, Hamel J. Librium for patients in labor. Obstet Gynecol 1968;32:188–194.

461. Stirrat GM, Edington PT, Berry DJ. Transplacental passage of chlordiazepoxide. Br Med J 1974; 2:729.

462. Duckman S, Spina T, Attardi M, Meyer A. Double-blind study of chlordiazepoxide in obstetrics. Obstet Gynecol 1964;24:601–605.

463. Kanto JH. Use of benzodiazepines during pregnancy, labour and lactation, with particular reference to pharmacokinetic considerations. Drugs 1982;23:354–380.

464. Scanlon JW. Effect of benzodiazepines in neonates. N Engl J Med 1975;292:649.

465. Gillberg C. "Floppy infant syndrome" and maternal diazepam. Lancet 1977;2:244.

466. Haram K. "Floppy infant syndrome" and maternal diazepam. Lancet 1977;2:612–613.

467. Speight AN. Floppy-infant syndrome and maternal diazepam and/or nitrazepam. Lancet 1977;1:878.

468. Wesson DR, Camber S, Harkey M, Smith DE. Diazepam and desmethyldiazepam in breast milk. J Psychoactive Drugs 1985;17:55–56.

469. Hauptmann A. Luminal bei epilepsie. Munchen Med Wochenschr 1912;59:1907–1908.

470. Gupta C, Yaffe SJ. Reproductive dysfunction in female offspring after prenatal exposure to phenobarbital: critical period of action. Pediatr Res 1981; 15:1488–1491.

471. Yaffe SJ, Dorn LD. Critical periods of neuroendocrine development: effects of prenatal xenobiotics. In: Timiras PS, ed. Plasticity and regeneration of the nervous system. New York: Plenum Press, 1991:81–89.

472. Valaes T, Kipouros K, Petmezaki S, Solman M, Doxiadis SA. Effectiveness and safety of prenatal phenobarbital for the prevention of neonatal jaundice. Pediatr Res 1980;14:947–952.

473. Hill RB. Teratogenesis and anti-epileptic drugs. N Engl J Med 1973;289:1089–1090.

474. Bodendorfer TW. Fetal effects of anticonvulsant drugs and seizure disorders. Drug Intell Clin Pharm 1978;12:14–21.

475. Committee on Drugs, American Academy of Pediatrics. Anticonvulsants and pregnancy. Pediatrics 1977;63:331–333.

476. Nakane Y, Okoma T, Takahashe R, et al. Multi-institutional study of the teratogenicity and fetal toxicity of anti-epileptic drugs: a report of a collaborative study group in Japan. Epilepsia 98;21:633–680.

477. Andermann E, Dansky L, Andermann F, Loughnan PM, Gibbons J. Minor congenital malformations and dermatoglyphic alterations in the offspring of epileptic women: a clinical investigation of the teratogenic effects of anticonvulsant medication. In: Epilepsy, pregnancy and the child. Proceedings of a Workshop in Berlin, September 1980. New York: Raven Press, 1981.

478. Dansky L, Andermann E, Andermann F. Major congenital malformations in the offspring of epileptic patients. In: Epilepsy, pregnancy and the child. Proceedings of a Workshop in Berlin, September 1980. New York: Raven Press, 1981.

479. Janz D. The teratogenic risks of antiepileptic drugs. Epilepsia 1975;16:159–169.

480. Hanson JW, Buehler BA. Fetal hydantoin syndrome: current status. J Pediatr 1982;101:816–818.

481. Janz D. Antiepileptic drugs and pregnancy: altered utilization patterns and teratogenesis. Epilepsia 1982;23(suppl 1):S53–S63.

482. Desmond MM, Schwanecke RP, Wilson GS, Yasunaga S, Burgdorff I. Maternal barbiturate utilization and neonatal withdrawal symptomatology. J Pediatr 1972;80:190–197.

483. Spiedel BD, Meadow SR. Maternal epilepsy and abnormalities of the fetus and the newborn. Lancet 1972;2:839–843.

484. Bleyer WA, Skinner AL. Fatal neonatal hemorrhage after maternal anticonvulsant therapy. JAMA 1976;235:826–827.

485. Lawrence A. Anti-epileptic drugs and the foetus. Br Med J 1963;2:1267.

486. Kohler HG. Haemorrhage in the newborn of epileptic mothers. Lancet 1966;1:267.

487. Mountain KR, Hirsh J, Gallus AS. Neonatal coagulation defect due to anticonvulsant drug treatment in pregnancy. Lancet 1970;1:265–268.

488. Evans AR, Forrester RM, Discombe C. Neonatal haemorrhage during anticonvulsant therapy. Lancet 1970;1:517–518.

489. Margolin FG, Kantor NM. Hemorrhagic disease of the newborn. An unusual case related to maternal ingestion of an anti-epileptic drug. Clin Pediatr (Phila) 1972;11:59–60.

490. Srinivasan G, Seeler RA, Tiruvury A, Pildes RS. Maternal anticonvulsant therapy and hemorrhagic disease of the newborn. Obstet Gynecol 1982;59:250–252.

491. Payne NR, Hasegawa DK. Vitamin K deficiency in newborns: a case report in a-1-antitrypsin deficiency and a review of factors predisposing to hemorrhage. Pediatrics 1984;73:712–716.

492. Lane PA, Hathaway WE. Vitamin K in infancy. J Pediatr 1985;106:351–359.

493. Pritchard JA, Scott DE, Whalley PJ. Maternal folate deficiency and pregnancy wastage. IV. Effects of folic acid supplements, anticonvulsants, and oral contraceptives. Am J Obstet Gynecol 1971; 109:341–346.

494. Hiilesmaa VK, Teramo K, Granstrom ML, Bardy AH. Serum folate concentrations during pregnancy in women with epilepsy: relation to antiepileptic drug concentrations, number of seizures, and fetal outcome. Br Med J 1983;287:577–579.

495. Biale Y, Lewenthal H. Effect of folic acid supplementation on congenital malformations due to anticonvulsive drugs. Eur J Obstet Reprod Biol 1984;18:211–216.

496. Shankaran S, Cepeda EE, Ilagan N, et al. Antenatal phenobarbital for the prevention of neonatal intracerebral hemorrhage. Am J Obstet Gynecol 1986;154:53–57 .

497. Morales WJ, Koerten J. Prevention of intraventricular hemorrhage in very low birth weight infants by maternally administered phenobarbital. Obstet Gynecol 1986;68:295–299.

498. De Carolis S. Antenatal phenobarbital in preventing intraventricular hemorrhage in premature newborns. Fetal Ther 1988;3:224–229.

499. Kuban KCK, Leviton A, Krishnamoorthy KS, et al. Neonatal intracranial hemorrhage and phenobarbital. Pediatrics 1986;77:443–450.

500. Donn SM, Roloff DW, Goldstein GW. Prevention of intraventricular haemorrhage in preterm infants by phenobarbitone; a controlled trial. Lancet 1981;2:215–217.

501. Bedard MP, Shankaran S, Slovis TL, Pantoja A, Dayal B, Poland RL. Effect of prophylactic phenobarbital on intraventricular hemorrhage in high-risk infants. Pediatrics 1984;73:435–439.

502. Espinoza J, Barnafi L, Schnaidt E. The effect of phenobarbital on intrahepatic cholestasis of pregnancy. Am J Obstet Gynecol 1974;119:234–238.

503. Laatikainen T. Effect of cholestyramine and phenobarbital on pruritis and serum bile acid levels in cholestasis of pregnancy. Am J Obstet Gynecol 1978;133:501–506.

504. Heikkinen J, Maentausta O, Ylostalo P, Janne O. Serum bile acid levels in intrahepatic cholestasis of pregnancy during treatment with phenobarbital or cholestyramine. Eur J Obstet Gynecol Reprod Biol 1982;14:153–162.

505. Tyson RM, Shrader EA, Perlman HN. Drugs transmitted through breast-milk, II: barbiturates. J Pediatr 1938;13:86–90.

506. Kaneko S, Sata T, Suzuki K. The levels of anticonvulsants in breast milk. Br J Clin Pharmacol 1979;7:624–627.

507. Nau H, Kuhnz, Egger HJ, Rating D, Helge H. Anticonvulsants during pregnancy and lactation: transplacental, maternal and neonatal pharmacokinetics. Clin Pharmacokinet 1982;7:508–543.

508. Horning MG, Stillwell WG, Nowlin J, Lertratanangkoon K, Stillwell RN, Hill RM. Identification and quantification of drugs and drug metabolites in human breast milk using GC-MS-COM methods. Mod Probl Paediatr 1975;15:73–79.

509. Reith H, Schafer H. Antiepileptic drugs during pregnancy and the lactation period. Pharmacokinetic data. Dtsch Med Wochenschr 1979;104:818–823.

510. Product information. Questran. Bristol Laboratories, 1992.

511. Innis SM. Effect of cholestyramine administration during pregnancy in the rat. Am J Obstet Gynecol 1983;146:13–16.

512. Koda S, Anabuki K, Miki T, Kahi S, Takahashi N. Reproductive studies on cholestyramine. Kiso to Rinsho 1982;16:2040–2094. Cited by Shepard TH. (61, p. 146).

513. Lutz EE, Margolis AJ. Obstetric hepatosis: treatment with cholestyramine and interim response to steroids. Obstet Gynecol 1969;33:64–71.

514. Shaw D, Frohlich J, Wittman BAK, Willms M. A prospective study of 18 patients with cholestasis of pregnancy. Am J Obstet Gynecol 1982;142:621–625.

515. Vanjak D, Moreau R, Roche-Sicot J, Soulier A, Sicot C. Intrahepatic cholestasis of pregnancy and acute fatty liver of pregnancy: an unusual but favorable association? Gastroenterology 1991;100:1123–1125.

516. Product information. Cuprimine. Merck Sharp & Dohme, 1992.

517. Crawhall JC, Scowen EF, Thompson CJ, Watts RWE. Dissolution of cystine stones during D-penicillamine treatment of a pregnant patient with cystinuria. Br Med J 1967;2:216–218.

518. Mjolnerod OK, Rasmussen K, Dommerud SA, Gjeruldsen ST. Congenital connective-tissue defect probably due to D-penicillamine treatment in pregnancy. Lancet 1971;1:673–675.

519. Laver M, Fairley KF. D-Penicillamine treatment in pregnancy. Lancet 1971;1:1019–1020.

520. Scheinberg IH, Sternlieb I. Pregnancy in penicillamine-treated patients with Wilson's disease. N Engl J Med 1975;293:1300–1303.

521. Marecek Z, Graf M. Pregnancy in penicillamine-treated patients with Wilson's disease. N Engl J Med 1976;295:841–842.

522. Solomon L, Abrams G, Dinner M, Berman L. Neonatal abnormalities associated with D-penicillamine treatment during pregnancy. N Engl J Med 1977;296:54–55.

523. Walshe JM. Pregnancy in Wilson's disease. Quart J Med 1977;46:73–83.

524. Lyle WH. Penicillamine in pregnancy. Lancet 1978;1:606–607.

525. Linares A, Zarranz JJ, Rodriguez-Alarcon J, Diaz-Perez JL. Reversible cutis laxa due to maternal D-penicillamine treatment. Lancet 1979;2:43.

526. Endres W. D-penicillamine in pregnancy—to ban or not to ban? Klin Wochenschr 1981;59: 535–537.

527. Harpey JP, Jaudon MC, Clavel JP, Galli A, Darbois Y. Cutis laxa and low serum zinc after antenatal exposure to penicillamine. Lancet 1983;2:858.

528. Beck RB, Rosenbaum KN, Byers PH, Holbrook KA, Perry LW. Ultrastructural findings in the fetal penicillamine syndrome [Abstract]. Presented at the 13th Annual Birth Defects Conference, March of

Dimes and University of California, San Diego, June 1980.

529. Gal P, Ravenel SD. Contractures and hydrocephalus with penicillamine and maternal hypotension. J Clin Dysmorphol 1984;2:9–12.

530. Gregory MC, Mansell MA. Pregnancy and cystinuria. Lancet 1983;2:1158–1160.

531. Ostensen M, Husby G. Antirheumatic drug treatment during pregnancy and lactation. Scand J Rheumatol 1985;14:1–7.

26

Drug Therapy in Pediatric Gastrointestinal Disease

ANGEL R. COLÓN

ANGEL R. COLÓN

GENERAL PRINCIPLES OF PEDIATRIC PHARMACOLOGY

The principles of pediatric pharmacodynamics are not surprisingly size related, but there are additional mitigating factors that include the physiologic immaturity of the infant, delivery vehicle, and parental-patient compliance. As a generalization, the problem of immaturity resolves by 2–3 months of age, and at the longest by 3–4 years. But the other factors remain considerations for years.

The concerns with neonatal pharmacology begin at birth and include agents the mother may have received during parturition. It is known that the human fetus has deficiencies or frank absences of drug metabolizing enzymes in the oxidative, reductive, and conjugative pathways, and the postnatal maturation of these systems is age variable. The perinatal effects of drugs given to pregnant women can be measured in cord blood, and is reflective of transplacental transfer.

Transplacental transfer is primarily dependent on lipid solubility and ionization (1). High lipid solubility and poor ionization facilitate placental transfer as can be seen with caffeine, for example. Other factors influencing placental transfer are molecular weight and protein conjugation. As a generalization, molecular weights less than 500 cross with facility, and those more than 1000 cross with difficulty. The degree of albumin conjugation decreases transfer because unconjugated drugs tend to cross first. For the pediatric gastroenterologist consulting on a newborn, signs of jaundice, coagulopathy, neuropathy, diarrhea, or vomiting, should prompt questions regarding placental drug transfer.

The newborn commonly demonstrates a prolonged plasma half-life for many drugs. For example, indomethacin in the neonate has a half-life of 14–20 hours (adult 2–11), for diazepam 25–100 hours (adult 15–25), and for theophylline 24–36 hours (adult 3–9) (2). Some drugs have significant hepatic maturational variances. For example, phenobarbital's half-life in the immediate newborn is up to 200 hours, for the 2 week old 100 hours, and for the 6 week old it is down to 50 hours but still significantly greater than the adult 12–18 hour value.

The four basic phases of drug metabolism involve absorption, distribution, biotransformation, and excretion. All are altered in the newborn and infant (3) (Fig. 26.1).

Absorption of oral drugs can be altered in the newborn due to delayed gastric emptying and intestinal dysmotility. However, once infancy and childhood are reached, absorption attains adult levels. Liquid preparations may enhance absorption in the child and is often the only form in which a child will comply with medication. However, its use may be limited by drug solubility and it precludes certain microencapsulation media such as those used for omperazole.

Distribution is seldom altered in the newborn. The neonate has increased extracellular water, but it does not ordinarily play a significant role in pharmacodynamics. However, it should be remembered that distribution in the nursing mother includes mammary circulation and that drugs commonly appear in breast milk. Some gastrointestinal *drugs secreted in breast milk* are cascara, danthron, and senna, all of which can produce diarrhea in the

519

Pediatric pharmacodynamics

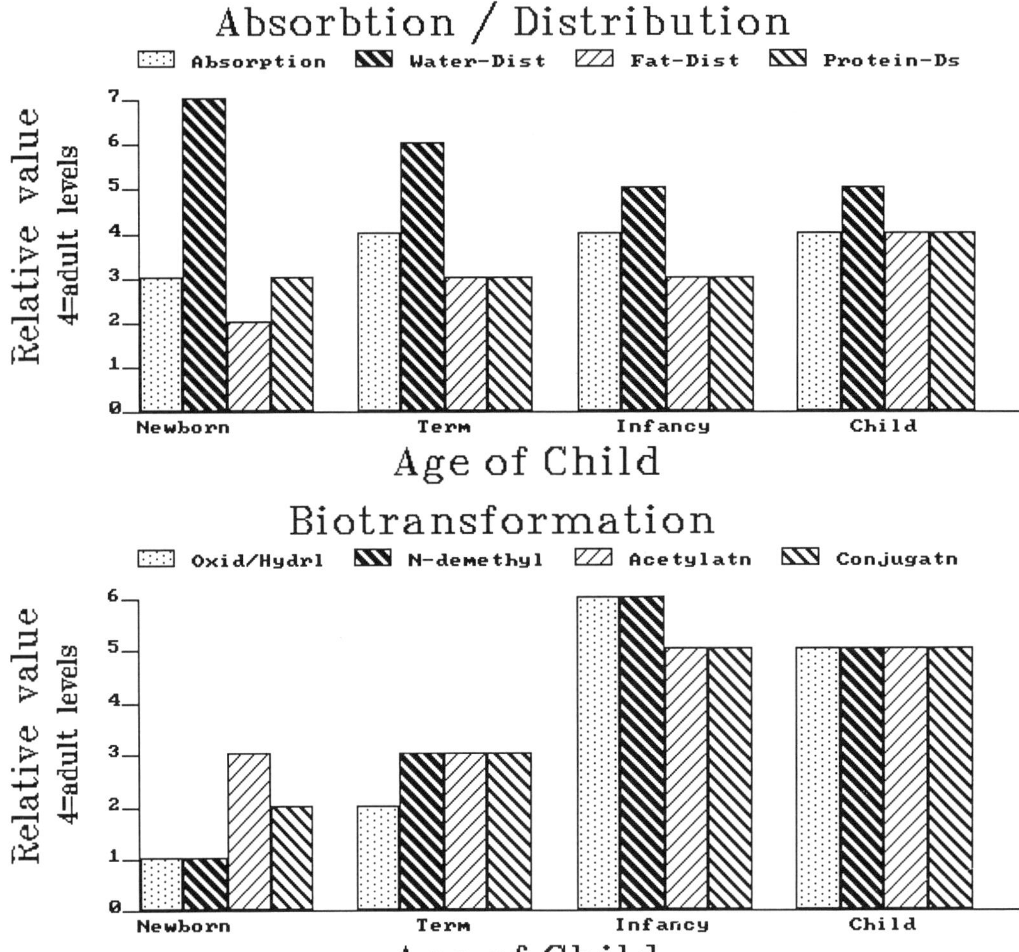

Figure 26.1. Summarizes the overall observations of pediatric pharmacodynamics and is adapted from Rylance (8).

infant; additionally bethanechol, clindamycin, metronidazole, and phenobarbital are commonly secreted (4), and may have secondary effects on the infant. Bethanechol has been reported to cause abdominal pain and diarrhea, diazepam jaundice, chlorpromazine drowsiness and lethargy, dicyclomine arrhythmias, and vancomycin both ototoxicity and nephrotoxicity. Additionally, the following drugs commonly used by gastroenterologists are known to be secreted in breast milk although their effects on the infant are uncertain: azathioprine, carbamazepine, hyoscyamine, colchicine, prednisone, and pyrantel (5, 6). Caution in their use with respect to a nursing mother is warranted.

Biotransformation is slow in the newborn, particularly premature infants. Oxidation and glucuronidation are especially affected. By 1 month of age, both pathways reach adult levels.

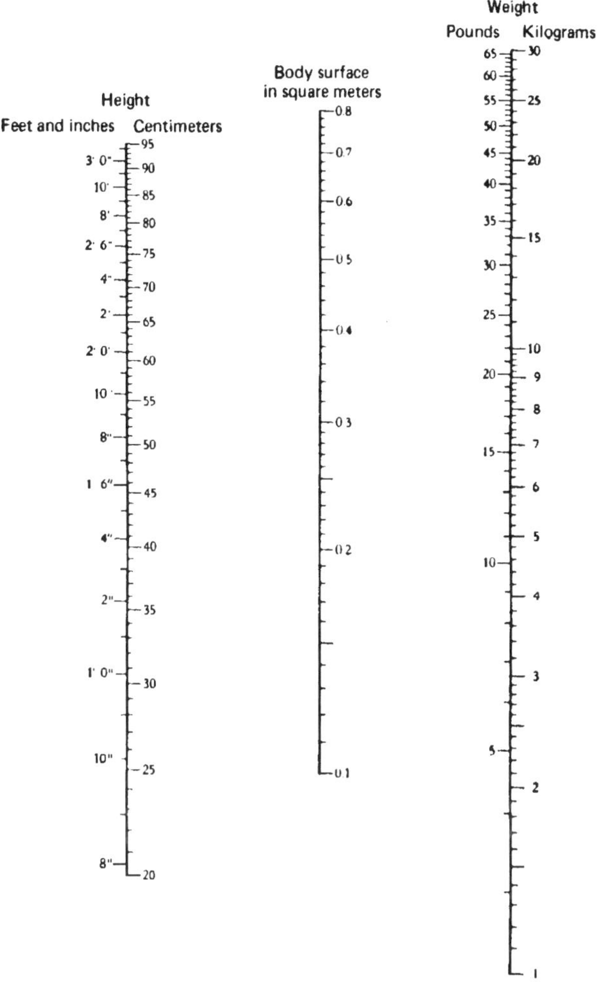

Figure 26.2. Nomogram for estimation of body surface.

Excretion is affected by nature of the neonatal glomerular filtration rate which is only about 50% of adult levels. Mature levels are not reached until 3–6 months of age.

A fifth factor, which is not properly part of pharmacodynamics, but which clearly affects the child, is compliance. Compliance is both pediatric patient and parent dependent. Additionally, it can be influenced by the drug form. For children liquids are generally formulated either as elixirs or suspensions. Elixirs are commonly alcohol vehicles—evenly dissolved, requiring no shaking. However, suspensions generally require vigorous shaking to assure even dosing. A measuring device is recommended for children. The common "teaspoon" volume can vary from 3–7 ml.

When a pediatric dosage schedule is not available, the most accurate method of estimating a dose can be extrapolated by using body surface area. A surface area nomogram (Fig. 2) facilitates this calculation (7), for example: Calculate the dosage of cimetidine for a child of 1 year, weighing 15 kg and measuring 75 cm. Plotting out these parameters on a surface area nomogram yields a surface area of 0.5 M. The average adult of 177 cm² and 76 kg has a surface area of approximately 2.0 M. Therefore, the child's dose will be approximately 25% that of the adult. If the adult dose is 1200 mg/24 hours, then the child's will be 300 or 20 mg/kg/day.

If a nomogram is not available, Clark's rule can be applied: This rule should serve only as rough guide and should be used conservatively.

Clark's rule: Dose for child

$$= \text{Adult dose} \times \frac{\text{Wt of child}}{150}$$

The tables that follow list the drugs and drug schedules commonly used in pediatric gastrointestinal disorders. Table 26.1 categorizes the drugs and Table 26.2 gives appropriate dosages. However, as with most pharmacologic agents, the admonition and generalization holds true that the physician should master the use of a few drugs rather than dabble in polypharmacy. The author has more than a score of years of caring for gastrointestinal disorders in children, and has evolved patterns of treatment that are commonly successful and reasonably free of side effects. They are regimens of personal choice and do not necessarily exclude others, and there are offered in the spirit of Walter Harris:

> There can be no Doubt but that a perfect Cure of the Disease of Children is as much to be desired by all, as any Thing else whatsoever in the whole Art of Physick . . . Wherefore I shall think myself happy, if I can strike out a few Hints, which others of greater Abilities may improve, and bring to Perfection. . . .
>
> *De morbis acutis infantum* (1689)

SPECIFIC THERAPY IN PEDIATRIC GASTROENTEROLOGY

The most common gastrointestinal disorders for which pharmacologic interventions are requested for children include anorexia, emesis, diarrhea, constipation, gastroesophageal reflux, peptic ulcer disease, colic, and inflammatory bowel disease. Less frequently en-

Table 26.1

Categorization of Commonly Used Gastrointestinal Pharmacologic Agents Used in Children (Some Agents Can Be Found in More Than One Category)

Acid-Peptic Disease/Gastroesophageal Reflux Disease
1. H₂-blockers
   cimetidine
   ranitidine
   famotidine
   nizatidine
2. Antacids
   aluminum hydroxide
   magnesium hydroxide
   magnesium trisilicate
   calcium carbonate
3. Demulctants
   bismuth subsalicylate
   suculfrate
   misoprostol ?
4. Pump blockers
   omeprazole
5. Prokinetics
   metoclopramide
   bethanechol
   domperidone
   cisapride

Antiemetics
1. Central
   chlorpromazine
   dimenhydrinate
   hydroxyzine
   ondansetron
   prochlorperazine
   promethazine
   trimethobenzamide
2. Local
   phosphorate carbohydrate

Diarrheal Disease
1. Adsorbents
   kaolin
   pectin
   attapulgite
2. Toxin binders
   charcoal
   cholestyramine
3. Antisecretories
   octreotide
4. Antimotility
   loperamide
   diphenoxylate
   paregoric
5. Bacteriostatics
   bismuth
   colistin
   metronidazole
   acidophilus, bifidus
6. Antibiotics (as per *genera*)
   Campylobacter spp—erythromycin
   Clostridia spp—vancomycin, metronidazole

Table 26.1 Continued
Categorization of Commonly Used Gastrointestinal Pharmacologic Agents Used in Children (Some Agents Can Be Found in More Than One Category)

Salmonella spp—ampicillin, chloramphenicol
Shigella spp—trimethoprim/sulph
Yersinia spp—trimethoprim/sulph

Flatulence
1. Antisurfactants
   simethicone
   charcoal
2. Disaccharidases
   lactase

Hypermotility States
1. Antispasmodics
   atropine (i.e., Donnatal)
   dicyclomine
   scopolamine
   hyoscyamine
2. Antianxiety drugs
   diazepam
   hydroxyzine

Inflammatory Bowel Disease
1. Steroids
   corticotropin
   hydrocortisone
   prednisone
   prednisolone
2. Salicylates
   5-amino-salicylic acid
   sulfasalazine
   osalazine
3. Antibiotics
   metronidazole
   nystatin
   fluconazole
4. Immunosuppressives
   azathioprine
   6-MP
   methotrexate
   cyclosporin

Allergic Enteropathy
1. Antihistamines
   hydroxyzine
   cyproheptadine
2. Kinin-blockers
   cromolyn sodium
3. Calcium supplements (milk-free diet)
   calcium carbonate
   calcium glubionate

Parasitic Diseases
1. Antiprotozoal
   metronidazole
   iodoquinol
   quinacrine
   trimethoprine sulfa
   furazolidone

Table 26.1 Continued
Categorization of Commonly Used Gastrointestinal Pharmacologic Agents Used in Children (Some Agents Can Be Found in More Than One Category)

2. Antihelminthics
   thiabendazole
   mebendazole
   pyrantel
   praziquantel
   niclosamide

Analgesics
1. Oral agents
   aspirin
   acetaminophen
   codeine
   ibuprofen
   meperidine
   morphine

Acute Hepatopathies/Fulmancy
1. Antiviral agents
   acyclovir
   gancyclovir
2. Antiammonemias
   lactulose
   neomycin
3. Cerebral edema drugs
   mannitol
   glycerol
4. False neurotransmitters
   L-Dopa
   bromocriptine
5. Coagulopathy
   fresh frozen plasma
   cryoprecipitate
   vitamin K

Chronic Liver Diseases
1. Cholestasis
   phenobarbital
   cholestyramine
2. Antivirals
   interferon
3. Nutritional deficiency
   albumin
   vitamins A, D, E, K
   carnitine
4. Chelation therapy
   pencillamine
   trientine

Cirrhotic States
1. Diuretics
   chlorothiazine
   furosemide
   spironolactone
   triamterene
2. Antipruritics
   ursodesoxycholic acid
   carbamazepine
   cholestyramine

Table 26.1 Continued
Categorization of Commonly Used Gastrointestinal Pharmacologic Agents Used in Children (Some Agents Can Be Found in More Than One Category)

3. Portal hypertension
   propranolol
5. Antifibrotics
   colchicine

Immunoprophylaxis
1. Globulins
   ISG
   HBIG
2. Vaccines
   hepatitis B vaccine
3. Post-transplant
   cyclosporin
   FK-506
   OKT3

Pancreatic Disease
1. Insufficiencies
   pancreatic enzymes
2. Mucolytics
   acetylcysteine

Constipation/Dyskesia/Dysmotility
1. Bulk agents
   psyllium
   calcium polycarbophil
2. Lubricants
   mineral oil
   glycerin
3. Osmotics
   lactulose
   sodium phosphate
   magnesium citrate
   milk of magnesia
   polyethylene glycol
4. Secretory agents
   senna
5. Prokinetics
   bisacodyl
   phenolphthalein
   casanthranol
   castor oil
6. Softeners
   docusate

Oral Lesions
1. Antifungal
   gentian violet
   nystatin
   ketokonazole
   fluconazole
2. Analgesics
   clove oil
   eugenol
   menthol
   phenol
   benzocaine

Table 26.1 Continued
Categorization of Commonly Used Gastrointestinal Pharmacologic Agents Used in Children (Some Agents Can Be Found in More Than One Category)

Procedural Sedation
   chloral hydrate
   diazepam
   fentanyl
   meperidine
   midazolam
   naloxone
   phenobarbital

countered are parasitosis, allergic enteropathy, cirrhosis, cholestasis, and pancreatic insufficiency. Treatment recommendation for each of these disorders follows in detail. Table 26.2 provides specific information on the drugs and doses available for use in children in a wider variety of disease states. The reader is also referred to general references on pediatric drug therapy (8–10).

TREATING GASTROINTESTINAL SYMPTOMS

Anorexia is a common complaint of parents rather than the child. More often than not, documenting normal growth curves will allay parental anxiety—but the complaint is commonly a cultural one. For some ethnic mothers unless the child consumes three times his weight in food, he is accused of "eating like a bird." Given normal nutrition, good growth, and normal psychosocial development, it is the pediatrician's task to hold the line on "over-nutrition." However, when confronted with a child who does not meet the above criteria, who is truly in evidence of hypocaloric nutrition, and for whom there is no organic explanation of anorexia, a trial of *cyproheptadine* is not unreasonable. Most commonly this intervention is used for the child between 2 and 6 years of age. Several observations are in order and must be explained to the parents: (a) The appetite stimulation effect begins on or about day 4, and begins to wane about day 20. Therefore, cycle its use, 3 weeks on, 10 days off. (b) In my experience, about 85% get the appetite stimulation. If not evident by day

Table 26.2
Dosages of Drugs Used in Pediatric Gastrointestinal Diseases[a]

Drug	Indication	Route/Dose	Comments
Acetaminophen	Analgesia	PO 10–15 mg/kg/dose q4hr	$T_{\frac{1}{2}}$ 1–3 hr, hepatotoxic.
Acetylcysteine	Mucolytic	PO, PR 5–30 ml of 10% sol	Start with 10 ml q6hr.
Acidophilus	Diarrhea	PO 1 capsule daily	
ACTH	IBD	IV 1.6 μ/kg/day	Give in D5W over 6–8 hr.
Acyclovir	Viremia	NB 30 mg/kg/day ÷ q8hr	Give over 1 hr, keep well hydrated, crystalization in renal tubules possible
		C 7.5 mg/kg/day ÷ q8	
Albumin	Hypoprotein	IV 1 gm/kg/dose in 3 hr	Comes as 5 and 25% concentration
A1 Hydroxide	Antacid	PO 0.5 ml/kg/dose 1 and 3 hr PC and HS	Usual concentration is 320 mg/ml.
5-Amino salicylic acid	IBD	PR 2 g/M²/HS	Comes as 4 g/60 ml enemas and suppositories, RSP.
Ampicillin	Antibiotic	PO 50 mg/kg/day ÷ q6hr	
Aspirin	Analgesic	PO 10 mg/kg/dose q4hr	RSP
Atropine	Antispasmodic	PO 0.01 mg/kg/dose q6hr	Commonly found in combination drugs.
Attapulgite	Antidiarrheal	PO 40 mg/kg/dose q6hr	
Azathioprine	IBD	PO 3 mg/kg/day M 1 mg/kg/day	Experimental, watch for toxic immunosuppression.
Benzocaine	Analgesia for oral mucous membranes	PO topical 7.5% sol PRN	Commonly compounded with phenol, menthol, clove oil, or eugenol.
Bethanechol	Antireflux	PO 0.1 mg/kg/dose 30 min AC and HS	
Biscodyl	Laxative	PO 0.3 mg/kg/day × 1	Crampy distress common.
Bismuth subsalicylate	Antidiarrheal	PO 5 mg/kg/dose	Pepto-Bismol has 17 mg/ml. Makes stools black. RSP
Bromocriptine	Hepatic coma	PO 70 μg/kg/day	Experimental, watch for hypotension.
Ca carbonate	Ca supplement	PO 500 mg/dose 4–6 × day	RDA for Ca 800–1000 mg
Ca glubionate	Ca supplement	PO 35–40 ml/day	Comes as 115 mg Ca/5 ml.
Ca polycarbophil	Laxative	PO 500 mg qd or bid	No liquid form available
Carbamazepine	Antipruritic	PO 5 mg/kg/day ÷ q6hr	Experimental. Hemo- and hepatotoxic.
Carnitine	Deficiency	PO 50 mg/kg/day	
Casanthranol	Laxative	PO 0.5 mg/kg/HS	Usually given combined with docusate.

Table 26.2 Continued
Dosages of Drugs Used in Pediatric Gastrointestinal Diseases[a]

Drug	Indication	Route/Dose	Comments
Castor oil	Laxative	PO 0.5 ml/kg/dose	
Charcoal	Antidiarrheal	PO 25 mg/kg/day ÷ q6hr	No liquid preparation for diarrhea.
Chloral hydrate	Sedation	PO 30 mg/kg/dose	
Chlorothiazide	Diuretic	PO 20 mg/kg ÷ q12hr	
Chlorpromazine	Antiemetic	PR 1 mg/kg/dose q8hr	Extrapyramidal effects, hypotension.
Chloramphenicol	Antibiotic	PO 50 mg/kg/day ÷ q6hr	Hematotoxic.
Cholestyramine	Antipruritic Antidiarrheal	PO 240 mg/kg/day ÷ q8hr	May constipate, give other Rx, 1 hr before.
Cimetidine	H_2 blocker	PO 20 mg/kg/day ÷ q6hr	
Cisapride	H_2 blocker	PO 0.2 mg/kg/dose ÷ q8hr	
Clove oil	(see Benzocaine)		
Codeine	Analgesia	PO 0.5 mg/kg/dose	Do not use <2 yr old. May CNS depression. Can constipate.
Colchicine	Antifibrogenic	PO 15 umg/kg/day ÷ q8hr	Experimental
Colistin	Antidiarrheal	PO 5 mg/kg/day ÷ q8hr	Use for enteropathic *Escherichia coli*
Cromolyn	Allergic enteropathy	PO 3 mg/kg/dose 30 min AC	
Cyclosporin	Post-transplant immunosuppress	PO 5–10 mg/kg/day	Nephrotoxic, hirsuitism, hypertension, tremors, Trough levels at 200 to 800 ng/ml (RIA).
Cyprohepatadine	Antihistamine	PO 0.25/kg/day ÷ q8hr	Appetite stimulation, sedation, do not use <6 mo old.
Diazepam	Procedural sedation	IV .01 mg/kg/dose PO .5 mg/kg/day ÷ q8hr	Respiratory suppression
Dicyclomine	Antispasmodic	PO 5 mg/dose/q6hr	Do not use <6 mo old
Dimenhydrinate	Antiemetic	PO 5 mg/kg/day ÷ q6hr	
Diphenoxylate	Antidiarrheal	PO 0.3 mg/kg/day ÷ q6hr	Do not use <2 yr.
Docusate	Constipation	PO 3 mg/kg/day ÷ q6hr	
Domperidone	Prokinetic	PO 0.6 mg/kg/dose q6hr	
L-Dopa	Hepatic coma	PO 15 mg/kg/day ÷ q8hr	Experimental. Give for 24 hr, if no improvement, discontinue.
Enprostil	Antisecretory	PO 1 μg/kg/day ÷ q12hr	Experimental.
Erythromycin	Antibiotic	PO 4 m mg/kg/day ÷ q6hr	
Eugenol	(see Benzocaine)		

Drug	Indication	Dose	Comments
Famotidine	H2 blocker	PO 0.5 mg/kg/day	
Fentanyl	Precedural sedation	IV 1 μg/kg/dose	Given over 3–5 min and watch for respiratory depression.
FK-506	Posttransplant immunosuppress	IV PO	Side-effects IV >> PO; headache, nausea, hyperesthesia.
Fluconazole	Antifungal	PO 5 mg/kg/day	
Furazolidone	Anti-Giardia	PO 6 mg/kg/day ÷ q6hr	Do not use <1 mo old
Furosemide	Diuretic	PO 2 mg/kg/dose q8hr	
γ-Globulin	Immune serum globulin	IM 0.06 ml/kg/dose q6mo.	HAV prophylaxis
	HBIG	IM 0.06 ml/kg/dose	HBV prophylaxis
Gancyclovir	Antiviral	IV 5 mg/kg/dose q12hr	Give for 21 days.
Gentian violet	Anti-*Candida*	Topical solution of 0.5% painted on q6hr	Stains clothes
Glycerol	Hepatic coma	IV 0.25–0.5 g/kg/hr	Osmotic therapy for cerebral edema.
Hydrocortisone	Anti-inflamatory	PO 2 mg/kg/day ÷ q6hr	
Hydroxyzine	Antianxiety	PO 2 mg/kg/day ÷ q6hr	
Hyoscyamine	Antispasmodic	PO 25 μg/ml 1 gtt/kg q4-6hr	
Interferon	Antiviral	SQ 40000 μ/kg/dose	Give 3×/wk. Experimental in children, indication HCV. Thrombocytopenia.
Iodoquinol	Antiprotozoa	PO 40 mg/kg/day ÷ q8hr	Do not use >28 days, can produce SMON
Ibuprofen	Analgesic	PO 20 mg/kg/day ÷ q8hr	
Kaolin (pectin)	Antidiarrheal	PO 1 cc/kg/dose	
Ketoconazole	Antifungal	PO 5 mg/kg/day	Monitor LFT
Lactase	Enzyme	PO 4500 μ/250 cc milk	
Lactulose	Laxative	PO 0.4 ml/kg/dose q8hr	
Loperamide	Antidiarrheal	PO 0.5 mg/kg/day ÷ q8hr	
Magnesium citrate	Laxative	PO 4 ml/kg/dose	Caution in renal disease
Magnesium hydroxide	Antacid	PO 0.5 ml/kg/dose	Give 1 and 3 h PC
Mannitol	Cerebral edema	IV 0.25 g/kg/dose push over 2–3 min	Osmotic therapy, watch renal function.
Mebendazole	Antihelminth	PO 100 mg/dose	For pinworm ×1, other roundworms q12hr × 3 days
Meperidine	Analgesia	PO, IV. IM 1 mg/kg/dose	Watch CNS depression.
Mercaptopurine	Severe Crohn's	PO 2 mg/kg/day	Experimental, potent multisystem toxicity.

Table 26.2 Continued
Dosages of Drugs Used in Pediatric Gastrointestinal Diseases[a]

Drug	Indication	Route/Dose	Comments
Methotrexate	Severe Crohn's	PO 0.1 mg/kg/q wk	As above.
Metoclopramide	Prokinetic	PO 0.1 mg/kg/dose AC, HS	Extrapyramidal effects
Metronidazole	Antiprotozoa antiflagellate antianerobe	PO 15 mg/kg/day ÷ q8hr	
Midazolam	Procedural sedation	IV 0.035 mg/kg/dose	Give over 2 min, watch O_2 saturation.
Mineral oil	Laxative	PO .25 ml/kg/dose	
Misoprostol	Antisecretory	PO 3 μg/kg/day ÷ q6hr	Analog of PG E_1, can be abortifacient, in children experimental.
Morphine	Analgesia	IM, IV 0.1 mg/kg/dose	CNS depression, not recommended PO.
Naloxone	Opiate antagonist	IM. IV 5 μg/kg/dose	Repeat as necessary
Neomycin	Gut sterilizer	PO 50 mg/kg/day ÷ q6hr	Renal and ototoxic.
Niclosamide	Tapeworms	PO 40 mg/kg/day	
Nystatin	Antifungal	PO 7500 μ/kg/dose ÷ q6hr	
Octreotide	Anti-VIP	SQ 3.5 μg/kg/day ÷ q8hr	
OKT3	Graft rescue	IV 0.1–1.0 mg/kg/day	Potent drug. Requires experienced physician.
Omeprazole	Antisecretory	PO 0.3 mg/kg/day	Not generally advised for children, no liquid formulary.
Ondansetron	Antiemetic	IV, PO 0.15 mg/kg/day ÷ q6–8 hr or 5 mg/m²	For chemotherapy and radiotherapy-induced emesis
Osalazine	IBD	PO 15 mg/kg/day ÷ q12hr	
Pancreatic enzymes	Insufficiency	PO general guidelines 1500 μ lipase/kg/meal	Must be individualized
Paregoric	Antidiarrheal	PO 0.25 ml/kg/dose q6hr	
Pencillamine	Chelator	PO 250 mg/dose q12hr	For Wilson's disease, add pyridoxine.
Phenobarbital	Hepatic enzyme induction	PO 5 mg/kg/day ÷ q8hr	Use for cholestasis
Phenol	(see Benzocaine)		
Phenolphthalein	Laxative	PO 2 mg/kg/dose	Not commonly used in children <2 yr.

Phosphorated carbohydrate	Antiemetic	PO 0.6 ml/kg/dose	May use up to 3–4 doses over 1–2 hr.
Plasma	Coagulopathy	IV 10 ml/kg/dose	
Polyethylene glycol (PEG)	Procedural purgative	PO 50 ml/kg/dose	May require NG tube for rapid administration in children.
Praziquantel	*Schistosoma taenia*	PO 75 mg/kg/day ÷ q8hr	Use for 1 day.
Prednisolone	Anti-inflammatory	PO .5 mg/kg/day ÷ q8hr	Methylated prednisone
Prednisone	Anti-inflammatory	PO 1 mg/kg/day	
Prochlorperazine	Antiemetic	PO, PR 0.4 mgk/kg/day ÷ q8hr, IM 0.1 mg/dose	Do not use IV
Promethazine	Antiemetic	PR .25 mg/kg/dose q6hr	
Propranolol	Portal hypertension	PO .5 mg/kg/day ÷ q8hr	Hypotension, and hypoglycemia possible.
Psyllium	Laxative	PO 100 mg/kg/dose	
Pyrantel	Antihelminth	PO 11 mg/kg/dose × 1	
Quinacrine	Anti-*Giardia*	PO 6 mg/kg/day ÷ q8hr	Use for 7 days.
Ranitidine	H_2 blocker	PO 3 mg/kg/day ÷ q12hr	
Scopolamine	Antiemetic	SQ. IV 6 μg/kg/dose	Available as transdermal patch for children >12 yr
Senna	Laxative	PO 5 mg/kg/dose	
Simethicone	Antiflatulent	PO 5 mg/kg/dose 4 × day	
Sodium phosphate	Laxative	PO 0.3 ml/kg/dose	Do not use in infants and toddlers.
Spironolactone	Diuretic	PO 1–2 mg/kg/day ÷ q8hr	
Suculfrate	Mucosal demulctant	PO 50 mg/kg/day ÷ q6hr	Can be made in slurry with water.
Sulfasalazine	IBD	PO 50 mg/kg/day ÷ q8hr	
Thiabendazole	Antihelminth	PO 50 mg/kg/day ÷ q12hr	
Thymosin	Antiviral	SQ .02 mg/kg/dose	Given 2×/wk, for HBV experimental.
Triamterene	Diuretic	PO 3 mg/kg/day ÷ q8hr	
Trientine	Chelator	PO 15 mg/kg/day ÷ q8hr	
Trimethobenzamide	Antiemetic	PO, PR 3.5 mg/kg/dose q8hr	
Trimethoprine sulfa	Antibiotic	PO 6–12 mg/kg/day ÷ q12hr	
Urosdeoxycholic acid	Antipruritic Antifibrogenic	PO 15 mg/kg/day ÷ q8hr	Experimental, diarrhea common.

Table 26.2 Continued
Dosages of Drugs Used in Pediatric Gastrointestinal Diseases[a]

Drug	Indication	Route/Dose	Comments
Vitamin A	Cholestatic disease, use PO 400–1000 μg/day		
Vitamin D	Cholestatic disease, use PO 10 μg/day		
Vitamin E	Cholestatic disease, use PO 5–10 mg/day, may require 10-fold		
Vitamin K	Cholestatic disease, use PO 5 mg/day		
Vaccine HBV	Prophylaxis	IM 5–10 μg/dose	Give 0, 1, 6, mo
Vancomycin	Antibiotic	PO 1–50 mg/kg/day ÷ q6hr	

[a]SQ, subcutaneous; PO, oral; IM, intramuscular; IV, intravenous; PR, per rectum; AC, before meals; PC, after meals; HS, at bedtime; NB, newborn; C, child; M, maintenance; PRN, as needed; IBD, inflammatory bowel disease; RSP, Reye's syndrome precautions (14, 15).

7, discontinue the drug. (c) Ninety-five percent of the patients will get a sedative effect from the drug. (d) Take advantage of the stimulation to deliver good nutrition and calories. Provide the parents with nutritional education.

Vomiting is a common gastrointestinal symptom in children which may be non-specific and not necessarily related to gastric distress or obstructive phenomenon. Children can vomit with mild head trauma, headache, earache, pharyngitis, coughing, crying, abdominal trauma, falls, hepatitis, car riding, sepsis, lead poisoning—the spectrum is legion, and need not be gastroenteritis, appendicitis, pancreatitis, obstruction, or cerebral edema.

Most nonsurgical vomiting in children is self-limited and requires only judicious oral rehydration, 20–30 ml every 20–30 minutes, and treatment of the primary cause until the symptom clears. Once assured that the cause of vomiting is not of a serious organic nature, then tincture of time is preferable to anti-emetics, all of which can complicate the observations with extrapyramidal side effects. However, given the child with vicious idiopathic cyclic vomiting, then careful use of a pharmacologic agent conjoined with intravenous hydration can be used. *Hydroxyzine* is generally safe, time-proven, and has the least extrapyramidal effects of all the agents. It has the additional benefits of some sedation and antihistaminic activity. If the patient fails this agent, then the stronger central antiemetic drugs such as *promethazine, chlorpromazine,* or *trimethobenzamide* can be tried.

Ondansetron has been used to prevent chemotherapy- and radiotherapy-induced emesis in several pediatric studies (11) as well as to treat vomiting from a variety of other conditions (12). As prophylaxis for chemotherapy-induced nausea and vomiting, a dose of 5 mg/m² up to 8 mg administered intravenously or orally three times daily resulted in a marked reduction in emetic episodes in more than 400 children aged 6 months–17 years receiving a wide variety of chemotherapy regimens (including conditioning therapy for bone marrow transplantation) (11). The drug was well-tolerated with a low incidence of side effects, headache being the most common (49). Anecdotal sucess has also been reported in a pediatric ICU setting in a dose of 0.15 mg/kg administered intravenously every 6 hours (12).

Diarrhea is a troublesome symptom for which treatment will depend on the cause or mechanism of action. With an obvious infectious cause, known allergic enteropathy, or known ingested stimulant, the treatment is easy and more often than not, specific. It is the persistent chronic diarrhea with a negative workup that poses the therapeutic dilemma. In my experience, adsorbents are useless in this setting and the following drugs are suggested: a short trial of *bismuth subsalicylate* (13), 5 mg/kg/dose four times daily for 5 days, followed by 2.5 mg/kg/dose four times daily for 5 days, and ending with 1.0 mg/kg/dose four times daily for 5 days. If this fails, then conjoined *metronidazole* and *cholestyramine* (14) for 10 days can be used. Almost all nonspecific childhood diarrhea will cease with these regimens. *Loperamide* and a histamine-2 receptor antagonist may have to be added to diarrhea with a secondary secretory component. If the symptoms return, then a more invasive workup is in order. The chronic prolonged use of clays, antimotility, and bacteriostatic agents without a thorough effort at making a diagnosis is not recommended.

Constipation like diarrhea requires knowledge of normal defecation patterns, as well as knowledge of the responsible mechanism, to institute proper treatment. Newborns generally have two to five mushy mustard-like stools/day, infants two to three soft stools/day, and children-adolescents one to two firm stools/day (15).

The constipated child may be stool-withholding because of defecation pain (dyskesia) and therefore profits primarily from the healing of any perianal lesions and the use of a stool softener. *Zinc oxide*-based emollients and *docusate* without stimulant are recommended from infancy on up. Infrequent defecation may be due to discoordinate colonic propulsion (dysmotility). If the constipation is non-syndromic, bulk agents conjoined with lubricants are most effective. Syndromic causes such as pseudo-obstruction, megacystic-microcolon, or Hirschsprung disease, etc. may respond to pharmacologic intervention, but always in consort with surgical consultation. Prokinetic agents cause cramping and are not generally recommended. Bulking agents and lubricants can be used from about 9 months of age on. In younger infants dysmotility often responds to external sphincter stimulation with glycerin suppositories.

True constipation marked by increased colonic water salvage responds well to secretory and osmotic agents; *senna* and *lactulose* are particularly effective and safe in children when used for controlled periods of time. Often encopresis is a component of chronic constipation. These children additionally require evaluation for megarectum, normal innervation processes, and the initiation of a behavioral modification program. If a dilated bowel is found on barium enema, then daily mineral oil and/or enemas are required to allow for a gradual normalization of bowel tone. In addition, a behavioral program that promotes a regular defecation time, daily exercise, and rewards are essential.

TREATING SPECIFIC CONDITIONS

Gastroesophageal reflux (GER) in infants is marked by recurrent spitting-up and vomiting. In addition, it can be associated with failure to thrive, aspirations, apnea/bradycardia, and reactive airway disease. Once proven by either radionuclide study, upper gastrointestinal series, or esophageal pH-probe, conservative measures should be tried first. These include elevation of the infant's head 30–45°, thickened formula (1 teaspoon of cereal/oz formula), and frequent-smaller volume feedings (16). Should these fail, then pharmacologic agents should be tried. *Metoclopramide* at a dose of 0.1 mg/kg per dose four times daily is effective but in the author's experience is associated with troublesome irritability in about 10% of infants. In these infants, *bethanechol* can be tried, but those infants who are not responsive to metoclopramide, also commonly are unresponsive to bethanechol. The

role of *cisapride* in infants has not been well studied. *Cimetidine* as an adjunct is very helpful in the infant who is irritable with GER. *Ranitidine* or *famotidine* may be more useful if polypharmacy and dosing schedule pose a problem. All three are available in a liquid formulation. *Omeprazole* is not available in a medium amenable to children.

Treatment should generally be continued for about 6 weeks. Those infants who continue to require medication after this period of time, will commonly "outgrow" their dose, but ordinarily the dose should not be changed if accompanied by appropriate weight gain. Fundoplication recommendations are reserved for those children who fail all medical therapy, and who demonstrate failure to thrive, recurrent pneumonias, erosive esophagitis and strictures, or intractable pain.

Colic is a common problem seen by the pediatrician, occurring in 20–30% of infants. Therefore, only the most troublesome of colic is referred to the gastroenterologist. It consists of recurrent paroxysms of abdominal pain beginning at about 2–6 weeks of life, which can be difficult to treat. Often a combination of dietary controls, environmental manipulation, and drug therapy must be used (17). The dietary controls may call for the suspension of cow-defined proteins, the environmental controls may call for warmth, motion, or better parenting skills, and the pharmacologic intervention may be antispasmodic and antiflatulent. In the author's opinion, *hyoscyamine* is the safest antispasmodic to use in infants, with better dose control and fewest side effects. *Simethicone* can be a useful adjuvant.

Inflammatory bowel disease (IBD) is generally treated in the same manner as is the adult disease. The same range of intestinal and extraintestinal complications are found in pediatric disease, however, arthritis, arthralgia, and growth failure are particularly troublesome in children with IBD. Growth failure can be seen in up to 30% of children and herein are required the skills of a pediatrician. Together with the nutritionist, the physician needs to establish programs that will conjoin enteral elemental nutrition, hypercaloric supplementation, and parenteral nutrition. It is critical to remember that growth arrest can be prevented and even reversed if considered early in the course of therapy. Catch-up growth is possible only before bone maturation.

Steroids are generally given on a every-other-day dosage schedule to minimize linear growth suppression. *Prednisone* is the preferred form and is given as a single morning dose. *Sulfasalazine* and *osalazine* are used with the same rationale as in the adult patient. Children, in general, tolerate sulfasalazine better than adults, with little in the way of headache or exanthem side effects. Osalazine, in the author's experience, produces more frequent diarrheal side effects in children. *Metronidazole*, when used in a dose of 15 mg/kg/day, has few side effects and is well tolerated by children. It is however, remarkably distasteful, and requires special concessions for children. A preparation in USP syrup with collegel and chocolate flavoring can facilitate compliance. The use of more potent immunosuppressives, such as *cyclosporine* or *azathioprine*, is reserved for severe, intractable, and non-responsive disease. Their use must be individualized from child to child. These agents should be considered before resorting to colectomy or significant bowel resection.

Allergic enteropathy can be a simple clinical disorder marked by the obvious sensitivity to a particular food such as the strawberry or chocolate. But the child referred to the gastroenterologist more commonly has dietary protein intolerance (DPI) an often enigmatic clinical syndrome encountered in the infant or young child. Symptoms are variable and can run the gamut from mild colic-like pain to grossly bloody stools with the one constancy that the elimination of the offending dietary protein(s)—be it of plant or animal origin—alleviates the symptoms. The problem becomes difficult when polyprotein intolerance is evident. This is the child that often requires a chemically defined diet, antisecretories, kinin-blockers, and dietary supplements. There is *no one* proper approach to this clinical situation, but the author's regimen with the most consistent benefits revolves around us-

ing a chemically defined *amino acid* nutrition combination plus oral *cromolyn sodium*. In the older child, *hydroxyzine, cyproheptadine*, and *loperamide* are often useful adjuncts. Despite pharmacologic intervention, tincture of time and patience are crucial, with the admonition to the parents that DPI can persist for up to a year or more.

The facilitation of worldwide travel and migration has made *parasitosis* in North American children a genuine consideration in gastrointestinal differential diagnosis. The most common protozoal infections encountered on this continent are *Giardia lamblia, Cryptosporidium muris*, and *Endoamoeba* spp. The most common roundworms are *Enterobius vermicularis* (pinworms) and *Ascaris lumbricoides*. Other less commonly reported organisms include protozoal *Entamoeba histolytica* and *Blastocytis hominis*, and among the worms *Necator americanus, Ancylostoma duodenale, Trichuria trichuris*, and the *Taenia* spp. Zoonoses include the dog and cat hookworms causing cutaneous larva migrans and the roundworm causing visceral larva migrans.

As a generalization, *metronidazole* serves best for most protozoal infections and *thiabendazole* for roundworms. A few observations with respect to children are in order. In the author's experience cutaneous larva migrans can be treated quite effectively with topical thiabendazole applied twice a day. The larva begins to die and involute almost immediately and in most cases dies within 72–96 hours. Heavy ascariasis in children requires precautions against worm migration. The author has seen the worms migrate per mouth and nose and even into in the biliary tree, in attempts to elude vermifuge. The worms can be sedated with *promethazine*, 45 minutes before the vermifuge is administered, facilitating a more natural defecation route of elimination. Remember the worms are flesh-pink, and a large female exiting per rectum is not infrequently thought by parents to represent evisceration. A word of caution about their appearance can save a panicked phone call. Taenia infections are commonly asymptomatic and discovered by the patient when a "moving white ribbon" is seen in the stools. *Niclosamide* is available in a chewable form.

Chronic liver diseases are treated with the same rationale and pharmacologic agents used in adults. However, with respect to children, several caveats are in order. The cholestatic infant is always at risk for developing vitamin E-deficient neuropathy. In its most severe form this spinocerebellar syndrome is marked by ataxia, nystagmus, areflexia, pigmentary retinopathy, decreased proprioception, and ophthalmoplegia. This is a progressive syndrome with areflexia appearing first, and unless corrected by 3 years of age, the symptoms advance inexorably and are not reversible. The cholestatic infant must have *vitamin E* levels checked frequently and supplementation with large doses ranging up to 100 IU/kg/day provided. The other fat-soluble vitamins should be assessed concomitantly.

Some cholestatic children can become secondarily carnitine deficient and demonstrate hypotonia, failure to thrive, recurrent infections, and cardiomyopathy. In these patients serum carnitine levels should be assayed and deficiency corrected with oral *carnitine* 50 mg/kg/day.

Both carnitine and vitamin E deficiency syndromes are peculiar to children and rarely reported in the adult.

REFERENCES

1. Cohen MS. Principles of drug disposition and therapy in infants and children. In: Rudolph AM, ed. Pediatrics. Norwalk, CT: Appleton & Croft, 1982:777–786.
2. Rane A, Thomson G. Prenatal and neonatal drug metabolism in man. Eur J Clin Pharmacol 1980;18:9–15.
3. Roberts RJ. Pharmacologic principles of drug therapy. In: Oski FA, ed. Principles and practice of pediatrics. Philadelphia: Lippincott, 1990:52–57.
4. Buchanan N. Speight TM, ed. Paediatric clinical pharmacology and therapeutics. In: Drug treatment. Baltimore: Williams & Wilkins, 1987.
5. Pruitt AW, Anyan WR, Hill RM, et al. The transfer of drugs and other chemicals into human breast milk. Pediatrics 1983;72:375–383.
6. Platzker A, Lew CD, Stewart D. Drug administration via breast milk. Hosp Prac 1980;15:111–122.
7. Shirkey HC. Pediatric dosage handbook. Washington, DC: American Pharmaceutical Association, 1980.
8. Rylance G. Prescribing for infants and children. Br Med J 1988;296:984–986.
9. Benitz WE, Tatro DS, eds. Pediatric drug handbook. Chicago: Year Book, 1981.
10. Serrano-Murphy VA, Bubica G. General pediatric therapy. In: Applied Therapeutics. Vancouver, WA: Applied Therapeutics, 1988.
11. Jurgens H, McQuade B. Ondansetron as prophylaxis for chemotherapy- and radiotherapy-induced emesis in children. Oncology 1992;49:279–285.
12. Tobias JD. Ondansetron: indications and applications in the paediatric intensive care unit. Anaesth Intens Care 1992;20:504–506.
13. Marshall BJ. The use of bismuth in gastroenterology. Am J Gastroenterol 1991;86:16–25.
14. Bowie MD, Mann MD, Hill ID. The bowel cocktail. Pediatrics 1981;67:920–921.
15. Colon AR, Jacob LJ. Defecation patterns in American infants and children. Clin Pediatr 1977;16:999–1000.
16. DiPalma JS, Colon AR. Gastroesophageal reflux in infants. Am Fam Physician 1991;43:857–864.
17. Colón AR, DiPalma JS. Colic. Am Fam Physician 1989;40:122–124.

27

Drug Interactions of Gastrointestinal Drugs

PHILIP D. HANSTEN

Drug interactions occur when one drug alters the response to another drug, or when the two drugs result in additive organ toxicity. Although drug interactions have been recognized since at least the early part of the 19th century, it has only been during the past 25 years that they have been given serious consideration in medical practice. Well over 1000 drug-drug interactions have been reported in the clinical literature, many of which have involved drugs used in gastroenterology. It is important to realize that most of the time that patients receive potentially interacting drug combinations, there is no overt adverse response. Although a few drug interactions result in adverse outcomes in almost everyone who receives the combination, the outcome of most drug interactions is highly situational. Thus, a given interacting pair of drugs can produce a serious adverse outcome in a predisposed patient, and be totally innocuous in another patient who does not have the appropriate risk factors.

Most drug interactions involve one drug that is *affected* by the interaction (the "object drug"), and another drug that *causes* the interaction (the "precipitant drug"). Drugs used in gastroenterology act primarily as precipitant drugs when they are involved in drug interactions.

Object Drug:	The drug whose effect is altered by the interaction.
Precipitant Drug:	The drug that causes the altered response in the object drug.

MECHANISMS OF DRUG INTERACTIONS

Drug interaction mechanisms can be divided into three main categories: pharmacokinetic, pharmacodynamic, and combined toxicity. The vast majority of known drug interactions involving medications used in gastroenterology are of a pharmacokinetic nature.

Pharmacokinetic Drug Interactions

Pharmacokinetic drug interactions involve alteration in the absorption, distribution, metabolism, or excretion of one drug by another.

ABSORPTION

Some drugs are capable of inhibiting the absorption of other drugs through adsorption on a large surface area, binding (e.g., through complexation or chelation), altering gastric acidity, and by affecting gastrointestinal motility. It is important to distinguish between alterations in *rate* of absorption and alterations in *extent* of absorption. Alteration in absorption rate with no change in extent of absorption is seldom clinically important because the steady-state serum concentration of the object drug is not affected. Changes in extent of absorption may be clinically important if the magnitude of the interaction is sufficient to place the steady-state serum concentration of the object drug in the subtherapeutic or toxic range. A number of clinically important drug interactions of medications used in gastroenterology involve altered absorption.

535

DISTRIBUTION

Distribution drug interactions occur when one drug affects the plasma protein binding or tissue binding of another drug, increasing the free plasma level of the displaced drug. Although increasing the free concentration enhances its pharmacologic response, the effect tends to be transient because the unbound drug is also more available for hepatic metabolism and/or renal excretion. Thus, protein-binding drug interactions are not likely to result in adverse effects in most cases.

METABOLISM

The hepatic metabolism of many medications can be enhanced or inhibited by concurrent administration of other drugs. Enhanced metabolism (enzyme induction) of drugs is known to follow the use of drugs such as barbiturates, carbamazepine, phenytoin, primidone, and rifampin. Enzyme induction is a gradual process, taking up to 7–10 days or more for maximal stimulation of metabolism. Inhibition of metabolism can be produced by a much wider variety of drugs than enzyme induction, including allopurinol, chloramphenicol, cimetidine, ciprofloxacin, diltiazem, disulfiram, erythromycin, fluconazole, fluoxetine, ketoconazole, metronidazole, propoxyphene, quinidine, sulfonamides, and verapamil. Enzyme inhibition tends to take place much more quickly than enzyme induction, and is probably maximal as soon as steady-state concentrations of the inhibitor are achieved in the liver. The time required to achieve a new steady-state plasma concentration of the object drug, however, can vary from a day or two up to several weeks, depending on the new prolonged half-life of the object drug. Altered metabolism is probably the most clinically important pharmacokinetic mechanism by which drugs interact.

RENAL EXCRETION

Inasmuch as most drugs are metabolized (and thus inactivated) in the liver before being excreted by the kidneys, altered renal excretion of unchanged drug is not a common mechanism of clinically important drug interactions.

Some drugs undergo active renal tubular secretion, a process that may be inhibited by concurrent administration of other drugs, thus increasing the serum concentration of the object drug. The renal elimination of some drugs that are weak acids or weak bases can be affected by drug-induced alterations in urinary pH. This results from changes in the proportions of ionized versus nonionized concentrations of the object drug, which in turn affects its ability to be absorbed back into the systemic circulation from the renal tubular urine. For many other drug interactions resulting from altered renal excretion, the precise mechanism of the interaction has not been determined.

Pharmacodynamic Drug Interactions

Most pharmacodynamic drug interactions occur when two drugs have additive or antagonistic pharmacologic properties. This may or may not result from effects on the same drug receptor. Knowledge of the pharmacologic properties of the two drugs usually allows prediction of this type of interaction. Moreover, additive pharmacodynamic drug combinations are often used intentionally, as with the use of multiple antihypertensive or antineoplastic drugs. Pharmacodynamic drug interactions do not appear to be common for drugs used in gastroenterology.

Combined Toxicity Interactions

Some drugs have in common an ability to adversely affect certain organ systems, and additive toxic effects may occur. For example, the concurrent use of two potentially hepatotoxic drugs may result in additive (or in some cases perhaps synergistic) damage to the liver. This, however, is not a common mechanism of drug interactions for drugs used in gastroenterology.

The remainder of this chapter deals specifically with a variety of drug interactions seen with medications used in the practice of gastroenterology.

ANTACID DRUG INTERACTIONS

Antacid drug interactions have been known for many years, and usually involve antacid-induced inhibition of gastrointestinal drug absorption (1, 2). It is important to realize that some antacid drug interactions occur with virtually all antacids, whereas other antacid interactions involve only certain antacids. This is at least partly because antacids can vary with one another regarding their alkalinizing potency, cation content, ability to alter urine pH, and ability to alter gastrointestinal motility.

Antacid-Binding of Other Drugs in the Gastrointestinal Tract

Most antacids appear to be able to bind with other drugs in the gastrointestinal tract. The exact nature of this antacid binding is not established for most interactions, and may involve processes such as complexation, chelation, and the adsorption of drugs on the high surface area of small antacid particles. Most of the studies involving the administration of antacids with other drugs have shown only a modest (and in most cases clinically important) reduction in the absorption of the object drug (e.g., the effect of antacids on cimetidine (3)). However, the absorption of some drugs (such as quinolone antibiotics and tetracyclines) may be markedly reduced by concurrent antacid administration. One theory consistent with these observations is that the large surface area of antacids modestly and nonspecifically adsorbs many drugs (resulting in only small reductions in their absorption) although antacids bind certain drugs in a more specific manner (e.g., complexation, chelation) that can markedly reduce their absorption.

Antacid-Induced Increases in Gastrointestinal pH

It was earlier thought that antacid-induced increases in gastrointestinal pH would alter the absorption of many drugs that are weak acids or weak bases by altering their ionization and hence their lipid solubility. It was theorized that antacid-induced increased alkalinity would shift weak bases more into their nonionized form, thus increasing their lipid solubility and their gastrointestinal absorption. Weak acid drugs were believed to behave in the opposite way, with increased gastrointes-

tinal pH reducing their absorption. The absorption process turned out to be much more complicated than that; however, it became clear that altered gastrointestinal pH could affect not just ionization, but also the dissolution rate of the object drug, an important rate limiting factor in drug absorption. Altered gastrointestinal pH can also affect other determinants of drug absorption, such as the rate of degradation of drugs by gastric acid, and gastrointestinal motility.

Gastrointestinal absorption of the antifungal agent ketoconazole is affected by gastrointestinal pH. Ketoconazole requires a relatively acidic gastric contents in order to go into solution. Inasmuch as drugs must be in solution before they can be absorbed, alkalinization of the gut with antacids or antisecretory agents may substantially reduce ketoconazole absorption (4, 5). The gastrointestinal absorption of the related antifungal drug, fluconazole, does not appear to be significantly affected by increases in gastric pH. Other effects of gastric acidity on the absorption of drugs are listed in Table 27.1.

It is commonly held that increasing gastrointestinal pH through the use of antacids or other drugs results in premature dissolution of enteric coated dosage forms. There is some clinical evidence that this may occur, e.g., with enteric coated aspirin (6). Nonetheless, there is little evidence that the magnitude of any such effect on enteric coating would result in a clinically important unwanted outcome. Moreover, many sustained release products do not rely on pH as the primary determinant for the release of the drug.

Antacid-Induced Changes in Urinary pH

Many commonly used antacids (e.g., magnesium-aluminum hydroxides) can increase urinary pH, usually by about one pH unit (7). For a small number of drugs that are weak acids or weak bases, this modest antacid-induced alteration in urinary pH affects the ratio of ionized to nonionized drug in the tubular urine. Nonionized drug is more lipid soluble than ionized drug and thus are more readily reabsorbed back into the blood from the tu-

Table 27.1
Effect of Increased Gastric pH[a] on the Absorption of Drugs

Drug	Effect of increased gastric pH on absorption
Cephalosporins	Moderate reduction in the gastrointestinal absorption of cefuroxime axetil and cefpodoxime proxetil—Little is known regarding the effect of gastric pH on the absorption of other cephalosporins
Enoxacin	Considerable reduction in the gastrointestinal absorption of enoxacin, but ciprofloxacin and ofloxacin do not appear to be affected
Glipizide	Increased absorption *rate* of glipizide with antacids, but extent of absorption may not be affected
Ketoconazole	Marked reduction in the gastrointestinal absorption of ketoconazole—fluconazole does not appear to be similarly affected
Nifedipine	Possible increase in bioavailability with H_2-receptor antagonists—other agents that increase gastric pH might produce a similar effect
Penicillin G	Variable increase in the gastrointestinal absorption of penicillin G—Most other penicillins are relatively acid stable and would not be expected to be significantly affected by increases in gastrointestinal pH

[a]As caused by drugs such as antacids, H_2-receptor antagonists, and omeprazole (12).

bular urine. In order for the renal elimination of an object drug to be affected in a clinically important way to alterations in urinary pH, it must have a pKa or pKb within a certain range, and a sufficient amount (e.g., at least 20%) of active drug must be eliminated unchanged in the urine. Fortunately, most drugs do not appear to possess both of these properties, and there are relatively few examples of drugs that are susceptible to alterations in urinary pH. Moreover, occasional doses of antacids are not likely to result in more than minor changes in the serum concentrations of the object drug.

Weak acids, such as salicylates, are more ionized and thus less lipid soluble when the tubular urine is more alkaline. Thus, antacid-induced increases in urinary pH shifts more salicylate to the ionized (and more readily excreted) form. In patients taking large doses of salicylate (e.g., several grams daily) elimination of unchanged salicylate in the urine is an important route of elimination due to saturation of hepatic metabolic pathways. Thus, urinary alkalinization can reduce the serum salicylate concentration substantially (8). In patients taking small or infrequent doses of salicylates, however, a much smaller percentage of the drug is eliminated unchanged in the urine, and alkalinization is unlikely to have a clinically important effect on salicylate serum concentration.

For weak bases such as quinidine and sympathomimetics, increasing the alkalinity of the urine shifts more of the drug to the more lipid soluble *nonionized* form. Thus, antacid-induced elevations in urinary pH tend to increase renal tubular reabsorption of such drugs resulting in elevated serum concentrations of the object drug. As with weak acids discussed above, the dose and duration of the object is an important determinant of the clinical importance of these interactions.

H_2-RECEPTOR ANTAGONIST DRUG INTERACTIONS

H_2-receptor antagonists are among the most widely used drugs in clinical medicine, and they are frequently used by patients who have disorders requiring the use of several other medications. Thus, it is important to identify those patients who are potentially at risk of clinically significant interactions with H_2-receptor antagonists.

Table 27.2
Relative Ability of H_2-Receptor Antagonists to Inhibit Hepatic Drug Metabolism

H_2-Receptor antagonist	Inhibitor of drug metabolism?	Amount of documentation
Cimetidine	Yes	Extensive. Numerous drug interaction studies involving both patients and healthy subjects
Ranitidine	Unlikely	Extensive. Numerous drug interaction studies involving both patients and healthy subjects
Famotidine	Unlikely	Moderate. Considerably fewer studies than with cimetidine or ranitidine. With few exceptions, they have consistently shown no effect on drug metabolism
Nizatidine	Unlikely	Limited. Only a few studies have been conducted, but they suggest no effect on drug metabolism.

H_2-Receptor Antagonist Effects on Drug Absorption

Unlike antacids, H_2-receptor antagonists are not known to bind with other drugs in the gastrointestinal tract. Current evidence suggests that there are few clinically important drug interactions of H_2-receptor antagonists that involve alteration of absorption. The ability of H_2-receptor antagonists to increase gastric pH may affect the absorption of some drugs, but as mentioned above under antacids, relatively few drugs have shown altered absorption due to altered gastrointestinal pH. The antifungal agent ketoconazole requires a relatively acidic gastric contents to go into solution. Inasmuch as drugs must be in solution before they can be absorbed, increasing gastric pH can markedly reduce ketoconazole absorption. Other drugs that may be affected by increases in gastric pH are listed in Table 27.1.

H_2-Receptor Antagonist Effects on Drug Metabolism

H_2-receptor antagonists differ regarding their ability to inhibit the hepatic metabolism of other drugs (Table 27.2). They will each be dealt with individually in the next section.

CIMETIDINE

Most clinically important drug interactions involving H_2-receptor antagonists result from inhibition of hepatic drug metabolism by cimetidine (9–11). Cimetidine binds with cytochrome P-450 enzymes in the liver, and may inhibit the metabolism of a large number of drugs (11–13) (Table 27.3). Cimetidine has an imidazole nucleus, a five-membered ring that appears to confer the ability to inhibit hepatic drug metabolism. Other drugs with an imidazole ring that are known to act as inhibitors of hepatic oxidative drug metabolism include ketoconazole, metronidazole, miconazole, and omeprazole (12).

Metabolic Pathways Affected

Cimetidine primarily affects oxidative metabolism in the liver (phase I reactions); conjugation (phase II reactions) do not appear to be affected. For example, cimetidine inhibits the hepatic oxidative metabolism of warfarin, but not the glucuronide conjugation of another oral anticoagulant, phenprocoumon (9). Similarly, cimetidine inhibits the oxidative metabolism of diazepam and several other benzodiazepines, but does not affect the metabolism of benzodiazepines that undergo glucuronide conjugation such as lorazepam, oxazepam, and temazepam (9).

Time Course

As with most drug interactions involving inhibition of hepatic metabolism, the interfer-

Table 27.3
Drugs Whose Elimination Is Inhibited by Cimetidine[a]

Adinazolam	Alprazolam	Amitriptyline
Bromazepam	Carbamazepine	Caffeine
Chlordiazepoxide	Chlormethiazole	Chloroquine
Cifenline	Clobazam	Desipramine
Diazepam	Diltiazem	Doxepin
Felodipine	Femoxetine	Flecainide
5-Fluorouracil	Flurazepam	Flurbiprofen
Glipizide	Glyburide	Imipramine
Labetalol	Lidocaine	Meperidine
Metoprolol	Metronidazole	Midazolam
Moricizine	Nicotine	Nifedipine
Nomidipine	Nitrazepam	Pentoxifylline
Phenytoin	Piroxicam	Procainamide
Propranolol	Quinidine	Quinine
Sulindac	Theophylline	Tolbutamide
Triamterene	Triazolam	Valproic acid
Verapamil	Warfarin	

[a]After Reference 13.

ence with drug metabolism begins as soon as sufficient concentrations of cimetidine appear in the liver (i.e., within the first day of cimetidine therapy). However, the time required to achieve a new steady-state serum concentration of the object drug depends on the half-life of the object drug (i.e., the new *prolonged* half-life of the object drug). For example, a patient receiving theophylline who is started on cimetidine will usually reach a new steady-state serum theophylline concentration within 2 days of starting cimetidine. This is because theophylline has a relatively short half-life, even after it is prolonged due to cimetidine. However, with patients on chronic warfarin therapy, a new steady-state prothrombin time is not achieved until about 10 days after cimetidine is started. This is because warfarin has a much longer half-life than theophylline, and its effect on the prothrombin time is somewhat delayed (12).

Variability

Most drug interactions are highly variable from one person to another, and cimetidine interactions are no exception. It is not unusual to see a two- to three-fold or greater inter-subject variation in the magnitude of the changes in the object drug due to an interaction with cimetidine. In some cases the presence or absence of risk factors (see below) can explain much of the variation, but in other cases there is no obvious explanation.

Risk Factors

When possible, it is generally preferable to use an alternative to cimetidine when the patient is receiving one or more drugs that are known to interact. When the decision is made to use cimetidine with interacting drugs, it is important to address possible risk factors to identify patients for whom preventive measures are indicated (12).

1. Larger doses of cimetidine. When the mechanism of a drug interaction is inhibition of metabolism, the dose of the inhibitor is usually a critical determinant to the magnitude of the interaction. Accordingly, large doses of cimetidine tend to produce greater effects on the object drug than small doses; cimetidine doses of 400 mg/day or less generally do not produce clinically important increases in serum concentration of object drug.

2. Impaired renal function. A substantial portion of cimetidine is excreted unchanged in the urine, and patients with severe renal impairment tend to accumulate cimetidine. If the dose of cimetidine is not reduced to compensate for the reduction in renal function, the resultant higher serum cimetidine concentrations would tend to increase the mag-

nitude of cimetidine-induced inhibition of drug metabolism.

3. Object drug with narrow therapeutic index. Adverse cimetidine drug interactions are more likely to occur when the object drug has a relatively narrow therapeutic range and potentially serious toxic effects when the therapeutic range is exceeded (e.g., theophylline, warfarin).

4. High pre-existing serum concentration of the object drug. When the serum concentration of the object drug is at the high end of the therapeutic range, even a modest increase in the serum concentration may be enough to result in a "toxic" level. Consider two patients, one with a serum theophylline concentration of 11 μg/ml and the other with a concentration of 18 μg/ml. A cimetidine-induced 40% increase in the serum theophylline concentration of each patient will increase the concentrations to 15.4 and 25.2 μg/ml, respectively. Thus, one patient would end up in the middle of the therapeutic range, while the other would be clearly in the toxic range.

5. Response to object drug is not being monitored closely. Close monitoring of the serum concentration and/or response to the object drug may substantially reduce the risk, because the interaction can be detected and adjustment made before an adverse effect occurs. For example, in a hospitalized patient on warfarin who is having daily prothrombin time determinations, an increased hypoprothrombinemic response due to cimetidine is likely to be detected quickly. Conversely, an outpatient whose prothrombin times are being monitored monthly would tend to be at greater risk because his excessive anticoagulation may remain undetected for weeks. Before deciding to use more frequent monitoring of the object drug as a way to reduce risk, consider substituting a non-interacting alternative to the precipitant drug. Even if the alternative medication is more expensive, the overall health care cost is usually less when one considers the cost of increasing the intensity of laboratory and clinical monitoring, and the cost of prolonged hospitalization should a serious complication of a drug interaction occur. Moreover, using a noninteracting alternative may reduce medicolegal liability; a toxic response to the object drug is likely to be blamed on the interacting drug

whether or not it was the primary cause of the excessive object drug response.

6. Changes in cimetidine therapy. Drug interactions are most likely to occur during "transition periods" when the precipitant drug is started, stopped, or changed in dosage. It is during these times that the effect of the object drug is increased or decreased. It is not unusual for cimetidine to be started and stopped, particularly when being used intermittently for peptic ulcer disease. Moreover, converting the patient from full dose cimetidine therapy to maintenance doses or vice versa also represents a "transition period" and is likely to affect the magnitude of the effect on the object drug.

Clinical Importance

Cimetidine has been shown to decrease the elimination of more than 50 drugs metabolized by the hepatic P-450 system (Table 27.3). For some drugs whose metabolism is inhibited by cimetidine, only pharmacokinetic data are available, and it is not known how often the interactions result in adverse outcomes. For other cimetidine interactions, however, the documentation includes both pharmacokinetic data and adverse clinical effects. Examples of such interactions are included in Table 27.4. More complete discussions of these well-described individual interactions are provided elsewhere (13).

An increasingly recognized interaction is that which occurs with cyclosporine. Puff and Carey (14) have recently demonstrated that oral cimetidine administration significantly alters the early metabolism of cyclosporine in liver transplant recipients. However, this did not appear to appreciably change cyclosporine through levels and thus cimetidine did not appear unsafe for use in orthotopic liver transplant patients. In their study, cimetidine elevated cyclosporine levels at 60 and 120 minutes but had no effect on levels drawn at 240 and 480 minutes. The dose of cimetidine used was 800 mg given 26, 14, and 2 hours before acute phase studies with cyclosporine and then over a 4-week period at a dose of 400 mg four times daily. D'Souza et al. (15) found that cimetidine prolonged the half-life and

Table 27.4
Cimetidine Drug Interactions That Have Resulted in Adverse Clinical Outcomes

Drug	Potential adverse effects
Antidepressants (tricyclic)	Antimuscarinic effects,[a] excessive sweating, inappropriate secretion of ADH
Carbamazepine	Drowsiness, vertigo, ataxia, diplopia, blurred vision, nausea, vomiting
Ketoconazole	Therapeutic failure[b]
Lidocaine	Sleepiness, dizziness, paresthesias, altered mental status, coma, seizures
Phenytoin	Nystagmus, ataxia, diplopia, vertigo, hyperactivity, increased seizure frequency, gastrointestinal symptoms
Procainamide	Prolongation of Q-T interval,[c] anorexia, nausea, vomiting
Theophylline	Tachycardia, restlessness, agitation, vomiting, headache, seizures
Warfarin	Hemorrhagic complications
Cyclosporine A	Renal allograft rejection

[a]Dry mouth, metallic taste, epigastric distress, constipation, dizziness, tachycardia, blurred vision, urinary retention.
[b]Although clinical evidence of cimetidine-induced reduction in antifungal response to ketoconazole in patients is limited, the magnitude of the reductions in ketoconazole serum concentrations due to cimetidine suggest that therapeutic failure of ketoconazole is possible.
[c]Seen less commonly than with quinidine and usually occurs in renal failure.

Table 27.5
Drugs Whose Metabolism Is *Not* Significantly Inhibited by Ranitidine[a]

Acetaminophen	Adinazolam	Amitriptyline
Bupivacaine	Carbamazepine	Chlordiazepoxide
Chlormethiazole	Chloroquine	Cifenline
Cyclophosphamide	Diazepam	Diltiazem
Doxepin	Flurbiprofen	Glipizide
Glyburide	Ibuprofen	Imipramine
Isoniazid	Lidocaine	Meperidine
Metoprolol	Mexiletine	Midazolam
Nicotine	Nifedipine	Nimodipine
Nitrendipine	Nortriptyline	Phenytoin
Piroxicam	Prednisone	Procainamide
Propranolol	Quinidine	Quinine
Sulindac	Theophylline	Tolbutamide
Valproic acid	Warfarin	

[a]After Reference 19.

clearance of cyclosporine in rats but had no effect on the volume of distribution. These authors suggest that cimetidine inhibits the metabolism of cyclosporine rather than altering its absorption. In vitro studies have demonstrated that cimetidine can reverse cyclosporine-induced inhibition of interleukin-2 production, and rejection of renal allografts in patients receiving cimetidine have been reported (16). However, larger studies of chronic use of cimetidine have not found an association between rejection or allograft function (17). Before a definitive conclusion can be made, it has been recommended that larger numbers of patients be studied.

RANITIDINE

Ranitidine is an H_2-receptor antagonist with a furan nucleus that appears to bind with considerably less affinity to cytochrome P-450 enzymes in the liver than cimetidine. As a consequence, it has only minimal effects on drug metabolism (9–11, 18, 19). Numerous controlled studies in both patients and healthy subjects suggest that ranitidine does not affect the pharmacokinetics of more than 40 drugs,

Table 27.6
Metabolism *Not* Significantly Inhibited by Famotidine or Nizatidine[a]

Famotidine	Nizatidine
Theophylline	Theophylline
Warfarin	Warfarin
Phenytoin	Phenytoin
Diazepam	Diazepam
Nifedipine	Chlordiazepoxide
	Lidocaine
	Metoprolol

[a]After References 20 and 21.

including amitriptyline, diazepam, doxepin, imipramine, lidocaine, mexiletine, phenytoin, propranolol, theophylline, tocainide, and warfarin (12, 18, 19) (Table 27.5). Isolated case reports have appeared in which ranitidine purportedly increased the serum concentration of drugs such as phenytoin, theophylline, and warfarin. Many of these cases were not credible due to factors such as a lack of challenge or rechallenge, or to the presence of other factors that could have been responsible for the changes in the object drug. Other cases were disproven when the cases were subjected to more intense scrutiny (19). Nonetheless, one cannot strictly rule out the possibility that ranitidine can, under special circumstances, alter the metabolism of other drugs. If such inhibition does occur, however, it is clear that is rare.

FAMOTIDINE

Famotidine is an H_2-receptor antagonist with a thiazole nucleus. As with ranitidine, it appears unlikely to affect hepatic drug metabolism. Although much less extensively studied (Table 27.6), famotidine does not appear to affect the metabolism of diazepam, phenytoin, nifedipine, theophylline, or warfarin (12, 20). Isolated case reports suggesting famotidine-induced inhibition of drug metabolism have appeared (e.g., theophylline), but if such inhibition does occur it must be quite rare (12).

NIZATIDINE

Nizatidine is the most recently introduced H_2-receptor antagonist in the United States.

Although it has not been used nearly as much as cimetidine, ranitidine, or famotidine, and although it remains much less extensively studied for drug interactions (Table 27.6), available evidence suggests that it does not inhibit hepatic drug metabolism (12, 21). As with ranitidine and famotidine, isolated case reports suggesting inhibition of drug metabolism have appeared, but inhibition is probably rare if it occurs.

H_2-Receptor Antagonist Effects on Renal Drug Elimination

For most drugs in clinical use today, drug metabolizing enzymes in the liver render the drug molecule more polar so it can be eliminated by the kidneys. Some drugs, however, are eliminated in substantial amounts as unchanged drug without alteration by the liver. One of the mechanisms by which the kidney eliminates unchanged drug involves a process of active tubular secretion. Drug interactions can occur when one drug interferes with or competes with the active tubular secretion of another (22). This may result in increased serum concentrations of one or both agents. A classic example of this type of interaction is the use of probenecid to prolong the serum concentration of penicillins, a favorable interaction still used today. Although most examples of this type of interaction have involved acidic drugs, there is growing evidence that there is also an active tubular secretion process for basic drugs (such as H_2-receptor antagonists) as well (12).

PROCAINAMIDE

Cimetidine appears to inhibit the active renal tubular secretion of procainamide and its active metabolite, N-acetylprocainamide (23, 24). In a study of healthy subjects, cimetidine increased the area under the procainamide plasma concentration time curve by 44%; procainamide renal clearance was reduced by 43%, whereas N-acetylprocainamide clearance was reduced by 24% (23). There is also some clinical evidence to suggest that cimetidine may increase the risk of procainamide toxicity, especially in the elderly (25, 26).

Some evidence suggests that ranitidine also can reduce the renal clearance of procainamide and N-acetylprocainamide, but the results are conflicting (19). In healthy subjects, pretreatment with ranitidine (150 mg twice daily) increased the area under the procainamide plasma concentration-time curve by 14% following a 1 g oral dose of procainamide; the AUC of N-acetylprocainamide increased by 13% (27). A higher dose of ranitidine (750 mg over a 12-hour period) resulted in a 21% increase in the procainamide AUC. In another study, however, ranitidine (150 mg twice daily for 4 days) did not affect the renal clearance of procainamide or N-acetylprocainamide (28). Thus, the evidence suggests that normal therapeutic doses of ranitidine are unlikely to affect the pharmacokinetics of procainamide to a clinically significant degree. The effect of supra-therapeutic doses of ranitidine on procainamide requires further study.

Famotidine does not appear to interfere with the renal clearance of either procainamide or N-acetylprocainamide (29), but little is known regarding a potential effect of nizatidine on procainamide pharmacokinetics.

TRIAMTERENE

In six healthy subjects receiving triamterene (100 mg/day for 4 days), cimetidine reduced triamterene renal clearance by 28%, and also appeared to inhibit the hepatic metabolism and gastrointestinal absorption of triamterene (30). This interaction is probably of minimal clinical importance, however, because cimetidine did not affect either the potassium-sparing or the natriuretic effects of triamterene. Ranitidine also has been reported to inhibit the renal elimination of triamterene (31) but, as with cimetidine, it does not appear likely that patients receiving the combination would be adversely affected. Little is known regarding the effect of famotidine or nizatidine on triamterene pharmacokinetics.

H_2-Receptor Antagonist Effects on Nonsteroidal Anti-inflammatory Drugs (NSAIDs)

The H_2-blockers are frequently used to heal acute ulcers and prevent ulcer relapse in patients receiving a variety of NSAIDs. They are undoubtedly used as well to prophylax against the development of upper gastrointestinal tract ulceration in NSAID users, although only misoprostol is approved by the FDA for the primary prevention of gastric ulcers in this setting. Given the widespread use of these agents, it is important to know whether or not clinically important pharmacokinetic or pharmacodynamic drug interactions might take place. Hepatic metabolism is the main route of elimination of most NSAIDs, with a majority undergoing oxidative metabolism by cytochrome P-450. Not surprisingly therefore, cimetidine has been shown to interact with many commonly used NSAIDs, including indomethacin, ibuprofen, piroxicam, aspirin, flurbiprofen, and sulindac (32), although the clinical significance of these interactions is unknown. Similarly, misoprostol may interact with diclofenac (33) although the results with indomethacin have been conflicting (34, 35). In contrast, ranitidine has no effect on any of these NSAIDs (32, 36).

H_2-RECEPTOR ANTAGONISTS AND ALCOHOL METABOLISM

Although an effect of cimetidine on blood alcohol levels was reported more than a decade ago (37), the possibility that these medications may have an important effect on alcohol metabolism has been receiving renewed interest. A series of studies performed by Lieber and co-workers (38–40) on the effects of H_2-blockers on gastric mucosal alcohol dehydrogenase activity (ADH) culminated in a recent report that suggested certain of the H_2-receptor antagonists might interfere with the first pass metabolism of alcohol through inhibition of gastric ADH, resulting in increased absorption and hence increased blood levels of alcohol (41). Based on these findings it has been implied by these investigators, and others (42, 43), that certain H_2-receptor antagonists might lead to "unexpected functional impairment" in patients consuming alcohol in amounts that were previously considered safe (41). As this interaction has been the subject of considerable attention, the following sections will attempt to summarize the pertinent clinical studies that have examined this potentially important phenomenon and the mechanisms by which it might occur.

Do H_2-Receptor Antagonists Elevate Blood Alcohol Concentrations?

Nearly three dozen publications (37–70), comprising more than 70 separate study arms with individual H_2-receptor antagonists, at varying doses, and given concomitantly with varying amounts of alcohol, have been published as of 1992 (Table 27.7). These studies also have varied in regard to the fed and fasting state of the test subjects. As a result, very few of the studies are directly comparable in terms of their methodology, and it is often difficult to draw direct conclusions concerning the effects of H_2-blockers on alcohol metabolism. In general, however, the bulk of these studies suggest that even if an H_2-blocker does lead to increased blood alcohol levels, the increase is very small in absolute terms. Perhaps more importantly, to date no study has demonstrated a clinically relevant effect (e.g., impaired psychomotor performance) from any alleged interaction (see below).

Of the approximately two dozen individual "studies" performed in *fasted* subjects, only two have shown any statistically significant elevation in blood alcohol concentration (BAC) (37, 55); and both were after relatively high oral doses of alcohol (0.7–0.8 g/kg). In both studies, the mean peak BAC exceeded 100 mg/dl, although the accuracy of the alcohol measurements in one of the studies has been criticized (71).

Pharmacokinetic studies of alcohol in *fed* subjects must be interpreted with care, as the size, type, and timing of the meal and other factors can control the rate of delivery of alcohol from the stomach into the small intestine (the major site of alcohol absorption) and hence the liver, which is now considered the

major site of alcohol metabolism (72). In addition, there is a large intersubject variability in the fed state, with blood alcohol levels varying by as much as 40% (61). Thus, large sample sizes and carefully standardized experimental procedures must be used to overcome this potential bias. It should be noted, that most of the studies reporting an increase in BAC from the concomitant use of H_2-receptor antagonists have used small numbers of test subjects and different methodologies. Seven of the 10 "positive" studies were seen with low doses of alcohol (three using 0.3 g/kg (40, 41) and four with 0.15 g/kg (39, 56, 70)). Palmer and colleagues (56) reported that ranitidine and nizatidine both enhanced the absorption of alcohol given in a dose of 0.15 g/kg in the morning, and that these effects were similar to those reported by others for cimetidine. In contrast, the effect of ranitidine on alcohol consumed in the evening was not significant in terms of peak concentration, and AUC was reduced to approximately one-third of the value seen in the morning. These investigators concluded that the increase in the actual amount of alcohol absorbed was actually quite small and was demonstrable only under special conditions (56, 73). Indeed, 25 of 35 studies with individual H_2 blockers in fed subjects have revealed no significant effect on mean peak blood alcohol concentrations (Table 27.7, Figs. 27.1 and 27.2).

Fraser et al. (61) have performed several studies with H_2-receptor antagonists using high and low doses of alcohol in the fed state. Their first study (61) showed no significant differences in BAC after the ingestion of 0.3 g/kg of alcohol with ranitidine, cimetidine, or famotidine compared with placebo. In a second study, using a larger dose of alcohol (0.6 g/kg), no difference in alcohol absorption was seen when ranitidine was compared with placebo (57). In a third trial using a smaller dose of alcohol (0.15 g/kg) after a course of ranitidine, only a trend toward a higher two hour plasma alcohol concentration was observed compared to placebo (3.89 mg-H/dl compared with placebo 3.17 mg-H/dl), but a statistically significant increase in mean peak

Table 27.7
Alcohol Interaction Studies with H_2-Antagonists and Other Agents (Descending Order of Alcohol Dose)[a]

Author	Subjects	Fed/fasting	Dose of alcohol/ type	Time given	Design	Treatment	C_{max} (mg/dl)	AUC (mg/dl/hr)	Comments
Holtzman et al. (44)	7 M 5 F	Fasting	45 g/d for 3 wk	Morning (8 AM)	XO	No treatment R 150 mg bid for 3 d C 300 mg qid for 3 d	N/A N/A N/A	N/A N/A N/A	No effect on distribution or clearance of alcohol
Johnson et al. (45)	4 M 4 F	Fed	1.5 g/kg	Fed meal 6 PM	Serial	Placebo C 400 mg bid for 3 d C 400 mg tid for 3 d	110 110 106	570 580 557	No effect on PK
Norpoth et al. (46)	12	Fed	1.4 g/kg Vodka in water or orange juice	AM? 30 min after meal	XO	Placebo R 150 mg bid for 2 d C 400 mg bid for 2 d	127 124 130	N/A N/A N/A	No effect on alcohol kinetics "No evidence that alcohol kinetics are affected"
Jonsson et al. (47)	12 M	Fasting	0.8 g/kg Ethanol in orange juice	Morning	XO	No drug R 300 mg/d for 7 d C 800 mg/d for 7 d O 20 mg/d for 7 d	104.9 103.0 100.7 101.7	400.2 400.2 381.8 391.0	No effect C_{max}, AUC, or any other values
Tanaka & Nakamura (48)	6 M	Fasting	0.8 g/kg Whisky	Morning (9.30–10 AM)	XO	Placebo R 150 mg bid for 7 d C 200 mg qid for 7 d F 20 mg bid for 7 d	112 110 111 114	517 516 523 515	No effect C_{max} or AUC
D'Ambrosi et al. (49)	10	Fed	0.8 g/kg Wine	Morning (10 AM)	XO	Placebo R 300 mg hs for 7 d C 800 mg hs for 7 d	N/A N/A N/A	N/A N/A N/A	Results not clear Study conducted circa 12 hr after last dose
Seltz et al. (50)	8 M	Fed	0.8 g/kg Gin in orange juice	Morning (1 hr after breakfast)	XO	Placebo R 150 mg bid for 7 d C 1 g/day for 7 d	73.0 75.5 85.9	304 308 350	No effect C_{max} or AUC C_{max} & AUC ↑ with C (73 to 86 mg/dl − $P < .02$; 304 to 350 mg/dl/h − $P < .05$)
de Pretis et al. (51)	12	Fasting (4 hr)	0.8 g/kg Wine	Unknown	XO	No treatment R 150 mg bid for 7 d C 400 mg bid for 7 d	N/A N/A N/A	N/A N/A N/A	No effect C_{max} or AUC

Reference	n	Fed	Dose	Timing	Design	Treatment			Comment
Roine et al. (89)	5 M	Fed	0.3 g/kg 9–14 % w/v orange juice over 10 min 200 ml	Morning (1 hr after breakfast)	XO	No treatment Aspirin 1000 mg with food (single dose)	25.1 34.9	40.64 51.27	C_{max} ↑ AUC ↑ during dosing aspirin ($P <$ .01) 39% and 26% resp. No iv dosing used. Random XO
Roine et al. (82)	7 M	Fed	0.3 g/kg orange juice over 10 min	Morning (1 hr after breakfast)	Serial	No treatment Alcohol 1 hr pB Omeprazole 20 mg 7 d	23.5 28.1[b]	38.4 42.9	C_{max} & AUC NS ↑ 20% and 12% resp
	3 M	Fed		Morning (2 hr after breakfast)	Serial	No treatment Alcohol 2 hr pB Omeprazole 20 mg 7 d	47.4	58.4 65.8	AUC NS ↑ 13%
Roine et al. (88)	5 M	Fed	0.3 g/kg Orange juice over 10 min 200 ml	? (1 hr after meal)	XO	Placebo single dose Cisapride 10 mg	24.0 32.3	36.5 45.2	C_{max} & AUC ↑ $P <$ .05 35% and 24% resp
Fraser et al. (61)	48 M	Fed	0.3 g/kg Absolute alcohol to 200 ml orange juice	Evening (7 PM)	PG	Placebo R 300 mg hs for 7 d C 800 mg hs for 7 d F 40 mg hs for 7 d	22.9 25.0 23.4 23.5	32.7 35.1 33.5 32.6	No effect C_{max} or AUC Additional dose taken 1.5 hr before alcohol
Terpin et al. (62)	12 M 4, 4, 4 M	?	0.3 g/kg Unknown	Unknown	PG	No treatment R 150 mg bid for 7 d No treatment C 1 g/d for 7 d No treatment O 20 mg bid for 7 d	N/A N/A N/A N/A N/A N/A	5.8[c] 9.0[c] 5.7[d] 14.7[d] 5.1[d] 5.2[d]	AUC ↑ during dosing with R & C Significant ↓ gastric first pass metabolism (from 43–15% & 19%, resp)
Roine et al. (40)	3	Fed	0.3 g/kg	Unknown	XO	Before R R 150 mg bid for 7 d Before C C 1 g/d for 7 d C 20 mg/d for 7 d	25.8 33.6 20.7 57.0 N/A	26.2 42.8 28.5 53.4 N/A	C_{max} ↑ & AUC ↑ during dosing with R & C (Significance not stated) Significant ↓ gastric first pass metabolism
Fraser et al. (63)	20 M	Fed	0.3 g/kg Orange juice over 1–2 min 200 ml from 100% orange juice	Morning (1 hr after meal)	XO DB	Placebo for 7 d R 150 mg bid for 7 d	18.0 21.1	27.8 32.4	No effect on C_{max} or AUC 17 and 17% ↑ resp
Raufman et al. (64)	23 M	Fed	0.3 g/kg in 500 ml orange juice over 8 min	Evening (1 hr after meal)	XO	No treatment for 7 d R 150 mg bid for 7 d C 400 mg bid for 7 d N 150 mg bid for 7 d F 20 mg bid for 7 d 7 d washout between each	13.5 14.1 14.0 13.5 13.2	18.3 18.1 19.9 19.4 17.6	No effect on C_{max} or AUC

Table 27.7 Continued
Alcohol Interaction Studies with H_2-Antagonists and Other Agents (Descending Order of Alcohol Dose)[a]

Author	Subjects	Fed/fasting	Dose of alcohol/ type	Time given	Design	Treatment	C_{max} (mg/dl)	AUC (mg/dl/hr)	Comments
Holtmann et al. (65)	3 M 3 F	Fasting (6 hr)	16 g Alcohol −0.23 g/kg 70 kg man 500 ml beer or 250 ml wine	?	XO DB	Placebo F 40 mg single dose	N/A	N/A	No significant effects; no data given; graph indicates ↑ levels at 15 min (NS) AUC ↑ (NS)
Holtmann et al. ?same study (66)	6	Fasting (6 hr)	16 g Alcohol −0.23 g/kg 70 kg man 500 ml beer	?	XO DB	Placebo F 40 mg single dose	N/A	N/A	No significant effects; no data given; graph indicates ↑ in levels at 15 min (NS) AUC ↑ (NS)
	6	Fasting (6 hr)	16 g Alcohol	?	XO DB	Placebo C 400 mg single dose	N/A N/A	N/A N/A	No data given; graph shows ↑ levels 15–45 min (NS) AUC ↑ (NS)
Etienne et al. (67)	5 M	Fed	0.2 g/kg in orange juice over 10 min	Morning (1 hr after meal)	XO?	Placebo for 7 d O 40 mg 7 d Misoprostol 800 µg 7 d C 800 mg bid	N/A	223.1[d] 182.5[a] 163 251.4	AUC ↑ NS 13% for C
Dobrilla et al. (52)	5 M 1 F	Fasting (4 hr)	0.8 g/kg Wine	Unknown (midday?)	XO	No treatment R 150 mg bid for 7 d C 400 mg bid for 7 d	82[e] 72[e] 91[e]	N/A N/A N/A	No effect C_{max} or AUC
Fraser et al. (53)	47 M	Fed	0.8 g/kg 100% Alcohol to 300 ml with orange juice	Evening (7 PM)	PG	Placebo R 300 mg hs for 7 d C 800 mg hs for 7 d F 40 mg hs for 7 d	85 87 86 86	358 348 361 341	No effect C_{max} or AUC Additional dose taken 1 hr before alcohol
Feely & Wood (37)	5 M	Fasting	0.8 g/kg 95% Alcohol in orange juice over 20 min	AM	XO	Placebo for 7 d C 300 mg qid for 7 d	140 163	717 771	Small increase in peak/AUC (NS) Subjects rated more intoxicated on cimetidine at peak

Study	Subjects	State	Dose	Time	Design	Treatment			Comments
Guram et al. (43)	6 M	Fed	0.75 g/kg Ethanol in 400 ml of orange juice	Afternoon/evening (4–8 PM)	XO	Control R 300 mg hs for 7 d C 800 mg hs for 7 d F 40 mg hs for 7 d N 300 mg hs for 7 d O 20 mg hs for 7 d	75.9 80.8 100 75.9 90.3 74.1	7122[f] 7821 8934 7121 8556 6833	AUC ↑ for R, C & N ($P < .05$) R—no effect C_{max} C_{max} ↑ for C & N ($P < .01$)
Papke et al. (54)	8 M 2 F	Fasting	0.75 g/kg 20% Alcohol over 20 min	Morning 2 hr after drug	?serial	Control C 1000 mg single dose C 200–400 mg for 7 d	95 94 102	325 304 352	No effect on any parameter
Webster et al. (55)	4 M 3 F	Fasting	0.7 g/kg Ethanol 25% v/v in orange juice	Morning	XO	No treatment R 150 mg bid for 2 d C 1 g/day for 2 d	116 148 136	296 349 337	C_{max} ↑ and AUC ↑ during dosing with ranitidine Trend for CNS
Palmer et al. (56)	12 M 12 F PU pts	Fasting/fed	0.67 g/kg Cocktails & wine	PM before and w/dinner	XO	Placebo C 300 mg qid	67.8 69.7	183 183	No significant effects
Fraser et al. (57)	24 M	Fed	0.6 g/kg 37.5% Vodka to 275 ml w/orange juice	Evening (7 PM)	PG	Placebo R 300 mg hs for 7 d	53.8 57.9	142.5 147.2	No effect C_{max} or AUC Additional R dose 1.5 hr before alcohol
Toon et al. (58)	18 M	Fed	0.5 g/kg 40% Vodka w/orange juice	Breakfast (8.30 AM) Lunch (1.30 PM) Dinner (6.30 PM)	XO	Placebo R 300 mg qid for 3 d Placebo R 300 mg qid for 6 d Placebo R 300 mg qid for 8 d	43.7 46.4 45.4 48.7 41.3 43.8	111.5 112.3 109.6 112.8 94.9 100.7	No effect C_{max} or AUC No effect C_{max} or AUC No effect C_{max} or AUC
Kleine & Ertl (59)	16 M	Fed	0.5 g/kg (3 Drinks over 60 min)			Placebo R 150 mg bid for 6 d R 300 mg bid for 6 d	15.3 14.0 15.5	17485[a] 14448[a] 15803	No effect C_{max} or AUC Last dose taken 15 min after first dose of alcohol
Palmer et al. (Dauncey et al.[h]) (56)	7 M 3 F	Fasting	0.5 g/kg Before breakfast	Morning	?	Control C 400 mg single dose C 400 mg bid Control R 150 mg single dose R 150 mg bid	62 61 65 66 59 67	N/A N/A N/A N/A N/A N/A	No effect on C_{max}

Table 27.7 Continued
Alcohol Interaction Studies with H_2-Antagonists and Other Agents (Descending Order of Alcohol Dose)[a]

Author	Subjects	Fed/fasting	Dose of alcohol/ type	Time given	Design	Treatment	C_{max} (mg/dl)	AUC (mg/dl/hr)	Comments
	7 M 3 F	Fasting	0.5 g/kg	Before dinner		Control R 150 mg bid Control C 400 mg bid	66 65 62 58	N/A N/A N/A N/A	No effect on C_{max}
Hindmarch & Gilburt (60)	10 F		0.5 g/kg			Placebo N	No data		No effect on psychomotor function
Edelbroek et al. (90)	8 M	Fed	0.5 k/kg in 400 ml orange juice	w/meal	XO	Saline before meal Erythromycin 3 mg/ kg iv single dose	55 77	6658 7614	C_{max} ↑ & AUC ↑ during dosing with erythromycin 40% and 14%, resp ($P < .05$)
DiPadova et al. (41)	20 M 8, 6, 6 M	Fed	0.3 g/kg 9–13% w/orange juice or 5% dextrose	Morning (1 hr after breakfast)	PG	Before R R 150 mg bid for 7 d Before C C 1 g/d for 7 d Before F F 40 mg hs for 7 d	31.6 41.8 29.6 56.9 28.0 29.8	38.9 52.9 29.7 58.2 40.9 36.8	C_{max} ↑ & AUC ↑ during dosing with R and C ($P < .01$) Significant ↓ gastric first pass metabolism with R and C (n = R [8], C [6], F [6])
Tan et al. (68)	3	Fasting	0.18 g/kg 1 ml/kg Sherry	Morning	?	No treatment C 200 mg single dose Chlorpheniramine	34 30.6 N/A	N/A N/A N/A	No effect of C on parameters Combination reduced levels
Palmer et al. (56)	24 M	Fed	0.15 g/kg 95% Ethanol in 120 ml of orange juice	Morning (1 hr after starting, 30 min after finishing breakfast)	XO	No treatment R 300 mg for 3 d	8.2 12.1	5.2 8.5	↑ C_{max} and ↑ AUC w/R ↑ C_{max} and ↑ AUC w/N
	19 M	Fed				No treatment N 300 mg for 3 d	8.3 12.8	5.6 9.2	
	23 M	Fed	0.15 g/kg 95% Ethanol in 120 ml of orange juice	Evening (1 hr after starting, 30 min after finishing dinner)	XO	Placebo R 300 mg dinnertime for 3 d C 800 mg hs for 3 d C 400 mg bid for 3 d	9.8 10.6 9.75 8.8	5.8 7.0 5.5 5.0	↑ AUC with R No effect of C

Fiatarone et al. (69)	9	Fed (error in abstract)	0.15 g/kg Ethanol in 200 ml of orange juice	Unknown	PG	No treatment R 300 mg/d	N/A N/A	N/A N/A	Significant ↓ gastric first pass metabolism
Fraser et al. (70)	20 M	Fed	0.15 g/kg 100% alcohol to 275 ml w/orange juice	Evening (7 PM)	XO	Placebo R 300 mg hs for 7 d	4.92 6.47	3.17 3.89	C_{max} ↑ (significant) AUC—no effect Additional dose taken 1.5 hr before alcohol
Hernandez-Munoz et al. (39)	6 M (methods N = 5, graph N = 6)	Fed	0.15/kg PO & IV	Morning (1 hr after breakfast)	Serial	Control C 400 mg bid for 7 d F 20 mg bid for 7 d	6.92[a] 10.4[a] 6.92[a]	4.25 7.52 5.26	77% AUC ↑ during dosing with C; C_{max} ↑ no data 24% AUC ↑ during dosing w/F; apparent faster rise compared w/placebo (graph)
Caballeria et al. (38)	6 M	Fed	0.15/kg PO & IV	Morning (1 hr after breakfast)	Serial	Control C 400 mg bid for 7 d	7.0[j] 11.0[j]	4.1 7.6	C_{max} ↑ & AUC ↑ during dosing with C 57% and 85% resp Significant ↓ gastric first pass metabolism 20%

[a]C, cimetidine; R, ranitidine; F, famotidine; N, nizaridine; O, omeprazole; AUC, area under the procainamide plasma concentration time curve; XO, cross-over; PG, parallel group; resp, respectively; bid, twice daily; aid, four times daily; hs, at bedtime; iv, intravenously; PO, orally, w/v, weight-to-volume; w/w, weight-to-weight; NS, not significant.
[b]Estimated from graph. No intravenous dosing was done.
[c]Baseline value for R.
[d]Units undefined.
[e]Estimated from graph.
[f]AUC in milligrams per decalite per minute.
[g]Data expressed as AUC 0.240 mg/l.
[h]Dauncey et al. (unpublished data) quoted by Palmer et al. (56).
[i]May be same as study in reference 59.
[j]Estimated.

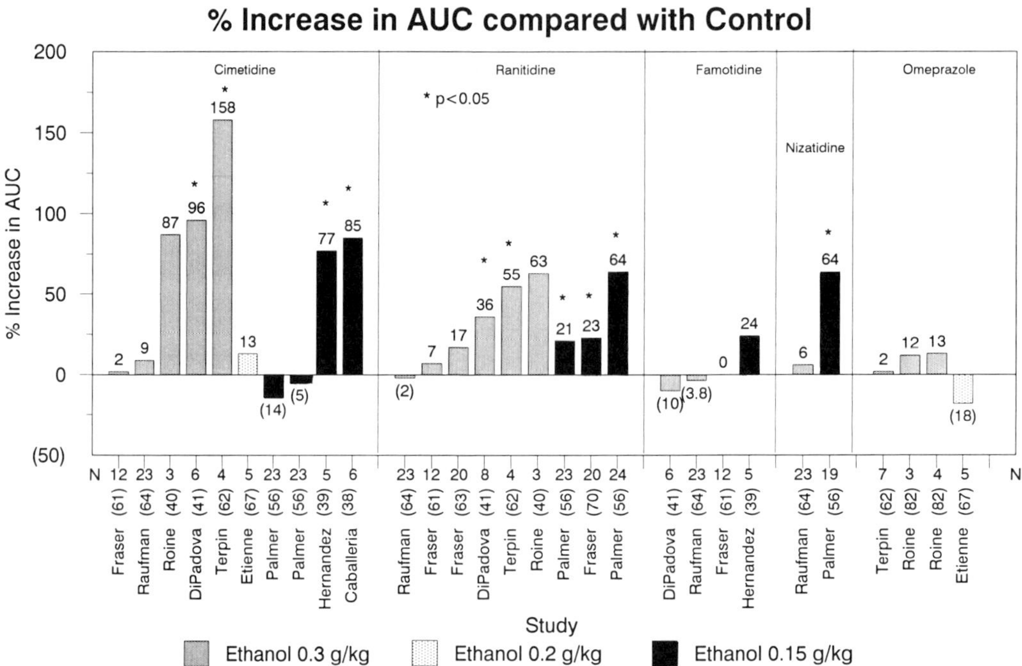

Figure 27.1. Percentage increases in blood ethanol AUC seen with H_2-receptor antagonists and omeprazole taken in conjunction with three doses of alcohol (0.15, 0.2, and 0.3 g/kg) as reported in the literature.

plasma alcohol concentration (6.47 versus 4.92 mg/dl) was observed (70). These investigators noted, however, that none of the volunteers reported any intoxication at the peak levels which ranged from undetectable to 13.1 mg/dl. They considered that the very small absolute increase in mean peak BAC was not of any clinical relevance. In a fourth study involving 47 men, the effect of ranitidine, cimetidine, and famotidine on plasma alcohol concentrations in the range of the legal driving limit for most countries (80–100 mg/dl) was studied and compared to placebo (53). Subjects received 0.8 g/kg of alcohol after 7 days' dosing with ranitidine 300 mg, cimetidine 800 mg, famotidine 40 mg or placebo given once daily. Mean plasma alcohol concentrations, mean peak alcohol concentrations, and the time to reach peak alcohol concentrations were not significantly different among any of the treatment groups or compared with placebo. Similarly, the AUC also

showed no differences. Individual results, however, showed a wide variation in alcohol absorption. This was interpreted as confirming the variable absorption of alcohol that occurs after a meal in a given individual. In an effort to replicate the study design of DiPadova et al. (41), Fraser et al. (63) performed a fifth study but were unable to demonstrate any significant effect of ranitidine 150 mg twice daily BID for 7 days on 0.3 g/kg of alcohol given in the fed state in the morning in 20 male volunteers. In another study that also attempted to replicate the work of Lieber's group, Raufman et al. (64) were also unable to confirm any significant effect of ranitidine, cimetidine, or famotidine on alcohol concentrations after 0.3 g/kg alcohol given in 500 ml of orange juice over an 8-minutes period in the evening after a meal.

The conflicting results reported by Lieber's group, that of Fraser, Pounder, and coworkers, and more recently of Raufman and col-

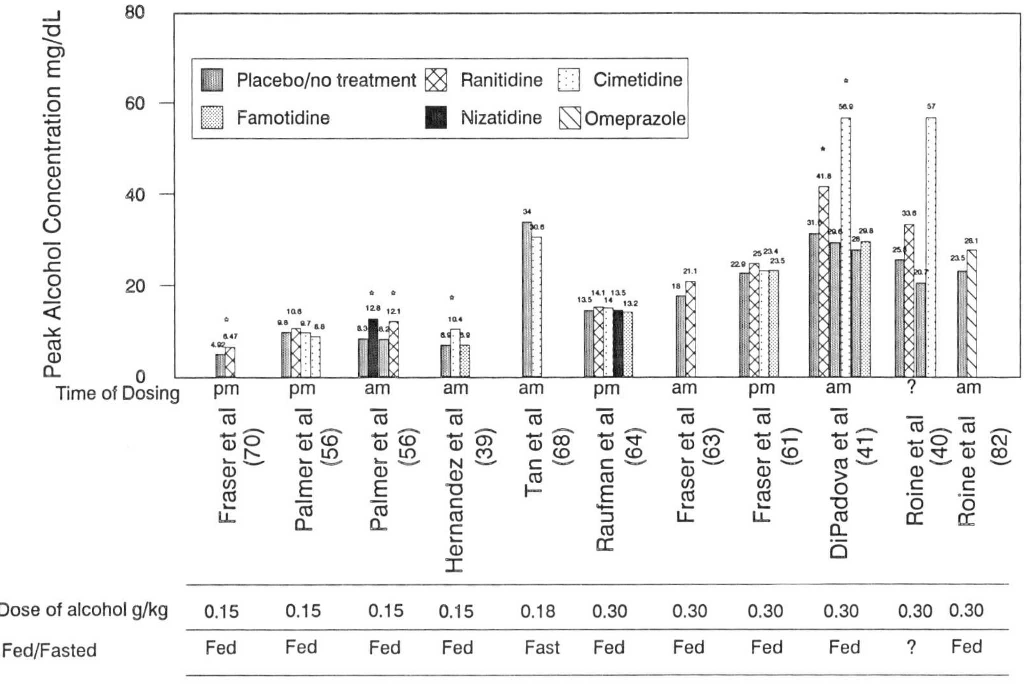

Figure 27.2. Mean peak alcohol concentrations reported in H_2-receptor antagonist and omeprazole-alcohol interaction studies. The legal limit of intoxication in most countries is 80 to 100 mg/dl (a value not exceeded by reports in the literature).

leagues may be best explained by methodologic differences in their studies, and have engendered an active debate (74–78). Lieber's studies involved morning dosing with alcohol after a breakfast meal. In contrast, Fraser et al. and Raufman et al. studied their subjects in the more clinically realistic evening setting. But perhaps most importantly, in contrast to Lieber's open, uncontrolled studies using very few subjects, the negative results observed by Fraser and Pounder (63) and by Raufman et al. (64) were based on placebo-controlled, double-blind, randomized trials using larger numbers of subjects. A recent study by Kleine and colleagues (59) adds to the list of reassuringly negative studies. Using doses of ranitidine that included 300 mg twice daily, no effect on alcohol in a dose of 0.5 g/kg (equivalent to three drinks over a 60-minutes period) was demonstrated. Furthermore, Holtzman et al. (44) have found that neither ranitidine nor cimetidine had any effect of the absorption or metabolism of alcohol in chronic alcohol users (both men and women). However, they did show a slightly increased first pass effect corroborating reports that alcohol is metabolized more rapidly in alcoholics.

Gastric ADH and Alcohol Metabolism

The scientific foundation supporting the theory that H_2-receptor antagonists might enhance the absorption of ethanol, is the ability of certain of these agents to inhibit gastric mucosal ADH (79–81). Until recently, it had-been widely assumed that gastric ADH could metabolize between 20 and 80% of an ingested dose of alcohol, based on studies in non-alcoholic, fed male subjects (38, 39). This effect was supposedly most evident at low doses of ingested alcohol (i.e., 0.15–0.3/kg; corresponding to one to two drinks). Data from an open, non-randomized study showed that cimetidine (but not famotidine) elevated blood ethanol levels in six subjects given 0.15 g/kg alcohol 1 hour after breakfast (38). In a follow-up study, a similar interaction was reported with ranitidine and cimetidine, again in an open, non-randomized study after an oral dose of 0.3 g/kg alcohol given one hour after breakfast (41). These investigators have assumed in these and subsequent publications (82) that their observations were explained by the inhibitory effect of cimetidine and ranitidine on gastric ADH, and that their observations confirmed the first pass metabolism role of this enzyme.

More recently, it has been shown that gastric ADH has a very low affinity for ethanol with ADH activity of rat gastric mucosa calculated to be only a small fraction of the ADH activity of the liver (0.07 units/g of tissue vs. 0.54 units/g of tissue, respectively) (83). In addition, the overall capacity of the liver to metabolize alcohol is estimated to be about 50 times greater than that of the stomach, based on the fact the liver weighs many times more than the gastric mucosa. In vitro measurements, even when carried out under highly unphysiologic conditions to optimize gastric ADH activity, indicate there is insufficient activity of the ADH enzyme to account for the observed first pass metabolism reported by Lieber and co-workers. In a study by Smith, Levitt, and their co-investigators (72), it was demonstrated that gastric metabolism in the rat (the model used by Lieber) is negligible, and that hepatic ADH is the major factor in the first pass metabolism of alcohol. Given what is known of rat and human Km values for gastric ADH, Smith et al. calculated that alcohol metabolism by human gastric ADH is also negligible (approximately 0.4% of a dose in 1 hour).

In an extension of this work, Levitt and Levitt have developed a model for human hepatic ethanol metabolism (84). Simulations of the time courses of blood ethanol concentrations using this model demonstrate that at the doses of alcohol used in clinical studies (0.15, 0.30, 0.90 g/kg), the hepatic first-pass metabolism is extremely dependent on the rate of delivery of ethanol to the liver. These investigators have concluded that "the known ability of the liver to metabolize ethanol explains published observations with regard to first pass metabolism and there is no need to postulate gastric metabolism of ethanol" (84). Thus, the exact role, if any, of gastric ADH in the metabolism of alcohol has been called into question.

What Is the Medical Significance of Any H₂-Receptor Antagonist-Alcohol Interaction?

As mentioned, this debate has become highly charged (74–78). Those who imply that the large percentage increase in BAC from baseline values could potentially lead to "unexpected functional impairment" (41) are countered by others who claim that these very small absolute value increases are very unlikely to produce any psychomotor or other impairment (61, 73). Moreover, statements that an H₂-alcohol interaction might lead to social or medical/legal consequences have been made without data to substantiate the claim (85). In contrast, several studies have been specifically conducted to examine psychomotor function in patients receiving cimetidine, ranitidine, and nizatidine with alcohol. In all of these studies, psychomotor responses to alcohol were unaltered by the concomitant use of any of these H₂-blockers (46, 58, 60). In addition, the early report by Feely and Wood (37) that cimetidine increased a subjective measure of inebriation could not be confirmed by Johnson et al. (45) using a similar analog scale.

Palmer (73) stressed the fact that while percentage increases in peak levels and total absorption as measured by AUC are often referred to as being statistically significant and therefore as "impressive increases," the absolute increases from most of these studies including his own are very small. For example, assuming that metabolism was similar in his test subjects and that 8 g of alcohol were metabolized by gastric ADH in the controlled setting and 2.5 g were absorbed, the increases in absorption due to ranitidine and nizatidine were rather trivial (63% of 2.5 g = 1.6 g or less than one-fourth of a tablespoon of 90-proof liquor). His findings also stressed the marked variability in the effect of H_2-blockers on alcohol disposition depending on the timing of alcohol and whether or not the patients were fed or fasting. In general, alcohol absorption was markedly diminished or absent when alcohol was given after dinner. For example, although ranitidine caused a 48% increase in C_{max} and a 63% increase in AUC when alcohol was given after breakfast, after dinner, the same dose of ranitidine produced only an 8% increase in C_{max} and a 21% increase in AUC, with only the later value still being significant (56). Thus, in what they term "real-life situations" concerning alcohol, the effects appear to be much less than in the artificial setting of an early morning dose of alcohol, and the absolute increases in blood alcohol levels remain well below any threshold for inebriation (73).

Although a diurnal variation in the metabolism of alcohol has been described (73), Sharma et al. (86) did not observe any diurnal variation on the first pass metabolism of alcohol in a recent study. Of the relatively few studies that have shown a significant effect of H_2-receptor antagonists on alcohol absorption, nearly all have been performed in the morning (either fasting or after breakfast) and these studies are in the minority compared to a much larger number where no significant increases were seen in absorption after the morning dosing of alcohol and these agents. Similarly, only one study has shown any significant increase after alcohol given at noon or at dinner time. Clearly the overall trend is that there is little or no significant effect of H_2-receptor antagonists on alcohol disposition after morning, noon, or evening dosing of alcohol.

Although the literature does not support a significant increase in blood alcohol levels with famotidine, it is important to note that relatively few studies (comprising a very limited number of subjects) have investigated the effect of famotidine's interaction with alcohol, and the drug has not been specifically studied in conjunction with psychometric testing (Table 27.7). Although it is correct to state that no statistically significant increases have been published with famotidine, estimates of numerical increases in AUC (as much as 24%) have been seen in some studies (39) (Fig. 27.2).

In summary, although a few small studies have demonstrated a statistically significant increase in mean peak blood alcohol concentrations or AUC levels after treatment with cimetidine, ranitidine, and nizatidine, these have all been small absolute value increases and have been observed only under experimental conditions. The clinical and medical/legal relevance of any of these observations appears to be negligible, especially in light of larger, controlled trials using similar designs and methodology that have been unable to replicate the positive findings reported by Lieber's group and a few others. Indeed, the FDA's Gastrointestinal Drugs Advisory Committee took up this issue in March 1993 and concluded that no change in the package labeling of any of the H_2-receptor antagonists was necessary with respect to alcohol (86a). Nevertheless, it is important to remember that alcohol remains a major social problem in our society and that no one should drink and drive or operate sophisticated machinery under the illusion that any particular medication will be "protective" against the effects of over indulgence. It is probably safe to conclude however, that whereas alcohol remains a socially relevant problem, the concomitant use of H_2-receptor antagonists is not part of that problem.

Effect of Other Agents on Alcohol Elimination

In addition to the H_2-receptor antagonists, a number of studies have examined the possible

Table 27.8
Drug Metabolism Significantly Affected by Omeprazole[a]

Diazepam	Nifedipine
Phenytoin	Warfarin
Cyclosporine	Disulfiram
Digoxin	

[a]After Reference 91.

effect of several other agents on the elimination of ethanol (87). As illustrated in Table 27.7, no significant effect on peak alcohol blood levels or AUC has been observed using a variety of doses of alcohol given with 20 mg of omeprazole (40, 43, 62, 67, 82). Similarly, no effect of misoprostol was observed in one study (67).

In contrast, significant increases in alcohol blood levels and AUC have been observed when alcohol is taken after cisapride (88), aspirin (89), and erythromycin (90). Both cisapride and erythromycin are promotility agents that most likely exert their effect on alcohol by increasing gastric emptying and therefore, increase absorption of alcohol from the small intestine. Additionally, erythromycin is known to be an inhibitor of the P-450 hepatic cytochrome system. However, its role in the inhibition of gastric ADH is unclear. Salicylic acid, acetaminophen, propranolol, and ethacrynic acid have all been shown to inhibit rat gastric ADH in vitro, although again, whether or not these compounds influence alcohol disposition by their role on gastric ADH remains unclear (56, 73).

OMEPRAZOLE DRUG INTERACTIONS

Omeprazole is a proton pump inhibitor that markedly inhibits gastric acid secretion. It has been used particularly in the treatment of refractory gastroesophageal reflux disease, ulcer disease, and hypersecretory states such as Zollinger-Ellison syndrome. Its potential to be involved with drug-drug interactions relates to its effect on gastric acidity, as well as both an inhibitory and possibly an inductive effect on the hepatic P-450 system.

Omeprazole Effects on Drug Absorption

The ability of omeprazole to dramatically reduce gastric acid secretion would be expected to affect the bioavailability of those drugs whose gastrointestinal absorption is pH dependent. However, as discussed above in antacids, relatively few drugs have demonstrated altered absorption due to changes in gastric acidity. Table 27.1 lists some drugs whose absorption may be affected by the increased gastric pH produced by antacids or H_2-receptor antagonists; omeprazole would be expected to interact in the same way.

Omeprazole Effects on Drug Metabolism

Like cimetidine, omeprazole has an imidazole nucleus and can inhibit the hepatic metabolism of other drugs. However, the clinical evidence available suggests that omeprazole is a weaker metabolic inhibitor than cimetidine, and does not affect as many drugs (91) (Table 27.8). Early studies using 40 mg/day of omeprazole demonstrated that it can substantially reduce diazepam clearance, and modestly reduce phenytoin clearance (92, 93). Subsequent studies using 20 mg/day of omeprazole indicate that such doses have smaller effects on diazepam metabolism and no effect on phenytoin metabolism (94, 95). Although in vitro evidence suggested that omeprazole would markedly inhibit the metabolism of coumarin anticoagulants (92), a study in 21 healthy subjects demonstrated only a slight increase in the hypoprothrombinemic response of warfarin after 2 weeks of concurrent omeprazole therapy (20 mg/day) (96). Nonetheless, one should keep in mind that larger doses of omeprazole may be more likely to interact with warfarin in a clinically important way.

Other drugs for which a possible interaction with omeprazole has been described include nifedipine (97), cyclosporine (98), digoxin (99), and disulfiram (100). Interestingly, omeprazole does not appear to affect the pharmacokinetics of propranolol or theophylline, two drugs that are clearly susceptible to inhibition of hepatic metabolism (101, 102). Neither has any significant effect of omeprazole on alcohol been seen (as discussed in *H₂-Receptor Antagonists and Alcohol Metabolism*).

Diaz et al. (103) recently reported that in primary hepatocyte culture, omeprazole induced hepatic cytochrome P-450 IA proteins. Although the clinical relevance of this observation remains unknown, the possibility that induction of this isoenzyme might increase the risk of acetaminophen-induced hepatotoxicity as well as alter the metabolism of certain carcinogens has been raised (104, 105).

In summary, available evidence suggests that omeprazole can act as an inhibitor of hepatic oxidative drug metabolism, and that the dose of omeprazole is an important determinant to the magnitude of the effect. Doses of more than 20 mg/day appear more likely to produce clinically important interactions than 20 mg/day or less. The possibility that omeprazole may induce P-450 cytochromes is intriguing and warrants further study.

SUCRALFATE DRUG INTERACTIONS

Sucralfate is an aluminum salt of sucrose that is minimally absorbed from the gastrointestinal tract, and thus is unlikely to have systemic interactions with other drugs. However, it can inhibit gastrointestinal drug absorption.

Sucralfate Effects on Drug Absorption

Sucralfate markedly inhibits the gastrointestinal absorption of orally administered quinolone antibiotics such as norfloxacin, ciprofloxacin, and probably other quinolones as well (106, 107). It is thought that the aluminum from the sucralfate chelates the quinolones, thus rendering them insoluble and incapable of being absorbed. Although the effect of spacing the doses of quinolines away from sucralfate has not been well studied, giving the quinolone at least 2 hours before or 6 hours after the sucralfate would probably minimize the interaction. Many other drugs do not appear to be as susceptible as quinolone antibiotics to the inhibitory effect of sucralfate on drug absorption. For example, sucralfate produces only a small reduction in the gastrointestinal absorption of digoxin, phenytoin, and

chlorpropamide, and has little or no effect on the absorption of many other drugs such as corticosteroids, erythromycin, H₂-receptor antagonists, NSAIDs, and procainamide (12). Evidence concerning the effect of sucralfate on warfarin absorption is conflicting. Isolated case reports suggest that sucralfate may inhibit the absorption of warfarin, but controlled studies suggest no effect (108–110). It is possible that the altered warfarin response in the case reports resulted from causes other than the sucralfate, but one cannot rule out the possibility that sucralfate does inhibit warfarin absorption in patients with specific predisposing factors. A recent report draws attention to a clinically significant reduction in thyroxine bioavailability that was not reversed by delaying levothyroxine ingestion for 2.5 hours after sucralfate (111). The authors speculated that binding occurred in the stomach and they recommend that levothyroxine be given a few hours before the first daily dose of sucralfate.

MISCELLANEOUS ANTIULCER AGENTS

Bismuth Preparations

Bismuth preparations in clinical use include colloidal bismuth subcitrate and bismuth subsalicylate. The systemic absorption of these agents after oral administration appears to be low; thus, like sucralfate, systemic interactions with other drugs appear unlikely. Bismuth subsalicylate has been shown to inhibit the gastrointestinal absorption of tetracyclines, and other bismuth preparations are expected to have a similar effect. Fifteen healthy subjects were given tetracycline 250 mg orally with and without 60 ml of bismuth subsalicylate, the bismuth was associated with a 34% reduction in tetracycline bioavailability (112). In another study of six healthy subjects, 60 ml of bismuth subsalicylate reduced doxycycline bioavailability by 22% when given 2 hours before the doxycycline, by 37% when given with the doxycycline, and by 51% when given every 6 hours for five doses with the doxycycline given with the last dose of bismuth (113). Giving the doxycycline 2 hours before the bismuth subsalicylate circumvented the interaction. It is possible that bismuth preparations also inhibit the absorption of other drugs, but little evidence is available. In a preliminary report, bismuth subsalicylate did not appear to affect the bioavailability of norfloxacin (114).

When using bismuth subsalicylate, one should keep in mind the substantial salicylate content of this product. This is unlikely to be a problem for people who take occasional salicylates for headaches and the like. However, in patients taking large antirheumatic doses of salicylates, one should calculate the amount of salicylate taken in the form of bismuth subsalicylate and reduce their salicylate intake by that amount. As of 1992, the "original" preparation of Pepto-Bismol contains 102 mg of salicylate per tablet (99 mg per tablet for cherry) and the "original" liquid contains 130 mg per tablespoonful; "maximum strength" Pepto-Bismol liquid contains 236 mg of salicylate per tablespoonful (115). However, manufacturers sometimes change their formulations, so it would be prudent to check the label of the bismuth subsalicylate product you are using for the salicylate content.

ANTICHOLINERGIC DRUG INTERACTIONS

Anticholinergic agents (more accurately termed "muscarinic antagonists") have been largely replaced by H_2-receptor antagonists and omeprazole when a reduction in gastric acid secretion is desired. When used in doses sufficient to reduce acid secretion, anticholinergics also tend to reduce gastrointestinal motility, which in turn can affect the absorption of some drugs. However, as mentioned above in Mechanisms of Drug Interactions, altered gastrointestinal motility tends to affect only the absorption rate of the object drug, and seldom has been shown to alter the *extent* of drug absorption. In patients on chronic digoxin therapy with a slowly dissolving digoxin preparation, the addition of propantheline (15 mg/day for 10 days) was associated with an increase in serum digoxin concentration in 9 of the 13 individuals (116). The proposed mechanism for this effect is that the slowed gastrointestinal motility allows this digoxin preparation to dissolve more completely, thus

enhancing its absorption. In subsequent studies propantheline did not affect the absorption of digoxin administered as a solution or as a more rapidly dissolving tablet preparation (Lanoxin) (117).

Anticholinergics can also be involved in pharmacodynamic drug interactions, such as when they are combined with other drugs that have anticholinergic effects. A number of commonly used drugs produce anticholinergic side effects and may be expected to add to the anticholinergic effects of anticholinergics used in gastroenterology (12). Examples of drugs with anticholinergic properties include antihistamines, disopyramide, phenothiazines, and tricyclic antidepressants.

PROKINETIC AGENT DRUG INTERACTIONS

Metoclopramide

The ability of metoclopramide to increase gastric emptying and enhance gastrointestinal motility has the potential for affecting the absorption of other drugs. Theoretically, drugs that are slowly dissolved in the gastrointestinal tract would be even less well absorbed due to metoclopramide-induced enhancement of gut motility (12). This may be partly responsible for the slight reduction in bioavailability of slowly dissolving digoxin preparations due to metoclopramide. For example, 11 patients on chronic therapy with such a digoxin product all developed a decrease in their serum digoxin concentrations (116). Digoxin capsules do not appear to be affected by metoclopramide (118) and it seems likely that rapidly dissolving tables (e.g., Lanoxin) would also be less likely to interact.

Metoclopramide has minor effects on the pharmacokinetics of a number of other drugs, probably through its effects on gastrointestinal motility (10, 119). Nonetheless, it is unlikely that the magnitude of the effects observed would be sufficient to result in adverse outcomes.

Cisapride

One would expect that the ability of cisapride to enhance gastrointestinal motility would affect the rate of gastrointestinal absorption of other drugs in a manner similar to that of metoclopramide; however, little information is available. In one study, cisapride and metoclopramide both slightly reduced the bioavailability of digoxin (120). If cisapride does affect the rate of absorption of other drugs, as with metoclopramide, it is unlikely that these effects would be clinically important in the vast majority of patients.

Cisapride appears to undergo substantial metabolism on its first pass through the liver (10). Agents with high first pass metabolism can be markedly affected by inhibitors of hepatic drug metabolism, which probably accounts for the substantial increase in cisapride bioavailability seen with concurrent cimetidine administration. In eight healthy subjects given cisapride (10 mg three times daily for 7 days) with and without cimetidine (400 mg three times daily for 7 days), cimetidine increased cisapride bioavailability by 45% (121). Inasmuch as cisapride appears to have relatively few adverse reactions, the clinical importance of this interaction is probably not great. Indeed, the combination of cisapride and cimetidine has been used with apparently good results in the treatment of severe gastroesophageal reflux disease (122).

ANTIDIARRHEAL DRUG INTERACTIONS

"Binding" Agents: Attapulgite, Kaolin-Pectin

Antidiarrheal agents such as attapulgite and kaolin-pectin have numerous small particles with a large surface area. Theoretically, drugs can bind on these particles, thus rendering the drug unavailable for absorption in the small intestine. There is limited evidence that attapulgite can impair the bioavailability of promazine, a phenothiazine agent (123). In another small study of four healthy subjects, 30 ml of kaolin-pectin reduced the absorption of quinidine (100 mg orally) by 59% (124). Kaolin-pectin can also reduce the bioavailability of chloroquine, digoxin, lincomycin, and quinidine; only slight reductions in bioavailability were observed when kaolin-pectin was given with aspirin or pseudoephedrine (12).

REFERENCES

1. Gugler R, Allgayer H. Effects of antacids on the clinical pharmacokinetics of drugs: an update. Clin Pharmacokinet 1990;18:210–219.
2. Hurwitz A. Antacid therapy and drug kinetics. Clin Pharmacokinet 1977;2:269–280.
3. Steinberg WM, Lewis JH, Katz DM. Antacids inhibit the absorption of cimetidine. N Engl J Med 1982;307:400–404.
4. Carlson JA, Mann HJ, Canafax DM. Effect of pH on disintegration and dissolution of ketoconazole tablets. Am J Hosp Pharm 1983;40:1334–1336.
5. Lelawongs P, Barone JA, Colaizzi JL, et al. Effect of food and gastric acidity on absorption of orally administered ketoconazole. Clin Pharm 1988;7:228–235.
6. Feldman S, Carlstedt BC. Effect of antacid on absorption of enteric-coated aspirin. JAMA 1974;227:660–661.
7. Gibaldi M, Grundhofer B, Levy G. Effect of antacids on pH of urine. Clin Pharmacol Ther 1974;16:520–525.
8. Hansten PD, Hayton WL. Effect of antacid and ascorbic acid on serum salicylate concentrations. J Clin Pharmacol 1980;20:326–331.
9. Powell JR, Donn KH. Histamine H_2-antagonist drug interactions in perspective: mechanistic concepts and clinical implications. Am J Med 1984;77:57–84.
10. Lauritsen K, Laursen LS, Rask-Madsen J. Clinical pharmacokinetics of drugs used in the treatment of gastrointestinal diseases. Clin Pharmacokinet 1990;19:11–31, 94–125.
11. Mitchard M, McIsaac RL, Bell JA. H_2-receptor antagonists. In: Damani LA, ed. Sulphur-containing drugs and related organic compounds: chemistry, biochemistry and toxicology, vol. 3, part A. Chichester: Ellis Horword, 1989:53–86.
12. Hansten PD, Horn JR. Drug Interactions and updates. Vancouver, WA: Applied Therapeutics and Lea & Febiger, 1993.
13. Somogyi A, Muirhead M. Pharmacokinetic interactions of cimetidine. Clin Pharmacokinet 1987;12:321–366.
14. Puff MR, Carey WD. The effect of cimetidine on cyclosporine A levels in liver transplant recipients. A preliminary report. Am J Gastroenterol 1992;87:287–291.
15. D'Souza MJ, Pollock SH, Solomon HM. Cyclosporine-cimetidine interaction. Drug Metab Disp 1988;16:57–59.
16. Primack WA. Cimetidine and renal allograft rejection. Lancet 1978;1:824–825.
17. Charpentier B, Fries D. Cimetidine and renal allograft rejection. Lancet 1978;1:1265.
18. Mitchard M, Harris A, Mullinger BM. Ranitidine drug interactions—a literature review. Pharmacol Ther 1987;32:293–325.

19. Klotz U, Kroemer HK. The drug interaction potential of ranitidine. an update. Pharmacol Ther 1991;50:233–244.

20. Somerville KW, Kitchingman GA, Langman MJS. Effect of famotidine on oxidative drug metabolism. Eur J Clin Pharmacol 1986;30:279–281.

21. Secor JW, Speeg KV, Meredith CG, Johnson RF, Snowdy P, Schenker S. Lack of effect of nizatidine on hepatic drug metabolism in man. Br J Clin Pharmacol 1985;20:710–713.

22. Kosoglou T, Vlasses PH. Drug interactions involving renal transport mechanisms: an overview. Drug Intell Clin Pharm 1989;23:116–122.

23. Somogyi A, McLean A, Heinzow B. Cimetidine-procainamide pharmacokinetic interaction in man: evidence of competition for tubular secretion of basic drugs. Eur J Clin Pharmacol 1983;25:339–345.

24. Rodvold KA, Paloucek FP, Jung D, et al. Interaction of steady-state procainamide with H_2-receptor antagonists cimetidine and ranitidine. Ther Drug Monit 1987;9:378–383.

25. Higbee MD, Wood JS, Mead RA. Procainamide-cimetidine interaction: a potential toxic interaction in the elderly. J Am Geriatr Soc 1984;32:162–164.

26. Bauer LA, Black D, Gensler A. Procainamide-cimetidine drug interaction in elderly male patients. J Am Geriatr Soc 1990;38:467–469.

27. Somogyi A, Bochner F. Dose- and concentration-dependent effect of ranitidine on procainamide disposition and renal clearance in man. Br J Clin Pharmacol 1984;18:175–181.

28. Rocci ML, Kosoglou T, Ferguson RK, Vlasses PH. Ranitidine-induced changes in the renal and hepatic clearances of procainamide are correlated. J Pharmacol Exp Ther 1989;248:923–928.

29. Klotz U, Arvela P, Rosenkranz B. Famotidine, a new H_2-receptor antagonist, does not affect hepatic elimination of diazepam or tubular secretion of procainamide. Eur J Clin Pharmacol 1985;28:671–675.

30. Muirhead MR, Somogyi AA, Rolan PE, Bochner F. Effect of cimetidine on renal and hepatic drug elimination: studies with triamterene. Clin Pharmacol Ther 1986;40:4000–4007.

31. Muirhead MR, Bochner F, Somogyi AA. Pharmacokinetic drug interactions between triamterene and ranitidine in humans: alterations in renal and hepatic clearances and gastrointestinal absorption. J Pharmacol Exp Ther 1988;244:734–739.

32. Dixon JS, Page MC. Interactions between non-steroidal anti-inflammatory drugs and H_2-receptor antagonists or prostaglandin analogues. Rheumatol Int 1991;11:13–18.

33. Dammann HG, Simon-Schultz J, Sallowsky E, Schmoldt A. The effects of misoprostol and of ranitidine on the pharmacokinetics of diclofenac. Gastroenterology 1992;102:A55.

34. Kendall MJ, Gibson R, Walt RP. Do ranitidine or misoprostol affect the systemic availability of indomethacin? Gastroenterology 1992;102:A96.

35. Rainsford KD. Effects of misoprostol on the pharmacokinetics of indomethacin in human volunteers. Clin Pharmacol Ther 1992;51:415–421.

36. Dixon JS, Lacey LF, Pickup ME, Langley SJ, Page MC. A lack of pharmacokinetic interaction between ranitidine and piroxicam. Eur J Clin Pharmacol 1990;39:583–586.

37. Feely J, Wood AJJ. Effects of cimetidine on the elimination and actions of ethanol. JAMA 1982;247:2819–2821.

38. Caballeria J, Baraona E, Rodamilans M, Lieber CS. Effects of cimetidine on gastric alcohol dehydrogenase activity and blood ethanol levels. Gastroenterology 1989;96:388–392.

39. Hernandez-Munoz R, Caballeria J, Baraona E, Uppal R, Greenstein R, Lieber CS. Human gastric alcohol dehydrogenase; Its inhibition by H_2-receptor antagonists, and its effect on the bioavailability of ethanol. Alcohol Clin Exp Res 1990;14:946–950.

40. Roine R, DiPadova C, Frezza M, Hernandez-Munoz R, Baraona E, Lieber CS. Effects of omeprazole, cimetidine and ranitidine on blood ethanol concentrations. Gastroenterology 1990;98:A114.

41. DiPadova C, Roine R, Frezza M, Gentry T, Baraona E, Lieber CS. Effects of ranitidine on blood alcohol levels after ethanol ingestion. Comparison with other H_2-receptor antagonists. JAMA 1992;267:83–86.

42. Holt S. Alcohol and H_2-receptor antagonists: over the counter, under the table? Am J Gastroenterol 1990;85:516–517.

43. Guram M, Howden CW, Holt S. Further evidence for an interaction between alcohol and certain H_2-receptor antagonists. Alcohol Clin Exp Res 1991;15:1084–1085.

44. Holtzman JL, Gebhard RL, Eckfeldt JH, et al. The effects of several weeks of ethanol consumption on ethanol kinetics in normal men and women. Clin Pharmacol Ther 1985;38:157–163.

45. Johnson KI, Fenzl E, Hein B. Influence of cimetidine on the elimination and effects of alcohol. Arzneimittelforschung 1984;34:734–736.

46. Norpoth T, Kneip M, Oehmichen M, et al. The effect of the administration of H_2-receptor blockers on alcohol kinetics and psychological fitness. Beitr Gerichtl Medizin 1986;44:1–4.

47. Jonsson K, Jones AW, Bostrom H, Andersson T. Lack of an effect of omeprazole, cimetidine, and ranitidine on the pharmacokinetics of ethanol in fasting male volunteers. Eur J Clin Pharmacol 1992;42:209–212.

48. Tanaka E, Nakamura K. Effects of H_2-receptor antagonists on ethanol metabolism in Japanese volunteers. Br J Clin Pharmacol 1988;26:96–99.

49. D'Ambrosi A, Greco A, Catellani A, Zangirolami A, Cinchini E, Alvisi V. The influence of therapy with oral cimetidine (C) and ranitidine (R) on ethanol metabolism. Proceedings of the Italian Society of

Gastroenterology, November 14–16; Milan, 1985:296.

50. Seitz HK, Bosche J, Czygan P, Veith S, Simon B, Kommerell B. Increased blood ethanol levels following cimetidine but not ranitidine. Lancet 1983;1:760.

51. de Pretis G, Piazzi L, Bonoldi MC, et al. Do H_2-antagonists influence the metabolism of ethanol in man. Presented at the VII Congress meeting, Italy, October, 1984:127.

52. Dobrilla G, de Pretis G, Piazzi L, et al. Is ethanol metabolism affected by oral administration of cimetidine and ranitidine at therapeutic doses? Hepatogastroenterol 1984;31:35–37.

53. Fraser AG, Sawyerr AM, Hudson M, Smith M, Rosalki S, Pounder RE. Ranitidine, cimetidine and famotidine have no effect on post-prandial high-dose (0.8 g/kg) alcohol absorption in healthy male volunteers. Gastroenterology 1992;102:A70.

54. Papke J, Borgmann VH, Dokert B, Bartels K, Krause D. Cimetidin und Ethanol Z Gesamt Inn Med 1989;44:731–733.

55. Webster LK, Jones DB, Smallwood RA. Influence of cimetidine and ranitidine on ethanol pharmacokinetics. Aust NZ J Med 1985;15:359–360.

56. Palmer RH, Rank WO, Nambi P, Wetherington JD, Fox MJ. Effects of various concomitant medications on gastric alcohol dehydrogenase and the first pass metabolism of ethanol. Am J Gastroenterol 1991;86:1749–1755.

57. Fraser AG, Prewett EJ, Hudson M, Sawyerr AM, Rosalki S, Pounder RE. Ranitidine has no effect on post-prandial absorption of alcohol (0.6 g/kg) after an evening meal. Eur J Gastroentol Hepatol 1992;4:43–47.

58. Toon S, Khan A, Langley S, Mullins F, Rowland M. Lack of effect of high dose ranitidine on the post-prandial absorption pharmacokinetics of alcohol. Gut 1992;33(Suppl):S10.

59. Kleine M, Ertl D. Comparative trial in volunteers to investigate ethanol (ETOH)-ranitidine (R) interactions. Gastroenterology 1992;102:A98.

60. Hindmarch I, Gilburt S. The lack of CNS effects of nizatidine with and without alcohol on psychomotor ability and cognitive function. Hum Psychopharmacol 1990;5:25–32.

61. Fraser AG, Prewett EJ, Hudson M, et al. The effect of ranitidine, cimetidine or famotidine on low-dose post-prandial alcohol absorption. Aliment Pharmacol Therap 1991;5:263–272.

62. Terpin MM, Frezza M, Buri L, et al. Antisecretive drugs and interactions of ethanol metabolism. Ital J Gastroenterol 1990;22:266.

63. Fraser AG, Sawyerr AM, Hudson M, Smith M, Rosalki S, Pounder RE. Ranitidine has no effect on post-breakfast ethanol absorption in male subjects. Am J Gastroenterol 1992;87:1268.

64. Raufman JP, Notar-Francesco V, Raffaniello R, Straus E. Histamine-H_2-receptor antagonists do not alter serum ethanol levels in fed, non-alcoholic men. Am J Gastroenterol 1992;87:1344.

65. Holtmann G, Knop G, Becker S, Singer MV. Does a single dose of famotidine influence the blood-alcohol level? Dtsch Med Wochenschr 1987;112:1619–1620.

66. Holtmann G, Singer MV. Histamine H_2-receptor antagonists and blood alcohol levels. Dig Dis Sci 1988;33:767–768.

67. Etienne M, Kremers P, Belaiche J. Influence of antisecretory drugs on gastric alcoholic dehydrogenase activity in man. Gastroenterology 1991;100:A521.

68. Tan OT, Stafford TJ, Sarkany I, Gaylarde PM, Tilsey C, Payne JP. Suppression of alcohol-induced flushing by a combination of H_1 and H_2 histamine antagonists. Br J Dermatol 1982;107:647–652.

69. Fiatarone JR, Bennett MK, Kelly P, James OFW. Ranitidine but not gastritis or female sex reduces the first-pass metabolism of ethanol. Gut 1991;32:A594.

70. Fraser AG, Hudson M, Sawyerr AM, Rosalki SB, Pounder RE. Short report: the effect of ranitidine on the post-prandial absorption of a low dose of alcohol. Ailment Pharmacol Therap 1992;6:267–271.

71. Sullivan JT, Sellers EM. Influence of cimetidine and ranitidine on ethanol pharmacokinetics. Aust NZ J Med 1986;16:414.

72. Smith T, DeMaster EG, Furne JK, Springfield J, Levitt MD. First-pass gastric mucosal metabolism of ethanol is negligible in the rat. J Clin Invest 1992;89:1801–1806.

73. Palmer RH. On: alcohol and H_2-receptor antagonists: over the counter under the table? [Letter]. Am J Gastroenterol 1991;86:112–113.

74. Fraser AG, Rosalki SB, Pounder RE. Effects of H_2-receptor antagonists on blood alcohol levels [Letter]. JAMA 1992;267:2469.

75. Hansten PD. Effects of H_2-receptor antagonists on blood alcohol levels [Letter]. JAMA 1992;267:2469–2470.

76. Palmer J, Powell JR, Euler A, McIsaac RL. Effects of H_2-receptor antagonists on blood alcohol levels [Letter]. JAMA 1992;267:2470.

77. Rowland M, Toon S. Effects of H_2-receptor antagonists on blood alcohol levels [Letter]. JAMA 1992;267:2470.

78. DiPadova C, Roine R, Gentry RT, Baraona E, Lieber CS. Effects of H_2-receptor antagonists on blood alcohol levels [Reply]. JAMA 1992;267:2470–2471.

79. Julkunen RJK, DiPadova C, Lieber CS. First-pass metabolism of ethanol—a gastrointestinal barrier against the systemic toxicity of ethanol. Life Sci 1985;37:567–573.

80. Julkunen RJK, Tannenbaum L, Baraona E, Lieber CS. First-pass metabolism of ethanol: an important determinant of blood levels after alcohol consumption. Alcohol 1985;2:437–441.

81. Caballeria J, Baraona E, Lieber CS. The contribution of the stomach to ethanol oxidation in the rat. Life Sci 1987;41:1021–1027.

82. Roine R, Hernandez-Munoz R, Baraona E, Greenstein R, Lieber CS. Effect of omeprazole on gastric first-pass metabolism of ethanol. Dig Dis Sci 1992;37:891–896.

83. Julia P, Farres J, Pares X. Characterization of three isoenzymes of rat alcohol dehydrogenase: tissue distribution and physical and enzymatic properties. Eur J Biochem 1987;162:179–189.

84. Levitt MD. Lack of clinical significance of the interaction between H_2-receptor antagonists and ethanol. Aliment Pharmacol Ther 1993;7:131–138.

85. Lewis JH, McIsaac RL. H_2-antagonists and blood alcohol levels. Dig Dis Sci 1993;38:569–572.

86. Sharma R, Gentry RT, Lim RT Jr, Lieber CS. First-pass metabolism of alcohol: absence of diurnal variation and its inhibition by cimetidine after an evening meal. Am J Gastroenterol 1992;87:1276.

86a. Anon. H_2-blocker interaction with alcohol is not clinically significant. FDC Reports "The Pink Sheet" March 22, 1993;55(12):10–11.

87. Guram MS, Howden CW, Holt S. Alcohol and drug interactions. Pract Gastroenterol 1992;16:47–54.

88. Roine R, Heikkonen E, Salapuro M. Cisapride enhances alcohol absorption and leads to high blood alcohol levels. Gastroenterology 1992;102:A507.

89. Roine R, Gentry T, Hernandez-Munoz R, Baraona E, Lieber CS. Aspirin increases blood alcohol concentrations in humans after ingestion of ethanol. JAMA 1990;264:2406–2408.

90. Edelbroek M, Horowitz M, Wishart J, Akkermans L. Erythromycin increases alcohol absorption by accelerating gastric emptying but slows small intestinal transit. Gastroenterology 1992;102:A924.

91. Andersson T. Omeprazole drug interaction studies. Clin Pharmacokinet 1991;21:195–212.

92. Gugler R, Jensen JC. Omeprazole inhibits oxidative drug metabolism: studies with diazepam and phenytoin in vivo and 7-ethoxycoumarin in vitro. Gastroenterology 1985;89:1235–1241.

93. Prichard PJ, Walt RP, Kitchingman GK, et al. Oral phenytoin pharmacokinetics during omeprazole therapy. Br J Clin Pharmacol 1987;24:543–545.

94. Andersson T, Andren K, Cederberg C, et al. Effect of omeprazole and cimetidine on plasma diazepam levels. Eur J Clin Pharmacol 1990;39:51–54.

95. Andersson T, Lagerstrom PO, Unge P. A study of the interaction between omeprazole and phenytoin in epileptic patients. Ther Drug Monit 1990;12:329–333.

96. Sutfin T, Balmer K, Bostrom H, Eriksson S, Hoglund P, Paulsen O. Stereoselective interaction of omeprazole with warfarin in healthy men. Ther Drug Monit 1989;11:176–184.

97. Soons PA, van den Berg G, Danhof M, et al. Influence of single-and multiple-dose omeprazole treatment on nifedipine pharmacokinetics and effects in healthy subjects. Eur J Clin Pharmacol 1992;42:319–324.

98. Schouler L, Dumas F, Couzigou P, Janvier G, Winnock S, Saric J. Omeprazole cyclosporine interaction. Am J Gastroenterol 1991;86:1047.

99. Oosterhuis B, Jonkman JHG, Andersson T, et al. Minor effect of multiple dose omeprazole on the pharmacokinetics of digoxin after a single oral dose. Br J Clin Pharmacol 1991;32:569–572.

100. Hajela R, Cunningham GM, Kapur B, et al. Catatonic reaction to omeprazole and disulfiram in a patient with alcohol dependence. Can Med Assoc J 1990;143:1207–1208.

101. Henry D, Brent P, Whyte I, Mihaly G, Devenish-Meares S. Propranolol steady-state pharmacokinetics are unaltered by omeprazole. Eur J Clin Pharmacokinet 1987;33:369–373.

102. Gugler R, Jensen JC. Drugs other than H_2-receptor antagonists as clinically important inhibitors of drug metabolism in vivo. Pharmacol Ther 1987;33:133–137.

103. Diaz D, Fabre I, Daujat M, et al. Omeprazole is an aryl-hydrocarbon-like inducer of human hepatic cytochrome P450. Gastroenterology 1990;99:737–747.

104. Farrell G. P450 IA2 and omeprazole. Gastroenterology 1992;102:1822–1823.

105. Lucier GW, Thompson CL, Hoel DG. Omeprazole, cytochrome P450, and chemical carcinogenesis. Gastroenterology 1992;102:1823–1824.

106. Parpia SH, Nix DE, Hejmanowski LG, Goldstein HR, Wilton JH, Schentag JJ. Sucralfate reduces the gastrointestinal absorption of norfloxacin. Antimicrob Agents Chemother 1989;33:99–102.

107. Van Slooten AD, Nix DE, Wilton JH, Love JH, Spivey JM, Goldstein HR. Combined use of ciprofloxacin and sucralfate. DICP Ann Pharmacotherapy 1991;25:578–582.

108. Braverman SE, Marino MT. Sucralfate-warfarin interaction [Letter]. Drug Intell Clin Pharm 1988;22:913.

109. Talbert RL, Dalmady-Israel C, Bussey HI, Crawford MH, Ludden TM. Effect of sucralfate on warfarin concentration in patients requiring chronic warfarin therapy [Abstract]. Drug Intell Clin Pharm 1985;19:456–457.

110. Neuvonen PJ, Jaakkola A, Totterman J, Penttila O. Clinically significant sucralfate-warfarin interaction is not likely. Br J Clin Pharmacol 1985;20:178–180.

111. Havrankova J, Lahaie R. Levothyroxine binding by sucralfate. Ann Intern Med 1992;117:445–446.

112. Albert KS, Welch RD, De Sante KA, DiSanto AR. Decreased tetracycline bioavailability caused by a bismuth subsalicylate antidiarrheal mixture. J Pharm Sci 1979;68:586–588.

113. Ericsson CD, Feldman S, Peckering LK, Cleary TG. Influence of subsalicylate bismuth on absorption of doxycycline. JAMA 1982;247:2266–2267.

114. Williams TW Jr, Yuk JH. Drug interaction with quinolone antibiotics in intensive care unit patients [Letter]. Arch Intern Med 1991;151:2485.

115. Pepto-Bismol. Physicians' desk reference for non-prescription drugs. Ed. 13. Montvale, NJ: Medical Economics Data, 1992:644.

116. Manninen V, Apajalahti A, Melin J, Karesoja M. Altered absorption of digoxin in patients given propantheline and metoclopramide. Lancet 1973;1:398–399.

117. Manninen V, Apajalahti A, Simonen H, Reissell P. Effect of propantheline and metoclopramide on absorption of digoxin [Letter]. Lancet 1973;1:1118–1119.

118. Johnson BF, Bustrack JA, Urbach DR, Hull JH. Effect of metoclopramide on digoxin absorption from tablets and capsules. Clin Pharmacol Ther 1984;36:724–730.

119. Yuen GJ, Hansten PD, Collins J. Effect of metoclopramide on the absorption of an oral sustained-release quinidine product. Clin Pharm 1987;6:722–725.

120. Kirch W, Janisch HD, Santos SR, Duhrsen U, Dylewicz P, Ohnhaus EE. Effect of cisapride and metoclopramide on digoxin bioavailability. Eur J Drug Metab Pharmacokinet 1986;11:249–250.

121. Kirch W, Janisch HD, Ohnhaus EE, van Peer A. Cisapride-cimetidine interaction: enhanced cisapride bioavailability and accelerated cimetidine absorption. Ther Drug Monit 1989;11:411–414.

122. Galmiche P. Combined therapy with cisapride and cimetidine in severe reflux oesophagitis: a double-blind controlled trial. Gut 1988;29:675.

123. Sorby DL, Liu G. Effects of adsorbents on drug absorption, II: effect of an antidiarrhea mixture on promazine absorption. J Pharm Sci 1966;55:504–510.

124. Moustafa MA, Al-shora HI, Gaber M, Gouda MW. Decreased bioavailability of quinidine sulphate due to interactions with adsorbent antacids and antidiarrheal mixtures. Int J Pharm 1987;34:207–211.

28

Drugs for Conscious Sedation for Gastrointestinal Endoscopy

GREGORY G. GINSBERG, CUONG C. NGUYEN, JAMES H. LEWIS,
DAVID E. FLEISCHER, FIRAS H. AL-KAWAS, and STANLEY B. BENJAMIN

Few would argue that the development of the flexible endoscope has had the single greatest impact on the practice of gastroenterology over the past two decades. The dramatic advances in endoscopy, however, have been closely tied to the incorporation of pharmacotherapeutic agents to allow safe and effective performance of a wide range of diagnostic and therapeutic procedures. Most patients undergoing endoscopy in westernized countries receive one or more premedications to facilitate the procedure (1, 2). It is critical that if we are to apply these medications in a wide variety of patients and circumstances, clinicians must have a thorough understanding of their pharmacology and use. This chapter will provide an overview of medications used in gastrointestinal endoscopy including topical anesthetics, agents for conscious sedation, and anticholinergics. Lastly, special situations such as paradoxical reactions, the "difficult to sedate patient," and reversal agents will be discussed.

CONSCIOUS SEDATION

Endoscopic conscious sedation refers to the altered level of consciousness frequently used to facilitate endoscopic procedures. Although mild to moderate sedation is produced, the patient is expected to independently and continuously maintain respiratory and airway control, respond to tactile stimulus, and co-operate with verbal commands. The goals of conscious sedation include relief of anxiety, improved patient tolerance to discomfort, and production of amnesia.

Deep sedation is a risk of conscious sedation, in which there is an increased level of sedation or hypnosis and partial or complete loss of the protective reflexes. In this setting, apparent ventilation, airway maintenance, and responsiveness are not reliable. The premeditated induction of deep sedation requires a physician other than the endoscopist (i.e., an anesthesiologist), committed to monitoring the patient's cardiopulmonary status. As a result, such deep sedation is not a required or desired level of consciousness for the performance of most endoscopic procedures.

Endoscopy is performed in a wide range of patients, from the otherwise quite healthy to those with multiple co-morbid diseases. Patient tolerance to endoscopy may vary considerably and may be effected by factors such as age, sex, and alcohol use (3). Additionally, body habitus, concomitant drug use, cigarette smoking, and personality may affect drug metabolism such that a dose that is insufficient in one patient may be excessive in another and vice versa (4). Therefore, a basic principle of conscious sedation is that its induction must be individualized.

Medication should be titrated to specific end-points that determine when a patient is appropriately sedated before beginning the procedure. These end-points help avoid over- or under-sedation. Observer end-points for endoscopic conscious sedation include visible relaxation, mild slurring of speech, glazed eyes, and tolerance to insertion of the endoscope.

Conscious sedation occurs along a spectrum. Some patients may appear fully awake and alert, whereas others may drift off to sleep, although they remain readily arousable and cooperative when stimulated. Mild slurring of speech is considered an appropriate end-point, however, marked slurring probably represents over-sedation.

The ideal drug or drug combination for endoscopic conscious sedation should have the following characteristics: provide rapid and reliable patient relaxation and cooperation; produce no local or systemic side effects; alleviate procedural discomfort; provide procedural amnesia; be short-acting with complete recovery of psychomotor function in time periods compatible with outpatient situations; and be inexpensive and easy to administer (5). In addition, its activity should not be affected by differences in patients sex, age, personality, concomitant diseases, or concomitant medications. The long list of agents that have been used to provide premedication for endoscopy is evidence that no single drug or drug combination satisfies all of these conditions. Benzodiazepines, opiate narcotics, neuroleptic hypnotics, and intravenous anesthetics, are all used to induce endoscopic conscious sedation.

INDICATIONS FOR ENDOSCOPIC PREMEDICATION

Most endoscopic procedures performed in the United States, Canada and in the United Kingdom use some form of local or systemic premedication (1, 2). The use of premedication, however, does not diminish the importance of adequate psychologic preparation (6, 7). A well-informed patient who understands the goals of the procedure and its performance techniques allows for the greatest cooperation, and may reduce or eliminate the need for premedication (8). Although endoscopy can,

in many instances, be carried out without the use of conscious sedation, most westernized patients believe or find endoscopic examinations and procedures to be uncomfortable and physically distressing. A patient's willingness to undergo repeated examinations often hinges on their previous endoscopic experiences. Many diagnostic and therapeutic endoscopic procedures would not be feasible without appropriate conscious sedation.

The benefits of avoiding conscious sedation are related to cost (based on a reduction of medication use and need for intravenous delivery systems), to a lessening of the intensity and duration of monitoring, and to a reduction in lost work hours as patients could resume normal activities (including driving an automobile) soon after completion of the procedure.

Serious cardiorespiratory events and deaths associated with endoscopic procedures are rare, occurring at the rates of 4.5 and 0.3/1000 procedures, respectively, in one recent large series (9). The relationship between the use of conscious sedation and complications or death is unclear. The main concern with the use of benzodiazepines, especially in combination with narcotics, is respiratory compromise leading to cardiac dysrhythmia (5). Conversely, the use of intravenous sedation may reduce cardiovascular stress during endoscopy as evidenced by a decreased incidence of arrhythmias (10, 11). The hopes that smaller diameter, more flexible endoscopes, might supplant the need for conscious sedation has not been borne out (11, 12).

Pound et al. (13) reported that patient tolerance was adequate or excellent in >90% of patients treated with topical Cetacaine alone undergoing esophagogastroduodenoscopy (EGD) with a 7.9-mm endoscope. The addition of oral diphenhydramine and acetaminophen elixir 30–60 minutes before the endoscopy improved patient tolerance slightly. However, 8.3% of patients required intravenous sedation to complete an adequate examination, and another 10% refused randomization, preferring to receive conscious sedation. Furthermore, this study excluded any complicated patients. Similarly, Ferrante et al. (14) found that 11% of screening endoscopies using a small diameter endoscope could not be completed without conscious sedation in patients who had received topical anesthesia and intramuscular atropine. Among patients who had previously undergone EGD with intravenous sedation, nearly one-half preferred sedation. In both studies, patients >60 years old tolerated endoscopy without sedation better than younger individuals.

Several reports in the literature, although not controlled trials, conclude that topical oropharyngeal anesthesia (TOPA) alone suffices as premedication for upper endoscopic procedures. Al-Atrakachi (15) reported no complications and a failure rate of only 0.2% during 2,000 EGDs performed in Iraq using only topical lidocaine spray and intramuscular atropine. Similarly, Boyacioglu et al. (16) reported a 0% failure rate using TOPA alone for 13,282 EGDs in Turkey. It is notable that these reports come from an area where the majority of upper endoscopies are normally performed without conscious sedation.

Conversely, Beavis et al. (17) evaluated 200 patients with a pediatric endoscope and the use of only topical pharyngeal anesthesia. The majority rated the experience as unpleasant or very unpleasant, with 11 examinations not completed because of patient intolerance. The majority of subjects (87%) preferred a barium upper gastrointestinal series over an upper endoscopy, and 6% said they would refuse a repeat examination. The authors concluded that such poor patient acceptance would greatly reduce patient willingness to undergo repeat examinations when necessary. In a prospective, controlled trial by Hoare and Hawkins (3), patients who received pharyngeal anesthesia only, compared to TOPA and intravenous diazepam, were more likely to find the procedure unpleasant, were worried about repeat examinations, or preferred a barium meal. Furthermore, failure to pass the instrument or to complete a thorough exam was significantly greater in patients receiving TOPA alone.

These studies strongly support the widely held opinion that the majority of patients in western society benefit from the use of parenteral conscious sedation in the performance of routine upper endoscopy, and that the routine use of TOPA as the only premedication for EGD is undesirable.

Few studies, surprisingly, have looked at the performance of colonoscopy without the use of premedication. Although flexible sigmoidoscopy rarely requires intravenous conscious sedation, the majority of physicians in the United States and the United Kingdom routinely administer intravenous conscious sedation for colonoscopy. However, two studies support the abandonment of routine use of conscious sedation for colonoscopy in favor of medication on demand for this procedure. Herman (18) performed colonoscopy in a prospective trial of 212 consecutive, nonselected patients, of whom 82% required no analgesia or sedation. Harrison and Sanowski (17), in a preliminary report, performed a comparative trial in which colonoscopy was begun on 104 veterans in whom one-third received standard premedication with meperidine and diazepam while the remaining two-thirds did not receive any premedication (but meperidine and diazepam were available on demand). Among those in the sedation-on-demand group, nearly one-half (48%) did not require any medication; the overall mean medication dose was lower, and there were fewer complications compared to the premedicated group. The authors, however, did not report the extent of the exams nor did they comment on the level of experience of the endoscopist. Interestingly, the patients' acceptance of the procedure did not differ between the groups. Although studies such as these suggest that initial routine sedation for colonoscopy may not be needed in all patients, we are of the opinion, that although conscious sedation is not always indispensable, pharmacologic premedication is desirable and should be offered to all patients undergoing endoscopic procedures to reduce both psychologic and cardiovascular stress and to enhance patient tolerance and compliance with subsequent exams (5).

TOPICAL PHARYNGEAL ANESTHESIA

Various local and topical anesthetics have been used to ease endoscope insertion, and improve patient tolerance for EGD. Agents used for TOPA include Astra spray (lidocaine 10%), Cetacaine spray (benzocaine 14%, butamben 2%, and tetracaine 2%), Hurricaine spray (benzocaine 20%), Pontocaine aqueous solution (tetracaine 2%), and viscous Xylocaine (lidocaine 10%). Clinical studies have demonstrated the superiority of a spray preparation over gargles (20) or lozenges (21).

Although topical anesthetics are generally thought to be safe, the potential for systemic absorption and toxicity exists. Patel et al. (22) described three cases of serious systemic toxicity including one death attributed to rapid absorption of tetracaine pharyngeal anesthesia. For tetracaine, which is readily absorbed, and other TOPA agents, systemic absorption is thought to be increased due to aspiration when gargling is encouraged. Lidocaine is readily absorbed from mucous membranes and excessive use can result in altered mental status, seizures, and cardiac dysrhythmias. The potential risk of acute methemoglobinemia has been reported with topical benzocaine and lidocaine (23). Otherwise, benzocaine is poorly soluble in water and, consequently too slowly absorbed to cause toxicity. True allergic reactions to TOPA agents are rare and often secondary to their paraben preservative (24). It has been suggested that anesthetizing the oropharynx may increase the risk of aspiration during and after the procedure (25).

As mentioned previously, in English-speaking countries, 85–90% of all upper gastrointestinal endoscopic procedures are performed using some form of intravenous conscious sedation (1, 2). Although the use of topical agents in addition to conscious sedation remains popular, their use has been questioned. Four double-blind controlled trials have been performed to evaluate this, with mixed results. Gordon et al. (26), in a double-blind trial,

showed the addition of a lidocaine gargle to parenterally administered meperidine, diazepam, and atropine improved patients' acceptance and physicians' assessment as to the ease of the procedure. However, Lachter et al. (27), in a double-blind, placebo-controlled trial, showed that the use of Cetacaine spray, in addition to parenteral diazepam did not reduce the amount of cough, gag, or degree of difficulty of intubation, except in the subgroup of patients being endoscoped for the first time, in whom the endoscope was passed more easily in those who received topical anesthesia. Chuah et al. (25), in a double-blind controlled trial, also found that in patients receiving intravenous midazolam for EGD, there was no added benefit when 15% lignocaine spray was compared to placebo. Finally, Canter and Baldridge (28) found no added benefit in using diluted viscous lidocaine gargle vs. placebo in patients undergoing EGD who were sedated with meperidine and diazepam.

Thus, in patients receiving adequate conscious sedation, and using modern endoscopes, the added benefit of topical oropharyngeal anesthetics remains controversial. Nonetheless, we routinely use TOPA, and in our large experience, it is both beneficial and without recognizable deleterious side effects. Benzocaine with its rapid onset, short duration of action, and virtually no systemic absorption, is our preferred agent. However, when upper endoscopy is performed for percutaneous endoscopic gastrostomy (PEG) placement or in the evaluation of acute upper gastrointestinal bleeding, we withhold TOPA to avoid any compromise of the gag reflex.

COMPLICATIONS OF CONSCIOUS SEDATION

Problems related to endoscopic conscious sedation include drug allergy, thrombophlebitis at the injection site, paradoxical reactions, and cardiopulmonary complications (Table 28.1). True hypersensitivity to benzodiazepines and opiates is unusual. However, individual patient intolerance is less uncommon, and often a drug substitution within

Table 28.1
Complications of Endoscopic Conscious Sedation

Oversedation
Overmedication
Hypotension
Cardiac arrhythmia
Respiratory insufficiency
Histamine liberation
Thrombophlebitis
Pain at injection site
Psychomimetic reactions

the same class is appropriate in such circumstances.

Thrombophlebitis

In patients receiving diazepam, which is poorly soluble in water, the incidence of thrombophlebitis is as high as 40% (29), and pain at the injection site as high as 78% (30). Diazemuls, a preparation of diazepam dissolved in soya bean oil and emulsified in water with monoglycerides and egg yolk phosphatides (available in Europe) has a reported lower incidence of thrombophlebitis (4–7%) (30). In contrast, midazolam, which is water soluble, has negligible local venous complications (31). The use of a running intravenous line likely further reduces the incidence of phlebitis from all medications (32).

Paradoxical Reactions

Paradoxical reactions denote those pharmacologic reactions of a drug that when administered within a therapeutic dosage range produce agitated excitement, mental confusion, and uncooperativeness. Patients tend to become more agitated—and even combative—as additional medication is given. The true incidence of paradoxical reactions, sometimes called idiosyncratic reactions, is unknown. The mechanism by which such reactions occur is not fully understood and identification of characteristics to identify patients at higher risk for paradoxical reactions is also lacking. However, it appears to occur more commonly, but not exclusively, in patients with a history of substance abuse.

Some authors (33) have postulated that benzodiazepine-mediated disinhibition causes increased aggressiveness when a patient has high levels of underlying anxiety. The relationship between underlying anxiety and vulnerability to disinhibition with benzodiazepines is still unclear (34). It is thought that disinhibition may be linked with long half-life benzodiazepines and is less frequent with short half-life compounds, however, paradoxical reactions are reported after midazolam (35).

Prompt recognition of a paradoxical reaction is important to avoid further medication and allow the undesirable effects to subside. However, it is even more important to distinguish an idiosyncratic (paradoxical) reaction from other causes of agitation during endoscopy, particularly the circumstance of inadequate analgesia during a painful procedure, and hypoxia. Other important concerns are avoiding injury to the patient, protecting the endoscopy assistant and the endoscopist from injury, and avoiding damage to equipment (e.g., from the biting the endoscope).

Management of a paradoxical reaction may require as little as waiting for the sedative effects of administered drugs to take full effect. Changing the class of drug used (i.e., a neuroleptic instead of a benzodiazepine) also may be beneficial. Flumazenil has been used to terminate a paradoxical reaction from midazolam (36). Finally, sedation with anesthesia support may be needed to provide deep sedation or general anaesthesia (37).

Cardiopulmonary Complications

Serious complications associated with diagnostic EGD have an incidence of 1 in 1,000 procedures, and mortality is estimated to be between 1 and 6 per 20,000 examinations (38). Although the total complication rate of EGD seems to have decreased by 40% over the past 15 years, this was accompanied by an apparently slight increase in cardiopulmonary complications and mortality (39).

Cardiorespiratory complications range from benign cardiac rhythm disturbances to pulmonary aspiration, respiratory depression

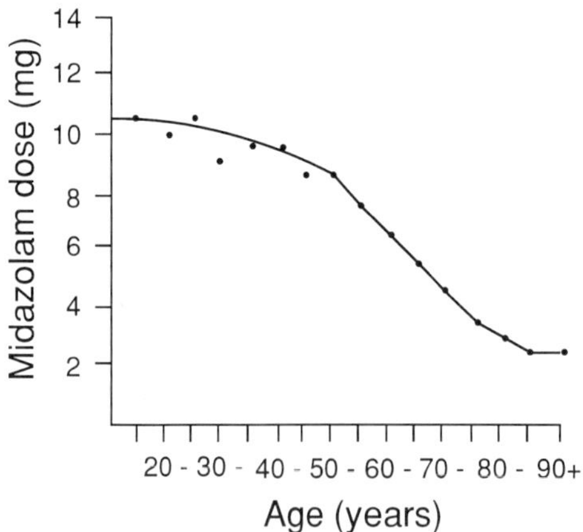

Figure 28.1. Dose of midazolam required to achieve conscious sedation in patients of increasing age. Reproduced with permission from Bell GD, Spickett GP, Reeve PA, Morden A, Logan RF. Br J Clin Pharmacol 1987;23:242.

with hypoxemia, apnea, hypotension, life-threatening dysrhythmias, myocardial ischemia and infarction, and death. The role of sedation in the development of cardiopulmonary complications is controversial (11, 40).

Both benzodiazepines and narcotics can cause respiratory depression. In therapeutic doses given intravenously, the benzodiazepines cause a central depression of respiration and blunt the ventilatory response to hypoxia and hypercapnia (41). Opioids produce a dose-dependent respiratory depression, the degree of which varies with the individual opioid (42). Oversedation can result in significant hypoventilation, hypercapnia, hypoxemia, and/or apnea. It is in this setting that cardiac arrhythmias and ischemia are more likely to occur (43).

Decreased oxygen saturation can be observed shortly after sedation, with a further fall to less than 90% during endoscopy (44). Oxygen desaturation may be accentuated in the elderly (45) and patients with chronic obstructive pulmonary disease (43). At the very least, patients with coronary artery disease should be monitored with pulse oximetry to identify early, critical falls in oxygen saturation to less than 90%. This value correlates

with a PaO_2 of less than 60 mm Hg. In this setting supplemental oxygen should be administered via nasal cannula to increase arterial oxygen tension (46).

Conversely, Lieberman et al. (10) demonstrated that the frequency of cardiac arrhythmias was significantly less in patients who received diazepam sedation vs. those who received no sedation. Others have also demonstrated that conscious sedation used during endoscopy reduces cardiovascular stress (11). True hypotension is not seen with benzodiazepines in doses used for endoscopic conscious sedation. In contrast, opiate narcotics and neuroleptics can cause hypotension, which may necessitate intravenous fluids, Trendelenburg positioning, termination of the procedure, use of naloxone (in the case of narcotics), and even pressor support to return the blood pressure to normal.

Endoscopists and endoscopy assistants should be familiar and facile with the basic and advanced elements of cardiopulmonary resuscitation. Ventilatory support equipment and reversal agents should be readily available. Judicious use of medications, supplemental oxygen, and cardiovascular monitoring will likely minimize the incidence and severity of cardiopulmonary complications.

TECHNIQUE OF ADMINISTERING CONSCIOUS SEDATION

The safety of endoscopy with conscious sedation will be improved by keeping the dosages of all drugs to the minimum amount allowing for patient comfort and successful performance of the procedure. It must be recognized that there is considerable variability in the pharmacokinetic and clinical drug response to various agents among patients. Particular attention to dosing limits is required for elderly patients and for those with coexisting medical illnesses. For midazolam, there is a direct inverse relationship between the age of the patient and the dose required to produce an adequate level of sedation (Fig. 28.1) (47).

Benzodiazepines should be administered slowly over 1–2 minutes, with the use of bolus

Table 28.2
American Society of Anesthesiology Physical Status Classification[a]

Class	Classification
1	A normal healthy patient
2	A patient with mild systemic disease
3	A patient with severe systemic disease that limits activity, but is not incapacitating
4	A patient with an incapacitating systemic disease that is a constant threat to life
5	A moribund patient not expected to survive 24 hours with or without an operation

[a]An "E" is added to the classification number if the scheduled procedure is an emergency.

injections to be avoided. Doses should not exceed the manufacturers' recommendations. It is equally as important to wait at least 2 minutes before giving additional doses, as the peak effect is generally apparent within 2–3 minutes for midazolam and diazepam. If additional sedation is required before the endoscopic procedure, we recommend titrating the dose by administering small increments until the proper level of sedation is reached. An additional 2 or more minutes after each incremental dose must be observed to fully evaluate the sedative effect. Delaying insertion of the endoscope 2–3 minutes after administration of sedation medication will attenuate the potential decrease in oxygen saturation (40).

Although commonly given together, the combination of a benzodiazepine and a narcotic analgesic can lead to an increased risk of adverse cardiorespiratory events (48). There is convincing evidence that the drug interaction between these two classes is synergistic and not simply additive (49). Even very small doses of a benzodiazepine and an opioid in combination may induce profound sedation and respiratory depression (50). The drugs should be administered separately, never mixed together in the same syringe, and at least 2 minutes should be allowed to pass between doses. In addition, the initial sedative dose of both drugs should be reduced. The opioid should be given first and the initial dose of the benzodiazepine should be reduced by approximately 30% (49).

Once an adequate level of sedation has been achieved, additional incremental doses may be titrated during the time it takes to complete the endoscopic procedure as needed to maintain proper sedation as well as to ensure a good analgesic and possibly amnestic effect. The use of a running intravenous line may, in addition to reducing the incidence of phlebitis, allow further dilution of the sedative medication, adding an even greater measure of safety.

MONITORING AND SUPPLEMENTAL OXYGENATION

For patients undergoing endoscopy with conscious sedation, monitoring refers to the clinical assessment of the patient during and after the procedure, including the measurement of various physiologic parameters, such as pulse, blood pressure, electrocardiographic rhythm, and oxygen saturation.

Adverse risk factors should be identified in the preprocedure interview. This will help to identify patients who might benefit from more intensive monitoring. Patients "at risk" for complications related to conscious sedation include: those classified as ASA grade III–V (Table 28.2); patients >60 years old; those with cardiac, cerebrovascular, pulmonary, hepatic, or renal disease; those with acute gastrointestinal bleeding, anemia, and morbid obesity (38).

Mere clinical observation for the early signs of respiratory depression and hypoxia has proven to be unreliable (2). The darkened room environment that is typical of most endoscopy suites makes this even more difficult. So, too, does patient positioning, which is often face down (as in endoscopic retrograde cholangiopancreatography [ERCP]) or away from the endoscopist (as in colonoscopy).

Continuous pulse oximetry, electrocardiogram, and blood pressure monitoring may improve the sensitivity of clinical monitoring of patients and may reduce the number of adverse cardiopulmonary events encountered during endoscopy (51, 51a, 51b). Although there is no direct controlled evidence that the routine use of monitoring equipment will reduce morbidity and mortality associated with gastrointestinal endoscopy, more intensive monitoring is certainly considered prudent in patients identified as being "at risk" (e.g., age >60, recent alcohol or drug withdrawal, patients undergoing ERCP, and any patient with a disease constituting an anesthesia risk [51b]).

In 1989 The American Society for Gastrointestinal Endoscopy (ASGE) developed guidelines for monitoring the risks associated with endoscopic conscious sedation. Fleischer (52) outlined several of these guidelines from the ASGE Standards of Practice Committee as follows: (a) A well trained gastrointestinal assistant is the most important part of the monitoring process; (b) the use of extracorporial equipment to monitor patients may be useful but is never a substitute for conscientious clinical assessment; (c) the amount of monitoring should be proportional to the perceived risk of the patient undergoing the procedure; (d) the minimal amount of clinical monitoring for all sedated patients should include heart rate, blood pressure, and respiratory rate before, during and after the procedure; (e) the proper role of continuous pulse oximetry, ECG, and blood pressure monitoring during endoscopy is controversial and remains unsettled; (f) the monitoring practice standards of free-standing office-based endoscopy units should not be different from those in hospital-based units.

Patient Recovery

Clinical monitoring must always be continued into the observation (recovery) period, and supplemental oxygen and noninvasive monitoring may be needed for occasional patients. Guidelines for evaluating residual effects and recovery from sedation before discharge are unsettled, and an accurate means to clinically assess post-anesthesia impairment and recovery to street fitness is lacking (53, 54). Considerable central nervous system depression may be present despite the patient appearing and feeling quite fully recovered. This has both practical and medicolegal ramifications. At the time of discharge, patients should be alert and communicative, able to take oral nourishment, and ambulate at their preprocedure level. Amnestic effects of midazolam and diazepam may extend beyond the normal recovery period. For this reason, written instructions should be provided to the patient to facilitate follow-up and therapy.

After the use of sedative drugs, it is recommended that patients not operate sophisticated machinery, drive a vehicle, or drink alcohol for up to 24 hours after the procedure. Outpatients should be accompanied (or driven) home by a responsible person. Inpatients should have orders written to continue frequent monitoring of vital signs, and verbal nurse-to-nurse contact should announce the patients arrival on the ward.

Supplemental Oxygen

Oxygen desaturation occurs frequently during upper endoscopy. The reasons are multifactorial and include compromise of the airway; aspiration; vagally mediated bronchospasm; as well as reduction in respiratory drive due to sedation (55). Other factors observed to influence oxygen desaturation include the level of experience of the endoscopist (56), the diameter of the endoscope used (10), and the presence of underlying pulmonary disease (40). The administration of supplemental oxygen before and during endoscopy has been shown to greatly diminish or prevent hypoxemia (40, 57). Supplemental oxygen via nasal cannula at 2–4 l/minute will not normally compromise respiratory function in patients with chronic obstructive airway disease. As previously discussed, it is recommended that supplemental oxygen be administered to patients undergoing endoscopic procedures who are considered to be at risk.

INDIVIDUAL DRUGS FOR CONSCIOUS SEDATION

Benzodiazepines

Benzodiazepines are the most commonly used medications for endoscopic conscious sedation (2, 9). Their broad acceptance is based on their anxiolytic, amnestic, sedative, and muscle relaxant properties. Among available benzodiazepines, diazepam (Valium) and midazolam (Versed) are the two agents most commonly used for conscious sedation for gastrointestinal endoscopic procedures (1, 58). They do, however, differ with regard to their potency and speed of onset of sedative effects as well as the quality of sedative effects, their amnestic response, their frequency of phlebitis and thrombophlebitis, and the time for recovery after conscious sedation.

Lorazepam (Ativan) has been evaluated for endoscopic premedication after both oral (58) and intravenous (59) administration. However, its delayed onset of effect (15–30 minutes), longer duration of action (12–24 hours), and unpredictable period of amnesia makes it a less desirable choice for short endoscopic procedures (60). Oral triazolam (Halcion), in one study, demonstrated only slight benefit over placebo for diagnostic upper endoscopy (61).

PHYSIOCHEMISTRY

Benzodiazepines are relatively small compounds and are lipid soluble at physiologic pH (Fig. 28.2). Midazolam is the most lipid soluble in vivo, but because of its pH dependent solubility, it is water soluble in a buffered acid medium (62). The high lipophilicity of diazepam and midazolam account for their rapid central nervous system effect and large volume of distribution. Midazolam's water solubility is responsible for its lower incidence of venous inflammation compared to diazepam.

METABOLISM AND CLEARANCE

Both diazepam and midazolam are metabolized in the liver by oxidation reduction. This pathway is susceptible to influences such as age, liver disease, obesity, and other drugs (63). Cimetidine inhibition of the oxidative enzyme function impairs diazepam clearance (64). Cigarette smoking increases the clearance of diazepam, but not midazolam (65). Chronic alcohol use increases the clearance of midazolam, and may translate into a higher dose required to provide sedation (66). In cirrhotics the half-life of diazepam is prolonged due to both decreased clearance and decreased plasma binding (66). Obese patients require larger doses for initial sedation owing to their greater volume of distribution (63).

Age reduces the clearance of diazepam significantly, and to a lesser degree that of midazolam. Therefore, benzodiazepines must be used cautiously in the elderly. Among 800 patients in whom midazolam was administered for endoscopic conscious sedation, the dose required for adequate sedation was markedly lower with age, with a 15% rate reduction per decade (67).

Either diazepam or midazolam is often given alone, but in many cases they are administered in combination with narcotic analgesics and atropine. They have additive effects with narcotics which allows one to reduce the dose of each medication. When diazepam or midazolam is used in combination with narcotics, the dose should be reduced significantly to avoid inducing respiratory depression as a consequence of their additive effects.

PHARMACOLOGY

Benzodiazepines exert their effect by binding to benzodiazepine receptors in the central nervous system that modulate γ-aminobutyric acid (GABA), the major inhibitory neurotransmitter in the brain. Binding is of very high affinity, stereospecific, and saturable. Midazolam has greater receptor affinity, and thus potency, than diazepam. The approximate relative potency is diazepam $(1\times)$ and midazolam $(3–4\times)$ (68).

It has been estimated that a benzodiazepine receptor occupancy of 20% is sufficient to produce anxiolysis, 30–50% for sedation, and unconsciousness occurs at 60% (65). According to Reves and Glass (65), an important aspect germane to the benzodiazepine receptor is that it can be occupied by two different kinds of ligands: agonists and antagonists (Fig. 28.3). Agonists (e.g., diazepam, midazolam) increase affinity for GABA leading to sedation. The antagonist (flumazenil) occupies the receptor but produces no activity and therefore blocks the actions of the agonists. The potency of the ligand is dependent on its af-

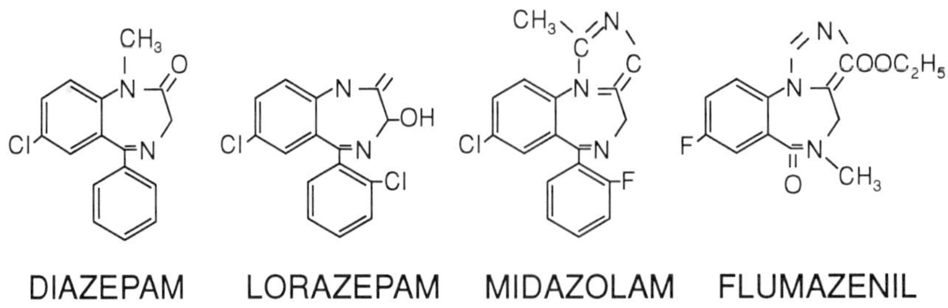

Figure 28.2. The structures of four benzodiazepines used in endoscopic conscious sedation.

finity for the benzodiazepine receptor and the duration of effect by the rate of clearance of the drug from the receptor.

DIAZEPAM

Diazepam has been the gold-standard to which all newer agents have been compared (69). Dating back to the early days of endoscopy, numerous studies have shown diazepam to facilitate examinations (47, 70). Diazepam may be given alone or in combination with a narcotic. After intravenous administration of diazepam the onset of action occurs in 1–5 minutes, the duration of action is 15 minutes–1 hour. The starting dose of diazepam is 0.10 mg/kg intravenously infused over a 2-minute period. The effect of a dose should be observed for 2–3 minutes before further medication is given. When additional medication is needed to initiate the procedure it should be titrated incrementally, using small doses (3–5 mg), administered over a 2-minute period and with ample time between successive doses to observe the full effect of the previously administered dose so as to avoid over medication.

Endoscopic studies show that diazepam is superior to topical oropharyngeal anaesthesia (3, 10), and has additive effects when combined with meperidine (71). Sedative effects are rated as high by patients and it produces partial or complete anterograde amnesia for the procedure in up to 73% of cases (72).

Two characteristics of diazepam may limit its use in endoscopic conscious sedation: resedation and venous irritation. Although initial plasma concentration falls rapidly because

of redistribution, drowsiness often returns with an increased concentration of diazepam in the plasma 6–8 hours later, the result of absorption from the gastrointestinal tract after excretion in the bile (73). Furthermore, diazepam metabolism forms active metabolites: desmethyldiazepam and oxazepam; the former achieving peak serum levels 10–15 hours postinjection with an elimination half-life of up to 200 hours. The incidence of thrombophlebitis is as high as 39% and pain at the injection site as high as 78% (30, 74).

Diazemuls is an oil emulsion formulation of diazepam with a reported decreased frequency of thrombophlebitis (30). However, in a prospective trial of diazemuls vs. diazepam for upper endoscopy, although the incidence of venous thrombosis was considerably less (3.6% vs. 25%, respectively), pain with injection occurred with the same frequency (75). It also produces significantly lower plasma levels than does diazepam (76).

MIDAZOLAM

Midazolam is a newer, relatively short-acting benzodiazepine that compares favorably with diazepam as premedication for endoscopy. It is approximately three to four times more potent than diazepam (67), with an onset of action that occurs 1–5 minutes after intravenous administration. The duration of action is usually less than 2 hours. Although midazolam has a more rapid onset of action compared to diazepam (77), recent studies have demonstrated that the peak drug effect occurs later for midazolam than for diazepam (78). After a single intravenous dose of either drug, maxi-

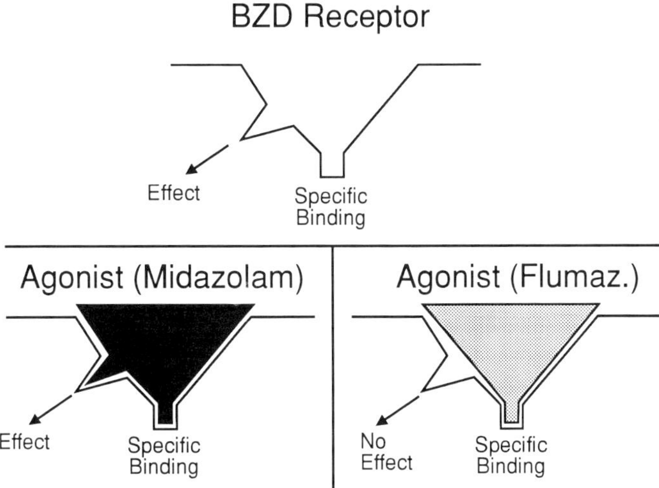

Figure 28.3. The benzodiazepine (*BZD*) receptor is an integral part of the GABA receptor complex. BZD agonists as well as antagonists bind specifically to the BZD receptor, but only BZD with agonistic properties are able to trigger an effect. Reproduced with permission from Amrein R, Hetzel W. Acta Anaesthesiol Scand 1990;34,S92:8.

mal central nervous system depression will be seen within 3–4 minutes. The risk of overmedication significantly increases if an inadequate period of time is allowed between multiple intravenous administrations. An increase in half-life has been demonstrated in the elderly and accounts for the enhanced sensitivity in that population (47, 63, 79).

After administration of equally potent doses of diazepam and midazolam, recovery time is consistently shorter for patients receiving midazolam, as demonstrated by psychomotor testing from (80). Plasma half-life of midazolam is 60–90 minutes with no active metabolites or intrahepatic circulation compared with an elimination half-life of up to 1 and 1.5 days for diazepam. The onset of amnesia occurs 2–5 minutes after midazolam administration and terminates 20 minutes after injection (81). Aside from the additive effects described when benzodiazepines are used in combination with a narcotic, no significant adverse drug interactions have been reported. Venous complications appear less frequently with midazolam than diazepam (82).

After the introduction of midazolam in 1986, an alarming number of cardiorespiratory complications, including some deaths

(potentially related to its use) were reported to the FDA (83). One-third of the complications occurred during endoscopic procedures. Investigation of this issue suggested the following situations contributed to undesirable outcomes: older age, combination with opioid, dose higher than manufacturer's recommendation, bolus injection, and lack of supplemental oxygen and monitoring.

An educational campaign was mounted that emphasized a titration method of administration, taking into account the patient's age, underlying cardiopulmonary status, and the concurrent use of other agents during endoscopy. These efforts led to a significant reduction in the frequency of reported cardiopulmonary events associated with midazolam (83). A recent American Society for Gastrointestinal Endoscopy/U.S. Food and Drug Administration study found no significant difference between the incidence of cardiopulmonary complications associated with the use of midazolam or diazepam. Concomitant use of a narcotic did, however, increase the risk (9).

The initial sedative dose of midazolam is 0.03 mg/kg. For otherwise healthy patients <60 years old, the rate of midazolam administration should be no more than 2.5 mg over

Table 28.3
Clinical Trials Comparing Midazolem and Diazepam for Endoscopic Conscious Sedation[a]

Author, year	Procedure	No. of patients	Mean dose (mg/kg)		Satisfaction		Amnesia	
			MDZ	DZP	Endoscopist	Patient	MDZ (%)	DZP (%)
Al-Khudhairi, 1982	EGD	100	0.10	0.15	NSD	NSD	92	54
Cole, 1983	EGD	40	0.12	0.20	NSD	NSD	51	38
Bergren, 1983[b]	EGD	60	0.05	0.15	NSD	MDZ[b]	60	7
Whitwam, 1983	EGD	100	0.07	0.15	NSD	NSD	74	44
Magni, 1983	EGD/ERCP	185	0.11	0.17	NSD	MDZ[d]	91	45
Bardham, 1984	EGD	149	10.3 mg	12.5 mg	NSD	MDZ[d]	96	73
Kawar, 1984	EGD	468	0.09	0.125	NSD			
Bianchi-Porro, 1988	EGD	23	0.07	0.15	NSD	MDZ[d]	91	39
Lee, 1988[b]	EGD	149	0.07	0.15	MDZ[e]	MDZ[d]	100	65
Brouilette, 1989[bd]	EGD/Col	60	0.09	0.14		MDZ[d]	63	23
Lewis, 1989[d]	Col	55	0.07	0.15	NSD	NSD	72	54
Ginsberg, 1992[d]	Col	53	0.06	0.17	NSD	NSD	55	32

[a]EGD, esophagotroduodenoscopy; ERCP, endoscopic retrograde cholangiopancreatography; MDZ, midazolam; DZP, diazepam; NSD, no significant difference.
[b]Diazemules.
[c]Patient who had previously undergone endoscopy preferred midazolam.
[d]In combination with meperidine.
[e]Preferred.

a 2-minute period. Some patients may respond to doses as small as 1 mg initially. In patients $\geq$60 years old or those with liver impairment, the titrated initial dose of midazolam should be no more than 1.5 mg initially given over at least 2 minutes. Age and poor liver function alter the pharmacokinetics of the drug. Such patients often require no more than 1.5 mg as an initial dose with many responding to as little as 0.5 mg. Similarly, in patients who are more prone to adverse outcomes in the setting of hypoxemia (i.e., those with pulmonary, cardiovascular, or cerebrovascular disease), the incremental dose of midazolam should be lowered. As with diazepam, and all drugs administered for endoscopic conscious sedation, an adequate time interval must be observed to assess the full sedative effect of the drug before administering additional doses.

Midazolam vs. Diazepam

In 12 trials comparing the use of midazolam vs. diazepam for endoscopic procedures (EGD, colonoscopy, and ERCP) the quality of the sedative effect of both drugs is similar (Table 28.3) (32, 67, 84–93). Physicians' assessment of the quality of endoscopic procedure demonstrated a preference for midazolam in one study by Lee et al. (91). Although patient evaluations were comparable in most studies, Berggen et al. (86) found that midazolam was favored by patients without prior EGD experience. Similarly, in the remaining studies that addressed patient acceptance, midazolam was also favored. However, there was no significant difference in recovery times. Amnesia for the procedure ranged from 51–96% with midazolam vs. 23–73% with diazepam. In all but one study (93) the difference in recall of the procedure or of discomfort was statistically significant. In two studies a significantly greater number of patients who received midazolam would agree to a repeat procedure if indicated (91, 92).

Narcotics

Narcotic analgesics provide pain relief, sedation, and euphoria. Two recent reports evaluating sedation practices of a subgroup of United States endoscopists revealed that meperidine (Demerol) was used in 76% and 87% of endoscopic procedures, fentanyl (Sublimaze) was used in 8.4%, other drugs mentioned were butomorphone (Stadol) and nalbuphine (Nubain) (1, 9). In the United

Kingdom only 13% of survey respondents used a narcotic, (meperidine) (2). In almost all cases narcotics are used in combination with a benzodiazepine for endoscopic conscious sedation. The great advantage of opioid narcotics is that their effects can be reversed with the opioid antagonist naloxone.

The narcotic analgesics, or opioids, behave similarly with respect to their physiochemistry, metabolism, and pharmacology. Aside from differences in their potency and duration of effect, other differences are based on preferential affinity for opioid receptors in different locations in the central and peripheral nervous systems. Analgesia is induced by μ-agonist opioids binding to μ-receptors in the central nervous system, which results in the inhibition of various nociceptive reflexes. The sedative effects are thought to be the result of interactions with GABA-ergic neurons. Meperidine is 0.1 times the potency of morphine; fentanyl is estimated to be 80 times as potent.

Peak analgesia occurs within 20 minutes of intravenous morphine administration, but may be sooner with the more lipid-soluble opioids. Metabolism takes place principally in the liver by conjugation with glucuronic acid. Seven to 10% of morphine is excreted via bile in the feces. The majority of elimination is via renal excretion of conjugated metabolites and a small amount of unchanged drug. The half-life of morphine is 2 hours; 90% of total excretion occurs within 24 hours.

Unwanted effects of opioids include respiratory depression, nausea, vomiting, mental clouding, increased pressure in the biliary tract, constipation, urinary retention, and hypotension. Liver disease will considerably increase the bioavailability of the drug. Renal impairment does not affect limited use for endoscopic sedation. Allergic reactions are uncommon and venous irritation is negligible. Respiratory depressant and hypotensive effects may be exaggerated and prolonged by phenothiazines, monoamine oxidase inhibitors, and tricyclic antidepressants, and the use of concomitant narcotics should be avoided. Although half-life and clearance are unaf-

fected by older age, an increased sensitivity among the elderly is observed with meperidine and other opioids (94).

Opioids produce a dose-dependent respiratory depression, the degree of which varies with the individual agent (95). Respiratory depression affects all phases of respiratory activity (rate, minute volume, and tidal volume), at least in part, by virtue of a direct effect on the brainstem respiratory centers (96). Maximal respiratory depression occurs 5–10 minutes after intravenous administration of morphine, but may affect respiration for up to 5 hours. These effects will be seen more rapidly with more lipid-soluble agents. Importantly, respiratory depression can occur with doses of narcotic too small to produce evidence of sedation. Opioids can also cause a delayed respiratory depression when the patient is in the recovery area postprocedure, and is no longer being stimulated (95).

Cardiovascular effects are due primarily to peripheral vasodilation and reduced peripheral resistance. This may result in hypotension with change in position or in patients with intravascular volume depletion. Vagally mediated bradycardia has been observed with all the opioids except meperidine (97).

MEPERIDINE

Meperidine is the most frequently used narcotic for endoscopic conscious sedation. Although it was shown to be superior to placebo in one study (98), it is most commonly used in combination with a benzodiazepine. Boldy et al. (99) noted that adding meperidine to diazepam for upper endoscopy significantly improved patient cooperation and caused a more profound sedation. In the reverse fashion, Castiglioni et al. (71) compared the addition of diazepam to intramuscular meperidine given 1 hour preprocedure and found the combination superior to meperidine alone. Chokhavatia et al. (100) compared meperidine to fentanyl, sufentanyl, and alfentanyl, in combination with midazolam, for endoscopic conscious sedation. Sedation and analgesia were comparable for upper endoscopy; however, meperadine was judged better than the other opioids with respect to patient comfort and amnesia during colonoscopy.

Although meperidine may offer greater efficacy and tolerability, and although many therapeutic endoscopic procedures could not be performed without a narcotic, its use is not without potential hazard. Arrowsmith et al. (9) reported that 94% of cardiopulmonary events reported in their sample were associated with administration of a narcotic or narcotic analog, whereas only 65% of the overall study population received a narcotic. Similarly, Daneshmend et al. (2) noted that adverse outcomes were reported more frequently by respondents who used other intravenous sedation, usually meperidine, in addition to a benzodiazepine.

Other narcotics have been evaluated in comparison with diazepam. Morphine was found to be inferior (101) whereas hydromorphone was found to be superior (102). One study showed phenoperidine to be superior to diazepam for upper endoscopy (103). In a double-blind randomized trial of meperidine versus butorphanol, in addition to diazepam, no considerable differences were observed (104).

FENTANYL

Fentanyl (sublimaze), is a more potent, shorter duration, synthetic opioid that may offer some advantages over meperidine for endoscopic conscious sedation (105). The onset of action is almost immediate with peak effect observed in minutes and a duration of 30–60 minutes. Doses of less than 200 μg produce analgesia, mild euphoria, and drowsiness. Although respiratory depression may exist beyond sedation, it is less than that of meperidine, and most of the drug is eliminated in 6 hours (106).

Fentanyl, when titrated to achieve its sedative effect in a controlled trial of upper endoscopy, improved patient tolerance and attenuated physiologic markers of endoscopy-induced cardiovascular stress (105). There was no difference in arterial oxygen saturation with routine continuous administration of oxygen at 2 ml/min via nasal cannula. In a study

comparing fentanyl to diazepam, the level of sedation, complications, and patient acceptance were similar. However, fentanyl was preferred by endoscopists and allowed for shorter recovery times (107). When fentanyl (0.05 mg) was compared to meperidine (50 mg) in combination with atropine 0.5 mg and diazepam 10 mg and to atropine and diazepam alone, there was significant depression of the arterial oxygen tension (PaO_2) immediately after premedication that included a narcotic, but not with diazepam alone (108). A significant reduction in the PaO_2 persisted in both narcotic groups if a standard diameter endoscope was used, but only in the meperidine group if a narrow diameter endoscope was used. The diameter of the endoscopes used was not provided.

Combining Narcotics and Benzodiazepines for Conscious Sedation

The theoretical advantage of using a narcotic in combination with a benzodiazepine is that the availability of naloxone allows for the reversal of at least one of the agents used for sedation. This concept is made more appealing because when a narcotic and benzodiazepine are used in combination, the dose of both can be lowered by 30–50% because of their additive sedative effects. Thus, less benzodiazepine would be on board should oversedation occur. The major risk is the additive respiratory depression possible when these drugs are used concurrently. Bailey et al. (109) have pointed out that "combining midazolam with fentanyl or other opioids produces a potent drug interaction that places patients at a high risk for hypoxemia and apnea." They recommend adequate precautions, including monitoring with pulse oximetry, and the administration of supplemental oxygen when these drugs are used in combination. Special consideration should be given to patients with increased age, obesity, COPD, sleep apnea, and liver disease; these require the dose of the narcotic to be decreased and the rate of administration also decreased. The narcotic should be given first, administered slowly over a 2-minute period. Time to achieve peak effect must be observed before adding the benzodiazepine with up to a fourfold reduction in total dosage (38).

For meperidine, a starting dose of 0.15–0.4 mg/kg is administered slowly. Additional dosing is titrated incrementally to obtain the desired level of sedation. We generally administer meperidine 10 mg, to be followed by midazolam 1.0 mg, each administered separately over 2 minutes, with 2–3 minutes between drugs.

Droperidol

Droperidol (Inapsine) is a potent neuroleptic of the butyrophone class. Its central nervous system depression is marked by apparent tranquility, disassociation with the surroundings, decreased motor activity, reduced anxiety, and mild sedation (65). Patients remain sensitive to pain and responsive to verbal commands, and there is no significant amnestic effect. When combined with a narcotic, the state of psychomotor sedation and analgesia is termed neuroleptanalgesia.

Droperidol produces its action centrally at sites where dopamine, serotonin, and norepinephrine act, possibly occupying the GABA receptors on the postsynaptic membrane. Similar action at the chemoreceptor trigger zone is responsible for its potent antiemetic effect.

The onset of action is within 3–10 minutes and duration of action from 3–6 hours. The short elimination half-life of 2 hours is at odds with the observance of residual effects for up to 12 hours, prompting some to postulate that droperidol has a propensity for central nervous system receptors. Metabolism occurs in the liver by hepatic microsomal enzymes.

Droperidol has little effect on the respiratory system. The predominant cardiovascular effect is vasodilation with hypotension, the result of moderate α-adrenergic blockade. Renal blood flow is not significantly altered, and there is little or no effect on myocardial contractility or conduction.

The experience with droperidol for use in endoscopic conscious sedation is limited. The first report on its use was by Le Brun (110), who used a combination of intramuscular and intravenous droperidol and fentanyl, along with intravenous diazepam. Although he reported positive results, significant hypotension (fall in systolic blood pressure >30 mm Hg) occurred in 25% of patients. Two comparative studies found the combination of droperidol with fentanyl (Innovar) provided better sedation than diazepam with a cholinergic (111, 112). More recently, Wilcox et al. (113) reported their retrospective experience with droperidol as an adjunct to conscious sedation with meperidine or meperidine and a benzodiazepine. They targeted a population of patients in whom standard sedation was inadequate or had resulted in paradoxic agitation, those with chronic alcohol and drug abuse, alcohol withdrawal, and young, anxious patients. The level of sedation was adequate in all but 2% of 1102 procedures. ERCP made up 15% (167) of their cases. Complications occurred infrequently (1.5%) consisting mostly of hypotension that responded to normal saline infusion and/or naloxone. Recovery time was not prolonged.

We have had similar positive experience with droperidol. The standard dose is 1.25 mg which is administered over a 2-minute period. Additional dosages can be administered not to exceed 5 mg. As the onset of action is 3–10 minutes, an adequate time interval must be observed between doses. Use of naloxone only reverses the narcotic-induced component of hypotension but does not counter that of droperidol. The emergence of droperidol as an adjunct to benzodiazepine and narcotic endoscopic premedication for the difficult to sedate group of patients is encouraging. The induction of neuroleptanalgesia should be accompanied by an increase in the intensity of monitoring in proportion to the risk of adverse outcome.

Propofol

Propofol (Diprivan) is an intravenous anesthetic recently approved for use in conscious sedation. Its current FDA approval requires the presence of an anesthesiologist for administration, monitoring, and airway management. The pharmacologic advantage of propofol is its ability to be rapidly titrated to the desired level of central nervous system depression and rapid "clear-headed" emergence. Propofol's rapid recovery is owed to its extremely high hepatic clearance. It is a short acting, potent hypnotic and mildly analgesic drug that is administered as a continuous infusion for maintenance of anesthesia (114). At subhypnotic doses propofol will provide sedation, amnesia, and a state of well being (115).

Several studies have evaluated the use of propofol sedation as a single agent by continuous infusion for endoscopic procedures with generally positive results (114, 116). Patterson et al. (117) evaluated single bolus injection of propofol and compared it to a single injection of midazolam for upper endoscopy. Although propofol provided more rapid recovery compared to midazolam, it was associated with pain on injection, a short amnesia span, and reduced patient acceptance. Church et al. (118) described the use of a computer-controlled infusion system designed to calculate and deliver a predicted target blood concentration of propofol during colonoscopy. They believe that with increased experience with such a system, an endoscopist might be able to control sedation with propofol.

Propofol, in the hands of an anesthesiologist, is capable of providing sedation for endoscopic procedures, with rapid recovery to "street-readiness." Its use should currently be reserved for situations when standard techniques for inducing conscious sedation are not available or are inadequate.

Barbiturates

Barbiturates, such as pentobarbital, secobarbital, and the shorter-acting, thiopental, provide good hypnotic effects and lack the nausea and vomiting that may occur with narcotics. However, the long duration of action and slow elimination half-life makes these agents poor choices for endoscopic premedication in adults. In addition, a lack of coordination and sleepiness persist for many hours after the procedure. Their use is generally confined to pediatric endoscopy.

ANTISECRETORY/ANTISPASMODIC DRUGS

Anticholinergic agents, such as atropine, are used as premedication by some endoscopists to reduce secretions and prevent vagal response during the procedure (2, 119). In most endoscopy suites, atropine is administered on an as needed basis for its vagolytic effects where bradycardia and hypotension result from the pain of visceral traction, as may occur during colonoscopy. In the past, anticholinergics were used to minimize secretions induced by irritating anesthetics that were used as premedications.

As an anticholinergic, atropine competes with acetylcholine at the cholinergic receptor sites, blocking parasympathetic impulses. These receptors are located throughout the body and thus atropine produces many different effects. Atropine can be given either as an intramuscular injection or intravenously before the procedure to reduce secretions and prevent vasovagal responses. Providing it is given at the recommended dose, atropine is not contraindicated in patients with glaucoma.

Although atropine decreases oral secretions and slows gastrointestinal motility; double-blind, randomized controlled trials have not demonstrated improvement in physician or in patient acceptance when atropine is added for upper endoscopy (120, 121). Similarly, Waxman et al. (122) failed to demonstrate a significant benefit when atropine was added routinely for colonoscopy. Furthermore, atropine has failed to effect the frequency of cardiac arrhythmias during endoscopy (123).

However, atropine is useful in treating sinus bradycardia accompanied by hemodynamic compromise, i.e., hypotension, signs of peripheral hypoperfusion such as confusion, or frequent ventricular ectopic beats. When bradycardia occurs during EGD or colonoscopy, efforts should be made to reduce the vagal tone by decompressing distended intestinal lumina, decreasing visceral traction, and reducing excessive looping. When bradycardia persists and results in hypotension, 0.4–0.6 mg of atropine should be administered intravenously. A dose of ≤0.3 mg may cause further sinus node slowing. A dose of ≥0.8 mg may produce sinus tachycardia with resultant myocardial ischemia and arrhythmia. The dose may be repeated every 5 minutes to a total of 2.0 mg (124).

Studies evaluating dicyclomine hydrochloride (Bentyl) (125), and glucagon (126) to facilitate colonoscopy failed to demonstrate a benefit from either drug in the opinion of the patients and the endoscopists. We occasionally use glucagon on an as-needed basis during ERCP to reduce duodenal motility and facilitate bile duct cannulation, or when removing gastric polyps via snare polypectomy to avoid peristaltic contractions carrying the polyp through the pylorus. Glucagon may be used on an as-needed basis to reduce spasm during colonoscopy. The dose of glucagon we use for these purposes is 0.2–0.5 mg.

Steiger et al. (127) concluded there was no advantage to using hyocine butylbromide (Buscopan) over placebo for routine upper endoscopy. However, their findings are contradicted in studies by Parente et al. (128) and Lazzaroni et al. (129) in which ease of examination was improved by cimetropil bromidum for upper endoscopy and timepidum bromide for duodenoscopy. The evolution of smaller caliber endoscopes and safe, effective medication for conscious sedation likely eliminates the need for routine use of antisecretory and antispasmodic medications.

REVERSAL AGENTS

The development of agents to reverse the effects of conscious sedation offers a major advantage to endoscopic practice. Naloxone has been available since the 1970s and reverses the effects of narcotic induced sedation. Efforts to extend its use to the benzodiazepines however, were unsuccessful (68). Before the development of flumazenil, there was an active search to identify available drugs that might reverse the sedative effects of benzodiazepines. Aminophylline and physostigmine were two such agents, however, neither convinc-ingly demonstrated efficacy for this purpose (68).

Naloxone

Naloxone (Narcan), an oxymorphone, is a pure opioid antagonist. It blocks narcotic effects by competitive inhibition at the μ-opioid receptors. In the absence of narcotics, naloxone in moderate doses has no discernable effects or side effects. The plasma half-life is 60–90 minutes; metabolism is by the liver (130).

Because of naloxone's short half-life, renarcotization is a risk when used to reverse long-acting opioids. Patients must be monitored closely for resedation (131).

Used clinically as a narcotic antagonist, naloxone completely reverses narcotic-induced ventilatory depression and sedation. As all opioid effects are reversed in parallel, pain and discomfort are suddenly unmasked as well. This may result in a sympathetic discharge leading to significant cardiovascular stimulation that may be detrimental to the patient. Hypertension, atrial and ventricular dysrhythmias, pulmonary edema, and cardiac arrest have been reported (132). Patients with underlying cardiac disease are at increased risk. However, there are cases of unexpected, sudden death in healthy patients receiving routine reversal of opiate anesthesia with naloxone (personal communication).

In some endoscopy centers naloxone is given routinely after an endoscopic procedure in which narcotic sedation was employed. Keefe and O'Connor (1) reported that 15% of survey respondents routinely, and 30% occasionally, reversed narcotics. Arrowsmith et al. (9) noted an increased use of naloxone among procedures with cardiopulmonary complications (48%) as compared with an entire study population (12%), in their evaluation of complication rates and drug use during endoscopy. It was inferred that the use of naloxone in this group was in response to concern about oversedation, rather than attributing the complication to naloxone.

Naloxone should be readily available wherever patients are receiving or recovering from endoscopic conscious sedation employing a narcotic agent. The starting dose is 1–2 mg intravenously for the reversal of narcotic induced respiratory depression or hypotension. This dose may be repeated at 2 to 3-minute intervals, up to 10 mg.

Vigilant clinical monitoring for early recognition and response to hypoventilation (stimulation, supplemental oxygen) and judicious use of narcotic analgesics, particularly in the elderly or debilitated, when used in combination with another drug, will minimize the need for naloxone use. Prolonged observation should be used to monitor for resedation after the use of naloxone to reverse medication-induced respiratory depression or hypotension.

Flumazenil

Flumazenil (Romazicon), an imidazobenzodiazepine, is a high affinity benzodiazepine antagonist that blocks the central effect of benzodiazepines by competitive inhibition at the receptor site (133). It reverses benzodiazepine-induced sedation, impairment of recall, and psychomotor dysfunction (134). However, it does not reverse sedation induced by narcotics, neuroleptics, or propofol.

It is relatively fast acting, attaining peak cerebral levels in 5–8 minutes, and is rapidly cleared by the liver. Antagonism is dependent on both the dose of flumazenil and the benzodiazepine. With large doses of a benzodiazepine, reversal may be only partial. Flumazenil's rapid elimination half-life of 40–80 minutes, while closer to that of midazolam than diazepam, is significantly shorter than that for both agents it is reversing; thus the potential for resedation exists (135).

Although flumazenil is very effective in reversing benzodiazepine CNS sedation, benzodiazepine-induced ventilatory depression is not consistently reversed. Gross et al. (136), found that although flumazenil reversed the sedative effects of midazolam, and the previously reduced tidal volume was increased, the decrease in the slope of the CO_2 curve was not increased. A study by Mora et al. (137) found that flumazenil only partially and variably reversed diazepam-induced respiratory depression. Similarly, Carter et al. (138) found that

although flumazenil clearly reversed the sedative effects of midazolam after upper endoscopy, the ventilatory effects were largely unaffected. Weinbrum and Geller (139) demonstrated that arterial oxygen saturation was improved after flumazenil reversal in patients sedated with a benzodiazepine alone, but not when a narcotic was added to sedation. Therefore, airway management and continued observation are essential after flumazenil reversal.

The drug is generally well tolerated with a "clear-headed emergence" from sedation (134). Side effects reported include pain at the injection site, dizziness, headache, blurred vision, nausea, vomiting, and agitation. Flumazenil may cause seizures in patients with multidrug overdose or a history of prior seizures. It may also cause withdrawal symptoms in patients with chronic benzodiazepine or alcohol abuse. Unlike naloxone, it is remarkably free of cardiovascular effects (134).

For reversal of the effects of benzodiazepine sedation, the initial dose is flumazenil 0.2 mg intravenously over a 15-second period. If the desired level of sedation is not observed in 45 seconds, an additional 0.2-mg dose can be given in the same manner and repeated every 60 seconds until the desired level of wakefulness is observed or until a total of 1 mg has been administered. If resedation occurs, dosing may be repeated at 20-minute intervals.

Several European studies have evaluated the use of flumazenil as an adjunct to endoscopic conscious sedation with similar results. All studies included tests of psychomotor function. In studies evaluating flumazenil vs. placebo, reversal of midazolam sedation was promptly seen within 5 minutes of flumazenil administration. Amnesia for the procedure was maintained but did not extend into the period after flumazenil administration, and no resedation was observed (140–143).

Three studies evaluated flumazenil reversal of midazolam and diazepam after upper endoscopy. Jensen et al. (144) and similarly, Birkenfeld et al. (145) reported a significant reduction in sedation in both groups without significant intergroup differences, and no resedation at 3 hours postprocedure. In contrast, in the study by Sanders et al. (146) in which psychometric assessment of four aspects of recovery over a 3-hour period showed attenuation, recovery from sedation was not complete. Baseline performance in accuracy of motor coordination, and cortical arousal were not reached after 3 hours in both groups. Patients in the diazepam group displayed persistent memory deficits after flumazenil administration.

U.S. studies to evaluate the use of flumazenil to improve memory of instructions given postprocedure, and to hasten the safe discharge of patients after endoscopic procedures are underway. The concept of administering flumazenil after endoscopic conscious sedation using a short-acting benzodiazepine, such as midazolam, is appealing, as it might allow the patient to spend the early part of recovery in a chair, rather than remaining supine on a stretcher, and may permit safe earlier discharge from the endoscopy area, with reductions in endoscopy unit costs and patient inconvenience.

Flumazenil is an essential emergency drug that should be readily available when bezodiazepine sedation is used. Its availability, however, is not an excuse for the administration of excessive doses of benzodiazepines (147). The routine use of flumazenil after outpatient endoscopy to facilitate earlier discharge is still being evaluated.

SUMMARY

It is possible to select and administer sedative and analgesic drugs that can produce a reliable level of sedation in most patients, to facilitate safe and effective gastrointestinal endoscopy. The availability of specific antagonists to both benzodiazepines and narcotics affords an additional level of safety. The emergence of neuroleptanalgesia for the difficult to sedate patient is welcomed, but requires further evaluation. Deep sedation provided by an anesthesiologist should be considered when standard conscious sedation measures fail.

An incremental titration technique of drug administration, with ample time between successive doses, and a dose reduction for elderly or debilitated patients and when medications are used in combination, will reduce the risks of oversedation, overmedication, and cardiopulmonary complications. Monitoring and the provision of supplemental oxygen should be individualized as dictated by the patients' needs.

REFERENCES

1. Keefe EB, O'Connor KW. 1989 A.S.G.E. survey of endoscopic sedation and monitoring practices. Gastrointest Endosc 1990;36:S13–S22.
2. Daneshmend TK, Bell GD, Logan RFA. Sedation for upper gastrointestinal endoscopy: results of a nationwide survey. Gut 1991;32:12.
3. Hoare AM, Hawkins CF. Upper gastrointestinal endoscopy with and without sedation: patient's opinions. Br Med J 1976;2:20.
4. Giles HG, MacLeod SM, Wright JR, Sellers EM. Influence of age and previous use on diazepam dosage required for endoscopy. Can Med Assoc J 1978;118:513.
5. Bianchi-Porro G, Lazzaroni M. Premedication for upper gastrointestinal endoscopy: still a matter for debate? Endoscopy 1991;23:32.
6. Shipley RH, Butt JH, Farbry JE, Horwitz B. Psychological preparation for endoscopy. Physiological and behavioral changes in patients with differing coping styles for stress. Gastrointest Endosc 1977;24:9.
7. Johnson JE, Morrissey JF, Levanthal H. Psychological preparation for an endoscopic examination. Gastrointest Endosc 1973;19:180.
8. Nelis GF. Preparation for endoscopy. Lancet 1980;2:861–862.
9. Arrowsmith JB, Gerstman BB, Fleischer DF, Benjamin SB. Results from the American Society for Gastrointestinal Endoscopy/U.S. Food and Drug Administration collaborative study on complication rates and drug use during gastrointestinal endoscopy. Gastrointest Endosc 1991;37:421–427.
10. Lieberman DA, Wuerker CK, Katon RM. Cardiopulmonary risk of esophagogastroduodenoscopy: role of endoscope diameter and systemic sedation. Gastroenterology 1985;88:468–472.
11. Sturges WF, Krone CL. Cardiovascular stress of peroral gastrointestinal endoscopy. Gastrointest Endosc 1973;19:119–122.
12. Thompson DG, Evans SJ, Murray RS, Leonnard-Jones JE, Cowen RE, Wright JT. Patients appreciate premedication for endoscopy. Lancet 1980;2:469–470.
13. Pound DC, et al. Oral medications for upper gastrointestinal endoscopy using a small diameter endoscope. Gastrointest Endosc 1988;34:327.

14. Ferrante WA, Balart LA, Burns TW, et al. Diagnostic screening endoscopy: an alternative to the barium meal [Abstract]. Gastrointest Endosc 1986;32:A143.

15. Al-Atrakchi HA. Upper gastrointestinal endoscopy without sedation: a prospective study of 2000 examinations. Gastrointest Endosc 1989;35:79–81.

16. Boyacioglu S, Ates B, Hilmioglu F. Upper gastrointestinal endoscopy without sedation [Letter]. Gastrointest Endosc 1989;35:581.

17. Beavis AK, LaBrooy S, Misiewicz JJ. Evaluation of one-visit endoscopic clinic for patients with dyspepsia. Br Med J 1979;1:1389.

18. Herman FN. Avoidance of sedation during total colonoscopy. Dis Colon Rectum 1990;33:70–72.

19. Harrison ME, Sanowski RA. Medication on demand during colonoscopy: a method to limit sedation and reduce complications. Gastrointest Endosc 1992;38:A227.

20. Smith JL, Opekun A, Graham DY. Controlled comparison of topical anesthetic agents in flexible upper gastrointestinal endoscopy. Gastrointest Endosc 1985;31:255–258.

21. Heuberger S, Weber KB, Sonnenberg A, et al. Topical anesthesia in preendoscopic medication: spray versus lozenges. Endoscopy 1979;2:131–132.

22. Patel D, Chopra S, Berman MD. Serious systemic toxicity resulting from use of tetracaine for pharyngeal anesthesia in upper endoscopic procedures. Dig Dis Sci 1989;34:882–824.

23. O'Donohue WJ, Moss LM, Angelillo VA. Acute methemoglobinemia induced by topical benzocaine and lidocaine. Arch Intern Med 1980;140:1508–1509.

24. Johnson WT, Destigter T. Hypersensitivity to pontacaine, tetracaine mepivacaine and methylparaben: a report of a case. JADA 1983;106:53–57.

25. Chuah SY, Crowson CP, Dronfield MW. Topical anaesthesia in upper gastrointestinal endoscopy. Br Med J 1991;303:695.

26. Gorden MJ, Mayes GR, Meyer GW. Topical lidocaine in preendoscopic medication. Gastroenterology 1976;71:564–569.

27. Lachter J, et al. Topical pharyngeal anesthesia for easing endoscopy: a double-blind, randomized, placebo-controlled study. Gastrointest Endosc 1990;36:19.

28. Canter DS, Baldridge ET. Premedication with meperidine and diazepam for upper gastrointestinal endoscopy precludes the need for topical anesthesia. Gastrointest Endosc 1986;32:339–341.

29. Kawar P, Dundee JW. Frequency of pain on injection and venous sequelae following the intravenous administration of certain anaesthetics and sedatives. Br J Anaesth 1982;542:935–939.

30. Olesen AS, Huttel MS. Local reactions to i.v. diazepam in three different formulations. Br J Anaesth 1980;52:609–610.

31. Fragen RJ, Gahl F, Caldwell N. A water-soluble benzodiazepine, RO 21-3981, for induction of anesthesia. Anesthesiology 1978;49:41–43.

32. Ginsberg GG, Lewis JH, Gallagher JE, et al. Diazepam versus midazolam for colonoscopy: a prospective evaluation of predicted versus actual dosing requirements. Gastrointest Endosc 1992;38:651–656.

33. Gardos C, Dimasco A, Salzman D, et al. Differential actions of chlordiazepoxide and oxazepam on hostility. Arch Gen Psychiatry 1968;18:757–760.

34. Binder RL. Three case reports of behavioral disinhibition with clonazepine. General Hospital Psychiatry, 1987;9:151–153.

35. Knaack-Steinegger R, Schou J. Therapy of paradoxical reactions to midazolam during regional anesthesia. Anaesthetist 1987;36:143–146.

36. Rodrigo CR. Flumazenil reverses paradoxical reaction with midazolam. Anesth Prog 1991;38:65–68.

37. Fleischer DE, Kidwell JA, Al-Kawas FH, Benjamin SB, Lewis JH, Nguyen CC. Sedation with anesthesiology support is appropriate for patients with mental retardation undergoing endoscopy. Gastrointest Endosc 1992;38:A282.

38. Bell GD, McCloy RF, Charlton JE, et al. Recommendations for standards of sedation and patient monitoring during gastrointestinal endoscopy. Gut 1991;32:823–827.

39. Hart R, Classen M. Complications of diagnostic gastrointestinal endoscopy. Endoscopy 1990;22:229–233.

40. Rimmer KP, Graham K, Whitelaw WA, Field SK. Mechanisms of hypoxemia during panendoscopy. J Clin Gastroenterol, 1989;11:17–22.

41. Alexander CM, Gross JB. Sedative doses of midazolam depress hypoxic ventilatory responses in humans. Anesth Analg 1988;67:377–382.

42. Philip BK. Opioids in outpatient anesthesia. Anesthesiol Rev 1991;18(S1):4–8.

43. Rostykus PS, McDonald GB, Albert RK. Upper intestinal endoscopy induces hypoxemia in patients with obstructive pulmonary disease. Gastroenterology 1980;78:488–491.

44. Bell GD, Reeve PA, Moshiri M, et al. Intravenous midazolam: a stud of the degree of oxygen desaturation occurring during upper gastrointestinal endoscopy. Br J Clin Pharmacol 1987;23:703–708.

45. Dhariwal A, Plevris JN, Lo NTC, Finlayson NDC, Heading RC, Hayes PC. Age-, anemia-, and obesity-associated oxygen desaturation during upper gastrointestinal endoscopy. Gastrointest Endosc 1992;38:684–688.

46. Bell GD, Morden A, Bown S, Coady T. Prevention of hypoxemia during upper gastrointestinal endoscopy by means of oxygen via nasal cannulae. Lancet 1987;1:1022.

47. Bell GD, Spickett GP, Reeve PA, Morden A, Logan RFA. Intravenous midazolam for upper gastrointestinal endoscopy: a study of 800 consecutive cases

relating dose to age and sex of patient. Br J Clin Pharmacol 1987;23:241–243.

48. Murray AW, Morran CG, Kenny GNC, Anderson JR. Arterial oxygen saturation during upper gastrointestinal endoscopy: the effects of midazolam/pethidine combination. Gut 1990;31:270–273.

49. Ben-Shlomo I, Abd-El-Khalim H, Ezry J, Zohar S, Tverskoy M. Midazolam acts synergistically with fentanyl for induction of anesthesia. Br J Anaesth 1990;64:45–57.

50. Lauven PM. Pharmacology of drugs for conscious sedation. Scand J Gastroenterol 1990;25(S179):1–6.

51. Cousins MJ. Monitoring—the anaesthetist's view. Scand J Gastroenterol 1990;25(S179):12–17.

51a. Fleischer DE, Al-Kawas F, Benjamin SB, Lewis JH, Kidwell J. Prospective evaluation of complications in an endoscopy unit. Gastrointest Endosc 1992; 38:414–424.

51b. Iber FL, Sutberry M, Gupta R, Kruss D. Evaluation of complications during and after conscious sedation for endoscopy using pulse oximetry. Gastrointest Endosc 1993;39:620–625.

52. Fleischer DE. Monitoring the patient receiving conscious sedation for gastrointestinal endoscopy: issues and guidelines. Gastrointest Endosc 1989; 35:262–266.

53. Drummond GB. The assessment of post-operative mental function. Br J Anaesth 1975;47:130–142.

54. Herbert M. Assessment of performance in studies of anesthetic agents. Br J Anaesth 1978;50:33–38.

55. Rimmer KP, Grahm K, Whitelaw WA, Field SK. Mechanisms of hypoxemia during panendoscopy. J Clin Gastroenterol 1989;11:17–22.

56. Lavis NG, Creasy MB, Harris K, Hanning CD. Arterial oxygen saturation during upper gastrointestinal endoscopy: influence of sedation and operator experience. Am J Gastroenterol 1988;83:618–622.

57. Griffin SM, Chung SCS, Leung JWC, Li AKC. Effect of intranasal oxygen in hypoxia and tachycardia during endoscopic cholangiopancreatography. Br Med J 1990;300:83–84.

58. Bader E, Lauttre G, Moshal MG, Baker LW. A trial of oral lorazepam as premedication for digestive endoscopy. S Afr Med J 1973;47:1361–1364.

59. Ramirez-Acosta J, Whizar-Lugo V, Cruz-Lozano C, Elizondo-Rivera J. A comparison of intravenous lorazepam and diazepam as endoscopic premedications. Gastrointest Endosc 1977;24:80–81.

60. George KA, Dundee JW. Relative amnestic actions of diazepam, flunitrazepam, and lorazepam in man. Br J Clin Pharmacol 1977;4:45.

61. Hedenbro JL, Ekelund M, Aberg T, Lindblom A. Oral sedation for diagnostic upper endoscopy. Endoscopy 1991;23:8–10.

62. Greenblatt DJ, Shader RI, Abernathy DR. Current status of benzodiazepines (first of two parts). N Engl J Med 1983;309:354–358.

63. Greenblat DJ, Abernathy DR. Midazolam pharmacology and pharmacokinetics. Anesthes Rev 1985;12(S3):17–20.

64. Locniskar A, Greenblat DJ, Harmatz JS, Zinny MA, Shader RI. Interaction of diazepam with famotidine and cimetidine, two H_2-receptor antagonists. J Clin Pharmacol 1986;26:299–303.

65. Reves JG, Glass PSA. Nonbarbituate intravenous anesthetics. In: Miller RD, ed. Anesthesia. New York: Churchill Livingstone, 1990:243–279.

66. Klotz U, Avant GR, Hoyumpa A, Schencker S, Wilkinson GR. The effects of age and liver disease on the disposition and elimination of diazepam in adult man. J Clin Invest 1975;55:347–359.

67. Bell GD, Spickett GP, Reeve PA, Morden A, Logan RF. Intravenous midazolam for upper gastrointestinal endoscopy, a study of 800 consecutive cases relating dose to age and sex of patient. Br J Clin Pharmacol 1987;23:241–243.

68. Whitwam JG, Al-Khudhairi D, McCloy RF. Comparison of midazolam and diazepam in doses of comparable potency during endoscopy. Br J Anesth 1983;55:773–777.

69. Ross WA. Premedication for upper gastrointestinal endoscopy. Gastrointest Endosc 1989;35:120–126.

70. Ticktin HE, Trujillo NP. Further experience with diazepam for preendoscopic medication. Gastrointest Endosc 1968;15:91–92.

71. Castiglioni LJ, Allen TS, Patterson M. Intravenous diazepam: an improvement in pre-endoscopic medication. Gastrointest Endosc 1973;19:134–136.

72. Bell GD. Premedication and intravenous sedation for upper gastrointestinal endoscopy [Review article]. Aliment Pharmacol Ther 1990;4:103–122.

73. Marshall BE, Longnecker DE. General anesthetics. In: Goodman Gilman A, eds. The pharmacological basis of therapeutics. New York: Pergamon Press 1990:304.

74. Hegarty J, Dundee JW. Sequelae after intravenous injection of three benzodiazepines—diazepam, lorazepam, and flunitrazepam. Br Med J 1977;2:1384–1385.

75. Gleeson D, Rose JDR, Smith PM. A prospective randomized controlled trial of diazepam vs. emulsified diazepam as a premedication for upper gastrointestinal endoscopy. Br J Clin Pharmacol 1983;16:448–450.

76. Fee JPH, Dundee JW, Collier PS, McClean E. Bioavailability of intravenous diazepam. Lancet 1984;2:813.

77. Reves JG, Fagen RF, Vinick HR. Midazolam: pharmacology and uses. Anesthesiology 1985;62:310–324.

78. Buhrer M, Maitre PO, Crevoisier C, Stanski DR. Electroencephalographic effects of benzodiazepines, II: pharmacodynamic modeling of the electroencephalographic effects of midazolam and diazepam. Clin Pharmacol Ther 1990;48:555–567.

79. Warning reemphasized in midazolam labeling. FDA Drug Bulletin 1987;17:5.

80. White PF. The role of midazolam in outpatient anesthesia. Anesth Rev 1985;12:55–60.

81. Dundee JW, Wilson DB. Amnestic action of midazolam. Anaesthesia 1980;35:456–461.

82. Galletly DC, Wilson LF, Treuren BC, Boon BP. Diazepam mixed micelle-comparison with diazepam in propylene glycol and midazolam. Anaesth Intensive Care Med 1985;13:352–354.

83. Lewis JH, Benjamin SB. Safety of midazolam and diazepam for conscious sedation. J Clin Gastroenterol 1990;12:716–717.

84. Al-Khudhairi D, McCloy RF, Whitwam JG. Comparison of midazolam and diazepam in sedation for gastroscopy. Gut 1982;23:A432.

85. Cole SG, Brozinsky S, Isenberg JI. Midazolam, a new more potent benzodiazepine, compare with diazepam: a randomized, double-blind study of preendoscopic sedatives. Gastrointest Endosc 1983; 29:219–222.

86. Berggen L, Eriksson I, Mollenholt P, Wickbom G. Sedation for fiberoptic gastroscopy: a comparative study of midazolam and diazepam. Br J Anaesth 1983;55:289–296.

87. Magni VC, Frost RA, Leung JWC, Cotton PB. A randomized comparison of midazolam and diazepam for sedation in upper gastrointestinal endoscopy. Br J Anaesth 1983;55:1095–1101.

88. Bardhan KD, Morris P, Taylor PC, Hinchliffe RFC. Intravenous sedation for upper gastrointestinal endoscopy: diazepam versus midazolam. Br Med J 1984;288:1046.

89. Kawar P, Porter KG, Hunter EK, McLaughlin J, Dundee JW, Brophy TO'R. Midazolam for upper gastrointestinal endoscopy. Ann R Coll Surg Engl 1984;66:283–285.

90. Bianchi-Porro G, Baroni S, Parente F, Lazzaroni M. Midazolam versus diazepam as premedication for upper gastrointestinal endoscopy: a randomized, double-blind, crossover study. Gastrointest Endosc 1988;34:252–254.

91. Lee MG, Hanna W, Harding H. Sedation for upper gastrointestinal endoscopy: a comparative study of midazolam and diazepam. Gastrointest Endosc 1989;35:82–84.

92. Brouillette DE, Leventhal R, Kumar S, et al. Midazolam versus diazepam for combined esophagogastroduodenoscopy and colonoscopy. Dig Dis Sci 1989;34:1265–1271.

93. Lewis BS, Shlien RD, Waye JD, Knight RJ, Aldoroty RA. Diazepam versus midazolam in outpatient colonoscopy: a double-blind randomized study. Gastrointest Endosc 1989;35:33–36.

94. Herman RJ, McAllister CB, Branch RA, Wilkinson GR. Effects of age on meperidine disposition. Clin Pharmacol Ther 1985;37:19–23.

95. Kallar SK. Conscious sedation in ambulatory surgery. Anesth Rev 1991;18(S1):9–12.

96. Jaffe JH, Martin WR. Opioid analgesics and antagonists. In: Goodman, Gilman A, ed. The pharmacological basis of therapeutics. New York: Pergamon Press, 1990:485–521.

97. Philip BK. Opioids in outpatient anesthesia. Anesth Rev 1991;18:4–8.

98. Dunn GD, Kubin RH, Laing RR, Sisk CW, Klotz AP. Double-blind study of endoscopic premedication. Gastrointest Endosc 1970;16:229–30.

99. Boldy DAR, English JSC, Lang GS, Hoare AM. Sedation for endoscopy: a comparison between diazepam and diazepam plus pethidine with naloxone reversal. Br J Anaesth 1984;56:1109–1112.

100. Chokavatia S, Nguyen L, Williams R, Kao J, Heavner JE. Sedation and analgesia for gastrointestinal endoscopy. Am J Gastroenterol 1993;88:393–396.

101. Ludlam R, Bennett JR, Comparison of diazepam and morphine as premedication for gastrointestinal endoscopy. Lancet 1971;2:1397–1399.

102. Peterson H, Myren J. Premedication for peroral endoscopy. Scand J Gastroenterol 1972;7:583–587.

103. Stephens MJ, Jakobovits AW, Dudley FJ. A controlled trial of phenoperidine and diazepam in gastrointestinal endoscopy. Gastrointest Endosc 1979; 25:127–129.

104. Bacon BR, Marshall JB, A randomized, prospective, double-blind clinical trial comparing butorphanol and meperidine in patients undergoing upper gastrointestinal endoscopy. Clin Anesth 1986;4:S67–S75.

105. Ishido S, Kinoshita Y, Kitajima N, et al. Fentanyl for sedation during upper gastrointestinal endoscopy. Gastrointest Endosc 1992;38:689–692.

106. Downes JJ, Kemp RA, Lamberstein CJ. The magnitude and duration of respiratory depression due to fentanyl and meperidine in man. J Pharmacol Exp Ther 1967;158:416.

107. Stephens MJ, Gibson PR, Jakobovits AW, Metz GL, Dudley FJ. Fentanyl and diazepam in endoscopy of the upper gastrointestinal tract. Med J Aust 1982;1:419–420.

108. Rozen P, Firman Z, Gilat T. The causes of hypoxemia in the elderly patient during endoscopy. Gastrointest Endosc 1982;28:243–246.

109. Bailey PL, Pace NL, Ashburn MA, Moll JW, East KA, Stanley TH. Frequent hypoxemia and apnea after sedation with midazolam and fentanyl. Anesthesiology 1990;73:826–830.

110. LeBrun HI. Neuroleptanalgesia in upper alimentary endoscopy. Gut 1976;17:655–658.

111. Rubin J, Bryer JV, Brock-Utne JG, Moshal MG. The use of neuroleptanalgesia for gastrointestinal endoscopy. S Afr Med J 1977;52:835–837.

112. Moshal MG, Rubin J, Greenberg MJ, Spitaels JM, Bryer JVO, White E. Variable premedication for upper gastrointestinal endoscopy. Am J Gastroenterol 1979;71:158–163.

113. Wilcox CM, Forsmark CE, Cello JP. Utility of droperidol for conscious sedation in gastrointestinal endoscopic procedures. Gastrointest Endosc 1990; 36:112–115.

114. Gepts E, Claeys MA, Camu F, Smekens L. Infusion of propofol as sedative technique for colonoscopies. Postgrad Med J 1985;61(S3):120–126.

115. Mackenzie N, Grant IS. Propofol for intravenous sedation. Anaesthesia 1987;42:3–6.

116. Dubois A, Balatoni E, Peters JP, Baudoux M. Use of propofol for sedation during gastrointestinal endoscopies. Anaesthesia 1988;43:S75–S80.

117. Patterson KW, Casey PB, Murray JP, O'Boyle CA, Cunningham AJ. Propofol sedation for outpatient upper gastrointestinal endoscopy: comparison with midazolam. Br J Anaesth 1991;67:108–111.

118. Church JA, Stanton PD, Kenny GNC, Anderson JR. Propofol for sedation during endoscopy: assessment of a computer-controlled infusion system. Gastrointest Endosc 1991;37:175–179.

119. Hedenbro JL, Frederickson SG, Lindblom A. Anticholinergic medication in diagnostic endoscopy of the upper intestinal tract. Endoscopy 1991;23:199–202.

120. Cook PJ, Bennett PN, Leonard-Jones JE, Warens TW. Premedication for endoscopy: a trial of atropine, pentazocine or pethidine as a supplement to diazepam. Scand J Gastroenterol 1978;13:33–39.

121. Cattau EL, Artnak CB, Castell DO, Meyer GW. Efficacy of atropine as an endoscopic premedication. Gastrointest Endosc 1983;29:285–288.

122. Waxman I, Mathews J, Gallagher J, et al. Limited benefit of atropine as premedication for colonoscopy. Gastrointest Endosc 1991;37:329–331.

123. Mccloy RM, Chiti CC. EKG changes during fiberoptic upper GI endoscopy and colonoscopy. Gastrointest Endosc 1976;22:231.

124. Morris DC, Walter PF, Hurst JW. The recognition and treatment of myocardial infarctions and its complications. In: Hurst JW, ed. The Heart, Arteries and Veins. ed. 7. New York: McGraw-Hill, 1990;53C:1062.

125. Bond JH, Chally CH, Blackwood WD. A controlled trial of premedication with dicyclomine hydrochloride (Bentyl) in colonoscopy. Gastrointest Endosc 1974;21:61.

126. Norfleet RG, Premedication for colonoscopy: randomized double-blind study of glucagon vs. placebo. Gastrointest Endosc 1978;24:164–165.

127. Steger AC, Galland RB, Murray JK, et al. The use of Hyocine in upper gastrointestinal tract endoscopy. Am J Gastroenterol 1986;81:615.

128. Parente F, Lazzaroni M, Imbimbo B, et al. The use of cimetropil bromidum as premedication for endoscopy of the upper gastrointestinal tract. a double-blind controlled trial. J Intern Med Res 1985;13:332.

129. Lazzaronni M, Parente F, Mailland F, et al. Timepidium bromide as premedication before duodenoscopy. Curr Ther Res 1985;37:277.

130. Ngai SH, Berkowitz BA, Yang JC, et al. Pharmacokinetics of naloxone in rats and in man. Anesthesiology 1976;44:398.

131. Longnecker DE, Grazis PA, Eggers GNN. Naloxone for antagonism of morphine-induced respiratory depression. Anesth Analg 1973;52:447.

132. Smith G, Pinnock C. Naloxone-paradox or panacea? Br J Anaesth 1985;57:547.

133. Nutt DJ, Cowen PJ, Little HJ. Unusual interactions of benzodiazepine receptor antagonists. Nature 1982;295:436–438.

134. Amrein R, Hetzel W. Pharmacology of Dormicum (midazolam) and Anexate (flumazenil). Act Anaesthesiol Scand 1990;34(S92):6–15.

135. Knudsen L, Lonka L, Sorensen BH, Kirkegaard L, Jensen OV, Jensen S. Benzodiazepine intoxication, treated with Anaexate. Anaesthesia 1988;43:274–276.

136. Gross JB, Weller RS, Conrad P. Flumazenil antagonism of midazolam-induced ventilatory depression. Anesthesiology 1991;75:179–185.

137. Mora CT, Torjman M, White PF. Effects of diazepam and flumazenil on sedation and ventilatory response. Anesth Analg 1989;68:473–478.

138. Carter AS, Bell GD, Coady T, Lee J, Morden A. Speed of reversal of midazolam-induced respiratory depression by flumazenil—a study in patients undergoing upper G.I. endoscopy. Acta Anaesthesiol Scand 1990;34(S92):59–64.

139. Weinbrum A, Geller E. The respiratory effects of reversing midazolam sedation with flumazenil in the presence or absence of narcotics. Acta Anaesth Scand 1990;92:65–69.

140. Pearson RC, McCloy RF, Morris P, Bardhan KD. Midazolam and flumazenil in gastroenterology. Acta Anaesthesiol Scand 1990;34(S92):21–24.

141. Bartelsman JFWM, Sars PRA, Tytgat GNJ. Flumazenil used for reversal of midazolam-induced sedation in endoscopy outpatients. Gastrointest Endosc 1990;36:S9–S12.

142. Dunk AA, Norton AC, Hudson M, Dundas CR, Ashley N, Mowat G. The value of flumazenil in the reversal of midazolam-induced sedation for upper gastrointestinal endoscopy. Aliment Pharmacol Ther 1990;4:35–42.

143. Rosario MT, Costa NF. Combination of midazolam and flumazenil in upper gastrointestinal endoscopy, a double-blind randomized study. Gastrointest Endosc 1990;36:30–33.

144. Jensen S, Knudsen L, Kirkegaard L, Krause A, Knudsen EB. Flumazenil used for antagonizing the central effects of midazolam and diazepam in outpatients. Acta Anaesthesiol Scand 1989;33:26–28.

145. Birkenfeld S, Federico C, Dermansky-Avni Y, Bruck R, Melzer E, Bar-Meir S. Double-blind controlled trial of flumazenil in patients who underwent upper gastrointestinal endoscopy. Gastrointest Endosc 1989;35:519–522.

146. Sanders LD, Piggott SE, Isaac PA, et al. Reversal of benzodiazepine sedation with the antagonist flumazenil. Br J Anaesthesiol 1991;66:445–453.

147. McCloy RF, Pearson RC. Which agent and how to deliver it?: a review of benzodiazepine sedation and its reversal in endoscopy. Scand J Gastroenterol 1990;25(S179):7–11.

29

Pharmacologic Management of Gastrointestinal Neoplasia

PAUL V. WOOLLEY and ROBERT DELAP

Cancer of the gastrointestinal tract is an important health problem in the United States and throughout the world. An estimated 11,100 cases of esophageal cancer, 24,000 cases of gastric cancer, 28,300 cases of pancreatic cancer, and 156,000 cases of colorectal cancer occurred in the United States in 1992 (Table 29.1) (1). The death rates from these cancers remain exceedingly high and surgery alone is often not sufficient therapy. Over the past two decades, cytotoxic drug treatment for gastrointestinal neoplasia has been extensively studied. Although the intrinsic drug resistance of these tumors presents formidable obstacles to complete cure, some significant advances have been made. This chapter reviews the current role of chemotherapy in gastrointestinal cancer.

GENERAL ASPECTS OF TREATMENT OF GASTROINTESTINAL CANCER

Treatment decisions in gastrointestinal cancer often depend upon tumor stage, that is, a description of the anatomic extent of disease progression. A widely used staging system is the TNM classification, which assesses a tumor by size in centimeters (T), spread to regional lymph nodes (N), and presence or absence of distant metastases (M). Stage grouping collects tumors of related TNM into groups of progressively increasing anatomic extent, usually from stage I to stage IV, that correlate with prognosis.

Table 29.1

Gastrointestinal Cancer Statistics in the United States for 1992

Site	No. of new cases	No. of deaths
Esophagus	11,100	10,000
Stomach	24,400	13,300
Pancreas	28,300	25,000
Liver/biliary tract	15,400	12,300
Colon	111,000	51,000
Rectum	45,000	7,300

Source: Boring et al. (1).

The currently available modalities to treat gastrointestinal cancer are surgery, cytotoxic drugs, biologic response modifiers, ionizing radiation, and combinations of these. Advances using genetically modified lymphocytes and other gene transfer techniques offer prospects for the future. Surgery is still the cornerstone of treatment and, whenever possible, a complete tumor resection is performed. The probability that this procedure is actually curative is related to disease stage. TNM staging at the time of diagnosis and initial treatment is a critical part of tumor management, but certain broad treatment principles can be stated by describing the tumor as either metastatic, locally advanced, or completely resected after surgery. Tumor progression is a combination of local and distant spread. A conceptual advance in the past two decades has been the recognition that local-

589

ized, surgically resectable disease may have spread systemically at the time of diagnosis, and that treatment failures result from micrometastases present at the time of surgery. This has lead to the incorporation into initial treatment of adjuvant chemotherapy to manage this disseminated microscopic residual disease. In the mid-1970s, randomized clinical trials established that postoperative adjuvant chemotherapy could diminish disease recurrence rates and prolong survival in women with breast cancer metastatic to axillary lymph nodes. Adjuvant chemotherapy has since become standard therapy for that clinical situation. Many research trials have been directed at prolonging disease-free survival and overall survival in gastric, pancreatic, colon, and rectal carcinoma by administration of chemotherapy after complete surgical resection. The success of these studies has varied and is discussed under the headings of the specific tumors.

Nonresectable, locally advanced gastrointestinal cancer presents two specific considerations. First, if the disease can be encompassed in a radiation port, then combined treatment with radiation and chemotherapy is a possibility. Whether it is actually used depends upon the exact extent of disease and whether clinical data exist that support its value. However, several trials have used this approach in gastric and pancreatic cancer. Second, initial treatment with chemotherapy may shrink a locally unresectable tumor sufficiently to allow surgical resection. Neoadjuvant chemotherapy refers to initial chemotherapy given to shrink a tumor and make it more accessible to radiation and/or surgery.

When a tumor has metastasized beyond its primary site, systemic therapy is essential to treatment, although surgery and/or radiation may still be required to manage local problems such as pain or obstruction. The initial evaluation of new drugs is done in patients with objectively measurable metastatic disease. Clinical activity of new agents is established by their ability to produce objectively verified tumor regression. Once this is established, a drug may be used further in combi-

nation, or in earlier stage disease. In the following discussion, the subjects of adjuvant therapy, locally unresectable disease, and metastatic disease will be addressed separately for each tumor site.

The effectiveness of cancer treatment is judged by several endpoints, including response, duration of response, disease-free survival, and overall survival. The term "response" specifically refers to objectively verifiable regression of tumor. A partial response is a 50% reduction in the product of the two largest perpendicular diameters of the tumor, and a complete response is the disappearance of all detectable disease. Although the view is widely held that partial responses correlate with improvement in survival, this is not necessarily the case. In particular, recent evidence indicates a poor correlation between partial regression of colon cancer and prolongation of survival.

ACTIVE DRUGS IN TREATMENT OF GASTROINTESTINAL CANCER

5-Fluorouracil

Some cytotoxic drugs that are useful in gastrointestinal cancer are listed in Table 29.2. The mainstay is 5-fluorouracil (5-FU), a fluorinated analog of the natural pyrimidine. This drug has been available clinically for over 30 years, but it is still the only agent that is effective for some neoplasms.

Thymidylate synthase (TS) is a key enzyme in thymidine nucleotide biosynthesis. Under physiologic conditions, it catalyzes the insertion of a methyl group at the 5-position of the pyrimidine ring of deoxyuridine monophosphate (dUMP) to form deoxythymidine monophosphate. This is an essential step in DNA synthesis. The methyl group for this reaction is donated from a reduced folate and the enzyme mechanism requires that the reduced folate cofactor, N^5,N^{10}-methylene tetrahydrofolic acid, bind to the enzyme-substrate complex to form a ternary structure.

Inhibition of TS can destroy cells that are synthesizing DNA (S-phase cells) by depleting their pools of thymidine nucleotide precursors. In the 5-FU metabolite 5-fluoro-

Table 29.2
Commonly Used Drugs in Gastrointestinal Cancer

Esophagus	5-FU, mitomycin C, cisplatin, bleomycin
Stomach	5-FU, nitrosoureas, mitomycin C, doxorubicin, cisplatin, etoposide, methotrexate
Pancreas (adenocarcinoma)	5-FU, biochemical modulators
Pancreas (islet cell tumors)	5-FU, streptozotocin, chlorozotocin, doxorubicin, cisplatin, etoposide
Colon/rectum (adenocarcinoma)	5-FU, leucovorin
Anal canal (squamous carcinoma)	5-FU, mitomycin C, cisplatin
Hepatocellular carcinoma	5-FU, doxorubicin, cisplatin

deoxyuridine monophosphate (FdUMP), the site of insertion of the methyl group is blocked by a fluorine atom. FdUMP inhibits TS by competing with dUMP for binding. By analogy with the native reaction, the binding of FdUMP to TS and its consequent inhibition of the enzyme depend upon the simultaneous binding of a reduced folate cofactor. This forms the basis of biochemical modulation of 5-FU in which administration of exogenous leucovorin can increase the in vivo pharmacologic activity of 5-FU (2).

In addition to its inhibition of TS, 5-FU is metabolized to 5-FU triphosphate and incorporated into RNA. This may interfere with RNA processing. However, most investigators believe that TS inhibition is the primary basis of its antineoplastic action. Recent evidence in rectal cancer indicates an inverse relationship between level of expression of TS and survival (3), i.e., higher levels of expression are associated with shorter survival. Other data (4) indicate that high levels of TS expression are associated with poor response of gastric cancer to chemotherapy. With continued exposure to 5-FU, both production of dUMP and intracellular TS levels can increase. Since the binding of FdUMP to TS is reversible, excess dUMP can compete with FdUMP for binding to TS and contribute to overcoming the TS inhibition. Treatment with 5-FU increases intracellular TS, appar-

ently by increasing synthesis at the translational level.

The biochemical modulation of 5-FU involves the coadministration of agents that may have no individual cytotoxic activity, yet can influence enzyme pathways that are important to the action of 5-FU (5). Examples include leucovorin (5-formyl tetrahydrofolic acid; folinic acid), N-(phosphonoacetyl)-L-aspartate (PALA), interferon, methotrexate, and hydroxyurea (Table 29.3). Leucovorin, for example, is metabolized to N^5,N^{10}-methylene-tetrahydrofolate, which then forms a stable ternary complex with FdUMP and TS. The result is effective and prolonged inhibition of TS. Extracellular leucovorin concentrations of 1–10 μM are necessary to stabilize the TS ternary complex. Leucovorin exists as both *d*- and *l*-stereoisomers and the *l*-isomer possesses biochemical activity while the *d*-isomer is inactive. This has led to clinical trials using only the *l*-isomer.

The other agents cited either inhibit enzymes besides TS in thymidine nucleotide synthesis, or interfere with thymidine salvage (5). Specifically, N-phosphonacetyl-L-aspartate (PALA) inhibits aspartate carbamoyltransferase (ACTase), while zidovudine (azidothymidine; AZT) and iododeoxyuridine (IUdR) interfere with the thymidine salvage pathway by competing with thymidine for binding to thymidine kinase. IUdR is also a

Table 29.3
Sites of Action of Biochemical Modulators of 5-FU

Leucovorin	Enhances FdUMP binding to TS
Methotrexate	Inhibits dihydrofolate reductase and depletes intracellular reduced folate
PALA	Inhibits L-aspartate transcarbamylase
Hydroxyurea	Inhibits ribonucleotide reductase and prevents the formation of excess dUMP
Interferon-α	Multiple mechanisms, including alteration of 5-FU pharmacology and immune modulation
Azidothymidine	Blocks the reutilization of thymidine by competing for binding to thymidine kinase
IUdR	Blocks the reutilization of thymidine by competing for binding to thymidine kinase; it is also phosphorylated by TK and incorporated into DNA as a fraudulent base

substrate for thymidine kinase, and is phosphorylated into products that are incorporated into DNA as fraudulent bases. Although AZT, PALA, and IUdR have limited activity as single agents, laboratory and animal studies suggest that combinations of 5-FU with these agents can improve treatment of a variety of tumors. One focus of current research is the coadministration of 5-FU, leucovorin, and these additional agents in an attempt to increase the efficacy of 5-FU.

Resistance to 5-FU and leucovorin is common, and clinical responses to this combination are often brief and produce only modest benefit. Major pathways of resistance include an increase in TS levels, an increase in other enzymes of de novo pyrimidine synthesis, and/or an increase in the salvage (recycling) of thymidine, which can lessen the dependence of the cell on de novo thymidine nucleotide synthesis.

Other Drugs

The other agents that are useful in gastrointestinal cancer are cisplatin, etoposide (VP-16), doxorubicin (Adriamycin), mitomycin C, streptozotocin, and interferon-α. They are used with different frequency in diseases at different sites. For example, colon cancer is resistant to virtually all drugs except 5-FU, but gastric cancer is responsive to many of the agents listed. The question of drug resistance in gastrointestinal cancer is an important one.

DRUG RESISTANCE IN GASTROINTESTINAL CANCER

All gastrointestinal tumors have limited sensitivity to cytotoxic drugs and none are as curable with chemotherapy as are responsive neoplasms such as lymphomas or testicular germ cell tumors. For example, colon cancer is resistant to drugs of almost every class except the fluorinated pyrimidines, and pancreatic cancer is one of the most resistant of all neoplasms. This resistance is a multifactorial phenomenon that depends not only on tumor doubling time, but also upon a variety of intrinsic cellular processes, including regulation of intracellular drug levels, drug and free radical detoxification, metallothioneins, enzymatic repair of DNA, and perhaps other mechanisms (6). Extensive research in the past 10 years has delineated several specific mechanisms that contribute to the drug-resistant phenotype. These include $P = 170$ glycoprotein-mediated multidrug resistance, expression of several antioxidant and detoxification enzymes, synthesis of intracellular glutathione, activity of O^6-methylguanine-alkyltransferase, and level of expression of nuclear topoisomerases I and II (7). The significance of understanding these processes is that many of them can be inhibited by pharmacologic methods, thereby sensitizing the tumor cell to drugs to which it is otherwise resistant. Not all of the following considerations have as yet been applied to gastrointestinal cancer, but they represent valid approaches.

Multidrug resistance refers to cross-resistance to drugs of several different structural classes. It was first identified as an in vitro phenomenon in which cells selected for resistance to a single agent became simultaneously resistant to several structurally unrelated compounds. On a molecular level, it results from the expression on the cell surface of a 170-kilodalton molecular weight protein that binds and hydrolyzes ATP and actively extrudes drugs and xenobiotics of a wide variety of molecular structures from the cell interior, thereby lowering their intracellular concentrations. This confers resistance to drugs of several classes, including anthracyclines and vinca alkaloids. The $P = 170$ glycoprotein is frequently expressed in gastrointestinal tumors, as has been particularly well documented in colon cancer. The $P = 170$ glycoprotein can be inhibited by various compounds including verapamil, cyclosporine, and certain phenothiazines. This has led to clinical trials in which the inhibitor is given in combination with a cytotoxic drug that is a substrate for $P = 170$.

Glutathione is a thiol-containing tripeptide that is present in millimolar concentrations within the cell and that serves several functions. It helps maintain a reducing environment and reacts directly with free radicals. It is also a substrate for glutathione peroxidase and the glutathione-S-transferases, which are detoxification enzymes that contribute to drug resistance. Reduction of intracellular glutathione levels can sensitize gastrointestinal cancer cells to some classes of drugs including melphalan (phenylalanine mustard), doxorubicin, and cisplatin (8). Buthionine sulfoximine is one drug capable of doing this. It interferes with glutathione synthesis by inhibiting γ-glutamylcysteine synthetase, an initial enzyme in the glutathione synthetic pathway. Buthionine sulfoximine is presently being used in clinical trials, but has not yet achieved a definite role in gastrointestinal cancer treatment.

Doxorubicin, bleomycin, and mitomycin C are among the antineoplastic drugs that produce intracellular oxygen free radicals. The antioxidant enzymes glutathione peroxidase, superoxide dismutase, and catalase catalyze the degradation of superoxide and hydrogen peroxide, and thereby contribute to the drug-resistant state. (7, 9). The glutathione-S-transferases detoxify various substrates, for example, the anticancer drug melphalan, by conjugating them with glutathione. A high level of expression of members of this enzyme family, especially glutathione-S-transferase-π may also contribute to the drug-resistant phenotype in colon cancer and other gastrointestinal neoplasms (10).

Some anticancer drugs, the nitrosoureas for example, exert their cytotoxic effects by reacting chemically with DNA and transferring alkyl groups to specific sites in the purine and pyrimidine bases. This is termed alkylation, and it can result in depurination and disruption of DNA strand pairing. The N7- and O^6-positions of guanine are among those susceptible to alkylation damage, with the latter resulting in strand disruption. The DNA repair enzyme O^6-methylguanine DNA methyltransferase catalyzes the removal of alkyl groups from guanine residues through a reaction which results in irreversible inactivation of the enzyme. The repair of high levels of acute methylation damage can deplete cells of O^6-methylguanine DNA methyltransferase activity to the extent that they become sensitized to other alkylating agents. This strategy has been used to sensitize colon carcinoma cells to nitrosoureas (11). Initial treatment in vitro with the highly reactive methylating agent streptozotocin sufficiently depletes colon carcinoma cells of enzyme activity that they become sensitized to the effects of the alkylating nitrosourea carmustine. Clinical trials have been conducted in colon cancer using sequential streptozotocin and carmustine (1,3-bis (2-chloroethyl)-2-nitrosourea [BCNU]) based on this rationale (12).

The nuclear enzymes topoisomerase I and II catalyze the formation and religation of single- and double-strand breaks during the replication of DNA. Some drugs used in cancer treatment inhibit these enzymes by stabilizing a reaction intermediate consisting of enzyme attached to a DNA strand at its point of interruption and preventing the religation process. The resulting persistence of DNA strand breaks leads by some mechanism to cell death. Anticancer drugs that are topoisomerase inhibitors include camptothecin (topoisomerase I) and etoposide and anthracyclines (topoisomerase II). Recent evidence indicates that although colon carcinoma is resistant to drugs that inhibit topoisomerase II, it is more sensitive to the camptothecins (13). Topoisomerases I and II thus can represent alternative drug targets, and development of the camptothecin family as antineoplastic agents in gastrointestinal cancer is an important area of research.

The clinical implications of these observations are not yet fully realized, and trials utilizing these principles are still being developed. The mechanisms of drug resistance mentioned here are among those being most actively studied at this time, but other pathways of resistance may also be important, such as those involving heat shock proteins. Complete tumor cell sensitization may require the simultaneous interference with more than one mechanism of drug resistance.

TREATMENT OF SPECIFIC DISEASES

As described earlier, the treatment of gastrointestinal tumors can be divided into the groups of advanced metastatic disease, locally advanced disease, and adjuvant therapy after complete resection. The following discussion of separate disease sites will consider each of these as appropriate.

Esophageal Cancer

Esophageal carcinoma may be of either squamous (epidermoid) or adenocarcinoma histology. In either case, it is a virulent disease. Adenocarcinomas often occur at the gastroesophageal junction and behave like gastric carcinomas. Those that arise above the gastroesophageal junction may originate in Barrett's esophagus. Metastatic squamous esophageal carcinoma is quite resistant to chemotherapy. It occasionally responds to combinations of 5-FU and cisplatin, but major disease regressions are not common and there is little evidence that chemotherapy can prolong survival in this situation. The traditional therapy of localized disease is surgery, when possible, or else radiation therapy. The results of both are unsatisfactory, however, with low cure rates and high mortality. The combined use of radiation therapy and surgery also fails to solve this problem. With the recognition that some cytotoxic drugs have activity in carcinoma of the esophagus, current research in localized esophageal cancer examines multimodality regimens that integrate chemotherapy with radiation and surgery. The general goals are to intervene early to prevent systemic metastasis, to shrink tumor and render it amenable to primary surgical resection, and to improve on the inadequate results obtained with surgery alone. Many of the data on responsiveness of esophageal carcinoma to chemotherapy originate in such trials.

The drugs that are most frequently employed in these studies include cisplatin, 5-FU, mitomycin C, and bleomycin. Etoposide and methylglyoxal-bis-guanylhydrazone have also been used occasionally. The protocols are of various designs. Some examine only one histology, others combine both squamous and adenocarcinomas. Many use both preoperative chemotherapy and radiation, and some incorporate postoperative chemotherapy as well. Some treat with a fixed number of drug cycles prior to surgery, while others treat to maximum response. Some have used chemotherapy alone in unresectable or poor risk cases. A summary of the currently published studies (14–26) is given in Table 29.4. No single regimen that is superior to all others has yet emerged and not all trials have shown a survival benefit to combined modality therapy. However, chemotherapy ± radiation can produce complete responses in some patients so that the surgical specimen contains no tumor. These patients are the ones who have the prolonged survival. The role of postoperative chemotherapy is not established.

A recent randomized trial (26) compared the following in patients with localized carcinoma of the thoracic esophagus: (a) four courses of 5-FU (1000 mg/m² daily for 4 days)

Table 29.4
Summary of Combined Modality Trials for Esophageal Carcinoma

Reference No.	No. of patients	Histology	Regimen	Results	Conclusion
Orringer et al. (14)	43	A 21 S 22	Cisplatin, vinblastine, 5-FU + radiation for 21 days. Transhiatal esophagectomy 21 days later	Surgery performed in 41 of 43, and 11 of 41 had no residual tumor in the surgical specimen. Median survival for all 43 patients 29 months. All complete responders disease-free at median follow-up of 36 months	The data suggest improved survival compared to earlier regimens
MacFarlane et al. (15)	22	A, S	Preoperative cisplatin and 5-FU, plus radiation. Mitomycin C added for adenocarcinoma	Complete responses in 36% of patients at time of resection. Three year survival 33%, compared with 21% in 114 patients treated with resection only	Data suggest improved survival
Hilgenberg et al. (16)	35	S	Preoperative 5-FU + cisplatin. Postoperative chemotherapy or radiation	Complete responses to chemotherapy in 37%. Survival for all patients at 42 months was 54%	Intermediate term survival improved
Popp et al. (17)	27	S	Two courses of preoperative 5-FU, cisplatin, mitomycin C or 5-FU, cisplatin, vincristine, + 30 Gy radiation	Complete response rate 24%. Survival at 30 months 21.4%, compared to 4.8% in 70 historical controls	Data suggest improved survival
Araujo et al. (18)	59	S	Radiation alone or radiation + 5-FU, mitomycin, bleomycin	Complete responses to radiation in 58%. Complete response to combined modality in 75%. Median duration of response 8 months for both groups. Median survival 6% RT, 16% RT/CT	No improvement in survival for combined modality treatment
Seydel et al. (19)	41	S	30 Gy radiation + 5-FU, cisplatin followed by esophagectomy	Survival at 3 years 8%	All 3 year survivors had tumor-free surgical specimens
Kelson et al. (20)	96	S	(a) Preoperative cisplatin, vincristine, bleomycin; or (b) Preoperative radiation 55 Gy	Objective response rate 64% for radiation, 55% for chemotherapy. Median survival of all patients 11 months, with 20% disease-free at 34 months	Surgery alone or radiation alone is standard therapy outside of a clinical trial setting
Roth et al. (21)	39	S	Pre- and postoperative cisplatin, vincristine, bleomycin or surgery only	Response rate to preoperative chemotherapy 47%. Median survival of responders >20 months, of nonresponders 6.2 months and for surgery only, 8.6 months	Overall survival prolonged for patients responding to chemotherapy

Table 29.4 Continued
Summary of Combined Modality Trials for Esophageal Carcinoma

Reference No.	No. of patients	Histology	Regimen	Results	Conclusion
Urba et al. (22)	24	A	Preoperative continuous infusion 5-FU + 49 Gy radiation. Transhiatal esophagectomy 3 weeks later	Radiographic improvement to the preoperative regimen in 41%. Median survival 11 months	No improvement compared to historical controls
Carey et al. (23)	15	A	2 cycles preoperative 5-FU, cisplatin	Tumor resectable in 11 of 15; 1 of 11 complete response and 10 of 11 with residual disease. Median survival time 10.47 months for all patients and 23.83 months for the resected patients	
Coia et al. (24)	9	A	60 Gy radiation + 2 courses of continuous infusion 5-FU for 96 hours + one bolus of mitomycin C	Seven complete responses in 8 evaluable definitively treated patients. Median disease-free interval 10 months and median survival 15 months in this cohort	A palliative or even curative regimen in patients who do not undergo surgery
Ajani et al. (25)	35	A	Preoperative and postoperative etoposide, 5-FU, and cisplatin	17 (49%) major responses to chemotherapy, with 6 complete responses. Projected median survival 23 months. After a median follow-up of 20 months, 15 patients alive with no evidence of relapse.	Need to use regimens that produce complete responses
Herskovic et al. (26)	121	A, S	Radiation alone, 64 Gy, or radiation, 50 Gy, plus infusional 5-FU and cisplatin in nonoperative disease of the thoracic esophagus	Median survival 8.9 months for radiation alone, 12.5 months for combined therapy. Survival at 2 years 10% for radiation only. 38% for combined therapy	Concurrent therapy with cisplatin and 5-FU and radiation superior to radiation therapy alone for localized carcinoma of the esophagus.

Table 29.5
Some Representative Regimens for Gastric Cancer

Combination	Acronym
5-FU Semustine	
5-FU Adriamycin Mitomycin C	FAM
5-FU Adriamycin Semustine	FAMe
Methotrexate 5-FU Adriamycin	FAMTX
5-FU Adriamycin Cisplatin	FAP
Etoposide Adriamycin Cisplatin	EAP

plus cisplatin (75 mg/m^2 on the first day) plus 5000 cGy of radiation therapy to (b) 6400 cGy of radiation therapy alone. The trial was stopped when the results in 121 patients demonstrated a significant survival advantage for those who received chemotherapy and radiation therapy. The radiation-treated patients had a median survival of 8.9 months and 10% survival at 24 months but, in the group treated with chemotherapy and radiation therapy, median survival was 12.5 months, with 38% survival at 24 months ($P < .001$). Those who received combined treatment had statistically fewer local and distant recurrences than those who received only radiation. However, severe side effects were more frequent in the patients who received combined therapy. Thus, although concurrent chemotherapy and radiation were superior to radiation therapy alone in controlling the primary tumor and distant metastases, and in prolonging survival, the combination had the greater toxicity.

This remains an important area for clinical research. Although a clear standard of care has not yet been defined by the available data, the possibility of a definitive role for chemotherapy as part of a multimodality approach to treatment is quite real. The demonstration of complete responses to initial chemotherapy, the favorable survival results in the complete responders, and the existence of randomized trials showing benefit to chemotherapy-containing programs are all encouragement for future efforts.

Gastric Cancer

GENERAL CONSIDERATIONS

Gastric cancer is somewhat unique among gastrointestinal neoplasms, because it regresses in response to several agents other than 5-FU. These include nitrosoureas, doxorubicin, mitomycin C, etoposide, and cisplatin. This has led to a succession of combination drug trials over the past two decades (Table 29.5). To date, a standard of treatment has not emerged, and despite the description of numerous active regimes, debate remains as to whether any of them is superior to a dose-intense schedule of 5-FU alone. Part of the controversy in this area centers around the relationship between the endpoints of objective response rate and survival. Although the disease regressions that occur when gastric cancer is treated with drug combinations can be dramatic and associated with improved performance status, appetite, and quality of life, they are usually partial responses of limited duration. When the survival curves of populations of patients treated in different fashions are compared, the differences are most notable in the interval between 6 and 18 months following start of treatment. Survival after 2 years is usually less than 10%, no matter what the quality of the initial response. A current goal is to develop regimens that can produce complete responses leading to survival past 2 years.

ADVANCED METASTATIC DISEASE

The questions that have arisen from the combination drug trials in gastric cancer include the relative value of multiple drug regimens and single agents, and the contribution of doxorubicin (Adriamycin) to treatment. One of the first combinations tested in the United States was 5-FU and a nitrosourea (27). In a randomized comparison of 5-FU and carmustine to each drug alone, the response rates were 41% for the combination, 29% for 5-FU, and 17% for carmustine. The median survivals of these groups were approximately the same, but survival at 18 months was 25% for the combination and 5–10% for the single agents. A subsequent four-arm randomized Eastern Cooperative Oncology Group trial (28) compared 5-FU plus semustine (methyl CCNU) to semustine alone in two of its arms. The two additional arms added an induction course of cyclophosphamide to these two regimens. The best response rate (40%) was obtained with 5-FU and semustine, as compared with 8% for semustine alone. The median survival of patients treated with the combination was 22 weeks compared with 10 weeks for those treated with the nitrosourea alone. Cyclophosphamide induction did not improve either regimen.

The FAM combination contains 5-FU, doxorubicin, and mitomycin C. In 62 patients treated with this regimen, the partial response rate was 42%, the median duration of response was 9 months, and the median survival of responders was over 12 months (29). Responses occurred both in local abdominal masses and in disease metastatic to liver, lungs, and lymph nodes. Hematologic toxicity was moderate and the combination was well tolerated. Objective responses were frequently accompanied by an improvement in performance status and sense of well-being that persisted for the duration of the response. Several cooperative groups reported comparable results with FAM. For example, the Southwest Oncology Group achieved a 37% response rate in 76 gastric cancer patients treated with FAM and reported that simultaneous use of the three drugs was superior to their sequential use (30). The Eastern Cooperative Oncology Group obtained similar results (31). The histologic subtype and cellular differentiation of the tumor did not seem to affect response rates. A number of variations of the FAM combination have been tested (32–34). Substitution of the fluorinated pyrimidine ftorafur for 5-FU produced excessive central nervous system and gastrointestinal toxicity without improving the outcome. Subsequent regimens that added the nitrosourea chlorozotocin to FAM, that substituted cisplatin for mitomycin C, or that combined FAM and triazinate were inferior to or equivalent to the parent combination without any clear benefit.

Several trials have examined the contribution of doxorubicin to combination drug therapy. The Gastrointestinal Tumor Study Group (GITSG) first compared doxorubicin alone to: (a) 5-FU, doxorubicin, and semustine (FAMe) and (b) 5-FU, mitomycin C, and cytosine arabinoside (FMC) (35). Single-agent doxorubicin produced objective responses in 24% of patients treated, but the response rate (47%) and survival values for FAMe were superior both to doxorubicin alone and to FMC. A second study (36) compared four regimens, two of which contained doxorubicin. Both 5-FU, doxorubicin, semustine and 5-FU, doxorubicin, mitomycin C showed statistically superior survival to 5-FU plus semustine, indicating that doxorubicin improved the effectiveness of treatment. These data indicate that doxorubicin-containing combinations are somewhat superior to those that lack it. The Eastern Cooperative Oncology Group reached a similar conclusion in a trial that compared 5-FU plus semustine alone to: (a) doxorubicin plus mitomycin; (b) 5-FU plus doxorubin plus mitomycin C; and (c) 5-FU plus doxorubicin plus semustine. The median survivals in the three doxorubicin-containing arms were 22, 18, and 30 weeks, compared with 13 weeks for 5-FU plus semustine.

Finally, Levi et al. (37) compared doxorubicin alone to 5-FU, doxorubicin, and semustine. Doxorubicin alone produced responses in 9 of 70 patients treated and the median survival was 19 weeks. In the combination arm, the overall response rate was 40% and the median survival was 33 weeks. Thus, the combination was superior, but the differences were small.

Despite the statistical significance of some of the comparisons in these trials, none of these regimens has truly increased the complete response rate or long-term survival of gastric cancer patients. Difficulty in interpreting these results can arise if response rates are emphasized over survival. In a study reported in 1985, 5-FU, FAM, and FA produced equivalent survival statistics even though the FAM combination produced the highest response rate (38).

These data suggest that only limited benefits result from combinations of 5-FU, doxorubicin, mitomycin C, and nitrosoureas. More recent combinations have studied biochemical modulation of 5-FU by methotrexate, or have incorporated cisplatin and etoposide. Three combinations of interest have been: (a) 5-FU, doxorubicin, and cisplatin (FAP); (b) etoposide, doxorubicin, and cisplatin (EAP); and (c) methotrexate sequenced with 5-FU plus doxorubicin (FAMTX). FAP has been the subject of at least four studies (33, 39, 40). EAP and FAMTX have been studied individually and also in randomized comparison with each other and with FAM.

The FAP combination was first reported by investigators at Georgetown (33) and was subsequently studied by the GITSG (39) and the North Central Cancer Treatment Group (40). It is logically attractive because of in vitro synergy between doxorubicin and cisplatin, but the clinical response rates and survival statistics resemble those of earlier regimens. A randomized comparison of FAP with 5-FU has shown no therapeutic advantage but increased toxicity for the combination (40).

Most recent attention has been directed at FAMTX and EAP, and their comparison with each other and with FAM. Initial trials of EAP suggested a high overall response rate, the occurrence of complete responses and improved survival compared with previous regimens. In 67 patients treated with EAP, the overall response rate was 64%, including 21% complete responses (41). Eight complete responses were pathologically confirmed (pCR). The

median response duration was 7 months for all patients, 16 months for the complete responders, 22 months for the pCR, and 6 months for partial responders. The median survival times were 9 months for all patients, 17 months for those who achieved complete response, 23 months for the pCR, and 9.5 months for the partial responders. The principal toxicities were leukopenia and thrombocytopenia, with 64% of patients developing grade 3–4 myelosuppression and 12% developing severe infections.

In a subsequent study (42), 36 patients were treated with the identical regimen. Four patients died of treatment-related sepsis or hemorrhage. Nine objective partial responses and three clinical complete responses were observed. The median time to progression was 4 months for all 36 patients and 8 months for the 12 who responded. Of the 13 patients with localized but unresectable disease, 5 subsequently underwent surgical resection, but only 1 was rendered disease free. The EAP regimen was quite toxic, but the response rates and survival times resembled those of more easily tolerated combinations.

The FAMTX combination was based on the concept of biochemical modulation of 5-FU by methotrexate (43). The 1982 description of the combination reported a 63% response rate (44). The European Organization for Research and Treatment of Cancer (EORTC) then conducted a Phase II study of FAMTX and found a 33% response rate (45). FAMTX was then compared to FAM in a randomized multicenter trial involving 213 patients (46). The response rate (41% vs. 9%) and survival (median, 42 weeks vs. 29 weeks) for FAMTX were statistically superior to FAM.

A study of a related regimen treated 23 patients with a combination of moderate-dose methotrexate, 250 mg/m^2, folinic acid rescue, and 5-FU, 600 mg/m^2. No complete responses occurred, but 5 patients had partial remissions. For responding patients, the median duration of remission was 6 months and the median survival was 11 months. The overall median survival was 6 months. The combination did not offer an advantage over single-agent therapy (47).

Finally, in a randomized comparison of EAP and FAMTX in 60 previously untreated patients (48), response rates were 33% for FAMTX and 20% for EAP. Three FAMTX and no EAP patients had complete remissions. The median survivals were 6.1 months for EAP and 7.3 months for FAMTX. At 1 year, 7% of EAP and 17% of FAMTX patients were alive. EAP caused significantly more myelosuppression than did FAMTX. Four EAP patients died of toxic side effects, but no FAMTX patients died of treatment-related causes. The conclusion was that FAMTX is at least as active as EAP and is significantly less toxic.

In summary, gastric cancer is responsive to more drugs and undergoes drug-induced partial regression more frequently than other gastrointestinal neoplasms. However, while response rate and survival are related, complete responses are infrequent and the partial responses are of limited duration. This limits the effects of treatment on overall survival. Drug combinations sometimes, but not always, produce superior survival to single agents in comparative trials. Most phase III studies show only small differences between regimens, and the median survival of advanced disease patients in different studies is often a remarkably constant 25 ± 5 weeks. These clinical data suggest that gastric cancer is a heterogeneous disease that is composed of both drug-sensitive and drug-resistant cell populations. Treatment that results in initial cell killing of the sensitive population simply selects a resistant population that regrows and kills the host. There is still no way to select patients who will respond to or most benefit from chemotherapy. A paramount concern is the design of approaches to circumvent inherent drug resistance.

MULTIMODALITY THERAPY OF LOCALLY ADVANCED DISEASE

Regional progression without distant metastases occurs frequently in gastric cancer (49). The clinical situation of locally advanced disease deserves special consideration for two reasons. First, if the disease can be encompassed in a radiation port, then it is logical to hypothesize that combinations of radiation therapy and cytotoxic drugs could simultaneously control local disease and prevent its systemic spread. Second, one can also hypothesize that initial chemotherapy could reduce the size of a locally advanced, unresectable tumor and render it operable. Both of these concepts have been tested in clinical trials.

For operational purposes, locally advanced gastric cancer means residual tumor that can be encompassed in a 400 cm^2 (20 $\times$ 20 cm) radiation port. Several groups have investigated radiation-chemotherapy combinations for locally advanced gastric cancer, but the results do not clearly show a benefit. A study of 62 patients treated at the Mayo Clinic between 1965 and 1974 (50) suggested that combined radiation and 5-FU improved survival. The regimen used 3750-rad external beam radiation and 15 mg/kg of 5-FU on each of the first 3 days of radiation. Thirty-nine patients randomized to treatment were compared with 23 untreated control subjects. Five-year survival rates were 23% in the treated group and 4% in the untreated group. However, 10 patients randomized to the treatment group did not actually receive treatment and yet had survival similar to the treated group.

Recent studies have used radiation in combination with either 5-FU and a nitrosourea or with FAM. Problems of patient tolerance occur with aggressive treatments. The Gastrointestinal Study Group compared chemotherapy with 5-FU and semustine alone to the same chemotherapy plus radiation (51). In the first year of follow-up, the death rate was 68% for the combined modality group and 44% for patients who received only chemotherapy. The differences in survival were most marked in the first 6 months of follow-up. Some deaths were attributed to the hematologic and nutritional complications of the radiation and chemotherapy. In the second through the fourth years, the survival curves of the combined modality group plateaued at about 20%, while that of the group treated with chemotherapy alone exhibited a sustained hazard for relapse.

FAM can be used in sequence with radiation without excessive toxicity (52). In one scheme, a cycle of FAM is given in the first 8 weeks, followed by two courses of external beam radiation, each of 2250 rads given over 3 weeks and accompanied on the first 3 days by 5-FU at a dose of 350 mg/m^2. Two weeks after completion of the radiation, FAM is resumed for six full cycles or to the point of tumor progression. The dose-limiting toxicity is moderate myelosuppression, but not cardiac or gastrointestinal toxicity. The median survival of 30 gastric cancer patients treated with the regimen is 14.5 months. The Southwest Oncology Group has reported favorable preliminary results with a similar regimen in which the chemotherapy dosage was lower (53). However, the Mayo Clinic has reported severe toxicity with 5-FU and doxorubicin induction followed by twice daily external beam radiation plus sensitizing 5-FU (54), followed by maintenance with 5-FU, doxorubicin, and semustine. The patients who received twice daily radiation experienced prolonged and severe anorexia, nausea, and decreased performance status. Three patients treated with once daily radiation plus 5-FU did not experience this complication. Survival figures were no better than those expected for moderate dose radiation and 5-FU, and relapse outside of the radiation port was frequent. These trials have not provided convincing evidence that local radiation therapy plus systemic chemotherapy markedly improves prognosis in locally advanced gastric cancer.

A newer strategy is to initiate chemotherapy before surgery in potentially resectable gastric carcinoma and then continue chemotherapy postoperatively. This approach is currently the subject of research at several institutions (55–58). Induction chemotherapy regimens have included: (a) 5-FU, leucovorin, and cisplatin (55); (b) 5-FU, leucovorin, interferon-α (56); (c) etoposide, 5-FU, and cisplatin (57); and (d) etoposide, doxorubicin, and cisplatin (58). Preoperative chemotherapy is reported to produce disease regression, to be associated with a high resectability rate, and to ameliorate subjective symptoms. These studies bear analogy to the preoperative trials in esophageal carcinoma, and are in some cases still in the feasibility stage. The issue is whether such early intervention can both increase resectability and prevent systemic spread of locally advanced disease.

ADJUVANT CHEMOTHERAPY FOR SURGICALLY RESECTED GASTRIC CANCER

Cure rates of gastric cancer with surgery alone are low once the disease has penetrated the muscular wall and spread to lymph nodes, and even complete resections are frequently associated with relapse. Many attempts have been made to improve the outcome of surgery in high-risk disease with postoperative adjuvant chemotherapy. The results of these studies have been inconsistent. Some indicate a benefit of adjuvant chemotherapy, but positive results have not been confirmed from one group to another. At this time, there is no compelling evidence that chemotherapy can reduce the systemic spread of gastric cancer after surgical resection (59).

Although early trials of adjuvant chemotherapy were performed both in the United States and Japan, the most pertinent studies have been reported in the last 10 years. The trials that began in the United States in the mid-1970s focused on 5-FU and nitrosourea combinations, based on data in advanced disease. Three randomized prospective trials of 5-FU and the nitrosourea semustine have been completed (60–63). The Gastrointestinal Tumor Study Group showed a positive effect of postoperative chemotherapy with a diminished relapse rate and a 20% increase in survival in treated patients over 5 years of follow-up (60). This occurred in patients both with involved lymph nodes and with negative nodes. However, neither of two other prospective trials, one by the Veterans Administrative Surgical Oncology Group and one by the Eastern Cooperative Oncology Group, confirmed these results (61, 62). Furthermore, a German trial that compared 5-FU plus carmustine to observation alone has not demonstrated a benefit of treatment (63). As a consequence, 5-FU/nitrosourea combinations are not proven as effective postoperative adjuvant treatment for gastric cancer.

Trials with adjuvant FAM have now been completed. Coombes et al. (64) described 315 patients randomized after surgical resection who received either FAM or were observed only. At a median follow-up of 68 months, there was no difference in disease-free survival or overall survival rates between the two arms of the study. Subgroup analysis suggested a benefit in patients with T3 and T4 tumors, but because the subgroups were retrospectively defined, this could have been a chance finding. Also, a randomized trial by the North Central Oncology Group (65) has not shown that adjuvant 5-FU and doxorubicin improves results over those with untreated control subjects. At this point, adjuvant chemotherapy for resected gastric cancer is not a standard of treatment, but remains an important area for research with the best available approaches. Randomization of study populations between a treatment arm and a control arm undergoing only follow-up observation remains an indispensable feature of such trials.

PANCREATIC CARCINOMA

Adenocarcinoma

The diagnosis of pancreatic carcinoma is often late, when surgical resection is not possible. Further treatment is greatly limited by the profound intrinsic resistance of pancreatic cancer to almost all cytotoxic drugs and to radiation. Unlike gastric carcinoma, a marked regression of an advanced pancreatic carcinoma following treatment with chemotherapy is distinctly unusual. The specific basis of this resistance has not been delineated, but it could include many of the mechanisms described in the section on drug resistance. Consequently, despite numerous attempts to develop effective drug combinations, no standard of treatment exists for pancreatic cancer at this time. The only agent that has consistently produced responses in over 20% of patients treated is 5-FU (66). In trials conducted during the 1970s, mitomycin C, streptozotocin, and doxorubi-

cin also appeared to have antitumor activity, and the initial results of studies using 5-FU, doxorubicin, and mitomycin C (FAM) showed some evidence of benefit, as did streptozotocin, mitomycin C, and 5-FU (SMF). However randomized studies in cooperative groups did not confirm a significant tumor response rate or any survival benefit (67). Both combinations produced objective responses in no more than 15% of previously untreated patients and those responses, with few exceptions, were of short duration. The median survival times of patients treated with FAM or with two schedules of SMF in this trial were 11.6, 13.3, and 17.7 weeks.

Because of the evidence that leucovorin can modulate the activity of 5-FU, it is logical to apply the principles of biochemical modulation to pancreatic cancer. However, in a recent study, 5-FU and high-dose leucovorin (68) produced only three objective responses in 42 patients with pancreatic cancer, and the median survival of the group was 6.2 months. These results were indistinguishable from those expected from 5-FU alone. Despite these data, it is possible that better results would be obtained by adding other biochemical modulators of 5-FU. A more recent investigational protocol employing the combination of 5-FU, leucovorin, and iododeoxyuridine (IUdR) has produced some encouraging results (69). IUdR is an inhibitor of the thymidine salvage pathway and may be synergistic with 5-FU (see earlier). It is also a radiation sensitizer. Laboratory and animal data indicate that combining IUdR with 5-FU could improve the response rate in pancreatic cancer. Current trials have examined only the drug combination, but future studies will integrate radiation into the regimen as well.

Some trials have examined the combined use of radiation and chemotherapy in locally advanced, unresetable pancreatic cancer. The results seem to show a weak additive effect of the two modalities. The Gastrointestinal Tumor Study Group compared 60-Gy external beam radiation therapy alone with either 40-Gy or 60-Gy radiation plus 5-FU (70). Median survival was 20 weeks in the radiation-only arm, 36 weeks for the 40 Gy plus 5-FU group, and 40 weeks for the 60 Gy plus 5-FU group. However, virtually all patients in the three arms had died at 2 years. The specific contribution of chemotherapy was not tested in that study and a later trial compared streptozotocin, mitomycin C, and 5-FU (SMF) alone with a regimen of radiation and sensitizing 5-FU followed by SMF (71). The group treated with combined modality therapy had a median survival of 42 weeks and an overall survival at 1 year of 41%, while the group treated with chemotherapy alone had a median survival of 32 weeks and 19% survival at 1 year. These differences were statistically significant. The conclusion was that SMF chemotherapy alone could not substitute for combined modality treatment and that the outcome of sequential trials of the GITSG had shown that combined modality treatment was superior to either radiation or chemotherapy alone. The combined use of FAM and external beam radiation has also been reported in clinically localized pancreatic cancer, but there was no clear advantage to the combination (52).

Few data exist regarding postoperative adjuvant therapy for resected pancreatic cancer. The Gastrointestinal Tumor Study Group reported a cohort of 43 patients who had undergone complete surgical resection of pancreatic carcinoma and then were randomized to either observation only or to postoperative radiation and weekly bolus of 5-FU (500 mg/m^2) for a total of 2 years of treatment (72). A statistically significant ($P = .05$) difference in 2-year survival occurred between the two groups. The treated group (21 patients) had a median survival of 21 months, and three patients were alive at 5 years; that of the control group was 11 months, and 1 patient was alive at 5 years.

In summary, advanced metastatic pancreatic cancer is, at present, an untreatable disease, aside from whatever palliative benefit can be obtained from 5-FU with or without leucovorin. Initial treatment with investigational drugs and protocols is justified whenever they are available. In a practice setting, expectations must be kept within bounds, and patients and families informed of the serious limitations of present therapeutic capability. Treatment is aimed at identifying those patients who are candidates for surgical resection. Postoperative treatment of surgically resected patients with radiation and 5-FU is justified by the GITSG data. Also, combined radiation and chemotherapy is justified in those with locally unresectable disease, but the minimal gains achieved by this approach should not obscure the fact that some patients who are older or in poor medical condition are candidates for supportive care only. This decision is a matter of judgment for the treating physician and for the patient.

Islet Cell Tumors

Pancreatic islet cell tumors arise from neuroendocrine cells that are biochemically related to the parent cells of carcinoid tumors. Islet cell tumors have a longer and more indolent natural history than adenocarcinomas of the pancreas, although their range of clinical aggressiveness can be quite variable. It is not unusual for patients to live for years with metastatic disease, unlike adenocarcinoma of the pancreas in which the expected survival is only 6–7 months. These tumors may secrete functional hormones that result in a wide array of endocrine syndromes associated with the hypersecretion of insulin, somatostatin, vasoactive intestinal polypeptide, glucagon, or gastrin. The endocrine manifestations of these diseases should not allow their malignant nature to be neglected. These tumors may be indolent and slowly progressive, but they are still cancers with the ability to invade, metastasize, and kill the host. Their long natural history may raise questions about the timing of chemotherapy.

The cytotoxic drugs that are useful in islet cell tumors include streptozotocin, 5-FU, doxorubicin, the streptozotocin analog chlorozotocin, cisplatin, and etoposide (VP-16). After a report in 1980 (73) of the superiority of streptozotocin plus 5-FU to 5-FU alone, the two-drug combination became regarded standard therapy for advanced islet-cell carcinoma. A recent randomized trial (74) compared: (a) streptozotocin plus 5-FU; (b) streptozotocin plus doxorubicin; or (c) chlorozotocin alone. Objective tumor regressions occurred in 69% of cases treated with streptozotocin plus doxorubicin, and 45% for streptozotocin plus fluorouracil ($P = .05$). Streptozotocin plus doxorubicin was also superior in time to tumor progression (median, 20 vs. 6.9 months; $P = .001$) and in overall survival (median, 2.2 vs. 1.4 years; $P = .004$). Chlorozotocin alone produced a 30% regression rate, with the time-to-tumor progression and the survival time equivalent to those observed with streptozotocin plus fluorouracil. Crossover therapy after the failure of either chlorozotocin alone or one of the combination regimens produced an overall response rate of only 17%, and the responses were transient. It was concluded that the combination of streptozotocin and doxorubicin is superior to the current standard regimen of streptozotocin plus fluorouracil.

Another recent study (75) used continuous infusion cisplatin and VP-16 in neuroendocrine tumors, including 20 pancreatic islet cell carcinomas. Only two partial objective tumor regressions were observed (7%) among 27 patients with well-differentiated carcinoid tumors or islet cell carcinomas. However, nine partial regressions and three complete regressions occurred among 18 patients who had anaplastic neuroendocrine carcinomas. The median duration of regression of the anaplastic tumors was 8 months and the median survival of all patients with anaplastic tumors was 19 months. Tumor response was not related to primary site of disease or endocrine hyperfunction. Possibly additional drug combinations using cisplatin and VP-16 together with streptozotocin, doxorubicin, and 5-FU will find application in the future.

COLORECTAL CANCER

The only drugs with clinically significant activity against colon cancer are the fluorinated pyrimidines, particularly 5-FU. This drug has been used on various schedules and doses, but while some benefits have been achieved, the outcomes are still imperfect. Colon carcinoma exhibits virtually complete intrinsic resistance to other cytotoxic drugs including alkylating agents, anthracyclines, vinca alkaloids, and epipodophyllotoxins. The complete mechanism of this resistance is not defined, but expression of the MDR phenotype and of the enzymes glutathione-S-transferase, O^6-methylguanine DNA methyltransferase, and topoisomerase II may play a role. Many, if not all, colon carcinomas express the MDR phenotype as determined by northern blotting, polymerase chain reaction, or protein expression (6–11).

Several approaches have been used to optimize the activity of 5-FU in colon cancer, which are addressed as follows: (a) bolus vs. loading schedules of administration; (b) combinations with other drugs; (c) prolonged infusion schedules; (d) biochemical modulation of 5-FU; and (e) locoregional infusion; particularly into the hepatic circulation. Work in the 1960s and 1970s emphasized the comparison of bolus and loading schedules. Data from the Mayo Clinic indicated that a weekly bolus administration schedule was as effective as monthly loading for colon cancer. The Central Oncology Group (76) compared four regimens of 5-FU administration: (a) a loading schedule of 12 mg/kg/day for 5 days; (b) weekly intravenous administration of 15 mg/kg; (c) a low dose schedule of 500 mg/day for 4 days; and (d) 15 mg/kg orally for 6 days followed by 15 mg/kg orally per week. Responses occurred in 33% of patients treated with the loading regimen and 12–18% of those treated with the other schedules. A modest survival benefit of 4–6 months was also projected for the patients treated with the loading regimen. This was also the more toxic regimen, with 18% of patients experiencing serious or life-threatening toxicities.

Combination chemotherapy has also been extensively studied in colon carcinoma but, at this time, it is simply not a viable approach (77–80). The concept of utilizing several drugs that have different mechanisms of action and different toxicities to achieve additive or synergistic results has been successful in many diseases, including leukemia, lymphoma, breast and ovarian cancer, small cell carcinoma of the lung, and testicular germ cell tumors. In colon cancer, large randomized trials comparing combinations of putative active single agents to 5-FU alone have not demonstrated any significant benefit to the combinations. The nitrosoureas and mitomycin C are among the agents that have been thought to have significant antitumor activity in colon cancer. They have been used both in metastatic disease and also as components of adjuvant treatment protocols, but this marginal clinical activity has never evolved into a significant therapeutic benefit. Conceivably newer active agents, for example, the camptothecins, will change this situation.

The schedule and dose intensity of 5-FU administration are among the determinants of its efficacy. Its in vivo half-life after bolus administration is about 10 minutes, but only those cells that are in S-phase are susceptible to 5-FU, so that prolonged exposure to the slowly cycling cells in the tumor is necessary to achieve significant cytotoxic effects. Most solid tumors have low S-phase fractions, of the order of 5% or less, and are proliferating slowly. For these reasons, schedules of repeated or prolonged administration are logically preferable to intermittent bolus schedules. The ways in which this concept have been applied include bolus administration on several sequential days, continuous infusion for 4–5 days, and prolonged continuous infusions of moderate daily doses for several weeks. Whether any of these approaches truly improves outcome remains controversial. A randomized trial that compared weekly bolus 5-FU to prolonged continuous infusion showed an increased regression rate with the continuous infusion, but the survival curves of the two groups were almost identical (81). Studies of a wide range of treatment schedules and doses show that 5-FU efficacy can vary unpredictably. If a tumor does not respond to treatment with 5-FU given on a 5-day bolus schedule, it may still respond to a prolonged continuous infusion. Toxicities of the different 5-FU treatment schedules also vary both

qualitatively and quantitatively. For example, a newer regimen utilizing a 24-hour infusion of 2.6 g/m^2 of 5-FU and 500 mg/m^2 of leucovorin on a weekly schedule produces less gastrointestinal toxicity and leucopenia than a conventional schedule of bolus injection for 5 consecutive days, even though the dose intensity is higher.

Biochemical modulation of 5-FU refers to the coadministration of agents that affect the pathways through which 5-FU acts, so as to produce additive or synergistic effects. The enzymatic basis of biochemical modulation has been discussed previously. The most important clinical modulation trials in colon cancer have utilized leucovorin, interferon, PALA, methotrexate, and hydroxyurea. Seven randomized trials have compared 5-FU/leucovorin to 5-FU alone and an eighth compared methotrexate/leucovorin/5-FU to 5-FU alone (5). These trials have varied in the dose and schedule of both the leucovorin and the 5-FU, and no single best regimen has yet been established. A trial by the North Central Oncology Group (82), which compared 5-FU alone to 5-FU plus high-dose leucovorin and to 5-FU plus low-dose leucovorin showed survival benefits for both leucovorin-containing regimens over 5-FU alone. However, only the patients in the low-dose arm reported improvement in quality of life indicators such as performance status, symptoms, and weight gain. A trial by the Gastrointestinal Tumor Study Group (83) also compared 5-FU alone to two arms containing either high-dose (500 mg/m^2) or low-dose (25 mg/m^2) leucovorin. The high-dose regimen had a response rate of 30.3%, which was statistically superior to 5-FU alone. However, severe diarrhea and stomatitis were encountered in this arm, leading to some toxic deaths. For these reasons, some regard 5-FU/low-dose leucovorin as the standard for comparison. However, this view is not universally accepted.

A recent meta-analysis (84) examined the completed trials that have compared 5-FU alone to 5-FU plus leucovorin. The data clearly show that the combination results in an increase in objective response rate (23% vs.

11%) and a change in the toxicity spectrum. However, there is no demonstrable survival advantage to the combination and the plots of survival against time for the two groups were virtually superimposable.

The combination of interferon-α and 5-FU has now been studied intensively. Early trials of interferon-α alone demonstrated that this agent lacked activity by itself in colon cancer, but several studies have examined 5-FU plus interferon and suggested beneficial effects. Two randomized studies were reported in 1993 (85, 86). One compared intensive 5-FU alone to the same dose of 5-FU plus interferon-α (85). The response rate was higher for the combination, but the response durations and survival times were approximately the same for both regimens. A second study compared 5-FU plus leucovorin with 5-FU plus interferon-α (86). The two combinations showed identical remission durations and overall survival times. It is unclear that the 5-FU and interferon-α combination is superior either to intensive 5-FU alone or to 5-FU plus leucovorin in extending overall survival.

POSTOPERATIVE ADJUVANT THERAPY OF COLON CANCER

Attempts to develop effective postoperative adjuvant treatment for colon cancer were unsuccessful for many years, but recent trials have given chemotherapy using 5-FU and levamisole an established place in the treatment of surgically resected colon cancer metastatic to lymph nodes and high-risk disease involving only the bowel wall.

Several early randomized studies comparing single-agent 5-FU with observation only failed to show statistically significant improvement in 5-year survival of patients receiving the adjuvant therapy. A meta-analysis of the completed studies involving over 3000 patients randomized between 5-FU and observation only showed only a 3.4% survival advantage for the group receiving 5-FU (87). Subsequent trials examined the combination of 5-FU and the nitrosourea semustine (methyl-CCNU). Randomized comparisons of this chemotherapy to no treatment were

performed by the Veterans Administration Surgical Oncology Group (88), the Gastrointestinal Tumor Study Group (89), and the Southwest Oncology Group (90). None showed any benefit to treatment.

This situation has now changed with the description of statistically significant benefits in disease-free survival and overall survival for high-risk colon cancer patients treated with 5-FU plus the immunomodulator levamisol (91). High risk includes disease metastatic to lymph nodes and also obstructing or perforating lesions that are otherwise confined to the bowel wall. The treatment consists of 5-FU, 450 mg/m²/day, for 5 days followed by weekly injections of 5-FU 450 mg/m² for 48 weeks. Levamisole is given as a 50-mg oral dose three times daily for 3 days, repeated every 2 weeks for 1 year. Two randomized trials have confirmed the benefit of this regimen. The larger trial observed a 19% improvement in disease-free survival and a 10% improvement in overall survival at 3 years (91).

These results have established the 5-FU and levamisole regimen as a standard of care. Now that this result has been achieved, further research is directed at refining and optimizing the regimen. Two questions that remain are: (a) Is a year of intermittent bolus 5-FU required, or could the time of treatment be shortened by more intensive treatment? and (b) Does the addition of leucovorin improve treatment? These questions have been addressed by a national trial that compared: (a) 1 year of standard 5-FU plus levamisole; (b) 5-FU plus low-dose leucovorin; (c) 5-FU plus high-dose leucovorin; and (d) 5-FU plus leucovorin and levamisole. This study has completed accrual and is now undergoing follow-up. The results of current trials will supply further definition to the appropriate agents for adjuvant therapy and the duration of treatment.

POSTOPERATIVE ADJUVANT THERAPY OF RECTAL CARCINOMA

The postoperative management of rectal cancer has evolved somewhat differently than that

Table 29.6
Recent Trials of Postoperative Radiation and Chemotherapy in Rectal Carcinoma

Group & Reference No.	Year	Randomization	Conclusion
Gastrointestinal Tumor Study Group (92)	1985	1. Observation 2. Radiation alone 3. 5-FU + semustine 4. Combined radiation and chemotherapy	Disease-free survival and overall survival improved in all treated patients compared with control. The greatest effect was with combination radiation and chemotherapy
National Surgical Adjuvant Breast Project (93)	1988	1. Observation 2. Chemotherapy with 5-FU semustine and vincristine 3. Radiation only	Improved disease-free survival and overall survival in males receiving chemotherapy, but not in females. Decreased locoregional recurrence in the radiation arm, but disease-free survival and overall survival not affected
North Central Cancer Treatment Group (94)	1991	1. Radiation only 2. Systemic chemotherapy with 5-FU and semustine + radiation and chemotherapy	Combination treatment significantly improved disease-free survival and overall survival compared with radiation
GITSG (95)	1992	1. Radiation + 5-FU and semustine 2. Radiation + higher dose 5-FU	The two arms are equivalent. The leukemogenic nitrosourea is not necessary

Note: The overall conclusion is that chemotherapy and radiation interact. The best results are formed with the two together. The next step is to optimize chemotherapy and to establish the value of continuous infusion 5-FU, leucovorin, and levamisole.

of colon cancer. Radiation therapy has been studied extensively because rectal carcinoma has a greater tendency than colon cancer to relapse locally, and because the rectum is a more fixed anatomic structure than the colon. The significant recent trials of adjuvant therapy in rectal cancer have emphasized the combined use of radiation and chemotherapy. Randomized studies comparing no treatment with radiation alone, chemotherapy alone, or with the combination of the two have demonstrated an additive effect of the combination (Table 29.6).

A trial by the Gastrointestinal Tumor Study Group (92) compared postoperative management of rectal carcinoma with radiation therapy alone, chemotherapy alone, or a combination of the two to observation only. The results showed improved disease-free survival and overall survival in all treated groups compared to control, but this was most striking in those receiving combination chemotherapy and radiation. A subsequent trial by the National Surgical Adjuvant Breast Project (93) compared radiation alone or chemotherapy with 5-FU, semustine, and vincristine with observation. There was improved disease-free survival and overall survival in males receiving chemotherapy, but not in females. Radiation only reduced loco-regional recurrences but did not affect disease-free survival or overall survival. The North Central Cancer Treatment Group (94) compared postoperative radiation alone with a program of combined chemotherapy and radiation plus chemotherapy and found an improved disease-free survival and overall survival in those receiving the combination. A second Gastrointestinal Tumor Study Group protocol (95) studied radiation in combination with two chemotherapy regimens: (a) 5-FU plus semustine and (b) 5-FU alone at a dose higher than in the two drug regimen. The results in the two arms were equivalent, indicating that the potentially leukemogenic nitrosourea is not necessary to achieve optimal results. Another intergroup trial that has asked a related question has closed and is undergoing follow-up. It compared bolus or continuous infusion 5-FU plus radiation therapy to bolus 5-FU plus semustine plus radiation therapy in resected rectal carcinoma. Complete analysis of this trial will be very useful in determining the need, if any, for the nitrosoureas in this setting.

Current research in postoperative adjuvant therapy of rectal carcinoma has demonstrated that chemotherapy and radiation interact, and that best results are achieved with the two together. Because research in colon carcinoma has taken a different course historically, it is still not possible to state whether levamisole and leucovorin have an additional role in the adjuvant therapy of rectal cancer. However, a recently closed randomized clinical trial compared standard radiation therapy in combination with four different chemotherapy regimens to address this question. The four arms were 5-FU alone, 5-FU plus levamisole, 5-FU plus leucovorin, and a combination of all three. This study closed in July 1992 and will require several years of follow-up to reach definite conclusions.

Carcinoma of the Anal Canal

Carcinoma of the anal canal includes several histologies, e.g., epidermal, basaloid, and cloacogenic. These are variants of poorly differentiated squamous carcinoma. These tumors are more responsive to chemotherapy and radiation than adenocarcinoma of the colon and rectum, and even bulky lesions may undergo complete regression. For this reason, combined chemotherapy and radiation is now the primary treatment of this disease. For many years, the treatment of carcinoma of the anal canal was abdominoperineal resection. Results using surgery as the only treatment were unsatisfactory with 5-year survival rates of only about 50% (96). Radical radiation was an alternative to this approach and produced 5-year survivals of 18–79% following radiation doses of 45–70 Gy. The introduction of

chemotherapy into the treatment of this disease began with a study by Nigro (97) using an infusion of 5-FU and mitomycin C to reduce tumor size prior to surgery. The combination was 5-FU, 1000 mg/m²/day, for 4 days and mitomycin C, 15 mg/m², as a single bolus, together with 30-Gy external beam radiation. One month later, the 5-FU infusion was repeated and subsequently the patients underwent abdominoperineal resection. The striking finding of the initial report was that six of nine patients were free of tumor at the time of surgery. This suggested that abdominoperineal resection could be avoided if the tumor underwent complete regression with combined chemotherapy and radiation. The criteria for complete regression included a negative biopsy of the residual scar in the anal canal. Several groups have since confirmed this hypothesis (98). The drug doses used in the various 5-FU/mitomycin C trials have been rather constant, but the radiation doses have ranged from 30–50 Gy in different studies. The rate of complete regression of local tumor following combined 5-FU/mitomycin C/radiation therapy treatment is >85% in almost all series, with local control and survival at 3–5 years ranging from 60–90%.

Because mitomycin C produces myelosuppression and occasionally hemolytic-uremic syndrome, some trials have examined radiation and 5-FU alone. The data from pilot studies are not conclusive, but suggest that regimens using only 5-FU in combination with radiation are effective. Preliminary results from an intergroup randomized trial indicate that a regimen of 45 Gy plus concomitant 5-FU infusion, 1000 mg/m²/day, for 4 days was, within statistical limits, as effective as the same regimen with mitomycin C added (99). Thus, mitomycin C may not be an obligatory component of the treatment. In newer trials, some groups are investigating cisplatin, which has cytotoxic effects of its own and is also a radiation sensitizer. It is probable that the emphasis of randomized trials in the next few years will be on determining the relative value of chemotherapy schedules containing

5-FU alone, or in combination with either mitomycin C or cisplatin.

Hepatocellular Carcinoma

Conventional intravenous single agent or combination drug therapy has no proven role in the treatment of hepatocellular carcinoma. This subject has been recently reviewed in detail (100). Some early studies suggested that doxorubicin was effective, but this has not been confirmed in subsequent practice and no standard therapy exists for this disease. One focus of recent efforts has been intra-arterial chemotherapy, given with the intent of shrinking the primary tumor and preventing metastatic spread. In a cohort of 83 patients treated with direct infusion of doxorubicin and cisplatin into the hepatic artery, the response rate was 60% and response was associated with prolonged survival compared with those who did not respond (101). Hepatocellular carcinoma exhibits high-level intrinsic drug resistance and this approach circumvents resistance by increasing the local drug concentration. Modifications of the method include adding the embolizing agent Lipiodol.

SUMMARY

The pharmacologic treatment of gastrointestinal cancer has been intensively studied for >20 years. Some of the significant advances have been in establishing postoperative adjuvant treatment for colon and rectal cancer and in developing multidisciplinary neoadjuvant approaches to esophageal, gastric, and anal canal cancer. In many areas, for example pancreatic cancer, standards of care do not exist, and use of investigational treatments is not only appropriate and ethical, but essential to any kind of progress. Nonetheless, rapidly increasing knowledge of drug resistance and of interactions between tumor and host immune system offer important areas for future research.

REFERENCES

 1. Boring CC, Squires TS, Tong T. Cancer statistics, 1992. CA-A Can J Clin 1992;42:19–39.
 2. Grem JL. Fluoropyrimidines. In: Chabner BA, Collins JM, eds. Pharmacologic principles of cancer treatment. Ed. 2. Philadelphia: Saunders, 1990:180–224.
 3. Johnston PG, Fisher E, Rockette HE, Fisher B, Wolmark N, Allegra CJ. Thymidylate synthase expression is an independent predictor of survival/disease-free survival in patients with rectal cancer. Proc Am Soc Clin Oncol 1993;12:202.
 4. Lenz HJ, Leichman L, Dananberg P, et al. Thymidylate synthase gene expression predicts response of primary gastric cancer to 5-fluorouracil-leucovorin-cisplatin. Proc Am Soc Clin Oncol 1993; 12:199.
 5. Kobayashi K, Schilsky R. Update on biochemical modulation of chemotherapeutic agents. Oncology 1993;7:99–109.
 6. McClean SM, Hill BT. An overview of membrane, cytosolic and nuclear proteins associated with the expression of resistance to multiple drugs in vitro. Biochim Biophys Acta 1992;1114:107–127.
 7. Redmond SMS, Joncourt F, Buser K, et al. Assessment of P-glycoprotein, glutathione-based detoxifying enzymes and O⁶-alkylguanine-DNA alkyltransferase as potential indicators of constitutive drug resistance in human colorectal tumors. Cancer Res 1991;51:2092–2097.
 8. Kramer RA, Zakher J, Kim G. Role of the glutathione redox cycle in acquired and de novo multidrug resistance. Science 1988;241:694–697.
 9. Mekhail-Ishak K, Hudson N, Tsao M-S, Batist G. Implications for therapy of drug-metabolizing enzymes in human colon cancer. Cancer Res 1989;49:4866–4869.
10. Shea TC, Kelley SL, Henner, WD. Identification of an anionic form of glutathione transferase present in many human tumors and human tumor cell lines. Cancer Res 1988;42:527–533.
11. Zlotogroski C, Erickson LC. Pretreatment of human colon tumor cells with DNA methylating agents inhibits their ability to repair chloroethyl monoadducts. Carcinogenesis 1984;5:83–87.
12. Micetich KC, Futscher B, Koch D, Fisher RI, Erickson LC. Phase I study of streptozotocin- and carmustine-sequenced administration in patients with advanced cancer. J Natl Cancer Inst 1992;84:256–260.
13. Giovanella BC, Stehlin JS, Wall MF, et al. DNA topoisomerase-targeted chemotherapy of human colon cancer in xenografts. Science 1989;246:1046–1048.
14. Orringer MB, Forastiere AA, Perez-Tamayo C, Urba S, Takasugi BJ, Bromberg J. Chemotherapy and radiation therapy before transhiatal esophagectomy for esophageal carcinoma. Ann Thorac Surg 1990;49:348–354.
15. MacFarlane SD, Hill LD, Jolly PC, Kozarek RA, Anderson RP. Improved results of surgical treatment for esophageal and gastroesophageal junction carcinomas after preoperative combined chemo-

therapy and radiation. J Thorac Cardiovasc Surg 1988;95:415–422.

16. Hilgenberg AD, Carey RW, Wilkins EW Jr, Choi NC, Mathisen DJ, Grillo HC. Preoperative chemotherapy, surgical resection, and selective postoperative therapy for squamous cell carcinoma of the esophagus. Ann Thorac Surg 1988;45:357–363.

17. Popp MB, Hawley D, Reising J, et al. Improved survival in squamous esophageal cancer. Preoperative chemotherapy and irradiation. Arch Surg 1986;121:1330–1335.

18. Araujo CM, Souhami L, Gil RA, et al. A randomized trial comparing radiation therapy versus concomitant radiation therapy and chemotherapy in carcinoma of the thoracic esophagus. Cancer 1991;67:2258–2261.

19. Seydel HG, Leichman L, Byhardt R, et al. Preoperative radiation and chemotherapy for localized squamous cell carcinoma of the esophagus: a RTOG Study. Int J Rad Oncol Biol Phys 1988;14:33–35.

20. Kelsen DP, Minsky B, Smith M, et al. Preoperative therapy for esophageal cancer: a randomized comparison of chemotherapy versus radiation therapy. J Clin Oncol 1990;8:1352–1361.

21. Roth JA, Pass HI, Flanagan MM, Graeber GM, Rosenberg JC, Steinberg S. Randomized clinical trial of preoperative and postoperative adjuvant chemotherapy with cisplatin, vindesine, and bleomycin for carcinoma of the esophagus. J Thorac Cardiovasc Surg 1988;96:242–248.

22. Urba SG, Orringer MB, Perez-Tamayo C, Bromberg J, Forastiere A. Concurrent preoperative chemotherapy and radiation therapy in localized esophageal adenocarcinoma. Cancer 1992;69:285–291.

23. Carey RW, Hilgenberg AD, Choi NC, et al. A pilot study of neoadjuvant chemotherapy with 5-fluorouracil and cisplatin with surgical resection and postoperative radiation therapy and/or chemotherapy in adenocarcinoma of the esophagus. Cancer 1991;68:489–492.

24. Coia LR, Paul AR, Engstrom PF. Combined radiation and chemotherapy as primary management of adenocarcinoma of the esophagus and gastroesophageal junction. Cancer 1988;61:643–649.

25. Ajani JA, Roth JA, Ryan B, et al. Evaluation of pre- and postoperative chemotherapy for resectable adenocarcinoma of the esophagus or gastroesophageal junction. J Clin Oncol 1990;8:1231–1238.

26. Herskovic A, Martz K, al-Sarraf M, et al. Combined chemotherapy and radiotherapy compared with radiotherapy alone in patients with cancer of the esophagus N Engl J Med 1992;326:1593–1598.

27. Kovach JS, Moertel CG, Schutt AJ. A controlled study of combined 1,3-bis-2-chloroethyl-1-nitrosourea and 5-fluorouracil therapy for advanced gastric and pancreatic cancer. Cancer 1974;33:563–567.

28. Moertel CG, Mittelman JA, Bakemeier RF, Engstrom P, Hanely J. Sequential and combination chemotherapy of advanced gastric cancer. Cancer 1976;38:678–685.

29. Macdonald JS, Schein PS, Woolley PV, et al. 5-Fluorouracil, doxorubicin, and mitomycin (FAM) combination for advanced gastric cancer. Ann Intern Med 1980;93:533–536.

30. Panettiere FJ, Haas C, McDonald B, et al. Drug combinations in the treatment of gastric adenocarcinoma: a randomized Southwest Oncology Group Study. J Clin Oncol 1984;2:420–424.

31. Douglass H, Lavin P, Goudsmit A, et al. An Eastern Cooperative Oncology Group evaluation of combinations of methyl-CCNU, mitomycin C, adriamycin and 5-fluorouracil in advanced measurable gastric cancer (EST 2277). J Clin Oncol 1984;2:1372–1381.

32. Gisselbrecht C, Smith FP, Macdonald JS, et al. The effect of sequential addition of the nitrosourea, chlorozotocin, to the FAM combination in advanced gastric cancer. Cancer 1983;51:1792–1794.

33. Cazap E, Gisselbrecht C, Smith FP, et al. Phase II trials of 5-fluorouracil, doxorubicin and cisplatin (FAP) in advanced, measurable adenocarcinoma of lung and stomach. Cancer Treat Rep 1986;70:781–783.

34. Ahlgren JD, Smith FP, Cazap E, et al. FAM (5-fluorouracil, doxorubicin and mitomycin-C) plus triazinate (FAM-T) in gastric carcinoma: a combined phase II trial of the Mid-Atlantic Oncology Program and the Pan American Health Organization. Cancer Treat Rep 1987;71:419–420.

35. The Gastrointestinal Study Group: Phase II–III chemotherapy studies in advanced gastric cancer. Cancer Treat Rep 1979;63:1871–1876.

36. The Gastrointestinal Tumor Study Group. A comparative clinical assessment of combination chemotherapy in the management of advanced gastric carcinoma. Cancer 1982;49:1362–1366.

37. Levi J, Fox R, Tattersall M, et al. Analysis of a prospectively randomized comparison of doxorubicin versus 5-fluorouracil, doxorubicin and BCNU in advanced gastric cancer: implications for future studies. J Clin Oncol 1986;4:1348–1355.

38. Cullinan S, Moertel CG, Thomas MD, et al. Comparison of three chemotherapeutic regimens in the treatment of advanced pancreatic and gastric carcinoma. JAMA 1985;253:2061–2067.

39. The Gastrointestinal Tumor Study Group. Triazinate and platinum efficacy in combination with 5-fluorouracil and doxorubicin: results of a three-arm randomized trial in metastatic gastric cancer. J Natl Cancer Inst 1988;80:1011–1015.

40. Cullinan S, Moertel C, Wieand H, Poon M. A randomized comparison of fluorouracil + adriamycin + cisplatin (FAP), fluorouracil + adriamycin + semustine (FAMe), FAMe alternating with triazinate and fluorouracil alone in advanced gastric cancer. A

North Central Oncology Group Study. Proc Am Soc Clin Oncol 1993;12:200.

41. Preusser P, Wilke H, Achterrath W, et al. Phase II study with the combination etoposide, doxorubicin and cisplatin in advanced, measurable gastric cancer. J Clin Oncol 1989;7:1310–1317.

42. Lerner A, Gonin R, Steele GD Jr, Mayer RJ. Etoposide, doxorubicin, and cisplatin chemotherapy for advanced gastric adenocarcinoma: results of a phase II trial. J Clin Oncol 1992;10:536–540.

43. Cadman E, Heimer R, Davis L. Enhanced 5-fluorouracil nucleotide formation after methotrexate administration: explanation for drug synergism. Science 1979;205:1135–1137.

44. Klein HO, Dias W, Dieterle F, et al. Chemotherapieprotokoll zur Behandlung des Metastasierenden Magenkarzinoms: Methotrexate, Adriamycin und 5-Fluorouracil. Dtsch Med Wochenshcr 1982;107:1708–1712.

45. Wils J, Bleiberg H, Dalesio O, et al. An EORTC Gastrointestinal Group evaluation of the combination of sequential methotrexate and 5-fluorouracil combined with adriamycin (FAMTX) in advanced measurable gastric cancer. J Clin Oncol 1986;4:1799–1803.

46. Wils JA, Klein HO, Wagener DJ, et al. Sequential high-dose methotrexate and fluorouracil combined with doxorubicin—a step ahead in the treatment of advanced gastric cancer: a trial of the European Organization for Research and Treatment of Cancer Gastrointestinal Tract Cooperative Group. J Clin Oncol 1991;9:827–831.

47. Dickinson R, Presgrave P, Levi J, Milliken S, Woods R. Sequential moderate-dose methotrexate and 5-fluorouracil in advanced gastric adenocarcinoma. Cancer Chemother Pharmacol 1989;24:67–68.

48. Kelsen D, Atiq OT, Saltz L, et al. FAMTX versus etoposide, doxorubicin and cisplatin: a random assignment trial in gastric cancer. J Clin Oncol 1992;10:541–548.

49. Gunderson LL, Sosin H. Adenocarcinoma of the stomach-areas of failure in a reoperation series (second or symptomatic looks). Clinicopathologic correlation and implications for adjuvant therapy. Int J Radiat Oncol Biol Phys 1982;8:1–11.

50. Moertel CG, Childs DS, Reitemeier RJ, Colby MJ, Holbrook MA. Combined 5-fluorouracil and supravoltage radiation therapy of locally unresectable gastrointestinal cancer. Lancet 1969;2:865–867.

51. Gastrointestinal Tumor Study Group. A comparison of combination chemotherapy and combined modality therapy for locally advanced gastric carcinoma. Cancer 1982;49:1771–1777.

52. Smith FP, Stablein D, Korsmeyer S, et al. Combination chemotherapy for locally advanced pancreatic cancer: equivalence to external beam radiation and implication for future management. J Clin Oncol 1983;1:413–415.

53. Haas CD, Mansfield CM, Leichman LP, Considine LP, Considine B, Bukowski RM. Combined nonsimultaneous radiation therapy and chemotherapy with 5-FU, doxorubicin, and mitomycin for residual localized gastric adenocarcinoma: a Southwest Oncology Group Pilot Study. Cancer Treat Rep 1983;67:421–424.

54. O'Connell MJ, Gunderson LL, Moertel CG, Kvols LK. A pilot study to determine clinical tolerability of intensive combined modality therapy for locally unresectable gastric cancer. Int J Rad Oncol Biol Phys 1985;11:1827–1831.

55. Leichman L, Silberman H, Leichman CG, et al. Preoperative systemic chemotherapy followed by adjuvant postoperative intraperitoneal therapy for gastric cancer: a University of Southern California Pilot Program. J Clin Oncol 1992;10:1933–1942.

56. Alexander HR, Grem JL, Pass HI, et al. Neoadjuvant chemotherapy for locally advanced gastric adenocarcinoma. Oncology 1993;7:37–42.

57. Ajani J, Ota DM, Jackson DE. Current strategies in the management of locoregional and metastatic gastric carcinoma. Cancer 1991;67:260–265.

58. Wilke H, Preusser P, Fink U, et al. Preoperative chemotherapy in locally advanced and nonresectable gastric cancer: a phase II study with etoposide, doxorubicin, and cisplatin. J Clin Oncol 1989;7:1318–1326.

59. Bleiberg H, Gerard B, Deguiral P. Adjuvant therapy in gastric cancer. Br J Cancer 1992;66:987–991.

60. The Gastrointestinal Tumor Studyd Group. Controlled trial of adjuvant chemotherapy following curative resection for gastric cancer. Cancer 1982;49:1116–1122.

61. Higgins GA, Amadeo JH, Smith DE, Humphrey EW, Keehn RJ. Efficacy of prolonged intermittent therapy with combined 5-FU and methyl-CCNU following resection for gastric carcinoma. Cancer 1983;52:1105–1112.

62. Engstrom P, Lavin P, Douglass HO, Brunner KW. Postoperative adjuvant 5-fluorouracil plus methyl-CCNU therapy for gastric cancer patients. Eastern Cooperative Oncology Group Study (EST 3275). Cancer 1985;55:1868–1873.

63. Schlag, P. Adjuvant therapy in gastric cancer. World J Surg 1987;11:473–477.

64. Coombes RC, Schein PS, Chilvers CE, et al. A randomized trial comparing adjuvant fluorouracil, doxorubicin, and mitomycin with no treatment in operable gastric cancer: International Collaborative Cancer Group. J Clin Oncol 1990;8:1362–1369.

65. Krook JE, O'Connell MJ, Wieand HS, et al. A prospective, randomized evaluation of intensive-course 5-fluorouracil plus doxorubicin as surgical adjuvant chemotherapy for resected gastric cancer. Cancer 1991;67:2454–2458.

66. Arbuck, SG. Overview of chemotherapy for pancreatic cancer. Int J Pancreatol 1990;7:209–222.

67. Gastrointestinal Study Group. Phase II studies of drug combinations in advanced pancreatic carcinoma: fluorouracil plus doxorubicin plus mitomycin C and two regimens of streptozotocin plus mitomycin C plus fluorouracil. J Clin Oncol 1986;4:1794–1798.

68. DeCaprio JA, Mayer RJ, Gonin R, Arbuck SG. Fluorouracil and high-dose leucovorin in previously untreated patients with advanced adenocarcinoma of the pancreas: results of a phase II trial. J Clin Oncol 1991;9:2128–2133.

69. DeLap R, Marshall J, Woolley P, Richmond E, Bodurian E, King D. Leucovorin, fluorouracil and iododeoxyuridine (LIF): a phase I study in patients with advanced cancer. Proc Am Soc Clin Oncol 1993;12:221.

70. Moertel CG, Frytak S, Hahn RG, et al. Therapy of locally unresectable pancreatic carcinoma: a randomized comparison of high dose (6000 rads) radiation alone, moderate dose radiation (4000 rads + 5-fluorouracil) and high dose radiation + 5-fluorouracil. Cancer 1981;48:1705–1710.

71. Gastrointestinal Tumor Study Group. Treatment of locally unresectable carcinoma of the pancreas: comparison of combined-modality therapy (chemotherapy plus radiotherapy) to chemotherapy alone. J Natl Cancer Inst 1988;80:751–755.

72. Gastrointestinal Tumor Study Group. Further evidence of effective adjuvant combined radiation and chemotherapy following curative resection of pancreatic cancer. Cancer 1987;59:2006–2010.

73. Moertel CG, Hanley JA, Johnson LA. Streptozotocin alone compared with streptozotocin plus 5-fluorouracil in the treatment of advanced islet cell carcinoma. N Engl J Med 1980;303:1189–1194.

74. Moertel CG, Lefkopoulo M, Lipsitz S, Hahn RG, Klaassen D. Streptozocin-doxorubicin, streptozocin-fluorouracil or chlorozotocin in the treatment of advanced islet-cell carcinoma. N Engl J Med 1992;326:519–523.

75. Moertel CG, Kvols LK, O'Connell MJ, Rubin J. Treatment of neuroendocrine carcinomas with combined etoposide and cisplatin: evidence of major therapeutic activity in the anaplastic variants of these neoplasms. Cancer 1991;68:227–232.

76. Ansfield R, Klotz J, Nealon T, et al. A phase III study comparing the clinical utility of four regimens of 5-fluorouracil. Cancer 1977;39:34–40.

77. Lavin P, Mittelman A, Douglass H, Engstrom P, Klaasen D. Survival and response to chemotherapy for advanced colorectal adenocarcinoma: an Eastern Cooperative Oncology Group Report. Cancer 1980;46:1536–1540.

78. Engstrom PF, MacIntyre JM, Mittelman A, Klaasen DJ. Chemotherapy of advanced colorectal cancer: fluorouracil vs. two drug combinations using fluorouracil, hydroxyurea, semustine, dacarbazine, razoxane and mitomycin. A phase III trial by the Eastern Cooperative Oncology Group. Am J Clin Oncol 1984;7:313–318.

79. Richards F, Case LD, White DR, et al. Combination chemotherapy (5-fluorouracil, methyl-CCNU, mitomycin C) versus 5-fluorouracil alone for previously untreated colorectal carcinoma. A phase III study of the Piedmont Oncology Association. J Clin Oncol 1986;4:565–570.

80. Windschitl H, Scott M, Schutt A, et al. Randomized phase II studies in advanced colorectal carcinoma: a North Central Cancer Treatment Group Study. Cancer Treat Rep 1983;67:1001–1008.

81. Lokich JJ, Ahlgren JD, Gullo JJ, Philips JA, Fryer JG. A prospective randomized comparison of continuous infusion fluorouracil with a conventional bolus schedule in metastatic colorectal carcinoma: a Mid-Atlantic Oncology Program Study. J Clin Oncol 1989;7:425–432.

82. Poon MA, O'Connell M, Moertel CG, et al. Biochemical modulation of fluorouracil: evidence of significant improvement of survival and quality of life in patients with advanced colorectal carcinoma. J Clin Oncol 1989;7:1407–1417.

83. Petrelli N, Douglass HO, Herrera L, et al. The modulation of fluorouracil with leucovorin in metastatic colorectal carcinoma: a prospective randomized phase III trial. J Clin Oncol 1989;7:1419–1426.

84. The Advanced Colorectal Cancer Meta-Analysis Project. Modulation of fluorouracil by leucovorin in patients with advanced colorectal cancer: evidence in terms of response rate. J Clin Oncol 1992;10:896–903.

85. York M, Greco FA, Figlin RA, et al. A randomized phase III trial comparing 5-FU with or without interferon alfa 2a for advanced colorectal cancer. Proc Am Soc Clin Oncol 1993;12:200.

86. Kocha, W. 5-Fluorouracil plus interferon alfa-2a (Roferon-A) versus 5-fluorouracil plus leucovorin in metastatic colorectal cancer: results of a multicentre, multinational phase III study. Proc Am Soc Clin Oncol 1993;12:193.

87. Buyse M, Zeleniuch- Jacquotte A, Chalmers TC. Adjuvant therapy of colon cancer: why we still don't know. JAMA 1988;259:3571–3578.

88. Higgins GA Jr, Amadeo JH, McElhinney J, McCaughan JJ, Keehn RJ. Efficacy of prolonged intermittent therapy with combined 5-fluorouracil and methyl CCNU following resection for carcinoma of the large bowel: a Veterans Administration Surgical Oncology Group Report. Cancer 1984;53:1–8.

89. Gastrointestinal Tumor Study Group. Adjuvant therapy of colon cancer: results of a prospectively randomized trial. N Engl J Med 1984;310:737–743.

90. Panettiere FJ, Goodman PJ, Costanzi JJ, et al. Adjuvant therapy in large bowel carcinoma: long-term results of a Southwest Oncology Group Study. J Clin Oncol 1988;6:947–954.

91. Moertel CG, Fleming TR, Macdonald JS, et al. Levamisole and fluorouracil for adjuvant therapy of

resected colon carcinoma. N Engl J Med 1990;322:352–358.

92. Gastrointestinal Tumor Study Group. Prolongation of the disease-free interval in surgically treated rectal carcinoma. N Engl J Med 1985;312:1465–1472.

93. Fisher B, Wolmark N, Rockette H, et al. Postoperative adjuvant chemotherapy or radiation for rectal cancer: results from NSABP Protocol R-01. J Natl Cancer Inst 1988;80:21–29.

94. Krook JE, Moertel CG, Gunderson LL, et al. Effective adjuvant therapy for high-risk rectal carcinoma. N Engl J Med 1991;324:709–715.

95. Gastrointestinal Tumor Study Group. Radiation therapy and fluorouracil with or without semustine for the treatment of patients with surgical adjuvant adenocarcinoma of the rectum. J Clin Oncol 1992;10:549–557.

96. Gordon PH. Current status-perianal and anal canal neoplasms. Dis Colon Rectum 1990;33:799–808.

97. Nigro, ND. An evaluation of combined therapy for squamous cell cancer of the anal canal. Dis Colon Rectum 1984;27:763–766.

98. Cummings BJ. Anal Cancer. Int J Rad Oncol Biol Phys 1990;19:1309–1315.

99. Flam MS, John MJ, Peters T, et al. Radiation and 5-fluorouracil vs radiation, 5-fluorouracil, mitomycin C in the treatment of anal canal carcinoma: preliminary results of a phase III randomized RTOG/ECOG Intergroup Trial. Proc Am Soc Clin Oncol 1993;12:557.

100. Lotze MT, Flickinger JC, Carr BI. Hepatobiliary neoplasms. In: DeVita VT, Hellman S, Rosenberg SA, eds. Cancer: principles and practice of oncology. Ed. 4. Philadelphia: Lipincott, 1993:883–914.

101. Carr BI, Iwatsuki S, Starzl TE, Selby R, Madariaga J. Regional cancer chemotherapy for advanced stage hepatocellular carcinoma. J Surg Oncol Suppl 1993;3:100–103.

30

Medical-Legal Aspects of Gastrointestinal Therapeutics

PETER A. PLUMERI

A physician may be held liable for failure to use appropriate drug therapy if the treatment of the patient falls below a reasonable standard of care. Any administration or prescription of drug therapy may precipitate a wide range of adverse effects. The general rules that govern liability for medical malpractice also apply to cases involving harmful reactions and interactions arising from drugs administered and prescribed. Similarly, pharmacists are increasingly being held to expanded clinical and dispensing functions and therefore increasing liability.

The goals of this chapter are to review several issues involving the medical-legal aspects of gastrointestinal therapeutics in order to develop a more knowledgeable and sensible approach for practicing physician-gastroenterologists, as well as for pharmacists. The Harvard Medical Practice Studies (1–3) reveal that 3.7% of hospitalizations result in an adverse event. Of these adverse events, approximately 27% are the result of negligence. Drug complications are the most common type of adverse events, representing 19% of the cases. Inasmuch as drug therapy often leads to untoward complications that result in malpractice action, several risk management strategies pertinent to drug-related malpractice will be discussed.

INTRODUCTION TO TORT LAW: MALPRACTICE DEFINED

Medical malpractice or negligence falls in the area of law known as torts. This is the area of civil wrongs. Civil wrongs are distinguished from criminal wrongs in two major respects.

First, the burden of proof is less (preponderance of the evidence versus beyond a reasonable doubt). Second, the punishment is less severe (monetary damages versus possible incarceration).

The plaintiff (the patient) must prove four essential elements in a negligence action against the defendant (the doctor) in order to prevail (4). These elements include the following: (a) A duty; (b) A breach of duty; (c) Proximate causation; and, (d) Damages.

DUTY

A legal duty is generally created through the physician-patient relationship. Typically, the relationship is created by an office visit, the performance of a consultation or the carrying out of a procedure. A duty may be created in circumstances when the physician never sees the patient. For example, a patient who is schedule to have a colonoscopy has a 95% obstruction of the sigmoid colon secondary to diverticular disease. He is given a prescription by a gastroenterologist's staff by telephone for

615

a 4-1 balanced electrolyte preparation, to be taken on the evening before the procedure. He sustains injuries by the precipitation of a complete colon obstruction as a result of using the electrolyte lavage solution. Even though the physician never saw the patient before the injury, a legal duty exists.

There are several unique duties relative to drug administration and prescriptions. These include the duty to warn, the learned intermediary doctrine, the duty to instruct, the duty to use the least dangerous drug, the duty to take an adequate history, and the duty to observe and monitor.

Duty to Warn

Generally courts have established a legal duty for physicians to warn patients of potential risks or reactions before administering or prescribing medications. For example, in Foley v. United States (5) the plaintiff was given medication to treat peptic ulcer disease and to induce sleep. The medication caused an exfoliative dermatitis, which precipitated latent depigmentation. The plaintiff's skin color was changed from black to white. The court stated that the physician was obligated to warn the patient of potentially harmful reactions when administering or prescribing a medication.

Arguments supporting the duty to warn include the patient's right to know the potential consequences of drug therapy, the increased likelihood of detecting adverse consequences, and enhanced patient compliance.

The physician's duty to warn patients about adverse drug consequences is further compounded by the pharmacist's duty to warn (6). A few recent cases are illustrative.

In Riff v. Morgan (7), the physician prescribed an ergotamine preparation for migraine headache. The physician did not warn the plaintiff of the potential adverse effects of this drug. The plaintiff subsequently had the prescription refilled four times by the defendant pharmacist. There was no authorization for the refills. The pharmacist also did not warn the plaintiff of the potential adverse effects. The plaintiff suffered permanent injuries as a result of the toxic properties

of ergotamine. Both the physician and pharmacist were found liable for prescribing and dispensing a potentially toxic and dangerous drug without instructions and warnings, respectively.

In Dooley v. Everett (8), the court found a pharmacist liable for failing to warn the patient of the risk of a drug interaction between theophylline and erythromycin. The pharmacist dispensed erythromycin to a child, who was already maintained on theophylline. The pharmacist has a duty to warn either the patient or the physician of foreseeable adverse effects.

Other recent cases (9–11), however, have held that a pharmacist has no duty to warn. Jurisdictions differ in their applicable legal standards and each practitioner needs to review the law in his or her place of practice.

As a practical matter, a practicing gastroenterologist must be mindful not only of his or her duty to warn the patient of potential adverse drug effects, but also that similar duty of the pharmacist exists (see below). In view of the complexities of their respective legal duties involved, the gastroenterologist needs to work cohesively with the pharmacist to minimize legal exposure.

Learned Intermediary Rule

The concept of the learned intermediary rule is applicable in most jurisdictions. It proposes that a pharmaceutical manufacturer discharges its duty to warn the ultimate user of its prescription drugs by supplying the physician with information about the dangerous propensities of its products (12). The physician acts as the intermediary between the manufacturer and the consumer. As such, the physician then has an independent duty to warn the patient of the inherent risks of the medication prescribed.

This rule has notable exceptions. When over-the-counter drugs are at issue, the manufacturer must give warnings directly to the consumer (13). Another example is that related to mass immunization programs. In Davis v. Wyeth Laboratories, Inc. (14), the manufacturer was held to have an independent duty to the consumer to warn. In this polio vaccination clinic there was no physician available to weigh the benefits and risks of treatment for each individual patient. Finally, in the case of oral contraceptives, the manufacturer must directly warn the consumer of risks. This warning is dependent on the consumer's involvement in the decision making process (15, 16).

Understanding the nature of the learned intermediary rule, the practicing gastroenterologist should view the manufacturer's information in a new light. The drug package insert is the principle means by which the manufacturer supplies the physician with information regarding its products' dangerous propensities. The insert, for the most part, effectively shifts the duty to warn the patient from the manufacturer to the physician. Although the package insert is considered "informational" by the Food, Drug and Cosmetic Act, it along with other communications from the manufacturer represents the labeling of the product. The insert and other communications serve to set the standard of care regarding a given product. Depending on the rules of evidence in effect, jurisdictions may allow the package insert to be admitted as an indicator of the applicable standard of care. The practicing gastroenterologist is best served by an awareness of the contents of the insert so that adequate warnings may be passed on to the patient. Such practice will satisfy the physician's duty to warn and will minimize malpractice risk.

Duty to Instruct

Physicians have a duty to instruct patients on drug usage. Instructions are necessary to assure the proper use of medication. In particular, warnings must be considered when prescribed drugs have known interactions with alcohol. In Kirk v. Michael Reese Hospital and Medical Center (17), the court found the physician liable for failing to instruct the patient on the effect of combining the prescribed drug with alcohol. Gastroenterologists should be careful to instruct the patient when prescribing medications such as metronidazole,

which has a well-known interaction with alcohol. (See Chapter 27 for a discussion of H_2-receptor antagonists and alcohol.)

Duty to Choose the Least Dangerous Drug

Physicians have a duty to use the least dangerous drug available to treat a patient's condition. The physician must balance the risks and benefits of the drug to the patient in making his or her selection (15).

In Marchese v. Monaco (16), the court held the physician liable for failing to use the least harmful drug. The patient was treated with neomycin injections which led to permanent hearing loss. Although the defendant could have used a safer antibiotic, he failed to do so. He failed to exercise reasonable care. This principle must be kept in mind when making pharmaceutical decisions.

Duty to Take an Adequate History

It is standard medical practice for the physician to obtain the patient's history before prescribing or administering drug therapy. Courts have also recognized the physician's legal duty to take a complete medical history. It is therefore incumbent upon the physician to inquire about past drug reactions or interactions, allergies, prior and present drug use (prescription, over-the-counter, and illicit), and the family history regarding adverse effects to drugs.

In Yorston v. Pennell (20), the patient was hospitalized for the treatment of a fractured leg. He reportedly told his physician of his penicillin allergy. This information was not recorded in the patient's written history. Although the chart contained a notation regarding the penicillin allergy, he was prescribed penicillin and suffered an adverse reaction. The court found the physician liable.

The failure to take an adequate history is a common shortcoming in medical malpractice litigation. It is critical for practicing gastroenterologists to take the time and expend the effort in obtaining an adequate history, particularly in the area of pharmaceutical use.

Careful history taking should prevent drug morbidity and mortality to a significant degree.

Duty to Observe and Monitor

Courts have recognized a physician's duty to observe the patient after the administration of a potentially dangerous drug so that reactions and complications may be promptly treated. During the course of an upper endoscopy the plaintiff complained repeatedly of pain and burning in his hand. At the completion of the procedure it was discovered that the hand with the intravenous line was swollen and edematous. The extravasation of diazepam led to an injury, which was only partially repaired by a surgical procedure. The court stated that the site should have been observed and inspected at the time of the patient's complaints (21).

Physicians who administer sedatives or narcotics in an outpatient setting must observe the patient for an appropriate period of time afterward. The early intravenous use of the benzodiazepine, midazolam, was implicated in the deaths of 81 patients (22). Most of the patients were elderly, and most of the deaths were related to cardiopulmonary complications. These occurrences precipitated an enhanced need to observe sedated patients (see Chapter 28).

The American Society of Gastrointestinal Endoscopy (ASGE) states, "Standard clinical monitoring for all sedated patients should include the determination of heart rate, blood pressure, and respiratory rate of the patient before sedation, immediately after the procedure, and at the time of discharge from the endoscopy area." Postprocedure comment includes the statement that "All patients receiving parental sedation should be given written instructions regarding the resumption of eating, medications and activities in addition to instructions on what to do if a complication develops." The role of continuous electrocardiographic monitoring and pulse oximetry remain controversial according to the ASGE (23). From a common sense legal perspective, there seems to be no reason to exclude these mechanical monitoring devices when using intravenous sedation.

Inasmuch as a major risk of conscious sedation is cardiopulmonary arrest, practicing gastroenterologists should be familiar with resuscitative techniques. This familiarity would include not only the mechanical aspects of intubation, chest compression, etc., but also the recognition of the pharmacology of effective resuscitation. Standards such as the certification in advanced cardiopulmonary life support (ACLS) would be useful benchmarks. Suffice it to say that the inability to resuscitate a patient, who has reacted adversely to conscious sedation, would likely prove detrimental in litigation.

Because most practicing gastroenterologists use intravenous sedation, the duty to observe and monitor these patient must be clearly understood. In the case of midazolam, it may be necessary to observe a patient's respiratory status for at least 2 hours (24). Steps taken on the part of the gastroenterologist to satisfy his or her duty to observe patients postsedation are effective risk management strategies.

BREACH OF DUTY

The element of "breach of duty" is a critical one for the gastroenterologist to comprehend. To prove this element, the plaintiff's attorney must show that the practice at issue deviated from a reasonable standard of care. A reasonable standard of care is considered to be good medical practice. It could be defined by traditional medical teachings, treatises, textbooks, and journal articles. The standard of care is not necessarily a singular practice or principle. The standard of care regarding prescribing and/or administering drugs requires that the physician obtain knowledge about the medication before its use.

The standard of care must be established in medical malpractice cases, especially in one involving a drug issue, by expert witnesses. The plaintiff's expert witness will attempt to show that the care rendered by the defendant fell below the standard of care. However, the defendant's expert will attempt to show that the care rendered met reasonable standards of practice. The jury, which is not usually competent to define a reasonable standard of care on its own, will evaluate the testimony of the experts (and other testimony) in defining the applicable standard of care (25).

In Incollingo v. Ewing (26), a child had been treated by a pediatrician several times in the past with chloramphenicol. At a later time, the child developed a respiratory infection. The child's mother requested another prescription for chloramphenical from the pediatrician. The request was denied. The mother obtained the prescription from her own physician. Several months later the child was diagnosed with aplastic anemia. The Supreme Court of Pennsylvania held that it was a jury question as to whether the physician's conduct fell below a reasonable standard of care.

Regarding pharmaceutical knowledge, physicians rely to a significant extent on the representations of the manufacturer in developing a reasonable standard of practice. This is both sensible and practical. If the physician chooses to ignore such information, the risks of malpractice increase. In Formella v. Ceiba-Geigy (27), the plaintiff alleged she was injured by oxyphenylbutazone. The physician testified that he had read *Physicians' Desk Reference* (PDR) the first time he used the drug, but not thereafter. The court concluded that the physician was negligent in assuming the drug was safe.

Depending on the jurisdiction, the PDR, drug treatises, pharmaceutical textbooks, journal articles, clinical studies, and other forms of "evidence" may or may not be entered to establish the standard of care. They may be considered hearsay and hence inadmissible (28, 29). In those jurisdictions prohibiting use of these materials as evidence, an expert witness may testify as to whether he or she agrees with the information in question or whether he or she considers it authoritative, but the contents may not be discussed.

The standard of care for a specialist such as a gastroenterologist is always national. The standard of care is also dynamic. Fast-paced and continual medical progress changes the applicable standard of care. The drug miso-

prostol is illustrative. According to its package insert, cotherapy with a nonsteroidal anti-inflammatory drug (NSAID) is indicated for the prevention of NSAID-induced gastric ulcers in patients who are considered to be at risk. These patients include the elderly, those with debilitating illnesses and those with a past history of ulcer disease (30).

In terms of practicing within a reasonable standard of care, does the physician ordering an NSAID without misoprostol cotherapy fail to meet it? Does the answer change if the patient is at "high risk"?

In reviewing the myriad medical, pharmacologic and legal issues surrounding misoprostol, this author concluded that a reasonable standard of care included the use of this agent in "high risk" patients receiving NSAID (31).

Walt in his recent review of misoprostol states,

> ". . . there is no convincing evidence to support the use of misoprostol cotherapy in any particular group of patients, including the elderly or these with a history of gastric or duodenal ulcer. Cotherapy has not been demonstrated to decrease rates of hospitalization, gastrointestinal bleeding or death. In practical terms, the excess risk associated with NSAID therapy can be countered only by stopping the NSAID. When this is not sensible, a full explanation of the risks and the evidence in favor of any cotherapy is required" (32).

In reconciling these different approaches (keeping in mind that the standard of care allows different therapies or solutions for the same problem), it appears that the failure to offer misoprostol cotherapy to a low-risk NSAID patient does not fall below a reasonable standard of care. With respect to the "high risk" patient, a prudent approach would allow the patient the option of misoprostol cotherapy after he or she is given sufficient information to make an informed decision.

Off-Label Drug Use

Many physicians choose to use a pharmaceutical product for unapproved indications or in unapproved dosage regimens. Although these actions are not illegal per se, they do put the physician in a precarious position regarding the standard of care. If a patient sustains damages as a result of such use, the plaintiff's attorney will undoubtedly attempt to establish liability on the part of the physician for not using the product in an indicated or approved manner. If another product is approved and available and has not been offered, the argument becomes more compelling.

For example, in treating inflammatory bowel disease, immunosuppressives ought not to be the first drug choice. Inasmuch as several other approved drug alternatives exist (33), they should be tried first. If the case is particularly vexing and unresponsive, immunosuppressives may become a reasonable option. When using an agent in an unapproved manner, the informed consent of the patient should be obtained (see below).

Black Box Warnings

The black box warning should be familiar to all practicing physicians and pharmacists. The Food and Drug Administration may require a manufacturer to highlight or stress certain warnings or precautions about its product in its drug information materials including the package insert. These special warnings are placed in a black box in bold black print.

When using a drug with a black box warning, a physician must understand that practice contrary to the black box prohibition is viewed as practice below reasonable standards of care. For example, the use of omeprazole as maintenance therapy for gastroesophageal reflux disease (34) or the use of misoprostol in pregnant women (30) is inappropriate. Further, intravenous midazolam should be used in settings that provide continuous monitoring of respiratory and cardiac function (35). In the event that a drug is used contrary to a black box warning, the patient's informed consent is essential (see below).

Informed Consent

The process of informed consent requires the interaction of the physician and patient in medical decision making. The essential elements of disclosure, which must be defined by the physician are the nature of the proposed treatment, its benefits, its risks, and its alternatives (36–38). Regarding drug therapy, jurisdictions vary as to their application of the informed consent process.

In Boyer v. Smith (39), the plaintiff was given phenylbutazone for back pain. The physician told the plaintiff about the associated risks of gastrointestinal ulcers, but no other risks. The plaintiff sustained a severe drug reaction (not an ulcer), which resulted in a 3-week hospitalization. In this case the court held that the doctrine of informed consent should not be expanded to include therapeutic drugs.

An opposite conclusion was reached in Niemera v. Schneider (40). The court ruled that the physician was obligated to inform the plaintiff of the risks of a DPT vaccination. He did not adequately warn the plaintiff of the risks of the dangerous side effect of seizure. Further, the court opined, this information would have helped the plaintiff recognize early signs of the risk and the gravity of the situation.

It is important for the practicing gastroenterologist to know the applicable standard in his or her jurisdiction. A prudent policy is to offer the patient sufficient information to meet the informed consent policy as a routine practice. Certain drugs appear to have a high potential of leading to litigation. Among the commonly used gastroenterologic drugs, the corticosteroid preparations are the most problematic. Corticosteroids are commonly used in inflammatory bowel disease and chronic liver disease. When using corticosteroids, the practicing gastroenterologist should obtain the patient's informed consent as a routine practice. A few cases are illustrative.

In United States v. Niblack (41), dexamethasone was used in decreasing doses over a 2-month period to treat the plaintiff's elevated intracranial pressure. He was suffering from pseudotumor cerebri and a sixth nerve palsy. He sustained aseptic necrosis of the hip as a result of the steroid treatment. In ruling that the defendant was not negligent, the court said that the plaintiff had been warned of the risks of dexamethasone (although not specifically of aseptic necrosis of the hip). The court delineated that the drug was indicated for the plaintiff's serious medical condition. It noted that aseptic necrosis was 1 of 50 potential side effects of corticosteroid therapy.

In Buckner v. Allergan Pharmaceuticals, Inc. (42), the court held that the manufacturer of a corticosteroid preparation had no duty to warn the ultimate consumer of the product of its risks. The court rejected the plaintiff's claim that the manufacturer had a duty to warn him of the risks of corticosteroid use. The court said that the manufacturer had a duty to warn the medical professional who prescribes, dispenses, or administers the product. The responsibility of warning and informing the patient was placed on the physician.

In Leyson v. Steuerman (43), the court held that the informed consent process was sufficient. It denied the plaintiff's claim for damages that resulted from the use of corticosteroids for the treatment of psoriasis. Although there was some issue as to whether the plaintiff had been informed of the risks of the drug before his first course of therapy, the court found the evidence sufficient that he had been informed during subsequent courses of treatment.

In Precourt v. Frederick (44), the trial court found an ophthalmologist liable for $1 million in damages. The damages were the result of aseptic necrosis of both hips related to corticosteroid treatment. The Massachusetts Supreme Judicial Court held that the verdict should be reversed in favor of the physician. If appears that the court believed that "the risk of aseptic necrosis was too remote to have required disclosure and culpability to the tune of $1 million." (45).

Informed consent should be obtained by practicing gastroenterologists as a routine practice when prescribing corticosteroids, when using drugs for off-label indications, and when using drugs in the face of black box warnings.

Therapeutic Interchange

Therapeutic interchange is a relatively new formulary policy that has significant potential impact on the pharmaceutical practice of the gastroenterologist (46). It represents a change in the standard of care.

Therapeutic interchange is a process wherein a pharmacist dispenses a drug different than the physician-prescribed drug. The drug selected is within the same chemical class as the physician prescribed drug but not the same chemical moiety. The American College of Physicians defines therapeutic interchange as the act of dispensing a drug different in chemical structure from the one originally prescribed. The substitute must be from the same therapeutic class and have the same pharmacodynamic and pharmacokinetic properties (47).

Therapeutic interchange is practiced in more than 50% of the nation's acute care hospitals and more than 30% of managed health care plans (48, 49). Its advantages include cost savings (50, 51), a more streamlined formulary, more rational drug policies, and better utilization of the pharmacist in health care delivery. The major disadvantage is potential liability for complications that may result from the use of the interchanged drug (which arguably would not have occurred with the physician-prescribed drug).

For example, a gastroenterologist prescribes the drug famotidine. Under the plan of interchange in effect, the pharmacist dispenses cimetidine. A drug interaction occurs between cimetidine and theophylline. Theophylline toxicity related seizures and other damages occur. The plaintiff will likely argue that the drug interaction would not have occurred if she had received the prescribed famotidine because the risk of such an interaction is much greater with cimetidine.

From the gastroenterologist's standpoint the two key provisions of the plan of interchange need to be understood. The first is the notification provision. These plans offer several alternatives including direct telephone calls from the pharmacist to the physician, hospital chart entries, medical staff informational meetings, and/or pharmacy newsletters. The physician needs to know when an interchange is made so it is imperative that the practitioner know how he or she will be notified. The second is the dispense as written (DAW) policy. Under this provision the physician has the right to obtain the prescribed drug if there is a valid clinical need for this agent.

Once the gastroenterologist is notified of the interchange of cimetidine for famotidine, for example, several options are available. These would include doing nothing, ordering more frequent serum levels of theophylline, lowering the theophylline dose, or entering a DAW order.

In short, therapeutic interchange represents a commonly applied, relatively new policy that changes the accepted standard of medical practice. Gastroenterologists need to know how to manage their practices in this regard to meet accepted standards of care.

CAUSATION

The element of causation or proximate cause requires that the plaintiff's attorney prove that there is some reasonable connection between the act or omission of the defendant and the damage that the plaintiff has suffered (52). Commonly applied tests of causation include the "but for" and "substantial factor test" tests. Under the former, the plaintiff must prove that "but for" the defendant's negligent act the damages would not have occurred. Under the later application, the plaintiff must prove that the defendant's negligent act was a "substantial factor" in the creation of the damages.

For example, a physician prescribes penicillin to a patient who is allergic to penicillin. The physician knew or should have known of the allergy. The patient dies 1 hour after the first intravenous dose. The patient, however, had end stage liver disease and was in stage IV hepatic coma. He was expected to live less than 24 hours at the time of the penicillin administration. The element of causation would be most difficult to prove under these circumstances. Would the patient's

death not have occurred "but for" the negligent act? Was the administration of penicillin a "substantial factor" in this patient's demise?

Proximate causation is at best unclear in its legal application. Nonetheless, it remains an important part of negligence law. From a practicing gastroenterologists's position, it is a point worth knowing, but of little use in structuring risk management strategies.

DAMAGES

Damages are the monetary awards given to successful malpractice plaintiffs, and are of three types. *Compensatory damages* are those designed to compensate the plaintiff for actual out-of-pocket expenses. Examples include physician's fees, hospital bills, rehabilitation expenses, medication costs, and funeral coverage. These damages are designed to place the plaintiff, insofar as it is possible, in the same position he would have been in if the negligent act had not occurred (53).

General damages are those for pain and suffering. These are less tangible, as illustrated by the decision of an appellate court in McLean v. United States (54) who awarded pain and suffering damages to the plaintiff who suffered anxiety and palpitations after mistakenly receiving a prescription for oxacillin instead of procainamide.

Punitive damages are rarely awarded in medical malpractice cases. They are designed to punish the tortfeasor. To prevail, the plaintiff must show willful, wanton, or reckless disregard or gross negligence on the part of the defendant (55). Some jurisdictions have adopted the principles of the "Restatement of Torts" (56) governing punitive damages. Generally, punitive damages may be awarded for conduct that is outrageous, because of the defendant's evil motive or reckless indifference to the rights of others.

The rules of punitive damages vary from state to state. For example, Pennsylvania and Ohio do not allow punitive damages in wrongful death actions. And Illinois and Massachusetts do not permit punitive damages in medical malpractice cases. The following cases are illustrative.

Punitive damages were awarded in Mulligan v. Lederle Laboratories (57). In this product liability action, the plaintiff alleged that Varidase caused chronic health problems (oral sores, microscopic hematuria, and glomerulonephritis). An award of $100,000 in punitive damages was upheld on the basis that there was sufficient evidence for the jury to conclude, under Arkansas law, that the defendant "knew or should have know that its course of conduct was about to inflict injury and yet continued its activities with conscious indifference to the consequences" (58). The court based its decision on physician-based complaints the company had received about the product, internal company correspondence, and published medical literature concerning the drug's dangers.

In McDaniel v. Merck, Sharp and Dohme (59), punitive damages were upheld against the manufacturer. The antibiotic cefoxitin had been used for approximately 1 month and the decedent developed fatal hemolytic anemia. The court found that the defendant knew of the serious risk of illness and death associated with long-term use of this drug and that it deliberately and negligently failed to communicate this knowledge to the medical community.

A physician was held liable for punitive damages in Hoffman v. Memorial Osteopathic Hospital (60). The plaintiff injured his back at work. He was examined by the defendant physician in the emergency room where at some point the patient fell on the floor. He was partially clothed and was crying for help. The physician informed him that there was nothing wrong with him and told him that he should go home. During this episode, the physician actually walked over the patient. He also instructed the staff not to pick the patient up from the floor. In remanding the case for a new trial on the punitive damage issue, the Pennsylvania Superior Court deemed the physician's actions sufficient for such a measure.

MEDICAL-LEGAL ASPECTS OF PHARMACY PRACTICE

A dispensing pharmacist's duty to warn patients that a prescribed drug may interact with alcohol or with another medication, and that there are limits on the number of doses that should be taken over a specified period of time, has been determined through several recent court decisions (7, 8, 10, 61). Moreover, the FDA Commissioner, the Office of the Inspector General, and the Health Care Financing Administration (HCFA) all have recently called for an expansion of pharmacy practice functions (62–66). These and other recommendations have resulted in the Omnibus Budget Reconciliation Act of 1990 (OBRA90) that mandates pharmacists to provide counseling for Medicaid patients (67). Although Congress passed this legislation with the expectation that such counseling on the part of pharmacists will lower the cost of pharmaceutical health care (while at the same time improving medical care), the wider legal implications of the OBRA90 bill for pharmacists have been the subject of several reviews (68). Several aspects of the OBRA90 legislation and their implications will be discussed below.

Patient Counseling Standards

OBRA90 requires drug use review (DUR) that pharmacists must perform to provide patients with sufficient information about their medications so as to avoid medication errors, to improve compliance and to warn about important side effects. Specifically, the law states:

"The pharmacist must offer to discuss with each individual—or care giver of such individual (in person, whenever practical or through access to a telephone service which is toll-free for long distance calls)—who presents a prescription, matters which in the exercise of the pharmacist's professional judgment (consistent with applicable state law respecting the provision of such information), the pharmacist deems significant including the following:

(aa) The name and description of the medication.

(bb) The dosage form, dosage, route of administration, and duration of drug therapy.

(cc) Special directions and precautions for preparation, administration, and use by the patient.

(dd) Common severe side effects of adverse effects or interactions and therapeutic contraindications that maybe encountered, including their avoidance and the actions required if they occur.

(ee) Techniques for self-monitoring drug therapy.

(ff) Proper storage.

(gg) Prescription refill information.

(hh) Action to be taken in the event of a missed dose."

Documentation by Pharmacists

The dictum "If you wrote it, you did it; if you didn't write it, you didn't do it!" applies as much to pharmacists as it does to physicians. OBRA90 specifically requires pharmacists to maintain a written record about their patients' drug therapy:

"A reasonable effort must be made by the pharmacists to obtain, record, and maintain at least the following information regarding individuals receiving benefits under this subchapter:

(aa) Name, address, telephone number, date of birth (or age), and gender.

(bb) Individual history where significant, including disease state or states, known allergies and drug reactions and a comprehensive list of medications and relevant devices.

(cc) Pharmacists' comments relevant to the individual's drug therapy."

Informed Refusal of Counseling

Much like informed consent and refusal in medical and surgical practice, pharmacists are partially protected from legal liability if a patient makes an informed refusal to accept their counseling advise. As stated in OBRA90:

"Nothing in this clause shall be construed as requiring a pharmacist to provide consultation when an individual receiving benefits of this subchapter or care giver of such individual refuses such consultation."

A patient who "refuses" counseling because the pharmacist is too busy to provide such advice in a timely fashion, or by means of some reasonable alternative (such as by letter or telephone call), will probably be found to be a invalid reason in the eyes of the state DUR boards or the courts.

DUR and Non-Medicaid Patients

The OBRA90 legislation as written currently applies only to Medicaid patients for the purpose of reducing pharmaceutical expenditures. However, as Brushwood and colleagues (68) have opined, it may become increasingly more difficult for a pharmacist to omit the same level of drug counseling for their other patients not covered by Medicaid. Once pharmacy practice has been elevated to a new set of practice standards (such as those mandated by OBRA90), these same standards must be upheld for all patients. To this end, it is expected that some state boards of pharmacy will probably require that the OBRA90 regulations be expanded to encompass a much broader range of patients. Thus, pharmacists, just as other health care professionals, will need to remain vigilant concerning the new standards of pharmacy care developed through legislation and court decisions.

Future Expectations

As Brushwood has written, consumer expectation for drug counseling is based on the expertise residing within pharmacy care. Furthermore, Brushwood notes that the patient-pharmacist relationship is contractually based on mutual pledges; that is, the patient pledges payment and the pharmacist pledges services. These services include the promise to deliver the patient's prescription and all information relevant to that prescription. In his knowledge-based model of professional responsibility to pharmacists, Brushwood concludes that the patient has a right to expect that these services will be provided to the best of the pharmacist's ability (61). As a result, pharmacists can no longer hide behind a shield of practice that falls below these new standards.

SUMMARY

The goals of this chapter were to review a number of aspects of medical-legal therapeutics for practicing physicians, including gastroenterologists. The fundamentals of malpractice law were reviewed in light of the most commonly used drugs in gastroenterologic practice, and appropriate risk management strategies delineated. The understanding of the concept of legal duty as well as the elaboration of the notion of the standard of care must be continuously emphasized as the most important legal principles.

REFERENCES

1. Brennan TE, Leape LL, Laird NM, et al. Incidence of adverse effects and negligence in hospitalized patients—results of the Harvard Medical Practice Study I. N Engl J Med 1991;324:370–376.
2. Leape LL, Brennan TE, Laird NM, et al. The nature of adverse events in hospitalized patients—results of the Harvard Medical Practice Study II. N Engl J Med 1991;324:377–384.
3. Localio AR, Lawthers AG, Brennan TA, et al. Relation between malpractice claims and adverse events due to negligence—results of the Harvard Medical Practice Study III. N Engl J Med 1991; 325:245–251.
4. Prosser W, and Keaton W. The law of torts. ed. 5. West Pub, 1984:160–164.
5. 314 F Supp 905 (Ohio 1970).
6. Brushwood DB. Medical malpractice: pharmacy law. New York: McGraw-Hill, 1986:228–229.
7. 353 Pa Super 21, 508 A2d 1247 (1986).
8. 805 SW2d 380 (Tenn Ct App 1991).
9. Stebbins v. Concord Drugs, 164 Mich App 204.
10. Ferguson v. Williams, 92 NC App 336, 374 SE2d 438 (1988).
11. McKee v. American Home Products, 113 Wash 2d 701, 782 P2d 1045 (1989).
12. Baccardi v. Holzman, 182 NJ Super 422 App Div (1981).
13. Forsiello v. Whitehall Laboratories, 165 NJ Super 311, 388 A2d 132 (1979).
14. 399 F2d 121 (9th Cir 1968).
15. Brushwood DB. Medical malpractice: pharmacy law. New York: McGraw-Hill, 1986:243.
16. MacDonald v. Ortho Pharmaceutical Corp., 394 Mass 131, 474 NE 2d 65 (1985).
17. 136 Ill App 3d 945, 483 NE 2d 906 (1985).
18. Leibowitz v. Ortho Pharmaceutical Corp., 224 Pa Super 418, 307 A2d 449 (1973).
19. 52 NJ Super 474 (1958).
20. 397 Pa 28, 153 A2d 255 (1959).
21. Horney v. Lawrence, 189 Ga App 376, 375 SE 2d 629 (1988).
22. Cardiovascular drug alerts. Midazolam and respiratory arrest. Nov. 1991.
23. Monitoring of patients undergoing gastrointestinal endoscopic procedures. ASGE publication 1022. American Society of Gastrointestinal Endoscopy, 1989.
24. Classen D. Intensive surveillance of midazolam use in hospitalized patients and the occurrence of cardio-respiratory arrest. Pharmacotherapy 1992;12:213–216.
25. Sanzari v. Rosenfeld, 34 NJ 128 (1971).
26. 444 Pa 263, 282 A2d 206 (1971).
27. 100 Mich App 649, 300 NW 2d 356 (1981).
28. Ruth v. Fenchel, 21 NJ 171 (1956).
29. Johnson v. Mountainside Hospital, 239 NJ Super 312 (App Div, certif den) 122 NJ 188 (1990).
30. Medical economic data. Physicians' desk reference. ed. 46. 1992:2160.
31. Walt AJJ. Misoprostol for the treatment of peptic ulcer and anti-inflammatory drug induced gastro-duodenal ulceration. N Eng J Med 1992;327:1575–1580.
32. Plumeri PA. NSAID gastropathy, misoprostol and the standard of care. J Clin Gastroenterol 1990; 12:470–474.
33. Hanauer SB, and Stathopoulos G. Risk-benefit assessment of drugs used in the treatment of inflammatory bowel disease. Drug Safety 1991;6:192–219.
34. Physicians' desk reference. ed. 46. Montvale NJ: Medical Economic Data. 1984:1531.
35. Physicians' desk reference. ed. 46. Montvale NJ: Medical Economic Data. 1984:1924.
36. Plumeri PA. Informed consent and the gastrointestinal endoscopist. Gastrointest Endosc 1985;31:218–221.
37. Plumeri PA. Informed consent—beware. J Clin Gastroenterol 1984;6:471–475.
38. Plumeri PA. The gastroenterologist and the doctrine of informed consent. J Clin Gastroenterol 1983; 5:185–187.
39. 497 A2d 464 (Pa Super 1985).
40. 114 NJ 550 (1989).
41. 438 F Supp 383 (Co 1977).
42. 400 So2d 820 (Fl App 1981).
43. 5 Haw App 504, 705 P2d 37 (1985).
44. 395 Mass 689 (1985).
45. Curran SJ. Informed consent in malpractice cases—a turn toward reality. N Eng J Med 1986;314:429–431.
46. Plumeri PA, and Crane VS. Legal and medical issues in therapeutic interchange: implications for pharmacists, physicians and P & T committees. Hosp Formul 1992;27:1040–1050.
47. American College of Physicians. Therapeutic interchange and formulary systems. Ann Intern Med 1990;113:160–163.
48. Stolar MH. ASHP national survey of hospital pharmaceutical services 1987. Am J Hosp Pharm 1988;45:801–818.
49. Doering PL, Russell WL, McCormick WC, et al. Therapeutic interchange in the health maintenance

organization outpatient environment. Drug Intell Clin Pharm 1988;22:125–130.

50. Guastella C. Cost savings realized from interchanging ceftizoxime for cefoxitin. Am J Hosp Pharm 1988;45:2376–2377.

51. Nolly RJ, and Skoutakis VA. Cost considerations of intravenously administered H-2 receptor antagonists. Drug Intell Clin Pharm 1989;23:S23–S28.

52. Prosser W, Keaton W. The law of torts. ed. 5. West Pub, 1984:263.

53. Prosser W, Keaton W. The law of torts. ed. 5. West Pub, 1984:6.

54. 613 F.2d 603 (5th Cir 1980).

55. Prosser W, Keaton W. The law of torts. ed. 5. West Pub, 1984: pp. 7–14.

56. Restatement of Torts (Second) Section 908(2).

57. 786 F2d 859 (8th Cir 1986).

58. Mulligan (cite 57) at 864.

59. 533 A2d 436 (Pa Super 1987).

60. 492 A2d 1382 (Pa Super 1985).

61. Brushwood DB. Pharmacist's duty to warn: toward a knowledge-based model of professional responsibility. Drake Law Rev 1991;40:1–60.

62. Kessler DA. Communicating with patients about their medications. N Engl J Med 1991;325:1650.

63. 42 CFR § 483.60 (1990).

64. Office of the Inspector General office of Analysis and Inspections. The clinical role of the community pharmacist. Dept Health and Human Service Publication OAI-01-89-89020 January 1990.

65. Office of the Inspector General State discipline of pharmacists. HHS publication OAI-01-89-89160 January 1990.

66. Office of the Inspector General medication regimens: Causes of noncompliance HHS publication OAI-04-89-89121 March 1990.

67. 42 USC § 1396–8, 1990.

68. Brushwood DB, Catizone CA, Coster JM. OBRA90: What it means to your practice. U.S. Pharmacist Oct. 1992.

Index

(Page numbers followed by *f* denote figures; those followed by *t* denote tables)